P9-BZC-920

Diagnosis of Diseases of the Breast

Diagnosis of Diseases of the Breast

Second Edition

Lawrence W. Bassett, MD
Iris Cantor Professor of Breast Imaging
Department of Radiological Sciences
David Geffen School of Medicine at UCLA
Los Angeles, California

Valerie P. Jackson, MD
John A. Campbell Professor of Radiology
Chairman, Department of Radiology
Indiana University School of Medicine
Indianapolis, Indiana

Karin L. Fu, MD
Medical Director
Eisenhower Lucy Curci Cancer Center Breast Center
Palm Desert, California

Yao S. Fu, MD
Senior Pathologist
Department of Pathology
Providence St. Joseph's Medical Center
Burbank, California

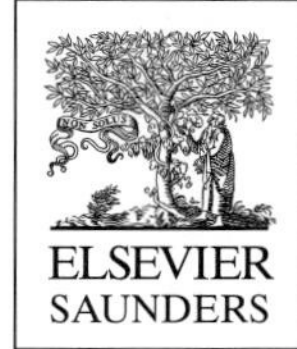

ELSEVIER
SAUNDERS

The Curtis Center
170 S Independence Mall W 300E
Philadelphia, Pennsylvania 19106

DIAGNOSIS OF DISEASES OF THE BREAST ISBN 0-7216-9563-9

NOTICE

Radiology is an ever-changing field. Standard safety precautions must be followed, but as new research and clinical experience broaden our knowledge, changes in treatment and drug therapy may become necessary or appropriate. Readers are advised to check the most current product information provided by the manufacturer of each drug to be administered to verify the recommended dose, the method and duration of administration, and contraindications. It is the responsibility of the licensed prescriber, relying on experience and knowledge of the patient, to determine dosages and the best treatment for each individual patient. Neither the publisher nor the author assumes any liability for any injury and/or damage to persons or property arising from this publication.

Library of Congress Cataloging-in-Publication Data

Diagnosis of diseases of the breast / Lawrence W. Bassett . . . [et al.].—2nd ed.
p. ; cm.
Includes bibliographical references and index.
ISBN 0–7216–9563–9
1. Breast—Diseases—Diagnosis. 2. Breast—Diseases. I. Bassett, Lawrence W. (Lawrence Wayne), 1942-
[DNLM: 1. Breast Diseases—diagnosis. 2. Breast—physiopathology. 3. Breast Diseases—therapy. 4. Diagnostic Imaging. WP 815 D5364 2005]
RG493.D54 2005
618.1'9075—dc22

2004046606

Acquisitions Editor: Allan Ross
Developmental Editor: Ed Pontee
Publishing Services Manager: Tina Rebane
Project Manager: Linda Van Pelt

Printed in the United States of America.

Last digit is the print number: 9 8 7 6 5 4 3 2 1

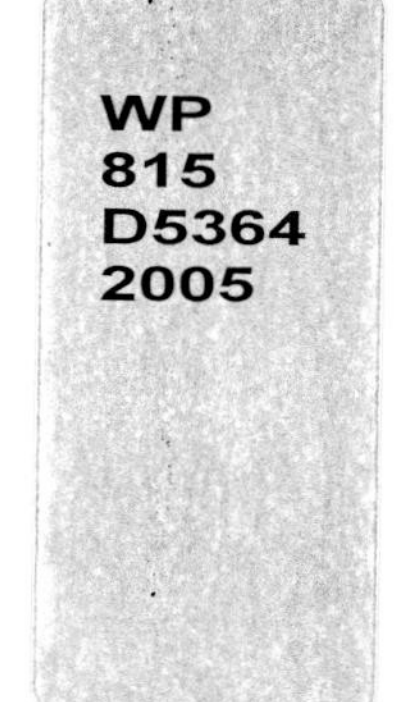

This book is dedicated to our families and friends, who supported us in this project.

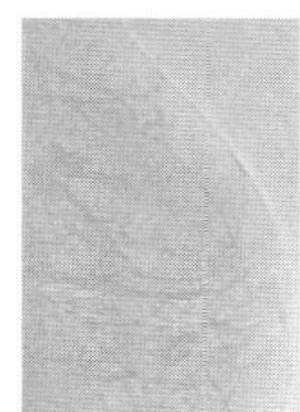

Contributors

Gary T. Barnes, PhD, FAAPM, FACR
Professor Emeritus, Department of Radiology, University of Alabama at Birmingham Medical Center; President, X-ray Imaging Innovations, Birmingham, Alabama
Mammography Equipment and Screen-Film Imaging Considerations

Lawrence W. Bassett, MD, FACR
Iris Cantor Professor of Breast Imaging, Department of Radiological Sciences, David Geffen School of Medicine at UCLA, Los Angeles, California
Positioning; Clinical Image Evaluation; Magnetic Resonance Imaging of Breast Tumors; Imaging-Guided Core Needle Biopsy of the Breast; After the Imaging-Guided Needle Biopsy; Galactography; The Normal Breast; Noninvasive Carcinoma; Invasive Malignancies; The Clinically Abnormal Breast; The Male Breast; The Augmented Breast

Robert S. Bennion, MD
Professor of Surgery, David Geffen School of Medicine at UCLA; Attending Surgeon, UCLA Medical Center, Los Angeles, California
Treatment of Breast Disease

Malcolm M. Bilimoria, MD
Assistant Professor of Surgery, Northwestern University, Feinberg School of Medicine, Chicago, Illinois
Clinical Examination of the Breast

R. James Brenner, MD, JD
Clinical Professor of Radiology, David Geffen School of Medicine at UCLA, Los Angeles; Director, Breast Imaging, Tower-St. John's Imaging, Joyce Eisenberg Keefer Breast Center, John Wayne Cancer Institute, St. John's Health Center, Santa Monica, California
Medicolegal Issues in Breast Imaging

Louise A. Brinton, PhD
Chief of Hormonal and Reproductive Epidemiology Branch, Division of Cancer Genetics and Epidemiology, National Cancer Institute, Rockville, Maryland
The Epidemiology of Breast Cancer

Priscilla F. Butler, MS
Adjunct Associate Professor, George Washington University School of Medicine and Health Sciences, Washington, DC; Senior Director, Breast Imaging Accreditation Programs, American College of Radiology, Reston, Virginia
Quality Control; The MQSA and the Accreditation Process

Seth Y. Cardall, MD
Transitional Year Resident, Mayo Clinic, Scottsdale, Arizona
The Normal Breast; Noninvasive Carcinoma; Invasive Malignancies

Helena R. Chang, MD, PhD
Professor of Surgery, David Geffen School of Medicine at UCLA; Director, Revlon/UCLA Breast Center, David Geffen School of Medicine at UCLA, Los Angeles, California
Treatment of Breast Disease

Prem K. Chantra, MD
Associate Physician Diplomat, Assistant Professor of Radiology, David Geffen School of Medicine at UCLA; Staff Radiologist and Director of Breast Imaging, VA Greater Los Angeles Healthcare System, Los Angeles, California
The Male Breast

Nanette D. DeBruhl, MD
Associate Professor of Radiological Sciences, David Geffen School of Medicine at UCLA, Los Angeles, California
Magnetic Resonance Imaging of Breast Tumors; The Augmented Breast

D. David Dershaw, MD
Professor of Radiology, Cornell University Joan and Sanford I. Weill Medical College and Graduate School of Medical Sciences; Director, Breast Imaging Section, Department of Radiology, Memorial Sloan-Kettering Cancer Center, New York, New York
The Conservatively Treated Breast

Carl J. D'Orsi, MD, FACR
Professor of Radiology, Oncology and Hematology, Emory University School of Medicine; Director of Breast Imaging, Winship Cancer Center, Atlanta, Georgia
Reporting and Communication

Victoria J. Edmond, MD
Assistant Professor of Radiology, Indiana University School of Medicine; Director of Breast Imaging, St. Margaret's Breast Center, Indianapolis, Indiana
Breast Ultrasonography

Stephen A. Feig, MD, FACR
Professor of Radiology, Mount Sinai School of Medicine of New York University; Director, Breast Imaging, The Mount Sinai Hospital, New York, New York
Digital Mammography, Computer-Aided Detection, and Other Digital Applications; Screening Results, Controversies, and Guidelines

Karin L. Fu, MD
Medical Director, Eisenhower Lucy Curci Cancer Center Breast Center, Palm Desert, California
Handling of Pathology Specimens; The Normal Breast; Benign Breast Lesions; Noninvasive Carcinoma; Invasive Malignancies

Yao S. Fu, MD
Senior Pathologist, Department of Pathology, Providence St. Joseph Medical Center, Burbank, California
Handling of Pathology Specimens; The Normal Breast; Benign Breast Lesions; Noninvasive Carcinoma; Invasive Malignancies

Richard H. Gold, BA, MD
Professor of Radiological Sciences, David Geffen School of Medicine at UCLA, Los Angeles, California
The History of Breast Imaging

David P. Gorczyca, MD
Director of Breast Imaging, Red Rock Radiology, Sunrise Hospital and Medical Center, Mountain View Hospital, and Southern Hills Hospital, Las Vegas, Nevada
The Augmented Breast

Randall A. Hawkins, MD, PhD
Professor of Radiology, Department of Radiology, University of California, San Francisco, School of Medicine; Chief of Nuclear Medicine, University of California, San Francisco, San Francisco, California
Nuclear Medicine Applications in Breast Imaging

Rita W. Heinlein, RT(R)(M)ARRT
Director, Mammography Consulting and Educational Services, Clarksville, Maryland
Positioning

Anne C. Hoyt, MD
Assistant Professor, Department of Radiological Sciences, Iris Cantor Center for Breast Imaging, David Geffen School of Medicine at UCLA, Los Angeles, California
After the Imaging-Guided Needle Biopsy

Valerie P. Jackson, MD, FACR
John A. Campbell Professor of Radiology and Chairman, Department of Radiology, Indiana University School of Medicine, Indianapolis, Indiana
Breast Ultrasonography; Presurgical Needle Localization; Other Ultrasonographically Guided Interventional Procedures; Galactography; Benign Breast Lesions; Reduction Mammoplasty

Ahmedin Jemal, PhD, DVM
Program Director, Cancer Surveillance, American Cancer Society, Atlanta, Georgia
The Epidemiology of Breast Cancer

Christine H. Kim, MD
Breast Imaging Radiologist, Torrance Memorial Medical Center, Torrance, California
Imaging-Guided Core Needle Biopsy of the Breast

Joan L. Kramer, PhD
Clinical Genetics Fellow, Clinical Genetics Branch, Division of Cancer Epidemiology and Genetics, National Cancer Institute, Rockville, Maryland
The Epidemiology of Breast Cancer

Michael N. Linver, MD
Clinical Associate Professor, Department of Radiology, University of New Mexico School of Medicine; Director of Mammography, X-ray Associates of New Mexico, P.C., Albuquerque, New Mexico
The Medical Audit; Coding and Billing in Breast Imaging

January K. Lopez, MD
Resident, Radiological Sciences, University of California at Los Angeles, Los Angeles, California
Normal Breast; Noninvasive Carcinoma; Invasive Malignancies

Susan M. Love, MD, MBA
Clinical Professor of Surgery, David Geffen School of Medicine at UCLA, Los Angeles; Medical Director, Dr. Susan Love Research Foundation, Pacific Palisades, California
Treatment of Breast Disease

Dawn Michael
Resident, Santa Clara Valley Medical Center, San Jose, California
Magnetic Resonance Imaging of Breast Tumors; The Augmented Breast

Mohan Ramaswamy, MD
Associate Medical Director, Biomedical Research Foundation, PET Imaging Center, Shreveport, Louisiana
Nuclear Medicine Applications in Breast Imaging

Handel E. Reynolds, MD
Radiology Associates of Atlanta, Atlanta, Georgia
Other Ultrasonographically Guided Interventional Procedures

Mark S. Shiroishi, MD
Radiology Resident, David Geffen School of Medicine at UCLA, Los Angeles, California
The Male Breast

Robert A. Smith, PhD
Director, Cancer Screening, American Cancer Society, Atlanta, Georgia
The Epidemiology of Breast Cancer

George J. So, MD, MSE
Staff Physician, Graziadio Radiology Center, Torrance Memorial Medical Center, Torrance, California
The Male Breast

Bao To, MD
Chief Resident, Nuclear Medicine, Department of Radiology, University of California, San Francisco; Associate Physician, Department of Radiology—Nuclear Medicine Division, Kaiser Permanente Vallejo Medical Center, Vallejo, California
Nuclear Medicine Applications in Breast Imaging

Lusine Tumyan, BS
Medical Student, David Geffen School of Medicine at UCLA, Los Angeles, California
The Clinically Abnormal Breast

David P. Winchester, MD
Professor of Surgery, Northwestern University, The Feinberg School of Medicine, Chicago; Chairman, Department of Surgery, Evanston Northwestern Healthcare, Evanston, Illinois
Clinical Examination of the Breast

Jerome S. Wollman, MD
Clinical Professor of Pathology, David Geffen School of Medicine at UCLA; Staff Pathologist, VA Greater Los Angeles Healthcare System, Los Angeles, California
The Male Breast

Martin J. Yaffe, PhD
Professor, Departments of Medical Biophysics and Medical Imaging, University of Toronto; Senior Scientist, Imaging Research Program, Sunnybrook and Women's College Health Science Centre, Toronto, Ontario, Canada
Digital Mammography, Computer-Aided Detection, and Other Digital Applications

Juanita Yun, MD
Department of Nuclear Medicine, Kaiser Permanente Walnut Creek Medical Center, Walnut Creek, California
Nuclear Medicine Applications in Breast Imaging

Preface

This book has been designed as a comprehensive work for all health care professionals who deal with breast disease and, in particular, breast imaging. Breast cancer is the second leading cause of cancer deaths in American women and a serious health problem in the United States. For many years, the mortality rate from this disease was stable, but in 1995 the mortality rate began to slowly decrease. This is attributed in part to the increased use of screening mammography. With the widespread use of screening mammography, most breast tumors are now first detected when they are very small. As a result, in 2002, the American Joint Committee on Cancer made substantial changes in their staging system for breast cancer to reflect the larger numbers of small cancers detected. These revisions focused on T1 stage tumors (≤2 cm in diameter), which were divided into four subcategories.

We have divided this book into seven sections, as follows:

Section I. This introductory chapter provides the history of breast imaging. It is a tribute to those early radiologists who devoted their careers to making breast imaging possible. They should not be forgotten.

Section II. This comprehensive section includes the full range of components of the mammography examination and audit results. The technical aspects and physical principles focus on conventional mammography; digital mammography is covered in detail in a subsequent chapter. Maintaining high-quality mammographic images depends on optimal positioning, clinical image evaluation, and quality control procedures. Mammography Quality Standards Act regulations and the accreditation process, which are discussed in this section, enforce quality standards. Once a high-quality image is obtained, the radiologist must use a systematic approach to evaluate the mammogram and communicate results effectively. This is expedited by using the standardized terminology and report organization of the American College of Radiology Breast Imaging Reporting and Data System (BI-RADS). Performing a medical audit allows radiologists and facilities to evaluate their overall performance. Therefore, we have included an in-depth chapter on the medical audit. It is also important for radiologists to understand the basics of coding and billing in breast imaging, especially when reporting the examination. The medicolegal issues in breast imaging are also covered in this section because these have become an important aspect of breast imaging.

Section III. Breast imaging has evolved beyond interpretation of conventional mammograms. The radiologist must also be familiar with the basics of clinical breast examination in the evaluation of symptomatic women or those with equivocal imaging findings. Ultrasonography remains the most important adjunctive imaging modality for the evaluation of mammographically and clinically detected breast abnormalities and is now undergoing clinical trials of its potential for screening. Mammography is moving into the digital era with the development of full-field digital mammography, computer-aided detection, and other digital applications. The chapter on digital mammography covers the technical and clinical aspects of this field. Magnetic resonance imaging of the breast is another technology with great potential; the evolution and status of this modality are covered in depth in this update. Finally, the applications of nuclear medicine in breast imaging are reviewed.

Section IV. Imaging-guided interventional procedures, which are now basic to the management of breast diseases, are covered in this section. In addition to employing presurgical needle localization, radiologists perform the majority of biopsies with ultrasound and stereotactic guidance for core needle biopsies. The chapters in this section go beyond the performance of the procedure and include management issues after the biopsy, such as determining concordance of imaging and pathologic examination results and deciding when open biopsy is indicated. This section includes a new chapter on the handling of pathology specimens. Other ultrasound-guided interventional procedures are also included. Finally, there is a chapter on galactography (ductography), including information on performance and interpretation of the examination.

Section V. An update on the status of screening mammography is provided in this section. It begins with a chapter on the epidemiology of breast cancer, followed by the results of screening trials, controversies about screening, and guidelines for screening, which are presented in depth.

Section VI. The emphasis is on pathologic and radiologic findings in the normal breast, benign breast lesions, noninvasive carcinomas, and invasive malignancies. The goal of this section is to provide an understanding of the pathologic basis of breast disease for radiologists performing breast imaging. A new chapter focuses on evaluation of the clinically abnormal breast, and the section ends with a chapter on the male breast.

Section VII. This section, written by dedicated breast surgeons, provides insights into the management of breast diseases and post-treatment evaluation. The final chapters address imaging evaluation of the conservatively treated breast, the augmented breast, and reduction mammoplasty.

We wish to thank our contributing authors for their excellent chapters. We also thank our families, friends, and coworkers for their help and patience in this endeavor. Finally, we thank our editor and staff at Elsevier for their guidance.

Lawrence W. Bassett, MD
Valerie P. Jackson, MD
Karin L. Fu, MD
Yao S. Fu, MD

Contents

Section I

INTRODUCTION

The History of Breast Imaging

Richard H. Gold

PIONEERS OF MAMMOGRAPHY

In 1913, Albert Salomon[1] (Fig. 1–1), a surgeon at the Surgical Clinic of Berlin University, became the first person to describe the usefulness of radiography in the study of breast cancer. He performed radiography on more than 3000 mastectomy specimens and correlated the radiographic, gross, and microscopic findings (Figs. 1–2 and 1–3). Salomon found that radiographs were useful to demonstrate the spread of tumor to the axillary lymph nodes and to distinguish highly infiltrating carcinoma from circumscribed carcinoma. In addition, he was the first person to observe on radiographs the microcalcifications associated with malignancy, although he did not then appreciate their significance or the usefulness of his observation.

After Salomon's paper on breast radiography, no related publications appeared until the late 1920s, when a number of articles on the use of radiography in the study of breast disease were published by various investigators working independently in different parts of the world. In Germany in 1927, Otto Kleinschmidt[2] reported the use of mammography as a diagnostic aid at the University of Leipzig Breast Clinic and credited the introduction of the technique in the clinic to his teacher, Erwin Payr, a noted plastic surgeon. In 1932, Walter Vogel,[3] also at the Leipzig clinic, published a paper on the mammographic differentiation of benign and malignant breast lesions. In Spain in 1931, on the basis of examinations of 56 patients, J. Goyanes and colleagues[4] described the mammographic features of the normal breast and distinguished inflammatory from neoplastic lesions. Furthermore, they emphasized the importance of breast positioning in mammography. South Americans Carlos Dominguez[5] of Uruguay, in 1929, and A. Baraldi[6] of Brazil, in 1934, described pneumomammography as a method to improve the delineation of lesions. The procedure required the injection of carbon dioxide into the retromammary and premammary spaces before radiography. Although J. Benzadon,[7] Baraldi's colleague, pursued this method of imaging, it failed to become generally accepted.

Great strides were made in the United States as well, mainly as a result of the work of Stafford Warren (Fig. 1–4), a radiologist at Strong Memorial Hospital in Rochester, New York. In 1930, Warren[8] reported the use of a stereoscopic technique for breast radiography, having performed it in 119 patients who subsequently underwent surgery (Fig. 1–5). In obtaining the mammograms, Warren used general-purpose radiographic equipment, "new" dual fine-grain calcium tungstate intensifying screens, a moving Potter-Bucky diaphragm (similar to today's reciprocating grids) to diminish scattered radiation, and the following technical factors: 50 to 60 kilovolt (peak) (kVp), 70 mA, a target-to-film distance of 63 cm, and an exposure time of 2.5 seconds. He wrote, "In many of the cases, there was no uniformity of opinion in the preoperative clinical diagnosis. . . . [T]he opinion from the mammogram on the other hand, was often very definite and most frequently correct."[8] In fact, in the 119 cases, only eight interpretative errors were made, including four false-negative diagnoses in the 58 cases of cancer.

Warren's accuracy in diagnosing breast cancer confirmed the usefulness of mammography as a diagnostic tool. In addition, Warren described the mammographic appearance of normal breasts and the mammographic features associated with pregnancy and mastitis. In 1931, another American radiologist, Paul Seabold,[9] reported the mammographic appearance of normal breasts in various physiologic states ranging from puberty to postmenopause, including changes seen during the menstrual cycle. In 1933, Ira Lockwood[10] published a review of mammographic diagnostic criteria.

Despite the surge of interest in mammography in the 1920s, progress in mammography had come to a halt in the United States by the mid 1930s. The most likely reasons were the unpredictable quality of the images and the inability to reproduce the high degree of accuracy reported by Warren.[11] Thus, during the 1930s, the majority of interested investigators were discouraged from pursuing mammography.

Jacob Gershon-Cohen (Fig. 1–6), a radiologist in Philadelphia, persisted in the study of mammography and made notable progress in diagnosis of breast cancer. In 1938, he and his colleague, Albert Strickler,[12] reported the range of normal radiographic appearances of the breast as a function of age and menstrual status, stressing the importance of understanding the appearance of the normal breast under all conditions of growth and physiologic activity before attempting the diagnosis of breast abnormalities. In the 1950s, Gershon-Cohen and pathologist Helen Ingleby[13] performed a roentgenologic-pathologic correlation of breast disease using whole-breast histologic sections, establishing mammographic criteria for the diagnosis of benign and malignant lesions. Gershon-Cohen[14] emphasized the

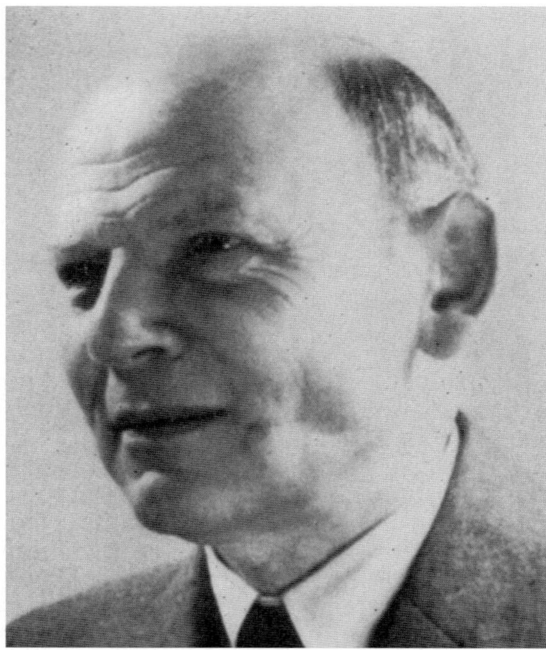

Figure 1–1. Albert Salomon. (Courtesy of Andre Bruwer, MD, Tucson, AZ.)

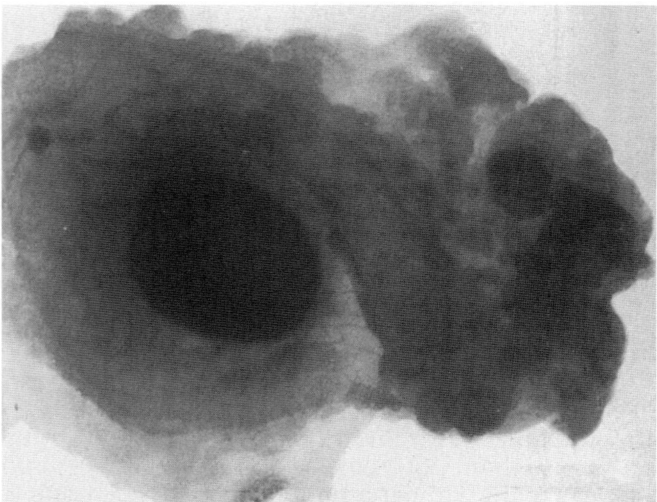

Figure 1–3. Another case from the radiographs of breast tissue specimens obtained by Salomon. The large mass on the left is an intracystic carcinoma, and the smaller masses on the right represent nodal metastases. (From Salomon A: Beitrage zur Pathologie und Klinik der Mammacarcinome. Arch Klin Chir 1913;101:573-668.)

use of high-contrast images and breast compression and recommended the simultaneous exposure of two juxtaposed films for adequate exposure of both the thinner peripheral and thicker juxtathoracic tissues.

During the 1950s, interest in mammography also grew outside the United States. In France in 1951, Charles Gros and R. Sigrist[15] published many articles related to mammography, emphasizing mammographic criteria for benign and malignant lesions and the indications for mammography. Later, Gros[16] developed the prototypic "dedicated" mammography unit containing a molybdenum anode and a device to compress the breast. In Uruguay, Raul Leborgne[17,18] (Fig. 1–7), a student of Dominguez, described the typical mammographic appearance of breast cancer and was the first person to emphasize the importance of microcalcifications in its diagnosis. He also stressed the usefulness of breast compression to immobilize the breast and diminish its

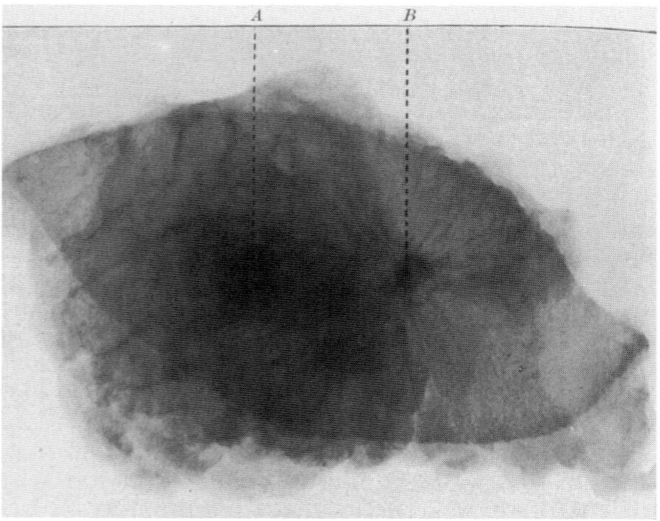

Figure 1–2. Radiographs of breast tissue specimens obtained by Salomon. Radiograph shows nipple (A) and carcinoma (B). (From Salomon A: Beitrage zur Pathologie und Klinik der Mammacarcinome. Arch Klin Chir 1913;101:573-668.)

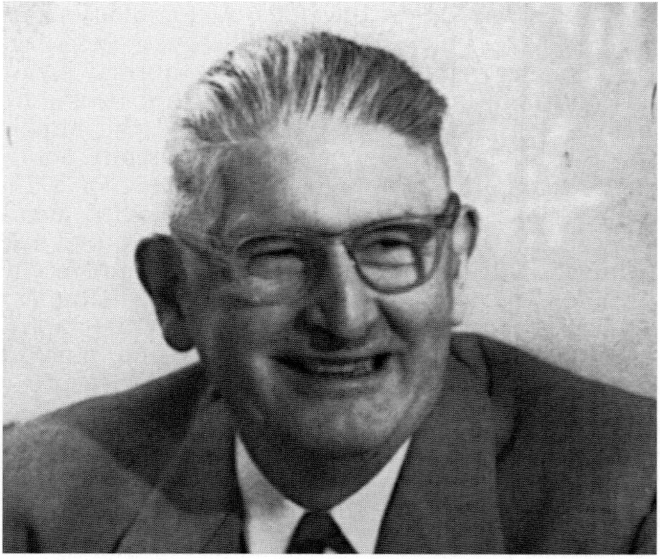

Figure 1–4. Stafford L. Warren. (Courtesy of Robert L. Egan, MD, Atlanta, GA.)

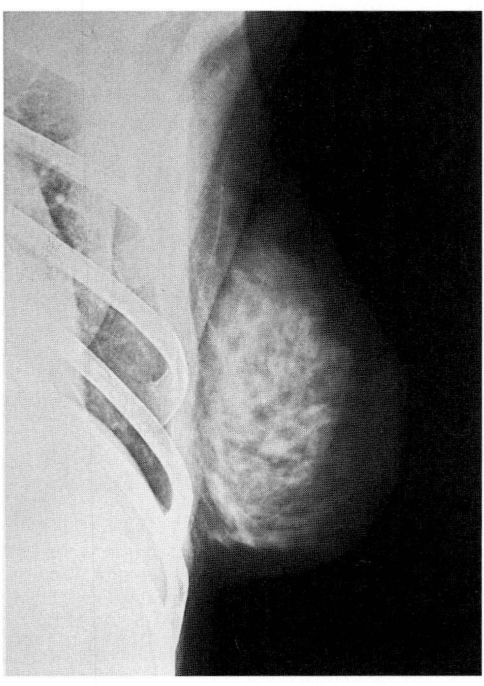

Figure 1–5. Mammogram obtained by Warren (circa 1939) of a normal dense breast. (Courtesy of Stafford L. Warren, MD, Los Angeles, CA.)

thickness to enhance image quality (Fig. 1–8). To achieve compression, he used a long cone with a flat surface at its distal end. Furthermore, he used a low–kVp technique (20 to 30 kVp), nonscreen film, a 60-cm target-to-film distance, and 5 mA for each

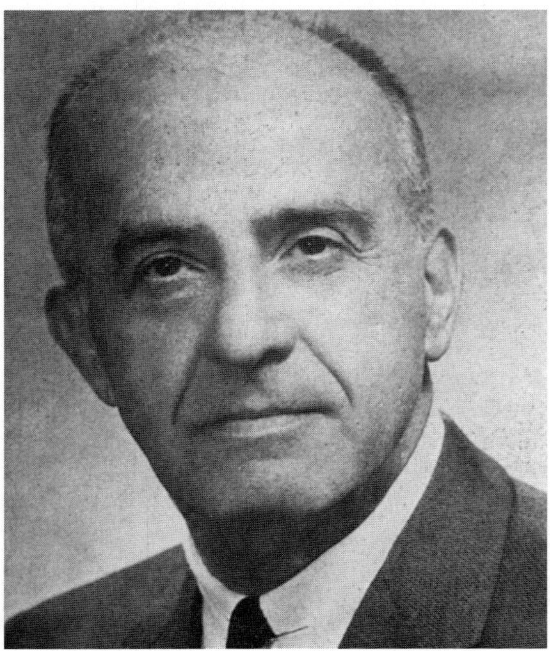

Figure 1–6. Jacob Gershon-Cohen. (From Obituary: Jacob Gershon-Cohen. Radiology 1971;99:455.)

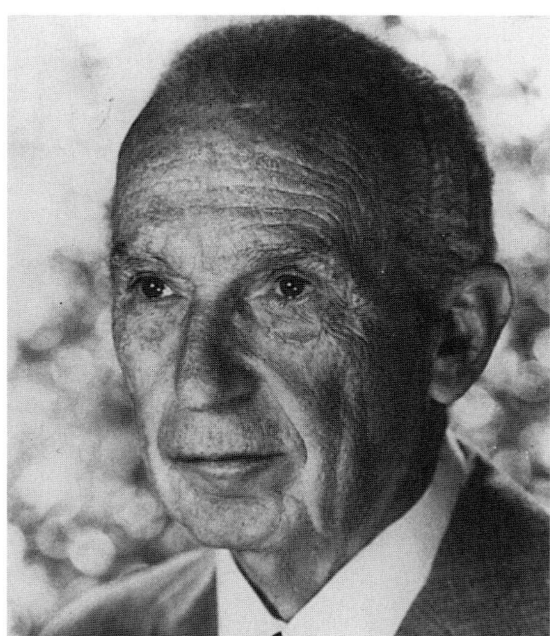

Figure 1–7. Raul Leborgne. (Courtesy of Felix Leborgne, MD, Montevideo, Uruguay.)

centimeter of compressed breast thickness. Leborgne also described the radiographic differences between benign and malignant calcifications and was the first person to report the significant association of microcalcifications with subclinical carcinoma, thus setting the stage for the use of mammography as a tool for cancer screening (Figs. 1–9 to 1–12).

Despite these advances, mammography was rarely used in the 1950s because of its perceived lack of clinical usefulness and technical reproducibility. Then, in 1960, Robert Egan (Fig. 1–13), a radiologist at the M.D. Anderson Hospital in Houston, Texas, described a high-milliamperage–low-kilovoltage technique that resulted in dependable, reproducible, diagnostic-quality mammographic images. Egan modified general-purpose radiographic equipment to optimize soft-tissue imaging by limiting the filtration of the x-ray beam to the inherent filtration of a conventional glass-window x-ray tube, adjusting the control panel of the generator to produce accurate values below 30 kVp, using type M (industrial) Kodak film for high detail and high contrast, and employing a cylindrical cone to reduce scatter. He used the following technical factors: 26 to 28 kVp, 300 mA, a 90-cm target-to-film distance, and a 6-second exposure time (Fig. 1–14).

Using this new technique, Egan[19] reported excellent imaging results for the first 1000 breasts that he studied (634 patients). In 1962, he described 53 cases of "occult carcinoma," which he defined as "one which remains totally unsuspected following examination by the usual methods used to diagnose breast cancer, including examination of the breast by an experienced and competent physician. To qualify for this definition, no symptoms or signs should be

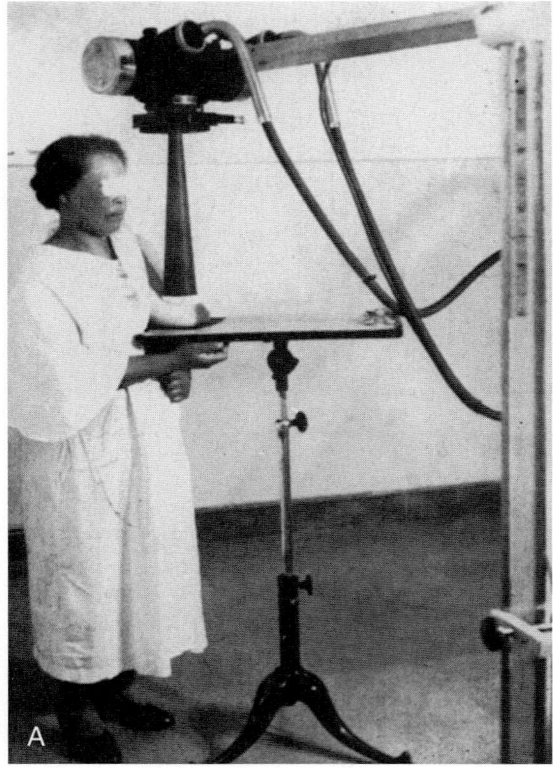

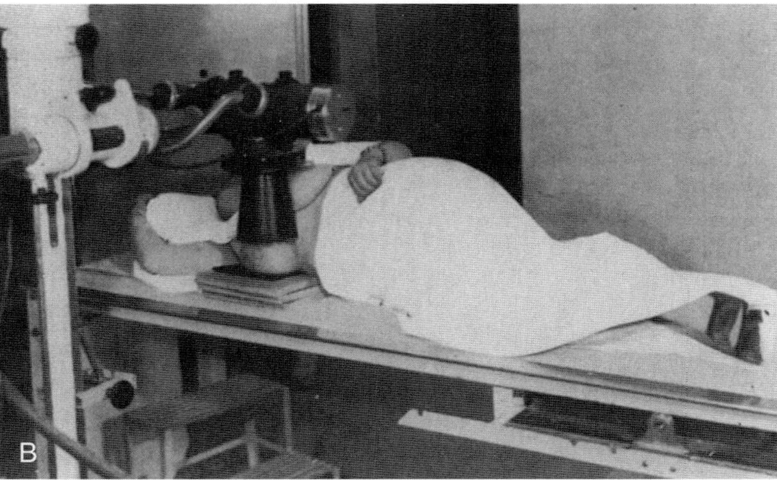

Figure 1–8. **A,** Leborgne's positioning of the patient for a craniocaudal mammogram. Leborgne's caption reads, "Observe the characteristics of the cone and the compression pad interposed between it and the breast." **B,** Leborgne's positioning for the lateral view. (**A** from Leborgne R: Diagnosis of tumors of the breast by simple roentgenography. AJR Am J Roentgenol 1951;65:1-11; **B** from Leborgne R: The Breast in Roentgen Diagnosis. Montevideo, Uruguay, Impresora, 1953.)

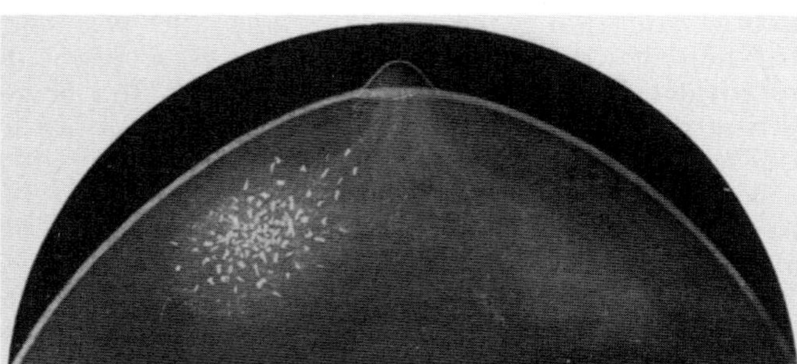

Figure 1–9. Leborgne's diagram of calcifications in carcinoma. His caption reads, "Scattering of countless, punctiform or elongated calcifications, very closely grouped, particularly in center." (From Leborgne R: The Breast in Roentgen Diagnosis. Montevideo, Uruguay, Impresora, 1953.)

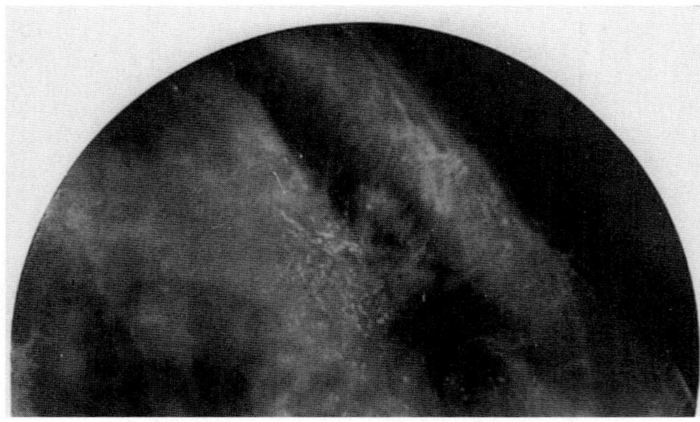

Figure 1–11. Leborgne's coned compression view shows calcifications in carcinoma. (From Leborgne R: The Breast in Roentgen Diagnosis. Montevideo, Uruguay, Impresora, 1953.)

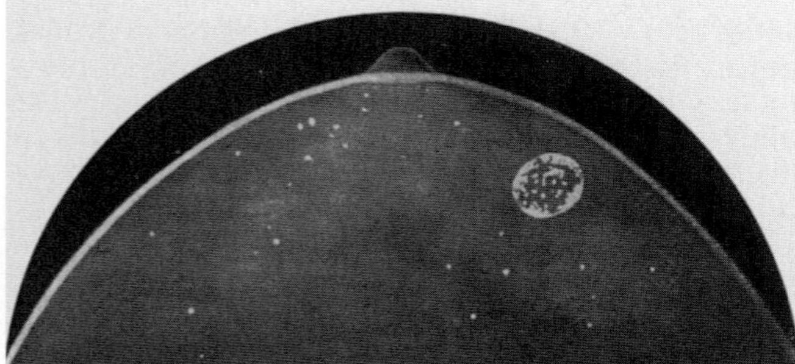

Figure 1–10. Leborgne's diagram of calcifications in fibrocystic disease. His caption reads, "Small calcifications in a circumscribed area, predominating in the periphery (calcifications in cyst); and tiny, punctiform, rounded calcifications scattered throughout the breast in ductal desquamation." (From Leborgne R: The Breast in Roentgen Diagnosis. Montevideo, Uruguay, Impresora, 1953.)

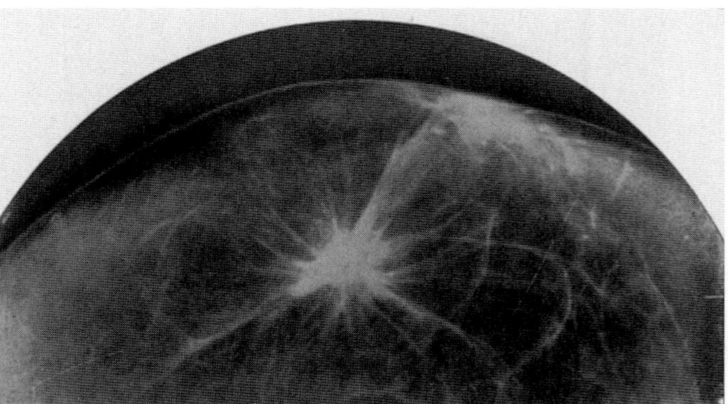

Figure 1–12. Leborgne's coned compression view reveals carcinoma with peripheral spicules. (From Leborgne R: The Breast in Roentgen Diagnosis. Montevideo, Uruguay, Impresora, 1953.)

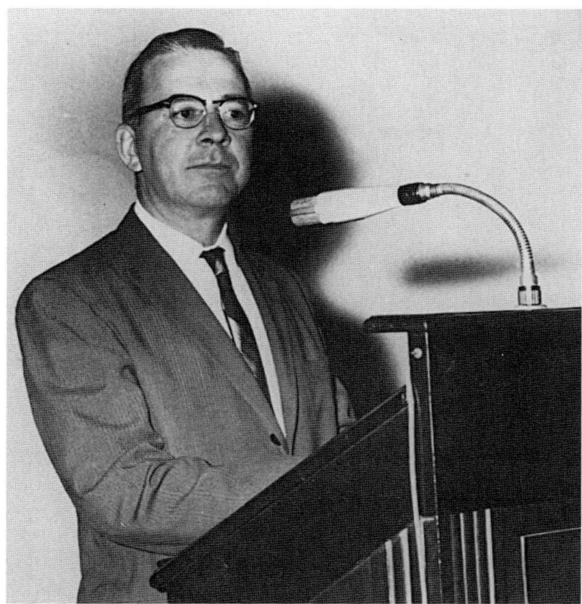

Figure 1–13. Robert L. Egan, spreading the mammography gospel in 1967. (Courtesy of Robert L. Egan, MD, Atlanta, GA.)

present."[20] The success of mammography in detecting these clinically occult carcinomas provided further support for its use as a screening tool.

Egan's success in making reproducible images not only led to the widespread use of mammography to detect breast cancer but also elevated its status to

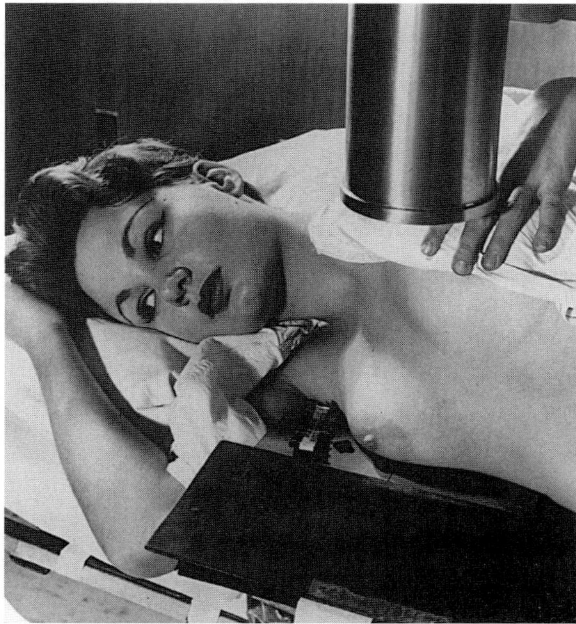

Figure 1–14. Egan's positioning for the mediolateral view. The patient lies on her side, her hand retracting her other breast. The cylindrical tube extending from the target was used to reduce scattered radiation. Technical factors used in obtaining the image included tungsten target, 2-mm focal spot, 28 kilovolt (peak), 300 mA, 6-second exposure, approximately 90-cm source-to-image distance, Eastman Kodak Industrial Type M film, no screen, and no grid. (Courtesy of Robert L. Egan, MD, Atlanta, GA.)

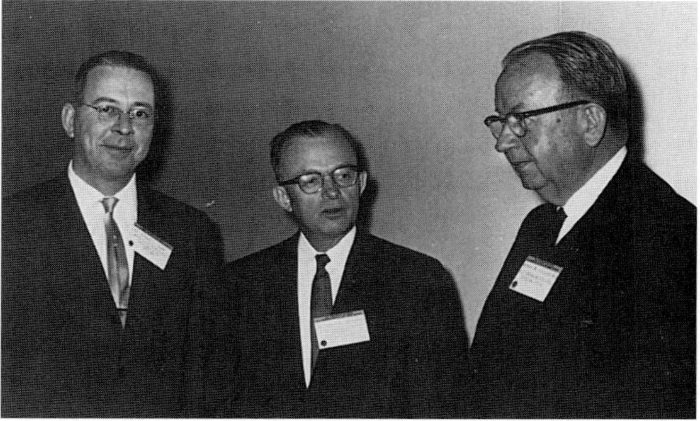

Figure 1–15. The three men responsible for the 1963 Conference on the Reproducibility of Mammography (*from left to right*): Robert L. Egan, MD, Lewis C. Robbins, MD (director of the U.S. Public Health Service Cancer Control Program), and Murray M. Copeland, MD (assistant director of M.D. Anderson Hospital). (Courtesy of Gerald D. Dodd, MD, Houston, TX.)

national recognition. In 1963, the Cancer Control Program of the U.S. Public Health Service, the National Cancer Institute, and the M.D. Anderson Hospital jointly conducted a nationwide investigation involving 24 institutions to verify Egan's results and to determine the possible clinical applications of mammography (Fig. 1–15).[21] The results of the study, presented in 1965, established that (1) the Egan technique of mammography could be learned by other radiologists, (2) mammograms of acceptable quality could be reliably produced, (3) mammography could enable differentiation between benign and malignant lesions, and (4) mammography could be used as a screening tool in asymptomatic women.[22] These results led the American College of Radiology (ACR) to establish a Mammography Committee, chaired by Wendell Scott, which initiated a nationwide training program for radiologists and technologists in the performance and interpretation of mammograms.[23]

The pioneers of mammography made three essential contributions to its evolution: They established a basis for future diagnostic criteria; they strove to improve image quality and reproducibility; and they stimulated widespread interest in mammography and its clinical uses. The wealth of insights and contributions of these pioneers set the stage for an uninterrupted period of intense technologic progress.

ERA OF TECHNOLOGIC PROGRESS

Until the mid-1960s, mammography was performed with general-purpose radiographic equipment. The inability of this equipment to produce finely detailed, high-contrast images led Charles Gros[16] (Fig. 1–16) in France to develop the prototype of the first dedicated mammography unit (Fig. 1–17). This x-ray unit contained two innovations. A molybdenum (rather than tungsten) target provided high subject contrast because of the prominent photoelectric effect of the low-energy x-rays it produced,

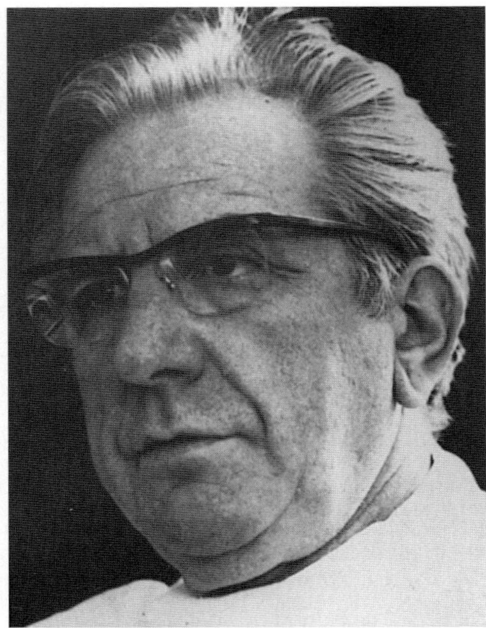

Figure 1–16. Charles Gros. (Courtesy of Dominique Gros, MD, Strasbourg, France.)

and a built-in cone compression device decreased the thickness of the breast and immobilized it during the exposure. In 1967, the Compagnie General de Radiologie (CGR), having developed the prototype with Gros, introduced the Senographe, the first commercially available dedicated mammography unit (Fig. 1–18). The molybdenum target, with its 0.7-mm focal spot, produced greater contrast among parenchyma, fat, and calcifications. The control

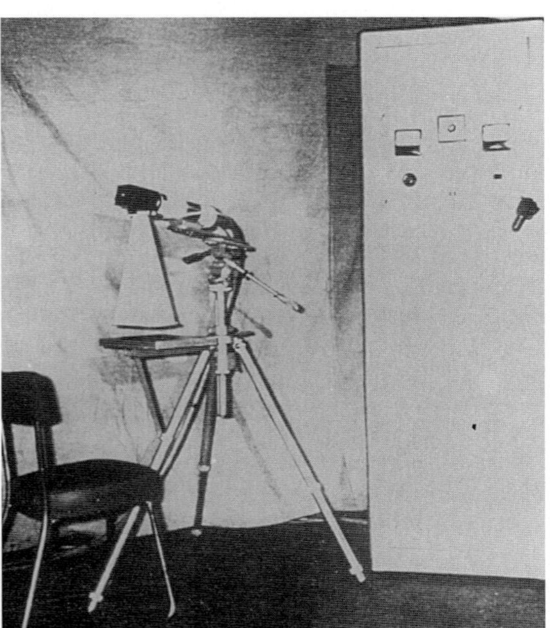

Figure 1–17. Gros's 1965 prototype of the Senographe, aptly called the Trepied ("three feet"). (Courtesy of GE Medical Systems, Milwaukee, WI.)

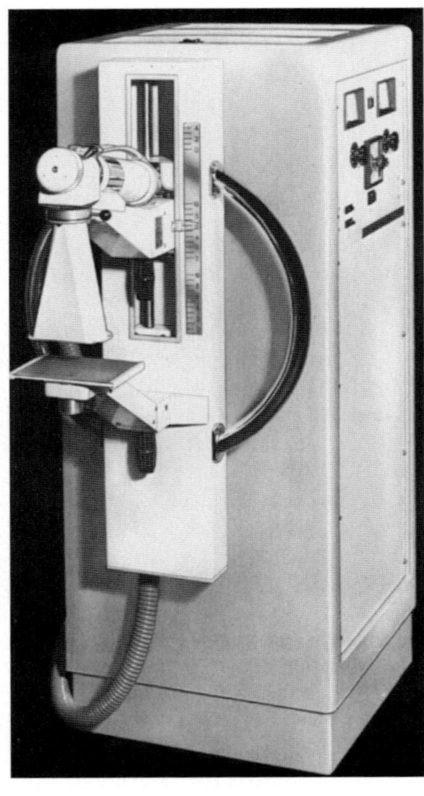

Figure 1–18. First production model of the CGR Senographe in 1966. (Courtesy of GE Medical Systems, Milwaukee, WI.)

panel, designed especially for mammography, offered exposure selections up to 40 mA and 40 kVp and exposure times up to 10 seconds. Built-in interchangeable compression cones decreased scattered radiation and motion unsharpness and separated overlapping breast structures. A rotating C-arm allowed patients to be examined in multiple projections while they sat upright. In the late 1960s, Gershon-Cohen[24] tested the Senographe and reported that contrast, sharpness, and depiction of calcifications were significantly better in Senographe images than in images produced by modified general-purpose radiographic units. However, the improved image quality was achieved at the expense of higher radiation dose. Another disadvantage was the unit's relatively short source-to-skin distance, which resulted in mild magnification and occasional distortion of the image.

In the early 1970s, other dedicated mammography units were introduced, including the Mammomat (Siemens), Mammodiagnost (Philips), and Mammorex (Picker), each incorporating various technical improvements. The Diagnost-U (Philips), introduced in 1978 in the United States, was the first mammography unit with a built-in reciprocating grid. Grids were used as early as 1930 by Stafford Warren,[8] but by the late 1970s, practitioners had a renewed appreciation for their usefulness in overcoming image degradation due to scattered radiation.[25] Investigators in the mid-1980s confirmed the effectiveness of grids in improving image quality.[26] Although they were effective in improving contrast and less expensive than reciprocating grids, stationary grids caused grid lines to appear in the image, a distraction to some radiologists.[27] The better contrast resulting from the use of grids was achieved, nevertheless, at the expense of higher radiation dose. In 1986, Edward Sickles and William Weber[28] reported that grids were most effective in imaging dense breasts but offered little benefit for imaging fatty breasts.

During the late 1970s to early 1980s, mammography x-ray units underwent additional improvements. A foot pedal to control breast compression permitted the technologist to have both hands free to position the breast more accurately. The addition of an automatic exposure timer made image quality more consistent from one examination to the next. Phototiming also helped to realize the screening of large populations because it allowed for the delayed batch processing of radiographs. In the late 1970s, a microfocal spot x-ray tube, which had already been used for magnified images of other organs,[29, 30] was placed into a mammography unit designed by Radiologic Sciences, Incorporated. Although magnification mammography provided highly detailed images of specific areas of interest, it required a higher radiation dose than standard mammography. Thus, the spot tube proved useful only as an adjunct to standard mammography.[31,32]

Higher image quality was achieved with the dedicated mammography unit but at the expense of a higher dose of radiation to the patient. In 1970, in an effort to reduce both radiation dose and exposure time without sacrificing image quality, J. L. Price and P. D. Butler[33] of Great Britain first used a high-definition intensifying screen and film held in intimate contact in an air-evacuated polyethylene envelope. Bernard Ostrum and colleagues[34] at the Albert Einstein Medical Center in Philadelphia, in association with the DuPont Company, conducted further experiments with screen-film combinations. In 1972, DuPont became the first manufacturer to market a dedicated screen-film system for mammography. A single-emulsion Cronex LoDose I film was placed in an air-evacuated, sealed polyethylene bag, with the film's emulsion side against a single Cronex LoDose calcium tungstate intensifying screen, thus reducing image blur by eliminating parallax unsharpness and image crossover. The new screen-film system allowed shorter exposures, thereby decreasing motion unsharpness and involving radiation doses 10 to 20 times lower than with direct film exposure.[35] A variety of mammographic screen-film combinations were soon being made by various manufacturers with the aim of further reducing radiation dosage.

In 1974, the 3M Company introduced rare-earth screens. Because such screens were more efficient than calcium tungstate screens in converting x-ray energy to light, they could be combined with fast-speed film.[36] In 1975, the Eastman Kodak Company introduced a complete mammographic image-recording system composed of a fast Min-R film and a rare-earth Min-R screen held tightly together in a special low-absorption Min-R cassette, thus eliminating the preparation time and vacuum-leakage problems associated with the polyethylene bag. In 1980, Eastman Kodak introduced the Min-R screen-Ortho-M film combination, which required half the radiation exposure required by the previous Min-R combination. In 1986, Eastman Kodak attempted to reduce the dose even further with the introduction of a two-screen dual-emulsion film system. Although this faster system did succeed in reducing radiation dosage, image resolution was decreased to an extent that many mammographers found unacceptable.[37]

Film processing also played a crucial role in the evolution of mammography. Before 1942, all radiographs, including mammograms, were processed manually (Fig. 1–19).[38] Image quality and reproducibility depended on strict adherence to protocols regarding timing, solution formulation, freshness and temperature, and darkroom maintenance. In 1942, the Pako Company introduced the first automated x-ray film processor, which processed films in approximately 40 minutes. In 1956, Eastman Kodak marketed the first roller transport processor (Fig. 1–20).[39] This processor accommodated all types of films, processing them in about 6 minutes. In 1960, film handling was made easier and drying more rapid with the introduction of polyester film base. In 1965, Eastman Kodak introduced 90-second processing. These advances in film processing brought an end to the variability in image quality that plagued manual processing.

While film mammography was continuing to evolve, xeromammography, an alternative method, emerged. In 1937, Chester Carlson developed the basic principles of xerography, which led to the commercial office copier in 1950.[40] In 1952, John

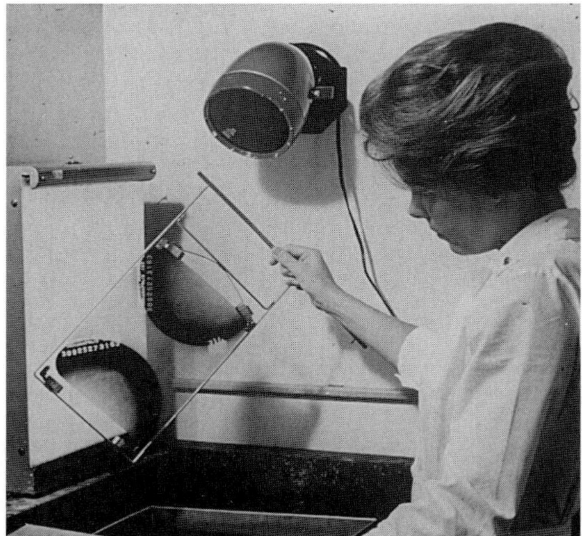

Figure 1–19. One of Dr. Egan's technologists hand-processing the nonscreen, industrial-grade mammography film used by Dr. Egan in the 1960s. (Courtesy of Robert L. Egan, MD, Atlanta, GA.)

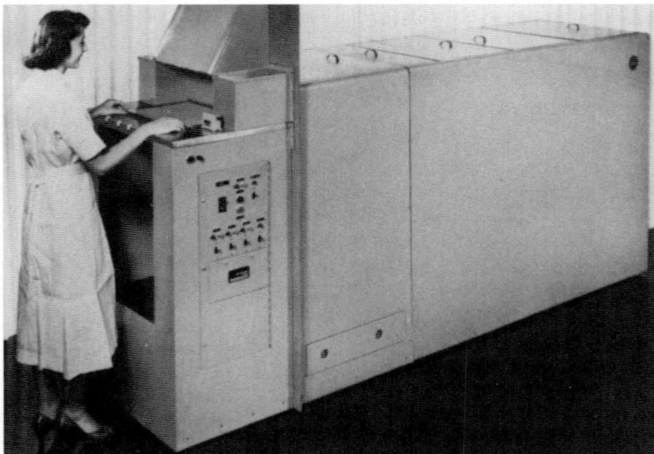

Figure 1–20. First automatic roller transport processor, introduced in 1956, accommodated all radiographic films designed for exposure with intensifying screens. It was approximately 10 feet long and weighed nearly three quarters of a ton. (Reprinted courtesy of Eastman Kodak Company, Rochester, NY.)

Roach and Herman Hilleboe[41] evaluated the medical potentials of xeroradiography, and in 1960, Howard Gould and associates[42] reported that xeroradiography provided images of the breast with greater detail than those produced by conventional film mammography. In 1964, John Wolfe[43] (Fig. 1–21) commenced his investigations of xeromammography using a primitive Xerox radiographic unit consisting of five bulky components (Fig. 1–22). With the cooperation of the Xerox Corporation, Wolfe made numerous modifications to the system, successfully condensing it into two components, a conditioner and a processor. In 1971, just before the introduction of the first dedicated screen-film system for mammography, the Xerox System 125 (Fig. 1–23) became commercially available.

When it was first introduced, positive-mode xeromammography produced high-contrast, high-resolution images at considerably lower radiation doses than were required for direct (nonscreen) film mammography. The superior image quality was attributed to a unique feature of xeroradiography, an edge enhancement phenomenon, whereby the edges of high-density structures, especially spiculations and calcifications, were accentuated (Fig. 1–24A). By 1987, in an effort to further reduce radiation exposure, radiologists had been encouraged to switch to negative-mode imaging and to use additional filtration of the x-ray beam, factors that degraded xeromammographic image quality (Fig. 1–24B). From the 1970s to the early 1980s, xeromammography and screen-film mammography were equally popular modes of breast imaging. However, by the 1980s, improvements in screen-film mammography led to better image quality and lower radiation dosage, resulting in its emergence as the dominant method of breast imaging. By 1988, the majority of facilities performing mammography in the United States were using screen-film systems, and 99% were using

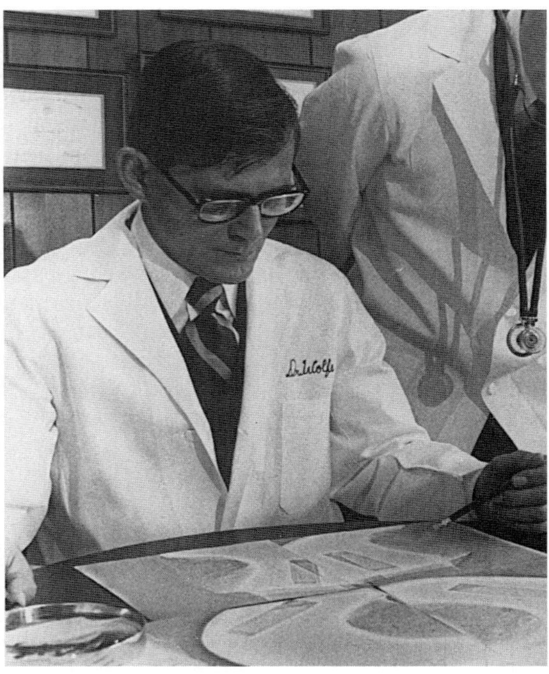

Figure 1–21. John Wolfe in 1970. (Courtesy of John N. Wolfe, MD, Detroit, MI.)

dedicated mammography equipment.[44] By 1989, the growing popularity of screen-film mammography had resulted in the diminution of sales of xeromammographic systems to the point that the Xerox Corporation, after introducing a black liquid toner for greater contrast (Fig. 1–24C), stopped producing them.

OTHER MODALITIES FOR BREAST IMAGING

While x-ray mammography was evolving, other methods of breast imaging were also undergoing development. Ultrasonography, employing high-frequency ultrasonic waves, became particularly successful in differentiating cystic from solid masses. Transillumination, or light-scanning, was a technique based on the imaging of patterns of absorption by the breast of applied near-infrared and red electromagnetic radiation. Thermography used instruments to record abnormal patterns of infrared radiation emitted by the diseased breast.

Breast Ultrasonography

In 1880, the French physicists Pierre and Jacques Curie discovered the *piezoelectric effect*, whereby an electrical charge is produced in response to the application of mechanical pressure on certain crystals.[45] The first attempt to develop a practical application for this effect was that of Paul Langevin, who was

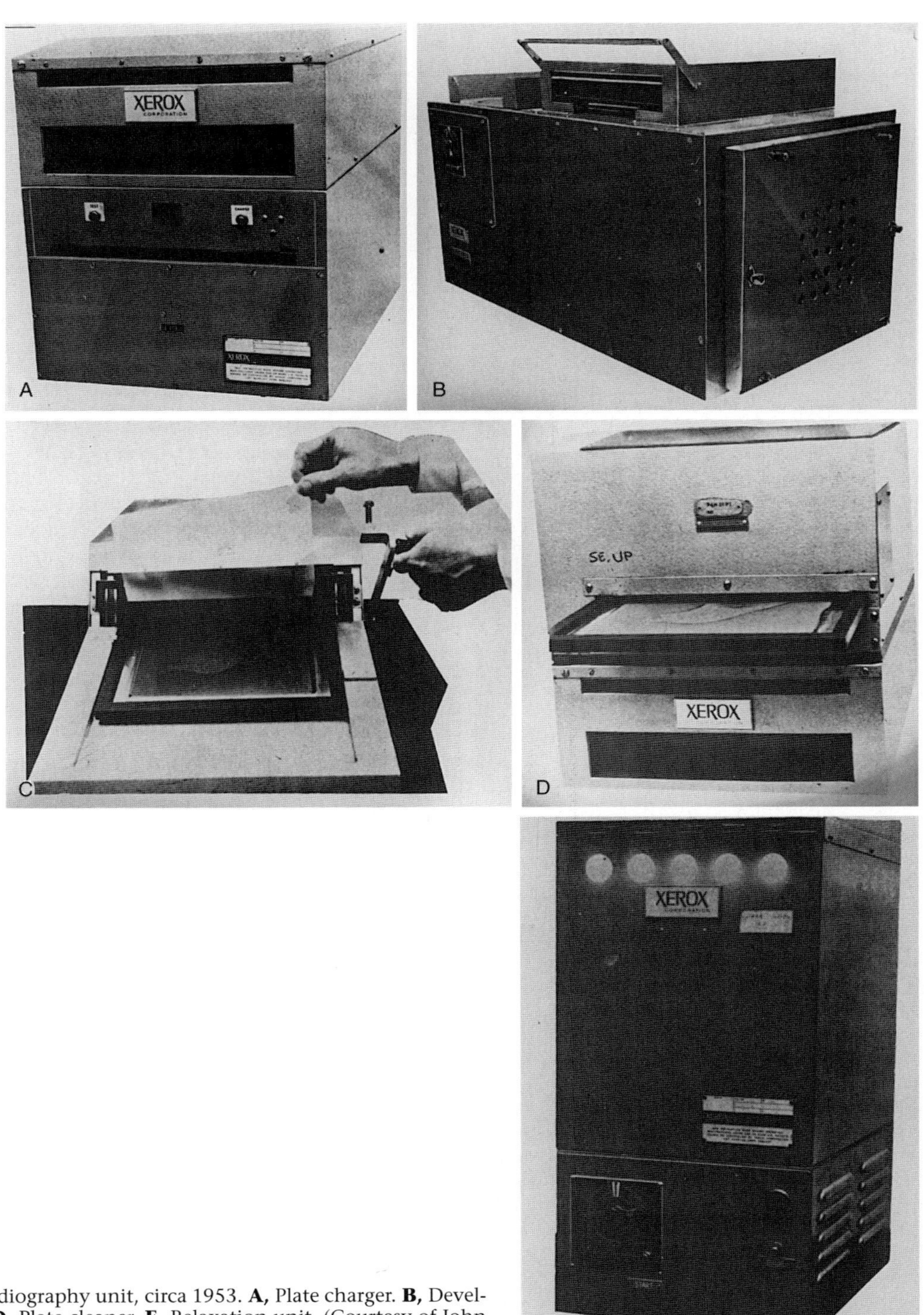

Figure 1–22. Components of xeroradiography unit, circa 1953. **A,** Plate charger. **B,** Development chamber. **C,** Transfer unit. **D,** Plate cleaner. **E,** Relaxation unit. (Courtesy of John N. Wolfe, MD, Detroit, MI.)

commissioned by the French government during World War I to investigate the use of high-frequency ultrasonic waves to detect submarines, leading to the development of SONAR (an acronym derived from "sound navigation ranging") during World War II.[46] In between the wars, other applications of ultrasound were explored, including its role in medicine. During the 1920s and 1930s, ultrasound was used therapeutically for physical therapy and was evaluated for treatment of cancer. During the late 1940s and 1950s, the efficacy of ultrasonography as a diagnostic tool was explored. Karl Dussik[47] of Austria ultrasonically depicted intracranial structures, becoming the first person to use this method for diagnosis. Other investigators, such as W. Guttner[48] in Germany, Andres Denier[49] in France, and Kenji Tanaka[50] in Japan, joined in the effort to explore the diagnostic capabilities of ultrasound.

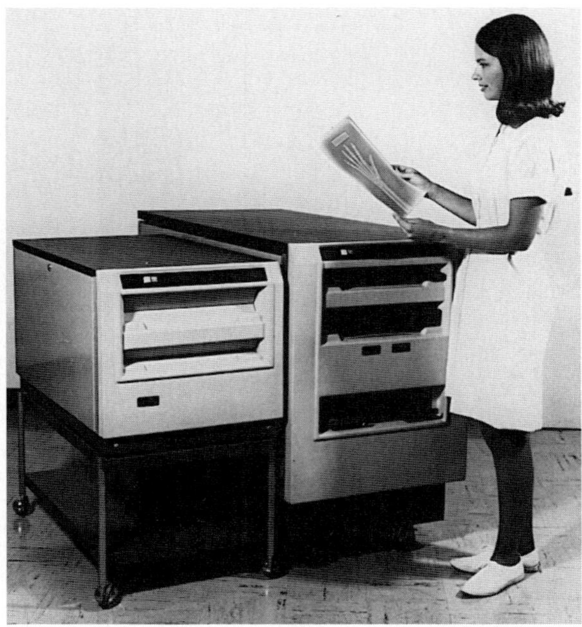

Figure 1–23. The 125/6 system developed by Xerox was the first commercial unit, marketed in 1971.

In the United States, George Ludwig[51] experimented with ultrasound, noting that the velocity of sound waves differed in various tissues, thus setting standards for later sonographic interpretation. In 1949, John Wild[52] used ultrasound to determine the thickness of the intestinal wall in various diseases. He determined that the echoes returning from tumors were different from those returning from normal tissues and suggested that these differences might make ultrasound useful for cancer detection. Later, Wild and John Reid[53,54] constructed several "echoscopes," or hand-held, direct-contact ultrasound scanners, including vaginal and rectal scanners, and even an experimental system for breast cancer screening (Fig. 1–25).

These early investigators used A-mode ultrasound technology, whereby returning echoes were displayed on an oscilloscope.[55] However, A-mode presentations were not anatomically based, and difficult anatomic correlations were required of the investigators. Technologic advances were made in the late 1940s and early 1950s, primarily by Wild and Reid and by Douglas Howry and colleagues, leading to the development of B-mode scanning. This new mode of scanning allowed for more accurate anatomic images because the interfaces of tissue planes and the outlines of organs could be visualized. Wild and Reid employed B-mode contact scanning (Fig. 1–26), but Howry developed a water bath system, which necessitated placement of the patient in an immersion tank made from the gun turret of a B-29 bomber (Fig. 1–27).[56,57] Although in 1950 Howry and his colleagues were successful in obtaining the first high-quality cross-sectional ultrasound images, their method proved impractical for very ill patients. In the early 1960s, the use of B-mode scanning, with its better image quality, led to the commercial marketing of ultrasonographic equipment

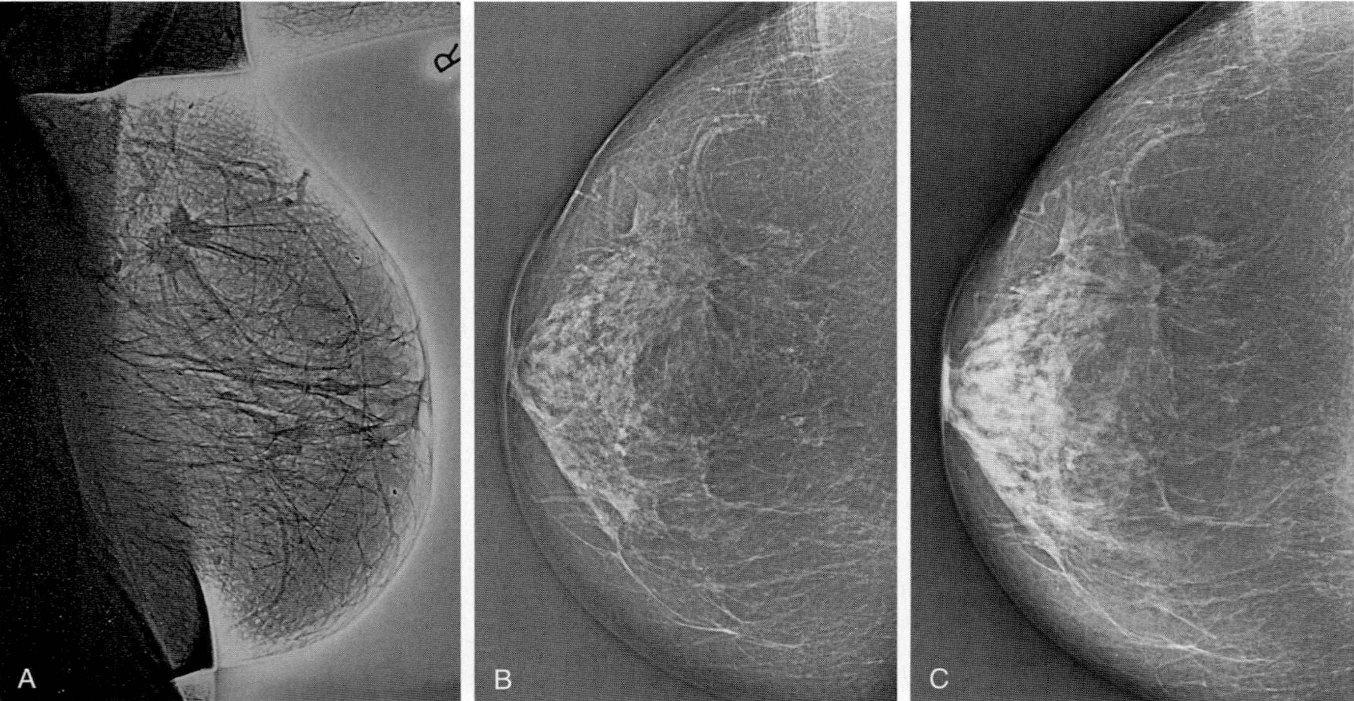

Figure 1–24. Evolution of xeromammography. **A,** Positive-mode xeromammogram reveals a carcinoma in the upper hemisphere of the breast. Note the sharply defined spiculations. **B,** Negative-mode xeromammogram of another spiculated carcinoma. The image is "flatter" in contrast and less detailed than in **A**. **C,** Image from the same projection as in **B,** but processed with liquid black toner.

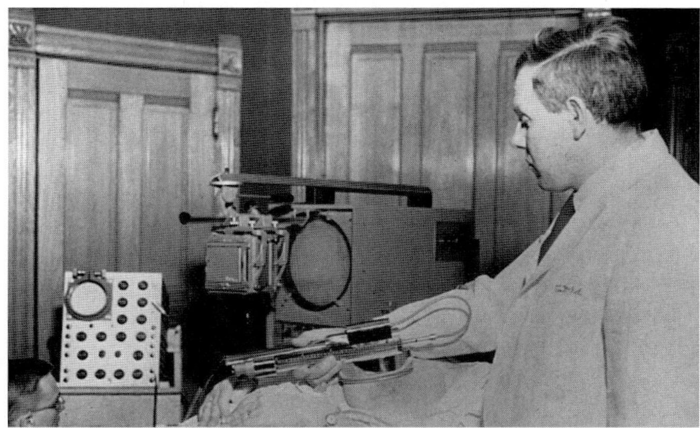

Figure 1–25. John Wild (*right*) and John Reid (*lower left*) employing their B-mode contact scanner to image patients' breasts. (Courtesy of Barry Goldberg, MD, Philadelphia, PA.)

specifically intended for medical diagnosis. As a result, new applications of diagnostic ultrasonography were explored, including echocardiography, echoencephalography, Doppler ultrasonography, obstetric ultrasonography, ophthalmologic ultrasonography, abdominal ultrasonography, and breast ultrasonography.

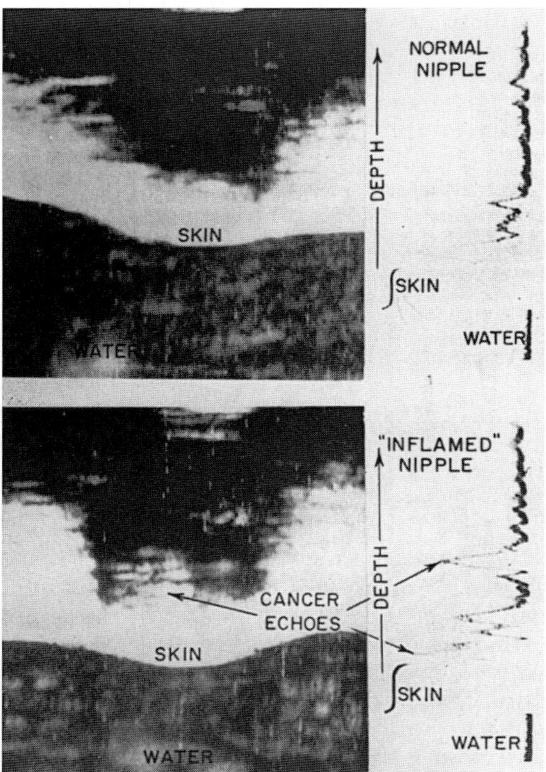

Figure 1–26. Both A-mode (*at right*) and B-mode scans of an "inflamed" nipple and a normal nipple of the same patient, obtained by Wild and Reid in 1953. In the same breast with the "inflamed" nipple, Wild and Reid diagnosed a malignancy, which was later confirmed pathologically. This was the first B-mode scan ever produced of a carcinoma in the living human breast. (Courtesy of Barry Goldberg, MD, Philadelphia, PA.)

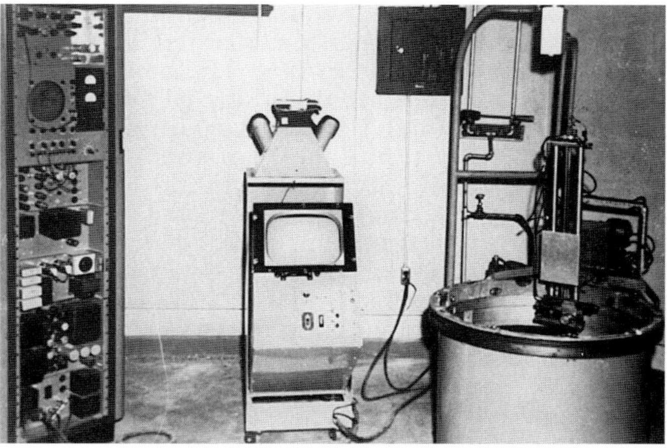

A

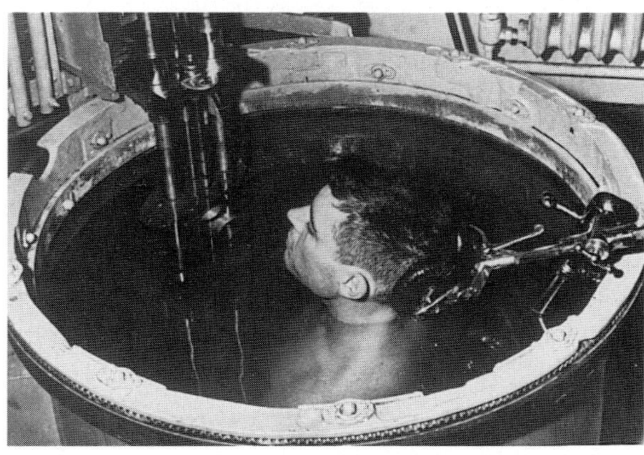

B

Figure 1–27. B-29 gun turret scanner developed by Douglas Howry and his team. **A,** The water-bath system necessitated placement of the patient in an immersion tank, with lead weights on the patient's abdomen for consistent immersion level. **B,** Close-up view with experimental subject. (Courtesy of Barry Goldberg, MD, Philadelphia, PA.)

Breast ultrasonography began in 1951 when Wild and Reid[53,54] in Minnesota and Toshio Wagai and his colleagues[58] in Japan independently produced ultrasonographic images of breast tumors. Wild and Reid[53, 54] were the first to develop equipment specifically designed for breast scanning and attempted to differentiate benign from malignant disease (see Fig. 1–26). They were able to detect some cancers as small as 2 to 3 mm and suggested that ultrasonography might prove beneficial in screening for early breast cancer. Furthermore, they were the first to differentiate between cystic and solid masses in the breast by means of ultrasonography.[53,54]

Recognizing the potential advantages of ultrasonography in breast cancer detection, investigators around the world worked to develop better techniques and equipment to improve breast imaging. Japanese investigators persisted in their investigations of breast scanning, evaluating diagnostic criteria for various breast lesions.[58] In 1968, British investigators P. N. T. Wells and K. T. Evans[59] reported their study of a large water-immersion breast scanner.

Although they were able to obtain high-quality, high-resolution images, immersion scanners were clinically unsatisfactory. Also in 1968, Elizabeth Kelly-Fry and her colleagues[60] in Illinois initiated a study, supported by the Cancer Control Program of the U.S. Department of Health, Education, and Welfare, on the usefulness of ultrasonography in the detection of breast cancer. They found that the modality not only was useful for detecting small cystic and solid masses but also had potential for detecting breast cancer before it became palpable.[60] In 1974, Jack Jellins, George Kossoff, and their associates,[61,62] at the Australian Ultrasonics Institute, developed the Octoson (Fig. 1–28), a multipurpose water bath scanner with eight large-aperture transducers, and developed a gray scale to produce high-quality images. In fact, gray-scale echography was introduced as a direct result of the investigations conducted at the Ultrasonics Institute. Advances in echocardiography led to the development of real-time imaging equipment, which allowed for continuous viewing and recording of images.[63]

Although the use of ultrasonography for breast cancer screening was first suggested by Wild in the 1950s, it was not until the late 1970s, as a result of nationwide concerns about the possibility of radiation-induced breast cancer from screening mammography, that this application was investigated on a large scale.[64-66] The resultant clinical studies showed that ultrasonographic screening was far less effective than screen-film mammographic screening of asymptomatic women.[64,67-69] For example, in 1983, Sickles and coworkers[69] reported that in a prospective study of 1000 women, only 58% of 64 pathologically proven cancers were detected by ultrasonography, compared with 97% by mammography. The limitations of breast ultrasonography in screening included inability to depict microcalcifications, difficulty in imaging of fatty breasts, inability to differentiate benign from malignant solid masses, and unreliable depiction of solid masses smaller than 1 cm.

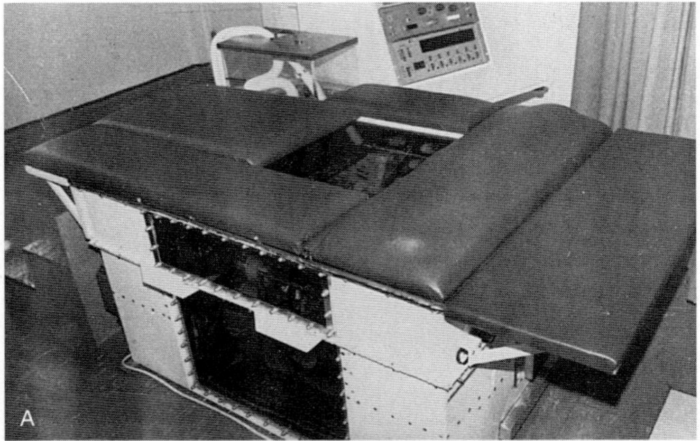

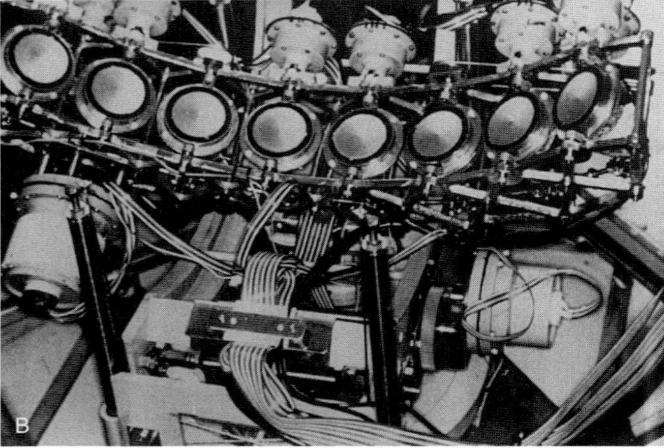

Figure 1–28. Octoson prototype, developed by Jack Jellins, George Kossoff, and others at Australia's Ultrasonics Institute in 1974. **A,** The patient lay on a plastic membrane covering the water bath, and ultrasonic coupling was achieved by the application of oil between the skin and the plastic. **B,** Eight transducers were mounted within the water bath. (Courtesy of Barry Goldberg, MD, Philadelphia, PA.)

The current role of breast ultrasonography is clearly not screening but the differentiation of cystic from solid masses, for which it has an accuracy rate approaching 96% to 100%.[70,71] Breast ultrasonography has evolved into an indispensable adjunct to mammography because the ultrasonographic diagnosis of a simple cyst precludes the need for further evaluation or follow-up, thus saving time, money, and anxiety.

Although ultrasonography currently has no role in screening for breast cancer and is used primarily to differentiate cystic from solid masses, features characteristic of malignant and benign solid masses have been described.[72] However, these criteria leave room for disagreement between observers, and false-negative interpretations still occur.[73] To be most effective, ultrasonography requires adequate time for the examination, real-time scanning, meticulous technique, and high-resolution equipment. Thus, a decision not to perform biopsy of a solid mass should not be based on its ultrasonographic features alone.

Light-Scanning (Diaphanography)

In the late 1920s, Max Cutler investigated transillumination of the breast to access masses.[74] His work stimulated a more refined technique by Charles Gros and his colleagues,[75] which they termed "diaphanography." They used "cold" light that could penetrate even dense breast tissue and obtained a photographic image of the transilluminated breast. Advances by Ernest Carlsen[76] combined cold light transillumination with an electronic system that analyzed light over a wide spectrum and stored the data for interpretation and retrieval.

Light-scanning of the breast was based on the concept that cancer, because of its greater blood supply, absorbs more near-infrared and red electromagnetic radiation than benign tissue. As a consequence, instead of real-time viewing by the human eye, which is totally insensitive to near-infrared rays, the evaluation was made of an image on infrared-sensitive photographic film (Fig. 1–29).[77] Alternatively, a television camera sensitive to near-infrared radiation displayed the image on a television monitor.

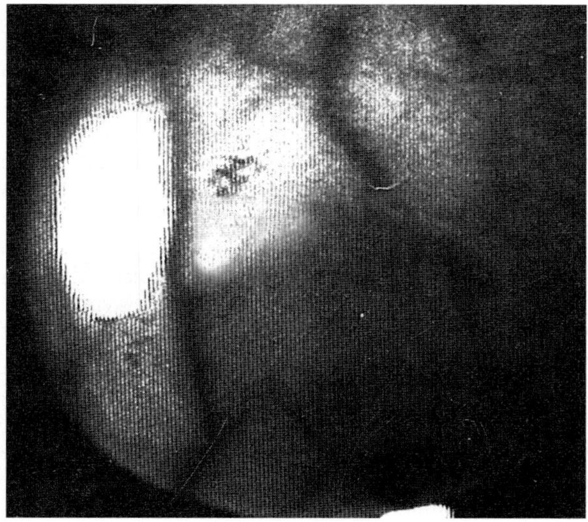

Figure 1–29. Transillumination, or light-scanning. Photograph of a transilluminated breast reveals a large cyst. Images were obtained by using a "cold" light probe that could penetrate dense breast tissue. (Courtesy of Christopher Merritt, MD, New Orleans, LA; reprinted from Merritt CRB, Sullivan MA, Segaloff A, McKinnon WP: Real-time transillumination lightscanning of the breast. Radiographics 1984;4:989-1009.)

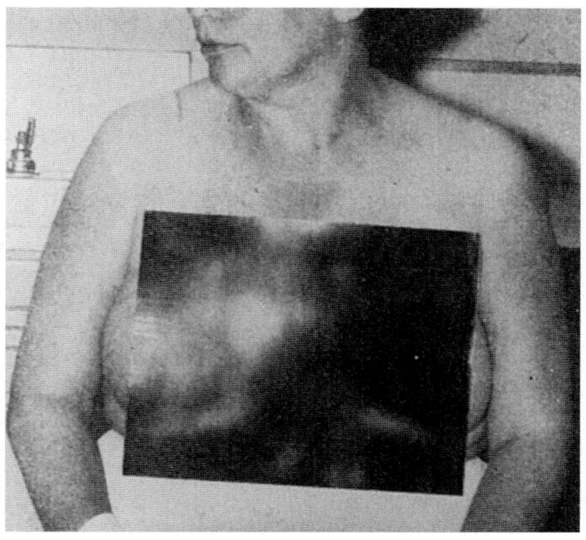

Figure 1–30. Lawson's thermogram of a patient's breast superimposed on a photograph of the patient. The infrared display shows a white focus that corresponds to the site of increased skin temperature over a carcinoma in the right breast. (From Lawson RN, Chughtai MS: Breast cancer and body temperature. Can Med Assoc J 1963;88:68-70.)

Electronic contrast enhancement of the video image increased the likelihood of visualizing subtle lesions. Although the technique was rapid, noninvasive, risk-free, and relatively inexpensive, prospective controlled feasibility studies showed light-scanning to be considerably less sensitive than mammography in the detection of nonpalpable cancer.[78-81]

Thermography

Galileo constructed the first thermometer in 1595, but it was not until the 18th century that Herman Boerhaave first used thermometry in a clinical setting. In 1851, Carl Wunderlich began to periodically measure the temperature of his patients, thus giving thermometry a permanent role in clinical examination.

Thermography was first investigated for evaluating breast disease in 1956, when Ray Lawson,[82] having observed that breast cancer was associated with elevation of the temperature of the overlying skin, used modified military heat scanners for breast evaluation (Fig. 1–30). Although the mechanisms of tumor thermogenesis and heat transfer are not understood completely, increased blood perfusion at the sight of the lesion is believed to be the primary factor responsible for the elevation in local skin temperature.[83] Lawson's early experiments evolved into telethermography, in which infrared radiation emitted from the body was focused by an optical mirror and displayed on a cathode-ray tube. The image was photographed for a permanent record.

A later method, contact liquid crystal thermography, involved placement of sheets of thin plastic containing heat-sensitive encapsulated liquid crystal cholesterol esters against the breast. Infrared radiation caused the black crystals to undergo changes of color, which varied with the infrared energies being emitted from the breast surface. A later method, computed thermography, employed multiple thermistors for infrared detection. The electronic signals were fed to a computer, which utilized various algorithms to determine whether the measurements were normal or abnormal without the necessity of imaging the breast.

Numerous objective analyses have found that thermography is unreliable in detecting subclinical cancer.[84,85] Indeed, the poorest results were obtained in women whose cancers were most amenable to therapy. Also, thermography could not be used as a prescreening examination to identify patients requiring mammography or reliably differentiate benign from malignant disease. In the Breast Cancer Detection Demonstration Project, the cancer detection rate for thermography was only 42%, a clinically unacceptable level, especially compared with rates of 57% for physical examination and 91% for mammography. Furthermore, thermography had an unacceptably high number of false-positive results.[86,87] Thus, thermography is not considered useful for breast cancer screening.

Radionuclide Imaging of the Breast

In 1966, Whitley and coworkers[88] described a single case of breast carcinoma in which intravenously administered technetium Tc 99m pertechnetate concentrated in the lesion. One year later, Bonte and associates[89] reported imaging breast carcinoma in 4 patients by means of iodinated (^{131}I) human serum albumin, but detail was poor.[89] In a chapter contained in a 1969 textbook, Buchwald and colleagues[90] described the visualization of the tumor in 18 of 26 patients with breast carcinoma through the use of Hg 197 mercuric chloride. Cancroft and Goldsmith[91] used technetium Tc 99m pertechnetate scintigraphy (Fig. 1–31) in 6 patients with palpable breast masses, of whom 4 had carcinoma (or "probable carcinoma" on the basis of physical examination or mammography), 1 had a biopsy-proven fibroadenoma, and the last had probable fibrocystic change that did not undergo biopsy. One of the 4 patients with presumed carcinoma refused biopsy and another, with bone metastases, was treated with radiotherapy to the primary lesion without biopsy. All of the biopsy-proven and presumed carcinomas showed increased radionuclide activity, and the benign lesions did not. However, any early enthusiasm generated for pertechnetate breast imaging was dissipated in 1974, when an investigation by Villarreal and associates[92] revealed significant numbers of false-negative and false-positive diagnoses of cancer with the modality. These investigators concluded that the procedure did not fulfill the requirements for a successful screening test.

In 1987, interest in radionuclide imaging of tumors was rekindled when technetium Tc 99m methoxyisobutyl isonitrile (MIBI), or sestamibi, was found to be taken up in a lung metastasis of a thyroid carcinoma.[93] The drug, originally designed as a myocardial perfusion tracer to assess coronary artery disease, has been investigated to determine its usefulness in the detection of breast cancer in patients scheduled to undergo breast biopsy. The results in these selected populations of women, most of whom had clinically suspicious lesions, have been variable; the modality shows good sensitivity for palpable lesions but more limited sensitivity for nonpalpable lesions.[94,95] The results of one preliminary investigation have suggested that scintimammography may be a valuable noninvasive complementary test in patients in whom mammography shows a low or indeterminate likelihood of cancer, especially when ACR Breast Imaging Reporting and Data System (BI-RADS) category III lesions ("probably benign findings") have been found.[96] As yet, there are no published studies of the efficacy of sestamibi scintigraphy for breast cancer screening.

Magnetic Resonance Imaging of the Breast

The concept of cancer detection by magnetic resonance imaging (MRI) was introduced by Damadian[97] in 1971. Four investigations published between 1975 and 1978 showed that T1 and T2 relaxation times differed between normal and malignant breast tissues in vitro.[98-101] In 1980, Mansfield and associates[102] reported the successful MRI localization of cancer in mastectomy specimens.[102] Two years later, Ross and colleagues[103] reported the results of an in vivo MRI investigation of the breasts of 65 women whose

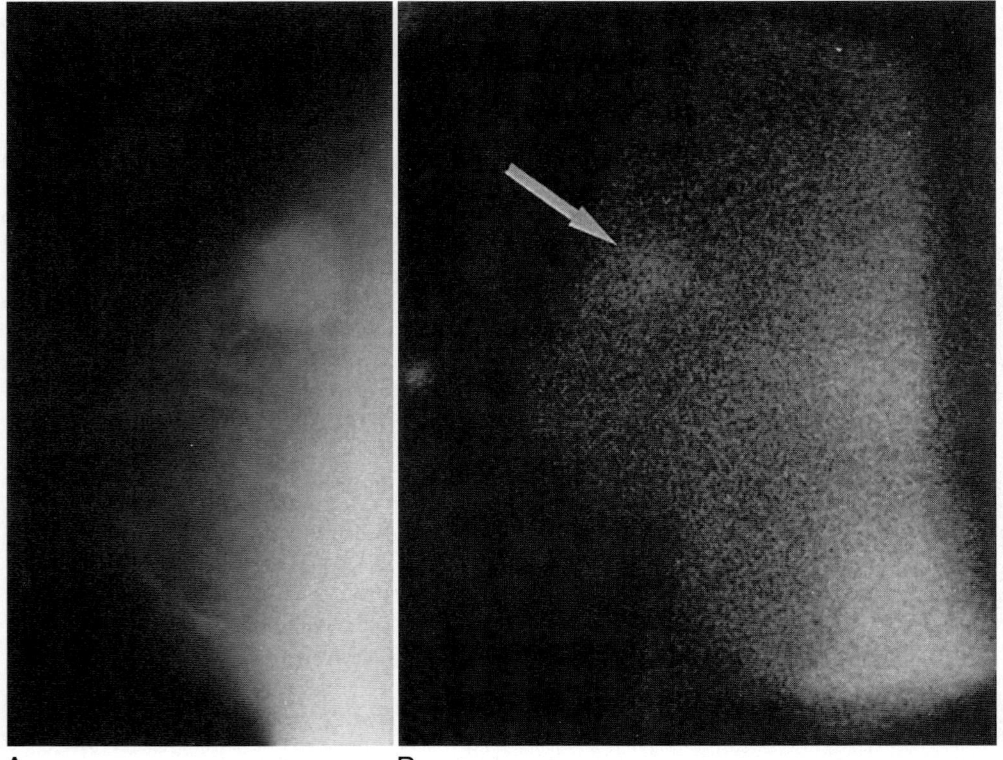

Figure 1–31. Technetium Tc 99m pertechnetate scintigraphy of breast carcinoma. **A,** Mediolateral mammogram demonstrates a mass with a spiculated margin. **B,** Gamma camera image shows focus of increased radionuclide activity (*arrow*). (From Cancroft ET, Goldsmith SJ: ^{99m}Tc-pertechnetate scintigraphy as an aid to the diagnosis of breast masses. Radiology 1973;106:441-444.)

tissue varied from normal to dysplastic to cancerous.[103] Seven of the women had carcinomas, two of which were clinically occult but mammographically suspicious. Using an early 0.045-tesla (T) FONAR QED 80 scanner, and imaging the patients in the supine position, these investigators found that the T1 relaxation times of dysplastic tissue and fibroadenomas overlapped those of malignant tissue.

In 1984, El Yousef and coworkers[104] published the results of an MRI study comparing the breasts of 10 normal volunteers with those of 45 patients with breast abnormalities (Fig. 1–32).[104] These researchers used a 0.3-T system, scanning the volunteers and 25 patients in the supine position and without a surface coil, and scanning 20 patients in the prone position and with a dedicated breast surface coil. Using both spin echo and inversion recovery pulse sequences, but obtaining only T1-weighted images, they compared their MR images with x-ray mammograms. Because they found considerable overlap in T1 relaxation times between cancer and benign breast lesions, El Yousef and coworkers[104] determined that the contour and configuration of the abnormalities provided the best differential diagnostic criteria. This preliminary experience in breast MRI emphasized morphology as the most useful criterion to distinguish benign from malignant breast disease.

In a scientific exhibit presented at the 1984 meeting of the Radiological Society of North America and an article published later, Alcorn and colleagues[105] reported their experience with a 0.5-T magnet and a dedicated breast surface coil used to image breasts with varied pathology.[105] These investigators blamed their necessarily imprecise calculations of T1 and T2 relaxation times for their lack of success in detecting breast cancer, and they were not optimistic about the value of morphology in detecting cancer that was surrounded by abundant parenchymal tissue. They ended their report with this prescient statement: "The future of MR imaging as an accurate modality for the detection of malignant breast neoplasms . . . will probably depend upon the use of appropriate paramagnetic contrast substances as well as other technical improvements."[105]

In 1986, Heywang and associates[106] evaluated the use of gadolinium enhancement (with intravenous gadolinium–diethylenetriamine-penta-acetic acid [Gd-DTPA]) to improve the differentiation between benign and malignant breast lesions. They found that most malignant tumors were enhanced but most benign lesions were not. The outgrowth of their work was the emergence of two different methods of contrast enhancement—dynamic, medium-resolution imaging *during* enhancement[107] and three-dimensional high-resolution imaging *after* enhancement.[108] The first method emphasized the value of information related to the time course of gadolinium enhancement, because malignant tumors theoretically enhance more rapidly than benign lesions. The proponents of this method maintained that clinically important enhancement was characterized by a 100% rise in signal intensity within the first 2 minutes after injection. The second method emphasized the value of whole-breast images for detecting unsuspected lesions. The investigators favoring this concept used ultimate signal intensity rather than dynamic information, with enhancement above 300 normalized units being considered clinically important.

Since these reports appeared, it has become clear that although cancers tend to enhance faster than benign lesions, there is overlap in their rates of enhancement. A major limitation of breast MRI remains its low specificity. The fact that most enhancing lesions are benign underscores the

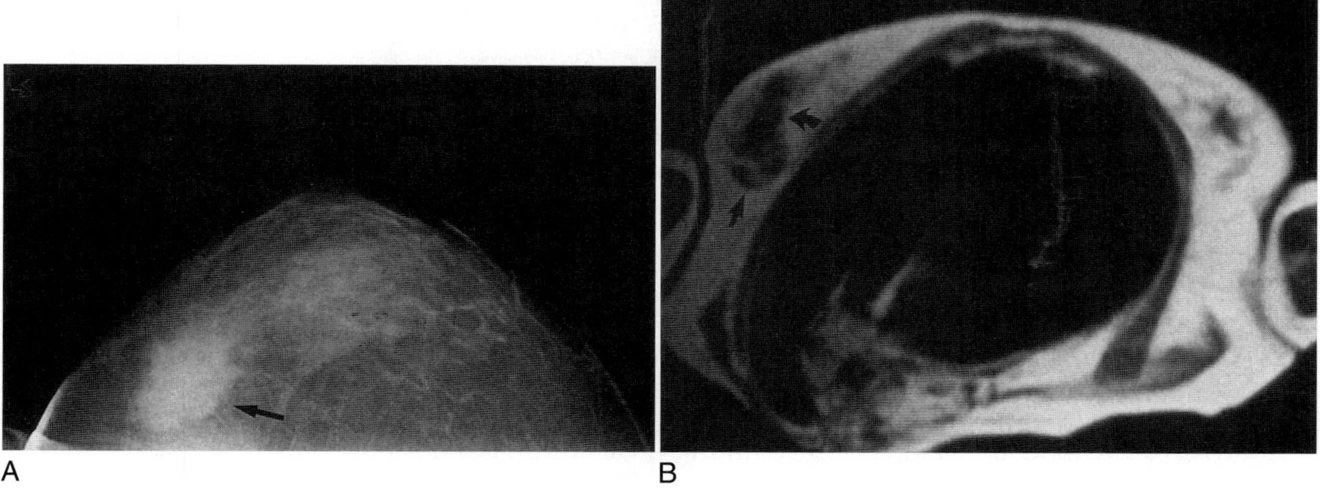

Figure 1–32. Early magnetic resonance (MR) image of breast carcinoma. **A,** Craniocaudal mammogram shows a spiculated mass (*arrow*). **B,** Axial spin-echo MR image (TR 500; TE, 30) of supine patient, obtained with cryogenic superconductive magnet (Teslacon) operating at 3.0 kilogauss. The cancer is marked by *arrows*. (From El Yousef SJ, Duchesneau RH, Alfidi RJ: Nuclear magnetic resonance imaging of the human breast. Radiographics 1984;4:113-121.)

importance of lesion morphology as a diagnostic criterion.[109] MRI of the breast has evolved to a state at which it is able to provide important information unavailable with other imaging methods, but as a method to detect, diagnose, and stage cancer, the modality remains in the investigational stage.

In 1993 and 1994, a flurry of articles appeared describing the use of MRI to detect abnormalities of breast implants, such as silicone gel "bleed," leak, and rupture. When the effectiveness of MRI in this regard was compared with that of ultrasonography, mammography, and CT, MRI was generally found to be the most accurate method.[110-112] When a question of breast implant integrity cannot be answered through the use of conventional imaging methods, MRI, although more costly than the other methods, is the one most effective in detecting implant failure.[113, 114]

SCREENING MAMMOGRAPHY

Of the variety of modalities available for breast imaging, x-ray mammography has proven to be the most efficacious for breast cancer screening. Although the concept of using mammography as a screening tool was hypothesized by many of its pioneers, Gershon-Cohen and Ingleby[115] were the first to actually investigate its use for screening, in 1958. They concluded that periodic mammograms of women older than 40 years would prove beneficial in reducing mortality from breast cancer.[116,117] However, because their studies did not include controls, their work was largely ignored.

In an effort to determine the efficacy of screening mammography, several prospective large-scale clinical trials were performed. The first of these was conducted from 1963 to 1967 under the auspices of the Health Insurance Plan (HIP) of New York.[118] Organized by Philip Strax, Louis Venet, and Sam Shapiro, the study was performed to determine whether periodic mammographic screening and physical examination could decrease mortality from breast cancer. The women in the study were equally divided into control and study groups. Those in the study group were requested to undergo annual physical examination and mammography for 4 consecutive years. The results of the study showed that the screened group had a 30% lower mortality overall than the control group of women; a 50% lower mortality was seen for those women who entered the study at 50 years or older.[119,120] Although mortality was 23% lower among the screened women younger than 50 years, this finding lacked significance because of an inadequate number of women in this age group.

Five of the eight randomized trials also found a lower mortality from breast cancer with screening for women aged 40 to 49 years.[121] The mortality reduction was 22% in the Edinburgh trial,[122] 23% in the HIP trial, 25% in the Kopparberg, Sweden, trial, 49% in the Malmö, Sweden, trial,[121] and 40% at 10 years in the Gothenburg, Sweden, trial.[123] Strengths of the benefit in the Gothenburg trial are its statistical significance and the fact that 30% of the women who died from breast cancer among those offered screening actually had refused to be screened but were still counted as having been screened.

The success of the HIP study led to the Breast Cancer Detection Demonstration Project (BCDDP), cosponsored by the National Cancer Institute (NCI) and the American Cancer Society (ACS). This program, designed to demonstrate the usefulness of annual mammography in women aged 35 to 74 years at the community level, began in 1973 and ran for 5 years. Although the lack of a control group prohibited definitive conclusions, the collected data reflected the advances made in mammography since the HIP study. Mammography detected 91% of all the cancers found during the course of the study. Of those cases, mammography of the cancers for which the physical findings were negative detected 42% (compared with 33% in the HIP study), whereas physical examination of the cancers for which the mammographic findings were negative detected only 9% (compared with 44% in the HIP study). One third of the cancers in the BCDDP study were noninfiltrating or infiltrating but smaller than 1 cm, whereas none of the cancers in the HIP study were smaller than 1 cm.[86,87] Moreover, these small cancers were detected in women of all ages.

Several studies in Europe also confirmed the value of mammographic screening. A Dutch case-control study of women older than 35 years who underwent single-view mammograms every 2 years found a 52% lower mortality in the screened group compared with the control group.[124] A second Dutch case-control study, limited to women 50 to 64 years of age screened initially and then at 12, 18, and 24 months, demonstrated a 70% lower mortality.[125] A larger population-based randomized control study conducted in Sweden involved women between 40 and 74 years who underwent single oblique-view mammography at 24- to 33-month intervals.[126,127] After 11 years, the data showed a 31% lower mortality and a 25% lower absolute number of cancers classified as stage II or more advanced.

The studies in the United States and Europe have clearly shown the value of screening mammography of asymptomatic women. Responding to the results of these studies, various medical groups have established screening guidelines. In 1976, the ACR became the first group to adopt such guidelines. The ACR recommended that mammograms be performed at 1- to 2-year intervals for women younger than 50 years and annually for women age 50 or older. However, controversy surrounded the efficacy of screening women younger than 50 years. In 1977, the NCI and the ACS recommended that women 39 years or younger enrolled in the BCDDP be screened only if they had a personal history of breast cancer and that women 40 to 49 years be screened only if they had a personal or family history of breast cancer.[128,129] In 1980, the ACS recommended a baseline mammogram for all women 35 to 40 years of age. As a result of the BCDDP's findings, that significant numbers of cancers were detected by mammography in women age 40 to 49 years, the ACS recommended mammography at 1- to 2-year intervals for women in that age group. In 1989, the ACS, NCI, and nine other organizations joined in issuing a uniform set of guidelines: Screening should commence at age 40 years, followed by a mammogram every 1 to 2 years until age 50, after which a mammogram should be performed annually.[130] Important differences from previous guidelines were the deletion of a baseline mammogram and greater support for screening women between 40 and 49 years old.

Widespread under-utilization of mammographic screening in the United States, first noted in 1955,[131] was still present in 1987, when studies showed that only 15% to 20% of American women older than 50 years had ever had a mammogram.[132] This finding led to attempts to identify barriers to screening mammography. In 1985, a study of 257 Michigan women demonstrated that only 19% of women 35 to 49 years old and 25% of women 50 years and older had ever had a mammogram, and that only 34% were aware of the recommended guidelines for mammography in women 50 years and older.[133] The study also indicated that 48% of the women planned to have mammograms solely on the basis of recommendations from their physicians, emphasizing the importance of physicians' attitude in the utilization of screening mammography. One study revealed that the primary reason that physicians did not recommend mammographic screening was a perceived risk of radiation.[134] Another study of physicians' attitudes found that some were unaware of the clinical benefits of screening mammography, and that 72% specified high cost versus low yield as the major reason for not recommending mammography to their patients.[135]

Efforts to overcome this widespread under-utilization of screening mammography have involved educating physicians and patients about the procedure and its usefulness in detecting early breast cancer and finding ways to reduce the cost of the procedure. Regarding its safety, physicians and patients have been reassured that with modern technology, the risk of radiation exposure with low-dose mammography is negligible.[136]

The high cost of screening mammography has been a persistent problem. In 1986, a survey of 58 facilities in Los Angeles found that the average cost of a mammogram was $125.[137] To reduce this cost, radiologists began to differentiate between diagnostic and screening mammographic examinations.[138] The *diagnostic examination* involves a more expensive and more complete examination of a symptomatic patient, with additional views obtained according to symptoms and clinical signs, whereas the *screening examination* is limited to asymptomatic patients and is less expensive, requiring only two views of each breast. A growing number of facilities now offer low-cost screening mammograms. Another approach to lowering costs is the use of mobile screening mammography vans (Fig. 1–33), first developed and successfully implemented by Philip Strax (Fig. 1–34) in the late 1960s.[139] Edward Sickles[140] has pointed out that the operating expenses for a van practice are considerably less than those for an office practice, primarily because no office rent is paid for the former. Moreover, mobile vans allow for mass screening in remote and socioeconomically depressed areas, thereby making screening mammography more accessible to more women. The result of these efforts has been to increase the use of screening and diagnostic mammography to the extent that in 1993,

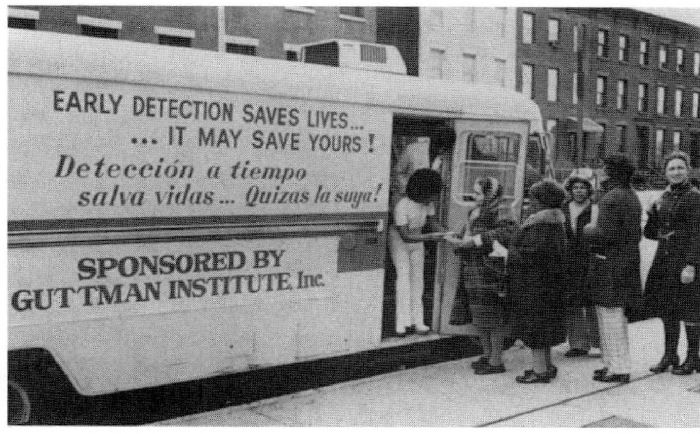

Figure 1–33. Self-contained mobile mammographic van used by Strax in the late 1960s. As many as 70 women per day underwent mammography in the van. The van contained facilities for obtaining a medical history and performing physical examination, mammography, and thermography. (Courtesy of Philip Strax, MD, Lauderhill, FL.)

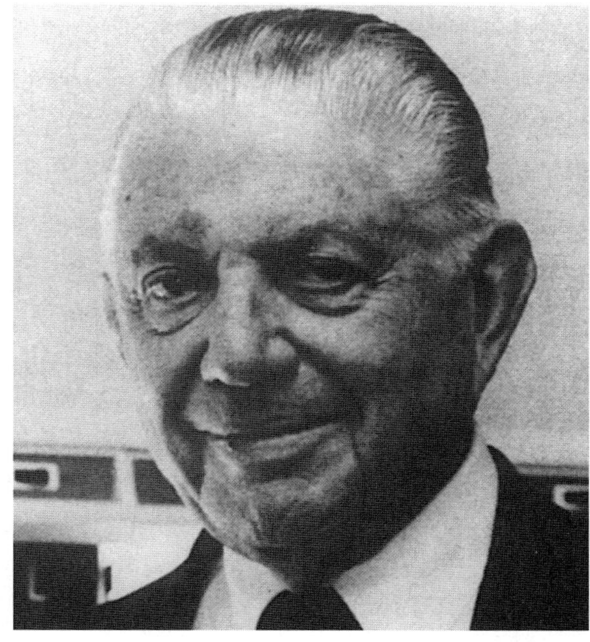

Figure 1–34. Philip Strax. (Courtesy of Philip Strax, MD, Lauderhill, FL.)

approximately 74% of all women 40 years and older were found to have had at least one mammogram.[141]

EDUCATION IN MAMMOGRAPHY

The usefulness of mammography depends highly on the proper use of dedicated mammography equipment and the diagnostic skills of the interpreter, which can be achieved only through proper education. In 1965, it was determined that the mammographic technique of Egan could be learned and used by other radiologists.[22] In 1967, the ACR established the Committee on Mammography, chaired by Wendell Scott, which undertook the responsibility of training radiologists and their technologists. With the assistance of Egan and with funding from the Cancer Control Program of the U.S. Public Health Service, 13 nationwide training centers using unique teaching aids were established (Fig. 1–35). Radiologists and their technologists were encouraged to participate in a 1-week period of training at the center of their choice, with travel expenses paid by the program, and to return to the center after 2 or 3 months for a 3-day refresher course.[23] By 1969, when the program was discontinued, 1300 radiologists and 2300 technologists had been trained.[142]

Despite growing interest and expanded training, the majority of radiologists remained unfamiliar with mammography. In an effort to increase its use, the ACR Committee on Mammography and Diseases of the Breast (formerly the Committee on Mammography) developed training tools that included a self-evaluation pre-test, a continuing education text, and a detailed technical evaluation of available dedicated mammography equipment. Funded by the NCI, several new centers of training for radiologists and their technologists were active from 1975 through 1978.

In 1980, a survey found that radiology residency programs lacked adequate training in mammography. Some residents had no exposure to mammography, and only a few had rotations devoted exclusively to mammography.[143] During the early 1980s, as breast cancer detection by mammography increased, so did related medicolegal actions and recognition of the need for more effective mammography training of radiology residents. In 1983, the American Board of Radiology began to include questions related to breast disease and mammography in its written examinations, and beginning in 1990, a section on mammography was incorporated into its oral examinations. These actions reflected the growing importance of mammography and were major factors in improving mammography training.

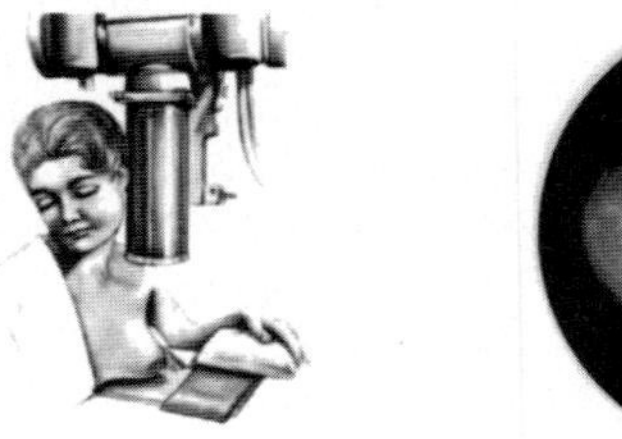

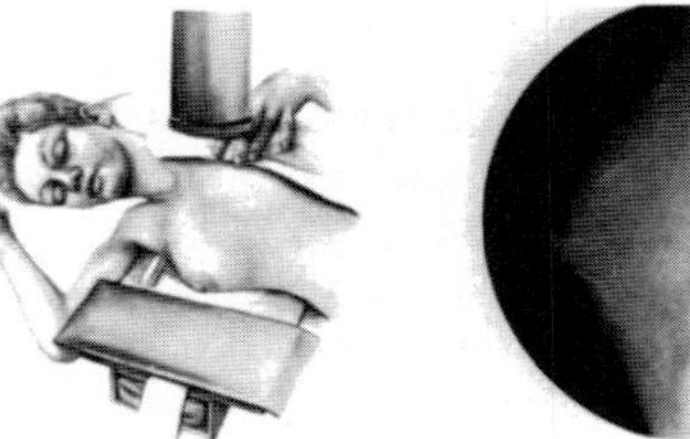

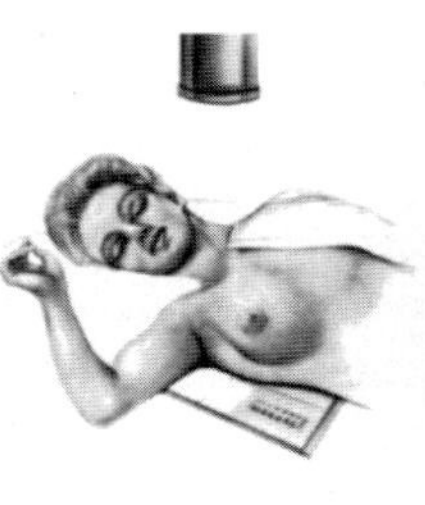

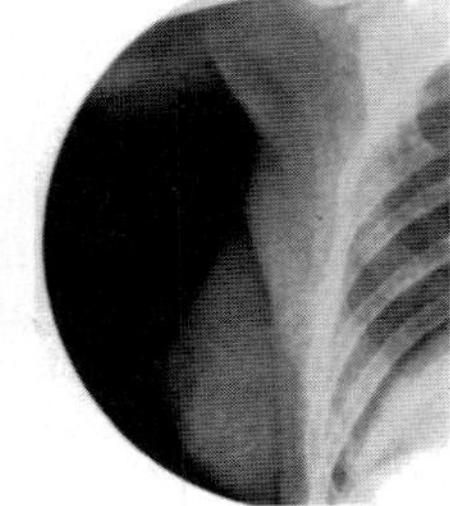

Film—Kodak Industrial X-ray Film, Type M (Estar Base), most satisfactory. Kodak Medical X-ray Film for Mammography (Estar Base) may be used.
Exposure Holder—Cardboard, with lead back.
Processing—Kodak Industrial X-ray Film, Type M. Process manually in fresh solutions. Development—5 to 8 minutes at 68 F, acid stop bath—30 seconds, fixation—12 to 15 minutes at 68 F, washing—20 minutes in running water.
Kodak Medical X-ray Film for Mammography. Designed to be processed in a Kodak X-Omat Processor for medical x-ray film using Kodak X-Omat chemicals.
Collimation—Extension cylinder, 4 by 12 inches.
Filtration—Inherent tube filtration only.
INDICATIONS FOR MAMMOGRAPHY
• Signs, Questionable Signs, or Symptoms of Disease of Breast
• Previous Radical Mastectomy
• High Familial Occurrence of Cancer of Breast
• Cancerophobia
• Previous Biopsy (Breast)
• Lumpy or Pendulous Breast
• Adenocarcinoma, Primary Site Undetermined
• Basis for Future Comparison

Figure 1–35. Radiographic projections and technical factors for performing mammography were developed by Egan and taught to radiologists throughout the United States during the 1960s. Teaching aids such as this chart were often used. (Courtesy of Eastman Kodak Co., Rochester, NY.)

HISTORY OF THE SOCIETY OF BREAST IMAGING

In 1984, Drs. Marc Homer, Carl D'Orsi, Stephen Feig, Harold Moskowitz, Myron Moskowitz, and Edward Sickles initiated a plan to create a society of radiologists who were committed to advancing research, teaching, and clinical work in breast imaging and who would meet periodically with their peers to present new ideas and to seek advice on all aspects of breast imaging (MJ Homer, MD, personal communication, March 14, 2001). Thus was born the Society of Breast Imaging (SBI). The organizational meeting of the Society was held in Boston on April 24, 1985, at which time the following objectives were established: (1) to improve and disseminate knowledge in the field of breast imaging, (2) to improve the quality of medical education in the field of breast imaging, (3) to foster research in all aspects of breast imaging, (4) to provide a medium for the exchange of ideas among professionals involved with breast imaging,

(5) to provide meetings for presentation and discussion of papers and for the dissemination of knowledge in the area of breast imaging, and (6) to establish a channel for publication of scientific reports in the field of breast imaging. In 1988, the SBI was welcomed as the newest member of the Intersociety Commission of the American College of Radiology. Although membership in the SBI was initially by invitation, a general membership category was established for radiologists in 1991, and an affiliate membership category for radiologic technologists in 1995. The first biennial meeting and Post-graduate Course of the Society occurred in 1993. The 4th Post-graduate Course, in 1999, hosted 860 registrants, exhibitors, and guests. The last Post-graduate Course was held in May 2001. A program to fund worthy research in breast imaging began in 1998. For the fiscal year 2000-2001, the SBI awarded $35,487 in grant support to young investigators mentored by senior investigators with established records in breast imaging research.[144] The SBI has also developed training curricula in breast imaging for residents and fellows.[145] By late 1999, the total membership of the SBI had reached 2019.

HISTORY OF THE REGULATION OF MAMMOGRAPHY

In 1975, Bicehouse[146] reported that surface radiation exposures delivered by mammography units in 70 medical facilities in eastern Pennsylvania ranged from 0.25 to 47 R! Obviously, some facilities were using radiation doses too low to obtain diagnostic images, whereas others were delivering excessive radiation. In 1975, the Bureau of Radiologic Health of the U.S. Food and Drug Administration (FDA), with the aid of state radiation control agencies, developed a mammography quality assurance program to minimize patient exposure while optimizing image quality. The purpose of the program, called Breast Exposure: Nationwide Trends (BENT), was to identify problems in dose and image quality and to help facilities improve mammography.[147] BENT consisted of four phases: During the first phase, mammography facilities were identified through a mailed questionnaire. During the second phase, the facilities were sent survey cards for recording the technical factors used in mammography. The cards also contained thermoluminescent dosimeters (TLDs), which were used to measure entrance skin doses. The program performed analysis of the technical factors and TLD exposures before proceeding to the third phase, in which state surveyors visited facilities with problems in exposure and recommended corrective procedures. During the fourth and final phase, another TLD survey card was sent to assess changes in the performance of mammography. By 1977, 42 states were enrolled in BENT. Although only 7% of the facilities performing film-screen mammography were found to have unusually high radiation exposures, 29% were identified as having unusually *low* exposures, suggesting that films were being underexposed. Of the film-screen units selected for follow-up, 89% had tungsten anodes, indicating that general-purpose radiographic units were being used rather than dedicated mammography units.

Concern had been growing among some scientists that breast cancer might be induced through the exposure of healthy breast tissue to ionizing radiation. In September 1975, Dr. John C. Bailar, III, editor of the *Journal of the National Cancer Institute*, met with the director of the NCI to discuss the possible radiation risks of mammography. Bailar expressed his concerns in an editorial, in which he concluded that "the overall benefits of mammography and screening of the general population have not been determined, and its hazards may be greater than are commonly understood. . . . There seems to be the possibility that the routine use of mammography in screening asymptomatic women may eventually take almost as many lives as it saves."[148] In October 1975, after a meeting among Bailar, NCI officials, and representatives of the American ACS, three experts were assigned to develop working groups to examine the pertinent issues. Dr. Lester Breslow was asked to determine the benefits of mammography in the HIP study, Dr. Arthur C. Upton to evaluate the possible radiation risks from mammography, and Dr. Louis B. Thomas to review the pathology of the cancers detected in the HIP study.[149] The Breslow working group concluded that the entire benefit of screening in the HIP study was realized in women older than 50 years.[150] The report of the Upton group on radiation risks disclosed an excess of breast cancer in three populations previously exposed to radiation: young American and Canadian women treated with radiation for postpartum mastitis, young American and Canadian women with tuberculosis subjected to multiple chest fluoroscopy procedures, and Japanese women 10 years and older who had survived atomic bomb irradiation.[151] This group used a linear dose-response curve to determine that the annual risk of development of breast cancer secondary to mammography was 3.5 to 7.5 new cases per 1 million women (at least 35 years old) at risk per rad to both breasts.[151] The concerns about the safety of mammography that were reported in the mass media in 1976 led to a "radiation scare" and a marked decline in the use of mammography. By the end of the 1970s, the future of mammography was uncertain.

The performance of mammography in the United States changed in the 1980s, when technologic advances allowed the reduction of radiation dose while simultaneously improving image quality. These advances resulted from the replacement of general-purpose radiographic equipment with tungsten anodes, used for film-screen mammography, by dedicated mammography units that used molybdenum anodes.[152] In 1979, 45% of all facilities performing mammography in the United States were using film-screen receptors, 45% were using xeromammography, and 10% were using direct-exposure (nonscreen) film.[147] By 1987, 54% of facilities used film-screen mammography, 30% xeromammography, 16% a combination of film-screen and xeromammography, and fewer than 1% direct film mammography.[153] By the end of the 1980s, film-screen mammography had become the predominant method, and fewer than 1% of film-screen mammography examinations were performed with general-purpose radiographic equipment, leading to a striking reduction in radiation doses.[38]

In 1986, specific guidelines for acceptable levels of radiation exposure in mammography were published by the National Council on Radiation Protection and Measurements.[154] The Council recommended that the average glandular dose for a two-view examination not exceed 800 mrad per breast. By the end of the 1980s, the combination of decreased x-ray dosage and validation of the mortality reduction through mammography screening in European clinical trials had restored confidence in mammography.[123-126] In 1989, 11 organizations including the ACS and the NCI endorsed screening mammography guidelines that included regular screening of women 40 years old and older.

Although concerns over radiation exposure from mammography had largely subsided, problems with image quality were resurfacing. In 1985 and 1988, the FDA and the Conference of Radiation Control Program Directors conducted nationwide assessments of phantom image quality and radiation doses under the National Evaluation of X-ray Trends (NEXT) program. The NEXT-85 survey reported that a significant number of facilities had image quality problems.[155] The NEXT-88 survey showed that there had been widespread replacement of general-purpose equipment by dedicated mammography units, a greater use of grids, and improvements in film processing; however, image quality was still variable, and 13% of facilities in the survey had unacceptable phantom image scores.[44] In 1988, a report on screening sites participating in an ACS Breast Cancer Awareness Program in Philadelphia identified marked variations in the performance of film processors as a source of unreliable image quality. Forty-one percent of the mammography sites evaluated had unacceptably wide variations in processor performance over intervals as short as 2 weeks.[156] The ACR responded to the problems in image quality and the need to identify community-based sites that would perform quality mammography for the ACS screening projects by developing the Mammography Accreditation Program (MAP).[157] ACR MAP began to accredit mammography facilities in August 1987. The accreditation program was voluntary and consisted of the following five parts: facility survey, phantom image evaluation, radiation dose measurement, clinical image evaluation, and processor performance. The program rapidly came to represent the standard for quality in mammography, and by the spring of 1991, a total of 4832 facilities had applied for accreditation.[158]

One of the impediments to the use of screening mammography had been its relatively high cost, which was not reimbursed by all health insurance plans.[135,159] In 1986, Maryland became the first state to pass legislation mandating screening mammography as a basic health insurance benefit.[160] The first mammography quality assurance legislation was included in the Maryland reimbursement law. By 1994, 41 states and the District of Columbia had legislation or regulations concerning mammography, including quality assurance standards. However, the legislated requirements and mandated standards did not always apply uniformly to all mammography facilities from state to state nor, for that matter, even within a state. A 1992 article in a law journal noted, "From a patient perspective, of course, practice guidelines or standards of care that differ from state to state merely heighten the confusion, fear, and risks surrounding mammography."[161]

Mammography regulations had reached the federal level in 1990, when the U.S. Congress passed the Omnibus Budget Reconciliation Act, creating the first budget to include federal funding for mammography screening. When the Health Care Financing Administration (HCFA) agreed to reimburse for screening mammography as a Medicare benefit for women 65 years and older and for disabled women between 35 and 64 years old, the administration also developed and imposed its own regulations and inspections as prerequisites for payment.[162] Although based largely on ACR MAP, the Medicare regulations included some controversial additional requirements, such as mandatory reports in lay language to examinees. The latter requirement was interpreted in varying ways by state inspectors. Some accepted a brief notification that the findings were normal or abnormal, whereas others demanded that a literal lay-language translation of the report that was sent to the referring health care provider be sent to the patient after her examination. Some states applied the requirement for the lay-language report to all women undergoing mammography, whereas others restricted the requirement to self-referred women. When inspections began in December 1992, these inconsistencies made it difficult for facilities to comply with Medicare regulations. Furthermore, inspectors in the different states had a variable range of expertise and training. Some Medicare inspectors were not employed by the Bureau of Radiologic Health. One report cited inspections by registered nurses whose experience came from inspecting long-term nursing care facilities.[163] The practice of making unannounced inspections added to the friction that developed between the facilities and the Medicare inspectors.

By 1992, the differing quality assurance recommendations, guidelines, and regulations established by professional organizations, federal agencies, and state agencies had resulted in a disturbing variability in the quality of mammography across the United States.[164] In response to media exposés, public pressure, and the growing evidence of problems in mammography quality, the ACR, ACS, Conference of Radiation Control Program Directors, American

College of Obstetricians and Gynecologists, and nearly 300 breast cancer support groups became united in their encouragement of federal standards and enforcement.[165] With solid support from consumers and professional organizations, the Mammography Quality Standards Act (MQSA) was passed by Congress and signed into law by President George Bush in October 1992.[166]

The responsibility for implementing MQSA was delegated to the FDA in June 1993. According to the MQSA, each of the approximately 10,000 facilities providing mammography would have to be certified by October 1, 1994, or cease performing mammography. The certificate would be issued for 3 years and would be renewable. The FDA was required to develop quality standards for accreditation bodies, personnel, equipment, record-keeping, reporting, and dose limits. Among other mandates, the new law required that all facilities be evaluated annually by a certified medical physicist and be inspected annually by approved inspectors. To accomplish this task within the time limit, the FDA established interim regulations that had to be met by October 1, 1994.[167]

In response to new data, primarily from Sweden, regarding the benefit of screening mammography for women between 40 and 49 years of age, NCI Director Richard Klausner requested that a consensus development conference be convened to develop a recommendation on the issue. In January 1997, this panel met to debate whether or not mammography screening should be recommended to women between 40 and 49 years of age. The panel concluded that the available data did not warrant a single recommendation for mammography for all women in their 40s, and that each woman should decide for herself whether to undergo mammography screening on the basis of information from her health care provider and her perception of the risks and benefits of mammography.[168] In February 1997, Dr. Klausner, testifying before the U.S. Senate Subcommittee on Labor, Health and Human Services, Education and Related Agencies, stated that the report of the panel overly minimized the benefits and overly emphasized the risks of screening mammography for women in their 40s. He maintained that a meta-analysis of eight randomized clinical trials involving about 180,000 women in their 40s from the United States, Sweden, Canada, and Great Britain showed a 15% reduction in mortality from breast cancer in the screened population.[169] Subsequently, a conference of experts organized by the American Cancer Society examined the new data and concluded that they supported a recommendation for screening women in their 40s on an annual basis, a recommendation that was supported by the ACR.[170,171]

One of the studies upon which the recommendation was based, the Swedish Two-County Trial of Breast Cancer Screening, had begun in 1975 and ended in 1985. Twenty years after its initiation, updated mortality results based on long-term follow-up led to new insights regarding the efficacy of screening.[172] The trial began in 1977 with 133,000 women randomly assigned either to regular periodic invitation to undergo screening or to no invitation. Because of fears about radiation exposure in the mid-1970s, screening was performed with single-view screen-film mammography, with a longer screening interval than is recommended today: An average of every 2 years for women 40 to 49 years old, and every 33 months for women 50 to 74 years old. The first mortality results, published in 1985, showed a 30% reduction in breast cancer mortality in the group invited to undergo screening.[126] Further follow-up continued to show about a 30% reduction in mortality in this group. Follow-up data for up to the end of 1998 showed a highly significant 32% reduction in breast cancer mortality in the group offered screening. The greatest effect on mortality was seen in women 50 to 59 years old. The results for women 40 to 49 years old were inconsistent between the two counties, with a substantial reduction in mortality observed in one county but not in the other. These latest follow-up data apply 20 years after randomization and 13 years after the end of the screening phase of the trial. Mammography screening for breast cancer continued to save lives even after 20 years. With improved imaging, two views instead of one per breast, and shorter inter-screening intervals, current screening programs have the potential to achieve even greater reductions in breast cancer mortality.

A later report evaluated the mortality from breast cancer in the Swedish women who underwent periodic mammographic screening.[173] The population of 6807 women diagnosed with breast cancer over a 29-year period was subdivided into three groups according to the period of their diagnosis: 1968 to 1977, before screening began; 1978 to 1987, the approximate period of the two-county randomized controlled trial of screening women aged 47 to 74 years; and 1988 to 1996, when *all* women in the two counties aged 40 to 69 years were invited to undergo screening. Analyzing breast cancer incidence and mortality within those time periods, the researchers in this study found that regular mammographic screening during the period 1978 to 1987 resulted in a 63% reduction in breast cancer deaths among the women who actually underwent screening. The mortality decline was 50% when breast cancer mortality among all women who were invited to undergo screening (non-attendees included) was compared with breast cancer mortality during the period when no screening was available (1968 to 1977).

The MQSA imposed a set of federal regulations on every facility and radiologist performing and interpreting mammograms. The interim regulations regarding accreditation were based on the ACR Mammography Voluntary Accreditation Program. The final regulations were published on October 28, 1997, in the *Federal Register*.[174] When the MQSA was re-authorized by Congress on October 9, 1998, a change was made in the final rule: A new requirement mandated that a report of the results of the screening procedure, prepared in lay language, be sent to each patient.[175]

References

1. Salomon A: Beitrage zur Pathologie und Klinik der Mammacarcinome. Arch Klin Chir 1913;101:573-668.
2. Kleinschmidt O: Brustdruse. In Zweife P, Payr E (eds): Die Klinik der Bosartigen Geschwulste. Leipzig, S. Hirzel, 1927, pp 5-90.
3. Vogel W: Die Roentgendarstellung der Mammatumoren. Arch Klin Chir 1932;171:618-626.
4. Goyanes J, Gentil F, Guedes B: Sobre la radiografiá de la glándula mamária y su valor diagnóstico. Arch Espano de Oncol 1931;2:111-142.
5. Dominguez CM: Estudio sistematizado del cancer del seno. Bol Liga Uruguay Contr Cancer Genit Femen 1929;4:145-154.
6. Baraldi A: Roentgen-neumo-mastia. Bol Soc Cir Buenos Aires 1934;18:1254-1267.
7. Benzadon J: Contribucion al estudio de la roentgen-neumomastia. Semna Med 1935;2:1085-1091.
8. Warren SL: Roentgenologic study of the breast. AJR Am J Roentgenol 1930;24:113-124.
9. Seabold PS: Procedure in roentgen study of the breast. Am J Roentgenol Radium Ther 1933;39:850-851.
10. Lockwood IH: Roentgen-ray evaluation of breast symptoms. Am J Roentgenol Radium Ther 1933;29:145-155.
11. Gershon-Cohen J: Breast roentgenology: Historical review. Am J Roentgenol Radium Ther 1961;86:879-883.
12. Gershon-Cohen J, Strickler A: Roentgenologic examination of the normal breast: Its evaluation in demonstrating early neoplastic changes. Am J Roentgenol Radium Ther 1938; 40:189-201.
13. Gershon-Cohen J, Ingleby H: Roentgenology of cancer of the breast: A classified pathological basis for roentgenologic criteria. Am J Roentgenol Radium Ther Nucl Med 1952;68: 1-7.
14. Gershon-Cohen J: Technical improvements in breast roentgenology. Am J Roentgenol Radium Ther Nucl Med 1960;84:224-226.
15. Gros CM, Sigrist R: Radiography and transillumination of the breast. Strasbourg Medical 1951;2:451-456.
16. Gros CM: Methodologie: Symposium sur le sein. J Radiol Electrol Med Nucl 1967;48:638-655.
17. Leborgne R: The Breast in Roentgen Diagnosis. Montevideo, Uruguay, Impresora, 1953.
18. Leborgne R: Diagnosis of tumors of the breast by simple roentgenography. AJR Am J Roentgenol 1951;65:1-11.
19. Egan RL: Experience with mammography in a tumor institution: Evaluation of 1000 cases. Radiology 1960;75:894-900.
20. Egan RL: Fifty-three cases of carcinoma of the breast, occult until mammography. Am J Roentgenol Radium Ther Nucl Med 1962;88:1095-1111.
21. Egan RL: Reproducibility of mammography: A preliminary report. Am J Roentgenol Radium Ther Nucl Med 1963; 90:356-358.
22. Clark RL, Copeland MM, Egan RL, et al: Reproducibility of the technic of mammography (Egan) for cancer of the breast. Am J Surg 1965;109:127-133.
23. Scott WG: Mammography and the training program of the American College of Radiology. Am J Roentgenol Radium Ther Nucl Med 1967;99:1002-1008.
24. Gershon-Cohen, J, Hermel MB, Birsner JW: Advances in mammographic technique. Am J Roentgenol Radium Ther Nucl Med 1970;108:424-427.
25. Barnes GT, Brezovich IA: The intensity of scattered radiation in mammography. Radiology 1980;136:641-645.
26. Egan RL, McSweeny MB, Sprawls P: Grids in mammography. Radiology 1983;146:359-362.
27. Dershaw DD, Masterson ME, Malik S, Cruz NM: Mammography using an ultrahigh-strip-density, stationary, focused grid. Radiology 1985;156:541-544.
28. Sickles EA, Weber WN: High contrast mammography with a moving grid: Assessment of clinical utility. AJR Am J Roentgenol 1986;146:1137-1139.
29. Genant HK, Doi K, Mall JC: Optical versus radiographic magnification for fine-detail skeletal radiography. Invest Radiol 1975;10:160-175.
30. Milne ENC: The role and performance of minute focal spots in roentgenology with special reference to magnification. CRC Crit Rev Radiol Sci 1971;2:269-310.
31. Haus AG, Paulus DD, Dodd GD, et al: Magnification mammography: Evaluation of screen film and xeroradiographic techniques. Radiology 1979;133:223-226.
32. Sickles EA, Doi K, Genant HK: Magnification film mammography: Image quality and clinical studies. Radiology 1977; 125:69-76.
33. Price JL, Butler PD: The reduction of radiation and exposure time in mammography. Br J Radiol 1970;43:251-255.
34. Ostrum BJ, Becker W, Isard HJ: Low-dose mammography. Radiology 1973;109:323-326.
35. Weiss JP, Wayrynen RE: Imaging system for low-dose mammography. J Appl Photogr Eng 1976;2:7-10.
36. Buchanan RA, Finkelstein SI, Wickersheim KA: X-ray exposure reduction using rare earth oxysulfide intensifying screens. Radiology 1976;118:183-188.
37. Haus AG: Technologic improvements in screen-film mammography. Radiology 1990;174:628-637.
38. Haus AG, Cillinan JE: Screen film processing systems for medical radiography: A historical review. RadioGraphics 1989;9:1203-1224.
39. Russell HD: Rapid processing of x-ray film. Photogr Sci Eng 1959;3:32-34.
40. Densdale A: Chester F. Carlson: Inventor of xerography. Photogr Sci Eng 1963;7:1.
41. Roach JF, Hilleboe HE: Xerography. Am J Roentgenol Radium Ther Nucl Med 1955;73:5-9.
42. Gould HR, Ruzicka FF, Sanchez-Ubeda R, Perez J: Xeroradiography of the breast. Am J Roentgenol Radium Ther Nucl Med 1960;84:220-223.
43. Wolfe JN: History and recent developments in xeroradiography of the breast. Radiol Clin North Am 1987;25:929-937.
44. Conway BJ, McCrohan JL, Reuter FG, Suleiman OH: Mammography in the eighties. Radiology 1990;177:335-339.
45. Curie P: Dévelopment, par pression, de l'électricité polaire dans les cristaux hémièdres à faces inclinées. Comptes Rendus Hébdomadaires des Séances de l'Academie des Sciences 1880;91:294.
46. Goldberg BB, Kimmelman BA: Medical Diagnostic Ultrasound: A Retrospective on Its 40th Anniversary. Rochester, NY, Eastman Kodak, 1988, p 3.
47. Dussik KT: Uber Moglichkeit hochfrequent mechanische Schwingungen als diagnostisches Hilfsittel zu verwenden. Ztschr f d ges Neurol u Psychiatr 1942;174:154.
48. Guttner W, Fiedler G, Patzold J: Uber Ultraschallabbidungen am menslichen Schadel. Acuistica 1952;2:148.
49. Denier A: Ultrasososcopie. CR Acad Sci 1947;222:758.
50. Tanaka K, Miyajima G, Wagai T, et al: Detection of intracranial abnormalities by ultrasound. Tokyo Med J 1952;69: 525.
51. Ludwig GD: The velocity of sound through tissues and the acoustic impedance of tissues. J Acoust Soc Am 1950;22:862.
52. Wild JJ: The use of ultrasonic pulses for the measurement of biologic tissues and the detection of tissue density changes. Surgery 1950;27:183.
53. Wild JJ, Reid JM: Echographic tissue diagnosis. In Proceedings of the 4th Annual Conference on Ultrasonic Therapy, Detroit, MI, Aug 27, 1955, p 47.
54. Wild JJ, Reid JM: Further pilot echographic studies on the histologic structure of tumors of the living intact human breast. Am J Pathol 1952;28:839-861.
55. Wells P: Physical Principles of Ultrasonic Diagnosis. New York, Academic Press, 1969.
56. Holmes J, Howry DH, Posakony G, Cushman CR: The ultrasonic visualization of soft tissue structures in the human body. Trans Am Clin Climatol Assoc 1955;66:208-225.
57. Howry DH, Bliss WR: Ultrasonic visualization of soft tissue structures of the body. J Lab Clin Med 1952;40:579-592.

58. Kikuchi Y, Ushidal R, Tanaka K, Wagai T: Early cancer diagnosis through ultrasonics. J Acoust Soc Am 1957;29:824.
59. Wells PNT, Evans KT: An immersion scanner for two-dimensional ultrasonic examination of the human breast. Ultrasonics 1968;6:220-228.
60. Kelly-Fry E, Kossoff G, Hindman HA: The potential of ultrasound visualization for detecting the presence of abnormal structures within the female breast. In Proceedings of the IEEE Sonics-Ultrasonics Symposium, Boston, MA, Oct 1972, p 25.
61. Jellins J, Kossoff G, Buddee FW, Reeve TS: Ultrasonic visualization of the breast. Med J Aust 1971;1:305-307.
62. Jellins J, Kossoff G, Reeve TS, Barraclough BH: Ultrasonic grey scale visualization of breast disease. Ultrasound Med Biol 1975;1:393-404.
63. Bom N, Lancee CT, Honkoop J, Hugenhotz PG: Ultrasonic viewer for cross-sectional analysis of moving cardiac structures. Biomed Eng 1971;6:500-503.
64. Cole-Beuglet C, Goldberg BB, Kurtz AB, et al: Clinical experience with a prototype real-time dedicated breast scanner. AJR Am J Roentgenol 1982;139:905-911.
65. Kobayashi T: Diagnostic ultrasound in breast cancer: Analysis of retrotumorous echo patterns correlated with sonic attenuation by cancerous connective tissue. J Clin Ultrasound 1979;7:471-479.
66. Kobayashi T, Takatani O, Hattori N, Kimura K: Differential diagnosis of breast tumors: The sensitivity graded method of ultrasonography. Cancer 1974;33:940-951.
67. Bassett LW, Kimme-Smith C, Sutherland LK, et al: Automated and hand-held breast ultrasound: Effect on patient management. Radiology 1987;165:103-108.
68. Cole-Beuglet C, Goldberg BB, Kurtz AB, et al: Ultrasound mammography: A comparison with radiographic mammography. Radiology 1981;139:693-698.
69. Sickles EA, Filly RA, Callen PW: Breast cancer detection with sonography and mammography: Comparison using state-of-the-art equipment. AJR Am J Roentgenol 1983;140:843-845.
70. Hilton SW, Leopold GR, Olson LK, Wilson SA: Real-time breast sonography: Application in 300 consecutive patients. AJR Am J Roentgenol 1986;147:479-486.
71. Jellins J, Kossoff G, Reeve TS: Detection and classification of liquid-filled masses in the breast by gray scale echography. Radiology 1977;125:205-212.
72. Stavros AT, Thickman D, Rapp CL, et al: Solid breast nodules: Use of sonography to distinguish between benign and malignant lesions. Radiology 1995;196:123-134.
73. Kahbar G, Sie AC, Hansen GC, et al: Benign versus malignant solid breast masses: US differentiation. Radiology 1999; 213:889-894.
74. Cutler M: Transillumination as an aid in the diagnosis of breast lesions. Surg Gynecol Obstet 1929;48:721-729.
75. Gros CM, Quenneville Y, Hummel Y: Diaphanologie mammaire. J Radiol Electrol Med Nucl 1972;53:297-302.
76. Carlsen EN: Transillumination lightscanning. Diagn Imaging 1982;4:28-33.
77. Ohlsson B, Gundersen J, Nillsson DM: Diaphanography: A method for the evaluation of the female breast. World J Surg 1980;4:701-705.
78. Bartrum RJ Jr, Crow HC: Transillumination lightscanning to diagnosis of breast cancer: A feasibility study. AJR Am J Roentgenol 1984;142:409-414.
79. Drexler B, Davis JL, Schofield G: Diaphanography in the diagnosis of breast cancer. Radiology 1985;157:41-44.
80. Geslien GE, Fisher JR, DeLaney C: Transillumination in breast cancer detection: Screening failures and potential. AJR Am J Roentgenol 1985;144:619-622.
81. Sickles EA: Breast cancer detection with transillumination and mammography. AJR Am J Roentgenol 1984;142:841-844.
82. Lawson R: Implications of surface temperatures in the diagnosis of breast cancer. Can Med Assoc J 1956;75:309-310.
83. Love TJ: Thermography as an indicator of blood perfusion. Ann N Y Acad Sci 1980;335:429-436.
84. Gold RH, Bassett LW, Kimme-Smith C: Breast imaging: State of the art. Invest Radiol 1986;21:298-304.
85. Moskowitz M, Milbrath J, Gartside P, et al: Lack of efficacy of thermography as a screening tool for minimal and stage I breast cancer. New Engl J Med 1976;295:249-252.
86. Baker LH: Breast Cancer Detection Demonstration Project: Five year summary report. CA 1982;32:196-225.
87. Beahrs OH, Shapiro S, Smart C, et al: Report of the working group to review the National Cancer Institute–American Cancer Society Breast Cancer Detection Demonstration Project. J Natl Cancer Inst 1979;62:639-698.
88. Whitley JE, Witcofski RL, Bolliger TT, Maynard CD: Tc99m in the visualization of neoplasms outside the brain. Am J Roentgenol 1966;96:706-710.
89. Bonte FJ, Curry TS III, Oelze RE, Greenberg AJ: Radioisotope scanning of tumors. AJR Am J Roentgenol 1967;100:801-812.
90. Buchwald W, Diethelm L, Wolf R: Scintigraphic delineation of carcinoma of the breast and parasternal lymph nodes. In McCready VR, Taylor DM, Trott NG, et al (eds): Radioactive Isotopes in the Localization of Tumours. New York, Grune & Stratton, 1969, pp 138-142.
91. Cancroft ET, Goldsmith SJ: ^{99m}Tc-pertechnetate scintigraphy as an aid to the diagnosis of breast masses. Radiology 1973;106:441-444.
92. Villarreal RL, Parkey RW, Bonte FJ: Experimental pertechnetate mammography. Radiology 1974;111:657-661.
93. Muller ST, Guth-Tougelides B, Crutzig H: Imaging of malignant tumors with MIBI-^{99m}Tc SPECT [abstract]. J Nucl Med 1987;28:562P.
94. Khalkhali I, Villanueva-Meyer J, Edell S, et al: Diagnostic accuracy of ^{99m}Tc-sestamibi breast imaging: Multicenter trial results. J Nucl Med 2000;41:1973-1979.
95. Khalkhali I, Cutrone JA, Mena IG, et al: Scintimammography: The complimentary role of Tc-99m sestamibi prone breast imaging for the diagnosis of breast carcinoma. Radiology 1995;196:421-426.
96. Polan RL, Klein BD, Richman RH: Scintimammography in patients with minimal mammographic or clinical findings. RadioGraphics 2001;21:641-655.
97. Damadian R: Tumor detection by nuclear magnetic resonance. Science 1971;171:1151-1153.
98. Medina D, Hazlewood CF, Cleveland DG, et al: Nuclear magnetic resonance studies on human breast dysplasia and neoplasms. J Natl Cancer Inst 1975;54:813-818.
99. Koutcher JA, Goldsmith M, Damadian R: NMR in cancer. X: A malignancy index to discriminate normal and cancerous tissue. Cancer 1978;41:174-182.
100. Goldsmith M, Koutcher JA, Damadian R: NMR in cancer. XIII: Application of the NMR malignancy index to human mammary tumours. Br J Cancer 1978;38:547-554.
101. Bouvee WMMJ, Getreuer KW, Smidt J, Lindeman J: Nuclear magnetic resonance and detection of human breast tumors. J Natl Cancer Inst 1978;67:53-55.
102. Mansfield P, Morris PG, Ordidge RJ, et al: Human whole body imaging and detection of breast tumours by NMR. Philos Trans R Soc Lond (Biol) 1980;289:503-510.
103. Ross RJ, Thompson JS, Kim K, Bailey RA: Nuclear magnetic resonance imaging and evaluation of human breast tissue: preliminary clinical trials. Radiology 1982;143:195-205.
104. El Yousef SJ, Duchesneau RH, Alfidi RJ, et al: Magnetic imaging of the breast. Work in progress. Radiology 1984; 150:761-766.
105. Alcorn FS, Turner DA, Clark JW, et al: Magnetic resonance imaging in the study of the breast. RadioGraphics 1985; 5:631-652.
106. Heywang SH, Hahn D, Schmidt H, et al: MR imaging of the breast using Gd-DTPA. J Comput Assist Tomogr 1986;10:199-204.
107. Kaiser WA, Zeitler E:. MR imaging of the breast: Fast imaging sequences with and without Gd-DTPA. Preliminary observations. Radiology 1989;170:681-686.
108. Heywang SH, Wolf A, Pruss E, et al: MR imaging of the breast with Gd-DTPA: Use and limitations. Radiology 1989;171:95-103.
109. Orel SG: Differentiating benign from malignant enhancing lesions identified at MR imaging of the breast: Are time-signal intensity curves an accurate predictor? Radiology 1999;211:5-7.

110. Berg WA, Caskey CI, Hamper UM, et al: Diagnosing breast implant rupture with MR imaging, US and mammography. RadioGraphics 1993;13:1323-1336.
111. Everson LI, Parantainen H, Detlie T, et al: Diagnosis of breast implant rupture: Imaging findings and relative efficacies of imaging techniques. AJR Am J Roentgenol 1994;163:57-60.
112. Monticciolo DL, Nelson RC, Dixon WT, et al: MR detection of leakage from silicone breast implants: Value of a silicone-selective pulse sequence. AJR Am J Roentgenol 1994;163:51-56.
113. Mund DF, Farria DM, Gorczyca DP, et al: MR imaging of the breast in patients with silicone-gel implants: Spectrum of findings. AJR Am J Roentgenol 1993;161:773-778.
114. Orel SG: MR imaging of the breast. Radiol Clin North Am 2000;38:899-913.
115. Gershon-Cohen J, Ingleby H: Roentgen survey of asymptomatic breasts. Surgery 1958;43:408-414.
116. Gershon-Cohen J, Hermel MB, Berger SM: Detection of breast cancer by periodic x-ray examination: A five-year survey. JAMA 1961;176:1114-1116.
117. Gershon-Cohen J, Ingleby H, Berger SM, et al: Mammographic screening for breast cancer: Results of a ten-year survey. Radiology 1967;88:663-667.
118. Shapiro S, Venet W, Strax P, Venet L: Evaluation of periodic breast screening with mammography: Methodology and early observations. JAMA 1966;195:731-738.
119. Shapiro S: Evidence on screening for breast cancer from a randomized trial. Cancer 1977;39:2772-2782.
120. Shapiro S, Strax P, Venet L: Periodic breast cancer screening in reducing mortality from breast cancer. JAMA 1971; 215:1777-1785.
121. King J: Mammography screening for breast cancer [letter to the editor]. Cancer 1994;73:2003-2004.
122. Moss S, Alexander F: Presentation to the International Union Against Cancer (UICC) Meeting on Breast Cancer Screening in Premenopausal Women in Developed Countries, Geneva, Switzerland, Sept 29-Oct 1, 1993.
123. Bjurstam N, Bjorneld L: Mammography screening in women aged 40-49 years at entry: Results of the randomized controlled trial in Gothenburg, Sweden. Presented at the 26th National Conference on Breast Cancer, Palm Desert, CA, May 8-14, 1994.
124. Verbeek AL, Hendricks JH, Holland R, et al: Reduction of breast cancer mortality through mass screening with modern mammography: First results of the Nijmegen project, 1975-1981. Lancet 1984;1(8388):1222-1224.
125. Collette HJA, Romback JJ, Dey NE, et al: Evaluation of screening for breast cancer in a nonrandomized study (the DOM Project) by means of a case-control study. Lancet 1984; 1(8388):1224-1226.
126. Tabár L, Fagerberg CJ, Gad A, et al: Reduction in mortality from breast cancer after mass screening with mammography: Randomized trial from the Breast Cancer Screening Working Group of the Swedish National Board of Health and Welfare. Lancet 1985;1:829-832.
127. Tabár L, Gad A: Screening for breast cancer: The Swedish Trial. Radiology 1981;138:219-222.
128. National Cancer Institute: Consensus Development Meeting of Breast Cancer Screening. (Publication No. NIH 78-1257.) Washington, DC, US Department of Health, Education and Welfare, Public Health Service, National Cancer Institute, 1977.
129. National Institutes of Health/National Cancer Institute consensus development meeting on breast cancer screening issues: Issues and recommendations. J Natl Cancer Inst 1978;60:1519-1521.
130. McIlrath S: Eleven medical groups endorse mammogram guidelines. Am Med News 1989;32:335.
131. Gershon-Cohen J, Ingleby H: Neglected roentgenography of breast disease. JAMA 1955;157:325.
132. Howard J: Using mammography for cancer control: An unrealized potential. CA 1987;37:33-48.
133. Fox S, Baum JK, Klos DS, et al: Breast cancer screening: The underuse of mammography. Radiology 1985;156:607.
134. Cummings KM, Funch DP, Mettlin C, Jennings E: Family physicians' beliefs about breast cancer screening mammography. J Fam Pract 1983;17:1029-1034.
135. Bassett LW, Bunnell DH, Cerny JA, Gold RH: Screening mammography: Referral practices of Los Angeles physicians. AJR Am J Roentgenol 1986;147:689-692.
136. Holleb AI: Guidelines for the cancer-related checkup: Five years later [editorial]. CA Cancer J Clin 1985;35:194.
137. Bassett LW, Fox SP, Pennington E, et al: Mammographic screening in Southern California: $2^1/_2$-year longitudinal survey of fees. Radiology 1989;173:61-63.
138. American Cancer Society: Proceedings of the workshop on cost of screening mammography. Cancer 1987;60:1669-1702.
139. Gold RH, Bassett LW, Widoff BE: Highlights from the history of mammography. RadioGraphics 1990;10:1111-1131.
140. Sickles EA, Weber WN, Galvin HB, et al: Mammographic screening: How to operate successfully at low cost. Radiology 1986;160:95-97.
141. Dodd GD: Screening for breast cancer. Cancer 1993;71:1038-1042.
142. Ross WL: A look into the past and into the future in cancer of the breast. Cancer 1969;63:762-766.
143. Homer MJ: Mammography training in diagnostic radiology residency programs. Radiology 1980;135:529-531.
144. SBI Grants. SBI News, October 2000, p. 6.
145. Feig SA, Hall FM, Ikeda DM, et al: Society of Breast Imaging residency and fellowship training curriculum. Radiol Clin North Am 2000;28:915-920.
146. Bicehouse HJ: Survey of mammographic exposure levels and technique used in Eastern Pennsylvania. Seventh Annual National Cancer Conference on Radiation Control, Hyannis, MA, April 27 to May 2, 1975 (DHEW Publication 76-8026). Bethesda, MD, DHEW, 1976.
147. Jans RG, Butler PF, McCrohan JL Jr, et al: Status of film/screen mammography: Results of the BENT study. Radiology 1979; 132:197-200.
148. Bailar JC: Mammography: A contrary view. Ann Intern Med 1976;84:77-84.
149. Gold RH, Bassett LW: X-ray mammography: History, controversy and state of the art. In Bassett LW, Gold RH (eds): Mammography, Thermography and Ultrasound in Breast Cancer Detection. New York, NY, Grune & Stratton, 1982, pp 3-11.
150. Breslow L, Henderson BE, Massey FJ, et al: Report of NCI ad hoc working group on the gross and net benefits of mammography in mass screening for the detection of breast cancer. J Natl Cancer Inst 1977;59:473-478.
151. Upton AC, Beebe GW, Brown JM, et al: Report of NCI ad hoc working group on the risks associated with mammography in mass screening for detection of breast cancer. J Natl Cancer Inst 1977;59:579-593.
152. Bassett LW, Gold RH, Kimme-Smith C: History of the technical development of mammography. Radiological Society of North America (RSNA) Categorical Course in Physics. Oak Brook, IL, RSNA, 1993, pp 9-20.
153. Bassett LW, Diamond JJ, Gold RH, McLelland R: Survey of mammography practices. AJR Am J Roentgenol 1987;149: 1149-1152.
154. Mammography: A user's guide. (NCRP Report No. 85.) Bethesda, MD, National Council on Radiation Protection and Measurements, 1986.
155. Reuter FG: Preliminary report—NEXT-85. National Conference on Radiation Control. Proceedings of the 18th Annual Conference of Radiation Control Program Directors. (CRCPD Publication 86-2). Charleston, WV, 1986, pp 111-120.
156. Galkin BM, Feig SA, Muir HD: The technical quality of mammography in centers participating in a regional breast cancer awareness program. RadioGraphics 1988;8:133-145.
157. McLelland R, Hendrick RE, Zinninger MD, Wilcox PA: The American College of Radiology Mammography Accreditation Program. AJR Am J Roentgenol 1991;157:473-479.
158. Hendrick RE: Quality assurance in mammography: Accreditation, legislation, and compliance with quality assurance standards. Radiol Clin North Am 1992;32:243-255.

159. American Cancer Society: Survey of physicians' attitudes and practices in early cancer detection. Cancer 1985;35:196-213.
160. McKinney M, Marconi K: Legislative interventions to increase access to screening mammography. J Community Health 1992;17:333-349.
161. Cocca SV: Who's monitoring the quality of mammograms? The Mammography Quality Standards Act of 1992 could finally provide the answer. Am J Law Med 1993;19:313-344.
162. U.S. Department of Health and Human Services: Interim final rules on conditions for Medicare coverage of screening mammography. 55 Federal Register 53511-53525, December 31, 1990.
163. Paquelet JR: Medicare, mammography and the Mammography Quality Standards Act of 1992. Radiology 1994;190:47A-49A.
164. U.S. General Accounting Office: Screening mammography: Federal quality standards are needed. (Publication No. GAO/T-HRD-92-39.) Washington, DC, General Accounting Office, 1992.
165. Reducing risk of faulty mammograms. Los Angeles Times October 28, 1991.
166. Mammography Quality Standards Act of 1992. Pub L No. 02-539.
167. U.S. Food and Drug Administration: Mammography facilities-requirements for accrediting bodies and quality standards and certification requirements; interim rules. 58 Federal Register 67558 and 58 Federal Register 67565 (1993).
168. National Institutes of Health Consensus Development Conference Statement: Breast cancer screening for women ages 40-49, January 21-23, 1997. National Institutes of Health Consensus Developmental Panel. J Natl Cancer Inst Monogr 1997;22:vii–xviii.
169. Klausner RD: Statement read before the Subcommittee on Labor, Health and Human Services, Education and Related Agencies, Senator Arlen Spector, Chairman, February 5, 1997.
170. Feig SA, D'Orsi C, Hendrick RE, et al: American College of Radiology guidelines for breast cancer screening. AJR Am J Roentgenol 1998;171:29-33.
171. Leitch AM, Dodd GD, Costanza M: American Cancer Society guide for the early detection of breast cancer: Update 1997. Cancer 1997;47:150-153.
172. Tabár L, Vitak B, Chen H-H, et al: The Swedish Two-County Trial twenty years later: Updated mortality results and new insights from long-term follow-up. Radiol Clin North Am 2000;38:625-651.
173. Tabár L, Vitak B, Chen H-H, et al: Beyond randomized controlled trials: Organized mammographic screening substantially reduces breast carcinoma mortality. Cancer 2001;91:1724-1731.
174. Quality Mammography Standards. Final Rule, Department of Health and Human Services, Food and Drug Administration. 21 CFR §16 and §900 (1997).
175. MQSRA (Mammography Quality Standards Re-Authorization Act of 1998). Pub L No. 105-248.

Section II

MAMMOGRAPHY: PERFORMING THE EXAMINATION

Mammography Equipment and Screen-Film Imaging Considerations

Gary T. Barnes

The formation of the screen-film (SF) mammographic image is depicted in Figure 2–1. Photons from the x-ray source are incident on the breast. Variations in tissue composition give rise to differences in attenuation, which in turn spatially modulates the transmitted x-ray beam (the x-ray image). The exiting x-rays are then captured by an intensifying screen. Spatial variations in the x-ray energy absorbed in the intensifying screen give rise to differences in screen response and light output. These differences in turn result in differences in film density (the mammographic image). Breast disease is manifested as small differences in subject contrast between lesions and their surroundings and by microcalcifications.

Visualization of these subtle subject contrast variations requires a high-contrast imaging system, in terms of both the x-ray spectrum incident on the breast and the image receptor. It is important not only to see the subtle lesions and microcalcifications but also to be able to delineate their borders to distinguish benign from malignant. This requires a sharp or high-resolution imaging system. Such borders are also easier to see if their sharpness is not degraded by graininess or artifacts. Image quality in screen-film mammography, and in medical imaging in general, depends on contrast, spatial resolution, noise, and artifacts.

Screen-film mammography is the most technically demanding radiographic examination. In clinical practice, the technical quality of the image depends on the adequate control of the following factors: (1) patient positioning and compression, (2) screen-film selection, (3) technique, (4) screen-film exposure, and (5) film development. Controlling and optimizing these factors in turn depend on equipment design and performance, film processing, technologists' training, and the assistance given to a site by the medical physicist. The objectives of this chapter are to review equipment design and performance considerations. Screen-film performance and processing are also discussed as well as acceptance testing and maintenance, along with differences in mammography unit design and performance that currently exist and their impact on image quality and patient dose.

X-RAY TUBE TARGET AND FILTER CONSIDERATIONS

X-Ray Spectra

Currently there are four target-filter combinations used in mammography: molybdenum-molybdenum (Mo/Mo), molybdenum-rhodium (Mo/Rh), rhodium-rhodium (Rh/Rh), and tungsten-rhodium (W/Rh). All screen-film mammography units currently being manufactured are equipped with a Mo/Mo target-filter combination, and in many, an Mo/Rh combination is also available. The GE DMR unit (GE Healthcare, Waukesha, WI) employs a dual-target (Mo and Rh) x-ray tube and has Rh/Rh available in addition to Mo/Mo and Mo/Rh. The Siemens Mammomat 3000 (Siemens, Malvern, PA) unit can be purchased with single (Mo) or dual (Mo/W) target x-ray tubes; the operator can select Mo/Mo or Mo/Rh target-filter combinations on the single-target unit and Mo/Mo, Mo/Rh, or W/Rh on the dual-target unit.

Since shortly after its introduction in 1966,[1] the Mo target, beryllium (Be) window, and Mo filter source assembly became (and still is) the "gold standard" target-filter combination used in mammography. The Be window (≈1.0 mm) minimizes beam hardening by the x-ray tube port and permits the spectra to be shaped by the added filtration. The Mo filter thickness employed varies from unit to unit, ranging from 15 to 30 μm, with 30 μm being the most common. Typical x-ray tube voltages range from 25 to 30 kilovolt peak (kVp) and occasionally higher in thick, dense breasts. The resultant x-ray spectra are rich in bremsstrahlung between 15 and 20 keV and Mo K-characteristic x-rays. X-rays 15 to 20 keV are optimal for imaging small to medium breasts.

The physical properties of Mo, Rh, and W are compared in Table 2–1. The atomic number of Rh is greater than the atomic number of Mo, and the K-edge and K-characteristic x-rays are ≈3 keV greater. The atomic number and K-edge of W are much greater than those of both Mo and Rh; as a result, the K-characteristic x-rays of W are not excited at mammography tube potentials. An appropriate spectrum for mammography is obtained by adding Rh filtration. The L-characteristic x-rays are present but too low in energy to be useful and so are filtered out by the added Rh filtration.

The 30-kVp spectra for Mo/Mo, Mo/Rh, Rh/Rh, and W/Rh target-filter combinations are compared in Figure 2–2. The Mo/Mo spectrum is rich in 15- to 20-keV x-rays. The increase in higher-energy x-rays in the 20- to 23-keV region with Mo/Rh is apparent. This increase is due to the differences in the absorption and K-edges of the Mo and Rh filters. There is an even greater increase in the 20- to 23-keV region with Rh/Rh and W/Rh combinations. The increase with Rh/Rh is due to the fact that the Rh K-characteristic X-rays are ≈3 keV higher than the Mo K-characteristic X-rays (see Table 2–1). The increase

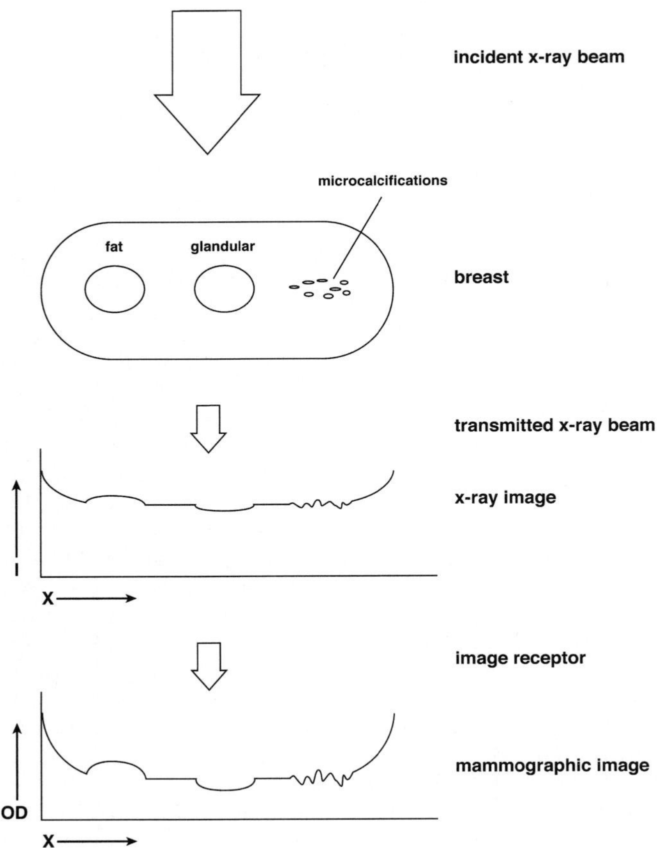

Figure 2–1. Formation of the screen-film mammography image. The incident x-ray beam is spatially modulated by the attenuation differences in the breast and forms the x-ray image. The x-ray image is in turn converted to a radiographic image by the screen-film processing system.

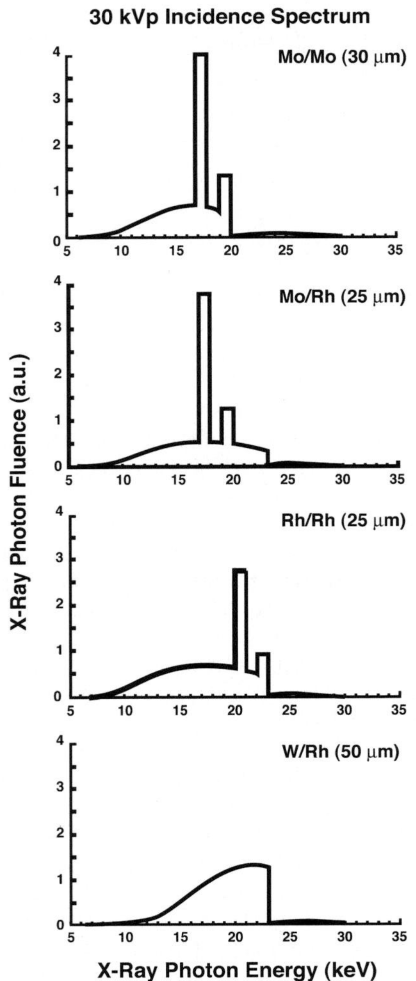

Figure 2–2. 30-kVp spectra for molybdenum-molybdenum (Mo/Mo), molybdenum-rhodium (Mo/Rh), rhodium-rhodium (Rh/Rh), and tungsten-rhodium (W/Rh) source assemblies incident on the breast. a.u., arbitary units. (Data from Gingold EL, Wu X, Barnes GT: Contrast and dose with Mo-Mo, Mo-Rh, and Rh-Rh target-filter combinations in mammography. Radiology 1995; 195:639-644; *and* Tucker DM, Barnes GT, Wu X: Molybdenum target x-ray spectra: A semiempirical model. Med Phys 1991;18: 402-407.)

with W/Rh is due to the greater thickness (50 μm) of Rh filtration employed with the tungsten target. Table 2–2 lists the radiation outputs at 30 kVp and the associated x-ray beam half-value layer (HVL) incident on the breast and transmitted by an 8-cm thickness of 50% adipose–50% glandular breast tissue.

Limitations of the Molybdenum-Molybdenum Target-Filter Combination

Figure 2–3 compares the 3-kVp Mo/Mo, Mo/Rh, Rh/Rh, and W/Rh spectra penetrating 8 cm of 50% adipose–50% glandular (50/50) breast tissue. This figure shows that at the higher tube potentials necessary to penetrate thick, dense breasts (i.e., 29 to 32 kVp), the Mo/Mo spectrum exiting the breast is bimodal, with a lower energy peak in the 17- to 20-keV range associated with bremsstrahlung and K-characteristic x-rays and a higher energy peak above 23 keV. Such bimodal spectra are not dose efficient; more homogeneous spectra with x-rays in the 20- to

Table 2–1. Physical Properties of Molybdenum, Rhodium, and Tungsten

Element	Atomic No.	Density (g/cm³)	Melting Point (°C)	K-edge (keV)	K_α (keV)	K_β (keV)
Molybdenum	42	10.2	2,610	20.0	17.4	19.7
Rhodium	45	12.4	1,966	23.2	20.2	22.8
Tungsten	74	19.3	3,360	69.5	58.6	68.2

Note: The L-edges of tungsten range from 10.2 to 12.1 keV and the L-characteristic x-rays from 8.3 to 10.2 keV.
Adapted from Lide DR (ed): Handbook of Chemistry and Physics, 72nd ed. Boca Raton, FL, CRC Press, 1991.

Table 2–2. 30-kVp Radiation Output and Half-Value Layer (HVL) Comparisons for Different Target-Filter Combinations

Target/Filter	R/100 mAs @ 0.5 m	HVL (mm of Al)	Transmitted HVL (mm of Al)*
Mo/30 μm Mo	2.35	0.37	0.89
Mo/25 μm Rh	2.05	0.43	0.89
Rh/25 μm Rh	1.96	0.44	0.94
W/50 μm Rh	0.82	0.55	0.94

*Transmitted by 8-cm-thick 50% adipose–50% glandular breast phantom. Al, aluminum.

23-keV energy range are preferable. Hence the introduction of Mo/Rh, Rh/Rh,[1] and W/Rh target-filter combinations.[2] The Mo/Rh, Rh/Rh, and W/Rh spectra penetrating 8 cm of 50/50 breast tissue have more x-rays in the 20- to 23-keV region than Mo/Mo and are more dose efficient—that is, the same or greater contrast can be obtained with a lower radiation dose.[2,3] This is apparent from a comparison of the incident and exiting HVLs of the 30-kVp Mo/Mo and Mo/Rh spectra in Table 2–2. The HVLs of the Mo/Mo and Mo/Rh x-ray beams transmitted or exiting 8 cm of 50/50 tissue (a thick, dense breast) are the same and would result in the same image contrast. However, the incident HVL of Mo/Mo is less (i.e., less penetrating) than the HVL of Mo/Rh, and a greater fraction of the incident Mo/Mo x-rays is absorbed in the breast. Thus, for a thick, dense breast, the same image contrast can be obtained with Mo/Rh as with Mo/Mo, with significantly less radiation.[3]

The Rh/Rh spectra and particularly the W/Rh spectra are even more dose efficient than Mo/Rh in imaging the thick, dense breasts. The problem with these newer target-filter combinations in screen-film mammography is that even though the spectra are very dose efficient, the contrast of the exiting beams is low (i.e., the HVLs of the exiting beams are too high; see Table 2–2). In a contrast-limited image receptor system such as screen-film, this feature is unacceptable, so these target-filter combinations offer little advantage for moderately thick breasts. The spectra penetrate very thick or inflamed breasts. Also, in digital mammography, which is not contrast limited, these spectra have more advantages and will be more widely used.

A disadvantage of Rh/Rh is that due to its lower melting point, the target cannot be operated at as high a tube current as an Mo target tube (i.e., 75 mA versus 100 mA), resulting in long exposure times when a high mA value is required. Also, the maximum permissible mA value is lower. This is not the case when a tungsten target is used with Rh filtration; this, along with the dose efficiency in imaging thick, dense breasts, is the reason why the W/Rh target-filter combination was introduced.[2] Tungsten has a higher melting point (3360°C) than Mo, so a tungsten target x-ray tube can be operated at a higher mA.

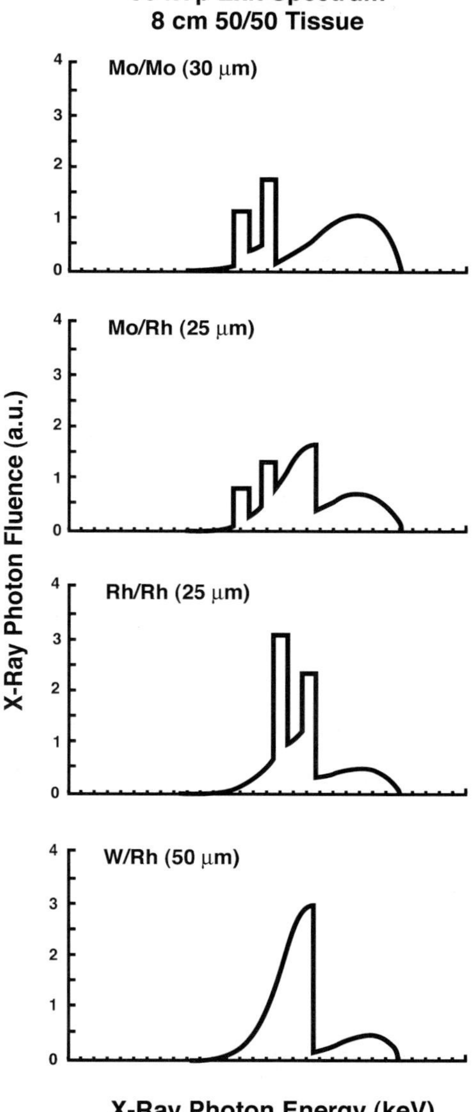

Figure 2–3. 30-kVp spectra for molybdenum-molybdenum (Mo/Mo), molybdenum-rhodium (Mo/Rh), rhodium-rhodium (Rh/Rh), and tungsten-rhodium (W/Rh) source assemblies exiting an 8-cm-thick, 50% adipose–50% glandular tissue breast phantom. (Data from Gingold EL, Wu X, Barnes GT: Contrast and dose with Mo-Mo, Mo-Rh, and Rh-Rh target-filter combinations in mammography. Radiology 1995;195:639-644; *and* Tucker DM, Barnes GT, Wu X: Molybdenum target x-ray spectra: A semiempirical model. Med Phys 1991;18:402-407.)

MAMMOGRAPHY EQUIPMENT

A screen-film mammography unit consists of an x-ray generator and control; U-arm; x-ray source assembly; collimator; compression device; breast support and grid assemblies; and automatic exposure control (AEC) subsystem (Fig. 2–4). Mammography Quality Standard Act (MQSA) regulations require that screen-film units be operated with both 18 × 24-cm and 24 × 30-cm image receptors and be equipped with

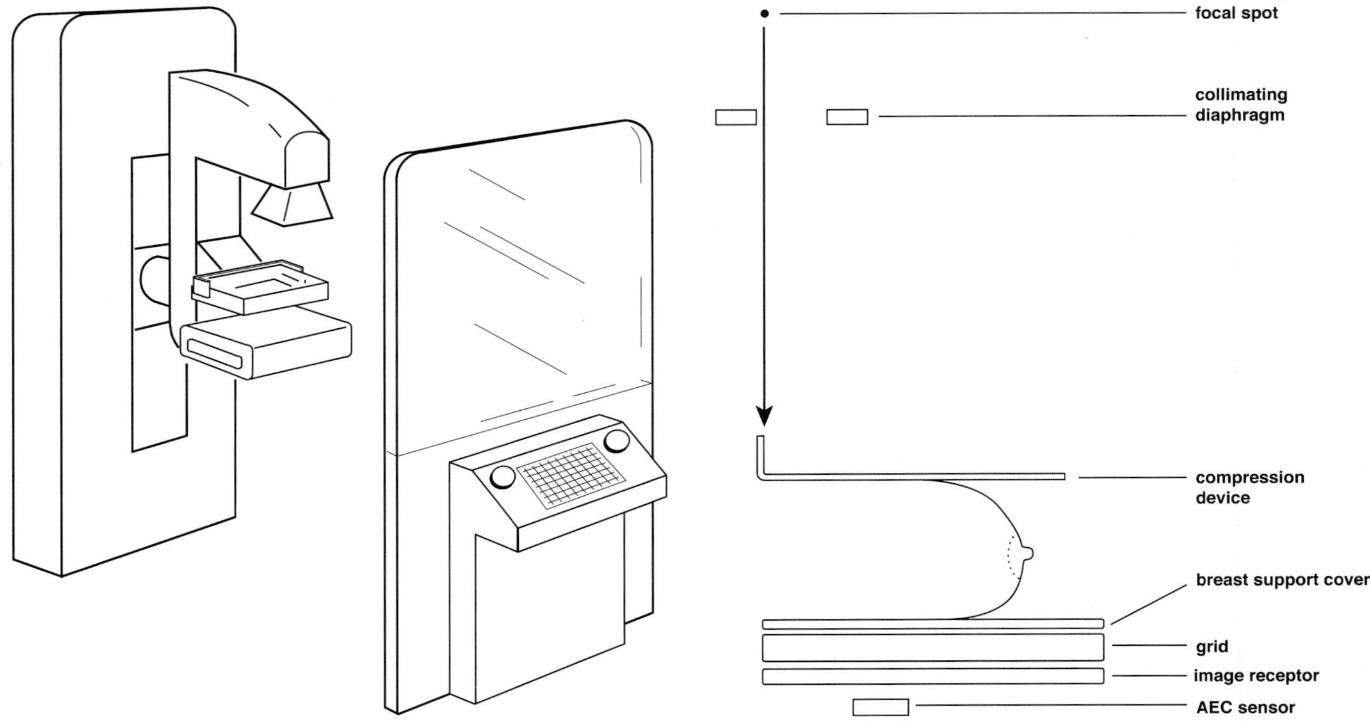

Figure 2–4. Screen-film mammography unit. Shown are the column, U-arm, radiation shield, and control. On some units, the control and shield are not separate and are attached to the column.

Figure 2–5. Geometry of a screen-film mammography unit. The focal spot is located directly above the chest wall edge of the compression paddle and cassette. The automatic exposure control (AEC) sensor is located below the screen-film cassette.

moving grids matched to the image receptor sizes.[4] In addition, diagnostic units have a magnification stand. The MQSA requires that in diagnostic units, the grid between the source and image receptor is removed for magnification procedures.[4]

The U-arm can be raised or lowered via a motor drive and can be rotated clockwise and counterclockwise. The x-ray source assembly (x-ray tube, tube housing, and filters) is mounted to the top of the U-arm and covered with a shroud. The collimator is mounted directly below the source assembly and is also covered by the source assembly shroud. The compression device is built into the vertical section of the U-arm. A horizontal mounting plate for attaching the grid assemblies and magnification stand is located at the bottom. The AEC subsystem consists of an AEC sensor and associated electronics. The sensor is built into the mounting plate and can be positioned at different locations from the chest wall to well back toward the nipple. Figure 2–5 shows the geometry of a screen-film mammography unit and the relative locations of the x-ray tube focal spot, collimator, compression paddle, grid cover, grid, screen-film cassette, and AEC sensor.

X-Ray Generator

All mammography units currently being manufactured use high-frequency x-ray generator technology. A block diagram of a high-frequency x-ray generator is shown in Figure 2–6. The input is typically single phase, which in turn is rectified and capacitor smoothed to achieve a direct current (DC) voltage waveform. The DC output is fed to an inverter circuit, which converts DC to pulses of high-frequency alternating current (AC). The output of the inverter is capacitor coupled to the primary winding of the high-tension transformer, where the voltage is stepped up, is rectified, and charges a high-voltage

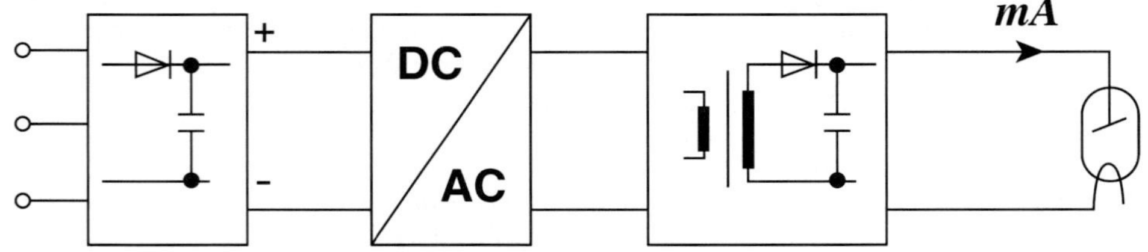

Figure 2–6. Block diagram of mammography high-frequency x-ray generator. Shown, from *left* to *right*, are the power circuit breaker connections, rectification circuit, inverter circuit, high-voltage transformer and rectification circuit, and x-ray tube.

capacitor that is in parallel with the x-ray tube. Often, a voltage doubling circuit is employed at this stage to reduce transformer cost. Typically, the cathode is grounded. On a few units, the anode is grounded. This latter arrangement is claimed to reduce off-focus radiation and improve image quality; however, there has been no peer-reviewed scientific publication documenting this claim.

A voltage divider is placed across the x-ray tube and used to obtain a kV feedback signal. The feedback signal is compared with the reference signal selected by the operator. If the feedback signal is less than the reference signal, the inverter pulsing rate is increased. Likewise, if the feedback signal is greater than the reference signal, the inverter pulsing rate is decreased. The inverter is pulsed at the maximum rate when an exposure is initiated and decreases as the high-voltage capacitor across the x-ray tube approaches the selected value. The inverter pulsing rate during an exposure stabilizes at a value that depends on the x-ray tube potential and mA selected and is greater at higher x-ray tube potentials and currents. A typical pulsing rate is 5000 to 10,000 Hz. In an alternative design, pulsing occurs at a constant frequency but the pulse width is modulated.

Closed-loop control, or kV and mA feedback, is inherent to high-frequency x-ray generator design. Its use results in a high degree of reproducibility that is independent of commonly experienced line voltage fluctuations. The on-off switching time of high-frequency mammographic generators is on the order of a millisecond, and the kV waveforms typically have very little ripple (<4%) and are essentially constant potential. Modern mammographic high-frequency x-ray generator designs are compact and offer exquisite exposure reproducibility. In the author's experience, the designs of the different manufacturers are competitive in performance, although there are differences in reliability.

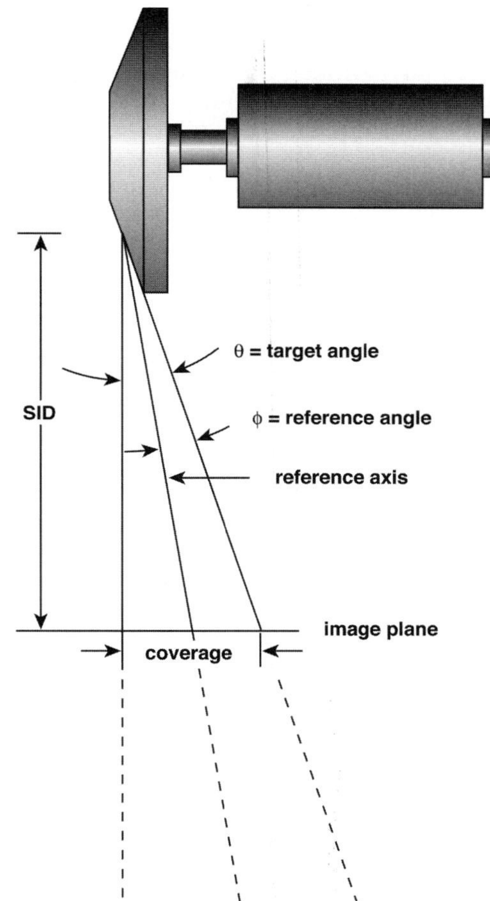

Figure 2–7. Geometry of a mammography x-ray tube. Illustrated are the rotor and target, focal spot, target angle, reference angle and axis, screen-to-image distance (SID), and coverage, or field of view (FOV). The size of the focal spot is specified by the mammography unit manufacturer as the projected dimensions (width and length) at the reference angle in a plane perpendicular to the reference axis.

X-Ray Tube

Mammography x-ray tubes typically have a large focal spot (0.3 mm) that is employed for grid work and a small focal spot (0.1 mm) that is used for magnification work. Screen-film mammography requires a beryllium window tube port. The target is molybdenum (Mo), and a user-selectable choice of 0.30 mm of Mo or 0.25 mm of rhodium (Rh) added filtration is common. As noted previously, two commercially available units employ dual-target x-ray tubes: The GE DMR has Mo and Rh targets, and the Siemens Mammomat 3000 can be equipped with a tube that has Mo and W targets. Only Rh or aluminum (Al) filtration can be selected with the Rh target of the GE DMR, and only Rh filtration with the W target of the Siemens Mammomat 3000. The clinical usefulness of the different target-filter options was discussed previously.

As illustrated in Figure 2–5, the x-ray tube focal spot or source is located directly above the chest wall edge of the screen-film cassette. The geometry of the x-ray tube target is illustrated in Figure 2–7. A number of factors depend on the x-ray tube target angle: heel effect (less radiation intensity on the anode side than on the cathode side along the x-ray tube axis); coverage (the cathode-anode field-of-view dimension before the radiation falls off to an unusable degree in the anode direction); and the effective or projected focal spot being smaller (in the tube axis direction) than the area of the target struck by high-speed electrons or line focus principle. These result in a number of practical tradeoffs. The smaller the target angle, (1) the smaller the coverage and the more pronounced the heel effect; (2) the greater the area struck by electrons; and (3) the greater the loadability (permissible kV × mA product). Loadability also increases with increasing focal spot size, anode disk diameter, and anode rotation speed.

To use the heel effect to best advantage and also to minimize equipment bulk in the vicinity of the patient's head, the cathode is positioned toward the chest wall and the anode toward the U-arm.

Radiation coverage depends on and increases with x-ray tube effective target angle. The effective target angle is equal to mechanical target angle plus the tube tilt angle. In screen-film mammography, the largest grid technique coverage is 24 cm (the smaller dimension of a 24 × 30-cm film). For a 65-cm source-to-image distance (SID) and typical mammography geometry (see Figs. 2–5 and 2–7), the effective target angle is 22 degrees, which is obtained either by employing a tube with a 22-degree target angle or by tilting a tube with a lesser target angle (i.e., 16-degree target angle on a 6-degree tilt).

For magnification work the coverage needed is less, and a number of manufacturers use a smaller effective target angle for the smaller focal spot, either by employing a biangular target x-ray tube or by changing the tube tilt. A sketch of a biangular tube is shown in Figure 2–8. The target has two angles; the larger effective target angle is used for the large focal spot and the smaller effective angle for the small focal spot. Employing a smaller target angle with the small focal spot increases its loadability, allowing one to obtain a higher mA at a given kVp and shorter magnification exposure times. High-speed anode rotation is also used to increase loadability of a small focal spot. The greater the x-ray tube current that can be achieved, the shorter the exposure time, resulting in less chance of patient motion. This issue is particularly important for magnification work, in which the exposure times are two or three times longer than grid technique exposure times.

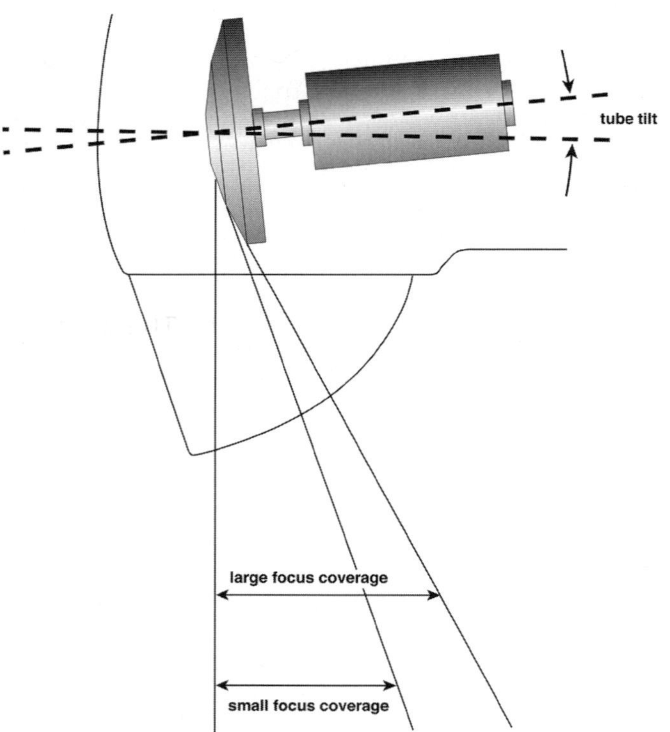

Figure 2–8. Bianglex mammography x-ray tube. Unlike the target shown in Figure 2–7, this target has two angles rather than one. The larger target angle is employed with the large focus and grid technique, for which a larger field of view (FOV) is needed. The smaller target angle is employed with the small focus and magnification technique, for which a smaller FOV is acceptable. Small focal spot loadability is improved with the smaller target angle.

According to MQSA regulations, the site's medical physicist must measure system resolution on installation of a mammography unit and annually thereafter.[4] The limiting system resolutions are measured at 28 kVp for grid technique, and also for magnification technique on diagnostic units. The resolution patterns are positioned 4.5 cm above the grid or magnification stand cover and 2 cm from the chest wall edge and are measured for all screen-film combinations employed with a given technique. For both grid and magnification techniques, the limiting spatial resolutions associated with the focal spot should be about 11 line pair per mm (lp/mm) for the length and about 13 lp/mm for the width. (The focal spot length is the projected focal spot dimension associated with the x-ray tube's cathode-anode axis, and the width is the projected dimension transverse to the tube's axis.) The primary factors determining the system resolution are the dimensions of the focal spot. Mammography units with smaller focal spots have better performance. It is not uncommon for focal spot system resolutions to exceed 15 lp/mm (length and width) for both large and small focal spots. There is a noticeable difference between mammography images obtained with system resolutions of 11 lp/mm and 15 lp/mm.

To minimize patient motion, the large focal spot should be capable of 100 mA or more over the clinically used range of tube potentials. Similarly, the small focal spot should be capable of 30 mA or more. There are marked differences between the x-ray tube loadability of different mammography units. A large focal spot limit of 100 mA over the useful range of tube potentials is common. In some units, the mA falls from 100 mA to 70 mA as the tube potential is increased above 28 kVp. This undesirable feature compromises one's ability to obtain high-quality images on thick, dense breasts. For one manufacturer's unit, the x-ray tube current remains relatively constant in the 140-mA range as the tube potential increases from 25 to 30 kVp. As a result, one is able to use a lower kVp and obtain higher-contrast images for a woman with thick, dense breasts than is possible with other units. The higher mA values are achieved when high-speed anode rotation is employed. With high-speed anode rotation,140 mA and 45 mA are achievable on the large and small focal spots, respectively, on widely used x-ray tubes over the clinical range of tube potentials.[5]

U-Arm and Imaging Geometry

The x-ray source assembly (x-ray tube, tube housing, and filter) and collimator are mounted at the top of the U-arm, and the image receptor is mounted at the opposite end or bottom. The U-arm can be raised or lowered via a motor drive and can be rotated

180 degrees from the vertical in both clockwise and counterclockwise directions. The MQSA regulations require that the motion of the tube–image receptor U-arm assembly be capable of being fixed in any position where it is designed to operate and, once fixed, that it not undergo unintended motion when the unit is energized or in the event of power interruption.[4] Two U-arm rotation designs are currently being manufactured. The simplest design is to counterbalance the U-arm, have it held in place with electromagnetic locks, then release the locks to manually rotate the U-arm. The alternative and more complex design is to use an electric motor to rotate the U-arm. Both designs work well and are reliable.

The SID on mammography units currently being manufactured is about 65 cm. This distance permits good patient access and flexibility in positioning. Longer SIDs increase tube loading, whereas shorter SIDs limit patient access and can compromise image quality, particularly when magnification is employed. The ray orthogonal to the image receptor should project along the chest wall and should be aligned with the chest wall edge of the compression paddle (see Fig. 2–5). This geometry maximizes the chest wall breast tissue imaged.

Collimator

The collimator determines the x-ray field of view (FOV). Two general approaches are employed. In high-end units, the collimator blades are automatically motor driven to the size of the image receptor, 18 × 24 cm or 24 × 30 cm, and for a given image receptor size, the operator can reduce (cone down) the FOV to two or more smaller sizes by pushing a button. In less expensive units, the collimator automatically switches between the 18 × 24-cm and 24 × 30-cm FOVs, and different diaphragms are manually switched out for the small focal spot and magnification as well as for coned-down views. On a number of less expensive units, the diaphragms are also manually switched between the 18 × 24-cm and 24 × 30-cm FOVs. From the technologists' perspective, because the grid and magnification stands are changed, there is little difference in terms of convenience, particularly for units on which the collimator automatically switches between the 18 × 24-cm and 24 × 30-cm FOVs. Reliability is better with the simpler approach, in which the small focal spot diaphragm is manually inserted for magnification techniques.

Compression Device

All mammography units are equipped with a compression device consisting of mechanical drive components located within the vertical section of the U-arm and a selection of paddles. MQSA regulations require that the compression initially be power driven and operable by hands-free controls on either side of the patient and that it have manual fine-adjustment controls that are also operable from both sides of the patient.[4] Also, a system must be equipped with different-sized compression paddles that match the sizes of all full-field image receptors provided with the system, the chest wall edge of the compression paddles must be straight and parallel to the edge of the image receptor, and paddles for special purposes (i.e., spot compression) may be provided. A diagnostic screen-film mammography unit is typically equipped with five or more compression paddles: 18 × 24-cm, 24 × 30-cm, and spot grid technique paddles, and 18 × 24-cm and spot magnification technique paddles. Only 18 × 24-cm and 24 × 30-cm grid technique paddles are needed on a screening unit. As illustrated in Figure 2–5, the central ray (the ray orthogonal to the image receptor) should project parallel to the chest wall, and the chest wall edge or lip of the paddle should be aligned with the central ray. According to MQSA regulations, the projection of the paddle lip must not be projected on the film and must not extend beyond the chest wall of the film by more than 6 mm (1% of the SID).[4] In practice, the paddle lip should not extend beyond the film's edge by more than 3 mm. If the paddle lip extends much beyond the chest wall edge of the film, tissue close to the chest wall will not be imaged. Also, the chest wall lip of the paddle should be about 3 cm high. If the lip is too short, the superimposition of tissue above the breast can be a problem on obese women.

MQSA regulations specify that the paddle must be flat and parallel to the breast support cover and must not deflect from parallel by more than 1 cm when compression is applied.[4] The compression force at which the deflection is checked is not specified. However, the maximum compression force for the initial power drive must be between 25 and 47 pounds[4]; presumably, if the paddle deflects 1 cm or less under 25 pounds of compression force, the regulation is satisfied. It should be noted that the regulations permit paddles that are not designed to be flat and parallel to the breast support cover during compression, and these paddles do not need to meet the deflection requirement but do need to meet the manufacturer's design specifications and maintenance requirements.[4] In clinical practice, a deflection of about 2 cm is not a problem because (1) a decrease of tissue thickness as one goes from the chest wall to the nipple tends to compensate for the heel effect and for the increasing x-ray beam path length through the breast due to beam angulation and (2) a compression paddle that deflects 1 to 2 cm results in a more comfortable experience for women undergoing the examination than a rigid paddle (i.e., one that does not deflect). Also important for comfort are the radius measurements of the compression paddle and grid cover chest wall edges. The radii of these edges should be about 4 mm. Smaller radii result in a more abrupt edge and greater patient discomfort. Larger radii, particularly for the grid cover, result in increased bulk and wasted space between the grid and grid cover.

Compression improves image contrast and reduces the radiation dose to the breast. Image contrast is increased because the thickness of the breast is reduced and there is less attenuation of the x-ray beam (less beam hardening), the relative intensity of scatter is less,[6] and a lower-kVp technique can be employed. An additional advantage is that breast tissue is spread out over a larger area, reducing the superimposition of overlying structures and increasing the number of x-rays employed to image the breast.[7] Breast thickness is more uniform, permitting the use of high-contrast films. Patient motion is reduced because the breast is constrained and, with decreased breast thickness, exposure time and radiation dose are reduced.

Radiation Output

MQSA regulations require that mammography units be capable of producing a minimum radiation output rate of 800 mR per second measured 4.5 cm above the grid breast support surface when operated at 28 kVp in the standard Mo/Mo target-filter mode. All mammography units currently being manufactured meet this requirement. However, measured radiation output rates vary from manufacturer to manufacturer, from 1000 to 2000 mR per second. The main reason for this factor of two in output rate is the loadability of the x-ray tube or the maximum mA the x-ray tube can achieve. Other factors, such as filter thickness, play a role. The radiation output rate is an important parameter to consider when purchasing a new mammography unit. Obviously, a unit with a higher radiation output rate will allow shorter exposure times on small and medium breasts and will have greater capability to penetrate thick, dense breasts without employing excessively high kVp values.

Antiscatter Grid Assembly

All screen-film mammography units must have small (18 × 24 cm) and large (24 × 30 cm) grid assemblies and moving grids.[4] The assemblies, which mount on the U-arm's mounting plate, consist of a grid, grid drive motor and associated electronics, and image receptor holder. From top to bottom, a grid assembly comprises a breast support plate or grid cover, grid, image receptor holder, and bottom plate. MQSA regulations also require that the grid assemblies fit snugly on the mounting plate with no side-to-side looseness and that screen-film cassettes are held securely by the image receptor holders.[4] It is of interest that at least two mammography units in widespread use and currently being manufactured do not hold cassettes securely, especially after a year or more of use.

Before the mid-1970s, because of the low kVp values employed and the small volume of tissue irradiated, scatter was thought to have little effect on mammography image quality. The work of Friedrich[8] and Barnes and Brezovich[6,9] corrected this impression. In clinical practice, the ratio of scatter to primary radiation emerging from the breast ranges from 0.3 to 1.5.[10] As a result, only 40% (thick, dense breast) to 75% (thin breast) of the possible contrast is imaged unless scatter is controlled.

In 1978, the improvement in contrast and image quality that could be obtained was demonstrated in patients with a scanning multiple-slit assembly[11] and with a special soft tissue grid developed by Philips and Smit-Röntgen.[12] Although scanning-slit techniques had superior performance, the approach is inherently bulky, and grids became the common means of controlling scatter in mammography.

A typical grid consists of lead lamellae separated by radiolucent spacers (Fig. 2–9). The height of the lead lamellae divided by the interspace thickness defines the grid ratio. In mammography, typical ratios are 4:1 or 5:1, and lamellae strip densities are 30 to 50 lines/cm. The grid is positioned as shown in Figure 2–10, so that the primary or information-carrying x-rays strike only the edges of the lead lamellae and only a small percentage are absorbed. Scattered x-rays do not travel in a straight line from the focal spot to the film. As a result, they strike a much greater area of lead and, compared with primary x-rays, are preferentially absorbed. The lamellae are projected by the primary beams as lines, and during an exposure, the grid is moved through a distance of 20 or more grid line spacings to blur out the lines. Ideally, a grid would transmit all the primary x-ray beam and absorb all the scatter. In practice, however, mammography grids transmit 60% to 75% of the primary x-rays and absorb 75% to 85% of the scatter.[10]

The performance of a grid depends on two factors: the improvement in contrast and the increase in dose that results when it is used. The factors are known as the contrast improvement factor (CIF) and the Bucky

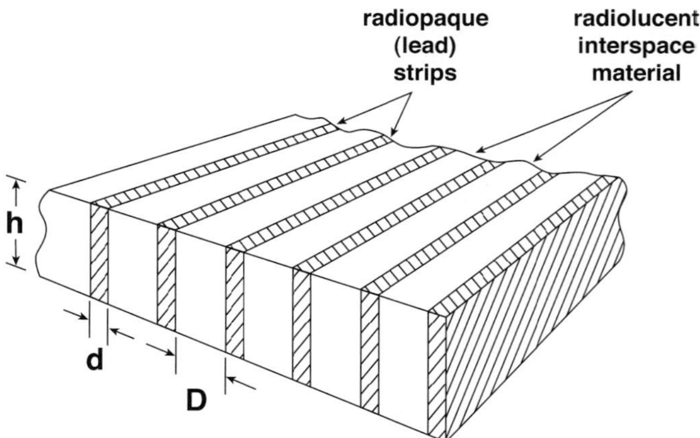

Figure 2–9. Conventional mammography grid. d, width of lead lamellae; D, width of radiolucent interspace material; h, height of grid. Not shown are the top and bottom carbon fiber covers.

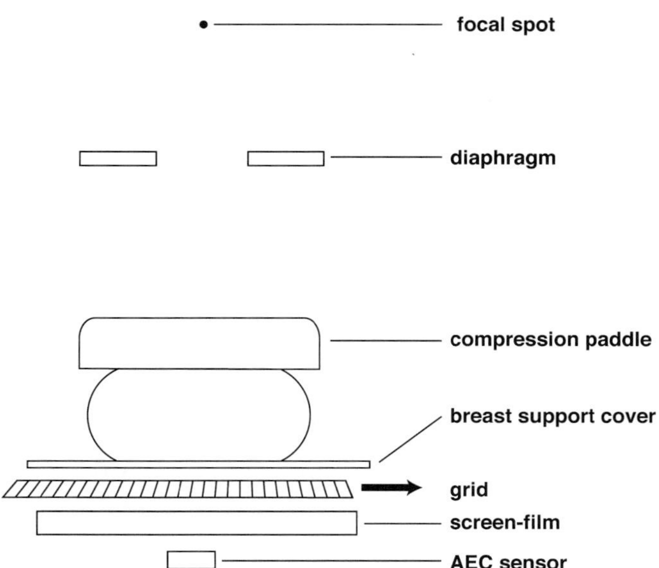

Figure 2–10. Mammography grid assembly. *Black lines* represent radiopaque lead strips that make up the grid. The lead strips are focused on the focal spot so that the primary and information-carrying x-rays "see" only the edges of the strips. The *arrow* at lower right indicates that the grid moves through a distance of more than 20 grid line spacings, i.e., >20 times the sum of the width of the lead lamellae plus the width of the radiolucent interspace material, or >20(d + D), during an exposure.

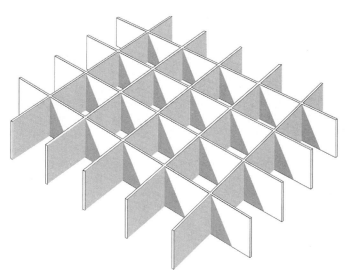

Figure 2–11. Principle of Lorad high-transmission cellular (HTC) grid. The grid controls scatter in two directions. A conventional linear grid controls scatter in only one direction.

factor. When one compares two grids, the grid that has the higher CIF and lower Bucky factor is better. Both the CIF and Bucky factor of mammography grids vary with the ratio of scatter to primary x-rays emerging from the breast and, thus, with breast thickness. It has long been realized that conventional mammography grids are limited in performance, and this knowledge has led a number of groups to investigate more efficient techniques.[13-16] Although improved efficiency has been demonstrated, the majority of systems achieving it have not been capable of conventional positioning flexibility or of accommodating both 18 × 24-cm and 24 × 30-cm cassettes. One approach that does not have these limitations is the cellular, air-interspace grid introduced by Lorad in the mid-1990s.[15] The grid, referred to as the HTC (high-transmission cellular) grid, is schematically shown in Figure 2–11. A linear grid controls scatter in one direction, and the cellular grid controls scatter in two directions. The specifications of the HTC grid and commonly used Smit-Röntgen grid are listed in Table 2–3. The experimentally measured CIFs and Bucky factors of the Smit-Röntgen and Lorad grids are compared in Table 2–4.[17] The HTC grid exhibits superior contrast improvement for all phantom thicknesses and tube potentials studied. It also has a lower (superior) Bucky factor for 2- and 4-cm phantom thicknesses and slightly higher Bucky factor (2.6% higher) for the 8-cm phantom thickness. In clinical practice, the HTC grid results in better contrast than a linear grid and is preferred by radiologists.

The lateral or left-to-right dimensions of the grid assemblies are of practical importance. An 18 × 24-cm film cassette measures 19.3 × 26.7 cm (i.e., chest wall–to-nipple dimension by lateral dimension). The lateral dimensions of the 18 × 24-cm grid assemblies of different mammography equipment manufacturers range from 28 to 30 cm. This dimension is important in imaging the axillary tail in the mediolateral oblique view. A grid assembly with a 28-cm lateral dimension is capable of imaging 1 cm more of axillary tail tissue than an assembly with a 30-cm lateral dimension.

Magnification Stand

MQSA regulations require that mammography systems used to perform noninterventional problem-

Table 2–3. Specifications of Smit-Röntgen and Lorad High-Transmission Cellular (HTC) Grids

Specification	Smit-Röntgen Grid	Lorad HTC Grid
Grid type	Linear	Cellular
Grid ratio	5:1	3.8:1
Interspace material	Fiber	Air
Septa material	Lead	Copper
Height of grid (h) (mm)	1.5	2.4
Width of lead lamellae (d) (mm)	0.016	0.03
Width of radiolucent interspace material (D) (mm)	0.30	0.64
Lines (cells) per cm	31	15
Lead or copper content (mg/cm²)	86 (Pb)	188 (Cu)

Data from de Almeida A, Rezentes PS, Barnes GT: Mammography grid performance. Radiology 1999;210:227-232.

Table 2–4. Contrast Improvement and Bucky Factors of Smit-Röntgen and Lorad HTC Grids

Tube Potential (kVp)	Phantom Thickness (cm)	Contrast Improvement Factor		Bucky Factor	
		Smit-Röntgen	Lorad HTC	Smit-Röntgen	Lorad HTC
25	2	1.08	1.13	2.18	2.00
	4	1.24	1.34	2.41	2.21
	8	1.46	1.56	3.62	—
30	2	1.08	1.14	1.98	1.91
	4	1.22	1.31	2.27	2.16
	8	1.52	1.62	2.70	2.77

Data from de Almeida A, Rezentes PS, Barnes GT: Mammography grid performance. Radiology 1999;210:227-232.

solving procedures have radiographic magnification capability available for use by the operator.[4] For magnification work, the grid is removed and replaced on the U-arm's mounting plate by the magnification stand and cassette holder. The regulations further require that at least one magnification value within the range of 1.4 to 2.0 be provided.[4] Implicit in this requirement and to meet the MQSA regulations system resolution, the unit must also have a small focal spot. For a 65-cm SID, space constraints limit the maximum magnification (2 cm above the breast support) to less than ×2.0. Although one or more manufacturers offer two magnification values (i.e., ×1.5 and ×2.0), the majority offer one value in the ×1.5 to ×2.0 range.

Magnification is employed to better delineate a region of interest of the breast. Image quality is improved because (1) system spatial resolution is better and (2) more x-ray photons are used to image the structure of interest and there is a 30% to 40 % decrease in effective noise.[18] Figure 2–12 compares the system modulation transfer function (MTF) responses for grid technique (large focal spot) and ×1.7 magnification technique with 0.1-mm and 0.2-mm focal spot sizes. Two important points of practical importance are demonstrated in the figure: First, magnification system resolution (0.1-mm focal spot) is better than grid technique, and second, the size of the small focal spot critically affects magnification system resolution. For example, at ×1.7, the system MTF response with a 0.2-mm focus is degraded compared with the 0.1-mm focal spot response. MQSA regulations are not overly stringent in this regard, requiring that the limiting spatial resolution associated with the width and length of the small focal spot be ≥13 lp/mm and ≥11 lp/mm, respectively.[4] Compared with a system with limiting resolutions of 13 lp/mm (width) and 11 lp/mm (length), images obtained with a system with limiting resolutions of 15 lp/mm appear sharper and microcalcification borders are better delineated. The measured system resolutions of a mammography unit are important parameters that have a direct impact on image quality, particularly the magnification system resolutions. Figure 2–12 does not show the effect of different magnification factors on system resolution. Provided that the small focal spot is sufficiently small (i.e., a true 0.1-mm focal spot), ×2.0 magnification gives better results than ×1.7, and ×1.7 gives better results than ×1.5.

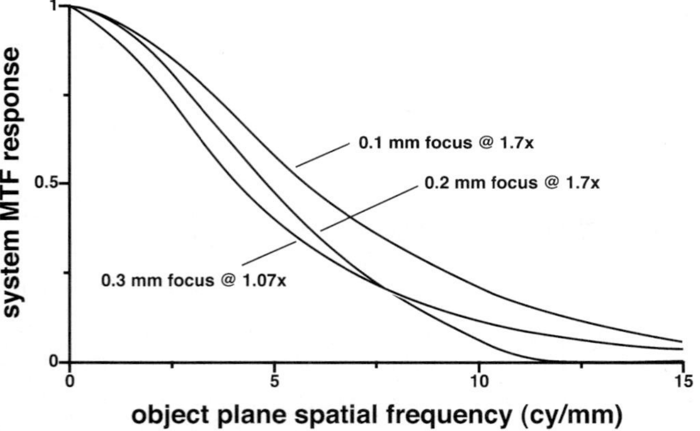

Figure 2–12. Comparison of system modulation transfer functions (MTFs) for grid technique and magnification technique with 0.1-mm and 0.2-mm focal spots. The published MTF for a Kodak Min-R 2000 screen was employed for the calculations (see Bunch PC: Advances in high-speed mammographic image quality. Proc SPIE 1999;3659:120-130). Rect function focal spot intensity distributions were assumed. The magnification MTF with a 0.1-mm focal spot is noticeably better than the grid technique MTF. Also, the magnification MTF with a 0.1-mm focal spot is noticeably better than with a 0.2-mm focal spot.

Additional factors affecting magnification image quality are kVp, exposure time, and FOV. If the small focal spot has sufficient loadability (i.e., ≥30 mA at 25 kVp), lower-kVp and shorter–exposure time techniques can be employed. Lowering the kVp increases subject contrast, and there is less chance of patient motion problems with shorter exposure times. Scatter depends on the FOV. Data for the dependence on the relative intensity of scatter on FOV in magnification mammography are limited, but fundamental imaging physics principles suggest that the smaller the FOV, the smaller the relative intensity of scatter imaged. The problem with decreasing the FOV too much is that it makes positioning difficult and also decreases the surround and the ability of the reader to orient himself or herself. A reasonable compromise is a 12 ×18-cm FOV at the image plane (≈7 cm × 10.5 cm at the object plane). A problem with a 12 × 18-cm FOV is that a significant region of the film is not exposed and must be masked for optimal viewing. However, the improvement in perceived image contrast more than compensates for this minor inconvenience.

Automatic Exposure Control

A fundamental requirement in screen-film mammography is that the film be properly exposed. If the film is too light or too dark, breast structures will not be displayed with maximum contrast, information will be lost, and cancers will be missed. Proper screen-film exposure depends on AEC performance. The AEC on a mammography unit should provide consistent film density as breast thickness is varied for the range of x-ray tube potentials employed clinically.

In screen-film mammography, the AEC sensor is located in the U-arm mounting plate behind the image receptor, as shown in Figures 2–5 and 2–10. The sensor detects x-rays that penetrate the breast and screen-film cassette and then generates a current proportional to the detected x-ray energy fluence. The current is amplified and charges a capacitor. The voltage across the capacitor is compared with a reference value, and when the two are equal, the exposure is terminated. Mammography units manufactured before 1990 did not achieved consistent film density because breast thickness and x-ray tube potential were varied.[7,19] Factors contributing to this unacceptable performance were greater beam hardening with increasing breast thickness, film reciprocity law failure, and AEC sensor dark current.[7] Modern AECs apply corrections for these effects and, if set up correctly, generally achieve acceptable performance. MQSA regulations require that the AEC track to within ±0.15 OD (optical density) of the average OD as breast phantom thickness is varied from 2.0 to 6.0 cm over the clinically used range of tube potentials, filters, and x-ray tube target materials.[4]

A mammography AEC should meet a number of other specifications, which are summarized in Table 2–5. The sensor should have a range of movement (≈8 cm) from close to the chest wall to out toward the nipple, so that it can be placed under the dense glandular tissue. A number of discrete positions are preferred, with the positions shown on the compression paddle (an MQSA regulation). A feature appreciated by technologists on one manufacturer's units is the additional ability to shift the sensor laterally about 2 centimeters on either side of the center line of the mounting plate. To assist the technologist, the lateral as well as the chest wall–to-nipple sensor positions are shown on the paddle.

The AEC sensor should sample an adequate region of the breast. If it is too small (i.e., 1 cm^2), only a small area of the breast will determine the screen-film exposure, and because breast tissue is highly variable, greater exposure (and density) variations will occur than with a larger sensor. Two solutions to this problem that work well in practice are (1) employing a D-shaped pickup with a sensitive area of ≥5 cm^2 and (2) using an array of three 1-cm^2 sensitive sensors and summing the results of the three. Two of the sensors are positioned 4 cm apart, and the third is located in the middle of the other two and 2 cm anteriorly. In either approach, a larger area of breast tissue is sampled, but not so large that it extends beyond the boundaries of small breasts encountered. Sampling a larger area of breast tissue results in greater consistency in clinical film OD.

The AEC should have a separate density calibration for grid and magnification techniques and two screen-film combination selections for each technique. (Several units also have a small and large grid assembly adjustment.) The unit should automatically select a default screen-film combination (programmable) for each technique—that is, a standard-speed screen-film system for grid technique and a faster screen-film system for magnification technique. It should also have 11 exposure steps (i.e., –5 to +5) with an exposure change of about 10% per increment. (The exposure change per increment should be programmable.) An exposure change of 10% corresponds to a film OD change of 0.15 to 0.20 for a typical mammography screen-film system. This is

Table 2–5. State-of-the-Art Mammography Automatic Exposure Control (AEC) Specifications

Sensor Location	Post Cassette
Sensor shape, active area	D-shaped, ≈5 cm^2 sensitive area
Sensor movement	Capable of being moved in 8 cm from the chest wall toward the nipple; a number of discreet positions are preferred, with the positions shown on the compression paddle
Technique calibration	Separate AEC density calibration for each technique—grid and magnification
Screen-film selections	There should be a choice of two screen-film combinations for each AEC technique
Technique selection	The unit should automatically select the proper AEC density calibration, focal spot size, and screen film when the unit is operated in a given mode—nongrid, grid, or magnification
AEC ± exposure settings	11 AEC exposure steps should be available for each AEC technique (i.e., –5 to +5) with ≈10% exposure change per increment; the exposure change per step should be adjustable by field service
Density tracking	AEC should be capable of holding film density within ±0.15 OD (optical density) as the kV is varied from 25 to 32 kVp and breast thickness from 2 to 8 cm for grid techniques and from 2 to 6 cm for magnification techniques
AEC modes	Auto Time and Auto kVp/filter/target—operator selectable: In the Auto Time mode, the operator selects the kVp and the unit determines the exposure time In the Auto kVp/filter/target mode, the unit has a test pulse at 25 or 26 kVp and increases the tube potential systematically by 1-5 kV (and changes the filter and target when appropriate) if the desired film density would not be achieved with a predetermined mA value, i.e., 250 mA
mA backup	500 mA for grid technique; 250 mA for magnification technique

a desirable degree of film OD control for the technologist. An OD change of 0.10 or less per increment is too fine, and a change of 0.30 or more is too great.

The operator should be able to select between two manual techniques: Auto Time and an Optimized Auto mode that selects the kVp or the kVp and filter. In the Auto Time AEC mode, the operator selects the kVp (and filter) and the unit determines the exposure time to achieve the correct film OD. In the Optimized Auto AEC mode, the unit selects the kVp and filter and determines the exposure time. On units that have dual targets, this latter mode also selects the target. Some manufacturers also offer an Auto kVp AEC mode, in which the Mo/Mo target-filter is selected by the operator and the unit selects the kVp and determines the exposure time.

SCREEN-FILM PROCESSING SYSTEM

Screen-Film Considerations

Currently, several manufacturers supply intensifying screen cassettes and film designed for mammography. To maximize spatial resolution, these are all single screen, single emulsion film systems. The film consists of silver bromide grains in a gelatin matrix (emulsion) coated onto a polyester base. The emulsion layer is typically 10 μm, and the polyester base 180 μm in thickness. The intensifying screen consists of Gd_2O_2S:Tb phosphor particles and binder layer coated on a polyester base. The phosphor particles are about 10 μm in size, the thickness of the layer is about 75 μm, and the thickness of the (polyester) base is about 225 μm. The coating weight of Gd_2O_2S:Tb phosphor is about 33 mg/cm^2. Gd_2O_2S:Tb is a bright phosphor that emits green light to which mammography film is sensitized (i.e., mammography film is orthochromatic).

The film is designed to have high contrast. This is accomplished with emulsions using a narrow silver bromide grain-size distribution of small cubic grains measuring approximately 1 μm. As illustrated in Figure 2–13, the x-ray beam is incident on the cassette and sequentially passes through the top of the cassette, the film base, and the film emulsion and then strikes the intensifying screen. Although a (very) small percentage of x-rays are absorbed by the emulsion's silver halide grains, the majority are absorbed in the intensifying screen and are converted to light, which in turn exposes the film. A small percentage penetrate the screen and strike the AEC sensor. The percentage of the x-rays absorbed per unit thickness in the phosphor layer is greatest close to the film and decreases with increasing depth in the screen. Less light diffusion and blur are associated with x-rays absorbed close to the film, and greater diffusion occurs for x-rays absorbed farther away from the film. For this reason, the film, screen, and cassette geometry shown in Figure 2–13 is employed rather than the reverse; this geometry maximizes screen-film spatial resolution.

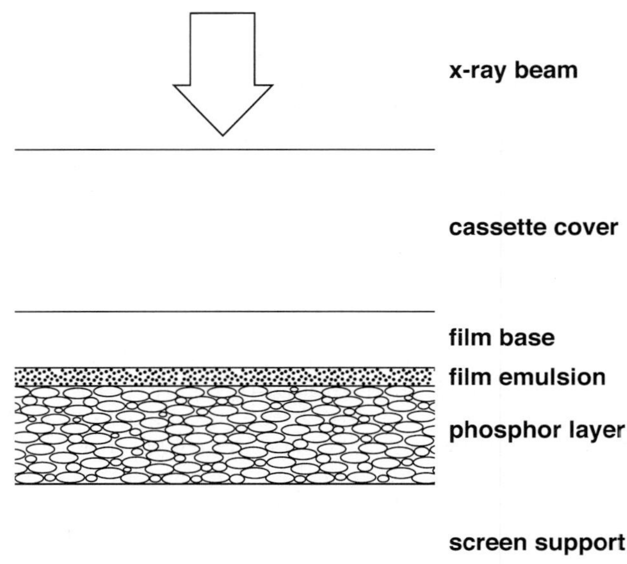

Figure 2–13. Screen-film system geometry. The x-rays transmitted by the patient (and grid) are incident on the cassette. They sequentially pass through the top (polycarbonate) cover of the cassette, the film base, and the film emulsion layer and are incident on the phosphor layer of the intensifying screen. Most are absorbed by the phosphor layer, and only a few pass through the cassette and strike the automatic exposure control (AEC) sensor positioned below the screen-film cassette. The x-rays absorbed by the screen's phosphor layer are converted to light, exposing the film.

Mammography screen-film manufacturers typically offer one film and two screen speeds—standard and medium. The medium-speed system has slightly less spatial resolution and slightly more noise than the standard-speed system. However, the differences are subtle. The standard-speed screen is commonly employed for the majority of work at most mammography centers. The medium-speed screen, however, can be employed to advantage in two areas—magnification techniques and grid work for imaging of thick, dense breasts. In these cases, one must increase the kVp and exposure time to obtain a properly exposed image with the standard-speed system. With the medium-speed system, the subtle decrease in spatial resolution and subtle increase in image noise are more than compensated for by the reduced exposure time and lower kVp techniques that can be employed.

Film Processing Overview

The exposure of film to light results in the formation of latent image centers on grains that have received a sufficient amount of light. A latent image center consists of 4 to 10 silver atoms clustered at a surface sensitivity speck on a grain. Film development consists of first immersing the film in the developing solution, where the organic developing agents reduce the silver halide grains with a latent image center to metallic silver. Grains that do not have a latent image center are not reduced. The developing solution is basic (pH ≈ 10.2). The fixing solution is acidic (pH ≈ 4.2), and development is stopped when the film is immersed in the fixing solution. In the fixing solution, the remaining undeveloped grains are removed from the emulsion. Fixation is followed by washing and drying the film. Film processing is important and has a significant impact on mammography image quality. If the processing is subpar, film speed and film contrast are compromised.

Automatic Film Processor Considerations

The automatic medical x-ray film processor transports the film through four processing stages just described. Each of these sections has transportation rollers associated with it and connection rollers to the next section. The film is placed on the feed tray and is transported by the feed rollers to the developer roller rack. After passing through the developing solution, the film is transported by the developer-fixer crossover roller rack to the fixer rack. After passing through the fixer solution, it is transported by the fixer-wash crossover rack to the wash rack and then to the dryer section, after which it exits the processor. As shown in Figure 2–14, there are two general classes of processors—shallow tank and deep tank. The shallow tank processors are less expensive (all tanks and roller racks are the same), more compact, and often recommended for mammography. However, deep tank processors have better chemistry agitation and, with the same chemistry, result in greater film speed and greater film contrast than shallow tank processors. As shown in Figure 2–15, the same film processed in a deep tank has noticeably greater speed and contrast compared with processing in a shallow tank processor with the same chemistry. Figure 2–16 compares the speed and gradient of film from the same box processed at four shallow tank and three deep tank processor sites. Films processed in deep tank processors have on the average 15% higher speed and 5% greater contrast than the films processed in shallow tank processors. Deep tank processors also have a greater volume of chemistry than the shallow tank processors, resulting in less variability and slower changes in chemistry performance.[20] The developer and fixer tanks have a smaller surface-to-volume ratio than the shallow tank processors, thereby limiting developer and fixer oxidation.

Whether deep tank or shallow tank, if the processor is not maintained properly, processing artifacts can be a problem. They can manifest as random wet pressure marks that increase the noise level of the resultant film or as more recognizable linear artifacts. As a general rule, rollers should be replaced and the racks completely rebuilt or replaced on a low-volume processor at 18-month intervals or sooner. On a high-volume processor, the rollers should be replaced and the racks rebuilt or replaced every year.

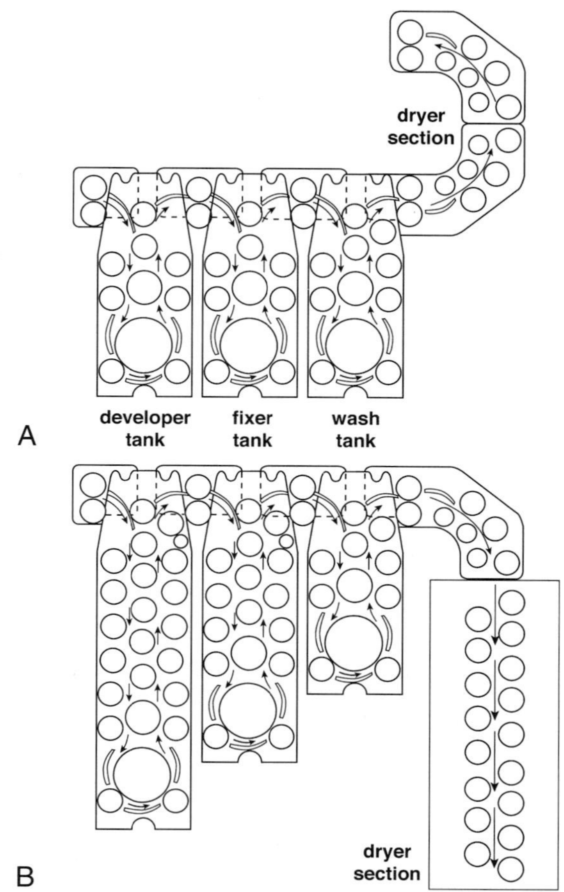

Figure 2–14. Shown are shallow tank (**A**) and deep tank (**B**) automatic film processors. Shallow tank processors are often recommended for mammography because of their low cost. However, fewer artifact problems and greater film speed and contrast are obtained with deep tank processors.

Chemistry Considerations

Chemistry has a major impact on film speed and contrast, and it is a good policy to follow the film manufacturer's recommendations. Film speed and contrast can be compromised when a chemical process not recommended by the film manufacturer is employed. In the author's experience and that of others (DJ Staton, personal communication, 2003), switching developer chemistry from "brand X" to the chemical process recommended by the film manufacturer leads to an approximately 15% increase in film speed.

It is also important that the chemicals are mixed correctly and that the replenishment rates are set to the film manufacturer's recommendations for the volume of film processed.[21] Cubic grain emulsions employed in mammography film are extremely sensitive to bromide ion concentration. If the processor developer tank's chemicals are not mixed correctly to start with (i.e., improper amount of start-up solution added for the volume of film processed), overdevelopment or underdevelopment can occur, and the

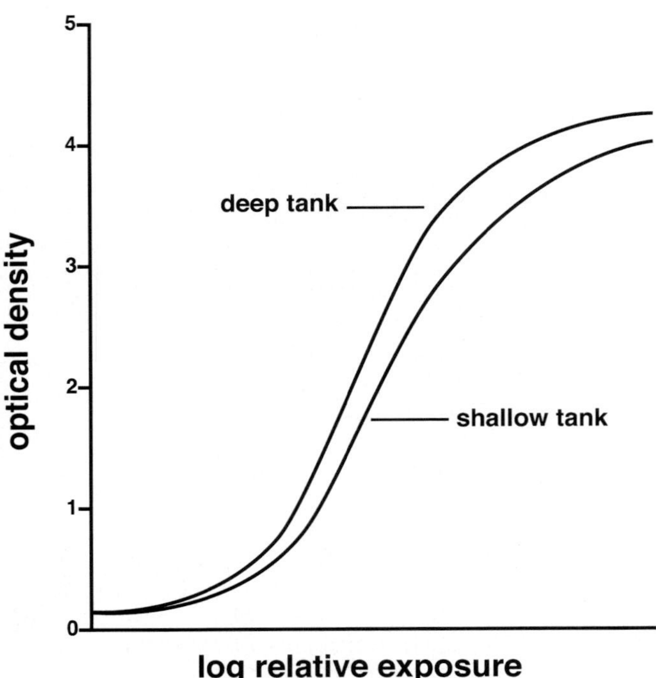

Figure 2–15. Comparison of the sensitometric response of Kodak Min-R 2000 film processed in shallow tank and deep tank Kodak automatic processors. In both cases, the same film emulsion was employed, the developer temperature was 95°F, and the chemistry was seasoned Kodak RP chemicals mixed and replenished to Kodak specifications. The film processed in the deep tank processor has noticeably greater speed and contrast than the film processed in the shallow tank processor.

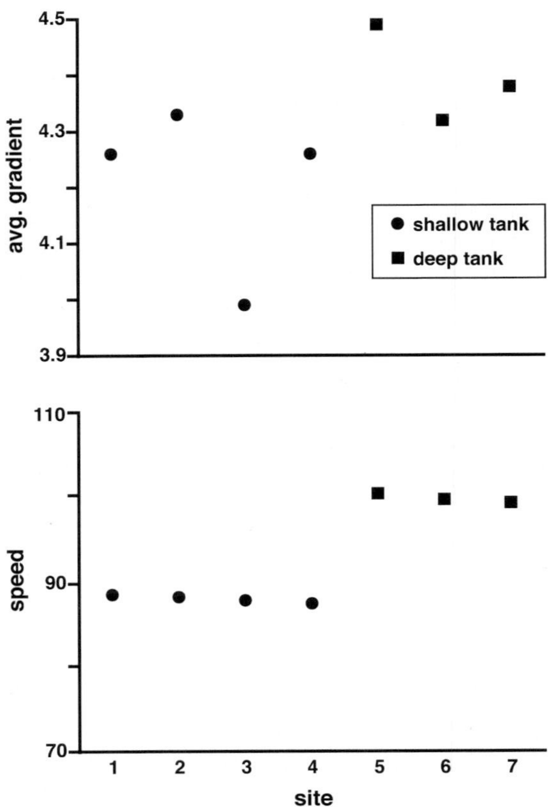

Figure 2–16. Comparison of Kodak Min-R 2000 film speed and contrast of three sites employing deep tank processors with five sites employing shallow tank processors. In all cases, the same film emulsion was employed, the developer temperature was 95°F, and the chemistry was seasoned Kodak RP chemicals mixed and replenished to Kodak specifications. The speed of the film processed in the deep tank processors is 14% greater, and the contrast 6% greater, than those of the same film processed in the shallow tank processors.

system will be unstable. Similarly, if the replenishment tank developer is not mixed correctly and the replenishment rate set appropriately for the volume of film being processed, film speed and contrast vary with time. Trends will be evident in the daily processor sensitometric QC chart.

TECHNIQUES AND SELECTION OF SCREEN SPEED

Grid Techniques

To keep breast dose and exposure times within reasonable limits, the penetrating quality of the x-ray beam should be increased as breast thickness is increased. With a unit that is equipped only with Mo/Mo, this goal is achieved by increasing the kVp. With more sophisticated units, one can change the filtration and, as noted previously, sometimes also the target. Techniques to achieve optimal contrast on the basis of the preceding dose and exposure time trends from the author's experience are presented in Table 2–6 for an Mo/Mo unit with a respectable radiation output rate (>1400 mR per second at 28 kVp). Table 2–7 presents techniques for a Mo/Mo

Table 2–6. Recommended Molybdenum/Molybdenum Grid Techniques*

	X-Ray Tube Potential		
Breast Thickness (cm)	Fatty Breast	Medium Breast	Dense Breast
<3	25 kVp	25 kVp	25 kVp
3-5	25 kVp	25 kVp	26 kVp
5-7	26 kVp	**26 kVp**	**27 kVp**
>7	**28 kVp**	**29 kVp**	**30 kVp**

***Boldface type** indicates medium speed screen-film system; regular type indicates standard speed screen-film system.

Table 2–7. Recommended Molybdenum/Molybdenum and Molybdenum/Rhodium Grid Techniques*

Breast	Fatty Breast		Medium Breast		Dense Breast	
Thickness (cm)	kVp	Filter	kVp	Filter	kVp	Filter
<3	25	Mo	25	Mo	25	Mo
3-5	25	Mo	25	Mo	26	Mo
5-7	26	Mo	**27**	**Mo**	**27**	**Mo**
>7	**28**	**Mo**	**27-28**	**Rh**	**28-29**	**Rh**

***Boldface type** indicates medium speed screen-film system; regular type indicates standard speed screen-film system.

and Mo/Rh unit. Both tables assume that one is using both standard-speed screen-film processing (standard-speed intensifying screen) and medium-speed systems (medium-speed intensifying screen). A standard-speed system typically results in an average glandular dose of 200 to 225 mrad for a 4.2-cm breast or for the American College of Radiology phantom, and a medium-speed system in an average glandular dose of 135 to 150 mrad. If only the standard-speed system is employed, the tube potentials would be about 2 kV higher for the table entries for which the medium-speed system is recommended. The medium-speed system can be employed to advantage in imaging the thick, dense breast, particularly on units that lower the mA above 28 kVp. The subtle decrease in spatial resolution and subtle increase in image noise are more than compensated for by the increase in contrast gained with the lower-kVp techniques that can be employed.

Magnification Techniques

With magnification, there is little or no decrease in system resolution when a medium-speed rather than a standard-speed screen is used. Similarly, there is little increase in effective image noise. However, there is a marked decrease in exposure time, and one can use lower kVp techniques and improve subject contrast. Medium-speed screens should always be used for magnification.

EQUIPMENT PERFORMANCE AUDITS AND MAINTENANCE

Acceptance Testing and Annual Performance Audits

According to MQSA regulations, performance evaluations of mammography units or image processors must be performed by (or under the direct supervision of) a qualified medical physicist whenever a new unit or processor is installed or whenever a unit or processor is dissembled and reassembled at either the same or at a new facility.[4] All problems found that do not satisfy MQSA regulations must be corrected, the correction documented, and the documentation reviewed by the medical physicist before the unit is put into clinical use. MQSA regulations also require that each facility undergo an annual equipment performance audit by a medical physicist. As with the initial or acceptance testing of a unit, problems found in meeting MQSA regulations must be corrected, the correction documented, and the documentation reviewed by the medical physicist. With an annual audit, however, the facility can continue to use the unit and has 30 days from the date of the audit (not the date of the report) to correct the problems. There are two exceptions: accreditation (ACR) phantom image quality and dose. If the phantom image made at the time of an annual audit does not satisfy the minimum standards of the accreditation body or if the average glandular phantom dose exceeds 300 mrad, the unit cannot be used for mammography until the problem is corrected.

Table 2–8. Initial and Annual Performance Audit Physics Tests Required by Mammography Quality Standards Act Regulations

Mammography unit assembly evaluation
Collimation assessment
Evaluation of system resolution (for both grid and magnification techniques)
kVp accuracy and reproducibility
Beam quality assessment (half-value layer measurement)
Breast entrance exposure and radiation output rate
Automatic exposure control (AEC) reproducibility
Uniformity of screen speed
AEC system performance
Artifact evaluation
Accreditation phantom image quality evaluation
Accreditation phantom average glandular dose
Assessment of site's quality control program

Table 2–8 lists the initial and annual medical physics performance tests. The initial or acceptance testing should be a more thorough evaluation than the annual performance audit. Compression paddle–cassette alignment should be checked for all paddles and techniques, grid Bucky factor or dose efficiency should be evaluated (this is not an MQSA requirement), and the check-out of the AEC performance should be more comprehensive and should be performed over a wider range of breast phantom thicknesses and x-ray tube potentials than required by MQSA regulations. MQSA requires that AEC performance should be checked for 2-cm, 4-cm, and 6-cm phantom thicknesses over the clinically used range of x-ray tube potentials. Acceptance testing should also use an 8-cm phantom thickness. (In my experience, most medical physicists routinely check AEC tracking for 2- through 8-cm phantom thicknesses during their annual performance audits.) For 2-cm and 4-cm phantom thicknesses, the acceptance testing AEC tracking evaluation should additionally include 1 kV above and 1 kV below the kVp value that would normally be checked. For 6-cm and 8-cm thicknesses, AEC tracking acceptance testing should include 2 kV above and 1 kV below the kVp value that would normally be checked. It has been documented in the literature for both mammography and general radiography that acceptance testing identifies problems and permits their correction before clinical use of a unit.[22,23]

During acceptance testing, special attention should be given to the grid and magnification technique system resolution tests. MQSA regulations require that the limiting system spatial resolution associated with the focal spot length be 11 lp/mm or higher and that the resolution associated with the focal spot width be 13 lp/mm or higher.[4] As noted previously, the primary factor determining the system resolution is the dimension of the focal spot, and mammography units that have smaller focal spots exhibit better performance. Furthermore, focal spot size and related performance tests do not improve with age. An x-ray tube that just meets the minimum requirements at one testing may not do so in a year or two, and replacing an x-ray tube after the warranty period is expensive. Magnification technique with limiting spatial resolutions of 11 lp/mm (length) and 13 lp/mm (width) would meet MQSA regulations. However, it would result in noticeably less sharp images than a unit with limiting spatial resolutions of 15 lp/mm. The borders of microcalcifications would not be delineated as well. The author believes that the acceptance testing limiting-system spatial resolutions should be 15 lp/mm or greater, especially for magnification technique. A new unit that just meets the MQSA limiting spatial resolution requirements would not be acceptable.

Another area in which MQSA regulations are not sufficiently strict, and a concession was made to manufacturers, is in the uniformity of screen (cassette) speed. The requirements are that the difference between the maximum and minimum OD values (for cassettes with screens of the same type) shall not exceed 0.30 when a homogenous, defect-free material (i.e., 4-cm thickness of methylacrylic plastic) is imaged.[4] This is an exceedingly generous tolerance and could yield films of the same patient for the same AEC settings that were acceptably and unacceptably exposed. A more reasonable criterion for acceptance testing of new cassettes is a maximum OD difference of 0.15, and 0.10 is preferable. In the author's experience, this criterion is achievable, especially at a large facility where one can group cassettes of a given speed and assign them to a given room or area. Differences between large and small cassettes are less critical and can be handled by having a different AEC density calibration for each size or noting the difference on the technique chart. A number of units are capable of different AEC density calibrations for the small and large grid assemblies and thus for the small and large cassette sizes.

Additional Medical Physics Equipment Evaluations

MQSA regulations require that evaluations be performed by a qualified medical physicist (or by an individual under the direct supervision of a qualified medical physicist) whenever major components of a mammography unit or processor are changed or repaired.[4] These evaluations are used to determine whether the new or repaired component meets MQSA Performance Standards. All problems are to be corrected before the new or repaired component is put into service. Examples of major equipment component replacement that require medical physics testing are the x-ray tube, collimation subassembly, compression subassembly, AEC sensor and associated circuitry, and grid assemblies. Examples of processor major components that require medical physics testing are replacement or rebuilding of processor racks (as opposed to routine cleaning and preventive maintenance).

Equipment Maintenance and Repair

The warranty on a new mammography unit is typically a year, during which the vendor maintains the unit and corrects problems. The quality and reputation of a vendor's service organization are an important consideration in purchasing a unit. After the warranty period, the five service options for a facility are a full service contract, partial service contract, no service contract, in-house service, and risk insurance with a third party. With no service contract, the facility pays time and materials for each repair and replaced component. Partial service contracts are variable but typically have most of the features of a full service contract, excluding glassware (x-ray tubes).

When one is purchasing a new unit, it is a good idea to require documentation of the costs of full service and the type of partial service contracts in which the facility is interested for a period of 5 years beyond the warranty period. This provides the purchaser a degree of price protection. Service contracts are an important cost consideration, and adding a 5-year full-service cost to the initial cost of the unit is known as its life cycle cost. If the service contract price for a mammography unit seems too high, either the equipment is not well engineered and requires an excessive amount of service or the service contract price is inflated. Either of these reasons detracts from the unit's desirability. Some equipment manufacturers sell new units at a relatively small profit margin with the intent of making a substantial profit on parts and service. Response time during regular working hours, evenings, and occasionally on weekends is also important; this issue should be documented before a unit or a service contract is purchased.

In-house service can be cost effective and provide timely response.[24] However, it is feasible only for larger facilities and must be well managed. Smaller facilities are limited to vendor or third-party equipment maintenance, either with or without a service contract. With in-house service replacement, parts can be a problem. Obtaining a purchase order for a part can take considerable time and effort at larger institutions. The process can be expedited with a parts contract, whereby the in-house service person need not obtain a purchase order before ordering a needed part.

There are at least two service risk insurance options. For one, the facility directly calls the service vender of choice to arrange for problems to be fixed, and the insurance company pays the service bill. For the other, the facility calls the third party risk insurer, which in turn arranges for the unit to be fixed with either the vendor or another service organization. Insurance options add a layer of bureaucracy, slow down repairs, and involve an additional party that is making money from the service. In the author's experience, risk insurance offers little or no advantage for mammography.

A cost-effective approach for a smaller facility is to expect to pay for time and materials, or to have no contract. To avoid a budget crisis, a service account should be set up and money added each year or each quarter to the account equal to the cost of a full service contract so as to pay for time and materials or repairs as needed. When the money in the account exceeds the cost of replacing the x-ray tube, the amount added the next year need only be equal to a service contract excluding glassware, and so on. With this approach, the facility is self insured and, provided that there is not a catastrophic equipment failure, saves money. Also, if a site is planning to not have a full service contract, it is advantageous on a new unit to schedule the medical physicist's annual performance audit a month or more before the end of the warranty period and request that the physicist send the report in immediately after completing the survey. The problems that are identified by the medical physicist and must be corrected are then covered by the warranty.

With any of the preceding service options, the original equipment manufacturer's preventive maintenance recommendations should be reviewed and the key points followed. For example, on some manufacturers' units, the automated AEC algorithms depend on the compressed breast thickness reading. If the reading is off by a centimeter or more, the wrong kVp and filter can be selected and image quality compromised. This is one of the many settings on a unit that must be checked and calibrated periodically. Preventive maintenance can minimize unnecessary and unexpected downtime.

References

1. Gabbay E: Mammography x-ray source. In Haus AG, Yaffe MJ (eds): Technical Aspects of Breast Imaging, 3rd ed. Oakbrook, IL, RSNA, 1994, pp 47-62.
2. Kimme-Smith CM, Sayre JW, McCombs MM, et al: Breast calcification and mass detection with mammographic anode-filter combinations of molybdenum, tungsten, and rhodium. Radiology 1997;203:697-683.
3. Gingold EL, Wu X, Barnes GT: Contrast and dose with Mo-Mo, Mo-Rh, and Rh-Rh target-filter combinations in mammography. Radiology 1995;195:639-644.
4. Part 900: Mammography. 21 CFR October 1997.
5. Integral M113R: Mammography X-Ray Source Assembly Product Description and Specifications. Salt Lake City, UT, Varian Medical Systems, Rev A, April 2003.
6. Barnes GT, Brezovich IA: Contrast: Effect of scattered radiation. In Logan WW (ed): Breast Carcinoma: The Radiologist's Expanded Role. New York, John Wiley & Sons, 1977, pp 73-81.
7. LaFrance R, Gelskey DE, Barnes GT: A circuit modification that improves mammographic phototimer performance. Radiology 1988;166:773-776.
8. Freidrich M: Der Einfluss der Streustrahlung auf die Abbildungsqualitat bei der Mammographie. Fortschr Rontgenstr 123;1975:556-566.
9. Barnes GT, Brezovich IA: The intensity of scattered radiation in mammography. Radiology 1978;126:243-247.
10. Barnes GT: Contrast and scatter in x-ray imaging. Radiographics 1991;11:307-323.
11. King MA, Barnes GT, Yester MV: A mammographic scanning multiple slit assembly: Design considerations and preliminary results. In Logan WW Muntz EP (eds): Reduced Dose Mammography. New York, Masson, 1979, pp 243-252.
12. Richter D: Evaluation of grid technique in mammography (paper B4). Presented to the 20th Annual Meeting of the American Association of Physicists in Medicine, San Francisco, July 30 to August 3, 1978.
13. Barnes GT, Wu X, Wagner AJ: Scanning slit mammography. Med Prog Technol 1993;14:7-12.
14. Jennings RJ, Fewell TR, Vucich J: Imaging and dose characteristics of a computer-optimized mammography system. Radiology 1991;181(P):234.
15. Pellegrino AJ, Lyke DN, Lieb DP, et al: Air cross grids for mammography and methods for their manufacture and use. US patent 5 606 589. February 25, 1997.
16. Robinson JD, Ferlic D, Kotula L, et al: Improved mammography with reduced radiation dose. Radiology 1993;188:868-871.
17. de Almeida A, Rezentes PS, Barnes GT: Mammography grid performance. Radiology 1999;210:227-232.
18. Barnes GT: Tube potential, focal spot, radiation output and HVL measurements on screen-film mammography units. In Barnes GT, Frey GD (eds): Screen-Film Mammography: Imaging Considerations and Medical Physics Responsibilities. Madison, WI, Medical Physics, 1991, pp 67-113.
19. Niklason LT, Barnes GT, Rubin E: Mammography phototimer technique chart. Radiology 1985;157:539-540.
20. Kimme-Smith CM: Screen-film selection, film exposure, and processing. In Barnes GT, Frey GD (eds): Screen-Film Mammography: Imaging Considerations and Medical Physics Responsibilities. Madison, WI, Medical Physics, 1991, pp 133-158.
21. Sobol WT: A model for tracking concentration of chemical compounds within a tank of an automatic film processor. Med Phys 2002;29:90-99.
22. Barnes GT, Hendrick RE: Mammography accreditation and equipment performance. Radiographics 1994;14:129-138.
23. Stears JG, Nelson R, Barnes GT, Gray JE: The need for acceptance testing: Experience from testing over 115 imaging systems at two major medical facilities. Radiology 1992; 183: 563-567.
24. Barnes GT, McDanal W: When is inhouse service cost effective? Proc SPIE 1980;233:286-290.

Chapter 3 Positioning

Rita W. Heinlein, Lawrence W. Bassett

In this chapter, we discuss the general principles of breast positioning, the maneuvers that the radiologic technologist uses to place the breast in the desired position on the film for a specific mammographic view. In addition, we have included the step-by-step approach used by the radiologic technologist for the most commonly performed mammographic views. A *view*, also called a *projection*, is defined as the image of the breast on the film resulting from the orientation of the x-ray beam and the breast positioning maneuvers performed by the radiologic technologist. A view is usually named according to the direction of the x-ray beam relative to the breast—for example, mediolateral or craniocaudal.

These positioning maneuvers should be of interest to radiologists because it is the interpreting physician who is ultimately responsible for the quality of the images. The American College of Radiology (ACR) has played a major role in educating practitioners about advances in breast positioning.[1] The methods described here are derived from the work of many radiologists and radiologic technologists who have taken a special interest in breast positioning. A Centers for Disease Control and Prevention (CDC)–ACR Cooperative Agreement for Quality Assurance Activities in Mammography, conducted from September 1990 to January 1995, brought together experienced radiologists and radiologic technologists to refine and then disseminate standardized methods for breast positioning in mammography.

The importance of the role of positioning in mammography cannot be overemphasized. Incorrect positioning of the breast was the most common problem encountered in the Mammography Accreditation Program peer review of clinical images.[2] Twenty percent of facilities failing the accreditation process for the first time had problems in positioning.[3] When mammography was performed with direct film techniques or with xeromammography using general-purpose x-ray equipment, positioning was limited to projections that depended on changing the position of the woman—for instance, from lying on the side on a table for the mediolateral projection to sitting on a chair for the craniocaudal projection.

The introduction of dedicated mammography units with rotating C-arms expanded the possibilities for obtaining different mammographic views of the breast without changing the position of the patient. With the continued evolution of dedicated equipment, the possibilities for breast positioning expanded even more. Today, because we do not have to rely on views limited to traditional radiographic projections (90-degree lateral and craniocaudal), breast positioning combines a better understanding of the breast's anatomy and mobility with the capability of modern dedicated equipment to achieve a large number of mammographic views. Screening is performed with a combination of two standard views that when performed properly can visualize all of a woman's breast tissue.[4] Diagnostic imaging uses additional views tailored to the patient's specific breast problem.

GENERAL PRINCIPLES

Dedicated Mammography Equipment

The introduction of rotational C-arms in dedicated mammography units has made it possible to obtain mammograms in almost any projection.[5] The addition of foot-controlled motorized compression, which allows the radiologic technologist to use both hands to position the breast, was another important advance. More effective compression devices have also improved positioning by holding the breast more effectively in the desired position, making the thickness of the breast more uniform, and reducing the possibility of motion during exposures. The availability of two sizes of image receptors for conventional mammography, 18 × 24 cm and 24 × 30 cm, makes it possible to more effectively position and compress small and large breasts.[6] Digital mammography receptors, currently in the development stages, will most likely enable a single receptor size to be used for all projections and patients.

Anatomy and Mobility of the Breast

The breast extends from the second rib superiorly to the sixth rib inferiorly and from the mid-axillary line laterally to the sternum medially. The base of the breast lies almost completely on the pectoral muscle, and a significant portion of the breast tissue may extend into the axilla. The latter portion of the breast, the axillary tail, can harbor breast carcinoma and should be visualized during screening mammography.[7] It is important to image as much breast tissue as possible for screening examinations. The mediolateral oblique (MLO), which includes the pectoral muscle and the axillary tail, is the primary view for screening because it shows the greatest amount of breast tissue in a single image.[7-9] However, medial tissue may be excluded on even a properly performed MLO.[9] The craniocaudal (CC) view, when properly performed, can visualize all of the medial tissue. Therefore, the standard views for screening, the MLO and the CC, are complementary.

The principle of mobile versus fixed tissue is used in breast positioning to maximize the amount of tissue that can be visualized.[10] The lateral and inferior aspects of the breast are mobile borders, whereas the medial and superior aspects are fixed (Fig. 3–1). The objective is to move the mobile tissues toward the fixed tissues and to avoid moving the compression plate against fixed tissues. The principle of fixed versus mobile tissues is discussed in presentations of maneuvers in the positioning for specific projections.

Tailoring the Examination to the Individual Woman

Before positioning is begun, it is important to evaluate the individual woman's body habitus and to determine whether she has any specific clinical problems or special requirements. "Routine" positioning may work for most women, but some women, such as those with kyphosis, those who use wheelchairs, or those with breast implants, require special attention, modifications of techniques, and more time to achieve the best results. When a palpable abnormality is present, it is important to identify the location on the surface of the breast with a lead marker (BB). The BB alerts the interpreting physician to the presence of the palpable abnormality and shows its location relative to other landmarks in the mammogram.

Profile View of the Nipple

Although it is desirable to have the nipple in profile on at least one of the routine views, the primary goal in breast positioning today is to show as much tissue as possible. Therefore, visualization of breast tissue should not be sacrificed to show the nipple in profile. When the nipple is not in profile on either standard view, an extra view can be performed specifically to show the nipple in profile. However, when proper positioning methods are used, this extra view is rarely necessary.[11]

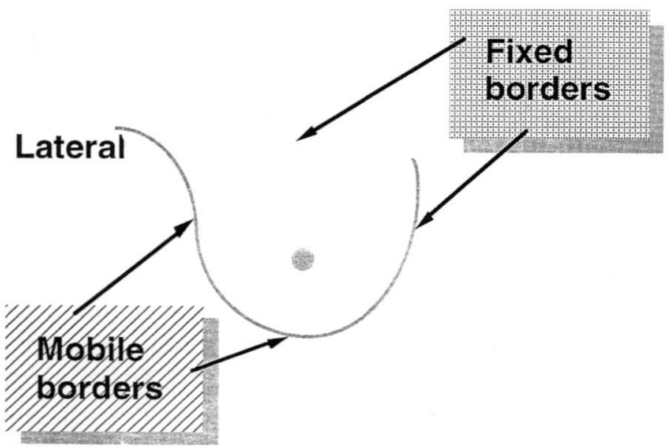

Figure 3–1. Fixed versus mobile borders. (From American College of Radiology Committee on Quality Assurance in Mammography: Mammography Quality Control. Reston, VA, American College of Radiology, 1992, pp 57-99.)

Breast Compression

Proper breast compression is a major factor in obtaining high-quality mammograms. Properly applied compression is one of the most neglected and yet most important factors affecting image quality in mammography. A primary goal of compression is to reduce the thickness of the breast so that it is more uniformly penetrated by the x-ray beam from the subcutaneous region to the chest wall (Fig. 3–2). This is achieved through the use of a rigid compression device with a 90-degree angle between the posterior and inferior surfaces. As compressive force is applied, the compression plate should remain parallel to the plane of the image receptor. This is particularly important with the low-energy (25 to 30 kV), less penetrating x-ray beams that are used in mammography.

There are other important reasons why proper compression is essential for mammography. Compression reduces the object-to–image receptor distance, for better resolution. Compression also separates structures within the breast, lessening the likelihood that a lesion will be missed because it is covered by other tissues or that the overlapping of normal tissues will be mistaken for an abnormality. Proper compression results in more uniform density by flattening the breast to a more two-dimensional structure, facilitating the distinction between more compressible, less dense benign structures, such as asymmetric normal tissue and cysts, and less compressible, denser lesions, such as malignancies. By reducing the breast thickness, proper compression lowers the dose needed for a proper exposure and improves contrast by decreasing scattered radiation. Furthermore, proper compression immobilizes the breast, lessening the possibility of unsharpness due to motion.

A well-designed and properly applied compression device, combined with a technologist's skill in gently but firmly pulling the breast onto the receptor, maximizes the amount of breast tissue that can be imaged. Because the use of proper compression is so critical, it is important to define the amount of compression desired in mammography today. In some cases, in an attempt to be "kind" to the patient, the technologist does not apply adequate breast compression, resulting in poor image quality and a higher radiation dose for the patient. The overall result is not beneficial to the patient. If compression is too "vigorous," however, women will find the

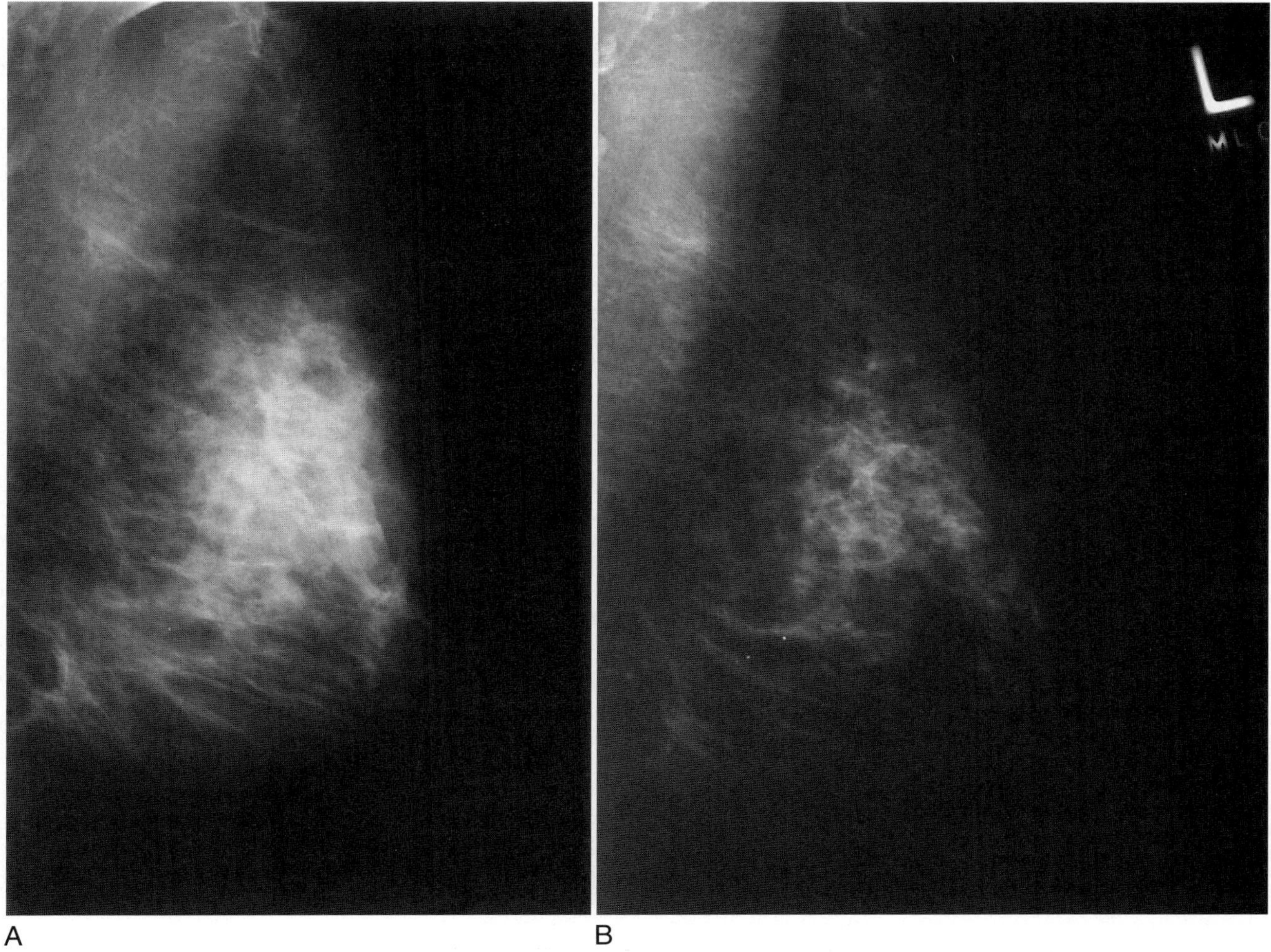

Figure 3–2. Effects of compression. **A,** Noncompressed breast. Tissues near the chest wall are not seen because they are underexposed; subcutaneous tissues are not seen because they are overexposed. **B,** Same breast compressed. More uniform thickness makes it possible to visualize tissues from the chest wall to the skin on the same image. (From American College of Radiology Committee on Quality Assurance in Mammography: Mammography Quality Control. Reston, VA, American College of Radiology, 1992, pp 57-99.)

examination unacceptable, a disincentive to their returning for periodic screening mammograms. Ideally, the amount of compression should be determined by two factors: the maximum extent to which the individual patient's breast can actually be compressed, and the amount of compression that the patient can tolerate at that time. At a minimum, the breast should be compressed until the tissue is *taut*—gentle tapping does not indent the skin when breast compression is taut. However, compression should be less than painful for most women. Therefore, proper compression falls within a range between taut and less than painful.

Patients can often tolerate more compression if they are prepared for it and if it is applied slowly, rather than unexpectedly and all at once.[4] Before beginning the examination, the technologist should establish rapport with the patient. The informed patient, educated as to what compression is, how long it will last, and why it is important, will tolerate more compression.[12,13] The technologist should explain that compression may be uncomfortable but should not be painful and that it will greatly improve the quality of the examination. For some women, the breasts may become very sensitive just before or during menstruation or occasionally at other times in the menstrual cycle.[14] Such women should schedule screening mammography for a time when their breasts are least sensitive. Women for whom the examination cannot be postponed or who are particularly sensitive can be told to take a medication that relieves breast tenderness, such as ibuprofen, before the mammographic examination.

Proper Maintenance of the Image Receptor

The Mammography Quality Standards Act (MQSA) final regulations require cleaning of the compression

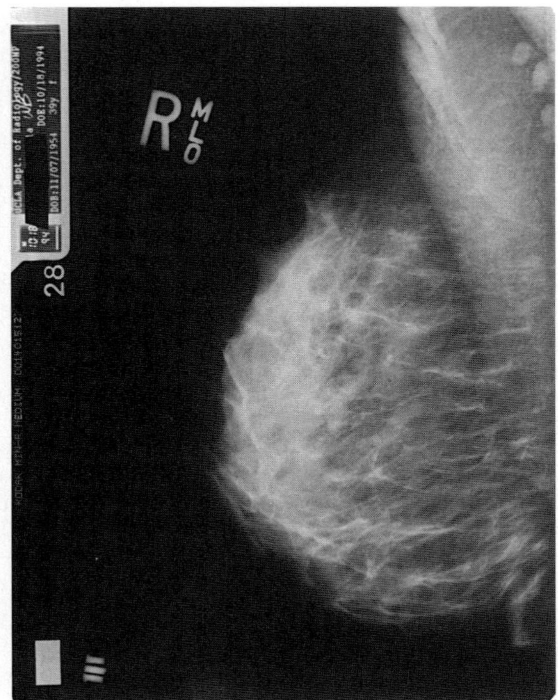

Figure 3–3. Properly labeled film. View and laterality. RMLO markers are placed near the axilla. 28, cassette/screen number; III, number of dedicated mammography unit. The woman's name and unique identification number, which also appear on a properly labeled film, have been masked here. (From American College of Radiology Committee on Quality Assurance in Mammography: Mammography Quality Control. Reston, VA, American College of Radiology, 1992, pp 57-99.)

device and top of the image receptor after use for each patient.[15] Selection of the disinfectant should follow manufacturer's specific recommendations to avoid damage to the equipment.

Labeling of Mammograms

Mammography films are important medical documents. Standardized labeling of mammography films ensures that films are not lost or misinterpreted. Except for labels specifying view and laterality, all labels should be placed as far from the breast as possible. Standardized labeling methods have been developed[16] (Fig. 3–3) and are presented in detail in Chapter 4.

MAMMOGRAPHIC PROJECTIONS

In addition to the standard views that are used in both screening mammography and diagnostic mammography, a variety of other positioning maneuvers and projections have been developed to address specific situations and problems. We have categorized mammographic views into three groups: (1) standard views, (2) views used to better define breast tissue and lesions, and (3) views used to better localize lesions. Table 3–1 lists the views described in this chapter, along with their standardized abbreviations and their purposes.

The remainder of this chapter addresses each of the projections and positioning commonly used for mammography, beginning with the standard projections. The names for views and the abbreviated codes used in this chapter are based on the ACR Breast Imaging Reporting and Data System (ACR BI-RADS) recommendations for standardized mammographic terminology.[17] Familiar synonyms for views are also given for some of the standardized terms.

Standard Views

The mediolateral oblique (MLO) and craniocaudal (CC) views are routinely obtained for all mammographic examinations, and these two views suffice for a screening examination of an asymptomatic woman. Because they may be the only views obtained, it is essential that they be performed as well as possible. Proper breast positioning is based on an understanding of the normal anatomy and the normal mobility of the breast.

Mediolateral Oblique View

The properly performed MLO view offers the best opportunity to image all of the breast tissue in a

Table 3–1. Mammographic Views: Standardized Labeling Codes and Purposes

View	Labeling Code*	Purpose
Mediolateral view	MLO	Standard view
Craniocaudal	CC	Standard view
90-degree lateral		
Mediolateral	ML	Localize, define
Lateromedial	LM	Localize, define
Spot compression	—	Define
Magnification	M†	Define
Exaggerated craniocaudal	XCCL	Localize
Cleavage	CV	Localize
Axillary tail	AT	Localize, define
Tangential	TAN	Localize, define
Roll		
Rolled lateral	RL‡	Localize, define
Rolled medial	RM‡	Localize, define
Caudocranial (from below)	FB	Define
Lateromedial oblique	LMO	Define
Superolateral-to-inferomedial oblique	SIO	Define
Implant displaced	ID	Evaluation of augmented breast

*R or L, indicating right or left breast, is used as a prefix (placed before the view code); for example, *R*MLO indicates a mediolateral oblique view of the right breast.

†Used as a prefix, located after the laterality (R or L breast) but before the projection; for example, R*M*MLO is a magnification mediolateral oblique view of the right breast.

‡Used as a suffix (placed after the view code); for example, LCC*RL* indicates a craniocaudal view of the upper tissue of the left breast rolled laterally.

single view (Fig. 3–4).[7-9] For this view, the plane of the image receptor is angled 30 to 60 degrees from the horizontal so that the receptor is parallel to the plane of the pectoralis muscle. The x-ray beam is directed from the superomedial aspect to the inferolateral aspect of the breast. It is imperative that the angle used be adjusted to the body habitus of the individual patient so as to image the maximum amount of tissue. Tall, thin patients require a steeper angle than short, heavy patients. Patients of average height and weight usually require an angle between 40 and 45 degrees. Using an angle that is not in the plane of the pectoral muscle results in less tissue on the image. It is rare for the proper angle for the MLO view to be different for the right and left breasts of the same patient. Some facilities record the angle used for the MLO view on the film so that it can be reproduced at the next examination.

The radiologic technologist performs the following maneuvers to position the patient for the MLO view:

1. Applying the principle of moving the mobile tissue toward the fixed tissue, lift the breast and then pull both breast tissue and pectoral muscle anteriorly and medially (see Fig. 3–4A). The patient's hand on the side being imaged should be resting on the handlebar.
2. Adjust the height of the image receptor to the level of the relaxed axilla so as to place the corner of the receptor behind the posterior fold of the axilla (see Fig. 3–4B).
3. Drape the patient's arm behind the receptor with the elbow flexed to relax the pectoral muscle (see Fig. 3–4C).
4. Rotate the patient toward the image receptor so that the edge of the receptor replaces your hand, maintaining the breast tissue and pectoral muscle

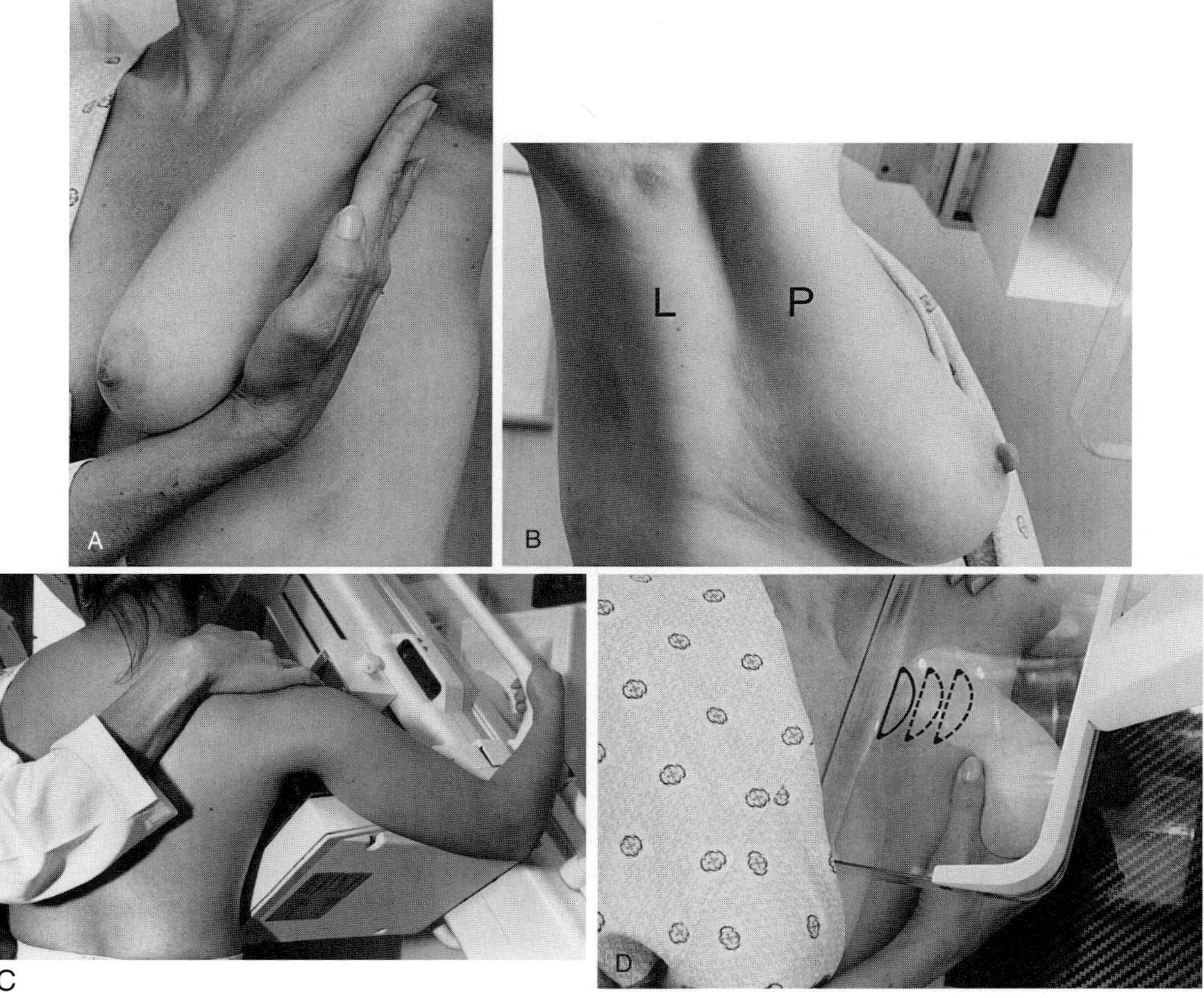

Figure 3–4. Mediolateral oblique (MLO) view. **A,** The radiologic technologist moves the breast and pectoral muscle anteriorly and medially. **B,** The image receptor is placed high in the axilla, bordered posteriorly by the latissimus dorsi muscle (L) and anteriorly by the pectoralis major muscle (P). **C,** The patient's arm is draped over the edge of the receptor in a relaxed position, and the image receptor is behind the axilla. **D,** The radiologic technologist uses her hand to position the breast so that it is not sagging.

Continued

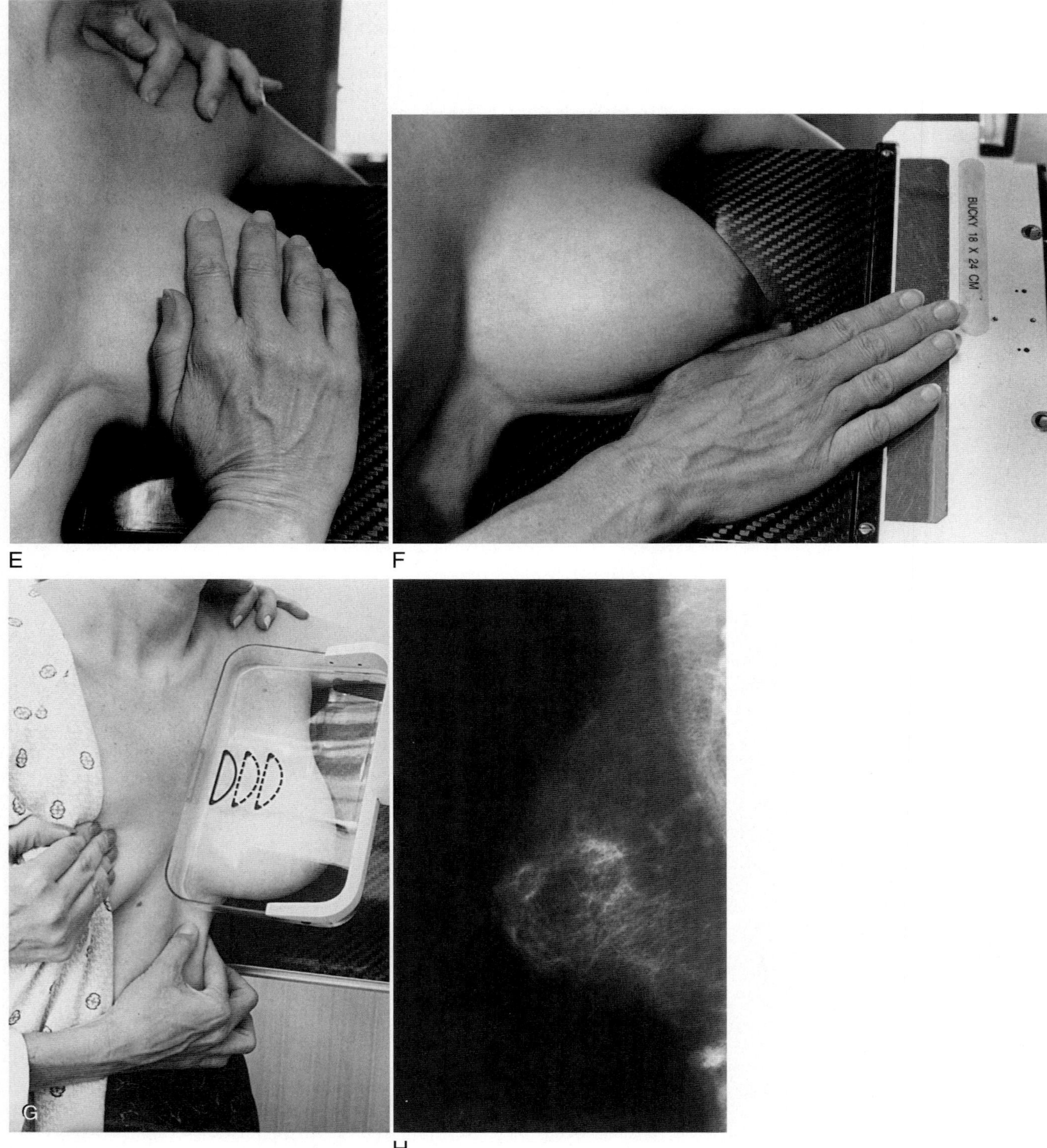

Figure 3–4, cont'd. E and **F,** As the compression tightens on the thicker posterior part of the breast (**E**), the radiologic technologist slowly moves her hand anteriorly (**F**) until the compression device is holding the breast up independently of her hand. **G,** The final step in positioning the MLO view is to open the inframammary fold (IMF). **H,** A lesion is seen in this well-positioned IMF.

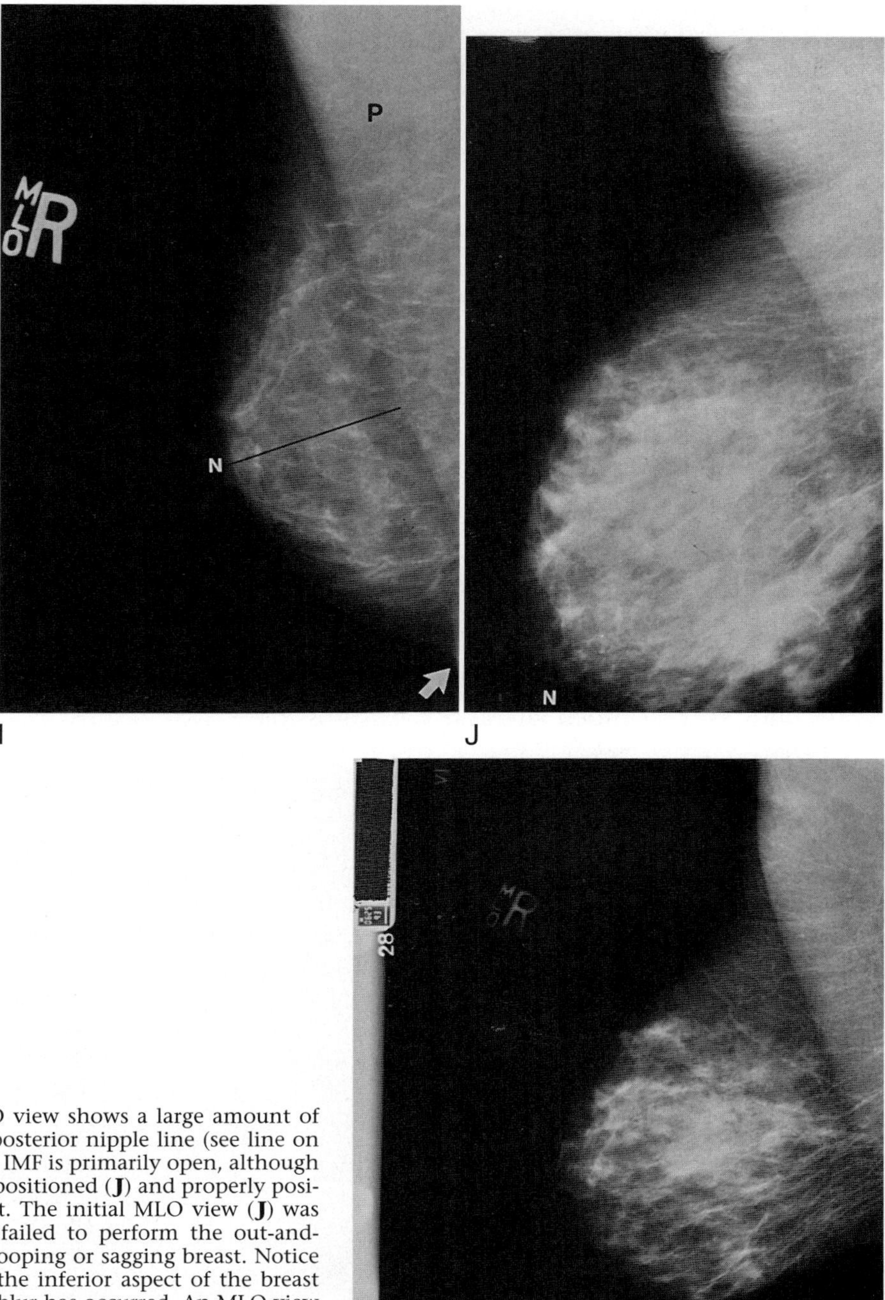

Figure 3–4, cont'd. I, Properly performed MLO view shows a large amount of pectoral muscle (P) extending well below the posterior nipple line (see line on **I**). The nipple (N) is high on the image, and the IMF is primarily open, although a small skin fold is present (*arrow*). Improperly positioned (**J**) and properly positioned (**K**) MLO projections of the same breast. The initial MLO view (**J**) was done by an inexperienced technologist who failed to perform the out-and-nipple-up maneuver correctly, resulting in a drooping or sagging breast. Notice that the nipple (N) is very low in the image, the inferior aspect of the breast extends below the image receptor, and motion blur has occurred. An MLO view (**K**) performed by a more experienced technologist was positioned properly. (From American College of Radiology Committee on Quality Assurance in Mammography: Mammography Quality Control. Reston, VA, American College of Radiology, 1992, pp 57-99.)

in its mobilized position. Hold the breast out away from the chest wall to prevent overlapping of tissues (see Fig. 3–4D).

5. Begin to apply compression. The upper corner of the compression paddle should be just below the clavicle. While moving your hand out of the field, continue to support the anterior breast with your hand under the nipple (see Fig. 3–4E and F).

   We call the combined hand movements the *out-and-nipple-up maneuver* (see Fig. 3–4D through F). The technologist should attempt to push the nipple toward the top of the image receptor until compression can maintain the breast in position (see Fig. 3–4F). If the hand supporting the breast is removed too soon, the breast will fall, resulting in inadequate separation of tissues. The importance of the out-and-nipple-up maneuver cannot be overemphasized.

6. The final step involves pulling abdominal tissue that is in front of the receptor inferiorly to open the inframammary fold (IMF) (see Fig. 3–4G).

If the following criteria are met, the MLO view has been properly positioned:

- The pectoral muscle is well visualized, wider superiorly than inferiorly with a convex anterior shape, and extends to or below the nipple line.
- The deep and superficial breast tissues are well separated.
- The breast is not sagging.
- Close inspection shows no evidence of motion blur.
- The IMF is open (see Fig. 3–4H).
- No posterior tissue is excluded.

Failure to execute the out-and-nipple-up maneuver properly results in sagging of the breast (see Fig. 3–4J).

Craniocaudal View

The CC view should be done in such a manner as to ensure that any tissue that may have been missed on the MLO view will be depicted on the CC view (Fig. 3–5). If any tissue is excluded from the MLO view, it is likely to be the medial tissue.[9] Therefore, the CC projection should demonstrate all of the medial tissue along with as much lateral tissue as possible.

To meet these goals without excessive exaggeration to the medial or lateral side, the radiologic technologist should position the patient for a CC projection in the following manner. As with the MLO view, the principle of mobile versus fixed margins is used.

1. Stand on the medial side of the breast being examined so as to have eye contact with the patient and to focus on the medial breast tissue.
2. Lift the mobile IMF as high as its natural mobility will allow (see Fig. 3–5A). This distance may range from 1½ to 7 cm from the neutral position.
3. Raise the image receptor to meet the level of the elevated IMF. Ask the patient to slouch. This allows the breast tissue to fall away from the thorax. With one hand under the breast and the other on top of the breast, gently pull breast tissue away from the chest wall and position the breast so that the nipple is in the center of the receptor (see Fig. 3–5B). This two-hands technique gently pulls the breast tissue away from the chest wall and maximizes the amount of superior as well as inferior breast tissue that is imaged.
4. With one hand on the posterior edge of the breast against the ribs, keep the breast in this position

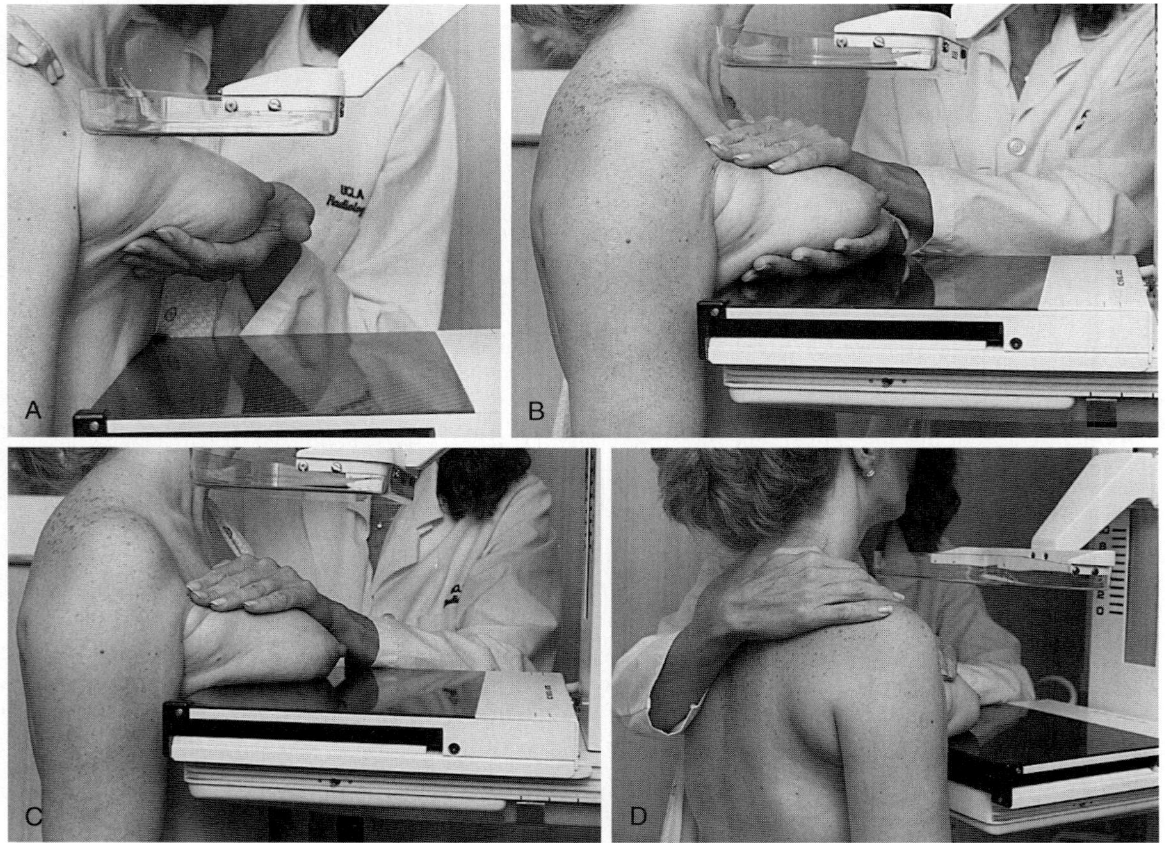

Figure 3–5. Craniocaudal (CC) view. The radiologic technologist positions from the medial side of the breast being imaged, to allow for eye contact and improved communication with the patient. **A,** The image receptor is at the neutral inframammary fold (IMF). The radiologic technologist lifts the IMF as high as its natural mobility will allow. **B,** With the receptor repositioned at the elevated IMF, a two-hands technique is used to place the breast. **C,** One hand is used to hold the breast in place. **D,** The other arm is placed around the patient's back to prevent her from backing away from the unit and to keep her shoulder down and relaxed. The radiologic technologist uses her fingers to pull the skin up over the clavicle so that subsequent compression will not result in a pulling sensation.

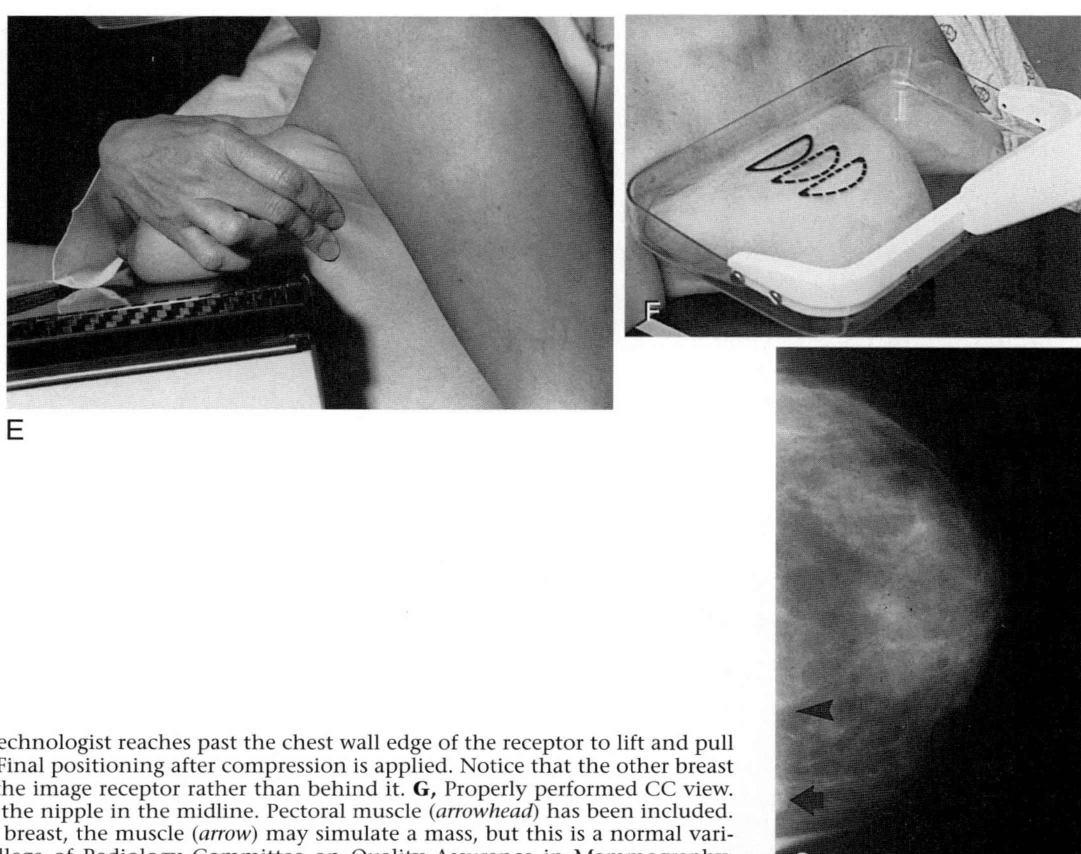

Figure 3–5, cont'd. **E,** The technologist reaches past the chest wall edge of the receptor to lift and pull posterior tissue forward. **F,** Final positioning after compression is applied. Notice that the other breast is draped over the edge of the image receptor rather than behind it. **G,** Properly performed CC view. The breast is centered with the nipple in the midline. Pectoral muscle (*arrowhead*) has been included. At the medial aspect of the breast, the muscle (*arrow*) may simulate a mass, but this is a normal variation. (From American College of Radiology Committee on Quality Assurance in Mammography: Mammography Quality Control. Reston, VA, American College of Radiology, 1992, pp 57-99.)

(see Fig. 3–5C). Bring the patient's head forward alongside the tube assembly. This will enable the patient to lean into the mammography unit, so that the superior breast tissue can be positioned near the chest wall over the image receptor.

5. Rotate the patient forward until her sternum touches the edge of the image receptor. This will require you to drape the breast not being imaged (the breast closer to you) over the corner of the receptor (rather than placing it behind the receptor). This last maneuver allows visualization of the posterior medial tissue.
6. Bring the patient's arm on the side not being imaged forward so she can hold onto the handlebar. Place your arm behind the patient's back with your hand resting on the top of the shoulder of the side being examined (see Fig. 3–5D). This allows you to use your hand to keep the patient's shoulder "relaxed down" while at the same time using your fingers to slide skin up over her clavicle to relieve any pulling sensation on her skin during subsequent compression (see Fig. 3–5E).
7. Reach past the chest wall edge of the image receptor to lift and bring the posterior lateral aspect of the breast onto the receptor. As compression is applied, move the hand holding the breast toward the nipple while continuing to pull lateral tissue forward to eliminate folds.
8. Have the patient allow her arm on the side being imaged to hang relaxed by her side, with the humerus externally rotated. This arm position also removes skin folds.

These maneuvers allow more breast tissue to be included in the CC view when compression is fully applied (see Fig. 3–5F).

If the following criteria are met, the CC view has been properly positioned:

- All medial tissue is visualized.
- The nipple is centered.
- Visualization of pectoral muscle (seen in approximately 30% of cases) or posterior nipple line measuring within 1 cm of the measurement on the MLO view (see Fig. 3–5G).

Additional Views

In addition to the standard views, many other views can be useful in the evaluation of a patient who has a palpable breast lump or an abnormality on screening mammogram.

90-Degree Lateral View

The 90-degree lateral (true lateral; straight lateral) view (Fig. 3–6) is the most commonly used additional view. The 90-degree lateral view is used in conjunction with the CC view to triangulate the exact location of lesions in the breast.

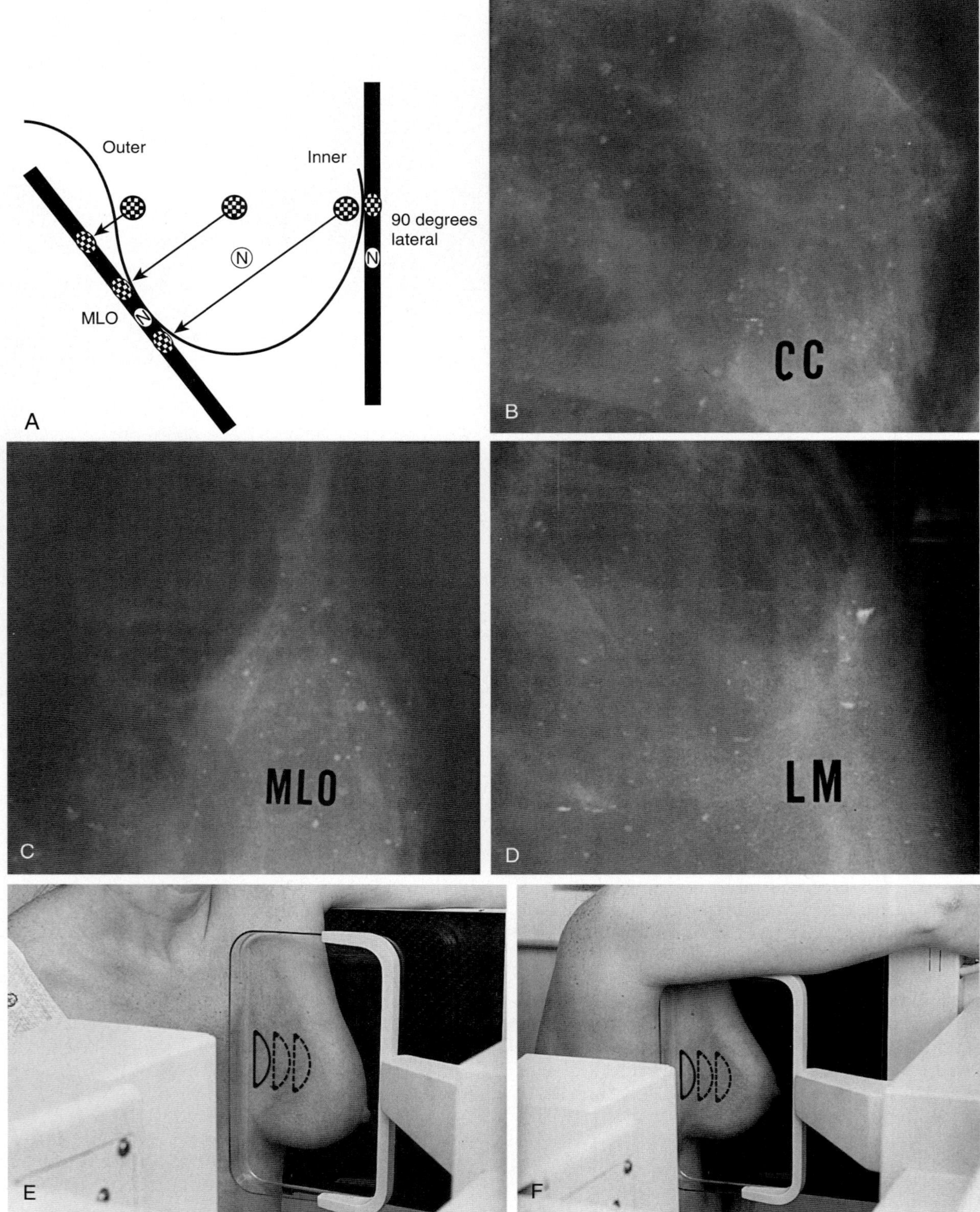

Figure 3–6. 90-degree lateral view. **A,** Relative to the nipple, lesions in the lateral (outer) part of the breast appear to be higher on the mediolateral oblique (MLO) view than on the 90-degree lateral view. Lesions in the medial (inner) part of the breast appear lower on the MLO than on the 90-degree lateral. **B** to **D,** Demonstration of milk of calcium with a 90-degree lateromedial (LM) view in a patient referred for biopsy of unilateral subareolar calcifications. Craniocaudal (CC) view (**B**) and MLO view (**C**) show numerous round amorphous calcifications. 90-degree LM (**D**) view shows layering of all of the calcifications. **E,** Positioning for the mediolateral view. **F,** Positioning for the LM view. (From American College of Radiology Committee on Quality Assurance in Mammography: Mammography Quality Control. Reston, VA, American College of Radiology, 1992, pp 57-99.)

When an abnormality is seen on the MLO view but not on the standard CC view, one must first determine whether it is a real abnormality, superimposed tissue, or an artifact on the film or in the skin. Sometimes repeating the MLO view with a slightly different angulation or obtaining a 90-degree lateral view will provide this information.

A change in location of a lesion relative to its distance from the nipple on the MLO and 90-degree lateral views can be used to determine whether the lesion is in the lateral, central, or medial aspect of the breast (see Fig. 3–6A). For example, if on the 90-degree lateral view the lesion moves up relative to the nipple or is higher than on the MLO film, the lesion is in the medial aspect of the breast. If on the 90-degree lateral view the lesion moves down relative to the nipple or is lower than on the MLO view, the lesion is in the lateral aspect of the breast. If the lesion does not shift significantly on the 90-degree view from its position on the MLO view, it is located in the central aspect of the breast.

The 90-degree lateral view is also used to demonstrate a fluid level, such as in the gravity-dependent calcifications of milk of calcium (see Fig. 3–6B through D).[18]

Mediolateral versus Lateromedial

When an abnormality has been identified, the more appropriate 90-degree lateral view—medial-to-lateral (mediolateral) or lateral-to-medial (lateromedial)—is the one that provides the shortest object-to-receptor distance, to reduce geometric unsharpness. For either view, the tube arm is rotated to 90 degrees.

For the mediolateral (ML) view (see Fig. 3–6E), the arm on the side being examined is draped behind the image receptor, with the elbow flexed and the hand resting on the handlebar to relax the pectoral muscle. The corner of the receptor is placed into the hollow of the axilla in front of the latissimus dorsi. Again using the principle of mobile versus fixed margins, the radiologic technician performs the following positioning maneuvers:

1. Pull breast tissue and pectoral muscle anteriorly and medially.
2. Lift the breast out and up while gently pulling the breast away from the chest wall.
3. Begin rotating the patient toward the receptor and start compression. When the compression paddle has passed the sternum, continue rotating the patient until the breast is in a true lateral position centered on the receptor.
4. Continue to apply compression until tissue is taut.
5. Open the IMF by gently pulling abdominal tissue down.

For the lateromedial (LM) view (see Fig. 3–6F), the tube arm is rotated 90 degrees, with the top of the image receptor at the level of the suprasternal notch. The patient is positioned with her sternum against the edge of the receptor, her neck extended, and her chin resting on the top of the receptor. The elbow should be flexed to relax the pectoral muscle. The radiologic technologist performs the following positioning maneuvers for the LM view:

1. Pull the mobile lateral and inferior tissue up and toward the midline.
2. Begin rotating the patient toward the image receptor.
3. Bring the compression paddle down past the latissimus dorsi.
4. Continue rotating the patient until the breast is in a true lateral position centered on the receptor.
5. Lift the arm on the side being imaged over the receptor.
6. Open the IMF by gently pulling abdominal tissue down.

Spot Compression

Spot or coned compression is a simple technique that merits more frequent application.[19-21] Spot compression views are especially helpful in evaluation of obscure or equivocal findings in areas of dense tissue. Compared with whole-breast compression, spot compression allows for greater reduction in thickness of the localized area of interest and improves separation of breast tissues (Fig. 3–7A and B). Spot compression does not require collimation to the area of interest. Variably sized spot compression devices, especially the smaller ones, can facilitate more effective localized compression.

Using the original mammogram, the technologist determines the placement of the small compression device by measuring the distance of the abnormality from the nipple (see Fig. 3–7E and F). A minimum of three measurements are taken: On a CC projection, the first measurement is posterior from the nipple to the level of the suspected abnormality; the second measurement is medial or lateral from the nipple line to the area of interest; and the third measurement is from the area of interest to the skin. On an MLO or 90-degree lateral projection, the first measurement is posterior from the nipple to the level of the suspected abnormality; the second measurement is superior or inferior from the nipple to the area of interest; the third measurement is from the area of interest to a skin border (see Fig. 3–7C and D). It is important for the radiologic technologist to use her hand to apply simulated breast compression while estimating the location of the abnormality, because the measurements taken from the image are from a compressed breast. Spot compression is often combined with microfocus magnification to improve resolution.

Magnification

A magnification (M) view can sometimes be helpful in differentiating benign from malignant lesions by permitting more precise evaluation of margins and other architectural characteristics of a focal density or mass. However, magnification views are most effective in the delineation of the number, distribution, and morphology of calcifications (Fig. 3–8A and

B).[22] This technique may also reveal unexpected findings that were not evident on routine views. An x-ray tube with a measured focal spot size of 0.1 mm or less is preferred to offset the geometric unsharpness resulting from the increase in the object-to-film distance. It also requires a magnification platform (see Fig. 3–8C) to separate the compressed breast from the cassette for a 1.5× to 2.0× magnification (the greater the magnification, the smaller the focal spot required).

With magnification mammography, it is critical that the patient remain still for the relatively longer exposure times that result from the air gap and the use of the microfocal spot. The air gap resulting from separation of the breast from the image receptor prevents a significant amount of scattered radiation

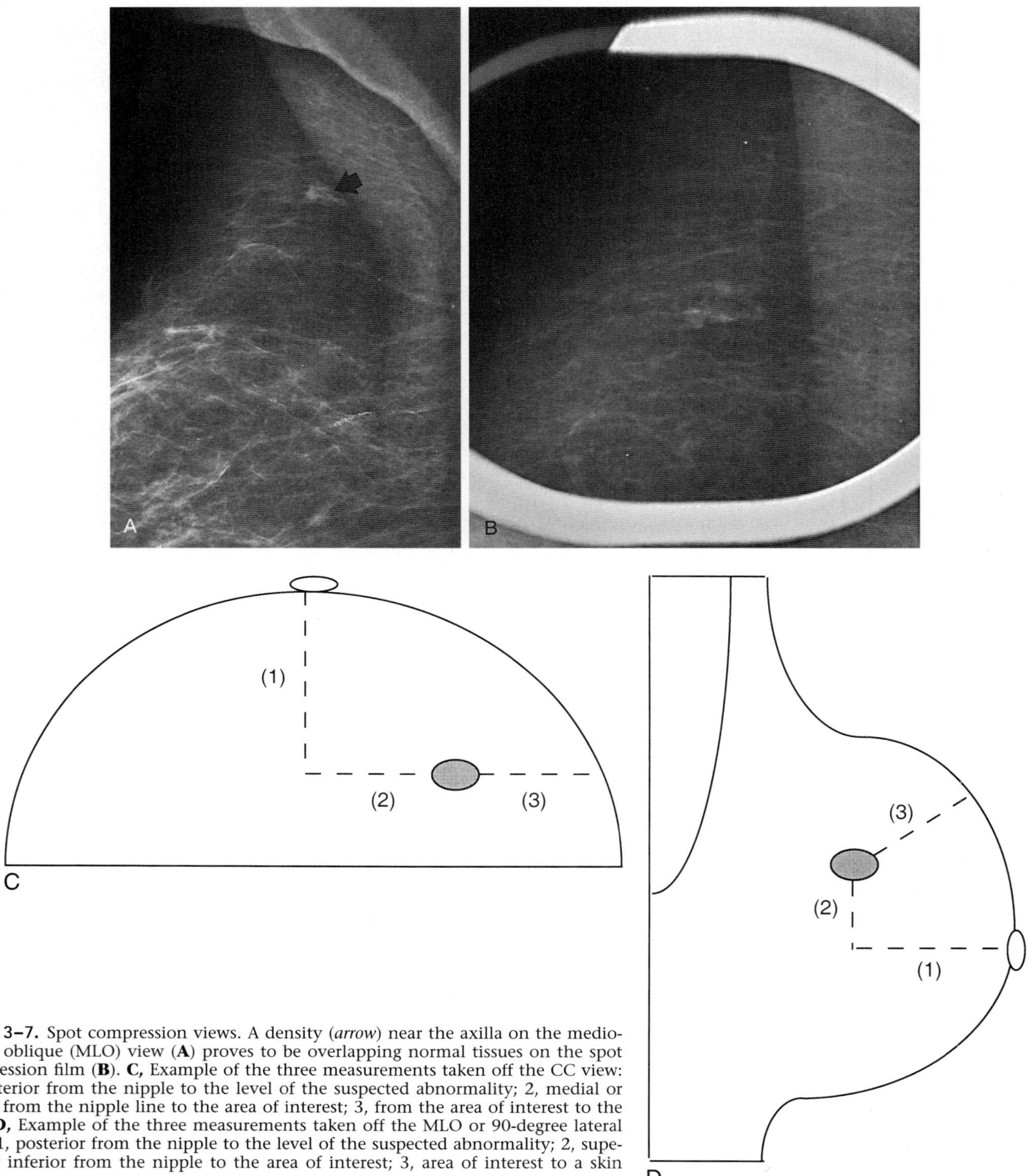

Figure 3–7. Spot compression views. A density (*arrow*) near the axilla on the mediolateral oblique (MLO) view (**A**) proves to be overlapping normal tissues on the spot compression film (**B**). **C,** Example of the three measurements taken off the CC view: 1, posterior from the nipple to the level of the suspected abnormality; 2, medial or lateral from the nipple line to the area of interest; 3, from the area of interest to the skin. **D,** Example of the three measurements taken off the MLO or 90-degree lateral view: 1, posterior from the nipple to the level of the suspected abnormality; 2, superior or inferior from the nipple to the area of interest; 3, area of interest to a skin border.

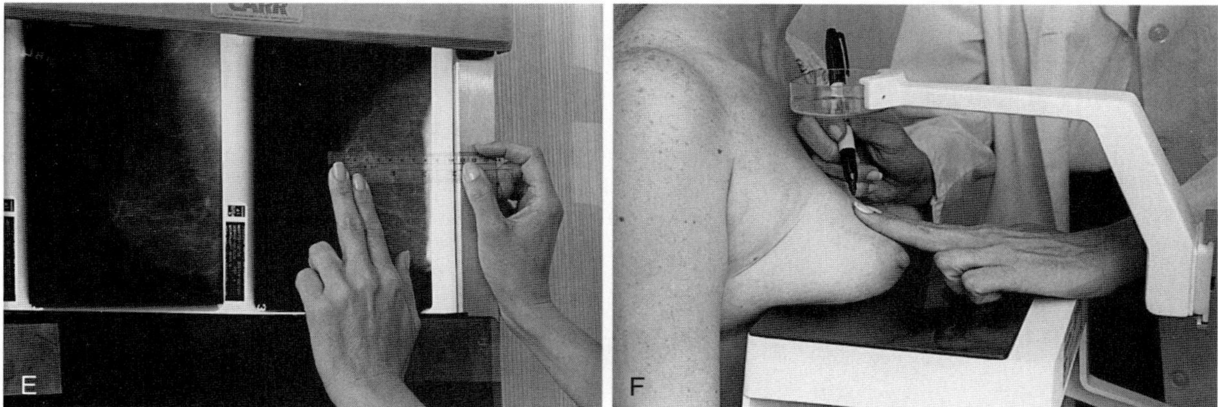

Figure 3–7, cont'd. E, The location of the lesion relative to the nipple is determined from the original films. **F,** Using her fingers to measure the distance from the nipple and the midline, the radiologic technologist marks the approximate location of the lesion on the overlying skin. She centers the spot compression device over that mark. (From American College of Radiology Committee on Quality Assurance in Mammography: Mammography Quality Control. Reston, VA, American College of Radiology, 1992, pp 57-99.)

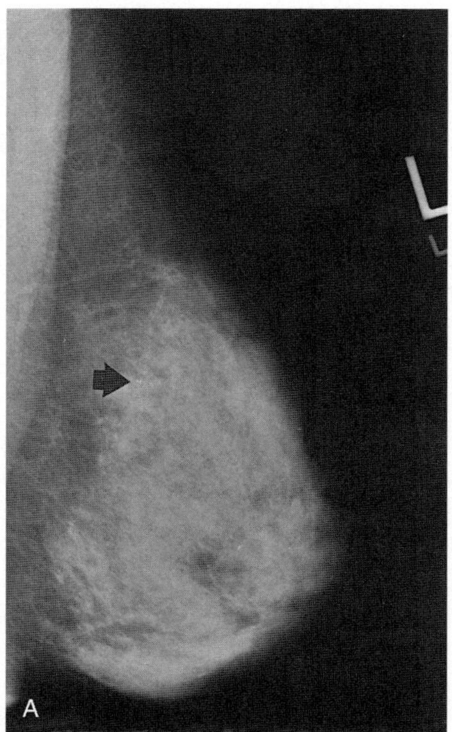

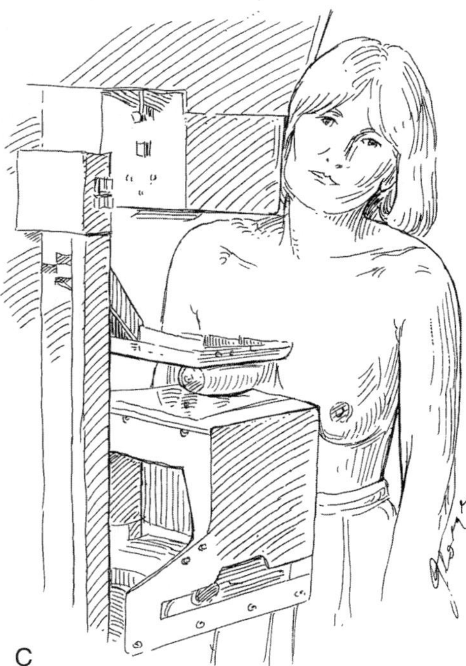

Figure 3–8. Magnification mammography. The mediolateral oblique (MLO) view (**A**) from a screening examination showed a small group of calcifications (*arrow*), but a spot magnification view (**B**) was required to demonstrate the true number of calcifications in the cluster, their heterogeneous morphology, and an adjacent cluster (*arrowhead*) located 1 cm inferiorly. **C,** Magnification stand separates breast from image receptor. (From American College of Radiology Committee on Quality Assurance in Mammography: Mammography Quality Control. Reston, VA, American College of Radiology, 1992, pp 57-99.)

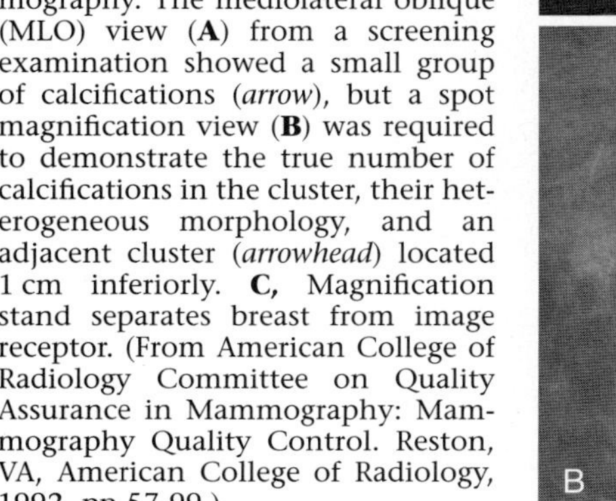

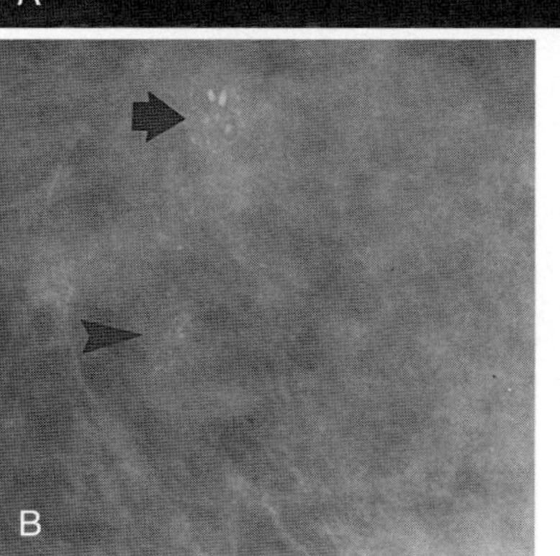

from reaching the film. Therefore, a grid is not necessary. In addition, the kilovolt (peak) (kVp) value should be increased by 2 to reduce the exposure time and the possibility of motion.

Exaggerated Craniocaudal View

The exaggerated craniocaudal (XCCL) view depicts lesions deep in the outer aspect of the breast. It visualizes the axillary aspect of the breast, including most of the axillary tail, in a craniocaudal projection. Often these lesions cannot be seen on the standard CC view but can be imaged by an XCCL view (Fig. 3–9B and C). The radiologic technologist positions the patient for a XCCL view as follows:

1. Begin positioning the patient as you would for the routine CC view.
2. After elevating the IMF, rotate the patient until the lateral aspect of the breast is in contact with the image receptor.

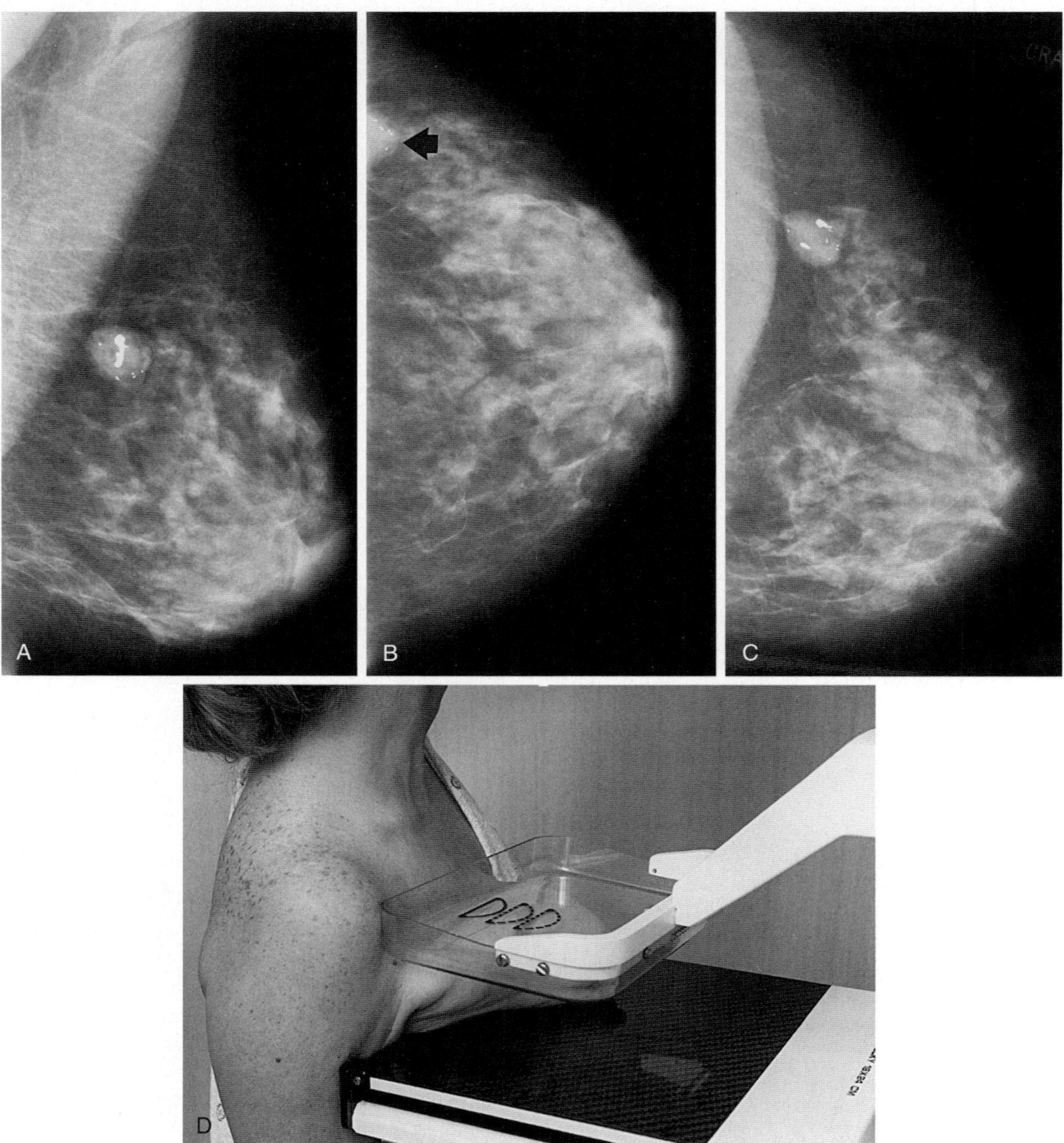

Figure 3–9. Exaggerated craniocaudal (XCCL) view. **A,** Mediolateral (MLO) view shows a calcified fibroadenoma in the superior aspect of the breast. **B,** On the standard craniocaudal (CC) view, only the anterior margin of the mass (*arrow*) could be seen in the lateral aspect of the breast, but the XCCL view (**C**) depicts the mass completely. **D,** Final positioning for the XCCL view. (From American College of Radiology Committee on Quality Assurance in Mammography: Mammography Quality Control. Reston, VA, American College of Radiology, 1992, pp 57-99.)

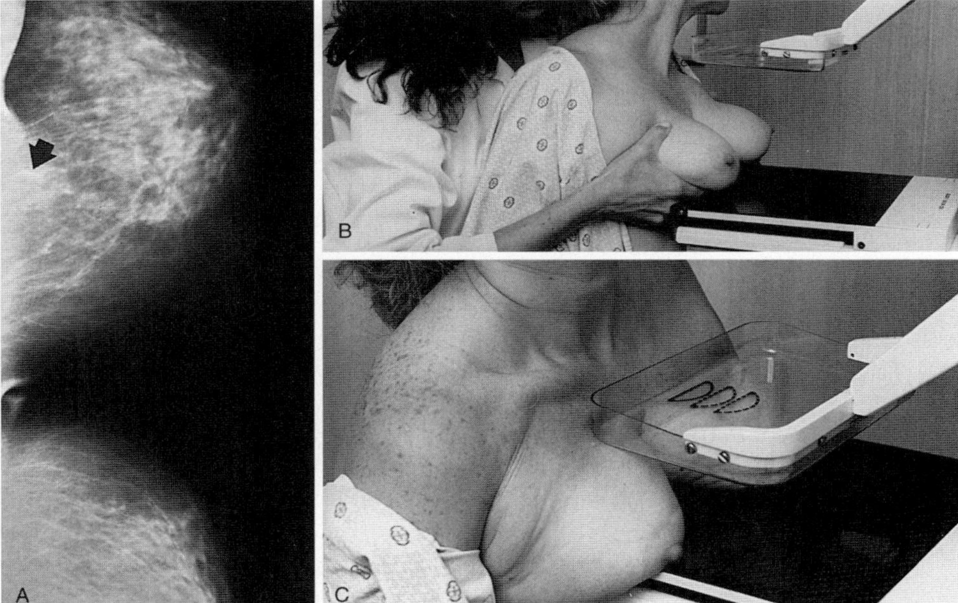

Figure 3–10. Cleavage view. **A,** Architectural distortion (*arrow*) near the chest wall in 11-o'clock position of the left breast was first identified on a mediolateral oblique (MLO) projection. It could not be visualized on the standard craniocaudal (CC) view. **B** and **C,** Positioning the breasts for the cleavage view. (From American College of Radiology Committee on Quality Assurance in Mammography: Mammography Quality Control. Reston, VA, American College of Radiology, 1992, pp 57-99.)

3. Center the lateral aspect of the breast with the nipple facing the opposite corner of the receptor (see Fig. 3–9D).
4. If the shoulder is in the way of the compression paddle, a 5-degree lateral tube angle can be used to allow the compression paddle to clear the humeral head.

Cleavage View

The cleavage view (CV), also called the valley view or double-breast compression view, is performed to visualize deep lesions in the posteromedial aspect of the breast (Fig. 3–10A). The patient's head is rotated away from the side of interest. To achieve this positioning, the technologist either (1) stands behind the patient and wraps her arms around the patient to reach the breasts (see Fig. 3–10B) or (2) stands in front of the patient on the medial side of the breast being imaged. Whether the technologist stands behind or in front of the patient, the IMFs must be elevated, and both breasts positioned on the image receptor. The technologist should remember to pull all of the medial tissue of both breasts anteriorly to image the cleavage. In order for the automatic exposure control (AEC) to be used, the breast of interest must be over the photocell with the cleavage slightly off center (see Fig. 3–10C). The manual technique must be used if the AEC is under an open cleavage.

Axillary Tail

The axillary tail (AT) view, previously referred to as the Cleopatra view, may be used to show the entire axillary tail as well as most of the lateral aspect of the breast in an oblique projection. The tube arm is rotated to an angle that will place the image receptor parallel to the axillary tail (Fig. 3–11). The patient

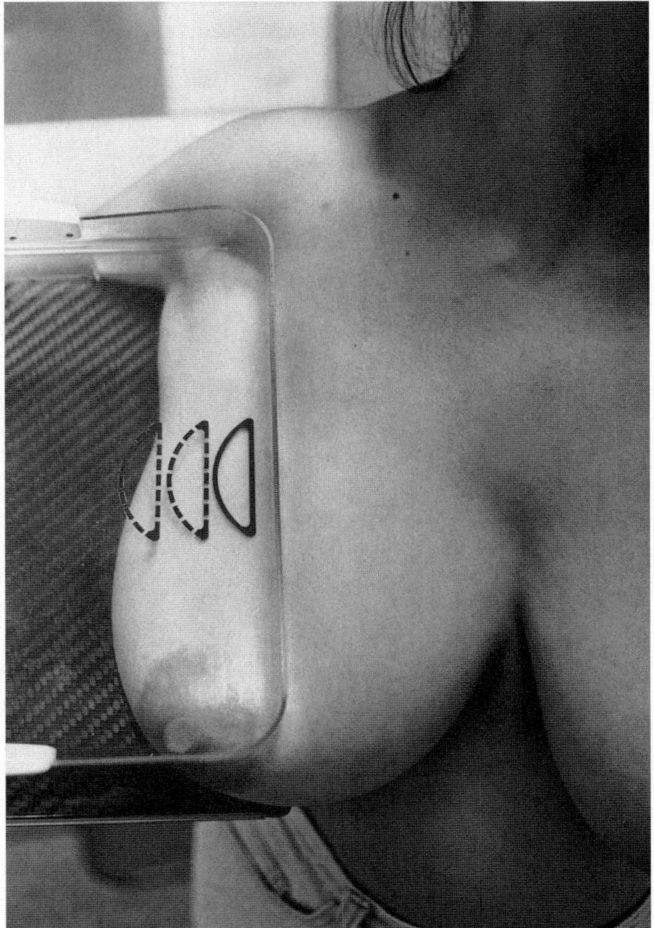

Figure 3–11. Axillary tail view. Final positioning. (From American College of Radiology Committee on Quality Assurance in Mammography: Mammography Quality Control. Reston, VA, American College of Radiology, 1992, pp 57-99.)

is turned to bring the axillary tail in contact with the receptor. The arm of the side being imaged is draped behind the top of the receptor with the elbow flexed and the hand resting on the handlebar. The axillary aspect of the breast is gently pulled out and away from the chest wall and placed on the receptor. This position of the axillary tail is maintained by the radiologic technologist's hand while compression is slowly applied.

Tangential View

A tangential (TAN) view can be used to image palpable lesions that are obscured by surrounding dense glandular tissue in the mammogram.[20] Performing the TAN view for this purpose can be facilitated by placing a lead marker (BB) directly over the palpable lump or mammographic abnormality (Fig. 3–12A). The C-arm is rotated, and the patient is turned so that the x-ray beam is tangential to the palpable lump or the BB (Fig. 3–12B). This maneuver places the palpable lump directly over the subcutaneous fat, which may allow visualization of the abnormality (Fig. 3–12C and D).

Tangential views can also be used to verify that calcifications seen on a mammogram are located within the skin (Fig. 3–12E-G).[23,24] With the use of a fenestrated plate with a radiopaque alphanumeric grid or a compression plate with multiple holes for guidance, a BB is placed on the skin of the breast directly over the calcifications. It is important to place the marker on the correct side of the breast—superior versus inferior, medial versus lateral surface. The C-arm or breast tissue (or both) is rotated until the BB is tangential to the x-ray beam. Seeing a

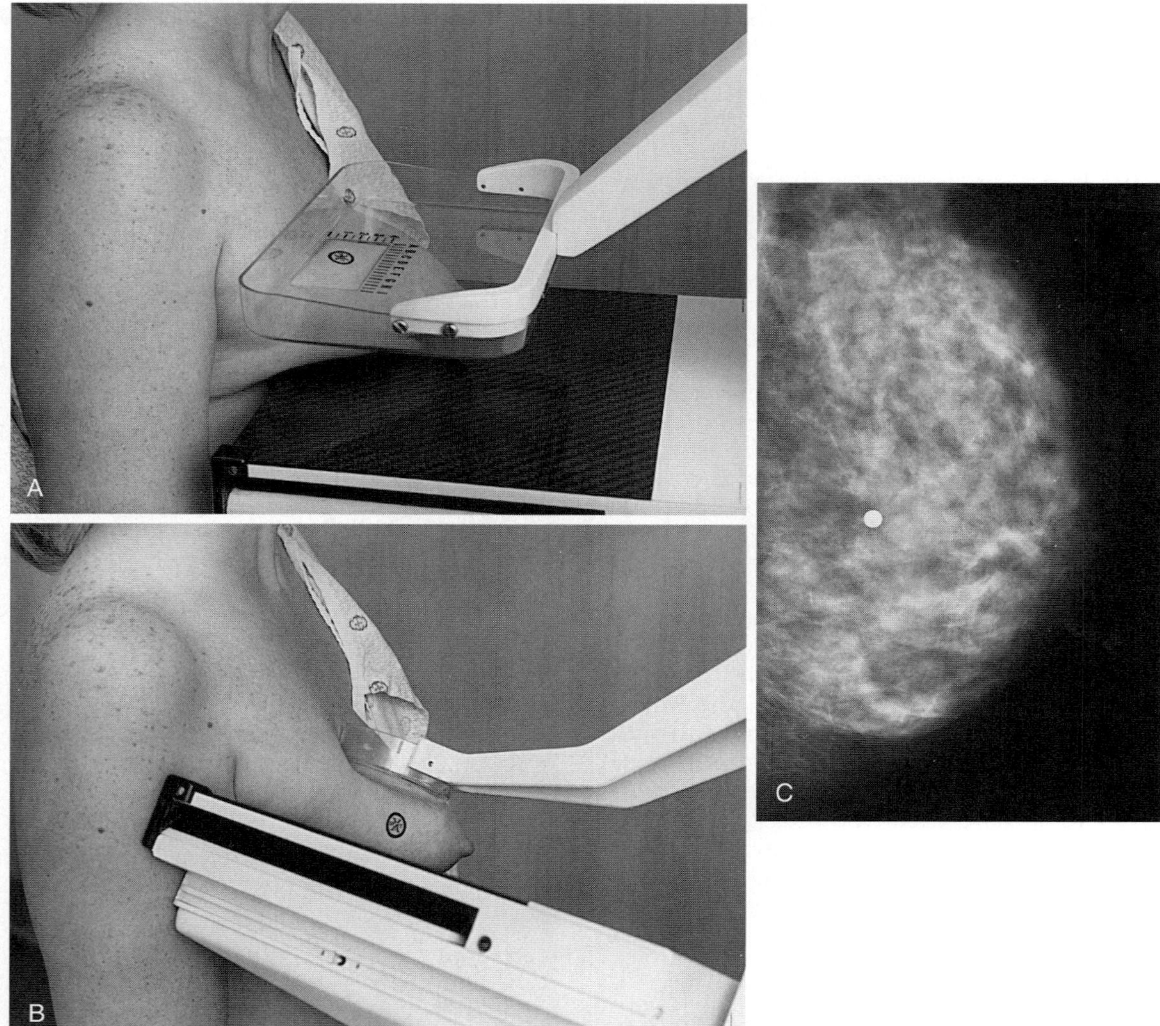

Figure 3–12. Tangential view. **A,** Placing lead marker (BB) on skin overlying nonpalpable lesion. Fenestrated compression plate with alphanumeric grid was placed on breast surface closest to abnormality, film was exposed while compression was maintained, then BB was placed on the skin on the basis of the relationship of the lesion to the image of the alphanumeric grid in the processed film. **B,** Final positioning for tangential view. **C** and **D,** Palpable mass, marked by the BB, was not visible on original mammogram (**C**).

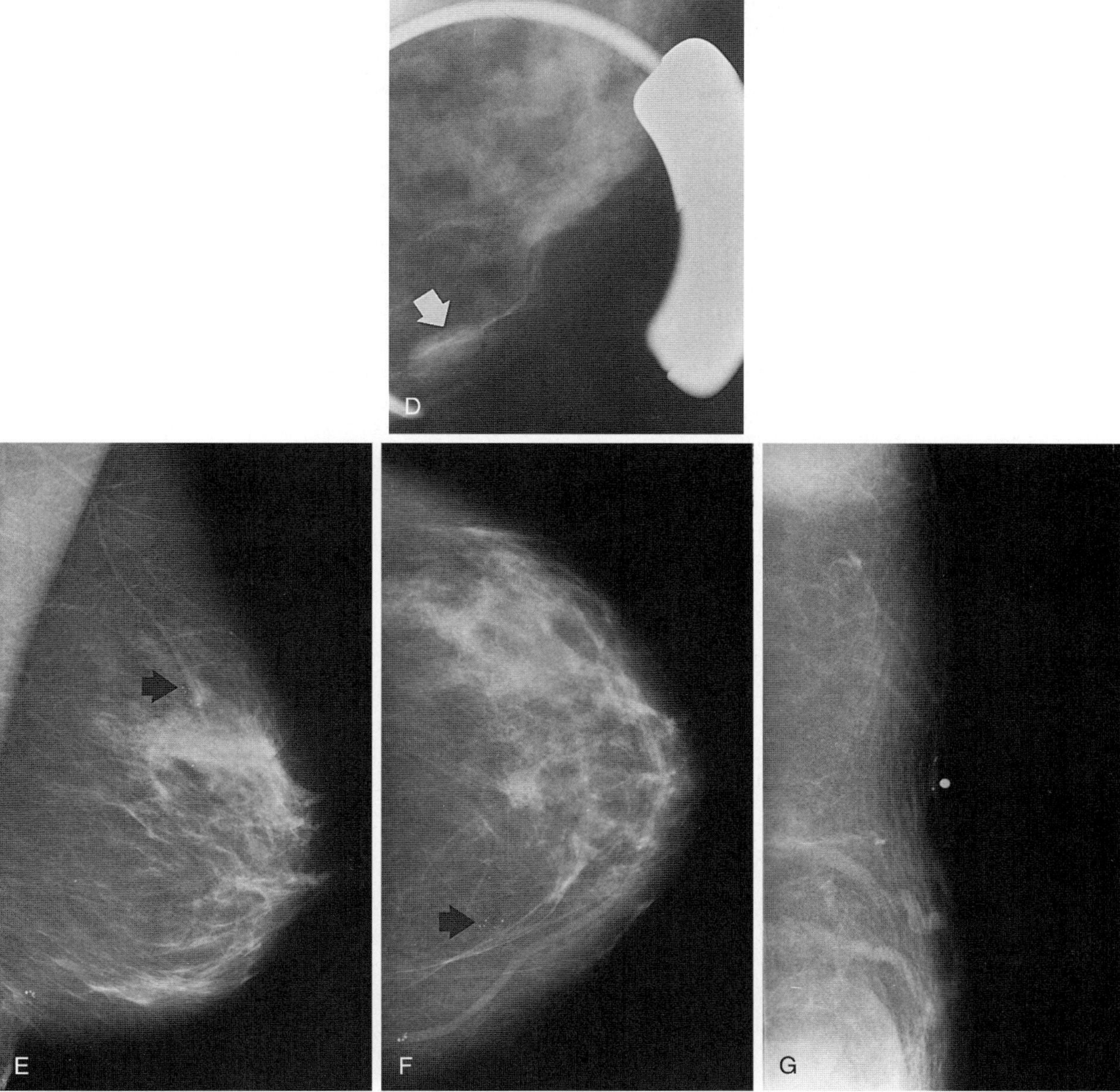

Figure 3–12, cont'd. Projection tangential to the palpable area (**D**) placed it over subcutaneous fat, allowing visualization of the oval mass (*arrow*) with circumscribed margins. Fine-needle aspiration cytologic findings were interpreted as fibroadenoma. **E** to **G,** This patient was referred for biopsy of "suspicious" calcifications (*arrow*) shown on MLO (**E**) and CC (**F**) views. A tangential view (**G**) shows the calcifications in the skin directly under the BB. Biopsy was canceled. (From American College of Radiology Committee on Quality Assurance in Mammography: Mammography Quality Control. Reston, VA, American College of Radiology, 1992, pp 57-99.)

shadow of the BB on the "bucky" (Potter-Bucky parallel scanning grid) indicates that the area of concern will be tangent to the x-ray beam.

Roll View

The roll view is used to separate superimposed breast tissues. The purpose is to confirm the presence of an abnormality, to better define a lesion, or to determine the location of a finding seen on only one of the standard views. The patient is repositioned so the same projection that demonstrated the abnormality is used. The technologist should place one hand on either side of the breast while the tissue is "rolled" in opposite directions (Fig. 3–13). Compression maintains the breast in the "rolled" position. Lead markers indicating the direction of the roll should be placed on the image (e.g., RL for rolled lateral, RM for rolled medial).

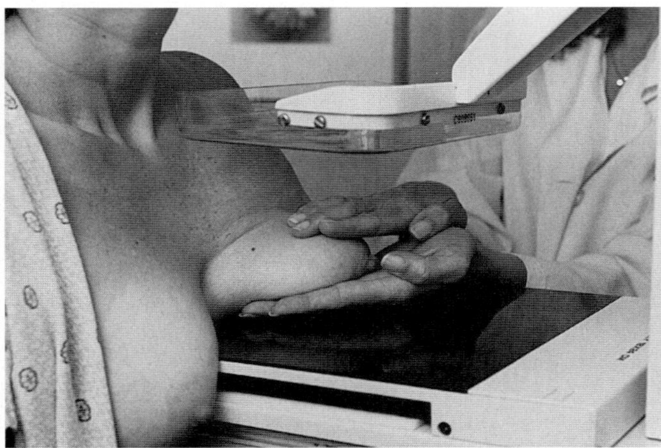

Figure 3–13. Roll view. (From American College of Radiology Committee on Quality Assurance in Mammography: Mammography Quality Control. Reston, VA, American College of Radiology, 1992, pp 57-99.)

Special Circumstances

Caudocranial View

The caudocranial view or from below (FB) view, also referred to as the reverse CC view, improves visualization of lesions in the uppermost aspect of the breast by providing a reduced object-to-film distance (Fig. 3–14A through C). Because the compression device comes from below, this view does not exclude the fixed tissues in the superior aspect of the breast and thus can show more posterior tissue. It can also be used during needle localization, to provide a shorter route to an inferior lesion, or to maximize the amount of tissue visualized in the male breast or in a woman with kyphosis. However, the FB view may not be possible in men or women with ascites or in those with a large, protruding abdomen.

For the FB view, the tube arm is rotated 180 degrees. The patient faces the unit with one leg on either side of the tube head. The IMF is elevated, and then the height of the tube arm is adjusted so that the superior border of the breast is in contact with the image receptor (Fig. 3–14D). With one hand on top of the breast and the other hand under the breast, the technologist gently pulls the tissue away from the chest wall and centers the breast on the receptor. Compression is applied slowly.

Lateromedial Oblique View

The lateromedial oblique (LMO) or reverse oblique view is performed with the x-ray beam directed from the lower-outer to the upper-inner aspect of the breast, the exact reverse of the MLO. This view improves visualization of the medial breast tissue by providing a reduced object-to-film distance. As for the MLO, the image receptor is placed parallel to the plane of the pectoral muscle, optimizing the amount

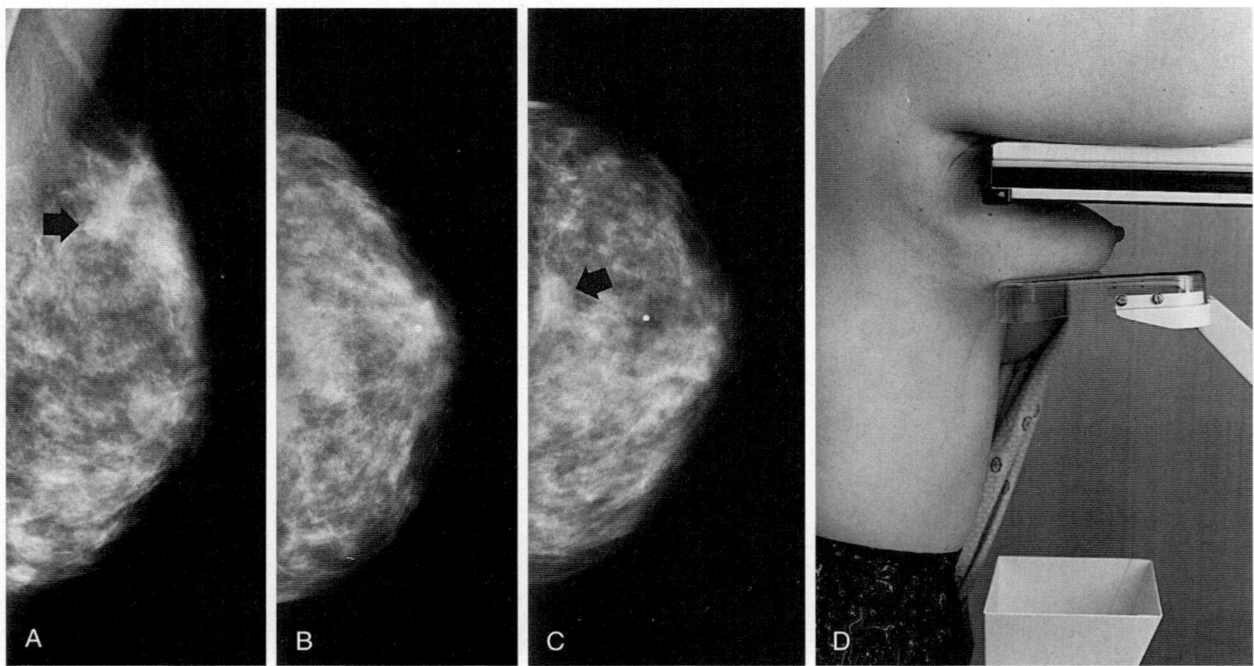

Figure 3–14. Caudocranial or from-below (FB) view. **A,** MLO view shows a possible mass and architectural distortion in a woman who thought she felt "thickening" in the upper part of her breast (lead marker [BB] is at this location). **B,** Standard craniocaudal (CC) view failed to show the abnormality. **C,** FB view showed the mass (*arrow*) directly posterior to the BB. Biopsy revealed invasive ductal carcinoma. **D,** Final positioning for caudocranial view. (From American College of Radiology Committee on Quality Assurance in Mammography: Mammography Quality Control. Reston, VA, American College of Radiology, 1992, pp 57-99.)

of breast tissue that is depicted. The reverse oblique view can be used to more comfortably position the breast, therefore allowing more tissue to be visualized in a patient with pectus excavatum, recent open heart surgery, or a prominent pacemaker.

The tube arm is rotated to the appropriate angle with the beam in an inferolateral-to-superomedial direction. The radiologic technologist positions the patient as follows (Fig. 3–15):

1. Adjust the height of the receptor so that the breast is centered.
2. Have the patient lean forward to place the edge of the receptor against the sternum.
3. Gently pull the breast up and out from the chest wall, making sure all medial tissue is in front of the receptor.
4. Begin to rotate the patient toward the receptor.
5. Bring the compression device down beyond the latissimus dorsi, and then finish rotating the patient forward until all the breast tissue is centered.
6. After the breast is fully compressed, open the IMF by gently pulling abdominal tissue down.
7. The patient's arm should be draped over the top of the receptor with the elbow flexed.

Superolateral-to-Inferomedial Oblique View

The superolateral-to-inferomedial oblique (SIO) view has sometimes been incorrectly referred to as a "reverse oblique." It is performed with the central ray directed from the upper-outer aspect of the breast to the lower-inner aspect (Fig. 3–16), and is *not* the reverse of the MLO. As a whole-breast projection, the SLO view has limited usefulness. Because it is taken at a 90-degree angle to the AT view, it can be used for pre-biopsy needle localization of lesions depicted on the AT view but not on the CC or XCCL views.

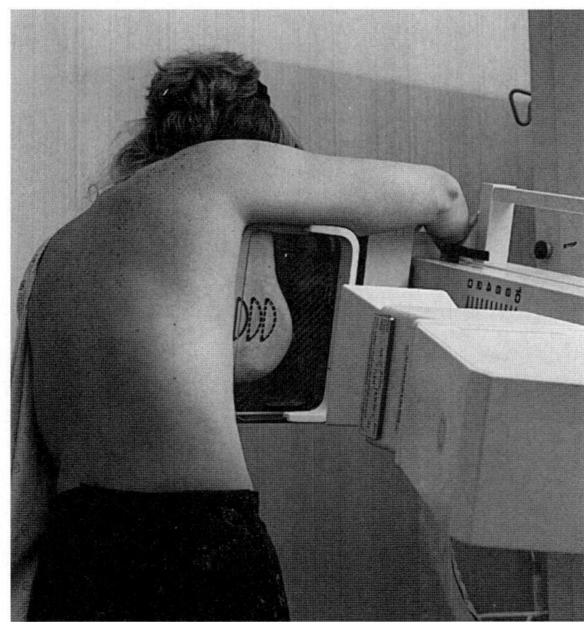

Figure 3–15. Final positioning for the lateromedial oblique (LMO) view. (From American College of Radiology Committee on Quality Assurance in Mammography: Mammography Quality Control. Reston, VA, American College of Radiology, 1992, pp 57-99.)

The Augmented Breast

Imaging the breast that has been augmented with saline or silicone implants presents special problems and challenges to the radiologist and radiologic technologist. The routine CC and MLO views require manually set exposure factors, and the amount of compression is limited by the compressibility of the implant. The purpose of compression on the implant-included view is to reduce motion unsharpness at the edge of the implant. Minimal pressure, enough to prevent the implant from moving during the exposure, is applied. The breast tissue will not be taut. In addition to the implant-included views in patients with augmented breasts, implant-displaced (ID) views in the CC and MLO or 90-degree lateral projections should be performed.[25]

For the ID view, the prosthesis is displaced posteriorly and superiorly against the chest wall while the breast tissue is gently pulled anterior to the prosthesis onto the image receptor and held in place with the compression device (see Fig. 3–17A through C). This allows for more compression of the anterior breast tissues than is possible when the implant is included in the field of compression (Fig. 3–17D). For a CC view, the tissue superior and inferior to the prosthesis, as well as all the anterior tissue, is pulled forward (Fig. 3–17E). For an MLO view, the tissue medial and lateral to the prosthesis, as well as the anterior tissue, is pulled forward with the anterior tissue.

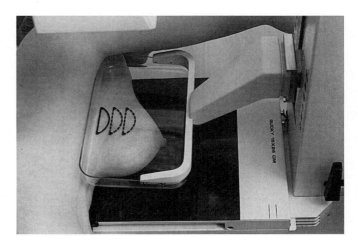

Figure 3–16. Final positioning for the superolateral-to-inferomedial oblique (SIO) view. (From American College of Radiology Committee on Quality Assurance in Mammography: Mammography Quality Control. Reston, VA, American College of Radiology, 1992, pp 57-99.)

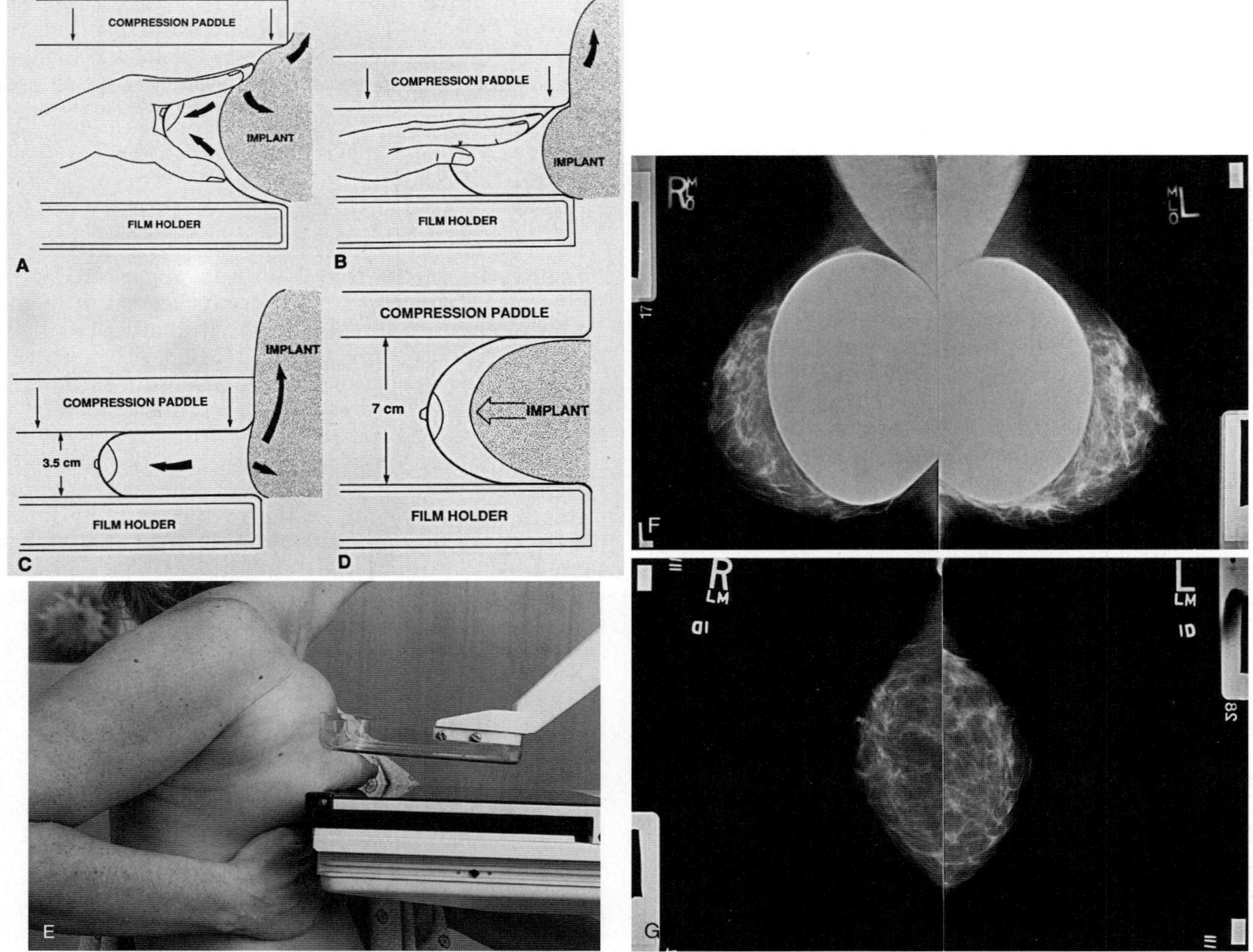

Figure 3–17. Augmented breast. Maneuvers for implant-displaced views (**A** to **C**) allow for better compression of anterior breast tissues than the implant-included view (**D**). **E,** Final positioning for right craniocaudal implant-displaced (RCC-ID) view. Right and left MLO implant-included (**F**) and 90-degree lateral implant-displaced (**G**) views of an asymptomatic woman with silicone implants who was referred for screening mammograms. (**A** to **D** from Eklund GW, Busby RC, Miller SH, et al: Improved imaging of the augmented breast. AJR Am J Roentgenol 1988;151:469-473; **E** to **G** from American College of Radiology Committee on Quality Assurance in Mammography: Mammography Quality Control. Reston, VA, American College of Radiology, 1992, pp 57-99.)

The radiologic technologist positions the patient as follows for the CC-ID view:

1. Have the patient bend forward as far as possible, to facilitate separation of anterior tissue from the implant. Gently pull the breast tissue forward while pushing the implant posteriorly with your fingers. Once the tissue is pulled forward, have the patient stand up.
2. Ask the patient to place her other hand on the rib cage directly under the breast to fill the gap between the edge of the image receptor and her ribs when the implant is displaced.
3. Position the breast tissue on the receptor. You should feel the edge of the receptor against your fingers holding the breast tissue forward.
4. Ask the patient to push her body against her hand. This causes the implant to move superiorly and posteriorly. Because the edge of the receptor is holding the inferior aspect of the implant back, remove the hand that was holding the inferior aspect of the implant.
5. Apply compression to the anterior tissue while slowing moving your fingers to the sides. The use of a spatula makes this last step easier. Before applying compression, place the edge of the spatula against the displaced implant. Then flip the spatula up, parallel to the chest wall.
6. Apply breast compression. Once the breast is compressed, slide the spatula out. Now the compression device has replaced the spatula in holding the prosthesis posteriorly.

Positioning for the MLO-ID view requires the following maneuvers. It is important to do the implant-included MLO first so that the patient will know how it feels to be positioned for an MLO.

1. Have the patient lean forward. Gently pull the breast tissue forward while pushing the implant posteriorly with your fingers. Once the tissue is pulled forward, have the patient stand up.
2. Ask the patient to place her hand on the handlebar with the corner of the image receptor behind her axilla, as she did for the implant-included MLO.
3. Place the breast against the edge of the receptor. Ask the patient whether she feels the edge of the receptor against her breast or against her ribs. If the patient feels the receptor against her breast, move on to step 4. If she feels the receptor against her ribs, start the positioning over again, because the implant is not sufficiently displaced.
4. Ask the patient to lean her body against the image receptor. You should see the implant bulge superiorly and medially. Now the receptor is displacing the implant medially and superiorly, so your hand can be removed.
5. Apply compression while sliding your fingers out. As for the CC-ID view, the use of the spatula makes this last step easier. Place the spatula against the displaced implant, and flip the spatula up parallel to the chest wall. With your free hand, try to pull more superior tissue into the field of view.
6. Apply compression. Once the tissue is properly compressed, slide the spatula out. Now the compression device has replaced the spatula in holding the medially and superiorly displaced prosthesis.

The MLO-ID view may be replaced with a 90-degree lateral ID view if the latter depicts more breast tissue. Both implant-included and implant-displaced views should be done for screening of asymptomatic women with breast implants (see Fig. 3–17F and G). Although the latter examination is designed for early detection of breast cancer in an asymptomatic woman, it should be considered a diagnostic examination, in that (1) a radiologist should be on site to answer questions or examine the woman if necessary, (2) additional views are needed, and (3) special expertise is required of the radiologic technologist.

Postmastectomy Mammography

The usefulness of imaging the postmastectomy side is controversial.[26] Proponents of this procedure might include an MLO projection of the skin over the mastectomy site, a spot view of any area of concern, and a view of the axilla.

References

1. American College of Radiology Committee on Quality Assurance in Mammography: Mammography Quality Control. Reston, VA, American College of Radiology, 1992, pp 57-99.
2. Hendrick RE: Quality assurance in mammography: Accreditation, legislation, and compliance with quality assurance standards. Radiol Clin North Am 1992;30:243-255.
3. Bassett LW, Farria DM, Bansal S, et al: Reasons for failure of a mammography unit at clinical image review in the American College of Radiology Mammography Accreditation Program. Radiology 2000;215;698-702.
4. Bassett LW, Hendrick RE, Bassford TL, et al: Quality Determinants of Mammography. Clinical Practice Guideline, No. 13. (AHCPR Publication No. 95-0632.) Rockville, MD, Agency for Health Care Policy and Research, Public Health Service, US Department of Health and Human Services, October 1994.
5. Gros CM: Methodologie: Symposium sur le sein. J Radiol Electrol Med Nucl 1967;48:638-655.
6. American College of Radiology: Recommended Specifications for New Mammography Equipment. Reston, VA, American College of Radiology, October, 1993.
7. Bassett LW, Gold RH: Breast radiography using the oblique projection. Radiology 1983;149:585-587.
8. Lundgren B, Jakobsson S: Single view mammography: A simple and efficient approach to breast cancer screening. Cancer 1976;38:1124-1129.
9. Sickles EA, Weber WN, Galvin HB, Ominsky SH: Baseline screening mammography: One vs two views. AJR Am J Roentgenol 1986;147:1149-1153.
10. Eklund GW, Cardenosa G: The art of mammographic positioning. Radiol Clin North Am 1992;30:21-53.
11. Bassett LW, Hirbawi IA, DeBruhl N, Hayes MK: Mammographic positioning: Evaluation from the viewbox. Radiology 1993;188:803-806.
12. Jackson VP, Lex AM, Smith DJ: Patient discomfort during screen-film mammography. Radiology 1988;168:421-423.
13. Stomper PC, Kopans DB, Sadowsky NL, et al: Is mammography painful? A multicenter patient study. Arch Intern Med 1988;148:521-524.
14. Brew MD, Billings JD, Chisholm RJ: Mammography and breast pain. Australas Radiol 1989;33:335-336.
15. Department of Health and Human Services. Federal Register 21 CFR Parts 16 and 900. Quality Mammography Standards. Final Rule, Department of Health and Human Services, Food and Drug Administration. 21 CFR §16 and §900 (1997).
16. Bassett LW, Jessop NW, Wilcox PA: Mammography film-labeling practices. Radiology 1993;187:773-775.
17. American College of Radiology: Breast Imaging Reporting and Data System (BI-RADS). Reston, VA, American College of Radiology, 1993.
18. Sickles EA, Abele JS: Milk of calcium within tiny benign breast cysts. Radiology 1981;141:655-658.
19. Berkowitz JE, Gatewood OMB, Gayler BW: Equivocal mammographic findings: Evaluation with spot compression. Radiology 1989;171:369-371.
20. Faulk RM, Sickles EA: Efficacy of spot compression-magnification and tangential views in mammographic evaluation of palpable breast masses. Radiology 1992;185:87-90.
21. Sickles EA: Combining spot-compression and other special views to maximize mammographic information. Radiology 1989;173:571.
22. Feig SA: Importance of supplementary mammographic views to diagnostic accuracy. AJR Am J Roentgenol 1988;151:40-41.
23. Berkowitz JE, Gatewood OMB, Donovan GV, Gayler BW: Dermal breast calcifications: Localization with template-guided placement of skin marker. Radiology 1987;163:282.
24. Kopans DB, Meyer JE, Homer MJ, Grabbe J: Dermal deposits mistaken for breast calcifications. Radiology 1983;149:592-594.
25. Eklund GW, Busby RC, Miller SH, et al: Improved imaging of the augmented breast. AJR Am J Roentgenol 1988;151:469-473.
26. Fajardo LL, Roberts CC, Hunt KR: Mammographic surveillance of breast cancer patients: Should the mastectomy site be imaged? AJR Am J Roentgenol 1993;161:953-955.

Chapter 4

Clinical Image Evaluation

Lawrence W. Bassett

Maintaining high-quality clinical images is one of the most important goals of quality assurance programs for mammography. Learning to recognize specific deficiencies in the clinical images and their possible causes allows the interpreting physician and radiologic technologist to correct image deficiencies as soon as possible. In addition to the ongoing daily assessment of clinical images by the interpreting physician and radiologic technologist, an external review of selected clinical images is mandated by the Mammography Quality Standards Act (MQSA).[1,2] The external clinical image evaluation is performed at least every 3 years and is done by specially trained radiologists under the auspices of accrediting bodies approved by the U.S. Food and Drug Administration (FDA).

The clinical image review of the American College of Radiology Mammography Accreditation Program (ACR MAP) requires that a screening examination of each breast of a woman with fatty breasts—ACR Breast Imaging Reporting and Data System (BI-RADS) type I or II—and of a woman with dense breasts—BI-RADS type III or IV—be submitted for each mammography unit.[3,4] Because of variations in body habitus and cooperation, it is not possible to attain ideal breast positioning and compression in all women.[5] Therefore, facilities are requested to submit what they consider to be representative images of their work.

Clinical image evaluation should consist of an assessment of the eight categories: positioning, compression, exposure, contrast, sharpness, noise, artifacts, and labeling. Each of these categories of mammography image quality is reviewed in detail in this chapter. In 1997, the initial clinical image evaluation submissions of 1034 units failed. In these failed initial applications, 6128 in various categories were cited by reviewers as deficient.[6] These deficiencies were as follows: 1250 (20%) problems in positioning; 944 (15%) in exposure; 887 (14%) in compression; 806 (13%) in sharpness; 785 (13%) in contrast; 703 (11%) in labeling; 465 (8%) in artifacts; and 288 (5%) in noise. A significantly higher proportion of failures was attributed to positioning deficiencies for fatty breasts than for dense breasts ($P = .028$). Higher proportions of failures in dense breasts were related to deficiencies in compression ($P < .001$) and exposure ($P < .001$). Table 4–1 summarizes the most common potential deficiencies of the eight clinical image categories.

POSITIONING AND COMPRESSION

Breast positioning has changed dramatically over the years. This change has arisen from a better understanding of the anatomy and mobility of the breast and improved capabilities of modern dedicated mammography equipment.[7,8] The standard views are the mediolateral oblique (MLO) and the craniocaudal (CC). Because these are the only views employed for screening examinations, the goal should be to image as much breast tissue as possible in each view.[5,9,10]

Image Receptor Size

Before beginning the actual positioning maneuvers, the radiologic technologist performing film-screen mammography determines which size image receptor is most appropriate for the woman being examined. Both 18 × 24-cm and 24 × 30-cm image receptors should be available for each film-screen mammography unit.[11] For digital mammography, there is now only one image receptor size, which will vary with manufacturers. If the receptor selected is too small, either the axillary or the inferior aspect of the breast is likely to be excluded from the image (Fig. 4–1). Furthermore, a receptor that is too large results in the interposition of other body parts between the large cassette and the breast, preventing adequate compression, which results in sagging of the breast on the MLO view, poor separation of structures, motion artifacts, and improper exposure (Fig. 4–2).[7] The effect of single-size image receptors for direct digital mammography is uncertain in terms of quality of positioning. For a small digital receptor used on a large breast, tiling of images must be performed. For example, an MLO view would include the upper breast on one image and the lower breast on a second image. Use of a larger image receptor to image a small breast may create other challenges in positioning.

Positioning for the Mediolateral Oblique View

The MLO view provides the best opportunity to show all of the breast tissue in a single image (Figs. 4–3

Table 4–1. Potential Deficiencies in Eight Clinical Image Evaluation Categories

Category	Potential Deficiencies
Positioning	Poor visualization of posterior tissues
	Sagging breast on MLO
	Inadequate amount of pectoralis major muscle on MLO
	Nonstandard angulation of MLO
	Breast positioned too high on image receptor on MLO
	Posterior nipple line on CC not within 1 cm of that in MLO
	Excessive exaggeration on CC view
	Portion of breast cut off
	Skin folds
	Other body parts projected over breast
Compression	Poor separation of parenchymal densities
	Non-uniform exposure levels
	Patient motion
Exposure	Generalized underexposure
	Inadequate penetration of dense areas
	Generalized overexposure
Contrast	Inadequate contrast
	Excessive contrast
Sharpness	Poor delineation of linear structures
	Poor delineation of feature margins
	Poor delineation of microcalcifications
	Poor film-screen contact
Noise	Visually striking mottle pattern
	Noise—limited visualization of detail
Artifacts	Punctate or lint
	Scratches or pickoff
	Roller marks
	Equipment-related artifacts, e.g., grid lines
	Hair, deodorant, etc.
	Image handling
	Image fogging
Labeling	Failure to properly identify: patient, facility, exam date, view at axillary side, RT, number of cassette and screen

CC, craniocaudal; MLO, mediolateral oblique; RT, radiologic technologist performing exam.

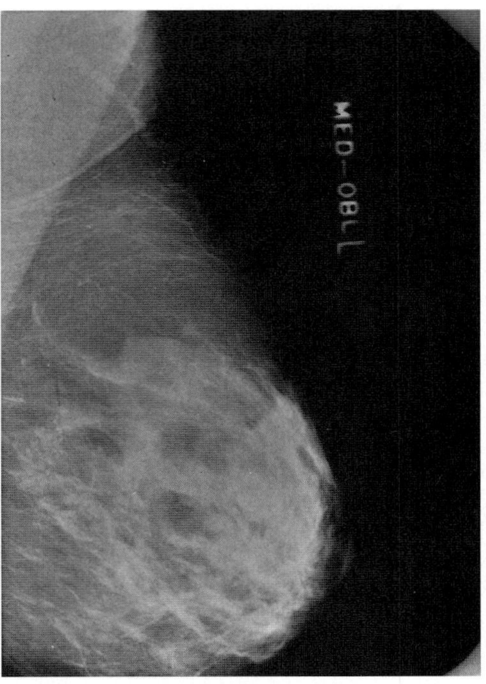

Figure 4–1. Image receptor too small for breast. The inferior aspect of the breast was excluded from the image.

and 4–4). Because the breast lies primarily on the pectoralis muscle, a generous amount of pectoralis muscle should be included to ensure that posterior breast tissues are shown. It is desirable for the muscle to extend inferiorly to the posterior nipple line (PNL) or below; this can be achieved in more than 80% of women.[5] On the MLO view, the PNL is drawn at an angle approximately perpendicular to the muscle, extending from the nipple to the pectoralis muscle or to the edge of the film, whichever comes first (see Fig. 4–4). Whenever possible, the fibroglandular tissue should not extend to the edge of the film, because such an extension would imply that additional posterior tissue was excluded from the image. Thus, it is desirable to see fat posterior to all the fibroglandular tissue.

Skin folds on the image should be avoided because they can obscure a lesion or mimic an abnormality (Fig. 4–5). Occasionally, skin folds in the axilla cannot be avoided, but they should not pose problems in interpretation.

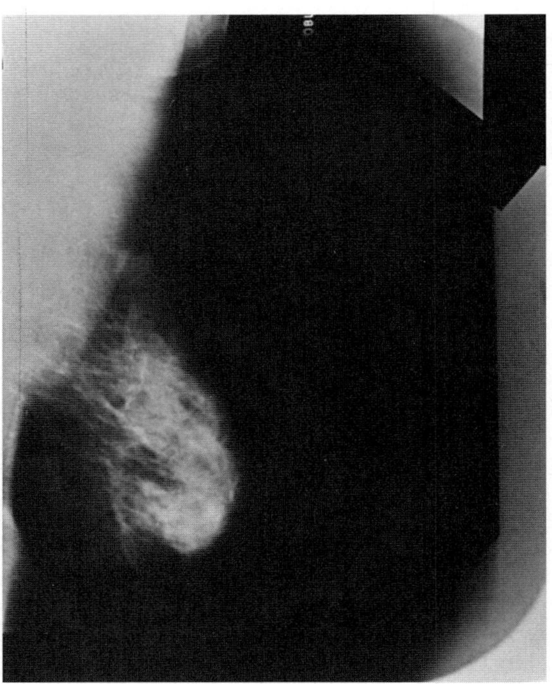

Figure 4–2. Image receptor too large for breast. Superimposition of shoulder and chest wall prevents proper positioning and compression. The breast is sagging, there is poor separation of fibroglandular tissues, linear structures in the inferior aspect of breast are blurred, fibroglandular tissue shows non-uniform exposure, and a large skin fold is present near chest wall.

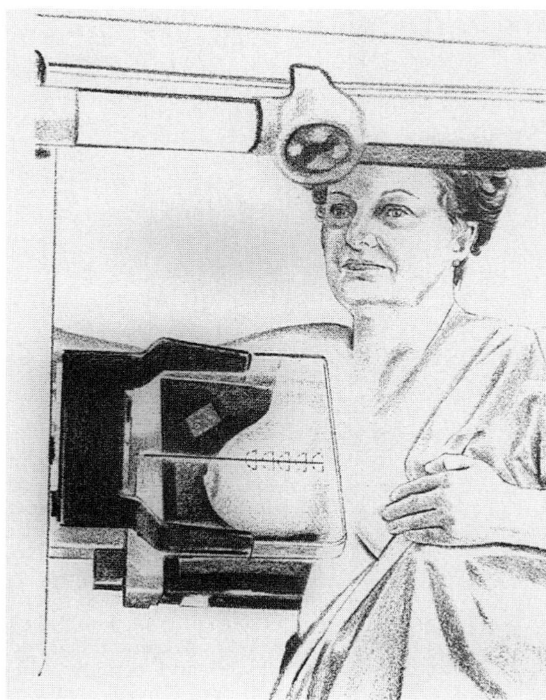

Figure 4–3. Woman properly positioned for mediolateral oblique view.

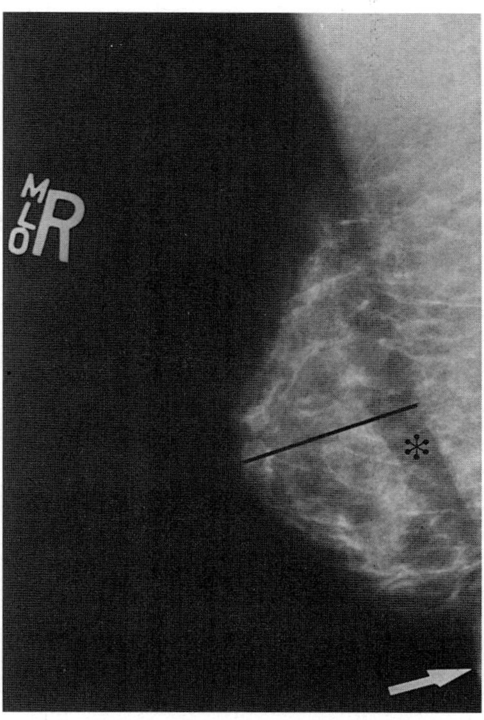

Figure 4–4. Proper positioning for the mediolateral oblique view: Note inclusion of a generous amount of pectoralis muscle, extension of the muscle below the posterior nipple line (a line drawn at a 45° angle from the nipple extending to the anterior edge of the pectoral muscle), visualization of retromammary fat (*asterisk*) posterior to the fibroglandular tissues, and open inframammary fold (*arrow*).

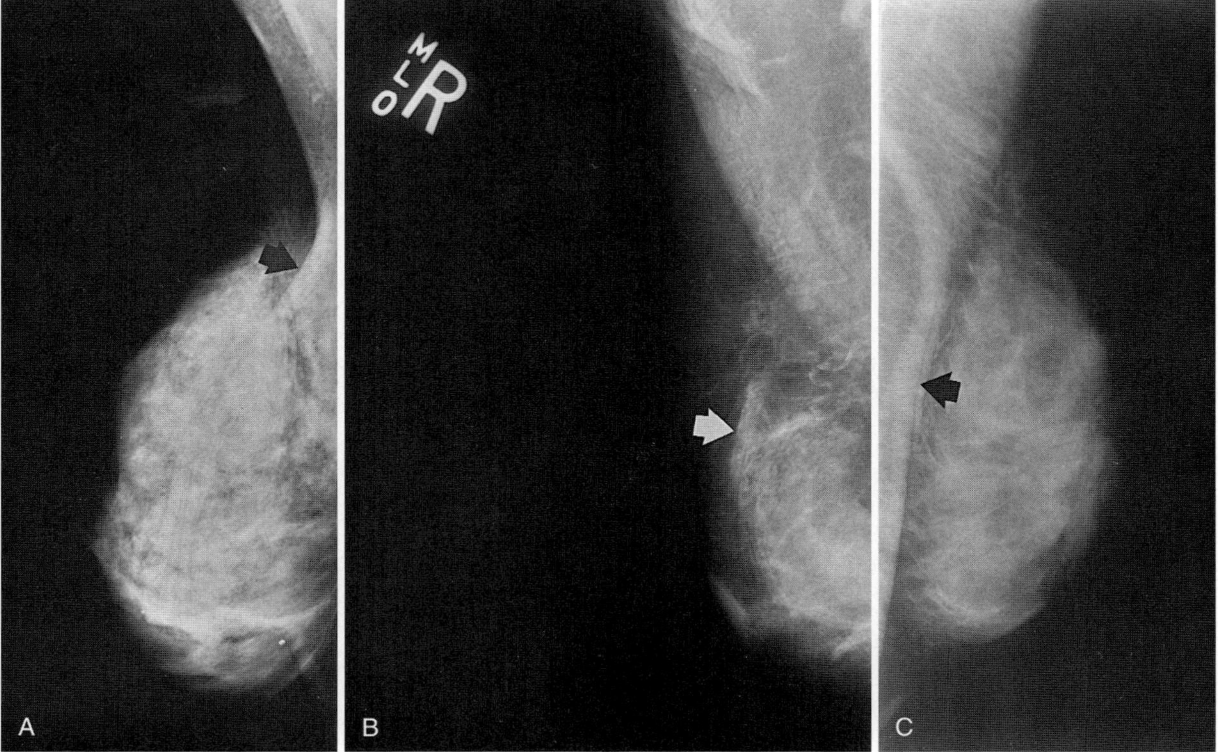

Figure 4–5. **A** to **C,** Deficiencies in positioning for mediolateral oblique view include prominent skin folds (*arrow*).

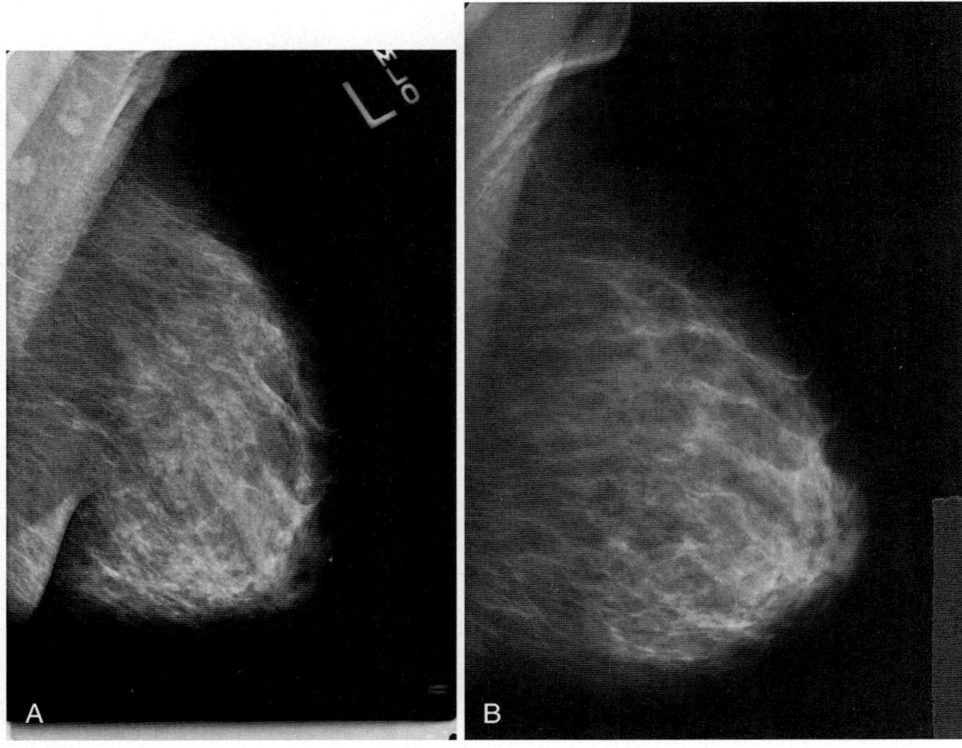

Figure 4–6. **A,** Deficiencies in positioning for mediolateral oblique: Sagging breast. The technologist did not hold the breast up and out as compression was applied. Note the low position of the nipple, overlapping of fibroglandular structures, and prominent inferior skin fold near the chest wall. **B,** Same breast, properly positioned and compressed. (From Bassett LW: Clinical image evaluation. Radiol Clin North Am 1995; 33:1027-1039.)

If proper positioning methods have been used during the initiation and application of compression, the breast should not be sagging (Fig. 4–6).[7]

Positioning for the Craniocaudal View

The overriding goal in positioning for the CC view should be to include all of the posteromedial tissue (Figs. 4–7 and 4–8), because the posteromedial tissue is the area of the breast most likely to be excluded in an MLO view. If proper techniques are used, the radiologic technologist can include all of the posteromedial fibroglandular tissue without resorting to exaggerated positioning of the CC view. Exaggerated positioning may result in unnecessary exclusion of posterolateral tissue (Fig. 4–9).[7] Although as much lateral tissue as possible should be included on the CC view, lateral tissue should never be included at the expense of medial tissue.

Visualization of the pectoralis muscle is evidence that sufficient posterior breast tissue has been included on the CC view. However, the pectoralis muscle is seen in only about 30% of properly positioned CC views.[5,8,10] When the muscle is not visualized, measurement of the PNL is a reliable index as to whether the CC view includes sufficient posterior tissue.[8] On the CC view, the PNL is drawn directly posterior from the nipple to the edge of the film. A good general rule is that the length of the PNL on the CC view should be within 1 cm of its length on the MLO view. The PNL is usually longer on the MLO view, but in approximately 10% of correctly positioned cases, the PNL is longer on the CC view.[5]

Compression

Compression decreases breast thickness and makes it more uniform. Decreased thickness reduces radiation dose, scatter radiation, and object unsharpness. Achieving uniform thickness means that film optical

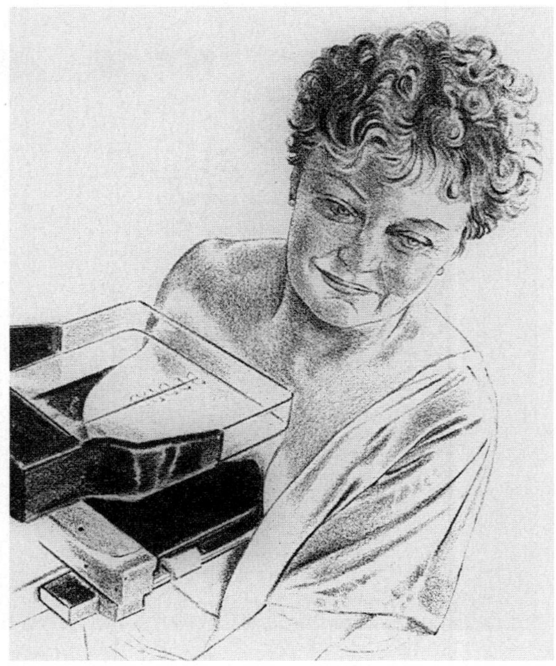

Figure 4–7. Woman properly positioned for craniocaudal view.

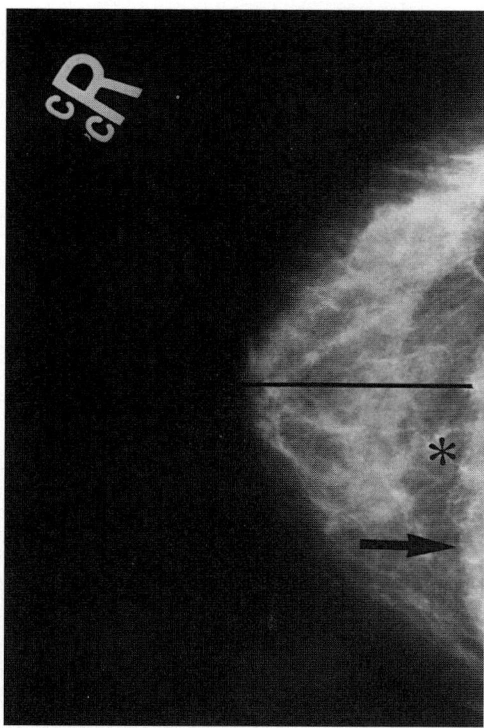

Figure 4–8. Evidence of proper positioning for the craniocaudal view includes presence of the pectoralis muscle (*arrow*) on the image, posterior nipple line (line from nipple to chest wall) within 1 cm of its length on the mediolateral oblique view, inclusion of retromammary fat (*asterisk*) posterior to all medial fibroglandular tissue, and location of the nipple in the midline of the image. Note that some posterior lateral tissue extends beyond the edge of the film.

densities are more likely to correspond to subtle attenuation differences rather than to thickness differences. Adequate compression also prevents motion unsharpness.

Inadequate compression manifests as overlapping of breast structures (Fig. 4–10), non-uniform tissue exposure (Figs. 4–2, 4–10 to 4–12), and motion unsharpness (Figs. 4–2, 4–10, 4–13 to 4–15). Motion due to inadequate compression is more commonly seen on the MLO view than on the CC view, because the breast is supported by the bucky (Potter-Bucky parallel scanning grid) on the CC view (see Fig. 4–15).

IMAGE QUALITY

Image quality, or the ability of the mammogram to portray diagnostic information clearly, depends on contrast, exposure, noise, and sharpness.

Contrast

Radiographic contrast can be defined as the degree of variation in optical density between different areas of the film. The different shades of gray on the film allow us to perceive attenuation differences in the breast tissues. Contrast in mammography image receptor systems has improved markedly over the

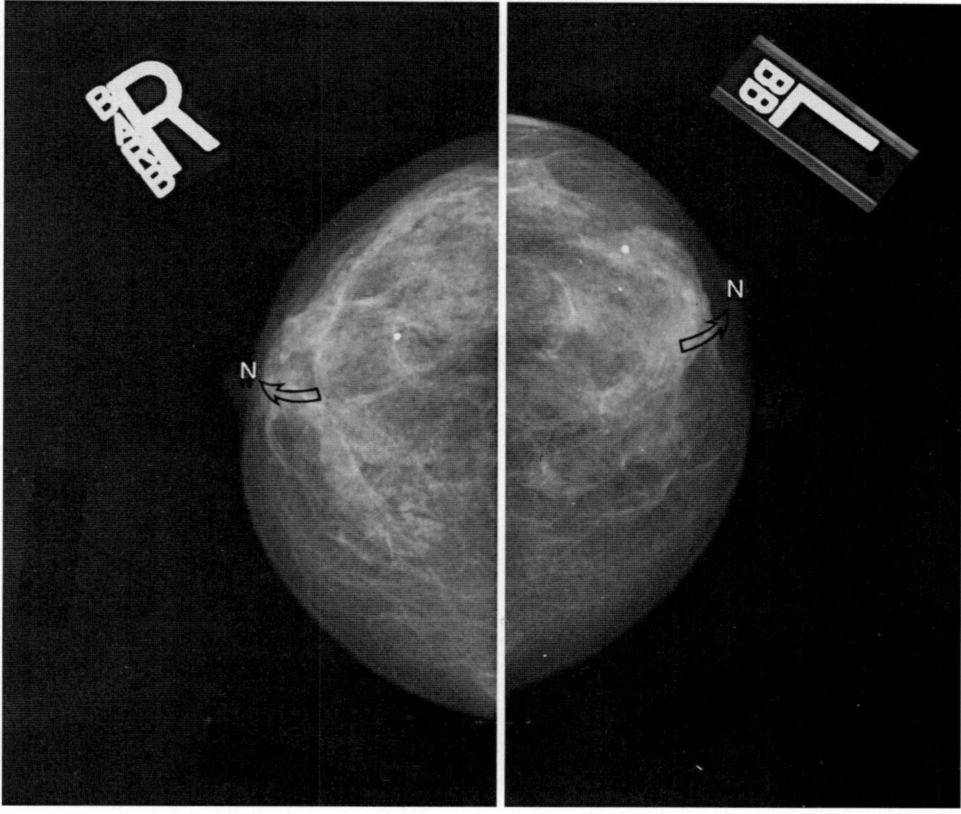

Figure 4–9. Exaggerated craniocaudal view positioning. The nipples (N) are rotated toward the lateral aspects of the breast rather than located in the midline, as in Figure 4–8. This exaggerated positioning might have been intentional to ensure that all of the posteromedial tissue was included but is unnecessary and results in the exclusion of posterolateral tissue. The labels "BARB" and "BB" should have included "MLO view."

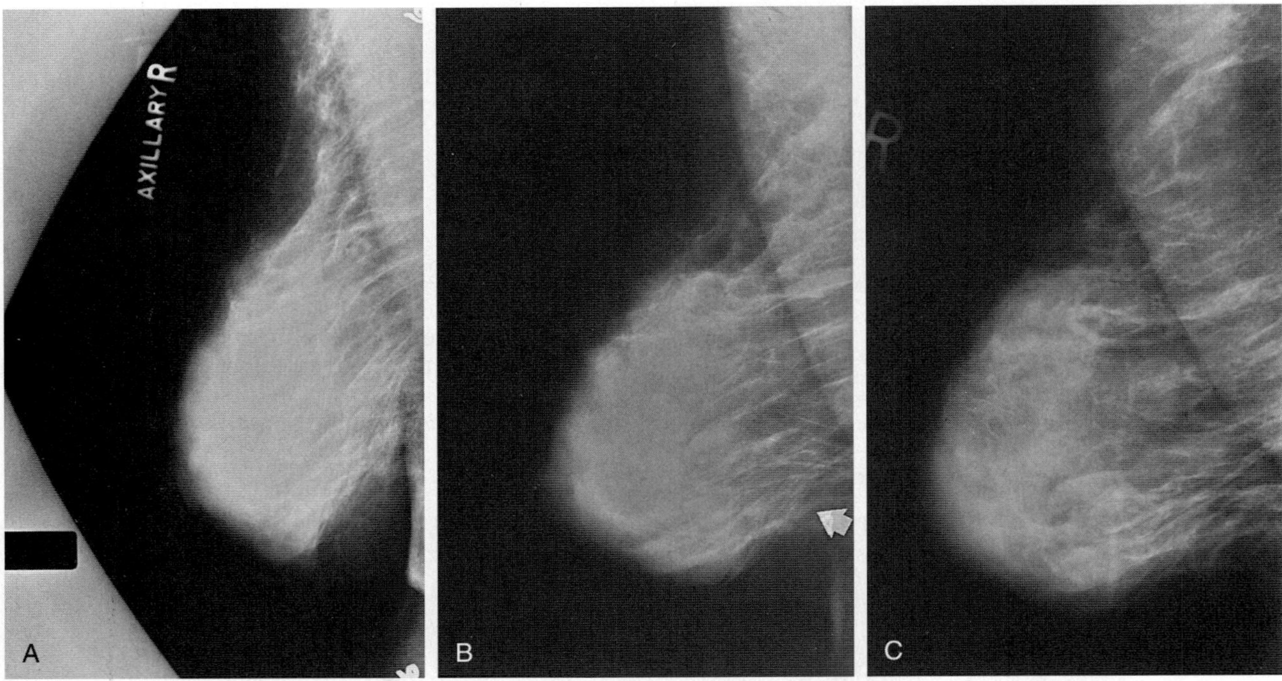

Figure 4–10. Improvements in positioning and compression of the same breast. **A,** Initial mammogram. The breast is sagging, and fibroglandular tissues are superimposed and underexposed. The pectoralis muscle is also underexposed. Also note that the screen identification number (6) is on the film twice and overlies the axilla and abdominal wall. The screen number should be on the opposite side of the screen. The laterality/view label should be "RMLO" rather than "AxillaryR." **B,** Mammogram taken 1 year later at the same facility. Positioning and compression are better than in the initial mammogram (**A**), but breast is still sagging, and fibroglandular tissues show inadequate separation, non-uniform exposure, and motion unsharpness (*arrow*). **C,** Mammogram another year later at a different facility. Improved positioning and exposure have resulted in presence of more pectoral muscle on the image, separation and uniform exposure of fibroglandular tissues, and minimal motion unsharpness.

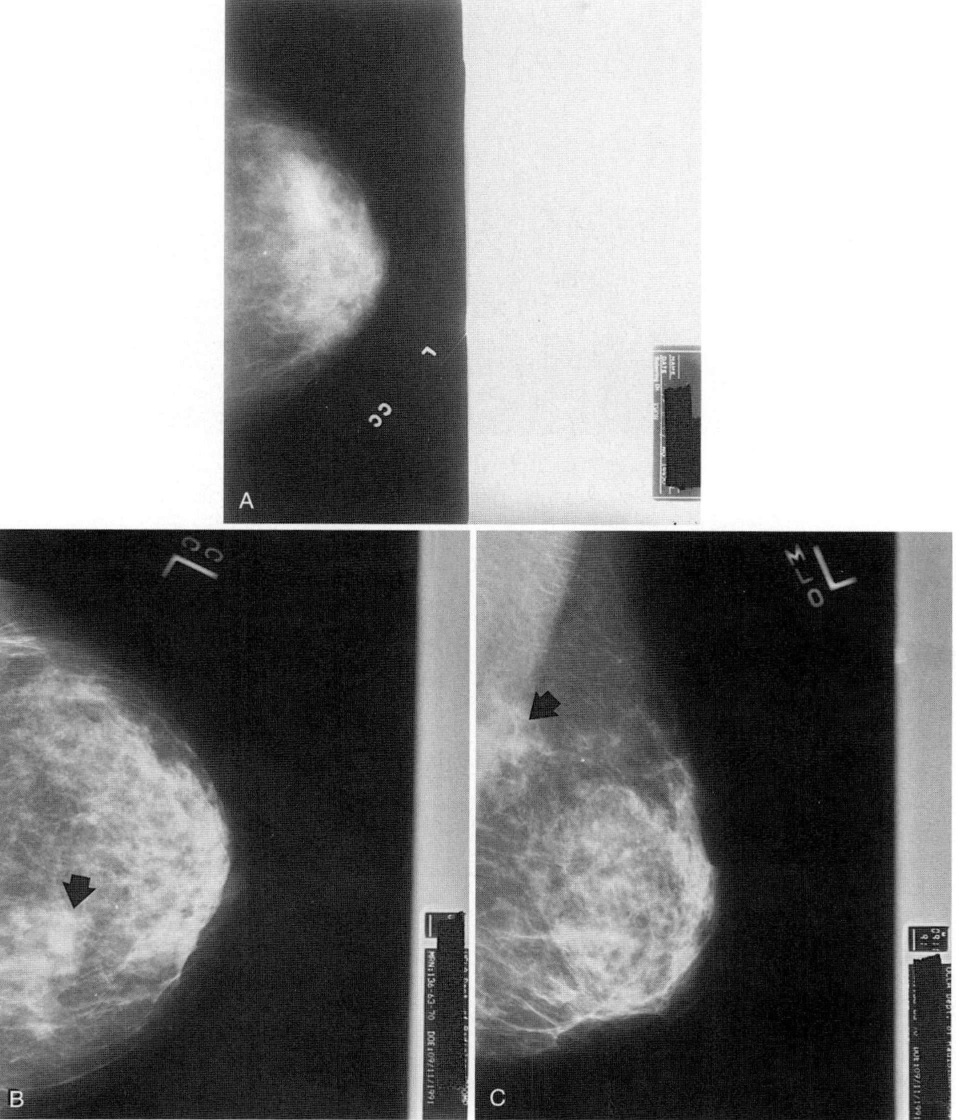

Figure 4–11. Inadequate positioning and compression versus proper positioning and compression of the same breast. **A,** Initial left craniocaudal (CC) view shows inadequate compression, resulting in non-uniform exposure of fibroglandular tissue. Note that the image receptor is too large and that the "LCC" marker was incorrectly placed at the medial aspect of the breast. There is excessive collimation. **B,** Left CC view obtained at another facility a few days later. Proper compression resulted in uniform exposure of fibroglandular tissue. Additional fibroglandular tissue (*arrow*) was depicted in the posteromedial aspect of the breast. **C,** Left mediolateral oblique view obtained at the second facility. The additional tissue (*arrow*) was located in the superior aspect of the breast and was probably excluded from the initial CC view because of failure to lift the inframammary fold as high as possible before positioning the breast.

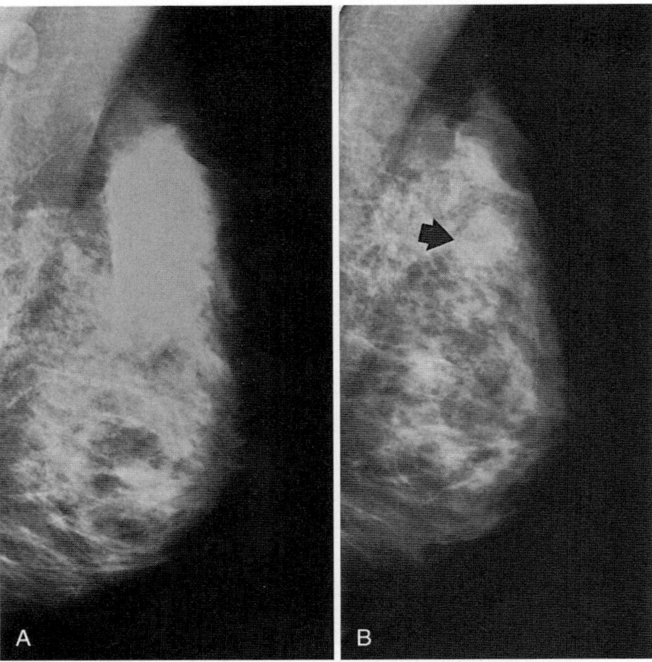

Figure 4–12. Inadequate compression and improved compression of the same breast. **A,** Non-uniform exposure of the fibroglandular tissues, with much of the superior tissue underexposed secondary to inadequate compression. **B,** Second film obtained with adequate compression reveals circumscribed mass (*arrow*) in the upper hemisphere of the breast. Ultrasonography showed the mass to be a cyst.

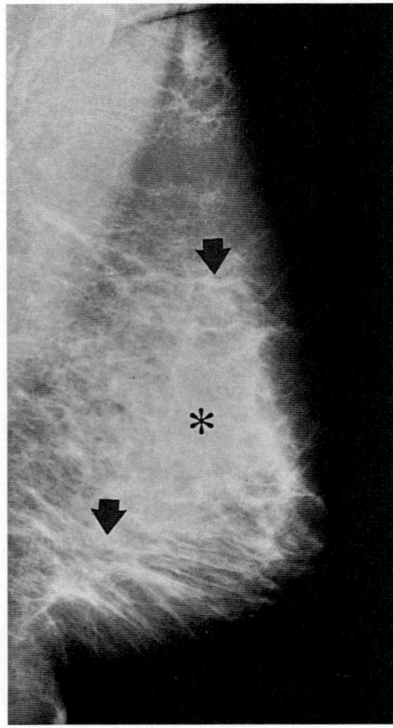

Figure 4–13. Motion unsharpness due to inadequate compression. Several linear structures (*arrows*) are blurred, and no structural details are seen in the center of the image (*asterisk*).

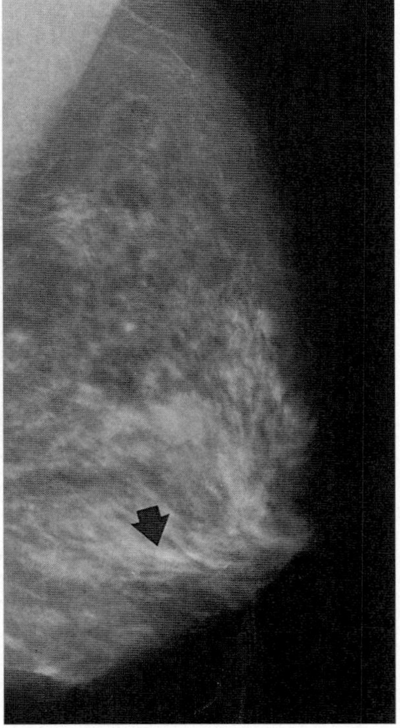

Figure 4–14. Motion unsharpness due to inadequate compression. Linear structures (*arrow*) are blurred throughout the lower half of the breast.

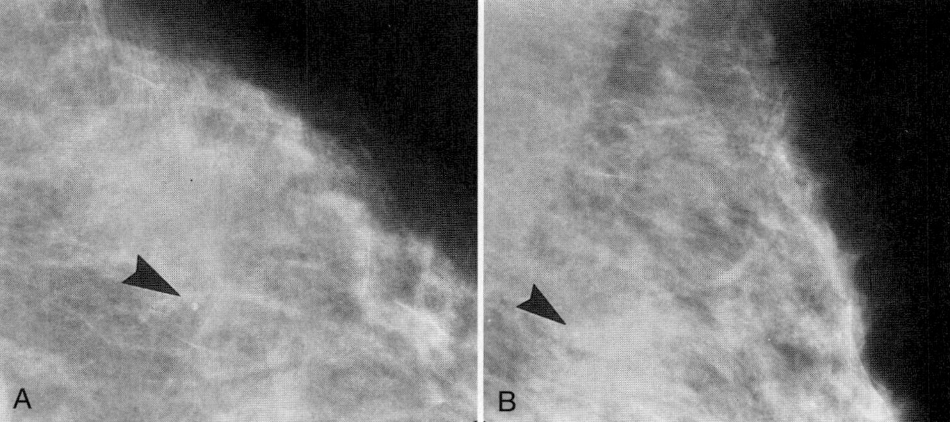

Figure 4–15. Blurring of calcification on mediolateral oblique (MLO) view due to motion secondary to inadequate compression. **A,** On craniocaudal view, calcification (*arrow*) has sharp margins. **B,** On MLO view, the calcification is blurred. (From Bassett LW: Clinical image evaluation. Radiol Clin North Am 1995;33:1027-1039.)

years (Fig. 4–16). In addition to the image receptor selected, radiographic contrast is also affected by subject contrast (radiation quality, kilovolt peak [kVp]) (Fig. 4–17), exposure (Fig. 4–18), film processing (darkroom conditions, processor development temperature, chemicals, and time), and scatter reduction (compression, grids). Film processing is one of the most important determinants of image contrast. Films should be developed according to the manufacturer's specifications. Longer processing times increase image contrast, although they also increase image noise because of the accompanying lower radiation exposure.[12] Processor temperature is also crucial, and the processor thermometer should be checked regularly for accuracy.[7]

High contrast is desirable, but it may be impossible to see both thick and thin parts on the same image if the contrast is too high. Thus, a balance must be reached between contrast and latitude when selecting the type of film to use for mammography.

The capacity for postprocessing allows for contrast adjustments in digital mammography. When digital films are to be printed out as hard copy, however, it is important to achieve the best contrast before the images are printed.

Exposure

The high-contrast films and low-kVp techniques used in film-screen mammography result in a small exposure latitude.[13,14] In other words, even small differences in kVp or milliamperes-second (mAs) result in large variations in optical density. Therefore,

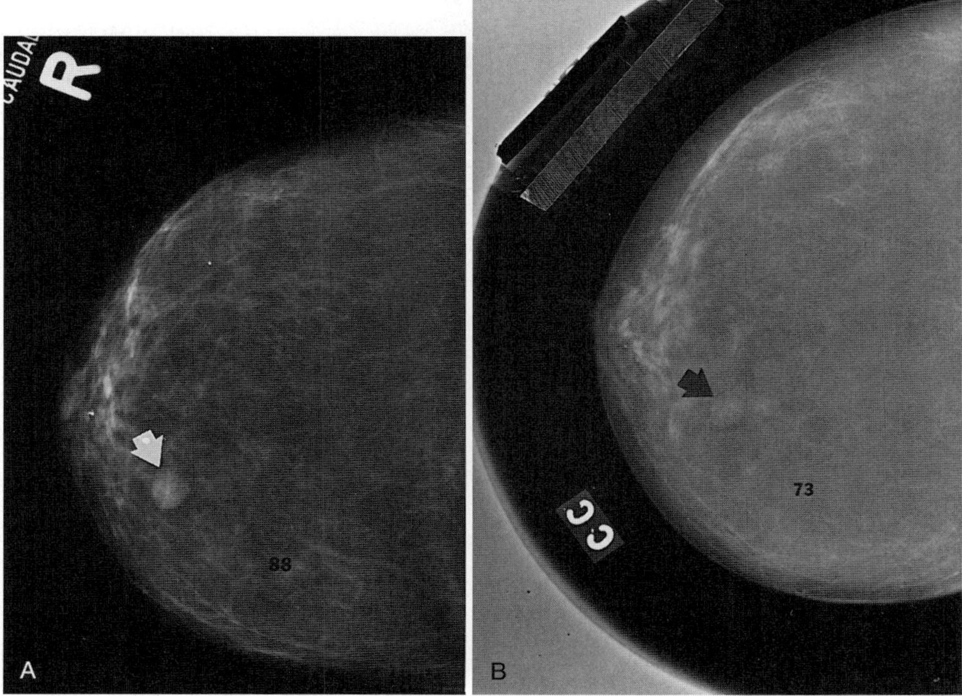

Figure 4–16. Improvements in radiographic contrast are signified by improved clarity of benign mass (*arrow*) in 1988 mammogram (**A**) compared with 1973 mammogram (**B**).

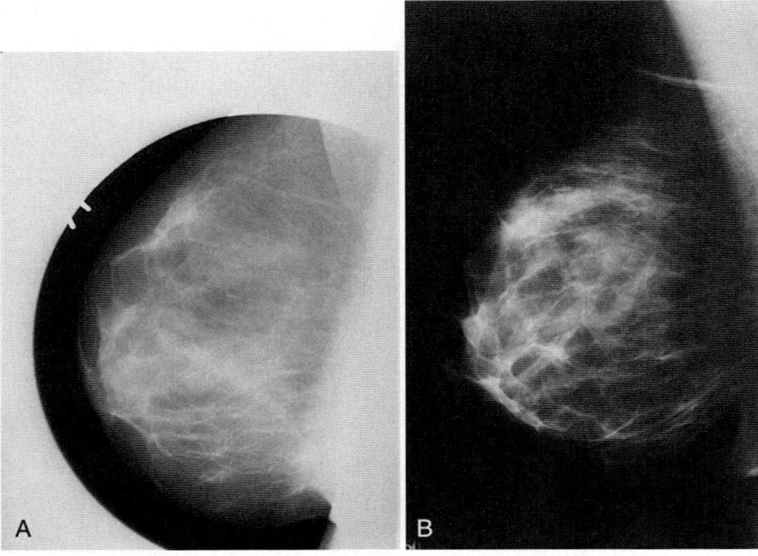

Figure 4–17. Effect of mammographic equipment on contrast. **A,** Initial mammogram shows inadequate contrast due to use of general-purpose radiographic equipment with a conventional tungsten target, an inadequate compression device, and no grid. Note the excessive collimation. **B,** Mammogram obtained 1 year later at facility with dedicated mammography equipment. Molybdenum target and filtration, proper compression, and antiscatter grid all contribute to better image contrast.

kVp and mAs must be carefully selected, and phototimer performance must be precise over the range of kVp, breast thickness, and density values encountered in clinical practice. Proper functioning of the phototimer should be evaluated through the use of varying thicknesses of breast-equivalent phantom material during initial calibration of the mammography unit, during the annual survey by the medical physicist, and at least monthly during the phantom image evaluation by the radiologic technologist.[7] The mammography generator should have sufficient output to adequately image large breasts and dense breasts with reasonably short exposure times (less than 2 seconds). The radiologic technologist can monitor exposures for each clinical image on the basis of the length of time of the audible exposure.

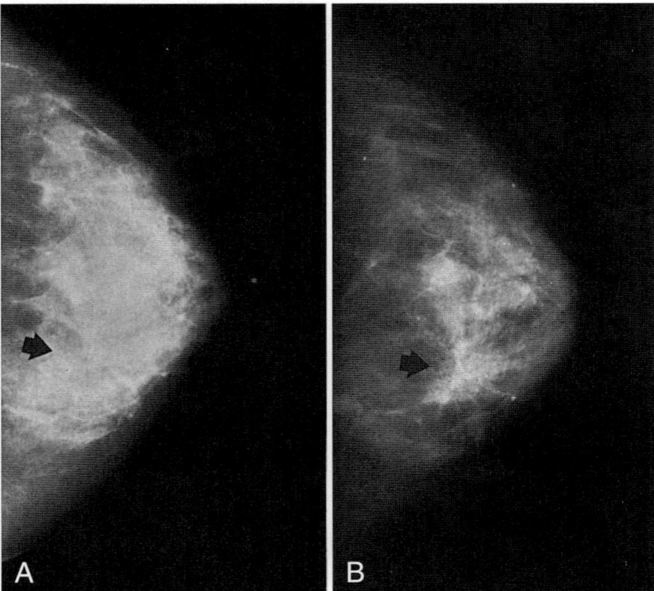

Figure 4–18. Effect of exposure on contrast. **A,** Initial left craniocaudal mammogram. An architectural distortion (*arrow*) in the medial aspect of the breast was noted only in retrospect. **B,** Mammogram obtained at another facility with adequate compression and exposure. Note the increased image contrast in the properly exposed image. The improved exposure and contrast made the carcinoma (*arrow*) obvious.

Proper mammographic exposure should be evaluated under correct viewing conditions. These viewing conditions, reviewed in the ACR *Mammography Quality Control* manuals, include adequate view box luminance, low ambient room light (illuminance) to minimize light reflected off the surface of the film, and masking of films to keep extraneous viewbox light that has passed through the unexposed area of the film from reaching the eye.[7] As indicated in previous chapters, appropriate viewing conditions for mammography are best achieved with dedicated mammography viewing equipment that provides adequate luminance, control of light intensity, and shutters or other masking devices. Ambient room light should be minimal. Obviously, similar recommendations apply for reading off soft copy monitors at workstations. In particular, the room light should be minimal and there should be no viewboxes or other strong light sources directly across the room, which would reflect on the monitor. It may be necessary to rearrange a room to achieve optimal conditions for soft copy reading.

Underexposure has been shown to be a more common image deficiency than overexposure (Fig. 4–19).[6] Underexposure manifests as inability to see details in dense fibroglandular tissue. Lesions can be obscured within underexposed dense tissue; underexposure is therefore a potentially more serious error because it can lead to false-negative findings (see Fig. 4–18). As a general rule, when images are properly exposed, the details within dense fibroglandular tissue are perceptible, but it may be difficult to see the skin and subcutaneous tissues unless all extraneous viewbox light is eliminated with masking. The

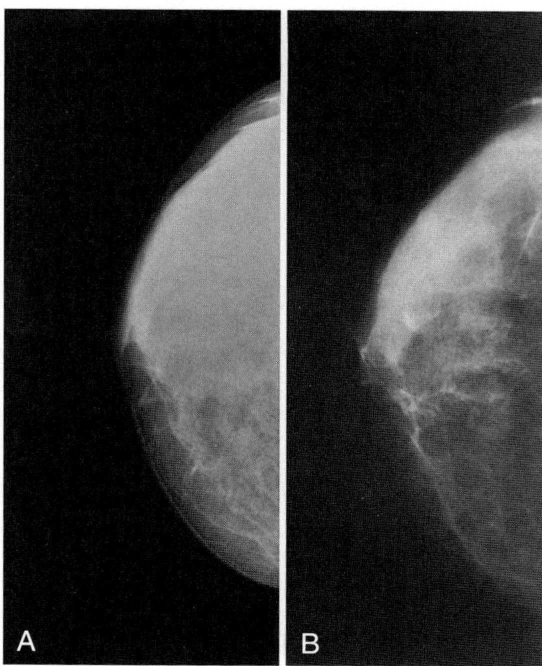

Figure 4–19. Underexposure and inadequate compression. **A**, The craniocaudal (CC) mammogram is underexposed so that details are not visible in the fibroglandular tissue. Inadequate compression contributed to the underexposure. Underexposed images are often deficient in contrast because the radiolucent tissues are also underexposed. **B**, CC mammogram obtained at another facility with proper compression and exposure has better detail in the dense tissues and higher contrast. More posterior tissue was also included as a result of improved positioning.

pectoralis muscle is one of the densest structures on the MLO view, and it is important that the muscle be exposed sufficiently to show superimposed breast tissue (see Fig. 4–10A).

Overexposure results in loss of details in the thin or fatty parts of the breast (Fig. 4–20). However, overexposure is frequently a "recoverable" error that can be compensated for through the use of dedicated mammography high-luminance viewboxes combined with masking of extraneous light or by "hot-lighting" overexposed areas of the film. Underexposure, on the other hand, is an unrecoverable error that requires imaging to be repeated.

For digital mammography, there is a wider exposure dynamic range (latitude). As a result, the range of exposure over which an acceptable image can be obtained is considerably wider.

Noise

Noise, or radiographic mottle, compromises the ability to discern small details, such as calcifications, in images. Quantum mottle is the major source of noise in mammography. Quantum mottle is caused by a statistical fluctuation in the number of x-ray photons absorbed at individual locations in the intensifying screen.[13] The fewer the total number of photons used to make the image, the greater the amount of quantum mottle observed. Thus, image recording systems that are faster, underexposed, or processed too aggressively have more noise. Ironically, noise is more likely to be present in high-contrast films because high contrast makes the mottle more evident.[13]

Sharpness

Sharpness is the ability of the mammographic system to define an edge. Unsharpness, often referred to as "blur," manifests as blurring of the edges of fine linear structures (see Fig. 4–4A), tissue borders, and calcifications. Types of unsharpness that may be encountered are geometric, motion (see Figs. 4–13 to 4–15), parallax, and screen as well as blurring due to poor film-screen contact (Fig. 4–21).[13]

An increase in focal spot size, a longer object-to-film distance, and a shorter source-to-image distance increase geometric unsharpness. Over the last decade, the focal spot sizes of dedicated mammography units have been reduced for both contact and magnification mammography. Today, the source-to-image distance should be at least 55 cm for contact mammography and 60 cm for magnification mammography.[11]

Parallax unsharpness refers to blurring due to the use of double-emulsion films. The image captured on each side of a dual-emulsion film is separated by the width of the film base. If the film is viewed from a distance different from the source-to-image distance,

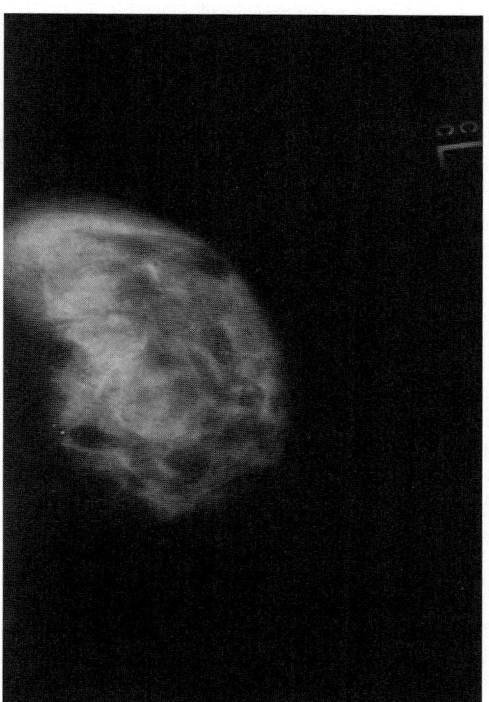

Figure 4–20. Overexposed craniocaudal mammogram. No details are visible in the subcutaneous or fatty tissues.

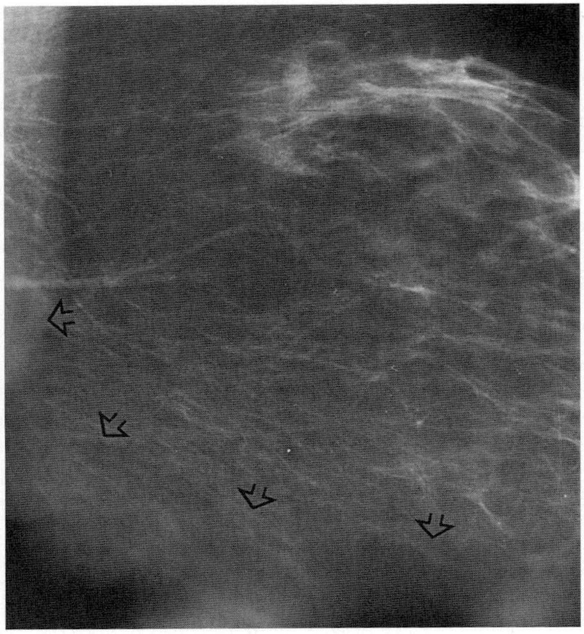

Figure 4–21. Loss of film-screen contact. Much of the detail is blurred (*arrows*) in the lower part of the image, a result of improper loading of the film into the cassette.

the slight offset of the two emulsions results in image blur. Because of the blur, double-emulsion films have not gained wide acceptance despite the benefits of lower radiation dose and longer tube life that they offer.

Screen unsharpness results from light diffusion; a single x-ray absorbed in the screen is converted to a large number of visible light photons. The spread of these photons from the point of x-ray interaction in the screen to where they are absorbed by the film creates blur. The production of faster screens, such as those that are thicker or have reflective coating behind them, yields greater photon spread and more screen unsharpness.

A loss of intimate contact between the screen and film results in the further spread of light from the screen before it reaches the film.[7] Poor film-screen contact can result from poorly designed or damaged cassettes, improper placement of the film in the cassette (see Fig. 4–21), dirt lying between the film and the screen, or air trapped between the film and the screen at the time the film is loaded. Complete elimination of the air after the cassette is loaded may take up to 15 minutes. Thus, it is recommended that the radiologic technologist wait at least 15 minutes before exposing cassettes after they are loaded.[7]

ARTIFACTS

An *artifact* can be defined as any density variation on an image that does not reflect true attenuation differences in the subject. Artifacts can result from problems in darkroom cleanliness, film handling, screen maintenance, processing, or the x-ray equipment. The presence of multiple artifacts on images suggests problems with quality control at a facility. Commonly encountered artifacts are dust or lint (Fig. 4–22), dirt, scratches, fingerprints (Figs. 4–23 and 4–24), and fog. Many artifacts can be avoided by

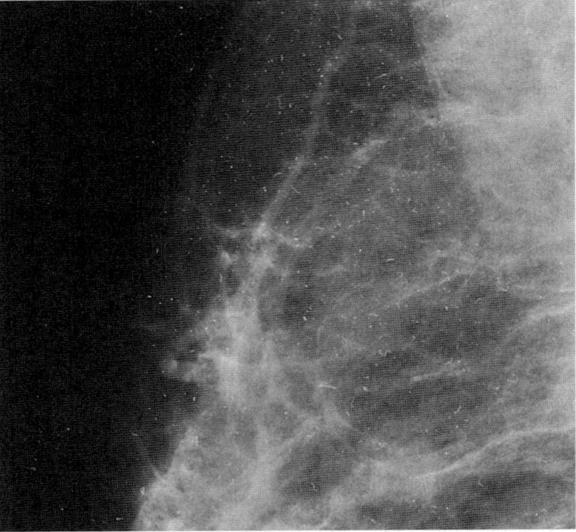

Figure 4–22. Poor screen maintenance. The artifacts represent dust and dirt on the screen.

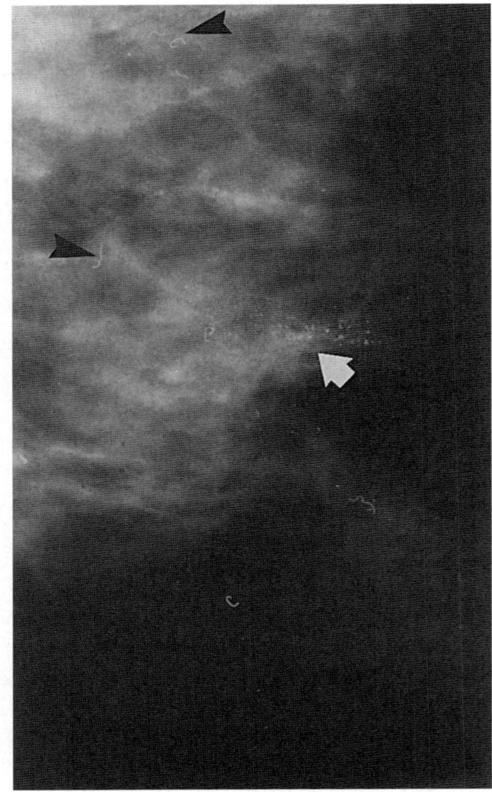

Figure 4–23. Poor screen maintenance. Fingerprints (*arrows*) on screen and dust (*arrowheads*).

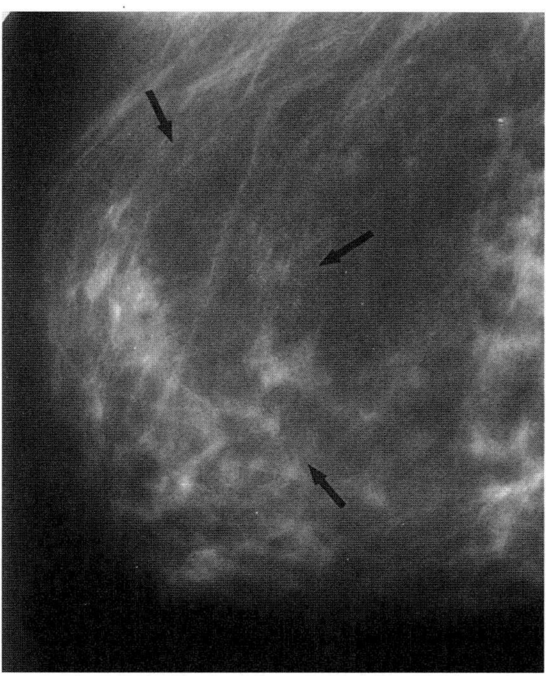

Figure 4–24. Poor screen maintenance. Three faint sets of fingerprints (*arrows*) were at first mistaken for microcalcifications.

careful attention to darkroom conditions, including cleanliness, film handling, and regular cleaning. The processor can be the source of many different types of artifacts—roller marks, loader marks, and chemical residues (Fig. 4–25). Routine processor maintenance, replenishment of chemicals, cleaning of rollers, and daily quality assurance activities are essential.

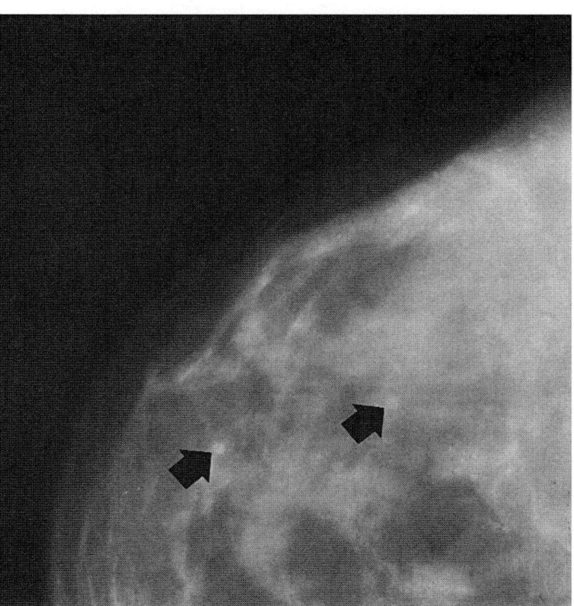

Figure 4–25. Multiple artifacts (*arrows*) visible on all of the films of this patient were due to residue of chemicals on the processor rollers, secondary to poor maintenance.

Equipment-related artifacts include grid lines and equipment parts superimposed on the image. When a moving grid is used, the grid lines should not be visible on the image. If grid lines are observed regularly, the drive mechanism should be repaired or replaced. Occasionally, it may be difficult to determine whether parallel linear artifacts are related to improper function of the grid or the processor rollers. Two images of a uniform phantom, such as the ACR mammography phantom, acquired with the same technical factors but introduced into the processor at right angles to each other can be used to determine whether linear artifacts are due to a faulty grid (the lines do not change direction relative to the properly positioned phantom) or to the processor (the lines do change orientation relative to the phantom).[7]

Improper size, design, or alignment of the compression device can result in inadequate visualization of deep tissues. If the device is improperly aligned with the image receptor, the posterior lip of the compression device may appear on the image (Figs. 4–26 and 4–27). For maximal effectiveness, the posterior edge of the compression device should be straight

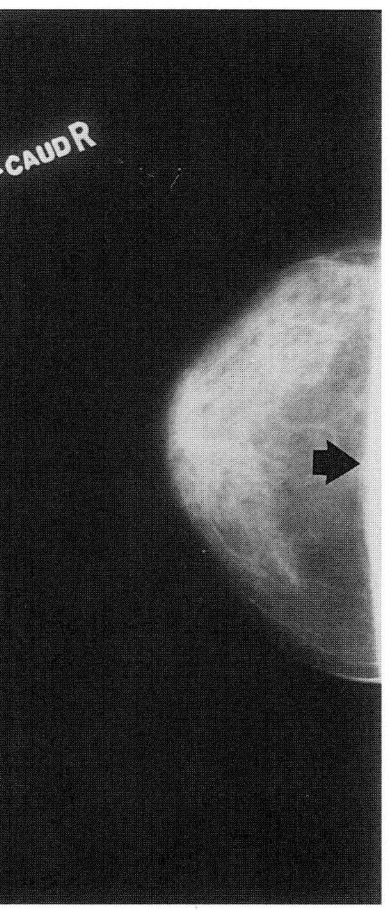

Figure 4–26. Improperly designed and aligned compression device. The curved opacity near the chest wall (*arrow*) is the posterior lip of the compression device, which is rounded and located anterior to the posterior edge of the film.

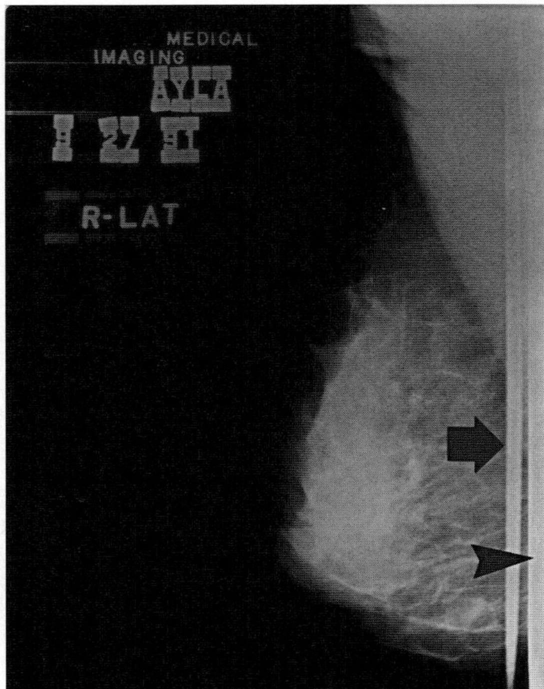

Figure 4–27. Improper alignment of compression device. The posterior lip of the compression device (*arrow*) is superimposed on the posterior aspect of the breast. Additional posterior breast tissue is excluded by excessive collimation (*arrowhead*). The following essential information was not provided in the film labeling: location of facility, patient's full name, ID number or birth date for patient, screen identification, and technologist's initials. View should be labeled "RMLO." Compression and exposure are also inadequate. (From Bassett LW: Clinical image evaluation. Radiol Clin North Am 1995;33:1027-1039.)

to match the posterior edge of the film, and the anterior aspect of the lip of the compression device should be posterior to the posterior edge of the film.[15] Exclusion of tissue near the chest wall can also be caused by the improper placement or poor fit of film in the cassette, poor fit of the cassette within the cassette tunnel of the bucky, or overcollimation of the image, especially at the chest wall (see Fig. 4–27).

COLLIMATION

Collimating close to the surface of the breast can preclude effective masking of images at the viewbox.[16] Excessive collimation can also result in exclusion of part of the breast from the image (Figs. 4–17A and 4–28). It is now understood that collimation to the surface of the breast provides no significant scatter reduction benefit. Thus, it is generally recommended that the x-ray beam be collimated to the edge of the film. However, posterior breast tissue would be excluded from the image if the collimation extended within the posterior edge of the film. Therefore, the collimation should be slightly posterior to the chest wall edge of the film. Recommendations for the maximum allowable posterior extension of the x-ray beam beyond the film have been put in federal regulations and in equipment specifications issued by the ACR.[11,15]

LABELING

Radiologists are frequently called on to review mammograms from other facilities. A review of mammograms from facilities across the country submitted for clinical image evaluation by the ACR MAP revealed that nonstandardized labeling practices were prevalent.[17] In addition to nonstandardized formats, films often did not contain enough information to adequately identify the facility or the examinee (Figs. 4–27 to 4–29). In many cases, eccentric methods for designating view and laterality resulted in confusion or incorrect information (Fig. 4–30).

Standardized methods for labeling films have been developed to ensure correct identification of facilities, patients, laterality, and view (Fig. 4–31). These labeling guidelines for mammography films can be divided into those that are considered essential or required, those that are highly recommended, and those that are merely recommended. Required items are identification label, view and laterality, cassette number (Arabic numeral), and initials of the radiologic technologist who performed the examination. The identification label should contain facility name

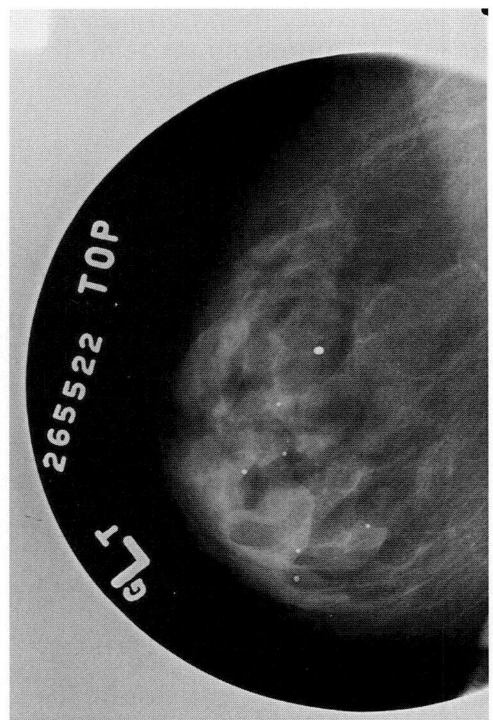

Figure 4–28. Round collimator results in exclusion of axillary tissue and precludes masking of extraneous light at viewbox. Labeling is incomplete and nonstandardized. Laterality designation and view should be located near axilla, making "TOP" unnecessary.

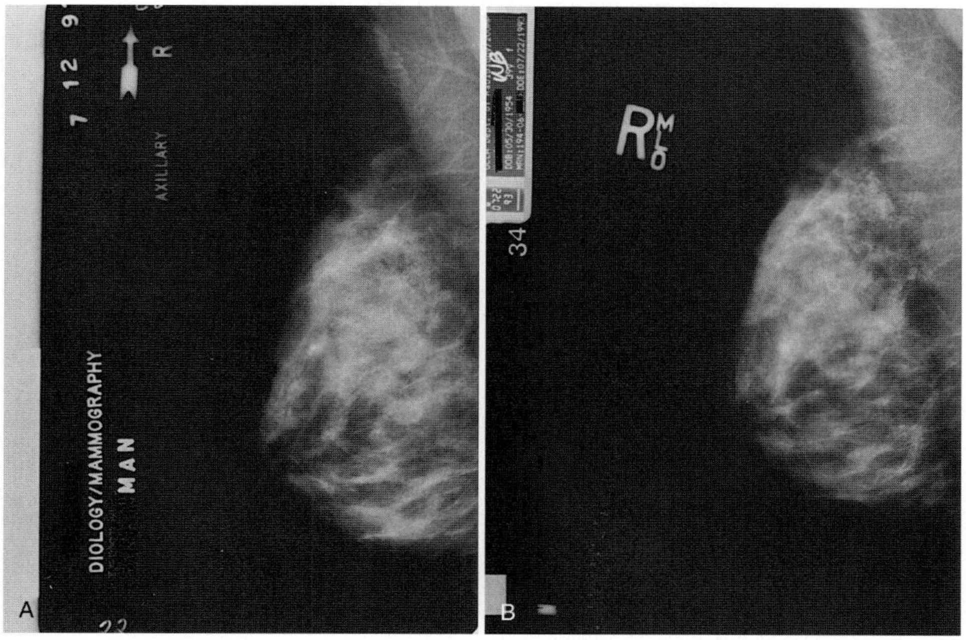

Figure 4–29. Different labeling of films for same patient. **A,** Mediolateral (MLO) view with nonstandardized labeling. Facility name (partially masked) is provided but no address. The patient's last name (partially masked) but no first name is given, and no unique ID number is provided. Designation for view is incorrect (should be "MLO," not "Axillary") and radiologic technologist is not identified. **B,** MLO view of same patient obtained 2 years later with standardized labeling (facility address partially masked, examinee name masked). Note improved positioning.

and address (at least city, state, and Zip Code), examinee's first and last names, and a unique additional identifier (e.g., medical record number, social security number, or date of birth). It is strongly recommended that the identification label be "flashed" on the image to make it as permanent as possible and enable it to be transferred onto copy films. Paper identification labels are not recommended. The laterality and view marker should be placed at the location on the image near the axilla to facilitate proper orientation of the image.[7] A list of standardized abbreviations for mammography views is provided in Chapter 3. The screen identification number should be located opposite the chest wall side of the film so that it is not superimposed on the image (see Fig. 4–10A).

Additional recommended film labeling methods include a date sticker that can be easily read with overhead light, a record of the technical factors used to make the image, and the number (Roman numeral) of the mammography unit employed. Date stickers expedite sorting of examinations because they can be read with overhead light and often are color coded by year. A label with image technical factors may be useful for clinical image evaluation and performance of future examinations.

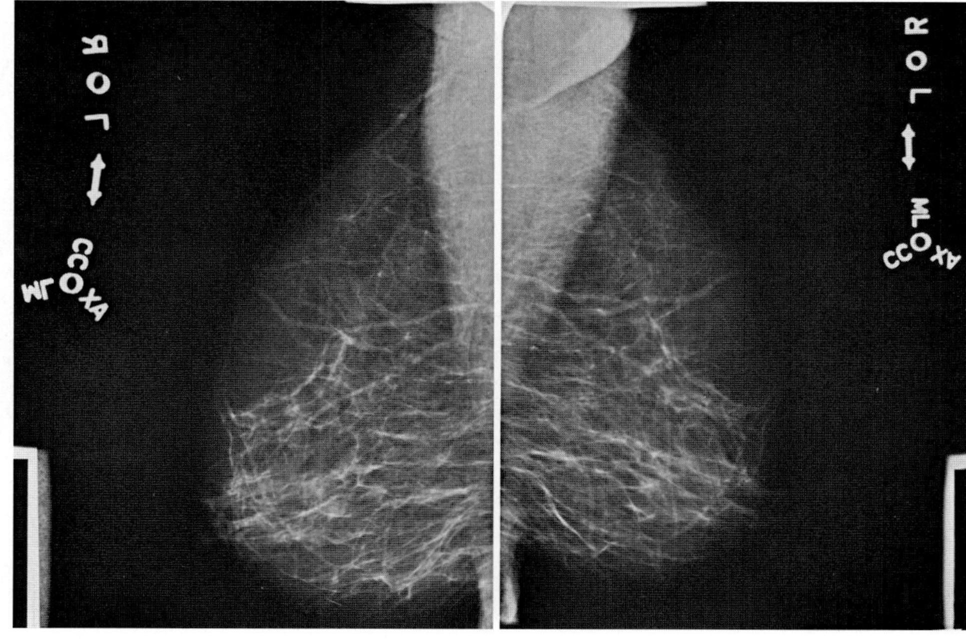

Figure 4–30. Confusion can result when facilities use eccentric labeling methods. In the system shown here, the laterality marker (L-R) and view marker (MLO-CC-AX) wheels were supposed to be rotated until the correct view and laterality were in direct opposition. The device results in the presence of both right and left laterality designations and three different view selections on every film. This was confusing to radiologists comparing these films with new mammograms. The system was apparently also confusing to the radiologic technologist spinning the wheels: The RMLO was incorrectly identified as "LCC"! One of the CC views was also labeled incorrectly.

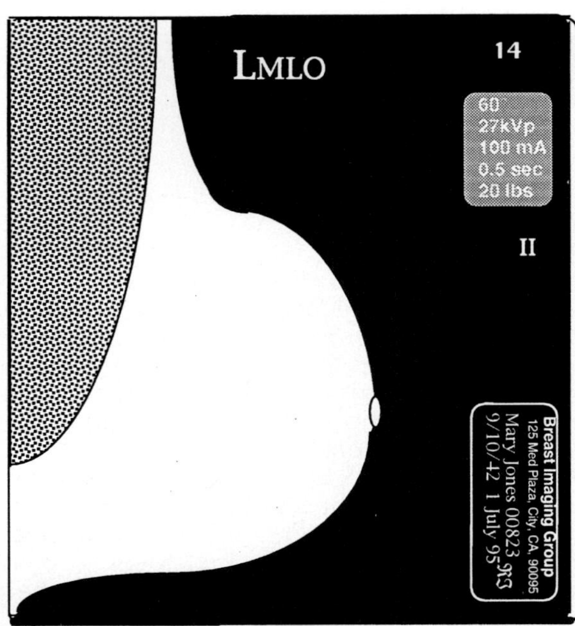

Figure 4–31. Recommendations for labeling of mammograms.

FULL-FIELD DIGITAL MAMMOGRAPHY: CLINICAL IMAGE EVALUATION

Procedures for clinical evaluation of images from full-field digital mammography (FFDM) units have been put in place in the ACR MAP. At least initially, clinical image evaluation will be based on submission of hard copy images. Each of these hard copy images must include the whole breast. In other words, tiled images of large breasts will not be accepted. The eight clinical image evaluation categories are the same as for film-screen mammography: positioning, compression, exposure, contrast, sharpness, noise, artifacts, and labeling. The ACR MAP radiologists who evaluate FFDM submissions must be qualified to interpret digital mammography in their practices and must interpret digital mammography on a regular basis. A pilot test conducted by the ACR revealed a failure rate for submitted digital mammograms essentially the same as that for film-screen mammography.

SUMMARY

Clinical image evaluation is an important quality control activity that should be performed on a daily basis by every radiologist who interprets mammograms. The radiologist's evaluation of the clinical images complements other quality assurance activities, such as phantom image evaluation. Ongoing feedback to the radiologic technologist about good quality or image deficiencies is recommended. Learning to recognize the most likely causes of image deficiencies expedites the rapid correction of problems and maintenance of high-quality procedures.

References

1. US Department of Health and Human Services, Food and Drug Administration: Mammography facilities—requirements for accrediting bodies and quality standards and certification requirements: Interim rules. 58 Federal Register No. 243, Tuesday, December 21, 1993.
2. Mammography Quality Standards Act of 1992, Publ L No 102-539.
3. Hendrick RE: Quality assurance in mammography: Accreditation, legislation, and compliance with quality assurance standards. Radiol Clin North Am 1992;30:243-255.
4. McLelland R, Hendrick RE, Zinninger MD, Wilcox PA: The American College of Radiology Mammography Accreditation Program. AJR Am J Roentgenol 1991;157:473-479.
5. Bassett LW, Hirbawi IA, DeBruhl N, Hayes MK: Mammographic positioning: Evaluation from the view box. Radiology 1993; 188:803-806.
6. Bassett LW, Farria DM, Bansal S, et al: Reasons for failure of a mammography unit at clinical image review in the American College of Radiology Mammography Accreditation Program. Radiology 2000;215:698-702.
7. American College of Radiology: Mammography Quality Control Manual. Reston, VA, American College of Radiology, 1999.
8. Eklund GW, Cardenosa G: The art of mammographic positioning. Radiol Clin North Am 1992;30:21-53.
9. Eklund GW, Cardenosa G, Parsons W: Assessing adequacy of mammographic image quality. Radiology 1994;190:227-307.
10. Helvie MA, Chan HP, Adler DD, Boyd PG: Breast thickness in routine mammograms: Effect on image quality and radiation dose. AJR Am J Roentgenol 1994;163:1371-1374.
11. American College of Radiology: Recommended Specifications for New Mammography Equipment. Reston, VA, American College of Radiology, October 1993.
12. Kimme-Smith C, Rothschild PA, et al: Mammographic film-processor temperature, development time, and chemistry: Effect on dose, contrast and noise. AJR Am J Roentgenol 1989; 152:35-40.
13. Curry TS, Dowdey JE, Murry RC: The radiographic image. In Curry TS, Dowdey JE, Murry RC (eds): Christensen's Physics of Diagnostic Radiology, 4th ed. Philadelphia, Lea & Febiger, 1990, pp 196-218.
14. Vyborny CJ, Schmidt RA: Mammography as a radiographic examination: An overview. Radiographics 1989;9:723-764.
15. Code of Federal Regulations, Title 21, Volume 8, Part 900, Subpart B, Section 900.12(e)(5)(vii).
16. Alter AJ, Kargas GA, Kargas SA, et al: The influence of ambient and viewbox light upon visual detection of low-contrast targets in a radiograph. Invest Radiol 1982;17:403-406.
17. Bassett LW, Jessop NW, Wilcox PA: Mammography film-labeling practices. Radiology 1993;187:773-775.

Chapter 5

Quality Control

Priscilla F. Butler

Quality control (QC) is defined as "the overall system of activities whose purpose is to provide a quality of product or service that meets the needs of the users; also, the use of such a system. The aim of quality control is to provide quality that is satisfactory, adequate, dependable, and economic."[1] Although the term quality assurance (QA) is often used interchangeably with QC, it has a broader meaning; quality assurance is "a system of activities whose purpose is to provide assurance that the overall quality control job is in fact being done effectively. The system involves a continuing evaluation of the adequacy and effectiveness of the overall quality control program with a view to having corrective measures initiated where necessary."[1] Quality control is an integral part of quality assurance. The definition of quality control for mammography that is used by the Agency for Health Care Policy and Research (AHCPR) is "The routine monitoring of performance and functioning of x-ray imaging and processing equipment."[2] That definition is the focus of this chapter.

Although the concepts of quality assurance and quality control were used by industry for some time, they were first applied to diagnostic radiology in the mid 1970s. A number of scientific papers were published then examining the benefits of implementing QC programs in terms of reduced radiation dose for the patient, improved image quality, and decreased facility costs.[3-6] Several film manufacturers introduced training programs in QC for their customers to ensure that they would obtain the best possible results. As far back as 1973, the Council of the American College of Radiology (ACR) approved resolutions encouraging quality imaging, quality assurance, and quality control by their membership.[7] In 1979, the U.S. Food and Drug Administration (FDA) published a recommendation that all diagnostic facilities implement quality assurance programs.[8] Several individuals and organizations published books and reports to serve as resources for diagnostic facilities implementing this new concept.[9-15]

In 1987, the ACR established the first voluntary, national program to accredit mammography facilities that demonstrated high-quality mammography. Dr. Gerald Dodd, MD, former Chairman of the ACR's Breast Task Force, recognized the need for a detailed instructional manual on quality control to aid facilities in achieving the necessary high quality for good patient care as well as accreditation. The ACR formed the Committee on Mammography Quality Assurance, chaired by R. Edward Hendrick, PhD, to develop the ACR's *Mammography Quality Control Manual*. The first version was published in 1990[16] as three separate manuals: one for the radiologic technologist, one for the medical physicist, and one for the radiologist. The ACR published an updated, single-manual version in 1992.[17] The 1992 Mammography Quality Standards Act (MQSA) significantly enlarged the impact of the ACR's QC manual. In 1993, the FDA's newly published interim rules for mammography facilities required them to conduct substantially the same QC tests and meet the performance criteria outlined in the 1992 manual.[18] The ACR revised the manual in 1994 to fit its new role as a regulatory document,[19] and the FDA adopted the 1994 manual by reference in a subsequent rule.[20] In 1997, the FDA published its final rule for mammography facilities, with specific details on required QC and performance criteria.[21] The ACR manuals were no longer referenced in the regulations. Consequently, in 1999,[22] the ACR's Committee on Mammography Quality Assurance modified the manual again to be consistent with the FDA's final rule requirements. Also, to encourage further improvements in image quality beyond the baseline standards set by the FDA, the manual recommends several additional tests and tighter performance criteria in some areas.

RESPONSIBLE INDIVIDUALS

Teamwork

Mammography QC takes a team approach. Officially, this team consists of radiologists (interpreting physicians), mammography technologists, and medical physicists. The team is often supplemented with the expertise of representatives and service personnel from x-ray equipment, film, and processor manufacturers. Under the FDA's final rule,[21] the facility must assign specific individuals to perform quality assurance and quality control activities who are qualified for their assignments and who will be allowed adequate time to perform these duties. The FDA's final rule spells out the regulated role of each official team member (Table 5–1), but in the hectic pace of health care today, many individuals do not realize the extent of their responsibilities.

All radiologists, medical physicists, and radiologic technologists working in mammography must meet the FDA-required minimum criteria for

Table 5–1. Quality Assurance (QA) Responsibilities of Mammography Personnel as Required by U.S. Food and Drug Administration (FDA)

Individual	Responsibilities
Lead interpreting physician	Has general responsibility to ensure that the QA program meets all FDA requirements Must ensure that individuals assigned to QA tasks are qualified to perform these tasks and that their performance is adequate
Reviewing (audit) interpreting physician	Must review and discuss the medical audit results with the other interpreting physicians (this may be the lead interpreting physician)
Interpreting physician	Follow the facility procedures for corrective action when asked to interpret images of poor quality Participate in the facility's medical outcomes audit program
Medical physicist	Must perform the facility's annual survey Must provide the facility with an annual survey report Is responsible for mammography equipment evaluations (when applicable)
Quality control technologist	Must be a qualified mammography technologist Responsible for all QA duties not assigned to the lead interpreting physician or the medical physicist. Normally, he/she is expected to perform these duties May assign other qualified personnel or may train and qualify others to do some or all of the tests Retains the responsibility to ensure that assigned duties are performed according to the regulations
Other personnel qualified to perform the QA tasks	Must have technical training appropriate for the assigned task(s) Training must be documented

qualification.[21] These requirements are summarized in Table 5–2. They apply to part-time or locum tenens staff as well. Mammography personnel should also be aware of the FDA's requirements for reestablishing qualifications if they no longer meet continuing education or continuing experience requirements.

Supervising Radiologist

The facility's supervising radiologist (or lead interpreting physician, as described in the FDA's final rule) has the responsibility for ensuring that all quality assurance requirements are met. He or she is ultimately responsible for the clinical image quality

Table 5–2. Summary of Mammography Personnel Qualifications as Required by the FDA

	Interpreting Physicians	Medical Physicist	Radiologic Technologist
Initial credentialing	Medical license *and* Certification by ABR, AOBR, or RCPS *or* Appropriate training (see text)	Certification by ABR or ABMP *or* State licensure *or* State approval	ARRT or ARCRT registered *or* State licensure
Initial training	60 hours Category I CME (40 hours if qualified before 4/28/99) 8 hours in each modality	Master's degree in physical science with 20 hours of physics and 20 hours of conducting surveys *or* If qualified before 4/28/99, BS in physical science with 10 hours of physics and 40 hours of conducting surveys 8 hours in each modality	If qualified after 4/28/99, 40 hours of training 8 hours in each modality
Initial experience	240 exams within 6 months of qualifying date *or* If board certified at first opportunity, 240 exams in any 6 months within last 2 years of residency	One facility and 10 mammography units *or* If qualified before 4/28/99 with BS in physical science, one facility and 20 units	If qualified after 4/28/99, 25 exams under direct supervision
Continuing experience	960 exams in 24 months	Two facilities and 6 mammography units in 24 months	200 exams in 24 months
Continuing education	15 hours Category I CME in 36 months (6 hours in each modality)	15 CEUs in 36 months (include training in each modality)	15 CEUs in 36 months (6 units in each modality)

ABMP, American Board of Medical Physics; ABR, American Board of Radiology; AOBR, American Osteopathic Board of Radiology; ARCRT, American Registry of Clinical Radiologic Technologists; ARRT, American Registry of Radiologic Technology; BS, bachelor of science degree; CEU, Continuing Education Units; CME, Continuing Medical Education in mammography; FDA, U.S. Food and Drug Administration; RCPS, Royal College of Physicians and Surgeons of Canada.

produced at the facility and the level of patient care provided. In addition, the supervising radiologist must ensure that the individuals he or she has assigned to conduct QA tasks are qualified to perform these tasks, have sufficient time to carry out these duties, and perform them adequately.

A single individual, who is an interpreting physician at the facility, must be designated as the supervising radiologist or lead interpreting physician; designating multiple lead interpreting physicians is not allowed and may lead to confusion. Although the supervising radiologist need not be on site, the ACR recommends that this individual review the QC technologist's results at least quarterly and the medical physicist's survey report annually to ensure that all required tests are being performed and that they meet minimum standards. The lead interpreting physician can easily document this by initialing the QC charts or report at the time of review.

Radiologist

The facility's radiologists (interpreting physicians) are an essential component of a strong QC program because they have an opportunity to evaluate the current clinical image quality with each film they interpret. In addition, by comparing current patient images with those done at the same facility the prior year (or with previous films taken at other facilities), radiologists can detect changes in quality over time.

The FDA's final rule requires all radiologists interpreting mammograms for the facility to follow the facility's procedures for taking corrective action when they are asked to interpret images of poor quality. An example of an appropriate procedure would be to provide written or verbal feedback to technologists on image quality parameters such as positioning, compression, optical density, contrast, patient motion, and technique factors. Radiologists typically have no problem providing timely feedback to technologists when they interpret the mammograms at the same site where the patients are imaged. However, this important feedback is often neglected when radiologists interpret images off site. Off-site radiologists should make special efforts to ensure that technologists receive appropriate and timely image quality critique to help improve their performance.

All radiologists interpreting mammograms must meet the following FDA requirements.[21]

Initial Qualifications. Every radiologist interpreting mammograms must:

- Be licensed to practice medicine.
- Be certified in diagnostic radiology by the American Board of Radiology (ABR), the American Osteopathic Board of Radiology (AOBR), or the Royal College of Physicians and Surgeons (RCPS) of Canada *or* have at least 3 months (2 months if initially qualified before April 28, 1999) of documented training in mammography interpretation, radiation physics, radiation effects, and radiation protection.
- Have 60 hours of documented Category I continuing medical education (CME) in mammography (40 hours if initially qualified before April 28, 1999), at least 15 of which must have been acquired in the 3 years immediately before the physician met his or her initial requirements.
- Have interpreted mammograms from examinations of 240 patients within the 6 months immediately prior to his/her qualifying date or in any 6 months within the last 2 years of residency if the physician becomes board certified at his or her first possible opportunity.
- Receive at least 8 hours of training in any mammographic modality (e.g., digital) for which he or she was not previously trained before beginning to use that modality.

Continuing Experience. Every radiologist interpreting mammograms must continue to interpret or multi-read at least 960 mammographic examinations over a 24-month period.

Continuing Education. Every radiologist interpreting mammograms must earn at least 15 hours of category I CME credit in a 36-month period, at least 6 of which must be related to each mammographic modality used.

Reestablishing Qualifications. Any radiologist who does not maintain the required continuing qualifications must reestablish his or her qualifications before resuming the independent interpretation of mammograms. A radiologist who does not meet the continuing experience requirements must either (1) interpret or multi-read at least 240 examinations under the direct supervision of an interpreting physician or (2) interpret or multi-read a sufficient number of examinations, under the direct supervision of an interpreting physician, to bring the total up to 960 examinations for the prior 24 months. These interpretations must be done within the 6 months immediately before the radiologist resumes independent interpretation. A radiologist who does not meet the continuing education requirements must obtain additional category I CME hours in mammography to bring the total up to the required 15 credits in the previous 36 months before resuming independent interpretation.

Medical Physicist

The medical physicist is responsible for performing the facility's annual survey. This includes evaluating the QC conducted by the facility's QC technologist as well as conducting the annual tests. Furthermore, the medical physicist must conduct a mammography equipment evaluation of the x-ray unit or film processors whenever a new unit or processor is installed, a unit or processor is disassembled and reassembled at the same or a new location, or major components of the unit or processor are changed or repaired. Although the medical physicist may not delegate these tests to unqualified individuals, he or she may directly supervise tests conducted by trainees.

Communicating survey and equipment evaluation results in a timely manner is an essential part of the medical physicist's responsibilities. The reports must eventually be in written form, but the physicist should either leave the facility a preliminary written report summary or provide a verbal summary immediately after completing the survey to reassure the facility that there are no problems or to allow the facility to quickly take corrective action.

In addition, "the medical physicist should be available to answer questions for the QC technologist carrying out the QC measurements listed" in the ACR Mammography QC Manual whenever problems are encountered. Radiologists and QC technologists should rely on the medical physicist as a resource for questions and problems regarding mammography image quality and quality control.

All medical physicists surveying mammography equipment must meet the following FDA requirements.[21]

Initial Qualifications. Every medical physicist who surveys medical equipment must:

- *Either* be licensed or approved by a state *or* be certified in Diagnostic Radiological or Imaging Physics by the ABR or the American Board of Medical Physics.
- Have a master's degree or higher in a physical science, 20 semester hours of physics, 20 contact hours of training in conducting surveys of mammography facilities, and experience in conducting mammography surveys of at least 10 units and at least one facility; *or*, if qualified before April 28, 1999, have qualified as a medical physicist under the interim regulations, and have a bachelor's degree or higher in a physical science, 10 semester hours of physics, 40 contact hours of training in conducting surveys of mammography facilities, and experience in conducting mammography surveys of at least 20 units and at least one facility.
- Have at least 8 hours of training with any mammographic modality (e.g., digital) before surveying units with that modality.

Continuing Experience. Every medical physicist who surveys medical equipment must survey at least two mammography facilities and a total of at least six mammography units within a 24-month period.

Continuing Education. Every medical physicist who surveys medical equipment must earn at least 15 CME hours or continuing education units (CEUs) in a 36-month period, including hours of training appropriate to each mammographic modality for which he or she provides physics services.

Reestablishing Qualifications. Any medical physicist who does not maintain the required continuing qualifications may not perform the surveys without the supervision of a qualified medical physicist. Before independently surveying another facility, the medical physicist must reestablish qualifications. Any medical physicist who does not meet the continuing experience requirement must complete a sufficient number of surveys under the direct supervision of a qualified medical physicist to bring the total surveys up to the required two facilities and six units in the previous 24 months. No more than one survey of a specific unit within a period of 60 days can be counted towards the total mammography unit survey requirement. Any medical physicist who does not meet the continuing educational requirements must obtain a sufficient number of continuing education units to bring the total units up to the required 15 in the previous 3 years.

Quality Control Technologist

The facility-designated QC technologist must be a qualified mammography technologist. She or he is responsible for conducting the daily, weekly, monthly, and semiannual QC tests. It is essential that this individual be given sufficient time to conduct these tests and take (or arrange for) appropriate corrective actions to address identified problems. Although a single designated QC technologist who has overall responsibility for routine QC generally allows for better management of the system, it is sometimes helpful to assign a backup QC technologist to cover the absence of the primary QC technologist. However, this backup person must be adequately trained to conduct and evaluate the tests in precisely the same way as the primary QC technologist in order to minimize artificial variations in results.

Normally, the QC technologist is expected to personally conduct each of the required QC tests. However, the FDA final rule allows the flexibility of assigning some QC tasks to other qualified individuals. For example, many hospitals designate a non-mammography technologist to conduct the processor QC testing and evaluation on each processor in the facility (both within and outside mammography). This practice is acceptable as long as (1) the individual is appropriately qualified and trained and (2) appropriate documentation of those qualifications and training are available. It is important to note, however, that the designated mammography QC technologist is responsible for ensuring that the tasks are done properly by standardizing test methodology, reviewing all data, overseeing repeat testing before calling the medical physicist or service personnel, and conferring with the radiologist and medical physicist.

All mammography technologists, including the quality control technologist, must meet the following FDA requirements.[21]

Initial Qualifications. Every mammography technologist must:

- Have general certification from the American Registry of Radiologic Technology or the American Registry of Clinical Radiologic Technologists *or* be licensed to perform general radiographic procedures in a state.
- Meet the mammography-specific training requirements by having at least 40 hours of documented training in mammography, including (1) training

in breast anatomy and physiology, positioning, and compression, QA/QC techniques, and imaging of patients with breast implants, (2) performance of a minimum of 25 mammography examinations under direct supervision of an appropriate MQSA-qualified individual, (3) at least 8 hours of training in the use of any mammographic modality (e.g., digital) before beginning to use that modality independently. (These criteria apply only to radiologists qualifying on after April 28, 1999.)

Continuing Experience. Every mammography technologist must perform at least 200 mammography examinations in a 24-month period.

Continuing Education. Every mammography technologist must earn at least 15 CEUs in a 36-month period that must include at least 6 CEUs in each mammographic modality used by the technologist in mammography.

Reestablishing Qualifications. Any mammography technologist who does not maintain the required continuing qualifications must reestablish her or his qualifications before performing unsupervised mammography examinations. A technologist who does not meet the continuing experience requirements must perform a minimum of 25 mammography examinations under the direct supervision of a qualified mammography technologist. Any technologist who does not meet the continuing education requirements must obtain a sufficient number of continuing education units in mammography to bring the total up to at least 15 in the previous 3 years, at least 6 of which must be related to each modality used by the technologist in mammography.

QUALITY CONTROL TESTS

The FDA clearly specifies the QC tests that must be performed on mammography equipment.[21] In the *1999 ACR Mammography Quality Control Manual*,[22] several additional tests are recommended to further address common image quality problems. These requirements and recommendations are summarized in Tables 5–3 and 5–4. Although performance of the recommended tests are *not required* for ACR accreditation, the ACR recommends that facilities follow the procedures and performance criteria outlined in the *1999* manual.

Table 5–3. FDA-Required and ACR-Recommended Mammographic QC Tests for Technologists

Test	FDA Required	Minimum Frequency	Required and Recommended Performance Criteria*	Time Frame for Corrective Action
Darkroom cleanliness		Daily	Few dust artifacts should appear on images.	
Processor QC	✓	Daily	Base + fog *must* be within ±0.03 of operating level. Mid-density and density difference *must* be within ±0.15 of operating level.	Immediately
Mobile unit QC	✓	Daily	Test *must* be passed each time unit is moved to a different location and before the unit is used on patients.	Immediately
Screen cleanliness		Weekly	Few dust artifacts should appear on images.	
Viewboxes and viewing conditions		Weekly	Marks on viewbox surfaces should be removed. Multiple-viewbox light should be uniform in color and intensity.	
Phantom images	✓	Weekly	Background optical density *must* be ≥1.20; the operating level should be ≥1.40. The density difference operating level should be ≥0.40. The 4 largest fibers, 3 largest speck groups, and 3 largest masses *must* be visible.	Immediately
Visual checklist		Monthly	Each item should function as appropriate.	
Repeat analysis	✓	Quarterly	Repeat rate should be <2% (or <5% if approved by radiologist and medical physicist). A change in rate of ±2% *must* be investigated.	Within 30 days of the test date
Analysis of fixer retention	✓	Quarterly	Residual fixer *must* be ≤0.05 g/m^2 (5 μg/cm^2).	Within 30 days of the test date
Darkroom fog	✓	Semi-annually	Fog *must* be ≤0.05.	Immediately
Screen-film contact	✓	Semi-annually	Large areas (>1 cm) of poor contact are unacceptable; cassettes with such areas *must* be repaired or removed from service.	Immediately
Compression	✓	Semi-annually	For initial power drive, maximum compression *must* be between 25 and 45 pounds.	Immediately

*Required criteria are designated by the use of *must*, and recommended criteria by the use of *should*.
ACR, American College of Radiology; FDA, U.S. Food and Drug Administration; QC, quality control.

Table 5–4. FDA-Required and ACR-Recommended Mammographic Annual Quality Control Tests for Medical Physicists

Test	FDA Required	Required and Recommended Performance Criteria*	Time Frame for Corrective Action
Mammographic unit assembly evaluation	✓	Systems with automatic decompression *must* have (1) override capability to allow maintenance of compression and (2) continuous display of the override status. Items that are hazardous or inoperative or that operate improperly should be repaired.	Within 30 days of the test date
Collimation assessment	✓	Both left + right and anterior + chest edge x-ray field–light field deviations *must* be ≤2% SID. X-ray field *must* not exceed any side of image receptor by >2% SID. X-ray field *must* not fall within chest wall side of image receptor. X-ray field should not fall within image receptor by >2% on the right and left sides or by >4% on the anterior side. Compression paddle edge *must* not extend beyond image receptor by >1% SID or appear on the image.	Within 30 days of the test date
Evaluation of system resolution	✓	For all focal spot sizes and anode materials: With the bars parallel to the anode-cathode axis, the system resolution *must* be ≥13 lp/mm. With the bars perpendicular to the anode-cathode axis, the system resolution *must* be ≥11 lp/mm.	Within 30 days of the test date
AEC system performance	✓	Over 2 to 6 cm, optical density *must* be maintained within ±0.15 of the mean. Over 2 to 8 cm and various modes, should maintain optical density within ±0.30 of the mean. Each density control step should result in a 12% to 15% change in mA or approximately a 0.15 increase in optical density.	Within 30 days of the test date
Uniformity of screen speed	✓	Density range (for same size cassette) *must* be ≤0.3.	Within 30 days of the test date
Artifact evaluation	✓	Artifacts *must* not be significant.	Within 30 days of the test date
Image quality evaluation	✓	Background optical density *must* be ≥1.20; the operating level should be ≥1.40. The density difference operating level should be ≥0.40. The 4 largest fibers, 3 largest speck groups, and 3 largest masses *must* be visible.	Immediately
kVp accuracy and reproducibility	✓	Measured kVp *must* be within ±5% of the indicated. Coefficient of variation *must* be ≤0.02 or ≤2%.	Within 30 days of the test date
Beam quality assessment (HVL)	✓	HVL (in mm Al) *must* be ≥ kVp/100. HVL (in mm Al) should be ≥ kVp/100 + 0.03. HVL (in mm Al) should be < kVp/100 + C (where *C* is 0.12 for Mo/Mo, 0.19 for Mo/Rh, 0.22 for Rh/Rh, and 0.30 for W/Rh).	Within 30 days of the test date
Breast exposure and AEC reproducibility	✓	Coefficient of variation for AEC reproducibility *must* be ≤0.05 or ≤5%.	Within 30 days of the test date
Average glandular dose	✓	Average glandular dose *must* be ≤0.3 rad (3.0 milligray) for a standard breast.	Immediately
Radiation output rate	✓	The radiation output rate at 28 kVp with Mo/Mo *must* be ≥800 mR/sec at any SID at which the system is designed to operate. System *must* be able to maintain this rate when averaged over 3 sec.	Within 30 days of the test date
Viewbox luminance and room illuminance		Viewbox luminance should be ≥3000 cd/m^2. Room illuminance should be ≤50 lux or preferably less.	

*Required criteria are designated by the use of *must*, and recommended criteria by the use of *should*.

ACR, American College of Radiology; AEC, automatic exposure control; cd, candela; FDA, U.S. Food and Drug Administration; HVL, half-value layer; kVp, kilovolt (peak); lp/mm, line pairs per millimeter; mm A1, millimeters of aluminum; Mo, molybdenum; QC, quality control; Rh, rhodium; SID, source-image distance; W, tungsten.

Although only minimum testing frequencies are specified in Tables 5–3 and 5–4, these tests should be performed whenever problems occur so that the causes may be identified before they affect clinical image quality or patient safety. In addition, if the QC program has just begun, the tests should be conducted more frequently for the first few months; this approach will give the QC technologist more experience in a shorter time and also provide better baseline data regarding the reliability of imaging equipment. Tests also should be conducted after service or preventive maintenance has been performed. It is particularly important that the processor QC test be performed any time the processor is serviced. The phantom image test should also be carried out at these times to test for processing artifacts.

The mammography facility must ensure that a medical physicist performs an equipment evaluation of the mammography unit and film processor at installation and conducts a complete survey at least annually. Under the FDA's final rule, the medical physicist is required to perform an equipment evaluation whenever a new unit or processor is installed, a unit or processor is disassembled and reassembled in the same or a new location, or major components of a mammography unit or processor equipment are changed or repaired (Table 5–5). The equipment evaluation must determine whether the new or changed equipment meets the applicable MQSA requirements for mammography equipment (Table 5–6) in addition to the applicable QC requirements for equipment (see Tables 5–3 and 5–4). All problems must be corrected before the new or changed equipment is put into service for examinations or film processing and before the facility may apply for accreditation of a mammography unit. In order to prevent scheduling delays, the facility should notify the medical physicist as soon as possible of upcoming equipment additions and changes so that an equipment evaluation may be scheduled immediately after installation

Table 5–5. Equipment Changes for Which Mammography Equipment Evaluations Are Required by the FDA*

Newly installed x-ray unit (even if used)
Newly installed processor (even if used)
X-ray unit or processor disassembled and reassembled at the same or new location
X-ray tube replacement
Collimator replacement
Filter replacement
Automatic exposure control replacement

*All problems must be corrected before the new or changed equipment is put into service for examinations or film processing.

Table 5–6. MQSA Requirements for Mammography Equipment

Feature	Requirement(s)	Rule Section	Effective Date
Motion of tube–image receptor assembly	The assembly shall be capable of being fixed in any position where it is designed to operate. Once fixed in any such position, it shall not undergo unintended motion.	3(i)	4/28/99
	This mechanism shall not fail in the event of power interruption.	3(ii)	4/28/99
Image receptor sizes	Systems using screen-film image receptors shall provide, at a minimum, for operation with image receptors of 18 × 24 cm and 24 × 30 cm.	4(i)	4/28/99
	Systems using screen-film image receptors shall be equipped with moving grids matched to all image receptor sizes provided.	4(ii)	4/28/99
	Systems used for magnification procedures shall be capable of operation with the grid removed from between the source and image receptor.	4(iii)	4/28/99
Beam limitation and light fields	All systems shall have beam-limiting devices that allow the useful beam to extend to or beyond the chest wall edge of the image receptor.	5(i)	4/28/99
	For any mammography system with a light beam that passes through the x-ray beam–limiting device, the light shall provide an average illumination of not less than 160 lux (15 ft-candles) at the maximum SID.	5(ii)	4/28/99
Magnification	Systems used to perform non-interventional problem-solving procedures shall have radiographic magnification capability available for use by the operator.	6(i)	4/28/99
	Systems used for magnification procedures shall provide, at a minimum, at least 1 magnification value within the range of 1.4 to 2.0.	6(ii)	4/28/99
Focal spot selection	When more than one focal spot is provided, the system shall indicate, prior to exposure, which focal spot is selected.	7(i)	4/28/99
	When more than one target material is provided, the system shall indicate, prior to exposure, the preselected target material.	7(ii)	4/28/99
	When the target material and/or focal spot is selected by a system algorithm that is based on the exposure or on a test exposure, the system shall display, after the exposure, the target material and/or focal spot actually used during the exposure.	7(iii)	4/28/99
Application of compression	Each system shall provide an initial power-driven compression activated by hands-free controls operable from both sides of the patient.	8(i)(A)	10/28/02
	Each system shall provide fine adjustment compression controls operable from both sides of the patient.	8(i)(B)	10/28/02

Continued

Table 5–6. MQSA Requirements for Mammography Equipment—cont'd

Feature	Requirement(s)	Rule Section	Effective Date
Compression paddle	Systems shall be equipped with different-sized compression paddles that match the sizes of all full-field image receptors provided for the system.	8(ii)(A)	4/28/99
	The compression paddle shall be flat and parallel to the breast support table and shall not deflect from parallel by more than 1.0 cm at any point on the surface of the compression paddle when compression is applied.	8(ii)(B)	4/28/99
	Paddles intended by the manufacturer's design to not be flat and parallel to the breast support table during compression shall meet the manufacturer's design specifications and maintenance requirements.	8(ii)(C)	4/28/99
	The chest wall edge of the compression paddle shall be straight and parallel to the edge of the image receptor.	8(ii)(D)	4/28/99
	The chest wall edge may be bent upward to allow for patient comfort but shall not appear on the image.	8(ii)(E)	4/28/99
Technique factor selection and display	Manual selection of mAs or at least one of its component parts (mA and/or time) shall be available.	9(i)	4/28/99
	The technique factors (kVp and either mAs or mA and seconds) to be used during an exposure shall be indicated before the exposure begins, except when AEC is used, in which case the technique factors that are set prior to the exposure shall be indicated.	9(ii)	4/28/99
	Following AEC mode use, the system shall indicate the actual kVp, and mAs (or mA and time) used during the exposure.	9(iii)	4/28/99
Automatic exposure control	Each screen-film system shall provide an AEC mode that is operable in all combinations of equipment configuration provided, e.g., grid, non-grid; magnification, non-magnification; and various target-filter combinations.	10(i)	4/28/99
	The positioning or selection of the detector shall permit flexibility in the placement of the detector under the target tissue. The size and the available positions of the detector shall be clearly indicated at the x-ray input surface of the breast compression paddle. [Note: This applies *only* to systems using screen-film image receptors.] The selected position of the detector shall be clearly indicated.	10(ii)	4/28/99
	The system shall provide means for the operator to vary the selected optical density from the normal (zero) setting.	10(iii)	4/28/99
X-ray film	The facility shall use x-ray film for mammography that has been designated by the film manufacturer as appropriate for mammography.	11	4/28/99
Intensifying screens	The facility shall use intensifying screens for mammography that have been designated by the screen manufacturer as appropriate for mammography and shall use film that is matched to the screen's spectral output as specified by the manufacturer.	12	4/28/99
Film processing solutions	For processing mammography films, the facility shall use chemical solutions that are capable of developing the film in a manner equivalent to the minimum requirements specified by the film manufacturer.	13	4/28/99
Lighting	The facility shall make special lights for film illumination, i.e., hotlights, capable of producing light levels greater than that provided by the viewbox, available to the interpreting physician.	14	4/28/99
Film masking devices	Facilities shall ensure that film masking devices that can limit the illuminated area to a region equal to or smaller than the exposed portion of the film are available to all interpreting physicians interpreting for the facility.	15	4/28/99

AEC, automatic exposure control; kVp, kilovolt (peak); MQSA, Mammography Quality Standards Act, Pub L No. 02-539; SID, source-image distance.

or modification and before the equipment is used for mammography.

Tests Performed by the Radiologic Technologist

Reaping the benefits of QC requires an investment of time. The mammography facility's supervising radiologist and management must give the QC technologist sufficient time each day to perform these important tests and evaluate their results. The approximate times needed to perform the QC tests are listed in Table 5–7.[23] Some of the technologist's QC tasks can be carried out simultaneously with other tests. For example, while waiting for the processor to warm up, the QC technologist can clean the darkroom and screens, check the viewbox and viewing conditions, review the visual checklist, or test the mammography unit's compression. Consequently, once an efficient routine is established, only a modest amount of time is required for a successful mammographic QC program.

Darkroom Cleanliness

For the production of high-quality clinical images, it is critical that artifacts on film images be minimized

Table 5–7. Amount of Time Required for Radiologic Technologist QC Tests

Nature of Procedure/Task and Minimum Performance Frequency	Time Required*
Daily	
Darkroom cleanliness	5 min
Processor QC	20 min
Weekly	
Screen cleanliness	10 min
Viewbox cleanliness	5 min
Monthly	
Phantom images	30 min
Visual checklist	10 min
Quarterly	
Repeat analysis	60 min
Analysis of fixer retention	5 min
Meetings with radiologist	45 min
Semiannually	
Darkroom fog	10 min
Screen-film contact	80 min
Compression	10 min
Total time for QC per year (5-day week)	160 hours

*Estimated times include setup, testing, and recording of results for a facility with two mammography units, one processor and 16 cassettes.
Adapted from Farria DM, Bassett LW, Kimme-Smith C, DeBruhl N: Mammography quality assurance from A to Z. Radiographics 14:371-385, 1994.

through maintenance of the cleanest possible conditions in the darkroom. The single-emulsion films that are currently in use for screen-film mammography are particularly sensitive to dust and dirt between the screen and film. Although the cause of the resulting prominent artifacts is obvious, the dust may degrade screen-film contact and produce image blurring, and the artifacts may mimic microcalcifications, leading to misdiagnosis. The QC technologist should minimize dust and dirt as much as possible.

Processor Quality Control

Processor QC procedures are designed to confirm and verify that the film processor and processor chemistry system are working in a consistent manner. Before conducting processor QC, the QC technologist should verify that the processor is performing consistently with the film manufacturer's specifications and then should establish baseline operating levels. This procedure should be carried out with new processors or whenever a significant change is made in imaging procedures (e.g., different film, a change in brand or type of chemicals, a change in processing workload). Once baseline operating levels are established, processor QC must be performed daily, at the beginning of the workday, before any patient films are processed but after the processor has warmed up. All levels falling outside the established performance criteria (described in Table 5–3) must be corrected before the processor is used to develop patient films.

Screen Cleanliness

The screen cleanliness procedure is similar to the darkroom cleanliness check, in that it ensures that mammographic cassettes and screens are free of dust and dirt particles that may degrade image quality or mimic microcalcifications.

Phantom Image

Routinely exposing a breast-simulating phantom and evaluating the image permits a facility to evaluate changes in image quality without exposing a patient to radiation. The phantom image test ensures that the film optical density, contrast (density difference), uniformity, and image quality due to the x-ray imaging system and film processor are maintained at optimum levels.

Darkroom Fog

Inappropriate darkroom safe-lights and other light sources inside and outside the darkroom can fog mammographic films. Fog reduces contrast. The darkroom fog test allows a facility to detect, identify, and eliminate the sources of fog that cannot be seen with the human eye.

Screen-Film Contact

Screen-film contact has a significant influence on image sharpness. Sharpness is essential in mammography for the detection of microcalcifications. The screen-film contact test ensures that optimum contact is maintained between the intensifying screen and film in each mammography cassette.

Compression

Appropriate compression is essential for high-quality mammography. Compression diminishes the thickness of tissue that must be penetrated by radiation, thereby reducing scattered radiation and increasing contrast, while limiting radiation exposure of the breast. Compression improves image sharpness by reducing the breast thickness, thereby minimizing focal spot blurring of structures in the image, and by minimizing patient motion. In addition, compression makes the thickness of the breast more uniform, resulting in more uniform image densities. The compression test determines whether the mammography system can provide adequate compression in both the manual and powered modes and ensures that the equipment does not allow too much compression to be applied.

Repeat Analysis

Repeating mammograms raises cost, decreases efficiency, and increases patient exposure. The repeat analysis allows the facility to determine the number and causes of repeated mammograms and rejected films so that problems may be identified and corrected.

Viewboxes and Viewing Conditions

Poor viewing conditions may impair the visibility of breast structures on even the highest-quality image. High ambient lighting and low viewbox brightness coupled with dirty viewbox surfaces can reduce the apparent contrast of films and obscure clinical information. Testing ensures that the viewboxes and viewing conditions are optimized and then maintained at an optimum level. If mammography technologists use a separate viewbox to check the density and quality of the mammography images and QC films, this viewbox should be similar to the reading viewbox in luminance and light color. In addition, the ambient lighting conditions should be similar to those used in the reading room.

Analysis of Fixer Retention in Film

Excessive residual fixer (thiosulfate, hyposulfite, or "hypo") can turn films brown and reduce their archival stability. This analysis determines the quantity of residual fixer in processed film.

Visual Checklist

The visual check ensures that the mammographic x-ray system's indicator lights, displays, mechanical locks, and detents are working properly and that the mechanical rigidity and stability of the equipment is appropriate.

Tests Performed by the Medical Physicist

Mammographic Unit Assembly Evaluation

The mammographic unit assembly evaluation ensures that all locks, detents, angulation indicators, displays, mechanisms, and mechanical support devices for the x-ray tube, compression device, and image receptor holder assembly are operating properly.

Collimation Assessment

If the x-ray field extends too far beyond the edges of the image receptor, the patient may be exposed to unnecessary radiation. If the x-ray field falls too far within the image receptor, breast tissue may be missed on the image, and the unattenuated light through large, unexposed portions of the film may degrade visibility of low-contrast structures. Collimation assessment ensures that that the x-ray field aligns with the light field, the collimator allows for full coverage of the image receptor by the x-ray field (but does not allow significant radiation beyond its edges), and the chest wall edge of the compression paddle aligns with the chest wall edge of the film.

Evaluation of System Resolution

The visualization of microcalcifications significantly depends on the resolving capability of a mammographic system. Therefore, the medical physicist evaluates the limiting resolution of the entire mammography system, including effects from geometric (focal spot) blurring and screen-film combination.

Automatic Exposure Control System Performance Assessment

A properly functioning automatic exposure control (AEC) system will allow the technologist to produce an appropriate and consistent film optical density for breasts of varying densities and thicknesses and with the use of various imaging modes. The performance of the mammography unit's AEC system should be assessed so that consistent image optical density can be maintained and optical density can be altered with the density control function.

Uniformity of Screen Speed

Variations among the speeds of intensifying screens can result in variations in image optical densities from cassette to cassette. The uniformity of the radiographic speed of image receptors routinely used for mammographic imaging therefore is assessed.

Artifact Evaluation

Excessive artifacts have the potential to obscure or mimic important clinical detail. Artifact evaluation assesses the severity and source of artifacts visualized on mammograms or phantom images so that they may be eliminated or minimized.

Image Quality Evaluation

Although the QC technologist performs an image quality evaluation weekly, the medical physicist is in the unique position to offer suggestions for image quality improvement on the basis of his or her experience evaluating phantom images from other units and facilities. In addition, the medical physicist can note changes that may have occurred from year to year. This evaluation allows the medical physicist to assess mammographic image quality and to detect temporal changes in image quality.

Accuracy and Reproducibility of Kilovolt (Peak)

Image contrast, exposure time, and patient exposure can be impacted by the selection and accuracy of the kilovolt (peak) (kVp). The medical physicist therefore ensures that the actual kVp is accurate (within ±5% of the indicated kVp) and that the kVp is reproducible, having a coefficient of variation equal to or less than 0.02.

Beam Quality Assessment (Half-Value Layer Measurement)

A low beam quality could be a cause for excessive radiation exposure; a high beam quality could be a cause of poor image contrast. Quality beam assessment ensures that the half-value layer of the x-ray beam is adequate.

Breast Entrance Exposure, Reproducibility of Automatic Exposure Control, Average Glandular Dose, and Radiation Output Rate

The medical physicist must also measure the typical entrance exposure for an average patient (approximately 4.2-cm compressed breast thickness; 50% adipose, 50% glandular composition), calculate the associated average glandular dose, assess short-term AEC reproducibility, and measure the air kerma (radiation output) rate.

Viewbox Luminance and Room Illuminance

The luminance of the viewboxes for interpretation or quality control of mammography images must be evaluated to ensure that they meet or exceed minimum levels, that the room illuminance levels are below prescribed levels, and that viewing conditions have been optimized.

Quality Control for Full-Field Digital Mammography Units

Full-field digital mammography (FFDM) is different from screen-film mammography in a number of ways. The detector is different, the image processing is different, and so is the QC. The FDA requires that the facility's QC technologist and medical physicist follow the QC procedures specified by the manufacturer of an FFDM unit. Although some of the tests specified by the various manufacturers are similar for different FFDM units, many are considerably different. Also different manufacturers specify different frequencies and performance criteria. The FDA final rule requires that facilities with FFDM units follow their manufacturer's current QA requirements.[24-26]

WHERE TO GO FOR HELP

High-quality mammography takes routine attention to producing quality mammograms, constant awareness of the performance of mammography equipment and chemistry, organizational skills, and, especially, knowing where to go for information and guidance. Currently a number of sources are available for help, whether one prefers reading information on paper, cruising the World Wide Web, or talking with an expert. This section summarizes some of the best sources:

Table 5–8 lists some of the governmental and organization contacts and has blanks for filling in contact information for specific mammography equipment and units. The QC technologist can photocopy the table, fill in contact names, addresses, and so on, and store it by the phone or computer so as to keep all essential QC contact information in one place.

Medical Physicists

The QC technologist should contact her or his medical physicist *first* whenever there are questions about how to perform or evaluate QC, if problems cannot be solved, or if they frequently reoccur. The medical physicist should serve as the facility's primary consultant on image quality.

Manufacturers' Representatives

Manufacturers' representatives or service personnel for the mammography unit, the film processor, the film, or the screen are typically specially trained to evaluate and address problems related to their products. Because it is sometimes difficult to identify the specific cause of a problem in a system that consists of many components, it may be useful to obtain the assistance of all the representatives at the same time. Many manufacturers maintain telephone "help" lines and Web sites to further assist customers.

Independent Consultants

Independent consultants in mammography may bring special expertise to the facility when researching specific issues such as problems with performance of QC or patient positioning.

Table 5–8. Contact Information for Quality Control Questions*

Source	Name	Phone Number	Web Site
Medical Physicist			
Mammography Unit Manufacturer			
Film and Screen Manufacturer			
Processor Unit Manufacturer			
Processor Service/Chemistry Company			
Consultant			
American College of Radiology	Mammography Accreditation Program Information Line	1-800-227-6440	www.acr.org
U.S. Food and Drug Administration	FDA Hotline	1-800-838-7715	www.fda.gov/cdrh/mammography

*This table may be photocopied and the relevant information filled in for each unit; the copy may then be kept by the telephone or computer for reference when questions arise.

The American College of Radiology's Mammography Accreditation Program

The ACR offers three sources of information and assistance with QC problems in mammography:

- *1999 ACR Mammography Quality Control Manual*: This "cookbook"-style manual[22] is the best source of information on how to perform and evaluate the QC tests required by the FDA and recommended by the ACR.
- The ACR Web Site (www.acr.org): This information-packed Web site is not for members only. The site contains Frequently Asked Questions, downloadable QC forms from the ACR's 1999 QC manual, information on stereotactic breast biopsy accreditation and breast ultrasound accreditation, the Breast Imaging Reporting and Data System (BI-RADS) lexicon, and the ACR's Breast Care Guidelines.
- The Breast Imaging Accreditation Information Line (800-227-6440): The phone line is staffed by experienced mammography technologists who can help with questions on accreditation, the FDA regulations, or other general mammography or QC issues.

U.S. Food and Drug Administration

The FDA also offers several resources for mammography QC.

- MQSA Web Site (www.fda.gov/cdrh/mammography): The FDA has developed an extremely useful and user-friendly Web site to help mammography facilities understand the current regulations and implement their requirements. Both the text of the MQSA and the Final Rule are available. Although no longer in print, the FDA had published a quarterly informative newsletter called *Mammography Matters*. Information about obtaining old issues is available on their Web site.
- The FDA's Policy Guidance Help System: This question-and-answer guidance document, updated several times a year, reflects the FDA's current thoughts on the regulations implementing the MQSA. Although it can be accessed directly though the FDA's Web site (www.fda.gov/cdrh/mammography), this system works best when downloaded to your own computer. (The FDA Web site has easy instructions for downloading.) The system is organized as a series of books or main topics.

SUMMARY

The radiologist, medical physicist, and mammography technologist, working together as a team, are the keys to providing optimum quality mammography images, which will ultimately give patients the best medical care possible.

References

1. Thomas W Jr: SPSE Handbook of Photographic Science and Engineering. New York, John Wiley & Sons, 1973.
2. Agency for Health Care Policy and Research: Quality determinants of mammography: Clinical Practice Guideline No. 13.

Rockville, MD, U.S. Department of Health and Human Services, 1994.
3. Trout ED, Jacobson G, Moore RT, Shoub EP: Analysis of the rejection rate of chest radiographs obtained during the coal mine black lung program. Radiology 1973;109:25-27.
4. Hall CL: Economic analysis of a quality control program. In Application of Optical Instrumentation in Medicine VI: Proceedings of the Society of Photo-Optical Instrumentation Engineers. 1977;127:271-275.
5. Patrylak J: Counting x-ray retakes reduces cost. Appl Radiol 1978;7:35-36.
6. Goldman L, Vucich JJ, Beech S, Murphy WL: Automatic processing quality assurance programs: Impact on a radiology department. Radiology 1977;125:591-595.
7. American College of Radiology: Digest of Council Actions. Reston, VA, American College of Radiology; 2001.
8. US Department of Health and Human Services, Food and Drug Administration: Quality assurance programs for diagnostic radiology facilities: Final recommendation. 44 Federal Register 71728-71740 (1979).
9. Gray JE: Photographic Quality Assurance in Diagnostic Radiology, Nuclear Medicine and Radiation Therapy. Volume I: The Basic Principles of Daily Photographic Quality Assurance. (HEW Publication [FDA] 76-8043.) Washington, DC, DHEW, 1976.
10. Hendee WR, Rossi RP: Quality Assurance for Radiographic X-Ray Units and Associated Equipment. (HEW Publication [FDA] 79-8094.) Washington, DC, DHEW, 1979.
11. Hendee WR, Rossi RP: Quality Assurance for Fluoroscopic X-Ray Units and Associated Equipment. (HEW Publication [FDA)] 80-8095.) Washington, DC, DHEW, 1980.
12. Gray JE, Winkler NT, Stears J, Frank ED: Quality Control in Diagnostic Radiology. Rockville, MD, Aspen Publishers; 1983.
13. National Council on Radiation Protection: Mammography—A User's Guide. (NCRP Report #85.) Bethesda, MD, National Council on Radiation Protection and Measurements, 1986.
14. National Council on Radiation Protection: Quality Assurance in Diagnostic Imaging. (NCRP Report #99.) Bethesda, MD, National Council on Radiation Protection and Measurements, 1988.
15. American Association of Physicists in Medicine (AAPM): Equipment Requirements and Quality Control for Mammography: AAPM Diagnostic X-Ray Imaging Committee Task Group # 7, College Park, Md, Report No. 29. 1990.
16. American College of Radiology. Mammography Quality Control Manual. Reston, VA, American College of Radiology; 1990.
17. American College of Radiology: Mammography Quality Control Manual. Reston, VA, American College of Radiology, 1992.
18. US Department of Health and Human Services, Food and Drug Administration: Mammography facilities—requirements for accrediting bodies and quality standards and certification requirements: Interim rules. 58 Federal Register 243 (1993).
19. American College of Radiology: Mammography Quality Control Manual. Reston, VA, American College of Radiology; 1994.
20. US Department of Health and Human Services, Food and Drug Administration: Quality standards and certification requirements for mammography facilities. 59 Federal Register 189 (1994).
21. American College of Radiology: Mammography Quality Control Manual. Reston, VA, American College of Radiology, 1999.
22. US Department of Health and Human Services, Food and Drug Administration: Quality mammography standards: Correction, final rule. 62 Federal Register 217 (1997).
23. Farria DM, Bassett LW, Kimme-Smith C, DeBruhl N: Mammography quality assurance from A to Z. Radiographics 1994;14:371-385.
24. GE Medical Systems Senographe 2000D QAP: Quality Control Tests for MQSA Facilities. Milwaukee, WI, QC Manual 2277390-100, Revision 3, 2001.
25. Fischer Imaging SenoScan Full Field Digital Mammography System Operator Manual, P-55933-OM Revision 1. Denver, August 2001.
26. Lorad Selenia Full-Field Digital Mammography System Quality Control Manual. Danbury, CT, December 2001.

The MQSA and the Accreditation Process

Priscilla F. Butler

The technical quality of mammography improved during the 1980s as conventional x-ray units were replaced with dedicated mammography systems. Grids were integrated with these dedicated systems, screen-film image receptors designed specifically for mammography were used, and xeromammography was phased out. In the mid-1980s, however, it became apparent that despite these technical advances, image quality and breast radiation dose from mammography varied greatly. Significant evidence of those problems came from the 1985 Nationwide Evaluation of X-ray Trends (NEXT) study that was conducted by the U.S. Food and Drug Administration (FDA) and the Conference of Radiation Control Program Directors (CRCPD).[1] This recognition led to the establishment of voluntary mammography quality standards through the American College of Radiology (ACR) Mammography Accreditation Program in 1987.[2] The Mammography Accreditation Program required a facility to perform a number of quality assurance activities and its personnel to meet certain qualification and continuing education standards. Furthermore, it required an evaluation of both phantom and clinical images produced in the facility by trained outside reviewers.

Several states passed legislation requiring mammography facilities to meet quality standards and submit to regular inspections by state radiation control inspectors.[3] In 1990, Congress passed legislation authorizing Medicare coverage of screening mammography; those facilities seeking Medicare reimbursement were required to register with the Health Care Financing Administration (HCFA) and meet quality standards similar to those of the ACR Mammography Accreditation Program.[4] Federal inspections of Medicare-registered screening facilities began in 1992.

THE MAMMOGRAPHY QUALITY STANDARDS ACT OF 1992

Recognizing the need for uniform national standards that would apply to both screening and diagnostic facilities, Congress passed the Mammography Quality Standards Act (MQSA) in 1992.[5] This Act, which became effective October 1, 1994, requires all mammography facilities to meet minimum quality standards for personnel, equipment, and recordkeeping, and to be certified by the FDA (or an FDA-approved state certifying body) in order to legally operate in the United States.

Requirements

The Act specifies the following eight requirements:

1. All mammography facilities must be accredited by private, nonprofit organizations or state agencies that have met both the standards established by the FDA for accreditation bodies and those that have been approved by the FDA. The MQSA requires a direct federal audit of the accreditation bodies through federal inspections by federal inspectors. It also requires that, as part of the overall accreditation process, actual clinical mammograms from each facility be evaluated for quality by the accreditation body.
2. A mammography facility physics survey, consultation, and evaluation must be performed annually by a qualified medical physicist.
3. An FDA-certified state or federal inspector must inspect mammography facilities annually. If state inspectors are used, the MQSA requires a federal audit of the state-inspected facilities.
4. Initial and continuing qualification standards for interpreting physicians, radiologic technologists, medical physicists, and inspectors must be established.
5. Boards or organizations eligible to certify the adequacy of training and experience of mammography personnel must be specified.
6. Quality standards for mammography equipment and practices, including quality assurance and quality control programs, must be established.
7. The Secretary of Health and Human Services (HHS) must establish a National Mammography Quality Assurance Advisory Committee (NMQAAC) to advise the FDA on issues including appropriate quality standards for mammography facilities and accreditation bodies.
8. Standards governing record-keeping for examinee files, requirements for mammography reporting, and examinee notification by physicians must be established.

In summary, from a mammography facility's point of view, MQSA requires three separate checks: *certification* by the FDA (or a state certifying body), *accreditation* by an approved body, and *inspection* by a state (or the FDA).

MAMMOGRAPHY QUALITY STANDARDS REAUTHORIZATION ACT OF 1998

Congress must periodically reauthorize the Act and its funding. The Mammography Quality Standards Reauthorization Act (MQSRA), signed by President Clinton in October 1998, made several significant changes that would affect mammography facilities.[6]

First, it included a requirement that "a summary of the written [mammography] report be sent to the patient [by the mammography facility] in terms easily understood by a lay person." This applies to every patient who undergoes mammography, not just self-referred patients. The intent of this law was to address women's concerns about breakdowns in communication that prevent timely and appropriate diagnosis and treatment of breast disease. Failure to comply with this reporting requirement would result in a citation by MQSA inspectors. Although the lay report need only be a summary, it must be in writing. It is important that any summary of abnormal results provide clear direction about the appropriate steps to be taken by the patient.

Second, the Secretary of HHS was instructed to conduct a demonstration project to study the effect of reducing the inspection frequency for compliant mammography facilities from annual to every other year. The FDA, in collaboration with the Conference of Radiation Control Program Directors, is currently conducting a program with 300 facilities to evaluate whether citation-free facilities can maintain their high standards without the scrutiny of annual inspections. FDA expects to have the final results of the demonstration project ready for publication in early 2005.

KEY PLAYERS IN THE MAMMOGRAPHY QUALITY STANDARDS ACT

The U.S. Food and Drug Administration

In 1993, the Secretary of HHS designated the FDA as the federal agency to implement the MQSA. The FDA's responsibilities are many; they include developing and promulgating the final standards; approving accrediting bodies; certifying all mammography facilities in the United States; training inspectors; inspecting facilities; evaluating the effectiveness of the program; and developing and implementing sanctions for noncompliant facilities. The MQSA program is administered by the Division of Mammography Quality and Radiation Programs of the FDA's Center for Devices and Radiological Health.

The State

A state's role can take many forms. The Act allows the Secretary of HHS to delegate inspections to a state agency, and most states have contracted with the FDA to do so. The Act also allows a state agency to apply to become an accrediting body. To date, four states are approved as accrediting bodies by the FDA: Arkansas, California, Iowa, and Texas. States may have stricter laws and regulations than the FDA, but if a state becomes an accrediting body, its regulations must be substantially similar to the MQSA regulations.

Finally, the Act allows the Secretary to authorize a state (upon application) to take on most of the FDA's roles in certifying mammography facilities within that state. The FDA has conducted a pilot test with Iowa and Illinois to serve as certifying bodies and, in 2002, issued final regulations allowing states to become certifying bodies.[7] Therefore, a state has the potential of serving not only as the inspecting organization but also as the accrediting body and certifying agency.

The Accrediting Body

Under MQSA, the accrediting body must have quality standards for both personnel and equipment that are equal to those established under MQSA. The accrediting body must review clinical images from each accredited facility not less than every 3 years and must conduct a random sample review of clinical images. It must ensure that these reviews are performed by qualified interpreting physicians who have no conflict of interest with the reviewed facility. The body must require an annual survey by a qualified medical physicist and must monitor and evaluate that survey.

The accrediting body must also make on-site visits annually to a sufficient number of facilities to evaluate the performance of its accreditation process. This body must develop a mechanism to investigate complaints, a system for reporting accreditation status to the FDA, and an adequate record-keeping system and must also maintain reasonable fees. The ACR is currently the only accrediting body that accredits mammography facilities nationwide. Arkansas, California, Iowa, and Texas currently perform accreditation only within their own jurisdictions.

The National Mammography Quality Assurance Advisory Committee

The NMQAAC was established to (1) advise the FDA on appropriate standards and regulations for facilities, accrediting bodies, and sanctions, (2) assist in developing procedures for monitoring compliance with MQSA quality standards, (3) assist in developing a mechanism to investigate consumer complaints, and (4) report on new developments in breast imaging that should be considered in the oversight of mammography facilities.

Furthermore, the Advisory Committee must determine the impact of the MQSA quality standards on access in rural areas and areas with a shortage of health professionals. It also must determine whether there will be an adequate number of qualified medical physicists after October 1, 1999, and assess the costs and benefits of compliance with MQSA. (The NMQAAC completed these studies prior to the implementation of the FDA's Final Rule and determined that MQSA would have little negative impact on access to mammography and that there were adequate qualified personnel to comply with MQSA.) The NMQAAC consists of 13 to 19 members, including radiologists, radiologic technologists, medical physicists, referring physicians, nurses, state radiation control personnel, and representatives from national breast cancer consumer health organizations.

THE INTERIM RULES

The Act required that all mammography facilities in the United States be certified before October 1, 1994. Recognizing the near impossibility of developing comprehensive regulations and providing initial certification of more than 10,000 mammography facilities within the same period, President Clinton signed legislation granting the FDA interim rule authority in 1993.

Because of the urgent public health need for national mammography standards, Congress decided to grant this interim rule authority rather than extend the deadline to develop standards. Under interim rule authority, the FDA could adopt appropriate existing standards from organizations such as the ACR and HCFA and from state regulations.

The FDA was not required to consult with the NMQAAC on the interim rules but was instructed to do so during the final rule-making process, as the Act stipulated. On December 21, 1993, the interim rules, entitled "Mammography Facilities—Requirements for Accrediting Bodies and Quality Standards and Certification Requirements," were published in the *Federal Register*.[8] The interim rules were divided into two subparts; the first dealt with accrediting bodies and the second with mammography facilities. They went into effect on February 22, 1994, and required that all facilities be certified by October 1, 1994.

MAMMOGRAPHY QUALITY STANDARDS: THE FINAL RULES

On April 3, 1996, the FDA published the proposed regulations for public comment.[9] Within the 90-day comment period, the FDA received approximately 1900 responses containing approximately 8000 individual comments from the health care community, state regulators, equipment manufacturers, and consumers. As a result, the FDA reworked the proposed rules to make them more performance based rather than proscriptive.

The final regulations for implementing the MQSA were released by the FDA on October 28, 1997.[10] In brief, the final rules established personnel requirements, clarified equipment standards, and shifted many of the proposed equipment requirements to performance outcomes in the quality assurance section of the regulations. Mammography facilities were also required to establish a system for communicating mammogram results and transferring the original mammograms at the request of the patient. The majority of the final regulations became effective on April 28, 1999. However, certain equipment regulations did not become effective until October 28, 2002. Some of the critical elements of the final rules are described in this section.

Requirements for Certification

To operate lawfully, a mammography facility must be MQSA certified as providing quality mammography services. In order to obtain an MQSA certificate, the facility must apply to an FDA-approved accrediting body. After the accrediting body decides to accredit the facility, the FDA (or state certifier) will issue a certificate to the facility or renew an existing certificate.

A new facility may apply for a provisional certificate. Effective for 6 months, the provisional certificate enables the facility to perform mammography and to obtain the clinical images needed to complete the accreditation process. A provisional certificate cannot be renewed, but a facility may apply for a 90-day extension of the provisional certificate.

To apply for a 90-day extension to a provisional certificate, a facility must submit to its accrediting body a statement of what the facility is doing to obtain certification as well as evidence that there would be a significant adverse impact on access to mammography in the geographic area served if such facility did not obtain an extension. The accrediting body forwards this request, with its recommendation, to the FDA (or state certifying body). If the FDA (or state certifying body) determines that the facility meets the criteria, a 90-day extension will be issued for a provisional certificate. A provisional certificate may not be renewed again beyond the 90 days.

A previously certified facility whose certificate has expired, that the FDA (or state certifying body) has refused to renew, or that the FDA (or state certifying body) has suspended or revoked may apply to have the certificate reinstated. The facility must contact its accrediting body and fully document its history as a previously provisionally certified or certified mammography facility. The FDA may issue a provisional certificate to the facility if the accrediting body determines that the facility has adequately corrected pertinent deficiencies. After receiving the provisional certificate, the facility may lawfully resume performing mammography services while completing the requirements for accreditation and certification.

Personnel Standards

Requirements for initial qualification, continuing education, and continuing experience for interpreting physicians, medical physicists, and radiologic technologists were also codified in the final rules. These requirements are summarized in Table 5–2.

Equipment

The final rules followed the direction set by the interim regulations in defining the practice of mammography as "radiography of the breast" using specifically dedicated equipment for the detection of breast cancer. However, the FDA excluded from the final regulations stereotactic and all other radiographic invasive procedures for localization and biopsy. Also exempted from the final regulations were investigational devices with an FDA-approved investigational device exemption (IDE). Table 5–6 summarizes the equipment requirements.

Medical Records and Mammography Reports

The final rules incorporate specific requirements related to reporting and record-keeping. The interpreting physician must prepare a written report containing the results of each examination in addition to the following information: the name of the patient and an additional patient identifier, the date of the examination, the name of the examination's interpreting physician, and an overall final assessment. The final assessment must be categorized in the report into one of the following categories: "negative," "benign," "probably benign," "suspicious," or "highly suggestive of malignancy." In cases in which no final assessment can be assigned because of an incomplete evaluation, the assessment must be labeled "incomplete: need additional imaging evaluation"; the reasons why no assessments can be made must be stated. This approach was primarily based on the ACR's 1993 Breast Imaging Reporting and Data System (BI-RADS) for reporting and tracking of mammography outcomes.[11] In 2003, the FDA approved alternative standards to allow "incomplete: need additional imaging evaluation and/or prior mammograms for comparison" and a new final assessment category of "known biopsy-proven malignancy" as described in the 2003 BI-RADS atlas.[12]

This written report, signed by the interpreting physician, must be provided to the patient's health care provider within 30 days of the date of the examination. If the assessment is "suspicious" or "highly suggestive of malignancy," reasonable attempts must be made to communicate this news to the health care provider (or his or her designee) as soon as possible.

The final rules also required that the facility send a written summary of the mammography report to the patient in terms easily understood by a layperson. This applies to every patient who receives a mammogram, not only self-referred patients. If the patient is self-referred and has not named a health care provider, the facility must also send a copy of the written report to the patient.

Current mammograms and records must be kept by the facility for at least 5 years. For a patient who has not had additional mammograms at the facility, the mammograms and records must be retained at least 10 years (or longer if required by state or local law). The mammograms may be retained as either hard copy (film) or as soft copy (if originally obtained as a digital image). However, if a facility ceases performing mammography and closes its doors, the FDA continues to hold the facility responsible for ensuring that there is a mechanism to release the films to the appropriate entity when requested. Finally, original film mammograms and copies of the reports must be transferred to the patient, another medical institution, or the patient's health care provider if requested by the patient. At this time, the FDA requires facilities with full-field digital mammography units to have the capability of providing the original mammograms on film.

Quality Assurance Standards

The final rules address equipment quality control in great detail. These are described in Chapter 5. In addition, the rules specify that each facility establish and maintain a mammography medical outcomes audit program to follow up positive mammogram assessments and to correlate pathology results with the interpreting physician's findings (see Chapter 8).

Mammographic Procedures and Techniques for Patients with Breast Implants

The final rules specify that facilities have a procedure in place to inquire whether or not patients have breast implants and use appropriate views to maximize the visibility of breast tissues of patients who do.

Consumer Complaint Mechanisms

A serious complaint is defined by the FDA as "a report of a serious adverse event," which means an "adverse event that may significantly compromise clinical outcomes or an adverse event for which a facility fails to take appropriate corrective action in a timely manner." Examples of serious adverse events include: poor image quality, missed cancers, the use of personnel that do not meet the applicable requirements of the regulations, and failure to send to the appropriate person(s) mammography reports or lay summaries within 30 days.[10] Facilities must have a written system for collecting and resolving consumer complaints and must maintain records of each serious complaint for at least 3 years. If a facility cannot resolve a serious consumer complaint to the satisfaction of the patient, the facility must report the complaint to its accrediting body as soon as possible.

AMERICAN COLLEGE OF RADIOLOGY MAMMOGRAPHY ACCREDITATION PROGRAM

The ACR is a professional society whose purpose is to improve the health of patients and society by maximizing the value of radiology and radiologists by advancing the science of radiology, improving radiologic service to the patient, studying the socioeconomic aspects of the practice of radiology, and encouraging improved and continuing education for radiologists and allied professional fields. Through its professional committees, the ACR has developed and implemented nine modality-specific accreditation programs since 1987 to encourage the use of high-quality imaging and radiologic procedures in medicine.[13]

In 1994, the FDA approved the ACR as an accrediting body under MQSA. The ACR is the country's oldest and largest accrediting body for mammography and accredits more than 90% of the mammography facilities in the United States as well as a number of facilities in other countries. Initially developed in 1987 by the ACR Task Force on Breast Cancer, the ACR program is currently directed by the Committee on Mammography Accreditation of the Commission on Quality and Safety. The ACR Mammography Accreditation Program offers radiologists the opportunity for peer review and evaluation of their facility's staff qualifications, equipment, quality control and quality assurance programs, image quality, breast radiation dose, and processor quality control. The requirements for accreditation are identical or equivalent to those in the FDA final rules.

Application for Accreditation

A new mammography facility must apply for accreditation on all active mammography units. Furthermore, a new facility must apply for accreditation even if it is to be opened with a previously accredited unit from a sister facility. The ACR mammography accreditation procedure is summarized by the flow chart shown in Figure 6–1. The facility must first complete an entry application to provide basic facility, equipment, and personnel information and must submit a summary of the pass or fail results from their medical physicist's Equipment Evaluation along with an application fee. No clinical or phantom images are submitted at this time.

If a facility fulfills the criteria evaluated for the entry application, the FDA (or state certifying body) is notified, and a provisional certificate is issued. The ACR then sends a full application with the appropriate testing materials to the facility to obtain information on the qualifications of radiologists, medical physicists, and radiologic technologists; quality control results; and other requirements of the MQSA. Image quality and dose evaluations are an important part of the process and are evaluated through the use of a specially designed breast phantom and thermoluminescent dosimeter (TLD). The facility must submit an image of the phantom as well as two sets of normal clinical films (one from a patient with fatty breasts and one from a patient with dense breasts), which will be scored by a review panel of ACR-trained mammography medical physicists and radiologists. Finally, processor (or laser film printer) quality control for a 30-day period must also be submitted for evaluation. Facilities must send all application and testing materials to the ACR within 45 calendar days of the date the full application was mailed.

Final Reports

When all stages of the evaluation are completed, the ACR issues a final report to the lead interpreting physician that contains specific assessments and recommendations. (The facility's original images are also returned with the report.) Every facility that successfully meets all of the criteria is awarded a 3-year accreditation certificate and a unit decal for each approved mammography unit. The ACR notifies the FDA (or state certifying body) of each unit's accreditation approval so that the body may issue the facility a 3-year MQSA certificate. Because the FDA (and state certifying bodies) certify facilities rather than units, each accredited unit within the facility must have the same expiration date, regardless of when it was accredited. The MQSA certificate has the same expiration date as the ACR accreditation expiration. The ACR lists each accredited facility on its Web site (www.acr.org).

For those facilities that do not meet the ACR's accreditation criteria, specific recommendations for improvement are made. These recommendations provide guidance so that a facility can meet the criteria after corrective action and re-application. Facilities may appeal any denial of accreditation (Table 6–1). The ACR strongly recommends that facilities take out of service any unit that fails to meet all of the accreditation requirements after two consecutive attempts. The unit may reinstate only after the facility submits a corrective action plan to the ACR, the ACR approves it, and the facility completes it. The FDA (or state certifying body) will provide the reinstating facility with a 6-month provisional MQSA certificate so that there is adequate time to complete the accreditation process.

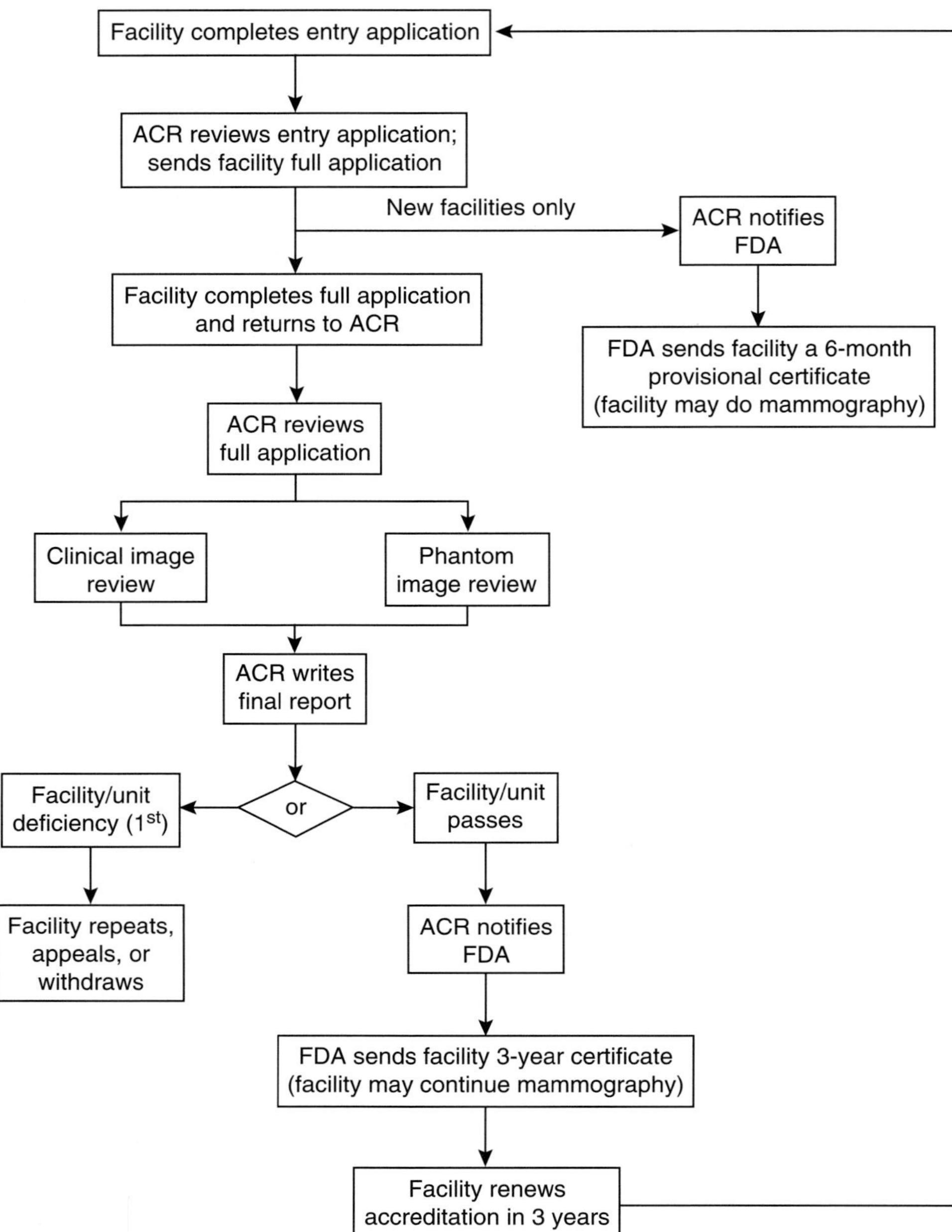

Figure 6–1. Mammography accreditation process of the American College of Radiology (ACR). FDA, U.S. Food and Drug Administration.

Renewal of Accreditation

The ACR sends a renewal application by mail to the accredited facility's lead interpreting physician approximately 8 months before the expiration of ACR accreditation. The renewal application process is the same as the process for new facilities.

New Units

When a facility installs a new unit (or a previously used or accredited unit that is new to the facility) after accreditation has been granted, the facility should contact the ACR for appropriate instructions. The FDA requires that all active mammography units be accredited. Furthermore, every facility must have an Equipment Evaluation performed by a qualified medical physicist and must submit the results to the ACR whenever a new unit is installed and before it is used for patient examination. All problems must be corrected, and documentation of correction provided to the ACR, before the new equipment is put into service.

If the facility has more than 13 months left on its current accreditation when the unit is installed, the ACR will ask the facility to complete a New Unit Addendum and submit a reduced fee. Facilities with new units that are applying in midcycle in this

Table 6–1. How a Mammography Facility Should Proceed if Accreditation Is Not Granted

Attempt at Accreditation	Accreditation Result	Facility Options
First	*NOT GRANTED:* First deficiency Facility may continue performing mammography with the unit as long as facility has a valid MQSA certificate	*REPEAT* testing for unacceptable area(s) (only if more than 60 days on MQSA certificate), *APPLY FOR REINSTATEMENT* by retesting all areas (if 60 days or less on MQSA certificate), *APPEAL* decision on original images, or *WITHDRAW*
Second	*NOT GRANTED:* Second deficiency = first failure ACR strongly recommends that the facility cease performing mammography with the unit	*APPLY FOR REINSTATEMENT* (after corrective action) by retesting all areas, *APPEAL* decision on original images, or *WITHDRAW*
Third	*NOT GRANTED:* Third deficiency = second failure ACR strongly recommends that facility cease performing mammography with the unit	*APPLY FOR REINSTATEMENT* after participating in Scheduled On-Site Survey, *APPEAL* decision on original images, or *WITHDRAW*

ACR, American College of Radiology; FDA, U.S. Food and Drug Adninistration; MQSA, Mammography Quality Standards Act.

manner will need to submit testing results only for the new unit (phantom image, dosimeter, clinical images, processor quality control, and the medical physicist's Annual Survey report) rather than the full application. Once accreditation is approved for that unit, its expiration date is the same as the expiration date for the other units at the facility (or the same as the expiration date of the unit it replaced).

If the facility has less than 13 months left on its accreditation when a new unit is installed, the ACR will instruct the facility to begin early renewal of accreditation on all units at the usual renewal fee. Once accredited, the new expiration date for all units will be the old expiration date plus 3 years.

Full-Field Digital Mammography Accreditation

The FDA approved the ACR to accredit GE Senographe 2000D full-field digital mammography (FFDM) units beginning February 15, 2003, the Fischer SenoScan beginning August 15, 2003, and the Lorad Selenia beginning September 15, 2003. At this time, the ACR accepts only hard-copy images for accreditation.

Once an accrediting body is approved for an FFDM unit, the FDA no longer accepts applications to extend existing MQSA certificates to include their use. All new applicants with such units must contact the ACR and apply for the accreditation of the units. Until FDA-approved accreditation is available for FFDM units other than the ones specified above, applicants must continue to apply to and be approved by the FDA for extension of their certificate in order to legally operate those digital units.

Quality Control

Each facility must submit documentation of compliance for all quality control tests as part of the application process. Documentation for the technologist testing must be provided on the Mammography Quality Control Checklist; documentation of the medical physicist Annual Survey results must be submitted on the Medical Physicist Mammography QC Test Summary (or in a similar format). These forms may be copied from the *1999 ACR Mammography Quality Control Manual*[14] or downloaded from the ACR Web site (www.acr.org). The radiologic technologist and medical physicist may use a different format for their in-house documentation of quality control, if they choose. Facilities must also submit processor (or laser film printer) quality control records for a 30-day period for evaluation with the clinical and phantom images.

Phantom Images and Radiation Dose

Image quality, radiation dose, and half-value layer are evaluated using thermoluminescent dosimeters and a specially designed breast phantom. The Lucite breast phantom with a wax insert containing fibers, specks, and masses simulates a 4.2-cm-thick compressed breast (Table 6–2).

A review panel of ACR-trained medical physicists scores the phantom image, which must meet the standards set by the Committee on Mammography Accreditation for the visualization of fibers, specks, masses, and artifacts. The four largest fibers, the three largest speck groups, and the three largest masses must be visualized in order for the image to pass. The ACR evaluation criteria are outlined in the *1999 ACR Mammography Quality Control Manual.*

Facility mammography personnel must expose the dosimeter on the phantom at the same time the accreditation image is produced. The dosimeter data are used to determine the average glandular dose for a breast of average size and density. The average glandular radiation dose may not exceed 300 mrad (3 mGy) per view.

Table 6–2. Sizes for Phantom Test Object of Mammography Unit

Fibers (mm diameter)	Specks (mm diameter)	Masses (mm thick)
1.56	0.54	2.00
1.12	0.40	1.00
0.89	0.32	0.75
0.75	0.24	0.50
0.54	0.16	0.25
0.40		

Clinical Images

The facility must submit two sets of negative clinical images (one from a patient with fatty breasts and one from a patient with dense breasts), which are scored by a review panel of ACR-trained radiologists. Each set of four clinical images must consist of two views, a craniocaudal (CC) view and a mediolateral oblique (MLO) view of the left and right breast of each patient. The parameters that are scored on the clinical images are positioning, compression, exposure level, sharpness, contrast, noise, exam identification, and artifacts. Clinical images should be examples of the facility's best work and are judged accordingly by the review panel. A Clinical Image Evaluation guide describing these eight parameters is available in the *1999 ACR Mammography Quality Control Manual.* Facilities may not submit images from models or volunteers.

Validation Procedures

Annual Updates

The ACR mails each accredited facility an annual update package to complete and return in order to verify that the facility is maintaining consistent quality during the 3-year accreditation period. Each accredited facility is required to submit a recent medical physicist's Annual Survey report summary for each unit and an update of the application data, identifying changes in address or certain personnel as part of this annual update.

Validation Film Checks

Under MQSA, the ACR is required to conduct "random clinical image reviews of a sample of facilities to monitor and assess their compliance with standards established by the body for accreditation." The ACR Committee on Mammography Accreditation has also specified that this accreditation program validation provide facilities with midcycle educational feedback on image quality.

The ACR recognizes that clinical images selected for this evaluation may be drawn from a relatively small sample of films in relation to the total number of mammograms performed at the facility. Furthermore, variations in clinical image quality may be attributed to the natural anatomical differences present in the female population. The ACR reviewers take these issues into consideration during their evaluation of validation film check images. The ACR provides a written report when the review is complete.

On-Site Surveys

The ACR Mammography Accreditation Program is required to conduct on-site surveys on a random sample of accredited facilities. These surveys validate

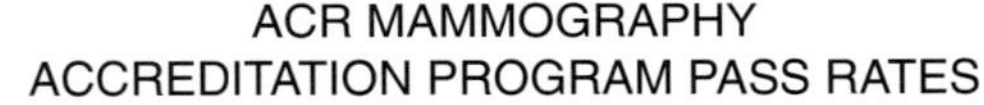

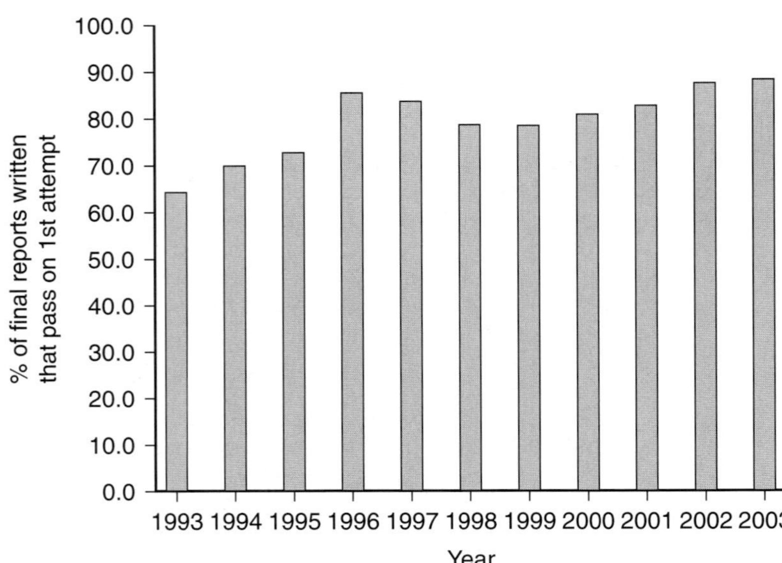

Figure 6–2. Pass rates for facilities participating in the American College of Radiology's Mammography Accreditation Program.

information submitted for accreditation and give facilities an educational opportunity through constructive criticism for quality improvement from direct interaction with the ACR reviewers. Any facility chosen for an on-site survey is notified in advance. Radiologist and medical physicist reviewers from the Mammography Accreditation Program serve as members of the survey team along with an ACR staff person. During this survey, the site visit team (1) reviews the quality assurance program, (2) reviews mammography policies and procedures, (3) reviews personnel qualifications, (4) reviews the facility's clinical images and mammography reports, and (5) works with the facility's staff to acquire and evaluate a phantom image along with a dose assessment of the x-ray unit.

SUMMARY

The quality of mammography performed in the United States has significantly improved since the ACR's accreditation program began in 1987 and Congress passed MQSA in 1992. In 1993, only 64.5% of mammography units applying for accreditation passed on their first attempt. Ten years later, 88.3% of units applying for (or renewing) accreditation passed on their first attempt (Fig. 6–2). This finding clearly illustrates the positive effects of the ACR Mammography Accreditation Program and the Mammography Quality Standards Act on the public health.

References

1. Conway BJ, McCrohan JL, Rueter FG, Suleiman OH: Mammography in the eighties. Radiology 177:335-339.
2. Hendrick RE, Haus AG, Hubbard LB, et al: American College of Radiology accreditation program for mammographic screening sites: Physical evaluation criteria. Radiology 1987; 165(P):209.
3. Hendrick RE: Quality assurance in mammography: Accreditation, legislation and compliance with quality assurance standards. Radiol Clin North Am 1992;30:243-255.
4. US Department of Health and Human Services (DHHS), Health Care Financing Administration, Medicare Program: Medicare coverage of screening mammography. 42 CFR Parts 405, 410, 413, and 494; 55 Federal Register 53510-53525 (1990).
5. Mammography Quality Standards Act of 1992, Publ L No 102-539.
6. Mammography Quality Standards Reauthorization Act of 1998, Publ L No105-248.
7. US Department of Health and Human Services, Food and Drug Administration: State certification of mammography facilities. 67 Federal Register 5446-5469 (2002).
8. US Department of Health and Human Services, Food and Drug Administration: Mammography facilities—requirements for accrediting bodies and quality standards and certification requirements: Interim rules. 58 Federal Register No.243, Tuesday, December 21, 1993.
9. US Department of Health and Human Services, Food and Drug Administration: Mammography quality standards: Proposed rules. 61 Federal Register 14855-14920 (1996).
10. US Department of Health and Human Services, Food and Drug Administration. Quality mammography standards: Final rule. 62 Federal Register 55852-55994 (1997).
11. American College of Radiology: Breast imaging reporting and data system (BI-RADS). Reston, VA, American College of Radiology, 1993.
12. American College of Radiology: Breast imaging reporting and data system (BI-RADS). Reston, VA, American College of Radiology, 2003.
13. American College of Radiology: Digest of Council Actions. Reston, VA, American College of Radiology, 2001.
14. American College of Radiology: Mammography Quality Control Manual. Reston, VA, American College of Radiology, 1999.

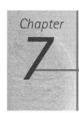

Reporting and Communication

Carl J. D'Orsi

Communication among health professionals and the people for whom they care plays a critical role in the delivery of health care, influencing the quality of care and its outcomes. Effective communication during the delivery of breast imaging services starts when a woman or her health care provider contacts an imaging facility to schedule a mammogram and ends with the tracking, monitoring, and follow-up of the patient. Strong lines of communication and clarification of the responsibilities of the referring provider, the personnel of the imaging facility, and the woman must be established at the outset and should continue through the entire imaging and reporting process. Effective communication is an essential part of quality assurance and risk management, promoting satisfaction among the women served, ensuring compliance with follow-up and long-term screening recommendations, and minimizing physician-patient conflict and the potential for malpractice claims.[1-3]

The very nature of the delivery of mammography services, especially screening mammography, is unique. Breast imaging, particularly screening mammography, is usually performed on healthy women who seek mammography as part of their regular regimen of health maintenance. The delivery of breast imaging services involves a host of health care professionals and support staff—the referring physician or referring health care provider, interpreting physician, pathologist, surgeon, radiologic technologist, radiologic physicist, nurse, and receptionist. Because many women receive their primary care from nonphysicians, such as nurses, nurse practitioners, and physicians' assistants, the term *health care provider* is used in this chapter to refer to all professionals who deliver primary care and who refer women for mammography.

Mammography, like any screening or diagnostic examination, has its limitations. Screening may have adverse consequences:

- The screening may fail to detect breast cancer.
- Normal mammographic findings may result in delay of appropriate care even when clinical signs of an abnormality are seen.
- Mammograms may be interpreted inaccurately.
- Mammography results and recommendation may not be received, or, if received, the recommendation may not be followed.
- A painful mammography experience may discourage a woman from participating in regular screening.

Optimal screening and diagnostic mammography mandates carefully designed policies of clinical practice and training for all personnel. Consistent implementation of activities to promote effective communication at each step of the process is imperative. The proliferation of mobile mammography facilities and the rapidly growing number of self-referred patients underscore this need.

Ideally, mammography is a partnership among the referring provider, the imaging facility and its personnel, and the woman. Effective communication lies at the core of this concept. Health care provider expertise does not automatically include the ability to elicit subjective information about patient values, needs, or sensitivities. In addition, a woman may not recognize the importance of combining mammography with a clinical breast examination, the need to convey her previous medical history and clinical signs and symptoms to the imaging personnel, or even the need to follow the recommendations of the interpreting physician. To combat potential misunderstanding by the patient, specific communication efforts must be made at every stage of the mammography process. Good communication at one stage increases the probability of improved communication at the next, with an enhanced opportunity to achieve early detection and effective treatment of breast cancer.

INITIAL CONTACT AND ACTIVITIES BEFORE THE EXAMINATION

A woman's initial contact with an imaging facility is usually through its support personnel, such as a scheduler or receptionist.[4] It is at this time that the interpersonal relationships by which care is delivered are first established.[1] Communication during the initial contact facilitates the identification of special needs related to language barriers or physical disability for which accommodations must be made throughout the examination, reporting, and follow-up processes.

A woman may be referred or scheduled for mammography by her referring health care provider. She may have a personal physician or other health care provider but request an appointment herself. Alternatively, she may not have a personal health care provider but may initiate her own appointment (self-referral). The patient's referral status should be determined when the appointment is made. The name, address, and telephone number of the woman's health care provider and the date when she was last seen by the provider should be obtained. Imaging facility personnel may wish to call the health care provider to confirm that the woman is the provider's patient. In addition, information about prior breast problems, surgery, abnormal mammograms, or cyclical pain should be obtained so that the woman can be appropriately scheduled for either screening or diagnostic mammography. Use of a standard scheduling form ensures that these inquiries are made of every patient by the imaging facility scheduler or other personnel (Fig. 7–1).

Information about the approximate length of the mammography visit, appropriate dress, and instructions not to use antiperspirants[5] or cosmetics near the area of the breasts should be given to the woman or referring provider by the scheduler when the appointment is made. Schedulers should also ask the woman to bring prior mammography films to the examination being scheduled. This exchange of information may help to ease any anxiety the woman may be experiencing and improves the quality of the examination.

When the woman actually comes for the examination, a clinical history questionnaire can be completed by her or by the mammography facility personnel (Fig. 7–2). This inquiry facilitates choosing the appropriate mammography examination and elicits information that may affect its interpretation. Receptionists may also give the woman a fact sheet on mammography, its limitations, and the importance of breast self-examination and clinical breast examination. The woman should also be informed, by facility personnel such as the receptionist or radiologic technologist, how much time it will take for her to receive the results of her examination and that if prior mammograms are needed for comparison, the report may be delayed. She should be instructed to call the facility or her health care provider if she does not receive the results within the stated time period or if she does not understand the results she has received. This step serves as an additional check on communication between the woman, her health care provider, and the imaging facility to ensure that the communication loop is not broken. It also reinforces the point that the woman has a responsibility for ensuring that she receives the results of her examination and understands the recommendations. However, except for the self-referred patient, the primary responsibility for communication of results to the patient rests with the referring health care provider.

The woman should also sign a release form for previous mammograms so that the facility can obtain them for comparison with the new examination (Fig. 7–3). The woman should leave the mammography facility satisfied that her questions have been answered and knowing the means by which the results of her examination will be communicated to her.

THE MAMMOGRAPHY EXAMINATION

The initial interaction between the woman and the scheduler or receptionist typically is followed by the mammography examination. The radiologic technologist's interaction with the woman expands on the initial communication bond established by the facility personnel and, in addition to facilitating a technically proficient examination, can contribute substantially to making the woman's examination a positive experience.

Before the examination, the technologist or technologist aide should confirm that the clinical history is complete. This information should be supplemented by any breast signs that the technologist observes, such as lumps, scars, or skin abnormalities, or by additional information from the woman (e.g., breast surgery).

Before the examination has begun, the technologist should explain to the woman, clearly and simply, what to expect.[4] This includes the views to be taken, the possible need for additional views, and the reasons why compression is required (i.e., to lower the radiation dose and improve image detail).[4] Simple, straightforward techniques such as making eye contact and pausing periodically to ask the woman whether she has any questions can help reassure her.

Education about breast compression decreases the likelihood that pain will adversely affect the performance of the examination. The anticipation of pain is the major predisposing factor to the experience of pain.[6] The technologist should try to maintain a dialogue with the woman during the examination. The technologist should indicate when compression will begin and should apply it gradually, allowing the woman to indicate the limit of her tolerance. Once informed of the reasons for compression of the breasts, most women understand and, even if they experience pain or discomfort, will not refuse future mammography.[7-9]

Other considerations for the technologist are the needs for sensitivity and for respecting the woman's right to privacy. The technologist should recognize that some women experience a level of distress related to having a mammogram that requires professional counseling beyond the scope of the radiologic technologist. The technologist should refer such women to the interpreting physician or to their health care providers.

AFTER THE EXAMINATION

Reporting the results of the mammography examination occurs at two levels: the technical or medical report (in technical language) to the woman's health care provider and the communication of results and recommendations (in lay language) to the woman.

Name: ______________________ Date of birth: ______________________

Address: ____

Telephone: (home) _______________ (work) ______________________

	(Screening)	(Diagnostic)
1. Do you have breast implants?	NO ______	YES ______
2. Is this a follow-up to an abnormal mammogram?	NO ______	YES ______
3. Do you have any breast problem such as a lump or discharge?	NO ______	YES ______
4. Have you had breast cancer without the removal of your breast?	NO ______	YES ______

(If any answer in 1–4 is yes, the mammogram should be scheduled as a diagnostic examination.)

5. What is your age? ______
(If screening and under 40, refer to radiologist or facility policy; if diagnostic and under 30, refer to radiologist for facility policy.)

6. Are you pregnant or nursing? NO ______ YES ______
(Ask only if woman is under 50.)

7. Do you have breast tenderness or pain at any time during the month? NO ______ YES ______
(If yes, schedule screening when breasts are least tender.)

If you have pain, is it in one spot? NO ______ YES ______
(If yes, refer to radiologist or facility policy.)

8. Have you had a mammogram before? NO ______ YES ______
If yes, when was it done? ________ Where? ______________________
____
(If outside films exist, ask the woman to bring the films with her at the time of the mammogram or provide the address where the previous films are kept.)

9. Information on health care provider:

Name: ______________________________

Address: ______________________________

Telephone: ______________________________

10. When was the last time you saw your health care provider? ______________

11. Do you have a written referral? NO ______ YES ______
(If yes, ask the woman to bring it with her to the facility.)

12. Does your health care provider know that you are scheduling mammography? NO ______ YES ______
(If no, ask the woman to inform her health care provider that she is scheduling mammography.)

Figure 7–1. Typical mammography scheduling questionnaire. (From Bassett LW, Hendrick RE, Bassford TL, et al: Quality Determinants of Mammography. [Clinical Practice Guideline, No. 13. AHCPR Publication No. 95-0632.] Rockville, MD: Agency for Health Care Policy and Research, Public Health Service, US Department of Health and Human Services, October 1994.)

Name: ______________________ Date of birth: ______________________

Address: ______________________

Telephone: (home) ______________ (work) ______________

1. Have you ever had a mammogram (x-ray exam of your breasts) before? NO ____ YES ____
   If no, please go to Question 3.
2. Where and when did you have a mammogram before?
   Where? ______________
   When? (month, year) ______________
3. Do you still have a period every month? NO ____ YES ____
   When did you have your last period? ______________
4. Are you pregnant? NO ____ YES ____
   How old were you when your first child was born? ______
   Are you nursing a baby? NO ____ YES ____
5. Do you take any medications? NO ____ YES ____
   Do you take hormones? NO ____ YES ____
6. Do you have breast implants? NO ____ YES ____
   Have you had any breast biopsies, surgeries, or reduction? NO ____ YES ____
7. Have you ever had a breast removed? NO ____ YES ____
   If yes: left ___ right ___
   Have you ever had radiation treatments to your breasts? NO ____ YES ____
   If yes: left ___ right ___
8. Did your natural mother have breast cancer? NO ____ YES ____
   If yes: Pre- or postmenopausal? ________
   Age at diagnosis: ________
   Do you have a sister or daughter who has breast cancer? NO ____ YES ____
   If yes: Pre- or postmenopausal? ________
   Age at diagnosis: ________
9. Have you recently found a lump in one of your breasts? NO ____ YES ____
   If yes: left ___ right ___
   Do you have any problems with your breasts? NO ____ YES ____
   If yes, please describe the problem(s): ______________________
   ____
10. When was the last time your doctor examined your breasts?
    (month, year) ______________
11. Referring health care provider:
    Name: ______________________
    Address: ______________________
    Telephone: ______________________

Figure 7–2. Example of information obtained at the time of mammogram.

Date: ____________________
Telephone: ____________________
Fax #: ____________________

Kindly release my ***original*** mammogram films and a copy of the report(s) to ____________________ at the above address. Your films will be returned by mail as quickly as possible.

Thank you for your cooperation.

Patient signature ____

(Print)
Patient name: ______________ ______________ ______________
First name Middle initial Last name

Date of birth: __________/__________/__________
(month) (day) (year)

X-Y-Z medical record # ____

Facility name/address (Where previous mammography was performed.)
____
____
____
____

Approximate date of mammography: ________/________/________
(month) (day) (year)

Figure 7–3. Release form for mammograms performed at other facilities.

The interpreting physician, the referring provider, and the woman are all responsible for ensuring that the mammography results are communicated in an effective and timely manner and that the accompanying recommendations are carried out.

Notifying the Woman of Mammography Results

The final regulations of the Mammography Quality Standards Act (MQSA) mandate that each facility send each patient a summary of the mammogram report in lay terms within 30 days of the mammographic examination. If the assessment is "suspicious" or "highly suspicious of malignancy," the facility must make reasonable attempts to ensure that the results are communicated to the patient as soon as possible. Similar attempts should be made to communicate suspicious findings to the woman's health care provider as soon as possible, in addition to the technical report.

Several studies have shown that direct communication of mammography results to the woman by the imaging facility affects compliance with follow-up recommendations in a positive manner.[3,10,11] Communication of the results of screening mammography only through the referring health care provider often leads to inadequate follow-up of abnormal results.[11] The impression that "no news is good news" can have adverse consequences for women with abnormal mammography results. Problems in communicating abnormal results have produced confusion about the next steps to be taken and have caused delays in diagnosis and treatment, with consequences that may limit treatment options and even hasten death.[11-14] Providing the results directly to the woman is a sound risk-management procedure and is a key component in facilitating communication between physicians and the women to whom they provide medical care. Many women, especially those who have little interaction with health care delivery systems, may be unaware of the need for follow-up with their regular health care providers or may make incorrect or unrealistic assumptions about the involvement of the imaging facility in this process. The fine points of physician interrelationships among the different specialties and their relative levels of responsibility for patient management are not as clear to the general public as they are to the provider community. The more explicit the instructions about follow-up, the greater the likelihood that they will be heeded. Improved physician-patient communication has also been shown to reduce the number of legal actions against the interpreting physician and the referring health care provider.[3,15-25]

Results should be communicated clearly, promptly, and in simple lay language. The written communication should document the name of the interpreting physician and, in the case of abnormal results, should detail the next steps the woman should take. Priyanath and colleagues[26] evaluated patient satisfaction, timely report delivery, anxiety, and follow-up on recommendations before and after the passage of the Mammography Quality Standards Reauthorization Act of 1998 (MQSA) using a telephone survey. Although the MQSA improved patient satisfaction and report delivery, it had no effect on reducing anxiety about or understanding of follow-up recommendations. This finding underscores the need for both patient and physician education about the expectations of mammography and its impact on breast cancer mortality.

Just as direct reporting of abnormal results has been shown to facilitate prompt and appropriate follow-up, direct reporting of normal results fosters the collaborative relationship among the woman, her health care provider, and the imaging facility by reinforcing the woman's role and responsibility in the health care delivery process. Table 7–1 summarizes a system for notification of results according to outcome. Communication of results can be achieved efficiently and at low cost through the use of form letters that use sensitive and thoughtful language (Fig. 7–4).

For a woman who comes for screening or diagnostic mammography on her own initiative and is able to name a personal physician or health care provider, the interpreting physician should try to document that the named provider accepts responsibility for the woman's breast care before sending the provider the mammography report. If the named provider declines to accept the mammography report, the facility should contact the woman directly to confirm that she indeed has a health care provider. For the woman who came for mammography but has no personal health care provider, the interpreting physician must assume responsibility for breast care, including education, physical examination, communication of mammography results directly to her, and follow-up care, until a health care provider accepts responsibility for her care.[14,27] The facility may supply the self-referred woman with a list of qualified providers. The interpreting physician should ensure that the clinician the woman chooses from this list will assume responsibility for her breast care. The name, address, and phone number of the provider chosen should be recorded in the woman's medical record, and a medical report of the results of the mammogram should be sent by the imaging facility to that provider. If the result of the examination is suspicious for cancer, imaging facility personnel should directly telephone the woman. Although self-referral has improved access to screening

Table 7–1. Reporting of Results by Mammography Facilities*

Outcome of Mammography Examination and Recommendation for Follow-Up	Communication to Women		Phone Communication to Health Care Provider in Addition to Standard Report	Always Necessary: Written Report to Health Care Provider
	Oral (On Site or by Telephone)	Written (On Site or Sent by Mail)		
Normal	Optional	Required	None	Required
Abnormal: schedule additional imaging and/or ultrasonography				
On-line†	Recommended‡	Required	Recommended‖	Required
Off-line†	Strongly recommended	Required	Recommended‖	Required
Abnormal: short-interval follow-up	Optional	Required	Optional	Required
Abnormal: biopsy	Optional; strongly recommended for self-referred women	Required¶	Facility is required to make reasonable effort to contact provider	Required

*"Required" indicates an element dictated by Mammography Quality Standards Act (MQSA). "Strongly recommended" applies to elements of mammography that are essential to good practice. "Recommended" applies to elements of mammography that are attainable in most but not all cases. "Optional" indicates an element of less compelling nature that cannot be justifiably "recommended."

†For an "on-line" study, the interpreting physician is present and reads the mammogram while the patient is there. For an "off-line" study, the mammogram may be read after the woman leaves, so the interpreting physician does not need to be present.

‡For any patient for whom additional views or ultrasonography is recommended, a telephone call or discussion on site with the patient may precede the written letter when the studies are to be performed immediately at that mammography facility. However, the results of the original and additional studies must be provided to the patient in writing.

‖A telephone call from the mammography facility to the woman's designated physician or other health care provider is recommended. A self-referred patient should be telephoned directly.

¶For any patient without a direct referral, the mammography facility may wish to send the letter via registered or certified mail.

Adapted from Bassett LW, Hendrick RE, Bassford TL, et al: Quality Determinants of Mammography. (Clinical Practice Guidelines, No. 13. AHCPR Publication No. 95-0632.) Rockville, MD: Agency for Health Care Policy and Research, Public Health Service, US Department of Health and Human Services, October 1994.

Date: ________________

Dear Ms.________________________:

We are pleased to inform you that the results of your recent mammography examination are **normal**. As you know, early detection of cancer is very important. Although mammography is the most accurate method for early detection, not all cancers are found through mammography. A thorough examination includes a combination of mammography, physical examination, and breast self-examination. Current American Cancer Society Guidelines recommend screening mammograms and physical breast examinations every year beginning at the age of 40. It is important to remember that a lump in the breast should never be ignored even if your mammogram is normal.

A report of your mammography results was sent to: (referring health care provider).

Your mammogram will become part of your medical file here at (facility name) for at least 10 years. You are responsible for informing any new health care provider or mammography facility of the date and location of this examination.

Thank you.

A

Date: ________________

Dear Ms.________________________:

Your recent mammography examination showed an area that we believe is **benign (not cancer)**. However, in six months, you should have a follow-up mammogram to confirm that this area has not changed.

As you know, early detection of cancer is very important. Although mammography is the most accurate method for early detection, not all cancers are found through mammography. A thorough examination includes a combination of mammography, physical examination, and breast self-examination. Therefore, if you have not had a recent physical examination of your breasts by your clinician, see your physician or other health care provider. It is important to remember that a lump in the breast should never be ignored even if your mammogram is normal.

A report of your mammography results was sent to: (referring health care provider).

Your mammogram will become part of your medical file here at (facility name) for at least 10 years. You are responsible for informing any new health care provider or mammography facility of the date and location of this examination.

Thank you.

B

Figure 7–4. **A,** Suggested form letter to women in lay language for regular follow-up. **B,** Suggested form letter to women in lay language for short-term follow-up.

Continued

mammography, it has increased the responsibilities of the interpreting physician and has led to a higher rate of failure to communicate and follow up abnormal results.

COMMUNICATION ISSUES AND THEIR RELATIONSHIP TO MALPRACTICE CLAIMS

The Physician Insurers Association of America (PIAA) reported results of malpractice claims related to breast cancer in 1990, 1995, and 2002.[20,28,29] Breast cancer is the second most expensive condition in terms of malpractice payments, exceeded only by claims associated with neurologically impaired newborns. Approximately 40% of claims involving breast cancer result in payment to the claimant, and the average payment exceeds $290,000 per claim. The average payment to claimants younger than 50 years is 63% higher than for patients 50 years and older.

Comparison of the latest PIAA study findings with previous study findings reveals important differences

Date: ______________

Dear Ms.______________________:

Your recent mammography examination showed a finding that requires additional imaging studies for a complete evaluation. Most such findings are benign (not cancer). Please call (telephone #) to schedule an appointment for these tests if you have not already done so.

A report of your mammography results was sent to: (referring health care provider).

Your mammogram will become part of your medical file here at (facility name) for at least 10 years. You are responsible for informing any new health care provider or mammography facility of the date and location of this examination.

Thank you.

C

Date: ______________

Dear Ms.______________________:

Your recent mammography examination showed an abnormality that requires further follow-up by your physician or other health care provider. The only way that you can be sure the abnormality is benign (not cancer) is to speak with your health care provider (if you have not already done so) and have follow-up tests. You should do this as soon as possible.

You and your physician or other health care provider will decide what additional tests are needed, based on the findings of your mammography examination, your breast physical examination, your medical history, and your concerns.

Your first priority now should be to complete testing of the abnormality seen on your recent mammography examination. Your health care provider has been sent a report of this examination and will be expecting your call. A report of your mammography results was sent to: (health care provider).

Your mammogram will become part of your medical file here at (facility name) for at least 10 years. You are responsible for informing any new health care provider or mammography facility of the date and location of this examination.

Thank you.

D

Figure 7–4, cont'd. C, Suggested form letter to women in lay language for additional imaging. **D,** Suggested form letter to women in lay language for biopsy recommended. (Courtesy of The American College of Radiology.)

and disturbing trends related to interpretation of mammograms. The current study shows that 33% of all defendants are radiologists, a 9% increase from the 1995 study, whereas the rates for general and family practitioners and surgical specialties as defendants showed drops of 8.5% and 2%, respectively. The most prevalent physician issue in the latest study was "mammogram misread," involving 38% of claims. However, the fifth most prevalent physician issue was "poor communication between providers," accounting for 8% of claims.

The latest PIAA data validate the need for improved communication among referring providers, imaging facilities, and women, especially premenopausal women. The vast majority of the claims analyzed in the 2002 study involved situations in which clinical signs and symptoms, including pain with or without a mass, were present. The risk-management recommendations by the PIAA echo the discussions in this chapter relative to the interdependent roles and responsibilities of the referring health care provider, imaging personnel, and patient regarding:

1. The need to obtain the results of clinical breast examinations and correlate them with the results of mammography.
2. The possible need to follow up with other diagnostic tests in the event of a normal mammogram.
3. The communication of results and follow-up recommendations.
4. The monitoring and tracking of patients.

The results from the 2002 PIAA study also show that there was no delay on the part of the patient in 67.3% of the cases. When the patient's behavior contributed to the delay in diagnosis, the most common cause was failure to keep follow-up appointments (13.8%). Implementation of a system for reporting results and follow-up recommendations, as well as communication of pertinent information to the women, beginning with information from the referring health care provider and followed by information from the imaging facility personnel, may help reduce the incidence of delayed diagnosis. Emphasizing to a woman that she has an important role in asking questions and following recommendations is vital to this communication process.

Many of the communication activities discussed in this chapter are intended to serve an educational function. A woman's interactions with her referring health care provider and the breast imaging facility may be her only opportunity to learn about mammography and breast health care. Women's perceptions of their risk for having breast cancer have been found to be more accurate when they are given their individual 10-year risk without being compared with women of their own age and race who were at lowest risk; counter to many theories, providing such information was not found to decrease the intention to seek mammography.[30] Pointing out the limits of mammography emphasizes the need for the woman to pay careful attention to lumps and other physical changes in her breasts and the possible need to obtain additional diagnostic tests or other medical care.[29] Many women are limited by economic constraints, poor access to medical care, and psychosocial dynamics as well as cultural factors.[31] These conditions make it difficult for a woman to advocate effectively for herself. However, optimal provider-patient communication can improve mutual understanding in the clinical setting.

Problems surrounding the sharing and delivery of information are among the most influential factors in the filing of malpractice claims.[1,19,21,23,24] Thus, integrating the principles of communication into every step of the mammography process is wise risk-management policy. Studies exploring the reasons, other than adverse outcome, that underlie medical malpractice claims have demonstrated the influence of failed communication on the decision of a patient to consult an attorney.[2,16] The most risk-laden behaviors were found to be dysfunctional delivery of information (i.e., lack of effectiveness in sharing diagnostic and prognostic information) and devaluing the patient or family perspective (i.e., discounting patient or family opinions).[32]

Similar findings about the direct relationship between malpractice claims and adverse interpersonal factors have been made in the birth outcomes, satisfaction with care, and malpractice project studies supported by the Agency for Health Care Policy and Research. Poor physician-patient communication (i.e., "would not talk, would not listen, rarely gave advice, did not explain reasons for tests") ranks highest among the interpersonal factors. Lack of communication was extremely high (27.6%) among physicians with a high frequency of malpractice claims, compared with the group of physicians who had no claims (8.2%).[11,33] Medical and demographic vulnerability was not a factor, because the populations served were similar for all the groups of physicians. A companion study did not reveal a relationship between prior claims experience and the technical quality of current practice. The researchers of this study concluded that if a difference among the physicians leads to different malpractice claims experiences, it relates to characteristics of practice that include the patients' perception of the physician's communication and interpersonal skills.[15]

Thus, communication is an essential part of quality assurance and risk management. Effective communication, which involves notifying women promptly of the results of their mammography examinations, promotes patient satisfaction and compliance with specific follow-up recommendations, including long-term regular screening, and also minimizes physician-patient conflict and the potential for malpractice claims.[3]

TECHNICAL REPORT

The written report to the referring health care provider should be concise and understandable. A well-written report increases the use of both screening and diagnostic mammography.[34] The American College of Radiology (ACR) has developed a Breast Imaging Reporting and Data System (BI-RADS) intended to standardize terminology in the mammography report as well as to outline the organization of the report.[33,35,36] The fourth edition is available, and this new edition includes terminology for use in breast ultrasonography and magnetic resonance imaging (MRI).

The use of standardized terminology and a system such as BI-RADS facilitates the medical audit and outcome monitoring, which provides important peer review and quality assurance data to improve the quality of patient care. Because this information is used in peer review, it is considered confidential and must be collected and reported in a manner that complies with applicable statutory and regulatory peer review procedures.

A major portion of the fourth edition BI-RADS consists of a breast imaging lexicon. A lexicon for ultrasonography and MRI is part of the new edition, as already mentioned. The terminology used in mammography has evolved over many years and has often led to confusion. The lexicon is an attempt to standardize the description of mammographic features in an effort to enhance understanding of the report and to simplify teaching and research in mammography. It is expected that as use of these terms increases, modifications, additions, and deletions will occur. A subcommittee has been established by the ACR to address possible changes in the lexicon.

The technical mammography report should begin with a brief statement concerning the reason for the examination, followed by a brief description of the composition of the breast; significant findings, if any, using standard terminology; results of comparison with prior examinations, if applicable; and, finally, an impression that encompasses an overall assessment and recommendation. In the mammography report, any clinical concern should be specifically dealt with, and all verbal communications with the woman, her health care provider, or both should be documented.

A brief description of overall breast composition should state whether a lesion might be hidden by dense parenchyma, as follows (Fig. 7–5):

- The breast is composed almost entirely of fat (<25% fibroglandular tissue).
- Scattered fibroglandular densities are present that could obscure a lesion (25% to 50% fibroglandular tissue).
- Heterogeneously dense breast tissue is present, which may lower the sensitivity of mammography (50% to 75% fibroglandular tissue).
- Extremely dense breast tissue is present, which lowers the sensitivity of mammography (>75% fibroglandular tissue).

A clear description and the location of any significant findings form the body of the report.

A *mass* is a space-occupying lesion seen in two different projections. If a potential mass is seen in only one projection, it should be called an *asymmetry* until it is confirmed to be three-dimensional. The description of a mass should include its size, shape (*round, oval, lobular,* or *irregular*), margin characteristics (*circumscribed, microlobulated, obscured, indistinct,* or *spiculated*), and a description of any associated calcifications (Fig. 7–6). The description of its location should be based on a clock face, quadrant, or both and should be further subdivided into anterior, middle, or posterior positions. *Subareolar* and *central* may also be used for locations.

Not only do the features listed here standardize language, but they also serve to categorize masses for appropriate follow-up. A round or oval mass suggests a benign finding, whereas an irregular mass suggests malignancy. A lobular mass may be thought of as intermediate in concern, demonstrating a degree of growth autonomy that may not be present with a round or oval mass. A circumscribed margin that sharply delineates a mass from surrounding tissue is at the benign end of the spectrum of margin characteristics, whereas a spiculated edge consisting of fine, thin radiating lines is in the malignant range of concern. Microlobulated and indistinct margins suggest early infiltration of breast tissue by a mass, but an obscured margin merely implies one that is concealed by surrounding glandular tissue.

When the finding is calcifications, a description of their morphology and distribution should be included (Fig. 7–7). Typically, *benign calcifications* include those with *vascular, coarse* (or *"popcorn"*), *lucent-centered,* or *sedimenting* appearances. Almost all such calcifications require no follow-up other than routine mammography. However, if the calcifications do not have these typically benign features, further evaluation may be necessary. For example, early vascular calcifications may not yet have assumed their typical thin, parallel linear forms.

Calcifications that are of intermediate concern are *amorphous* and *coarse heterogeneous*. Amorphous calcifications are typically hazy and irregular in appearance, whereas coarse heterogeneous calcifications are also irregular but are conspicuous, larger than pleomorphic calcifications, and not as large as dystrophic calcifications. The calcifications of greatest concern are those that are *pleomorphic*—those that are 0.2 to 0.3 mm in size, irregular, and denser than amorphous calcifications—and those that are *fine, linear,* and *branching*, indicating their presence in the small terminal ducts and features usually associated with malignancy. The latter two categories of calcification often require tissue sampling to exclude malignancy. The distribution of the calcifications may also be helpful in determining the further disposition of the patient. A *cluster* or *linear* arrangement of calcifications is worrisome, even in the presence of calcifications that may be only of intermediate concern or that appear benign. A linear arrangement of punctate calcifications may prompt biopsy. As the arrangement becomes less focal and assumes a *segmental, regional,* or *diffuse* distribution, concern about the malignant nature decreases. However, calcifications of greatest concern, such as those that are fine, linear, and branching, should be sampled even if diffusely distributed. In general, one should act on the most worrisome calcifications and not allow the presence of adjacent calcifications with benign characteristics to dissuade one from urging a biopsy.

Architectural distortion, asymmetry, and *focal asymmetry* should be described (Fig. 7–8). Although sometimes difficult to detect, *architectural distortion*—or tethering of the glandular tissue with the production of radiating, fine spicules unassociated with a mass—is often a feature of malignancy. *Global asymmetry*—the presence of glandular tissue in one part of the breast that is not found in a similar location in the contralateral breast—is often a normal finding and, if unassociated with a palpable mass or malignant mammographic features, requires no follow-up. *Focal asymmetry* is glandular tissue without the properties of a true mass, such as convex outward borders, but with a similar appearance on both craniocaudal and mediolateral oblique views. Although it may merely represent an asymmetrical focus of glandular tissue, further evaluation with a spot compression view or ultrasonography may be warranted. Other abnor-

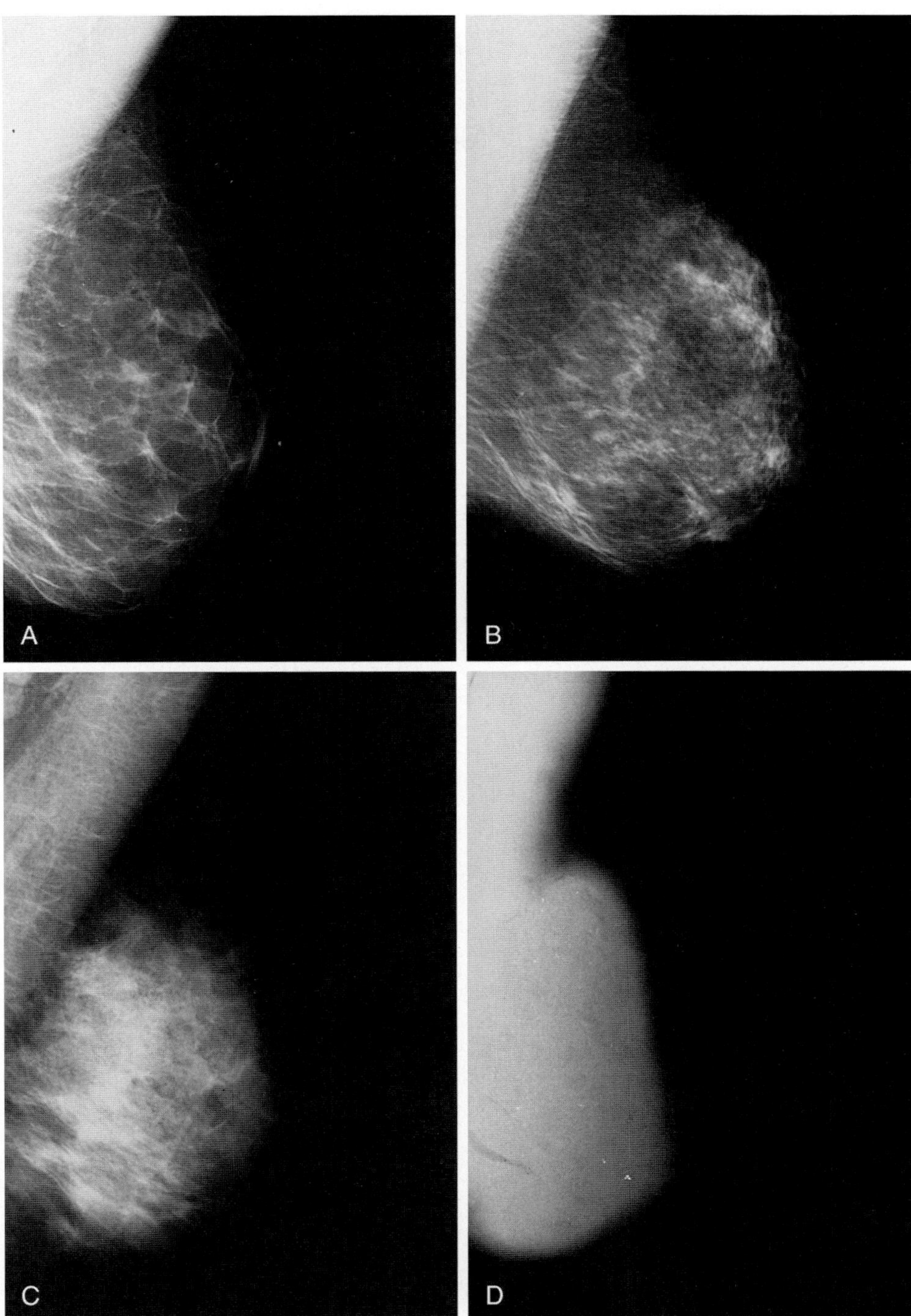

Figure 7–5. Fibroglandular composition of the breast, mediolateral oblique views. **A,** Breast almost completely replaced by fat (<25% fibroglandular tissue). **B,** Scattered fibroglandular densities (25% up to 50% fibroglandular density). **C,** Heterogeneously dense breast tissue (50% up to 75% fibroglandular density). **D,** Breast tissue is extremely dense (>75% fibroglandular density).

malities defined within the ACR BI-RADS system are *skin and nipple retraction, skin thickening, trabecular thickening, skin lesions,* and *axillary lymphadenopathy.* The reader is urged to consult the ACR BI-RADS document for a formal discussion of definitions and examples of each feature.[36,37]

Although the density of a lesion is often difficult to assess, it is an important feature because most breast cancers producing a visible mass are of equal or higher density than an equal volume of fibroglandular tissue in the same breast.[38] The *density* of a lesion may be defined as the x-ray attenuation of the lesion relative to the attenuation of an equal volume of fibroglandular breast tissue. Thus, densities can be described as *high, equal* (or *isodense*), or *low.* A particularly important category is a *fat-containing* or *radiolucent* circumscribed lesion, because breast cancers never contain fat, although they may entrap it. Fat-containing circumscribed masses include lipid cysts, lipomas, galactoceles, intramammary nodes, and hamartomas (fibroadenomalipomas).

Perhaps the most important part of the report consists of a clear summary of the findings, an assessment of what they mean, and a recommendation of

Masses

Shape:

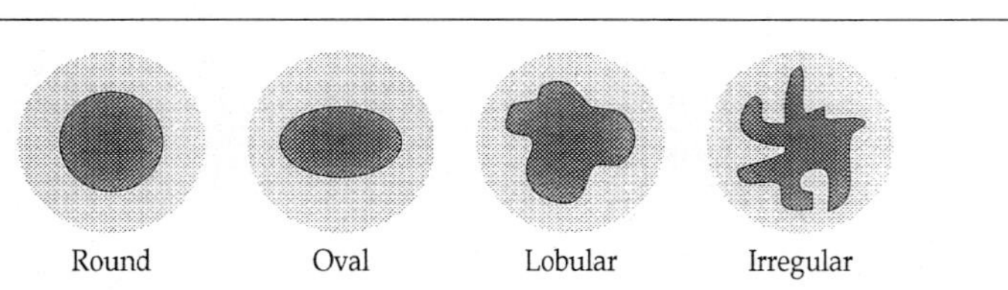

Margin

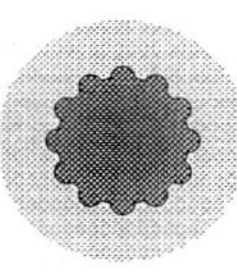
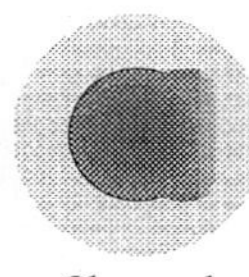

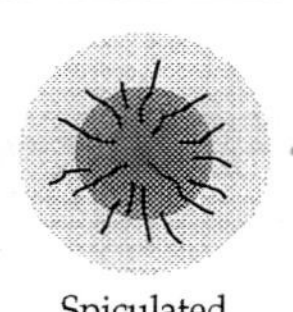

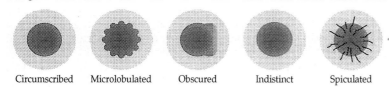

Figure 7–6. Shapes and margins of masses seen on mammograms.

Calcifications

Elements

Typically Benign: *Intermediate:* *Great Concern:*

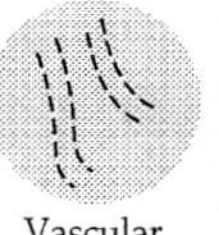
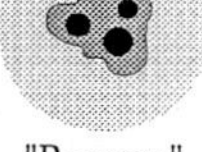
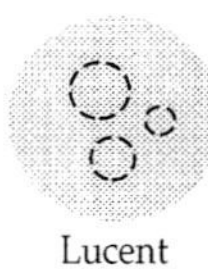
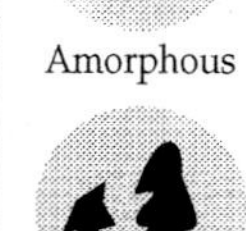
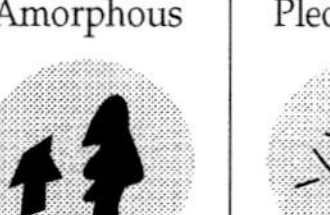
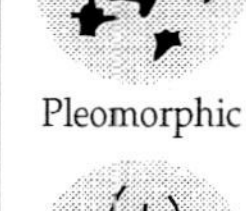

Distribution

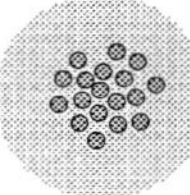

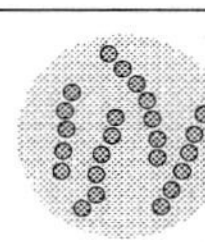
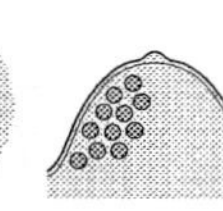
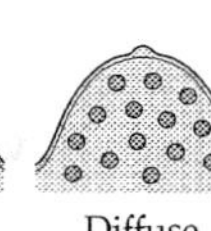
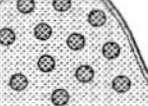

Figure 7–7. Element configuration and distribution of calcifications seen on mammograms.

Special Features

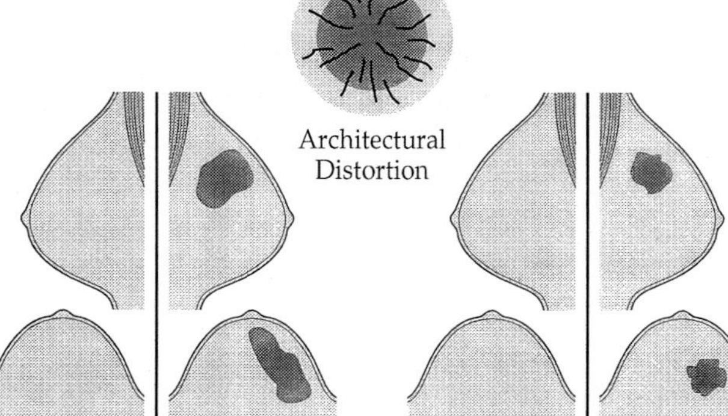

Figure 7–8. Architectural distortion and asymmetry of masses seen on mammograms.

the action to be taken. The final impression should be complete. An indeterminate impression is usually given only in the screening setting, for which additional evaluation is recommended. *Assessment incomplete* (category 0) is reserved for screening examinations in which an additional image evaluation, such as ultrasonography or special mammographic or spot compression views, is required. The following categories are those used for assessment of a diagnostic or screening examination that does not require additional investigation:

- Category 1: *Negative* is reserved for a mammographic examination with no findings.
- Category 2: An assessment of *benign* is used when the interpreter wishes to describe an obviously benign finding, such as an involuting fibroadenoma with coarse "popcorn" calcification, or multiple secretory calcifications.
- Category 3: A *probably benign* assessment includes findings that have a very high probability of being benign. Recent reports have validated the use of this category rather than biopsy, demonstrating that when the category is appropriately used, there is less than a 2% chance that a malignancy will be assigned to this category.[39-41] Of course, this requires the interpreter to routinely assess the outcomes of findings assigned to this category to ensure that there is not an inordinate amount of cancer discovered in this category. For a further discussion of this category, the reader is encouraged to address the new Fourth Edition of BI-RADS and the guidance chapter within.
- Category 4: A *suspicious abnormality* is not characteristic of breast cancer but has a reasonable probability of being malignant.
- Category 5: The *highly suggestive of malignancy* group includes lesions that have a high probability of being malignant. The lesions assigned to this category should have at least a 95% chance of malignancy, because category 5 was intended to identify lesions that could go directly to definitive therapy without prior tissue diagnosis. This scenario could possibly occur in rural or underserved areas where full diagnostic services may not be available.
- Category 6: *Known biopsy-proven malignancy*. This category is reserved for lesions identified on imaging before definitive therapy and known to be malignant.

Assessments of *negative* and *benign* require only routine follow-up, usually yearly mammograms. The *probably benign* category is best managed with a short-term follow-up examination, usually after 6 months for the involved breast, followed by a bilateral examination after a second 6-month interval, and then by one to two more bilateral examinations at 12-month intervals (coinciding with screening mammography) to establish the absence of a change (see Fig. 7–16). The *suspicious abnormality* requires biopsy, and any lesions that are *highly suggestive of malignancy* or a *known malignancy* require appropriate action, usually excisional biopsy or definitive therapy, or both.

SUMMARY

Clear and unambiguous communication by the interpreting physician to the woman and to the health care provider is essential. Communication along established guidelines, using standardized terminology, should greatly decrease cases of absent or inappropriate follow-up, with their inherent poor outcomes. Examples of several mammographic examinations and their reports are illustrated in Figures 7–9 through 7–15. Figure 7–16 is an algorithm for category 3 results.

Text continued on p. 134

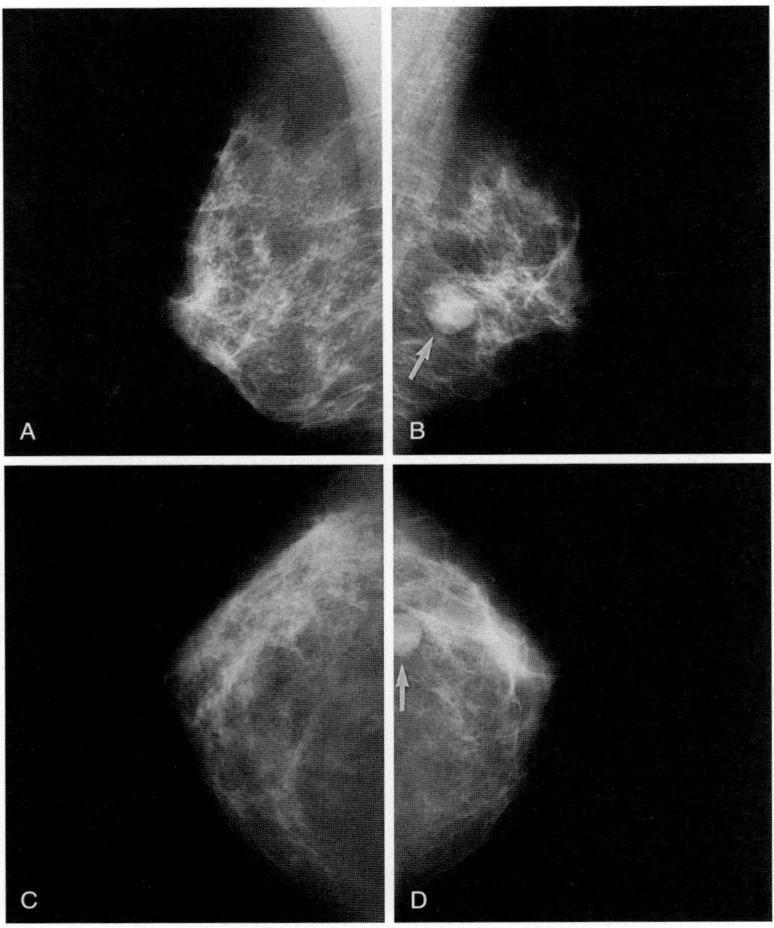

Mary Smith
DOB: 11/5/43
Referring Physician: Fred Jones, MD

BILATERAL SCREENING MAMMOGRAMS

March 1, 1996

Clinical History: Screen.

There are no prior films for comparison. There are scattered fibroglandular densities bilaterally. A 15-mm round circumscribed mass is present at the 5 o'clock position in the posterior third of the left breast. The right breast is unremarkable.

IMPRESSION:
15-mm mass at 5 o'clock in the left breast. Ultrasound is recommended for further evaluation. The woman will be contacted regarding the need for ultrasound and the date for this examination.

BI-RADS CATEGORY 0: NEED ADDITIONAL IMAGING EVALUATION.

Boris Breef, MD
Radiologist

E

Figure 7–9. Category 0, incompletely evaluated mass. Right and left mediolateral oblique (**A, B**) and craniocaudal (**C, D**) views demonstrate a circumscribed 15-mm mass (*arrows*). **E,** The report. The patient was subsequently recalled for additional imaging, including ultrasonography, which demonstrated a simple cyst. Routine screening mammography was then recommended.

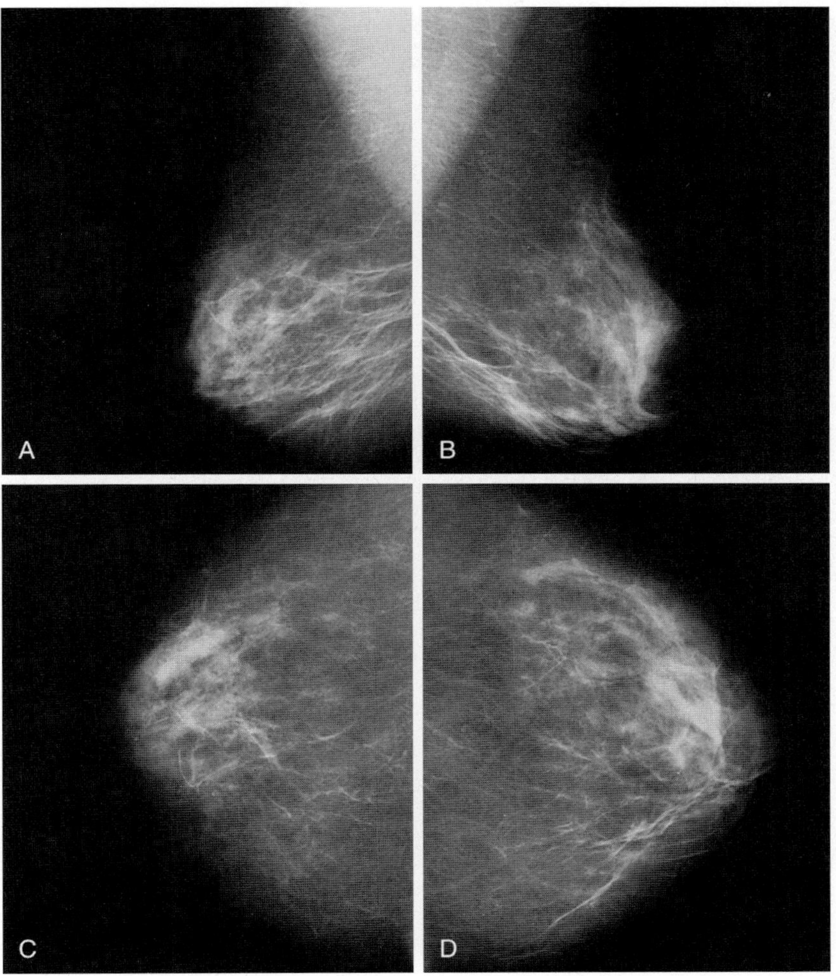

Martha Jones
DOB 10/10/36
Referring Physician: Mark Medicine, MD

BILATERAL SCREENING MAMMOGRAMS

June 3, 1995

Clinical History: Screen.

Compared with the prior study of 7/2/93, there are again scattered fibroglandular densities. No masses, significant calcifications, or other findings are seen.

IMPRESSION:
No change from prior examination. No mammographic evidence of malignancy. Yearly mammograms are recommended.

BI-RADS CATEGORY 1: NEGATIVE.

Steven Short, MD
Radiologist

E

Figure 7–10. Category 1: normal mammogram. Right and left mediolateral oblique (**A, B**) and craniocaudal (**C, D**) mammograms. **E,** The corresponding report.

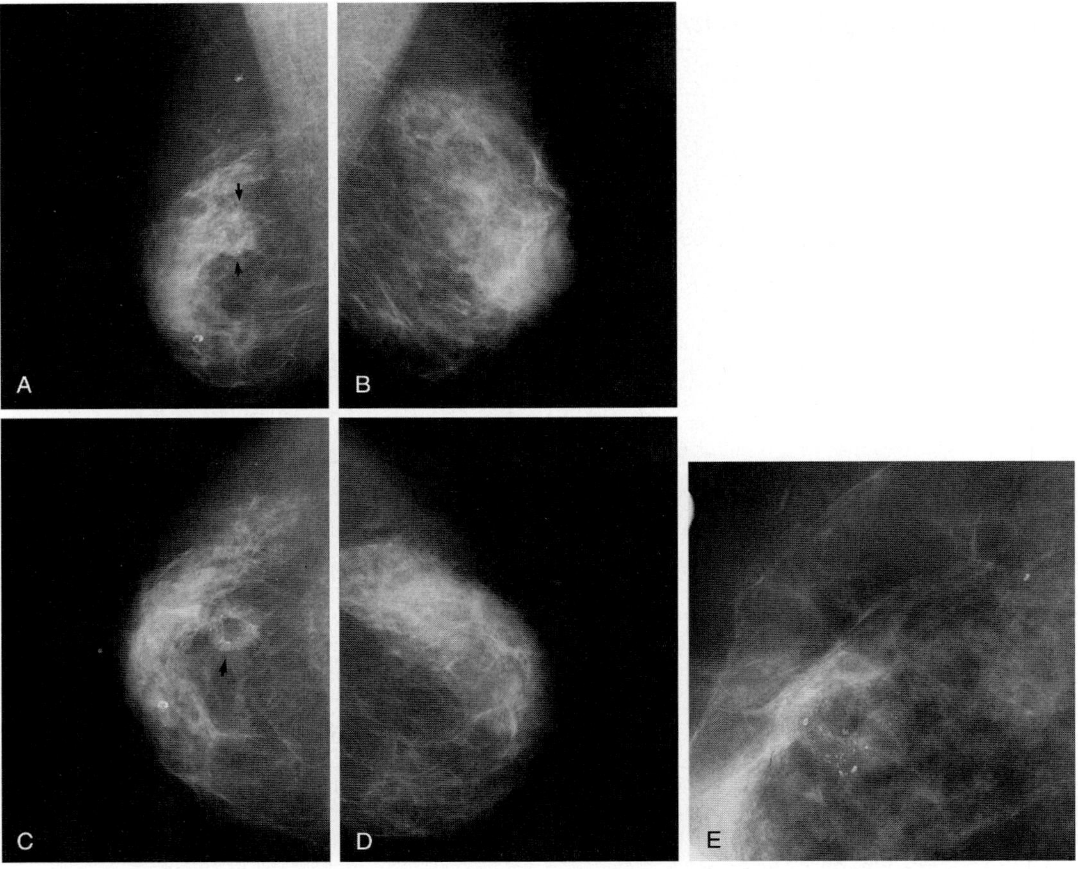

Freda Jones
DOB: 7/12/30
Referring physician: Frank Surgeon, MD

BILATERAL SCREENING MAMMOGRAMS

February 1, 1995

Clinical History: Prior history of chest trauma. Screen.

Compared with previous mammograms from St. Elsewhere Breast Center dated 6/10/92, scattered fibroglandular densities are again identified. There is an obscured 15-mm mass with a radiolucent center at the 12 o'clock position in the middle third of the right breast with no change from the prior exam. There are associated rim calcifications at its periphery. The left breast is unremarkable.

IMPRESSION:

Mass at 12 o'clock in the right breast, compatible with benign fat necrosis. Yearly mammograms are recommended.

BI-RADS CATEGORY 2: BENIGN FINDING.

Sebastian Katz, MD
Radiologist

F

Figure 7–11. Category 2: benign finding. Right and left mediolateral oblique (MLO) (**A, B**) and craniocaudal (**C, D**) views. **E,** Magnification right MLO view from a prior diagnostic examination. **F,** The corresponding report. This finding, which was unchanged for 3 years, represents post-traumatic fat necrosis.

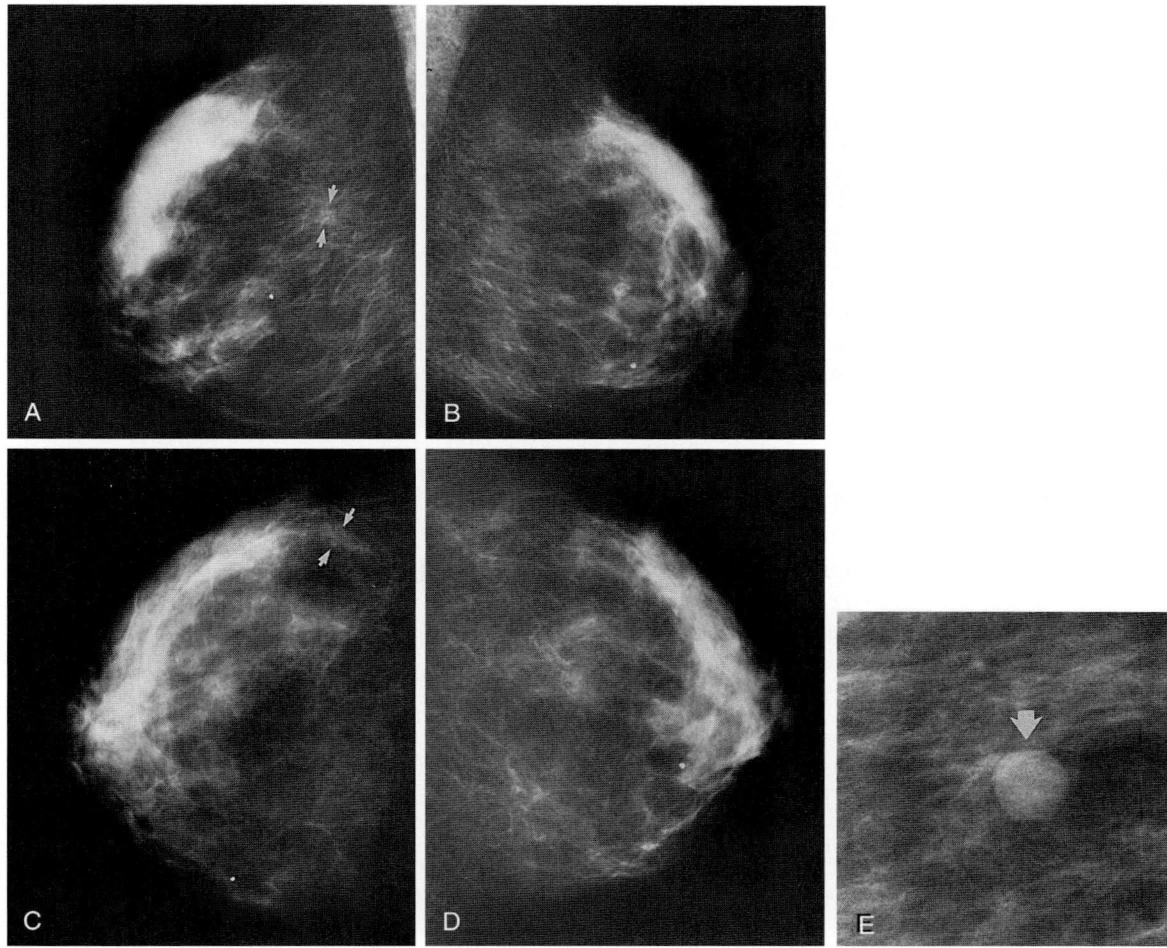

Figure 7–12. Category 0. Category 3. Right and left mediolateral oblique (**A, B**) and craniocaudal (**C, D**) views, and spot compression magnification mediolateral view (**E**).

Continued

Susan Jones
DOB: 9/21/40
Referring physician: Bill Williams, MD

BILATERAL SCREENING MAMMOGRAMS

March 15, 2002

Clinical History: Screen

There are no old films available for comparison. There are scattered fibroglandular densities bilaterally. There is a 9-mm partially circumscribed partially obscured mass at 9 o'clock in the posterior third of the right breast. The left breast is unremarkable.

IMPRESSION:

9-mm mass in the right breast. Patient requires further imaging evaluation. The woman will be contacted regarding the need for this follow-up and date for this appointment.

BI-RADS CATEGORY 0: FURTHER IMAGING ASSESSMENT.

Alexis Katt, MD
Radiologist

F

March 16, 2002

Clinical History: Diagnostic right mammogram

Spot compression views demonstrate a circumscribed asymmetry at 9 o'clock in the posterior third of the breast. There is no ultrasound counterpart.

IMPRESSION:

Mass as described above.

BI-RADS CATEGORY 3: PROBABLY A BENIGN FINDING—SHORT INTERVAL FOLLOW-UP IN SIX MONTHS IS SUGGESTED.

Alexis Katt, MD
Radiologist

G

Figure 7–12, cont'd. F and **G,** The corresponding reports. Positioning for the mediolateral oblique views was difficult. The 9-mm circumscribed asymmetry (*arrows* in **A**, **C**, and **E**) was subsequently monitored and remained stable for 4 years.

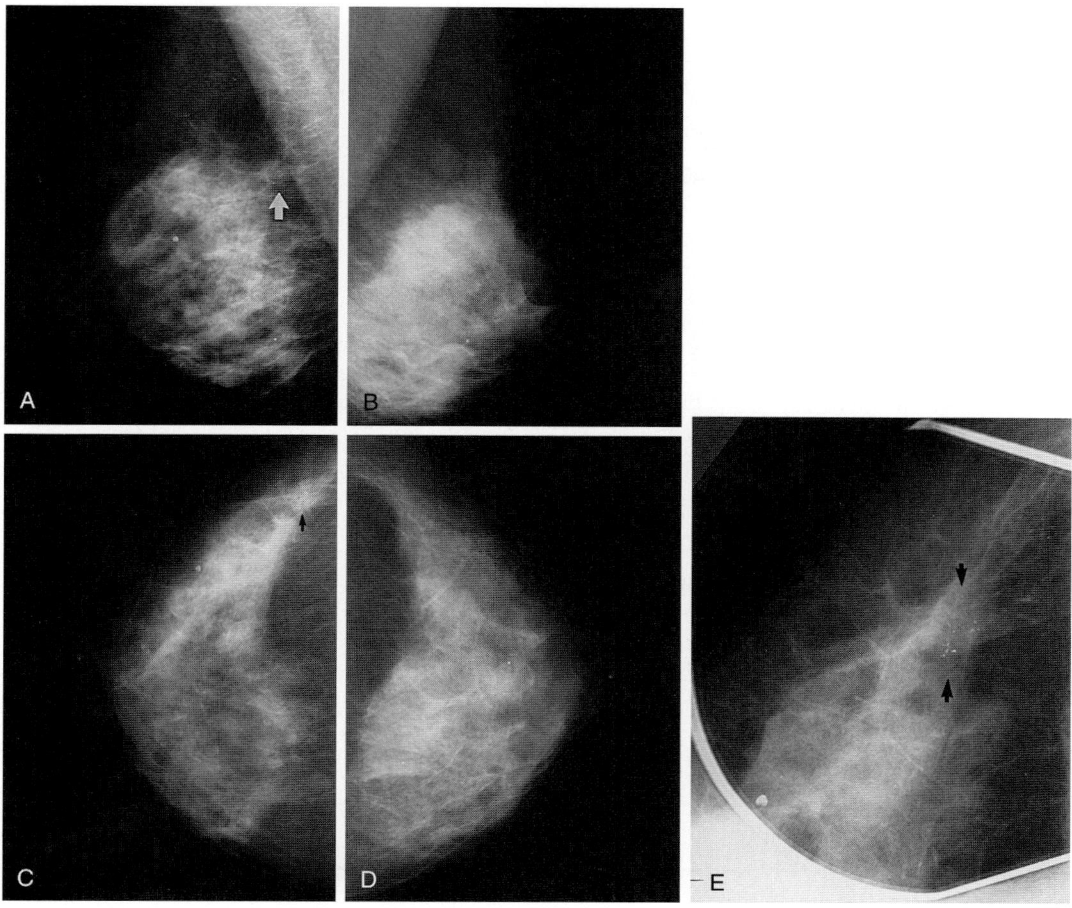

Figure 7–13. Category 4, suspicious calcifications (*arrows*). Right and left mediolateral oblique (**A, B**), craniocaudal (CC) (**C, D**), and spot compression magnification CC (**E**) views of a cluster of microcalcifications.

Continued

Maryann Smith
DOB: 2/2/26
Referring physician: John Adams, MD

BILATERAL SCREENING MAMMOGRAMS

August 19, 2002

Clinical History: Screen

Comparison with a prior study of 8/10/93. The breasts are heterogeneously dense. This may lower the sensitivity of mammography. There is a cluster of microcalcifications at 9 o'clock in the posterior third of the right breast new from the prior exam. There are other scattered benign calcifications bilaterally. No suspicious masses or areas of architectural distortion are seen.

Left breast is unremarkable.

IMPRESSION:

Cluster of new microcalcifications at 9 o'clock in the right breast.

BI-RADS CATEGORY 0: FURTHER IMAGING ASSESSMENT.

Sally Succinct, MD
Radiologist

F

August 20, 2002

Clinical History: Diagnostic right mammogram

Magnification spot compression view demonstrates a cluster of pleomorphic calcifications.

IMPRESSION:

Calcifications as described above suspicious for malignancy. Dr. Adams was notified of the results on August 20, 2002.

BI-RADS CATEGORY 4: SUSPICIOUS ABNORMALITY—BIOPSY SHOULD BE CONSIDERED.

Sally Succinct, MD
Radiologist

G

Figure 7–13, cont'd. F and **G,** The corresponding reports. Ductal carcinoma in situ was found at biopsy.

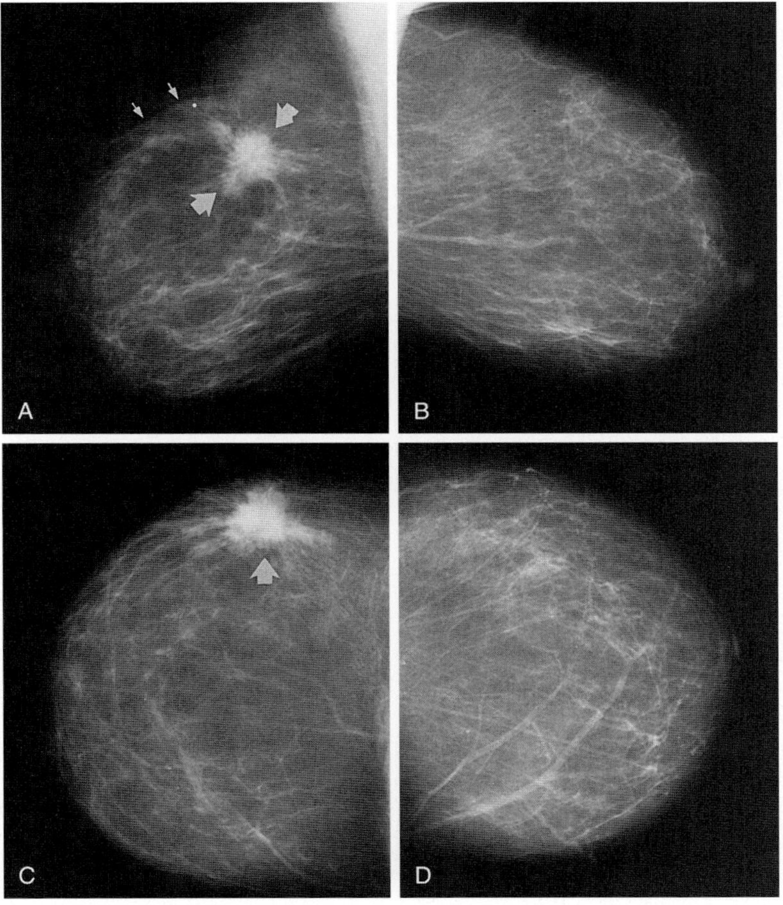

Joan Brown
DOB: 3/2/27
Referring Physician: Harry Martini, MD

BILATERAL DIAGNOSTIC MAMMOGRAMS

February 5, 1996

Clinical History: Palpable mass in the right breast.

There are scattered fibroglandular densities bilaterally. There is a 2.5-cm spiculated mass with associated skin retraction at 9 o'clock in the right breast. The left breast is unremarkable.

IMPRESSION:
2.5-cm mass in the right breast. Dr. Martini was notified of the results on February 5, 1996 at 11:30 am.

BI-RADS CATEGORY 5: HIGHLY SUGGESTIVE OF MALIGNANCY—APPROPRIATE ACTION SHOULD BE TAKEN.

Abe Normal, MD
Radiologist

E

Figure 7–14. Category 5, highly suggestive of malignancy. Right and left mediolateral oblique (**A, B**) and craniocaudal (**C, D**) mammograms of a woman with a palpable right breast mass (*large arrows*) with skin retraction (*small arrows*). Positioning was difficult because of the woman's debilitated condition. **E,** The corresponding report. At biopsy, this lesion was found to be invasive ductal carcinoma.

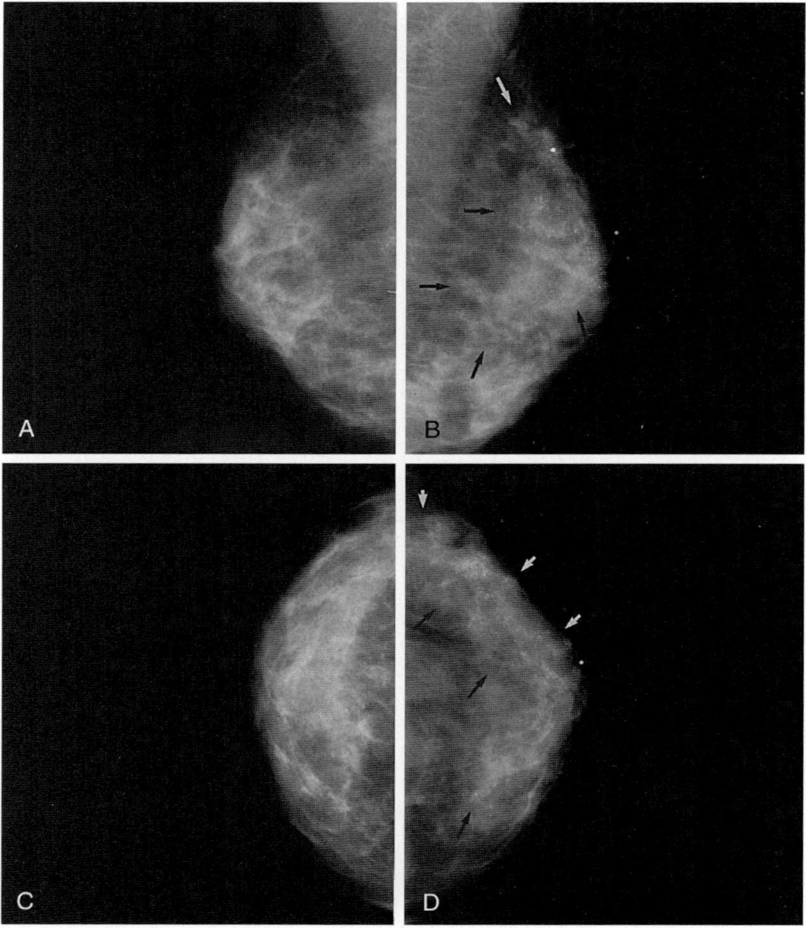

Barbara Smith
DOB:4/3/42
Referring Physician: William Smith, MD

BILATERAL DIAGNOSTIC MAMMOGRAMS

March 15, 1996

Clinical History: Palpable thickening in the left breast.

The breasts are heterogeneously dense, which may lower the sensitivity of mammography. There is an 8-cm regional distribution of pleomorphic microcalcifications extending from the 1 o'clock to the 7 o'clock position in the left breast. The right breast is unremarkable.

IMPRESSION:
Regional distribution of pleomorphic calcifications in the left breast. Dr. Smith was notified of the results on March 15, 1996 at 10:30 am.

BI-RADS CATEGORY 5: HIGHLY SUGGESTIVE OF MALIGNANCY—APPROPRIATE ACTION SHOULD BE TAKEN.

Cal Cium, MD
Radiologist

E

Figure 7–15. Category 5: highly suggestive of malignancy. Right and left mediolateral oblique (**A, B**) and craniocaudal (**C, D**) mammograms of a woman with palpable thickening in the left breast. A large region of pleomorphic microcalcifications is present in the left breast (*arrows*). **E,** The report. Biopsy identified this lesion as comedocarcinoma.

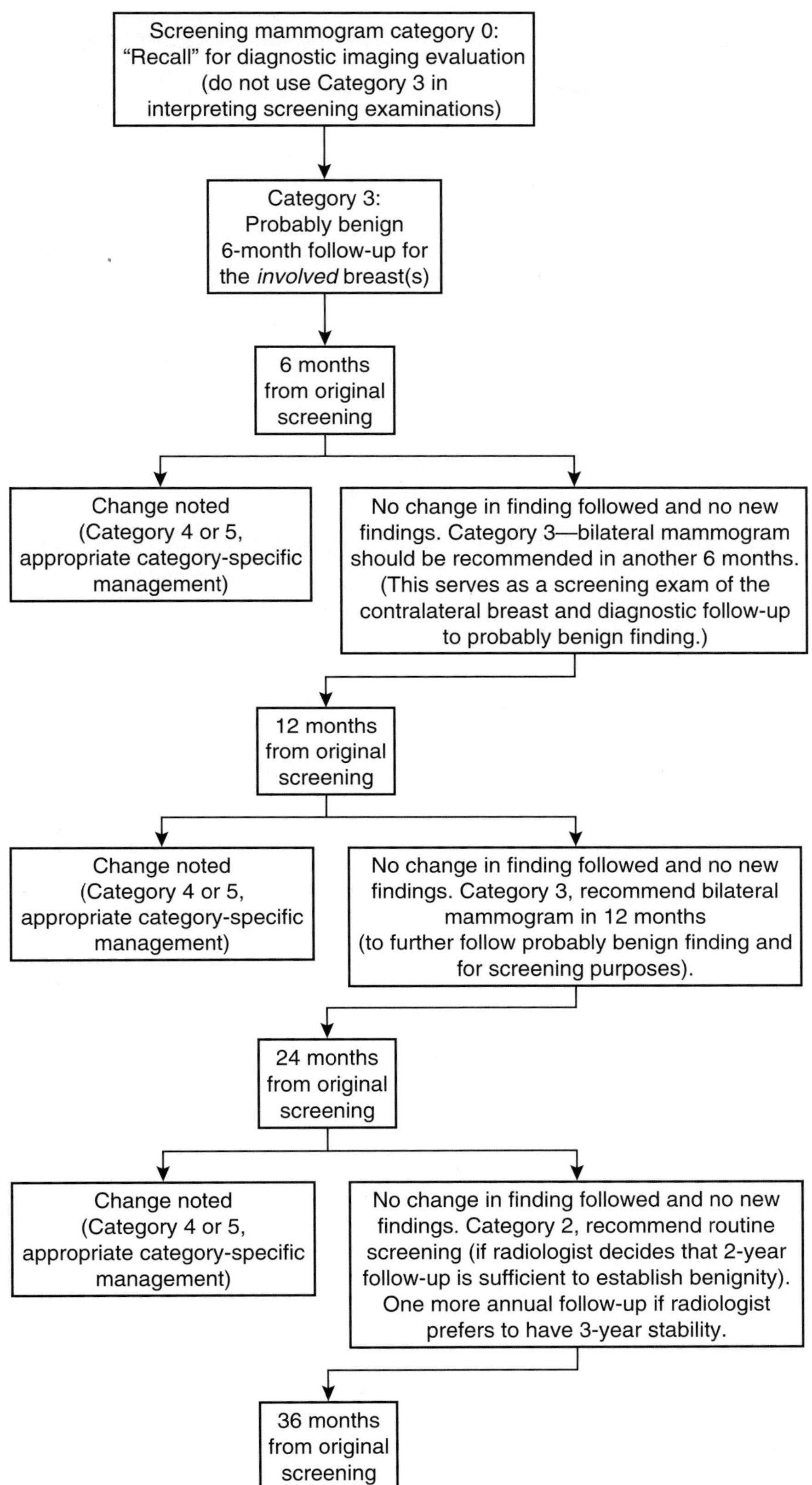

Figure 7–16. Category 3 algorithm. (From American College of Radiology [ACR]: ACR BI-RADS Mammography, 4th ed. In ACR Breast Imaging Reporting and Data System Atlas. Reston, VA: American College of Radiology, 2003.)

References

1. Beckman HB, Markakis KM, Suchman AL, Frankel RM: The doctor-patient relationship and malpractice: Lessons from plaintiffs' depositions. Arch Intern Med 1994;154:1365-1370.
2. Hickson GB, Clayton EW, Entman SS, et al: Obstetricians' prior malpractice experience and patients' satisfaction with care. JAMA 1994;272:1583-1587.
3. Rubin E, Frank MS, Stanley RJ, et al: Patient-initiated mobile mammography: Analysis of the patients and the problems. South Med J 1990;83:178-184.
4. Bassett LW, Hendrick RE, Bassford TL, et al: Quality Determinants of Mammography. (Clinical Practice Guideline, No. 13. AHCPR Publication No. 95-0632.) Rockville, MD: Agency for Health Care Policy and Research, Public Health Service, US Department of Health and Human Services, October 1994.
5. Barton JW, Kornguth PJ: Mammographic deodorant and powder artifact: Is there confusion with malignant microcalcifications? Breast Dis 1990;3:121-126.
6. Rutter DR, Calnan M, Vaile MS, et al: Discomfort and pain during mammography: Description, prediction and prevention. BMJ 1992;305(6851):443-445.
7. Brew MD, Billings JD, Chisholm RJ: Mammography and breast pain. Australas Radiol 1989;33:335-336.
8. Jackson VP, Lex AM, Smith DJ: Patient discomfort during screen-film mammography. Radiology 1988;168:421-423.
9. Stomper PC, Kopans DB, Sadowsky NL, et al: Is mammography painful? A multicenter patient study. Arch Intern Med 1988;148:521-524.
10. Cardenosa G, Eklund GW: Rate of compliance with recommendations for additional mammographic views and biopsies. Radiology 1991;181:359-361.
11. Monsees B, Destouet JM, Evens RG: The self-referred mammography patient: A new responsibility for radiologist. Radiology 1988;166:69-70.
12. Brenner RJ: Medicolegal aspects of breast imaging. Radiol Clin North Am 1992;30:277-286.
13. DeNeef P, Gandara J: Experience with indeterminate mammograms. West J Med 1991;154:36-39.
14. Robertson CL, Kopans DB: Communication problems after mammographic screening. Radiology 1989;172:443-444.
15. Adamson TE, Tschann JM, Guillon DS, Oppenberg AA: Physician communications skills and malpractice claims: A complex relationship. West J Med 1989;150:356-360.
16. Entman SS, Glass CA, Hickson GB, et al: The relationship between malpractice claims history and subsequent obstetric care. JAMA 1994;272:1588-1591.
17. Killilea B: Improving communications can prevent malpractice. Indiana Med 1990;82:272-273.
18. Messinger OJ: The patient's perception of care: A factor in medical litigation. Can Fam Physician 1989;35:133-135.
19. Miller RH, Williams PC, Napolitana G, Schmied J: Malpractice: A case-control study of claimants. J Gen Intern Med 1990;5:244-248.
20. Physician Insurers Association of America: Breast Cancer Study. Rockville, MD: Physician Insurers Association of America, 2002.
21. Shapiro RS, Simpson DE, Lawrence SL, et al: A survey of sued and non-sued physicians and suing patients. Ann Intern Med 1989;149:2190-2196.
22. Unger P: Failure to diagnose breast cancer—the communication dilemma. ACR Bull 1990;6:10.
23. Valente CM, Antlitz AM, Boyd MD, Troisi AJ: The importance of physician-patient communication in reducing medical liability. MD Med J 1988;37:75-78.
24. Wooley FR, Kane RL, Hughes CC, Wright DD: The effects of doctor-patient communication on satisfaction and outcome of care. Soc Sci Med 1978;12:123-128.
25. Ong G, Austoker J: Recalling women for further investigation of breast screening: Women's experiences at the clinic and afterwards. J Public Health Med 1997;19:29-36.
26. Priyanath A, Feinglass J, Dolan NC, et al: Patient satisfaction with the communication of mammographic results before and after Mammography Quality Standards Reauthorization Act of 1998. AJR Am J Roentgenol 2002;178:451-456.
27. Brenner RJ: Evolving medical-legal concepts for clinicians and imagers in evaluation of breast cancer. Cancer 1992;69(Suppl):1950-1953.
28. Physician Insurers of America: Breast Cancer Study. Lawrenceville, NJ: Physician Insurers of America, 1990.
29. Physician Insurers Association of America: Breast Cancer Study. Washington, DC: Physician Insurers Association of America, 1995.
30. Lipkus IM, Birdavolu M, Fenn K, et al: Informing women about their breast cancer risks: Truth and consequences. Health Communication 2001;13:205-226.
31. Meyer N, Fernadez M, Gold R: A report of the literature review: Effective and culturally sensitive health care provider communication and health promotion of Hispanic clients. Calverton, MD: MACRO International, 1994.
32. Hickson GB, Clayton EW, Githens PB, Sloan FA: Factors that prompt families to file malpractice claims following perinatal injuries. JAMA 1992;267;1359-1363.
33. Kopans DB: Standardized mammography reporting. Radiol Clin North Am 1992;30:257-264.
34. Hindle WH: Concise, clinically pertinent mammography requests and reports as an aid to increasing the utilization of screening and diagnostic mammography. Womens Health Issues 1991;1:86-89.
35. Kopans DB, D'Orsi CJ: ACR system enhances mammography reporting. Diagn Imaging 1992;14:125-32.
36. American College of Radiology (ACR): ACR BI-RADS Mammography, 4th ed. In ACR Breast Imaging Reporting and Data System, Breast Imaging Atlas. Reston, VA: American College of Radiology, 2003.
37. D'Orsi CJ, Kopans DB: Mammographic feature analysis. Semin Roentgenol 1993;28:204-230.
38. Jackson VP, Hendrick RE, Feig SA, Kopans DB: Imaging of the radiographically dense breast. Radiology 1993;188:297-301.
39. Sickles EA: Periodic mammographic follow-up of probably benign lesions: results in 3,184 consecutive cases. Radiology 1991;179:463-468.
40. Varas X, Leborgne F, Leborgne JH: Nonpalpable probably benign lesions: Role of follow-up mammography. Radiology 1992;184:409-414.
41. Varas X, Leborgne JH, Leborgne F, et al: Revisiting the mammographic follow-up of BI-RADS Category 3 lesions. AJR Am J Roentgenol 2002;179:691-695.

The Medical Audit

Statistical Basis of Clinical Outcomes Analysis

Michael N. Linver

Medicine is the art of dealing with uncertainty.
The practice of breast screening is the acme of that art.

—Moskowitz, 1988

The *mammography medical audit* can be defined in broad terms as a retrospective evaluation of the appropriateness and accuracy of mammographic image interpretation. The medical audit has been recognized by numerous experts in mammographic interpretation as the ultimate indicator of mammography performance.[1-4] It is the distillation of all of the quality assurance and quality control aspects addressed in mammography. It is the best measure of the interpretive ability of the mammographer. The medical audit removes the mystique and uncertainty of mammography and replaces them with a means to quantify and verify the value of the mammographer's work. It should therefore be an integral part of every practice.

I and other members of the multidisciplinary Clinical Practice Guideline Panel on Quality Determinants of Mammography, convened by the Agency for Health Care Policy and Research (AHCPR) of the U.S. Department of Health and Human Services, originally prepared much of the material on the medical audit in this chapter. The material was published by AHCPR as part of their Clinical Practice Guideline series.[5]

The medical audit of a mammography practice has numerous benefits. It evaluates the ability of mammography to detect very small cancers at the expected rate, one of the most important measures of success of any mammography practice.[2-4,6] Radiologists receive individualized feedback regarding their performance. This feedback provides confidence, if the results are within expectations, or identifies a need for additional training in interpretive skills for the mammographer or technical skills for the technologist, if they are not.[3,4,6-8] Longitudinal audits may detect the causes of false-negative errors, allowing for identification and correction of technical and interpretive shortcomings.[4,6,9-11] When audit data are reviewed and acted on appropriately, they become a powerful source of education for the mammographer.[9] Audit results within expected values can also be used to improve the compliance of both referring physicians and patients with screening mammography guidelines[3,6] as well as to indicate acceptable levels of performance to third-party payers and government agencies.[3,6]

Individual audit data may be useful for a medicolegal defense.[3,4,8,12] As a part of a risk management program, timely audits of abnormal mammograms promote optimal follow-up of patients.[2] Audit data such as the number of screening cases recalled for additional evaluation have been valuable for calculating costs per patient screened.[1] As capitation arrangements become more prevalent throughout the medical community, radiologists seeking to contain costs when vying for capitation contracts with health care organizations should find such information useful. A final benefit of the audit process is that pooling of the data may allow universal outcomes analysis to be performed through a national database.[3,4,13]

Another compelling reason to perform a mammography audit relates to federal law. In 1992, Congress passed the Mammography Quality Standards Act (MQSA). This legislation regulates the practice of mammography. Subpart 3 Section 354f21A calls for "standards that require establishment and maintenance of a quality assurance and quality control program at the facility that is adequate and appropriate to ensure the reliability, clarity, and accurate interpretation of mammograms." The final Rule of MQSA, which went into effect in 1999, mandates a limited form of the audit.[14] The specific audit requirements under MQSA are elaborated in more detail later.

Other regulatory organizations have also recognized the value of the medical audit. The Joint Commission on Accreditation of Healthcare Organizations (JCAHO) requires "periodic assessment by the radiology department/service of the collected information in order to identify important problems in patient care."[15] For compliance with its voluntary practice guidelines and technical standards, the American College of Radiology (ACR), in its document titled *ACR Practice Guideline for the Performance of Screening Mammography*, specifies the following: "Each facility shall establish and maintain a mammography medical outcomes audit program to follow up positive mammographic assessments and to correlate pathology results with the interpreting physician's findings. This program shall be designed to ensure reliability, clarity, and accuracy for the interpretation of mammograms. Analysis of these outcome data shall be made individually and collectively for all interpreting physicians at a facility at least annually. It is understood that in some practice situations it will not be possible to obtain follow-up information on all positive mammograms."[16] In the fourth edition of the American College of Radiology syllabus *Breast Imaging Reporting and Data System* (BI-RADS), a major chapter is devoted to follow-up and outcomes monitoring, describing the performance of the audit in detail.[17]

COLLECTION OF AUDIT DATA: WHAT SYSTEM SHOULD BE USED?

When one undertakes a medical audit, the volume of data that must be acquired for analysis can present an imposing challenge. Although the data can be gleaned manually,[3,4] specially designed computer software programs have been created to perform such tasks.[3,7,18-22] A variety of commercial software products are efficient, effective, and widely available. Most practices currently performing audits find these programs user friendly and affordable. These programs may include all the information recommended in "Follow-up and Outcomes Monitoring" chapter in the ACR BI-RADS syllabus,[17] or less information if only a limited audit is possible. A computer data collection program can be incorporated into a complete computerized reporting system.[17,20]

In deciding how best to collect audit data, one must consider the real cost of an audit in dollars and in time. Initiating and maintaining an audit requires a significant time commitment by at least one member of a mammography practice. For a small practice, use of a computer program to handle modest amounts of data is not essential, but for a large practice, it is a necessity. Careful assessment of needs before initiation of an audit can turn a data collection nightmare into a task that is manageable both fiscally and physically as well as one that is a rewarding educational experience.

THE DATA: WHAT SHOULD BE COLLECTED? WHAT SHOULD BE CALCULATED?

A variety of data can be collected that reflect the nature and quality of a mammography practice. To decide what data are most essential, one must consider the following three major questions, which directly measure a mammographer's performance:[23]

- Does the practice meet the primary goal of an effective screening program? In other words, is a high percentage of cancers being detected in the screened population? What are the detection rate and sensitivity for asymptomatic cancer?
- Is a large percentage of cancers being found with a favorable prognosis? That is, are the majority of mammographically detected cancers small and confined to the breast? What are the percentages of minimal cancers and lymph node–negative cancers being found?
- Are other important parameters reflecting screening and diagnostic success equivalent to those demonstrated in other screening programs? That is, are request rates for further imaging evaluation or biopsy in the acceptable range? What is the recall rate, and what is the positive predictive value (PPV)?

Table 8–1 lists the essential raw and derived data that are required to answer these questions (an exception is sensitivity, which is discussed later). *Raw data* refer to specific items of information, interpretive results and recommendations, and pathology findings collected directly from the mammography and pathology reports. *Derived data* refer to calculated measures of various mammographic and pathologic parameters based on the collected raw data. The raw data that are listed in Table 8–1 have been collected in most major audits reported in the literature.[1-4,6,7,18,24-26] They are all readily accessible and relatively easy to collect, regardless of the method used. Sources of these data are discussed later.

Additional data are listed as part of the more complete raw data list in Table 8–2. They are also of great value, although they can add considerable time and complexity to the audit process. These data have

Table 8–1. The Essential or Basic Mammography Audit: Minimum Desired Raw and Derived Data

A. Raw data:
   1. Dates of audit period and total number of examinations in that period.
   2. Number of screened examinations; number of diagnostic examinations.*
   3. Number of recommendations for further imaging evaluation (recalls) (ACR BI-RADS Category 0 = "Needs Further Evaluation").
   4. Number of recommendations for biopsy or surgical consultation (ACR BI-RADS Categories 4 and 5 = "Suspicious Findings" and "Highly Suggestive of Malignancy").†
   5. Biopsy results: malignant or benign (keep separate data for FNA or core biopsy cases).†
   6. Tumor staging: histologic type (in situ [ductal] or invasive [ductal or lobular]), grade, size, and nodal status.

B. Derived data (calculated from the raw data):
   1. True-positive results.
   2. False-positive results = three sub-definitions: FP_1, FP_2, FP_3 (see text).
   3. Positive predictive value:
      a. If a screening/diagnostic facility, can define any of three ways:
         (1) Based on abnormal screening examination (PPV_1).
         (2) Based on recommendation for biopsy or surgical consultation (PPV_2).
         (3) Based on result of biopsy (PPV_3 or positive biopsy rate).
      b. If screening facility only, can define only one way, based on abnormal screening examination (PV_1).
   4. Cancer detection rate for asymptomatic (true screening) cases.
   5. Percentage of minimal cancers‡ found.
   6. Percentage of node-negative invasive cancers found.
   7. Recall rate.
   8. Analysis of any known false-negative examinations.†

*Separate audit statistics should be maintained for asymptomatic and symptomatic patients.
†Collection of these data is required under MQSA final rules.
‡Minimal cancer: invasive cancer ≤1 cm or in-situ ductal cancer.
ACR BI-RADS, American College of Radiology Breast Imaging Reporting and Data System; FNA, fine-needle aspiration.

Table 8–2. More Complete Mammography Audit: Raw Data to Be Collected*

1. **Dates of audit period and total number of examinations in that period (usually a 6- or 12-month period).**
2. Risk factors:
   a. Patient age at the time of the examination.
   b. Breast cancer history: personal or family (especially premenopausal cancer in first-degree relative—mother, sister, or daughter)
   c. Hormone replacement therapy.
   d. Previous biopsy-proven lobular carcinoma in situ or atypia.
3. **Number and type of mammograms: screening (asymptomatic) or diagnostic (clinical breast signs or symptoms of possible abnormality or abnormal screening mammogram)**†
4. First-time examination or follow-up (repeat) study.
5. Mammographic interpretation and recommendation (try to conform to ACR lexicon).
   a. Further imaging evaluation (recall) [ACR BI-RADS Category 0 = "Needs Further Evaluation"].
   b. Routine follow-up (ACR BI-RADS Categories 1 and 2 = "Negative" and "Benign Findings").
   c. Early follow-up (ACR BI-RADS Category 3 = "Short-term Follow-up").
   d. Biopsy or surgical consultation (ACR BI-RADS Categories 4 and 5 = "Suspicious Findings" and "Highly Suggestive of Malignancy")‡
6. **Biopsy results: benign or malignant (keep separate data for FNA or core biopsy cases).**‡
7. Cancer data:
   a. Mammographic findings: mass, calcifications, indirect signs of malignancy, no mammographic signs of malignancy.
   b. Palpable or nonpalpable tumor.
   c. Tumor staging (pathologic): histologic type, grade, size, and nodal status.

***Bold type indicates data desired for the essential mammography audit.**
†Separate audit statistics should be maintained for asymptomatic and symptomatic patients.
‡Collection of these data required under final rules of the Mammography Quality Standards Act.
ACR BI-RADS, American College of Radiology Breast Imaging Reporting and Data System; FNA, fine-needle aspiration.

been useful in many studies as determinants of prevalent versus incident cancer rates (*prevalent cancers* are those found on the first mammogram; *incident cancers* are those found on a subsequent mammogram), predictive value of various mammographic findings, and significance of various risk factors.[1-3,6,7,18,24,25]

Although not required for calculation of the essential derived data listed in Table 8–1, the additional raw data listed in Table 8–2 are still worthwhile to collect because they provide information about certain variables that can cause marked fluctuation in audit results. For instance, if a large proportion of mammography examinations was performed on patients screened for the first time (those with prevalent cancers), the rate of cancers detected should be much higher than in a population that has been screened previously (incident cancers). Thus, knowledge of the proportion of initial screening mammograms to follow-up screening mammograms can be extremely useful in fine-tuning and interpreting the audit results.[3,7]

Table 8–3. The More Complete Mammography Audit: Derived Data to Be Calculated*

1. **True-positives, false-positives (three subdefinitions: FP_1, FP_2, FP_3),** true-negative, false-negative results (MQSA final rules require analysis of any known false-negative results)†
2. Sensitivity.
3. **Positive predictive value:**
   a. Based on abnormal screening exam result (PPV_1).
   b. Based on recommendation for biopsy or surgical consultation (PPV_2).
   c. Based on results of biopsy (PPV_3).
4. Specificity.
5. Cancer detection rate:
   a. Cancer detection rate for asymptomatic (true screening) cases.
   b. Prevalent vs incident.
   c. Overall.
   d. Rates within various age groups.
6. **Percentage of minimal cancers‡ found.**
7. **Percentage of node-negative invasive cancers found.**
8. **Recall rate.**
9. **Analysis of any known false-negative examinations.**†

***Bold type indicates data desired for the essential mammography audit analysis.**
†Collection of these data required under MQSA final rules.
‡Minimal cancer: invasive cancer ≤1 cm or in-situ ductal cancer.
MQSA, Mammography Quality Standards Act.

As with the raw data, the essential derived data can be supplemented with additional derived data of great value, as noted in Table 8–3. These additional data are also highly desirable, but time constraints and lack of accessibility of certain raw data, especially false-negative results (see the following list), may preclude their being calculated.

Before calculating any of the derived data in Table 8–1 or Table 8–3, one should categorize every mammographic examination result into one of four groups according to the following definitions (based on major audit studies in the literature):

1. True-positive (TP): Cancer diagnosed within 1 year after biopsy recommendation based on an abnormal mammogram (consensus).
2. True-negative (TN): No known cancer diagnosis within 1 year of a normal mammogram (consensus).
3. False-negative (FN): Diagnosis of cancer within 1 year of a normal mammogram result.[1,7,10,11,24,26,27] Although numerous other definitions of false-negative results exist, this definition historically has been the one most widely applied.
4. False-positive (FP): The literature supplies the following three different definitions:
   a. No known cancer diagnosed within 1 year of an abnormal screening mammogram result (i.e., a mammogram for which further imaging evaluation or biopsy is recommended) (FP_1).[1-3,24,26]
   b. No known cancer diagnosed within 1 year after recommendation for biopsy or surgical consultation on the basis of an abnormal mammogram result (FP_2).[1,7]

SCREENING TEST FOR CANCER	BIOPSY RESULTS: Positive	BIOPSY RESULTS: Negative
Positive	True positive (TP)	False positive (FP)
Negative	False negative (FN)	True negative (TN)

Figure 8–1. Graphic representation of relationship among true-positive (TP), false-positive (FP), false-negative (FN), and true-negative (TN) mammogram results. (See text for explanation.)

c. Benign disease found at biopsy within 1 year after recommendation for biopsy or surgical consultation on the basis of an abnormal mammogram result (FP_3).[3,7,24]

Another way to conceptualize the relationship among these four groups of results is expressed graphically in Figure 8–1.[28] Women screened for breast cancer with mammography were assigned to the top (positive) group if the result indicated a suspicion of breast cancer or in the bottom (negative) group if the result was judged to be normal. Each group was then subdivided according to whether patients were subsequently found to have breast cancer (left columns) or not (right columns). There are then four possible combinations:

- If results of both mammogram and biopsy are positive for cancer, the mammogram result is designated true-positive (TP).
- If both mammogram and biopsy results are negative for breast cancer, or if the mammogram result is negative and no clinical evidence of breast cancer is found in the absence of a biopsy, the mammogram result is designated true-negative (TN).
- If the mammogram result is positive and either the biopsy result is negative or no clinical evidence of breast cancer is seen within 1 year, the mammogram result is designated false-positive (FP).
- Conversely, if the mammogram result is negative for cancer and the biopsy result positive, the mammography result is designated false-negative (FN).

Given these definitions and raw data, one can now calculate the following derived data on the basis of major audit studies in the literature.

Sensitivity

Sensitivity is defined as the probability of detecting a cancer when a cancer exists or, alternatively, as the percentage of all patients found to have breast cancer within 1 year of screening whose mammograms were correctly diagnosed as suspicious for breast cancer.[2,6,7,9,18,24,26,29,30] Sensitivity can be expressed as follows:

$$\text{Sensitivity} = \frac{TP}{TP + FN}$$

Positive Predictive Value

The following three separate definitions of PPV may be applied on the basis of the three definitions of false-positive results given previously:

- PPV_1 (abnormal screening): The percent of *all abnormal screening examination results* (i.e., those for which biopsy, further imaging evaluation, or short interval follow-up examination was recommended) that lead to a diagnosis of cancer.[2,3,18,26,29]

$$PPV_1 = \frac{TP}{\text{number of abnormal screening examinations}}$$

or

$$PPV_1 = \frac{TP}{TP + FP_1}$$

- PPV_2 (biopsy recommended): The percentage of *all cases recommended for biopsy or surgical consultation* as a result of screening that resulted in the diagnosis of cancer.[1,7] PPV_2 can therefore be expressed as:

$$PPV_2 = \frac{TP}{\text{number of cases recommended for biopsy after abnormal screening examinations}}$$

or

$$PPV_2 = \frac{TP}{TP + FP_2}$$

- PPV_3 (biopsy performed): The percentage of *all biopsies actually performed* as a result of screening that resulted in the diagnosis of cancer. This is also known as the *biopsy yield of malignancy*, or the *positive biopsy rate*.[3,7,18,31] PPV_3 can therefore be expressed as:

$$PPV_3 = \frac{TP}{\text{number of biopsies}}$$

or

$$PPV_3 = \frac{TP}{TP + FP_3}$$

It should be noted that the various types of PPV just described are measures of completely different skills utilized by the breast imager. PPV_1 is considered a measure of one's perceptive skills at screening, whereas PPV_2 and PPV_3 are deemed measures of analytical skills utilized in diagnostic mammographic evaluation. Further, for interpretation and comparison of audit data from a particular mammography practice with published data to be accurate, it is important to know which definition of PPV is being used. For practices performing only screening mammography, only PPV_1 is of value in evaluating data. For practices performing both screening and diagnostic mammography, all three definitions of PPV can be applied.

Specificity

Specificity is defined as the probability of a normal mammogram report when no cancer exists or, alternatively, as the percentage of all patients with no evidence of breast cancer within 1 year of screening who were correctly identified as having normal mammograms at the time of screening.[1-3,18,24,26,29] Specificity can therefore be expressed as:

$$\text{Specificity} = \frac{\text{TN}}{\text{FP} + \text{TN}}$$

Some variation in the range of specificity exists, depending on the definition of false-positive results being applied, but the variations are small because of the very small number of false-positive results and the very large number of true-negative results in most audit series.

Overall Cancer Detection Rate

Defined as the overall number of cancers detected per 1000 patients examined by mammography, the *overall cancer detection rate* should be available in all basic audits.[1-3,7,10,18,24,29-31] Of even greater value is the cancer detection rate in asymptomatic patients, as this group represents the true screening population.[2,3,7,32] Therefore, all mammograms should be classified as screening or diagnostic so that the cancer detection rate in the asymptomatic group might be calculated.

The following cancer detection rates can be calculated only if the appropriate raw data are collected. Although not essential to a basic audit, such rates provide valuable audit information and should be calculated when possible.

- Prevalent versus incident cancer rates (i.e., rates of cancer in first-time versus follow-up examinations)[3,5,7,18]
- Cancer detection rates by age group[3,9,18]

In addition, separate sensitivities, PPVs, and specificities can be calculated for each of these subgroups, yielding yet another stratum of useful audit information. A summary of major articles that include medical audit data on mammography screening is shown in Table 8–4.

ANALYZING THE DATA: WHAT DO THE NUMBERS TELL YOU?

The real value of calculating the derived data as described in the previous section lies in creating quantitative measures of the six pieces of derived data that can address the three questions one must answer if mammography of high quality is to be achieved: By quantifying sensitivity and cancer detection rate, one can assess whether a high percentage of cancers are being detected in the screened population. By quantifying tumor size and node positivity, one can evaluate whether a high percentage of those cancers found at screening have a favorable prognosis. By quantifying recall rate and PPV, one can determine whether those cancers are being found through the use of acceptably efficient and appropriate performance criteria.

The relationship among these data can best be conceptualized using a representative receiver operating characteristic (ROC) curve for mammography,[28,33] as shown in Figure 8–2. An ROC curve for any individual mammographer can be generated by assessing his or her interpretive skills in predicting the likelihood of malignancy in a mixed set of positive and negative mammogram examinations with proven outcomes. The mammographer plots his or her performance as a series of graph points based on his or her answers to such an assessment, with each point representing that mammographer's perceived likelihood plotted against the actual findings. The resulting series of plotted points defines the ROC curve for that individual. Each mammographer's ROC curve is slightly different but should always be above the diagonal line in Figure 8–2 spanning the curve from lower left to upper right, which represents chance performance. Operators with greater mammographic interpretative skills generate ROC curves whose arcs span higher above that line (showing a higher percentage of true-positive and true-negative interpretations), and those with lesser skills generate curves coming closer to the line. Regardless of the height of

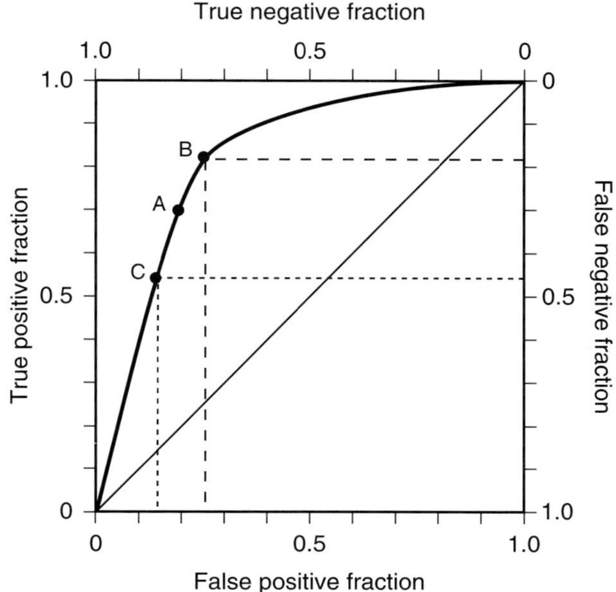

Figure 8–2. Representative receiver operation characteristics (ROC) curve for mammography. (See text for explanation.)

Table 8–4. Summary of Medical Audit Data from Mammography Screening Studies in the Medical Literature, 1987–1993

	Population Screened					Results									Tumor Data		
Study*	Total Patients	Asymptomatic (%)	Symptomatic (%)	Baseline (%)	F/U (%)	TN	FP†	TP	FN	PPV‡§	Sensitivity‡	Specificity‡	Recall Rate (%)	Cancer Detection Rate/1000	Median Size (cm)	Mean Size (cm)	Lymph Node Positivity (%)
Spring and Kimbrell-Willmot, 1987[4]	6430	NG	NG	NG	NG	5960	338 (3)	117	15	0.257_C (0.218, 0.300)	0.886 (0.820, 0.935)	0.946 (0.940, 0.952)	NG	18.19	NG	2.2	32.3
Bird, 1989[1]	21,716	NG	NG	NG	NG	19,402	2172 (1)	130	12	0.056_A (0.048, 0.067)	0.915 (0.857, 0.956)	0.900 (0.895, 0.903)	9.27	5.99	NG	1.7	29
Sickles, 1992[3]	37,093	94	6	61	39	36,399	456 (3)	220	18‖	0.325_C (0.290, 0.363)	0.924 (0.883, 0.955)	0.988 (0.986, 0.989)	5.66	5.93	1.2	1.5	11.2
Linver et al, 1992[7]																	
First year	18,706	86	14	39	61	18,215	340 (2)	121	30	0.263_B (0.223, 0.306)	0.801 (0.726, 0.860)	0.982 (0.980, 0.984)	5.34	6.47	1.5	1.7	2.6
Second year	19,927	88	12	29	71	19,232	487 (2)	181	27	0.271_B (0.238, 0.307)	0.870 (0.815, 0.912)	0.975 (0.973, 0.977)	8.12	9.08	1.2	1.6	18.5
Burhenne, 1992[18]	11,824	100	0	NG	NG	10,786	984 (1)	47	7	0.045_A (0.034, 0.061)	0.870 (0.751, 0.946)	0.916 (0.911, 0.921)	8.72	3.97	NG	NG¶	11
Lynde, 1993[30]	21,141	NG	NG	NG	NG	19,771	1263 (1)	98	7	0.072_A (0.059, 0.087)	0.933 (0.868, 0.973)	0.940 (0.937, 0.943)	6.44	4.64	NG	1.2	2.0
Robertson, 1993[2]	25,788	100	0	NG	NG	24,061	1539 (1)	170	18	0.099_A (0.086, 0.115)	0.904 (0.853, 0.942)	0.940 (0.938, 0.943)	6.63	6.59	NG	NG**	NG

*Superscript numbers indicate chapter references.

†Numbers in parentheses represent type 1, 2, or 3 FP, as defined in text.

‡For PPV, sensitivity, and specificity, the two sets of numbers in parentheses represent the confidence intervals for each.

§Subscripts$_A$, $_B$, and $_C$ represent PPV_1, PPV_2, and PPV_3, respectively, as defined in text.

‖Estimated from partial sample.

¶85% were stage 0 or stage 1.

**66% were stage 0 or stage 1.

FN, false-negative mammogram results; FP, false-positive mammogram results; F/U, patients receiving a follow-up mammogram, screening or diagnostic, at any time after their baseline mammogram; NG, not given; PPV, positive predictive value; TN, true-negative examination results; TP, true-positive examination results.

the arc of a mammographer's ROC curve, if he or she starts from a point in the middle of the curve (point A) and then increases his or her false-positive fraction to point B on the curve (which would be reflected in a relatively lower value for PPV or a higher recall rate), the mammographer would experience an obligatory decrease in the false-negative fraction; this change would be reflected in a higher sensitivity and a higher cancer detection rate. Conversely, if a mammographer decreases his or her false-positive fraction to point C on the curve (as reflected in an increase in PPV and a decrease in the recall rate), he or she would find an increase in the false-negative fraction; this would be reflected in a decrease in sensitivity and a lower cancer detection rate.

What the preceding discussion means, very simply, is that what we do in mammographic interpretation is a trade-off: To find every cancer present and have *no* false-negative results, we would necessarily have to recall virtually every patient and request surgery on a large majority—both of which are unacceptable scenarios if screening mammography is to be cost-effective and psychologically accepted by the women being screened. Indeed, if one is operating too close to the high end of the ROC curve, where the slope is shallow (e.g., to the right of point B in Fig. 8–2), the inefficiency is apparent: One can decrease the false-negative rate only minimally, while increasing the false-positive rate to an unacceptably high level. Therefore, one should operate closer to the middle of the ROC curve, where one can be the most efficient and yet still effective in detecting early breast cancer. By calculating and comparing the derived data described earlier, a mammographer can determine where he or she is operating on a representative ROC curve (or even on his or her own ROC curve, if known), and adjust his or her approach to mammographic interpretation accordingly.

It should be noted that those valuable parameters related to tumor size and node positivity are not reflected in this model of the ROC curve. However, the ROC curve still serves as a useful construct for understanding and utilizing the interrelationships among the other stated measures of interpretative quality. Desirable numerical goals designed to keep the mammographer operating near the middle of the ROC curve (those toward which the mammographer should strive) are as listed in Table 8–5. These numbers are based on a review of all major audits in the literature (most of which are listed in Table 8–4); they are discussed separately in this section.

Table 8–5. Analysis of Medical Audit Data: Desirable Goals

PPV based on abnormal screening examination (PPV_1)	5%–10%
PPV when biopsy (surgical, FNA, or core) recommended (PPV_2)	25%–40%
Tumors found—stage 0 or 1*	>50%
Tumors found—minimal† cancer*	>30%
Node positivity*	<25%
Cancers found/1000 cases*	2–10
Prevalent cancers found/1000 first-time examinations*	6–10
Incident cancers found/1000 follow-up examinations*	2–4
Recall rate	≤10%
Sensitivity (if measurable)	>85%
Specificity (if measurable)	>90%

*Screening cases only.
†Minimal cancer: invasive cancer ≤1 cm or in-situ ductal cancer.
FNA, fine-needle aspiration; PPV, positive predictive value.

Sensitivity

The published range of sensitivity in most mammography audits is between 85% and 90%, using the definition given in the previous section.[1-4,7,10,24,26,30] This range is therefore believed to be a desirable goal for which to strive (see Tables 8–4 and 8–5). Sensitivity may vary with patient age, appearing to decrease in younger populations with denser breast tissue,[18] but nonetheless remains an extremely valuable parameter. Unfortunately, sensitivity is often among the most difficult data to obtain, because it requires knowledge of the actual number of false-negative results for accurate calculation (see previous section). It is usually necessary to establish a direct link with a complete tumor registry to find the actual number of false-negative results.[2,7,10,18] Thus, it may not be possible to calculate "true" sensitivity. One may be forced instead to estimate the number of false-negative results so as to obtain an approximation of sensitivity. However, it is still desirable to make such an estimate.[3]

Positive Predictive Value

The PPV is virtually always measurable, through the use of one or more of the definitions described previously. As already shown, definitions in the literature vary considerably, but the most often quoted is the PPV for all cases recommended for biopsy, PPV_2. This number is greater than 25% and less than 40% in most reported series (see Tables 8–4 and 8–5).[3,6,7] This range is considered an achievable goal for which to strive. If a facility performs only screening mammography, then the PPV based on the number of abnormal screening examination results (PPV_1) is more relevant and should be applied instead. This number is greater than 5% and less than 10% in most reported series.[2,3,18,26,29] For screening examinations, this range is considered an achievable goal for which to strive. Facilities performing both screening and diagnostic mammography may also find this number of value, in addition to PPV_2. For cases in which core, fine-needle aspiration (FNA), or vacuum-assisted needle biopsy is recommended and performed, separate PPV statistics should also be maintained for each of these biopsy groups.

As with sensitivity, the PPV is subject to many variables. Among those that must be assessed in considering its true significance within a given practice situation are age distribution, percentage of palpable cancers, cancer detection rate, the size and lymph node positivity of cancers found, and the sensitivity.[25,27,33-36] The obligatory relationship of cancer detection rate, sensitivity, and PPV to individual mammographers' ROC curves was discussed earlier. The effect of the age distribution on PPV relates to findings by some researchers that PPV is directly proportional to the age of the population being screened and to the prior probability of disease within each age group.[3,27,35] The older the screened population, the higher the PPV. PPV varies directly with the size of tumors found in a screening mammography program: When most tumors are large, PPV tends to be higher; finding a greater number of small tumors can usually be accomplished only at the expense of a lower PPV.[27]

Tumor Size

In most reported series, more than 50% of tumors diagnosed by mammography are stage 0 or stage 1.[2,4,18] Even more importantly, most series have shown that more than 30% of cancers diagnosed by mammography were minimal cancers (i.e., invasive cancer ≤1 cm or in situ ductal cancer).[1,3,7,10,18,26,30,31] Because it has been well established that mortality from breast cancer is directly related to tumor size, the preceding percentages for small and early-stage tumors found by mammography should be considered desirable goals for which to strive (see Tables 8–4 and 8–5). Later published audit data from our practice, and from others' as well, show that tumors detected at screening that are stage 0 or stage 1 account for as many as 80% of all screening-detected tumors, and minimal cancers for as many as 60%.[34,35]

By reaching these goals, one can achieve the greatest impact on ultimate patient outcomes. Tumor size varies with the percentage of screening and diagnostic examinations in a mammography practice; examinations of symptomatic patients invariably yield larger tumors than do those of a pure screening population.[4,7,18,34]

Lymph Node Positivity

Tumor size should also be correlated with the rate of lymph node positivity, which in most reported series has been less than 25% in the screened population.[1,3,4,7,18,26,31] Because it has also been well established that mortality from breast cancer is directly proportional to node positivity, this rate for node positivity must also be considered a desirable goal for which to strive in one's practice (see Tables 8–4 and 8–5).

Cancer Detection Rate

The cancer detection rate is quite variable, with rates of 2 to 10 cancers per 1000 reported in most screening series (see Tables 8–4 and 8–5).[1-4,7,18,24-26,31,34,35] Variability in this rate is due to differing rates of detection in first-screened women versus already screened women (i.e., prevalent versus incident cancers). In most screening populations, prevalent cancer rates vary from 6 to 10 per 1000, and incident cancer rates from 2 to 4 per 1000.[7,18,24] The cancer detection rate also varies with age.[3,7,18,24,35,37] Despite these variables, the cancer detection rate serves as a measure of the relative threshold for abnormal that is being achieved. For example, even if an audit shows that sensitivity and PPV are both acceptably high, if the number of cancers found is less than 2 per 1000 asymptomatic patients, then the sensitivity value is suspect. The number of cancers eluding detection in that particular population is probably too great, and the overall quality of the mammography being practiced should be further evaluated.[25,36]

Recall Rate

It is of great value to assess the *recall rate*—the percentage of patients for whom further imaging evaluation (e.g., coned compression views, magnification views, ultrasonography) is recommended—for two reasons: First, the recall rate can be utilized to calculate one of the commonly used definitions of false-positive results (FP_1) and one of the definitions of PPV (PPV_1) (see previous section on derived data). Accordingly, the recall rate is of value to all facilities but especially to those performing only screening mammography. Second, the cost-effectiveness and credibility of mammography can be negatively affected by a disproportionately high recall rate.[1]

In most large reported series, the percentage of patients recalled for further imaging evaluation is 10% or less.[1-3,18,26,34] This value is therefore believed to be a desirable number for which to strive (see Tables 8–4 and 8–5). However, later data derived from more than 30 practices in North Carolina indicate that a rise in recall rates beyond 4.8% resulted in very little improvement in sensitivity, and that increasing recall rates beyond 5.8% was accompanied by a significant decrease in PPV_1. Therefore, it appears that the best trade-off between relatively high sensitivity and PPV_1 values may be accomplished with a recall rate of approximately 5% to 6%.[38] Many investigators have also noted that the recall rate decreases with growing experience over time.[1,3]

Specificity

Specificity is a measure of quality that is difficult to acquire. In fact, in many large studies, it is not even

Table 8–6. Outcomes Data for Case Mixes of Screening plus Diagnostic Mammography Examinations

Screening : Diagnostic Case Mix	Rate of Abnormal Findings (%)	Positive Biopsy Findings (%)	Cancer Detection Per 1000	Nodal Metastasis (%)	Stage 0 & Stage 1 Cancer (%)	Mean Size of Invasive Cancer (mm)
90:10	6	38	10	8	87	14.4
80:20	7	40	15	9	86	14.8
70:30	8	41	20	9	85	15.2
60:40	10	41	25	9	83	15.6
50:50	11	42	30	11	82	16.0
40:60	12	43	35	11	80	16.4
30:70	13	44	39	12	79	16.8
20:80	14	45	44	13	78	17.2
10:90	15	45	49	13	76	17.6

From Sohlich RE, Sickles EA, Burnside ES, et al: Interpreting data from audits when screening and diagnostic mammography outcomes are combined. AJR Am J Roentgenol 2002;178:681-686.

calculated.[1,2,4,7] When calculated, specificity is usually found to be greater than 90% (see Tables 8–4 and 8–5).[2,18,26] However, it is often difficult to obtain an accurate measure of specificity because its calculation requires knowledge of all true-negative results, a number that in turn is based on the number of false-negative results, the least accessible information in any audit. Consequently, specificity is not considered essential to a routine audit.

ANALYZING THE DATA WHEN SCREENING AND DIAGNOSTIC OUTCOMES ARE COMBINED

Many mammography practices cannot easily segregate screening and diagnostic mammography data to correctly and accurately calculate the requisite derived data for evaluating mammography performance outcomes. If the screening and diagnostic mammography cases remain mixed, the calculated derived data cannot be properly analyzed, because of the confounding effects of combining screening and diagnostic mammography data. For this reason, Sohlich and colleagues[39] have developed mathematical models based on comprehensive audit data from their own practice. These outcomes tables give approximate values for recall rate, PPV, cancer detection rate, tumor size, and lymph node positivity for screening-to-diagnostic case mix ratios ranging from 90:10 to 10:90, and are summarized in Table 8–6. In this table, "diagnostic mammograms" are defined as those performed because of: (1) abnormal findings at screening, (2) 6-month follow-up for probably benign findings, (3) follow-up in patients with previous lumpectomy for breast cancer, (4) presentation of a patient with a palpable lump, and (5) "other."

Another outcomes table, Table 8–7, was created for practices that do not separate screening and diagnostic examinations to any extent during auditing. In Table 8–7, comparison is made between screening mammogram cases and cases in which the diagnostic examination is performed solely to evaluate a palpable lump, again giving approximate values for the same derived data as in Table 8–6 over a spectrum of screening-to–palpable lump proportions, from 2% palpable lumps, to 50% palpable lumps. (Sohlich and colleagues[39] constructed several other tables for additional specific situations, consideration of which is beyond the scope of this discussion.)

Once individuals in a practice have estimated their own mix of cases, they can use the appropriate derived data numbers in these tables as benchmarks with which to compare their observed outcomes.

It should be understood that the data in these tables are from an academic institution with full-time

Table 8–7. Outcomes Data for Screening plus Diagnostic Mammography for Case Mixes Based on Percentage of Cases Evaluated for Palpable Masses

Palpable Mass (%)	Rate of Abnormal Findings (%)	Positive Biopsy Findings (%)	Cancer Detection Per 1000	Nodal Metastasis (%)	Stage 0 & Stage 1 Cancer (%)	Mean Size of Invasive Cancer (mm)
2	7	40	15	8	86	14.3
5	8	41	18	10	83	15.4
10	9	43	24	12	79	17.0
15	9	44	29	14	76	18.3
20	10	44	35	16	73	19.3
30	12	46	46	19	68	21.0
50	15	51	68	23	61	23.1

From Sohlich RE, Sickles EA, Burnside ES, et al: Interpreting data from audits when screening and diagnostic mammography outcomes are combined. AJR Am J Roentgenol 2002;178:681-686.

breast imaging specialists and therefore may not be achievable in the community practice setting. Nonetheless, they provide approximate goals for which practices that cannot separate their screening and diagnostic mammography data should strive.

FURTHER BENEFITS: THE AUDIT AS A TEACHING TOOL

The audit is an important teaching tool. The *group* audit is important because it provides great statistical power, which in turn allows for comparison with overall expected rates in other group audits, such as those listed in Table 8–5.[3,7] However, the multiple variables described previously (e.g., prevalent versus incident cancer rates, age of a population, ratio of screening to diagnostic mammograms) that markedly influence the results of a group audit may render comparisons with other group audits less valuable than a comparison of individual audits within a group practice.

A major advantage to an *individual* audit is in providing a valid relative comparison among group members. If certain group members show considerable variation in sensitivity and other performance standards, measures can be taken to improve the performance of those at variance and thus improve future outcomes.[3,7] Even so, individual audit data can still be unclear, especially when the numbers involved are so small as to show large statistical variation. For instance, a very competent mammographer interpreting a low volume of cases might find 10 cases of breast cancer one year and only 2 cases the next year, strictly on the basis of random chance, a phenomenon exaggerated when the numbers involved are small. This problem can be obviated in part as further data and larger numbers of cases for each individual accrue over the years, but should never be ignored when comparisons of audit data are being made.

As mentioned previously, false-negative results may be difficult to identify without access to a complete tumor registry.[3] However, if cases with false-negative results are available for review, they should be evaluated thoroughly to assess cause (technical versus interpretive error).[4,9-11] A critical review of such cases allows a group to take action to improve overall quality, thus improving future outcomes.

THE AUDIT AS REQUIRED BY THE MAMMOGRAPHY QUALITY STANDARDS ACT

As mentioned earlier, all practices are now mandated to perform an audit under MQSA, as outlined under the final rules effective April 28, 1999.[14] However, the final rules require only that all "positive" mammogram results (BI-RADS final assessment categories 4 and 5) be tracked for eventual pathologic outcome at biopsy, either cancer (TP) or benign (FP). This activity, although admirable, falls woefully short of measuring actual practice quality and efficiency as outlined in the preceding discussion. In fact, it allows for calculation of only one (PPV) of the six vital pieces of derived data required for such measurement.

The final rules do request, but do not mandate, that FNs be sought, and require that a lead physician oversee the entire quality assurance process and designate one individual to perform the audit activities at least yearly, take corrective actions as needed, and review data collectively and by individual.

The final rules further encourage, but do not require, radiologists to perform a more extensive audit. It is hoped that those radiologists truly serious about measuring their mammographic skills would do so through the collection and calculation of the more extensive parameters of practice quality and efficiency described here.

SOURCES FOR AUDIT DATA

Much of the patient demographic information and all of the pertinent mammographic findings should be readily available from a well-designed mammography reports record, especially if the reports are computerized.[3,7,18,22] Biopsy results are available from a variety of sources, as follows:[1-4,7,18,26,31]

1. If malignant, the results can be found through a complete regional or state-wide tumor registry. If such a registry does not exist or access to its data is not possible, a definitive diagnosis of cancer can be obtained from one or more of the following (in order of preference):
   a. The pathology report.
   b. The surgical report (if a frozen-section analysis was done).
   c. The referring physician or surgeon, by phone or letter.
   d. The patient herself (last resort), by phone or letter.
2. If benign, the results can be obtained from the pathology report.

Patients often receive care at outside institutions, making data collection more difficult. If hospital reports are not available, the diagnosis can usually be obtained by phone or letter from the referring physician or the surgeon. The patient herself should be considered as a possible last source. The importance of obtaining complete follow-up on every patient with suspicious findings cannot be stressed enough. Every effort should be made to obtain this information through the methods described.

THE VALUE OF THE AUDIT IN EVERYDAY PRACTICE: PERSONAL EXPERIENCE

In 1987, our group of 12 private practice radiologists elected to take measures to improve the overall quality and efficiency of mammography in our

Table 8–8. Summary by Year of Comparison of Initial Follow-Up Examinations, Screening Cases Only, 1988–1992

	1988	1989	1990	1991	1992	5-Year Total
Total screening examinations	16,067	17,627	20,415	25,180	31,164	110,453
Initial examinations	6185	5059	4981	5741	8682*	30,648
	(38.5%)	(28.7%)	(24.4%)	(22.8%)	(27.9%)	(27.7%)
Follow-up examinations	9882	12,568	15,434	19,439	22,482	79,805
	(61.5%)	(71.3%)	(75.6%)	(77.2%)	(72.1%)	(72.3%)

*Reason for slight increase in 1992 was that we began screening in remote rural areas with two mammography vans, performing approximately 5000 mammograms, virtually all of which were initial screening studies.

practice. To do so, we obtained additional mammographic training, developed our own computerized mammography reporting system, and began to evaluate our ongoing performance by conducting an audit of mammography results. The first 2 years of our audit experience have been previously reported[7] and are summarized in Table 8–4, along with other mammography audits in the literature. In the second year of our audit, the number of cancers diagnosed increased 50% (from 121 to 181), our sensitivity increased from 80% to 87%, and our PPV_3 and PPV_2 values remained essentially unchanged at 32% and 27%, respectively. Median tumor size decreased from 1.5 cm to 1.2 cm, and the rate of node positivity decreased from 26% to 18.5%. Our recall rate rose 50%, from 5.3% to 8.1%. We attributed the overall improvement in performance seen in the second year to, among other factors, an alteration in our overall interpretive approach learned through attendance at dedicated teaching courses during the first year of the audit. It was only through the audit process that we were able to assess our performance and obtain quantitative proof to support our belief that the quality of our mammography practice was improving.

Once its value to our practice was established, we continued to perform an extensive annual audit. Because of the unique combination of our computerized program and an accessible state-wide tumor registry, we have been able to obtain complete audit data on the more than 400,000 mammograms interpreted since the initiation of our computer program in 1988. In addition to the findings reported for the first 2 years, we have since identified several other trends of great value to us individually and as a group, some of which are worthy of mention here.

First, in evaluating our raw data, we found that the proportion of initial to follow-up screening mammography examinations has progressively diminished since 1988 (Table 8–8). Because a lower number of cancers is found in the follow-up group (incident cancers) than in the first-screened group (prevalent cancers) in screening populations, we therefore would have expected a slight decrease in the rate of screening-detected cancers over the years. This is indeed what we found: In 1989, we detected 6.24 cancers per 1000 screened patients; this value fell to 4.75 by 1992 (Table 8–9). Knowing that we were seeing a higher percentage of follow-up screening patients each year, we therefore had a ready explanation for the gradual drop in rate of screening-detected cancers we had observed.

A second trend we identified relates to four of the other major parameters of mammographic quality: tumor size, node positivity, percentage of minimal cancers, and PPV (Tables 8–10 to 8–12). As mentioned earlier, we noticed a significant decrease in tumor size and node positivity between 1988 and 1989 in both the combined (symptomatic and asymptomatic) tumor group and the asymptomatic tumor group. We attributed this decrease to an overall improvement in our interpretive skills during that time related to attendance at dedicated mammography courses.[7] Since then, we have noted a continued slight downward trend in tumor size and node positivity in both groups as well as a progressive rise in the percentage of minimal cancers (see Tables 8–10 and 8–11). These data added further support to our original hypothesis and boosted our conviction that we were continuing to achieve a measurable level of success in detecting early breast cancer. Moreover, we found that we accomplished these goals without requesting a greater percentage of unnecessary biopsies: The PPV_3 remained between 31% and 35%, and the PPV_2 between 26% and 29% (see Table 8–12).

Review of individual audit data has also proved helpful. We have observed some variation in sensitivity and PPV_3 in our group. Some members with acceptable sensitivity numbers have shown an inordinately low PPV_3. This would indicate that the thresh-

Table 8–9. Summary by Year of Surgical Consults Recommended, Number and Rate of Cancers Found, and PPV—Screening Cases Only, 1988–1992

	1988	1989	1990	1991	1992	5-Year Total
Total screening examinations	16,067	17,627	20,415	25,180	31,164	110,453
Total surgical consults recommended	282	433	446	542	513	2216 (2.0%)
Cancers found at biopsy	77	110	111	149	148	595 (0.54%)
PPV based on recommended surgical consults (PPV_2) (%)	27	25	25	27	29	27
Cancers found/1000 patients	4.79	6.24	5.44	5.92	4.75	5.36

Table 8–10. Summary by Year of Size and Nodal Status of All Cancers Found by Mammography, 1988–1991

	1988	1989	1990	1991	1992
Average tumor size (cm)	1.72	1.57	1.50	1.37	1.49
Median tumor size (cm)	1.5	1.2	1.3	1.0	1.1
Minimal tumors* (%)	36	41	43	47	50
Node-positive tumors (%)	26	18.5	23	21	16

*Minimal tumors: invasive cancer ≤1 cm or in-situ ductal cancer.

Table 8–11. Summary by Year of Size and Nodal Status of All Asymptomatic (Screening-Detected) Cancers Found, 1988–1992

	1988	1989	1990	1991	1992
Average tumor size (cm)	1.32	0.95	1.30	0.89	1.09
Median tumor size (cm)	1.2	0.9	1.0	0.8	0.8
Minimal tumors* (%)	50	62	55	60	63
Carcinoma in situ (%)	23	25	23	41	31
Node-positive tumors (%)	12.5	5.7	17	13	12

*Minimal tumors: invasive cancer ≤1 cm or in-situ ductal cancer.

old for the criteria for biopsy they were using was set too low. By reviewing their audit numbers, they have taken measures to slide a bit more toward the middle of the ROC curve, with considerable success.

Another audit activity that has proven extremely useful, as shown previously in other audit reports, has been the review of all identified cases with false-negative results.[4,9,10] We hold a group conference every 6 to 12 months to review each case in detail and to establish the cause of its false-negative status. This nonthreatening team approach has been highly successful and has firmly established the role of the mammography audit in our practice as a sophisticated and invaluable teaching tool.

MEDICOLEGAL CONSIDERATIONS

At this time, all states have statutes that protect from legal discovery all peer review records generated by a structured peer review committee in the hospital setting.[32,36] However, virtually no statutes exist to protect from discovery all other information generated in the hospital under the auspices of organized quality review activities or quality review information obtained in the outpatient setting.[40] Therefore, it is recommended that complete mammography audits be maintained primarily as internal audits. Interpreting physicians should not disseminate the audit data without being aware of confidentiality legislation in their state.

Model legislation does exist: Congress provided protection to participants of quality control programs and created a qualified immunity for the medical quality assurance records generated by the programs within the military health care system (10 USC 1102) and the Department of Veteran Affairs (38 USC 5705). Efforts have been made to enact legislation to protect audit material generated outside the military setting but have so far been unsuccessful.[40] Such legislation, if enacted, would encourage all mammography facilities to participate in the medical audit process without fear of increasing their medicolegal liability, allowing the facilities to more completely fulfill the quality assessment standards required by JCAHO, ACR, and MQSA and to provide audit information to benefit their radiologists and, if released publicly, the medical community and patients they serve. At this time, however, such broadly drawn legislation does not exist.

THE EXPANDING ROLE OF THE MEDICAL AUDIT: PROBLEMS AND PROMISE

With the promulgation of the MQSA Final Regulations, some limited mammography audit activities are now required components of each mammography practice. Many mammographers consider this development a mixed blessing. Although the virtues of the audit process are readily evident, the difficulties in collecting the necessary data, especially in smaller and rural practices, are just as obvious. The added time and work required to perform an audit and other quality assurance activities mandated under MQSA for the radiologist, technologist, and other personnel may discourage some facilities to the extent that they will discontinue performing mammography. Such an outcome would undermine the very purpose of the MQSA, that of improving access to high-quality mammography for women in all socioeconomic settings. Indeed, those women in greatest jeopardy of losing mammography services

Table 8–12. Summary by Year of PPV_2 and Positive Biopsy Rate (PPV_3) for All Tumors Found by Mammography, 1988–1992

	1988	1989	1990	1991	1992	5-Year Totals
Surgical consults requested	461	668	651	817	749	3346
Biopsies done in this group	368	570	526	704	670	2838
Benign results	247	389	341	485	456	1918
Malignant results	121	181	185	219	214	920
PPV_3 (positive biopsy rate) (%)	33	32	35	31	32	32
PPV_2 (all cases recommended for biopsy) (%)	26	27	28	27	29	27

are the ones in rural and low-income areas that are already underserved. It is hoped that the U.S. Food and Drug Administration and other empowered regulatory agencies will take the necessary measures to avoid such an outcome.

If mammography audits can be successfully established in all practices, if federal legislation is passed protecting audit data from discovery, and if patient confidentiality can be ensured,[42] then the promise these data offer can be realized. By pooling and entering these data in a national mammography database, we can provide more accurate answers to many of the vital questions concerning mammography today.[3,13,41] We must improve screening compliance and tumor detection regionally and within various age and ethnic groups; we need more accurate and more complete feedback of data results to individual mammography facilities; and we need to achieve the ultimate goal of screening mammography: reduction of mortality from breast cancer in all age groups. Toward these ends, the National Cancer Institute (NCI) has established the Breast Cancer Surveillance Consortium.[42] The Consortium, which focuses on community practices, comprises groups from eight states with a total population of more than 1 million women of screening age, and with a breast cancer rate of at least 3700 new cancers per year. The Consortium has already begun to analyze their pooled audit data to examine and, it is hoped, resolve many of the issues delineated here. If practices in other states not included in the Consortium could somehow contribute their mammography audit data as well, the attainment of the goals of screening mammography could be assessed even more completely.

CONCLUSIONS

The mammography medical audit is currently the only objective measure of the interpretive ability of the mammographer. It also offers a means of quantifying the success of mammography in detecting early breast cancer. Because it is such a vital component of mammography quality assurance, a limited form of the audit is now federally mandated by MQSA.

The appropriate collection, calculation, and analysis of raw and derived data for either a basic or a more complete audit should be performed to answer the three essential questions that determine a mammographer's success: (1) Are the cancers that exist being found, (2) are a large proportion of these cancers small and node negative, and (3) are these cancers being found with an acceptable number of patient recalls and biopsies? Answering these questions with quantitative data enables the performance of the mammographer to be compared with the range of desirable values found in other audits throughout the medical literature. Further, each mammographer can estimate where he or she is operating on the ROC curve and adjust his or her approach to mammographic interpretation accordingly. Additional audit activities, such as evaluating group audit versus individual audit statistics and reviewing false-negative results, can offer further benefit as teaching tools that improve clinical outcomes.

Certain medicolegal concerns regarding discoverability of audit records, particularly in the outpatient setting, must be kept in mind. These concerns, together with concerns about the feasibility of performing an audit in many practices, currently impede widespread collection of audit data. If these problems can be remedied and the data pooled in a national mammography database, ideally in collaboration with the NCI Breast Cancer Surveillance Consortium, the full potential for using audit data to answer unresolved questions about the early detection of breast cancer can be realized.

Acknowledgments

I thank Richard Bird, MD, Peter Dempsey, MD, Robert D. Rosenberg, MD, and Charles Kelsey, PhD, for their help in preparing the manuscript. I also thank the following fellow members and consultants on the AHCPR Panel on Quality Determinants of Mammography who helped me develop the section of the Clinical Practice Guideline on the medical audit: R. James Brenner, MD, JD, Janet R. Osuch, MD, Robert Smith, PhD, Victor Hasselblad, PhD, and Darryl Carter, MD.

References

1. Bird RE: Low-cost screening mammography: Report on finances and review of 21,716 cases. Radiology 1989;171:87-90.
2. Robertson CL: A private breast imaging practice: Medical audit of 25,788 screening and 1,077 diagnostic exams. Radiology 1993;187:75-79.
3. Sickles EA: Quality assurance: How to audit your own mammography practice. Radiol Clin North Am 1992;30:265-275.
4. Spring DB, Kimbrell-Wilmot K: Evaluating the success of mammography at the local level: How to conduct an audit of your practice. Radiol Clin North Am 1987;25:983-992.
5. Bassett LW, Hendrick RE, Bassford TL, et al: Quality Determinants of Mammography. (Clinical Practice Guideline No. 13. AHCPR Publication No. 95-0632.) Rockville, MD, Agency for Health Care Policy and Research, Public Health Service, US Department of Health and Human Services, October, 1994.
6. Sickles EA, Ominsky SH, Sollitto RA, et al: Medical audit of a rapid-throughput mammography screening practice: Methodology and results of 27,114 examinations. Radiology 1990; 175:323-327.
7. Linver MN, Paster S, Rosenberg R, et al: Improvement in mammography interpretation skills in a community radiology practice after dedicated teaching courses: 2-year medical audit of 38,633 cases. Radiology 1992;184:39-43.
8. Reinig JW, Strait CJ: Professional mammographic quality assessment program for a community hospital. Radiology 1991;180:393-396.
9. Bird RE, Wallace TW, Yankaskas BC: Analysis of cancers missed at screening mammography. Radiology 1992;184:613-617.
10. Burhenne HJ, Burhenne LW, Goldberg F, et al: Interval breast cancers in the Screening Mammography Program of British

Columbia: Analysis and classification. AJR Am J Roentgenol 1994;162:1067-1071.
11. Moskowitz M: Interval cancers and screening for breast cancer in British Columbia [commentary]. AJR Am J Roentgenol 1994;162:1072-1075.
12. Brenner, RJ: Medicolegal aspects of breast imaging. Radiol Clin North Am 1992;30:277-286.
13. Clark RA, King PS, Worden JK: Mammography registry: Considerations and options. Radiology 1989;171:91-93.
14. US Department of Health and Human Services, Food and Drug Administration: Mammography quality standards: Final rule. 62 Federal Register 55851-55994 (1997).
15. Joint Commission 1990 Accreditation Manual for Hospitals. Chicago, Joint Commission on Accreditation of Healthcare Organizations, 1989.
16. American College of Radiology: ACR Practice Guideline for Performance of Screening Mammography [adopted by the ACR Council, 1999]. In ACR Practice Guidelines and Technical Standards. Reston, VA, American College of Radiology, 2003.
17. American College of Radiology: ACR BI-RADS™—Mammography. 4th ed. In ACR Breast Imaging Reporting and Data System, Breast Imaging Atlas. Reston, VA, American College of Radiology, 2003.
18. Burhenne LJW, Hislop TG, Burhenne HJ: The British Columbia mammography screening program: Evaluation of the first 15 months. AJR Am J Roentgenol 1992;158:45-49.
19. Haug PJ, Tocino IM, Clayton PD, et al: Automated management of screening and diagnostic mammography. Radiology 1987;164:747-752.
20. Heilbrunn K, Graves RE: Increasing compliance with breast cancer screening guidelines: A clinician-oriented approach. Presented at American College of Radiology 24th National Conference on Breast Cancer, New Orleans, March 12-18, 1990.
21. Monticciolo DL, Sickles EA: Computerized follow-up of abnormalities detected at mammography screening. AJR Am J Roentgenol 1990;155:751-753.
22. Sickles EA: The use of computers in mammography screening. Radiol Clin North Am 1987;25:1015-1030.
23. Tabar L, Fagerberg G, Duffy SW, et al: Update of the Swedish two-county program of mammographic screening for breast cancer. Radiol Clin North Am 1992;30:187-210.
24. Braman DM, Williams HD: ACR accredited suburban mammography center: Three year results. J Fla Med Assoc 1989;76: 1031-1040.
25. Ciatto S, Cataliotti L, Distante V: Nonpalpable lesions detected with mammography: Review of 512 consecutive cases. Radiology 1987;165:99-102.
26. Lynde JL: A community program of low-cost screening mammography: The results of 21,141 consecutive examinations. South Med J 1993;86:338-343.
27. Kopans D: The positive predictive value of mammography. AJR Am J Roentgenol 1992;158:521-526.
28. D'Orsi CJ: Screening mammography pits cost against quality. Diagn Imaging 1994;16:73-76.
29. Baines CJ, Miller AB, Wall C, et al: Sensitivity and specificity of first screen mammography in the Canadian National Breast Screening Study: A preliminary report from five centers. Radiology 1986;160:295-298.
30. Margolin FR, Lagios MD: Development of mammography and breast services in a community hospital. Radiol Clin North Am 1987;25:973-982.
31. Moseson D: Audit of mammography in a community setting. Am J Surg 1992;163:544-546.
32. American Medical Association: A Compendium of State Peer Review Immunity Laws. Chicago, American Medical Association, 1988, p vi.
33. D'Orsi CJ: To follow or not to follow, that is the question. Radiology 1992;184:306.
34. Dee KE, Sickles EA: Medical audit of diagnostic mammographic examinations: Comparison with screening outcomes obtained concurrently. AJR Am J Roentgenol 2001;176:729-733.
35. Linver MN, Paster SB: Mammography outcomes in a practice setting by age: Prognostic factors, sensitivity, and positive biopsy rate. Monogr Natl Cancer Inst 1997;22:113-117.
36. Moskowitz M: Predictive value, sensitivity and specificity in breast cancer screening. Radiology 1988;167:576-578.
37. Moskowitz M: Breast cancer: Age-specific growth rates and screening strategies. Radiology 1986;161:37-41.
38. Yankaskas BC, Cleveland RJ, Schell MJ, et al: Association of recall rates with sensitivity and positive predictive values of screening mammography. AJR Am J Roentgenol 2001;177:543-549.
39. Sohlich RE, Sickles EA, Burnside ES, et al: Interpreting data from audits when screening and diagnostic mammography outcomes are combined. AJR Am J Roentgenol 2002;178:681-686.
40. American Medical Association: Report of AMA reference committee G, substitute resolution 722, "Medical peer review outside hospital settings." Chicago, American Medical Association, June, 1992.
41. Hurley SF: Screening: The need for a population register. Med J Austr 1989;153:310-311.
42. Linver MN, Rosenberg RD, Smith RA: Mammography outcome analysis: Potential panacea or Pandora's box? [commentary]. AJR Am J Roentgenol 1996;167:373-375.

Coding and Billing in Breast Imaging

Michael N. Linver

The dramatic success of mammography in bringing about a 20% decrease in breast cancer deaths in the United States since the mid-1980s[1] ironically has been accompanied by a precipitous drop in mammography reimbursement. The latter development has resulted in the curtailment and even elimination of mammography services in many radiology practices.[2] Those radiologists who perform breast imaging studies have become increasingly frustrated as fiscal disaster becomes the reward for their diligent effort and success in effectively changing the natural history of this disease. Even those most committed to the goal of driving down deaths from breast cancer through high-quality mammography now find that goal increasingly difficult to attain owing to inadequate reimbursement.

It is therefore more important than ever that the radiologist understand the workings of the reimbursement system as comprehensively as possible. With such an understanding, the radiologist can construct a strategic plan for financial survival in the breast imaging arena. Much of the following discussion centers on Medicare reimbursement, because Medicare sets the reimbursement precedents that most private payers follow.

CODING AND BILLING TERMINOLOGY: THE "LANGUAGE" OF REIMBURSEMENT

One must first have a thorough understanding of coding terminology. The code specified by the *International Classification of Diseases, 9th Revision: Clinical Modification*[3] (ICD-9-CM) for a service provided by the radiologist defines the medical indication for that service. This classification was begun and is overseen by the World Health Organization. With the receipt of a claim for payment, all payers initially evaluate the ICD-9-CM code to establish whether the service provided was appropriate for the medical condition being evaluated. For example, most providers consider ICD code 174.0 ("malignant neoplasm of the female breast") as an appropriate coding for performance and interpretation of a "diagnostic mammogram" and would allow coverage. More recently, the Centers for Medicare and Medicaid Services (CMS) has allowed radiologists to code certain findings from the radiology examination as the primary diagnosis on the CMS claim form (CMS Program Memorandum AB-01-144). Radiologists may now use, for example, ICD code 793.80, for "abnormal mammogram, unspecified," or ICD code 793.81, for "mammographic calcifications." Appropriate submission of the procedure code (CPT/HCPCS [see next paragraph]) would still be required before payment would be forthcoming for a covered diagnosis, however.

The Current Procedural Terminology (CPT) system was originally established by the American Medical Association (AMA) to identify procedures performed by physicians (CPT codes and descriptions only are copyrighted by the AMA; all rights reserved).[4] For more specificity, three additional modifying levels of CPT codes were added by HCFA (Health Care Financing Administration, the government body, now called CMS, that is responsible for overseeing Medicare payment).[5] These modifying codes are known as the CPT/HFCA Common Procedures Coding System (CPT/HCPCS) codes and are divided into three levels: level I HCPCS codes, which are listed in the AMA CPT codebook, and two lower levels—level II alpha-numeric codes (primarily nonphysician codes, or new technology) and level III local or regional codes. These three levels of modifying codes allow for more detailed reporting of various health care services. Selected codes, primarily diagnostic, are further divided into the global procedure (combined professional and technical component) and the separate professional and technical components of a procedure. For instance, for the performance and interpretation of a bilateral diagnostic mammogram of a Medicare patient (performed under ICD code 174.0, "malignant neoplasm of the female breast," as its indication), a CPT/HCPCS code of 76091 should be applied, with a current global reimbursement under the 2004 Final Medicare Fee Schedule (published in November 2003) of $95.58, representing a summation of the professional fee of $44.43 and the technical fee of $51.15.

MEDICARE REIMBURSEMENT: SETTING THE PRECEDENT; BACKGROUND AND PRESENT STATUS

First and foremost, one must have a complete understanding of the precedent-setting Medicare reimbursement system. Medicare reimbursement underwent a major overhaul in the early 1990s, when Congress directed the HCFA to study physician payment reform. The system that resulted, initiated by Medicare in 1992, became known as the Resource-Based Relative Value System (RBRVS).[6]

The RBRVS was created when the existing CPT codes were wed to a weighted system assigning a relative value to each physician procedure under what was to be known as the Medicare Fee Schedule (MFS). The MFS is regarded as resource-based, because the fee for a physician's service is based on the resources needed to provide that service: physician work, practice expenses, and professional liability insurance costs. All three components for a particular service are assigned a numerical value called a Resource Value Unit (RVU). These values then undergo regional adjustment for local differences in resource costs.[7]

To determine dollar reimbursement, one multiplies the respective geographic adjustments by the three RVU values assigned the service, adds them, and then multiplies the sum times the conversion factor. For 2004, the Medicare Fee Schedule conversion factor (as modified under the Prescription Drug/Medicare Reform Bill of 2003) is 37.3374, an increase of 1.5% compared with 2003. For current updates on the Physician Fee Schedule, one can consult the CMS Web site, at www.cms.gov/regulations/pfs/2004/

In April 2000, the HCFA published the final rules for a hospital outpatient prospective payment system (HOPPS) for hospital outpatient services.[8] HOPPS standardized Medicare reimbursement for procedures (technical component only) performed in outpatient facilities within a hospital and reduced patient out-of-pocket expenses as well. By prohibiting the "unbundling" of nonphysician outpatient services, the HCFA created instead 451 "bundled" Ambulatory Payment Classifications (APCs). The HCFA assigned a payment weight based on the factors for each APC. Payment is then determined through the use of a conversion factor and geographic adjustment factors. In general, the APC payment scale is similar to what existed before. However, two notable exceptions are the unilateral diagnostic mammogram (CPT code 76090) and the bilateral diagnostic mammogram (CPT code 76091), both of which have a proposed technical component payment for 2004 of $35.46, almost 30% less than the technical fee for a screening mammogram.[9] This particular instance of gross under-reimbursement should well be corrected, as the Prescription Drug/Medicare reform bill (H.R. 1 and S. 1) passed by Congress and signed by the President in late November 2003 was to include a substantial increase in the APC payment for both unilateral and bilateral diagnostic mammography (J Cooper, personal communication, 2003). This legislation authorized a rise in these rates to the same levels now being reimbursed by Medicare for the technical components of the same procedures performed in a nonhospital setting.

APC codes apply only to the technical components of radiology services for Medicare patients in a hospital setting. Professional fees are determined by the usual MFS based on the RBRVS.[10] For current updates on HOPPS, one can consult the CMS Web site, at www.cms.gov/regulations/hopps/2004p/changecy2004.asp.

Medicare payment rates do change on a regular basis: The CMS seeks input from the Resource Value System Update Committee (RUC) of representatives from the AMA and 22 specialty organizations, including the American College of Radiology, in order to update the physician work component of the RVU scale each year, and uses this information to conduct a comprehensive review of all relative values every 5 years. In their 1993 and 1998 reviews, the HCFA accepted approximately 90% of RUC recommendations. It is through the RUC that the greatest opportunity exists for an increase in reimbursement for breast imaging procedures in the near future.

The Medicare fee that is most critical to the success of every breast imaging facility is the reimbursement for screening mammography, originally set by congressional mandate in the Omnibus Budget Reconciliation Act of 1990.[11] Unfortunately for all financially struggling breast imagers, the initial reimbursement rate was set artificially low, at $55, and remained artificially low over the next decade. Congress did enlarge the pool of eligible women by extending yearly coverage to all Medicare-eligible women 40 years and older via the Balanced Budget Act of 1997[12] but did nothing to significantly improve reimbursement.

However, in December 2000, HR4577, the Medicare, Medicaid, and SCHIP Benefits Improvement and Protection Act (BIPA) was passed, returning screening mammography to the purview of the MFS. The global rate for screening mammography for 2003 under the MFS was $82.77, a slight increase over the 2002 rate but less than had been hoped for. As of December 2003, the final Medicare rate for 2004 is pegged only slightly higher, at $84.01. However, efforts to pass legislation further raising screening mammography reimbursement are still under way.[13]

CURRENT MEDICARE REIMBURSEMENT: ACCEPTABLE ICD-9-CM AND PROCEDURE CODES FOR MAMMOGRAPHY, AND PAYMENT RATES

The ICD-9-CM code for a screening mammogram, V76.12 ("special screening examination for malignant neoplasm, breast"), has been universally accepted by all regional Medicare carriers. However, acceptable reimbursement codes for diagnostic mammography vary tremendously from one Medicare carrier to the next. Although most payers adhere to the concept that "diagnostic mammography is generally indicated when there are signs or symptoms suggestive of malignancy,"[15] their individual interpretation of acceptable diagnosis codes is surprisingly diverse. Table 9–1 presents the ICD-9 codes for diagnostic mammography accepted for reimbursement by two large Medicare carriers, one in the Northeast and one in the Southwest.[14,15] As one can see, surprisingly few codes are accepted and reimbursed by

Table 9–1. Differences in Acceptance of Various ICD-9 Codes for Diagnostic Mammography by Two Separate Medicare Carriers, One in the Northeast United States and the Other in the Southwest United States

ICD-9 Codes for Diagnostic Mammography		Accepted by Medicare Carrier in Northeast	Accepted by Medicare Carrier in Southwest
172.5:	Malignant melanoma of skin of breast	Yes	No
173.5, 173.9:	Other malignant neoplasm	Yes	No
174.0-174.9:	Malignant neoplasm of female breast	Yes	Yes
175.0-175.9:	Malignant neoplasm of male breast	Yes	Yes
198.81:	Secondary neoplasm of breast	Yes	No
217.0:	Benign neoplasm of breast	Yes	No
232.5:	Carcinoma in situ of breast	Yes	No
233.0:	Carcinoma in situ of breast	Yes	Yes
238.3:	Neoplasm of breast soft tissue	Yes	Yes
239.2:	Neoplasm of uncertain behavior	Yes	No
239.3:	Neoplasm of unspecified nature of breast	Yes	Yes
451.89:	Thrombophlebitis of breast	Yes	No
610.0-611.9:	Other disorders of breast	Yes	Yes
793.8:	Nonspecific abnormal findings on radiological and other examination of body structure, breast	Yes	Yes
V10.3:	Personal history of malignant neoplasm, breast	Yes	Yes
V42.81-V42.9:	Organ or tissue replaced by transplant	No	Yes
V51.0:	Aftercare involving use of plastic surgery	No	Yes

both carriers, and a sizable number are reimbursed by only one of the two. It is therefore important to communicate with one's own Medicare carrier as to the acceptability of these or other ICD-9-CM codes for diagnostic mammography.

Table 9–2 lists examples of breast imaging–related procedural CPT codes and the corresponding reimbursement by Medicare for 2003 and the final Medicare reimbursement rates for 2004, as of December, 2003[9,16,17] (Granucci S, Kolb G, personal communication, 2003).

In assessing the Medicare payment rates in Table 9–2, one must keep in mind that these are national averages. They do not reflect geographic adjustments made by individual regional carriers. Reimbursement by local Medicare carriers may vary by as much as 30%.[18]

MEDICARE'S SPECIAL RULES RELATING TO MAMMOGRAPHY REIMBURSEMENT

Under Medicare, a screening mammogram is defined as a "preventive measure when a person has no history or personal history of breast cancer." It is "for routine screening of asymptomatic women, with or without a family history, and with or without a physician's recommendation." Thus, a Medicare-eligible woman does not need a written requisition to receive a screening mammogram. In essence, the screening mammogram for a Medicare-eligible woman has become a self-referred examination. If a woman needs a diagnostic mammogram because of clinical signs or symptoms of possible breast cancer, Medicare does require a written, telephone, or e-mail referral from the clinician, under Medicare Carrier Memorandum (MCM) #1725, section 15021(A)(5) (a-3). However, if a diagnostic mammogram is required for further evaluation of a screening-detected abnormality, no physician request is required.

As of 2002, Medicare allows reimbursement for both a screening mammogram and a diagnostic mammogram for the same patient, even if both are performed on the same day, with the proviso that the diagnostic mammogram was precipitated by an abnormal screening mammogram. Before 2002, Medicare would reimburse only for the diagnostic mammogram under these circumstances. Medicare does require the modifier "GG" to be attached to diagnostic mammogram CPT codes to ensure reimbursement in this situation.

Medicare reimburses for one baseline screening mammogram between ages 35 and 40 years, and for yearly screening mammograms beginning at age 40, in Medicare-eligible women. Under the "Lapsed Time Rule," a screening mammogram performed for a Medicare-eligible patient is not covered unless at least 11 months have elapsed since the last screening. Another Medicare rule relates to the "Advance Beneficiary Notice." Under this rule, the facility must notify the patient before the mammogram if the facility believes that Medicare may not pay for the mammogram and must explain to the patient the specific reason why Medicare may not pay (not enough time elapsed since last screening, patient does not meet Medicare age requirements, etc.). Further, the facility is required to obtain written acknowledgment of this notice, in writing, from the patient. If a facility fails to meet these requirements, any charges denied reimbursement by Medicare cannot be passed on to the patient; if the patient in such a case is "erroneously" billed, the action may constitute fraud and may subject the facility to heavy penalties. Also, the mammography center must be certified by the U.S. Food and Drug

Table 9–2. Selected Examples of Procedural CPT Codes and Medicare Reimbursements: National Average Fees, Unadjusted for Geography*

Services		2003 Fees ($) (Effective 3/1/03)				2004 Final Fees ($) (Effective 1/1/04)			
		Global	Professional	Technical	APC†	Global (Nonfacility)	Professional (Facility 26)	Technical (Facility TC)	APC†
1. Screening Mammogram									
76092	Bilateral	82.77	36.05	46.72	46.72	84.01	35.84	48.17	48.17
Diagnostic Mammograms									
76090	Unilateral	75.78	35.68	40.10	33.86	77.29	36.22	41.07	35.46
76091	Bilateral	94.17	44.14	50.03	33.86	95.58	44.43	51.15	35.46
2. Breast Biopsy: Stereotactic									
99241	E & M consultation code (i.e., provide opinion or advise on treatment to referring physician)	47.45	33.11	—	43.96	50.03	33.60	—	50.62
76095	Stereotactic localization code	355.35	81.66	273.68	206.17	361.80	82.52	279.28	241.64
19102	Needle core biopsy with imaging guidance	257.13	103.37	—	162.72	229.62	104.54	—	178.40
19103	Automated vacuum-assisted biopsy	594.82	188.71	—	274.90	601.13	191.17	—	304.34
76098	Specimen radiograph	24.65	8.46	16.19	39.92	24.64	8.21	16.43	42.57
19295	Placement of titanium clip for possible follow-up surgery or localized radiation	97.85	97.85	—	75.30	106.04	106.04	—	82.40
99211	E & M code (post-procedure, follow-up of patient, may not require presence of a physician)	20.60	8.83	—	43.96	22.03	8.96	—	50.62
99212	E & M brief physician visit with exam or counseling	36.42	23.17	—	43.96	38.46	23.52	—	50.62
3. Breast Biopsy: Ultrasound-Guided									
99241	E & M consultation code	47.45	33.11	—	43.96	50.03	33.60	—	50.62
76942	Ultrasound localization code	146.04	34.58	111.46	72.26	156.44	34.72	121.72	71.37
19102	Needle core biopsy with imaging guidance	257.13	103.37	—	162.72	229.62	104.54	—	178.40
76645	Echography, breast, with image documentation	67.69	27.59	40.10	51.04	69.07	28.00	41.07	56.14
99211	E & M code, post-procedure	20.60	8.83	—	43.96	22.03	8.96	—	50.62
4. Wire Needle Localization									
76096	Preoperative placement of needle localization wire (radiologist supervision & interpretation)	78.72	28.69	50.03	99.05	79.90	29.12	50.78	190.42
19290	Preoperative placement of needle localization wire	155.24	64.74	—	Bundled	162.79	65.71	—	Bundled
19291	Each additional lesion	86.45	32.00	—	Bundled	90.36	32.48	—	Bundled
76098	Radiographic examination of surgical specimen	24.65	8.46	16.19	39.92	24.64	8.21	16.43	42.57
5. Ductography									
76086	Superv. and interp., single duct	118.82	18.39	100.42	99.05	120.97	18.67	102.30	119.40
76088	Superv. and interp., multiple ducts	162.96	22.81	140.15	99.05	166.15	23.15	143.00	119.40
19030	Ductogram/galactogram inj. of contrast	189.81	77.99	—	Bundled	186.69	78.78	—	Bundled
6. Full-Field Digital Mammograms									
G0202	Screening mammogram, bilateral	132.06	36.79	95.27	95.27	133.29	35.84	97.08	91.63
G0204	Diagnostic mammogram, bilateral	140.15	45.98	94.17	46.49	140.76	45.18	95.58	49.15
G0206	Diagnostic mammogram, unilateral	112.93	37.15	75.78	46.49	113.88	36.59	77.29	49.15
7. Computer-Assisted Detection (CAD): New Codes for 2004									
76083	Screening mammogram—use with 76092	19.13	3.31	15.82	15.82	19.42	3.36	16.06	15.11
76082	Diagnostic mammogram—use with 76090-76091 (76085 has been deleted)	19.13	3.31	15.82	15.82	19.42	3.36	16.06	8.31
8. Breast Magnetic Resonance Imaging (MRI)									
76093	Breast MRI, unilateral	756.68	82.14	673.54		770.64	84.01	686.63	
C8905	Breast MRI, unilateral, without & with consultation (hospital only code)				482.08				502.37
76094	Breast MRI, bilateral	996.15	82.77	913.39		1015.20	84.01	931.57	
C8908	Breast MRI, bilateral, without & with consultation (hospital only code)				482.08				502.37
76393	MR guidance for needle placement	504.33	76.88	427.45	Bundled	511.89	78.03	433.86	346.46

*Medicare reimbursement rates do not contain local geographic adjustments for any of the fees noted in this outline.

†Bundled services are not payable by Medicare in the office or hospital setting and are packaged into the basic procedure; however, coverage by non-Medicare payers varies and may be paid by some.

APC, Ambulatory Payment Classification; CPT, Current Procedural Terminology; E & M, evaluation and management; facility = hospital, outpatient; Facility 26, Medicare modifier code for the professional component; Facility TC, Medicare modifier code for the technical component; non-facility = physician office.

Administration (FDA) to be eligible for Medicare reimbursement.

FOLLOWING MEDICARE'S EXAMPLE: THE REST OF THE PAYERS

Virtually all payers currently reimburse physicians using the same CPT coding for procedures that CMS (formerly HCFA) utilizes for Medicare reimbursement. However, there is considerable variability by payer group in the amount of reimbursement. For instance, many private payers are reimbursing full-field digital mammography at the same rate as film mammography, even though Medicare reimbursement rates for full-field digital mammography are fully 50% higher than those for film mammography. Even the conditions under which reimbursement is distributed vary considerably by payer. Each private company has its own interpretation of the "Elapsed Time Rule" and holds each patient responsible for establishing her own eligibility for a mammogram. However, like the Medicare carriers, the private insurers inevitably deny and delay payment for claims if they believe that their particular "rules" for reimbursement have not been strictly followed.

Health Maintenance Organizations (HMOs) usually reimburse at rates arrived at through negotiation with individual facilities. These rates are usually calculated as a percentage of Medicare rates and vary from one extreme to the other, depending on local competition. In general, the HMO rules for reimbursement are more convoluted than those of private insurers; one might be tempted to wonder whether the intent of such complications is to delay and deny payment for even the most legitimate claim for reimbursement.

Both HMOs and private payers often require pre-authorization for certain breast imaging procedures, especially interventional procedures. If pre-authorization is not requested and granted, most payers do not reimburse the costs, regardless of other circumstances. (Under Medicare rules, CMS does not require pre-authorization for interventional breast imaging procedures, but Medicare carriers reserve the right to deny claims for payment later if they deem the procedures inappropriate for any reason.) At present, no payers are reimbursing costs on a routine basis for screening breast ultrasonography and screening breast magnetic resonance imaging (MRI). Pre-authorization is required on a case-by-case basis for high-risk patients or others for whom these examinations are medically indicated.

The last significant, but nearly extinct, payer group is the cash-paying customer. Some states require that even a self-paying patient must present a signed referral from the clinician before a facility performs the examination. Aside from this minor exception, the facility dictates the rules for payment from self-paying patients.

MAXIMIZING REIMBURSEMENT: STRATEGIES FOR SUCCESS

Faced with the woefully low levels of reimbursement for most mammographic procedures, each mammography facility must adopt an aggressive and vigilant attitude to avoid financial loss. The strategy for success should focus on implementation of the following measures:

1. Know and diligently apply the preceding rules for reimbursement.
2. Appropriately combine the identification of the patient, the indication for the examination, and all applicable procedural codes with the report of the procedure itself.
3. Pay close attention to coding and billing habits.
4. Solicit and cultivate the cooperation of the clinicians.
5. Train all facility personnel to be knowledgeable regarding these same billing issues and to be fastidious in collecting all patient information relevant to billing.
6. Perform periodic internal data-quality audits.
7. Challenge payer denials and underpayments if they appear inappropriate or contradictory.
8. When negotiating with HMOs, use the facility's own mammography outcome data to demonstrate that finding earlier, smaller cancers with mammography translates into dollar savings for the HMO.
9. Do not forget about making services attractive for the cash-paying customers by offering a "discount."
10. Get involved politically by mobilizing patients and women's advocacy groups to support legislation increasing mammography reimbursement.

Knowing and Applying the Rules. According to a Medical Group Management Association survey conducted in 2001, more than one third of all claims submitted to payers are rejected or ignored, most often because of submission errors.[19] Therefore, one must do everything possible to beat the insurance carriers at their own game by preempting their anticipated denial of a claim. A basic but extremely effective first step is to identify and correct the most common causes of delay and denial:[20]

- Incorrect procedure ordered by the clinician
- Application of incorrect ICD-9-CM and/or CPT code(s) to the procedure
- Failure to obtain pre-authorization from the payer before the desired procedure
- Improper documentation for the procedure provided by the radiologist in his or her dictated report
- Provision of inadequate written documentation and/or incorrect billing information

Appropriate Combination of Information and Report and Applicable Procedural Codes. Verify that all the relevant information—patient identification, examination indications, and procedure codes—is accurately reflected in the dictated report. The report should have clear findings and conclusions and should include (1) correct identification of the mammogram as either screening or diagnostic, (2) listing of all views performed, and (3) the clinical history, because payment is based on the correct ICD-9-CM code in addition to all applicable CPT codes. For interventional breast procedures, it is important to include all applicable CPT codes, because these procedures always have more than one code (see Table 9–2). In addition, Medicare has assigned the interventional codes 19102 and 19103 a global period of 0 days. This means that other biopsy-related pre-procedure or post-procedure examinations, as well as any consultations with the patient before or after the procedure—E and M codes (see Table 9–2)—are not "bundled" with the original procedural code and may be billed separately. Although controversial, E and M codes can be successfully billed by breast imagers, provided that proper and complete documentation is performed. Because E and M codes have been successfully "unbundled" from the interventional procedures, one should be successful in billing for CPT codes 9924x and 992xx. However, one must meet the E and M Documentation Guidelines to do so. Additional documentation criteria for consultations (9924x) include a physician's request for an opinion or advice and a separate written report to the referring physician.

The 1995 and 1997 E and M Documentation Guidelines, as well as the proposed 2000 Guidelines released by HCFA, can be obtained from the HCFA Web site, at www.hcfa.gov/medicare.mcarpti.htm/ (the 1995 guidelines are preferred by most providers at this time). A strong word of caution is in order: If one does choose to bill the CPT E and M codes, one should be fastidious in following and documenting all the necessary steps required by the E and M Documentation Guidelines, including the appropriate history, mini-physical examination, and recommendations (Poller WR, personal communication, 2003). Failure to do so, if detected on Medicare review, may lead to charges of fraud and abuse.

Proper Coding and Billing Habits. If the radiologist is doing the coding and utilizing a short list of CPT codes (a "cheat sheet"), the listing must be verified as accurate and current, including all the newest codes. Otherwise, coding should be left in the hands of dedicated and well-trained staff personnel. One should monitor the local Medicare Review Policy (LMRP) portion of Medicare Part B bulletins for any local policy change.

Certain coding and billing practices should be avoided. In particular, one should not "up-code" (i.e., change a code to one with higher reimbursement) inappropriately, and one should try not to re-bill a patient for a procedure. If done too frequently, these actions create a "suspicious situation" that payers will target, setting up a potential "adverse profile" for the entire practice.[21]

Clinician Cooperation. One may have to educate clinicians and their staffs as to their contribution to proper reimbursement procedures. First, they should send or "fax" a signed referral before the examination is performed. Second, the clinician must provide the appropriate clinical diagnosis for each examination. For example, "fibrocystic disease" cannot be listed as the reason for a diagnostic mammogram if this diagnosis is not biopsy proven. Third, the clinician must fill out the requisition as correctly and completely as possible. This can best be accomplished with the help of a well-designed, user-friendly order form provided by the facility. Such a form should include: a checklist of possible procedures to be performed (screening mammogram, diagnostic mammogram, breast ultrasonogram, ultrasound-guided core biopsy, ductogram, etc.), a checklist of the patient's symptoms, if any (pain, lump, thickening, etc.), and a diagram of the breasts for the purpose of marking the location of pertinent physical findings. It is also useful for the form to contain all the facility's office phone numbers, including a fax number. Meeting regularly with all major clinician referrers, their respective staffs, or both, and apprising them of the importance of complying with the preceding conditions, enables one to avoid many reimbursement problems.[20]

Facility Personnel Training. If possible, designate one or two billing staff members as specialists in billing breast imaging procedures. The contributions of such individuals are invaluable. Not only do payers deny up to 35% of claims, but also a further 5% to 10% of claims are reimbursed at an inappropriately reduced rate.[19] Only through careful monitoring of claims by well-trained, specialized billing staff members can such situations be discovered in one's own practice. Important billing benchmarks, such as total charges, collections, number of days claims remain in Accounts Receivable, the distribution of the Accounts Receivable, and payer mix, should be monitored monthly for unexpected changes and trends. For instance, if a large and growing number of claims are suddenly remaining in Accounts Receivable and are not being resolved in 60 days or less, a more serious look at the entire billing system is in order. This kind of analysis can best be performed by billing specialists. If a practice does not allow for such individuals in-house, consideration should be given to utilizing a competent and proven outside billing service.[19]

Periodic Internal Audits of Data Quality. Every facility should compile and subdivide the causes for denials and delays of claims. Persons responsible for such problems, be they physicians or other staff members, should be identified and trained to minimize recurrences. Although time-consuming, this approach offers obvious and immediate benefits.[21]

Challenging Denials and Underpayments. A facility should make a habit of challenging denials of payments and underpayments. If necessary, one should arrange to meet with key payer personnel to review one's legitimate claims. A little well-placed explanation of what one actually does for customers (i.e., patients) may go a long way toward increasing reimbursement.

Using Outcome Data in HMO Negotiations. In negotiations with HMOs, a facility should use its own mammography outcomes data to demonstrate the savings to the HMOs of finding cancers at earlier stages, while they are smaller. Further, if one's call-back rate is low and positive biopsy rate appropriately high, one can argue even more effectively about the savings to the HMO. Through such demonstrations, one may be able to negotiate a "carve-out" for proportionally higher reimbursement from the HMO for breast imaging procedures than for other imaging modalities.

Discounts for Cash Payments. A facility can make its service more attractive to cash-paying customers by offering discounts. If not participating with Medicare, one can even negotiate individual contracts with patients (usually discounting 20% for cash payment). In doing so, one must also treat all patients the same, so the discount rate chosen must be consistent. Additionally, a facility cannot waive copays and must bill at least once. Professional courtesy discounts should not be offered.

Political Involvement. Mammographers should mobilize patients and women's advocacy groups to support legislation to increase reimbursement for mammography. Such groups potentially represent the single most powerful weapon in the battle for better reimbursement.

SUMMARY

Through high-quality breast imaging services, radiologists have contributed mightily to the dramatic drop in breast cancer deaths observed since the mid-1980s in the United States. Despite their medical success, however, breast imagers face the continuing problems of rising costs and falling reimbursement. Therefore, their understanding of coding and billing under the current reimbursement system is critical to the very survival of breast imaging services within their practices. By effectively transforming reimbursement information into a careful coding and billing strategy for success, radiologists can more realistically anticipate the day when their breast imaging facilities evolve from their present status as lifesaving "loss leaders" to true financial "profit centers."

References

1. Peto R, Boreham J, Clarke M, et al: UK and USA breast cancer deaths down 25% in year 2000 at 20-69 years. Lancet 2000; 355:1822-1830.
2. Brice J: Mammography in jeopardy. Diagn Imaging 2001; 23:50-55.
3. International Classification of Diseases, Ninth Revision: Clinical Modification, 6th ed. Salt Lake City, UT, Ingenix Publishing Group, 2000.
4. Current Procedural Terminology: CPT 2003 Professional Edition. Chicago, IL, American Medical Association, 2002.
5. HCPCS National Level II Codes 2003. Salt Lake City, UT, Ingenix Publishing Group, 2002.
6. Mitchell JB: Physician DRGs. N Engl J Med 1985;313:670-675.
7. U.S. Department of Health and Human Services, Health Care Financing Administration: Medicare Program: Revisions to payment policies and adjustments to the relative value units under the physician fee schedule for calendar year 1999: Final rule and notice. 63 Federal Register 211 (1999).
8. U.S. Department of Health and Human Services, Health Care Financing Administration: Prospective payment system for hospital outpatient services. 65 Federal Register 18433-18482 (2000).
9. U.S. Department of Health and Human Services: 2004 proposed Schedule for HOPPS. 68 Federal Register (155) (2003) (codified at 42 CFR §410 and 419, 47966-48248.
10. Farria DM: The Hospital Outpatient Prospective Payment System: An overview. Semin Breast Disease 2001;4:21-26.
11. U.S. Department of Health and Human Services: Interim final rules on conditions for Medicare coverage of screening mammograms. Federal Register 53511-53525 (1990).
12. Balanced Budget Act of 1997 (Medicare revisions), Section 4104. Publ L 105-33.
13. Assure Access to Mammography Act of 2001 ("Enhanced reimbursement for screening mammography under the Medicare program"). SB-548.
14. Radiology Coding Alert, sample issue 1999;1-3.
15. Medicare Providers' News. Part B: Oklahoma/New Mexico, November 1997.
16. U.S. Department of Health and Human Services: 2003 final Physician Fee Schedule. 67 Federal Register 251 (2002) (codified at 42 CFR §410, 414, and 485):79966-80184.
17. U.S. Department of Health and Human Services: 2004 Final Physician Fee Schedule. 68 Federal Register 63196-63395 (2003).
18. Brice J: Small change for big medicine. Diagn Imaging 2000; 22:42-49.
19. Cassel D, Brant-Zawadzke M, Dwyer C: Learn importance of billing carefully. Diagn Imaging 2003;25:49-55.
20. Ikeda DM, Linver MN: ICD-9-CM codes, CPT codes, billing and collection. SBI News October 2000:1, 7-9.
21. Yoder L, Anderson R: Assess your practice's coding intelligence. Imaging Economics July-August 1999;74-80.

Medicolegal Issues in Breast Imaging

R. James Brenner

The enthusiasm generated from clinical trials—many of which have been reviewed in this text—that demonstrate the impact of the use of screening mammography on case-fatality rates from breast cancer has prompted growing compliance with this procedure in both the United States and elsewhere. More sophisticated conventional imaging involving diagnostic mammography and ultrasonography, combined with experience and outcome data, has served to increase both sensitivity and specificity, thus decreasing both false-negative and false-positive results. New technologies such as magnetic resonance imaging have provided additional tools for definable circumstances, such as identification of primary breast cancer in women presenting with adenocarcinoma of the axillary lymph nodes but normal mammographic and physical findings,[1] enabling breast imagers to further improve both detection and diagnostic ability.

That success has also been embraced by the lay community. Women who undergo periodic mammography and whose cancers are not diagnosed at a sufficiently small size may believe that the care rendered them has not merely failed to realize the potential benefit they sought but has been substandard. The end result of that perception—accurate or not—is often the initiation of legal action against a woman's health care provider. In 1990, the Physicians Insurers Association of America (PIAA), a consortium of physician-owned liability carriers who often pool claims data, identified delay in diagnosis of breast cancer as the second leading cause of malpractice actions against physicians.[2] The study was repeated in 1995, at which time this problem was identified as the leading cause of malpractice actions. Furthermore, the most commonly named defendant was the radiologist.[3] Similar results were reported in 2002.[3a]

The dual role of screening and diagnostic (or problem-solving) mammography is peculiar to breast imaging; with most other studies performed by radiologists, examinations are usually ordered by treating physicians to help diagnose clinical problems. On the other hand, as screening strategies such as lung cancer screening with computed tomography become incorporated into clinical practice, the issues that relate to the dual nature of mammography may emerge in increasing importance. Such issues include cost-effectiveness, targeted populations at risk, and liability.

This chapter discusses issues of liability, incorporating principles that are germane to the practice of all imaging, but is focused on breast imaging and intervention. Risk management considerations are introduced to identify methods to mitigate circumstances that invite legal exposure. Historically, medical school curricula and postgraduate education programs have not explored such concepts, although their consideration is essential in providing strategic guidance and proper medical care in an era of cost containment and increased utilization review.[4]

BASIC LEGAL CONCEPTS

There are many different forms of law, each with different standards of proof and application. Criminal law, for example, is concerned with protecting society against certain acts. Criminal defendants are therefore prosecuted not by other individuals but by the state or federal government, and standards of proof are very high because of the loss of personal liberty resulting from conviction. Criminal law rarely applies to the practice of medicine, except for enforcement of "fraud and abuse" concerns related to the filing of false claims (e.g., billing) or violation of specific relationships that physicians and health care facilities enjoy. On occasion, decisions about termination of life may be subject to criminal prosecution.

Civil law governs disputes between individuals. The relationship between individuals affords its own standard of proof (preponderance of evidence) and legal proceedings. More specifically, tort law—a branch of civil law—applies to most circumstances involving physicians. As in 18th century English common law, American courts have seen the role of a physician as a public calling. Although physicians may be subject to certain tort law guidelines that are universal—such as the intentional tort of battery (discussed later)—malpractice issues generally derive from another type of tort law, the law of negligence.

The law of negligence is based on the conduct of a physician. Although an adverse outcome is the most likely event to trigger a malpractice action, it is the conduct of the defendant, not the outcome, that is at issue.[5] A trial is an attempt to establish the truth regarding questions of fact, not law, and is primarily focused on (1) whether the physician complied with a proper standard of care rendered to the patient ("liability") and (2) whether the departure from the standard of care actually caused injury ("causation"). These determinations are usually made with the assistance of expert witnesses who help the court to establish what the "standard of care" is, and the judge or jury then decides whether the defendant has complied with that standard of care.

Questions of law are established by appellate courts, which often review cases not to reconsider facts but to decide matters of legal concern. Thus, appellate decisions, as opposed to trial decisions, have precedent-setting importance. In the review of cases, published decisions often remark on issues of care ("dicta") that assist physicians in determining what is expected of them. Relatively few appellate decisions are made regarding the practice of medicine, and a review of such published decisions from 1970 to 1993 regarding breast cancer evaluation has been published in the medical literature.[6] Trial court decisions, which resolve particular issues in dispute and particular circumstances, have no precedent-setting value.

Fundamentally, the *standard of care* required of a physician is considered in a legal context to be an objective one, namely, what a reasonable and prudent physician would do under similar circumstances.[7] This definition derives from common law notions. However, standards of care may also be derived from laws passed by local, state, or the federal government. Most medical malpractice cases are governed under state law, provisions usually found in the Business and Professional Codes. The Mammography Quality Standards Act (MQSA) of 1992 and the Mammography Quality Standards Recertification Act of 1997[8] provide express statutory standards of care, reflecting societal consensus. This federal law pre-empts state law, meaning that it applies as a minimum standard, below which state laws are not applicable. These standards require no expert testimony to sustain and are essentially incontestable. The implications of such statutory standards are addressed subsequently.

There are hundreds of specialty society practice standards, practice guidelines, and other, primarily consensus-based protocols that have been used indirectly to establish standards of care. Because panels drafting such guidelines cannot be cross-examined by attorneys, they are not generally considered admissible as evidence in courts of law. However, experts establishing a basis or foundation for their testimony may refer to such guidelines that presumably reflect established principles. The effect of such guidelines is therefore important to recognize, especially if a given practice departs from such published statements.

In this context, it should be noted that most courts accept testimony regarding standard of care according to the "alternative school of thought" doctrine. If conduct has a rational basis, it may be considered reasonable even if it departs from given cited practice guidelines.[5] Such guidelines are not tantamount to standards of care. For example, different societies may prescribe different intervals for screening mammograms, and following one or the other prescription may be reasonable, depending on the circumstances. Note the emphasis on reasonable conduct, which is the benchmark for the requisite legal standard of care.

Traditionally, courts have emphasized the so-called locale rule, whereby a physician's conduct is best determined in terms of local standards of care. Since 1990, this approach has been de-emphasized in favor of a more universal application of standard of care. In the field of breast imaging, this trend is even more valid, given national standards propagated by federal legislation such as MQSA. Thus, experts from different parts of the country are commonly employed to provide testimony as to the applicable standard of care in a given case.[9]

The importance of a trial decision cannot be overemphasized. Physicians who believe that they may appeal their case to a higher court if they fail to prevail at trial should recognize the low likelihood of appellate review. Consider a West Virginia court admonition: "Where in the trial of an action of law before a jury, the evidence is conflicting, it is the province of the jury to resolve the conflict, and its verdict thereon will not be disturbed unless believed to be plainly wrong."[10] The court went on to comment that even when a juror claims to have been somewhat confused about the law or evidence, the verdict will not necessarily be impeached. Most legal actions do not even proceed to trial, usually being resolved by informal but legally binding settlements. Regardless of the type of resolution, if there is any exchange of consideration (e.g., tendering of money, forgiving of debt), the actions are reported to the National Practitioner Data Bank. Awards exceeding certain money amounts are usually reported to State Boards governing medical practice. Given the federal government's concern about patient safety after the Institute of Medicine's 2000 report *To Err Is Human*, public attention to such issues is not likely to wane.[11]

THE LAW OF NEGLIGENCE

As mentioned, most malpractice cases are considered from a standpoint of legal *negligence*, a part of civil law. Although the term has a pejorative connotation, its legal meaning is a term of art, denoting three and, more functionally, four elements that need to be satisfied in order for a plaintiff to prevail. The law of negligence is based on conduct, not outcome. On the other hand, it is an adverse outcome that usually triggers a lawsuit, designed to establish whether a physician's conduct satisfied that standard of care that a reasonable and prudent physician would satisfy under similar circumstances.[7] The standard for such conduct is "reasonable care," and the law recognizes mistakes that are not necessarily negligent. A formal statement of this concept is as follows: "One who undertakes gratuitously or for consideration to render services to another which he should recognize as necessary for the protection of the other person or things, is subject to liability of physical harm resulting from his failure to exercise reasonable care or perform his undertaking if his failure to exercise such care increased the risk of such harm."[12]

The first element of negligence is duty. It is the duty of the radiologist to obtain reasonable images, render a reasonable interpretation, and effectively communicate that interpretation according to the circumstances of the case. The second element is a breach of that duty. The third element is causation. When the conduct of the defendant bears a direct causative relationship to patient injury—often denoted as "cause in fact" and "proximate cause"—the third element has been satisfied. The terms of art regarding causation can be confusing, and the California Supreme Court has perhaps focused the issue by defining it in terms of "substantial factor"; namely, if the conduct of the defendant is a substantial factor in causing injury to the plaintiff, causation has been shown.

The establishment of negligent conduct, however, does not necessarily either prompt or sustain a lawsuit. Ordinarily, damages or consequences of that negligence must be shown. The purpose of the law of negligence is to, to the extent possible, "make the plaintiff whole" again; in other words, it is directed at restitution. A delay in the diagnosis of breast cancer cannot be undone, so that society has determined that money damages is a common denominator for compensating an aggrieved plaintiff. Loss of income, medical expenses, and pain and suffering are usually recognized as damages. As shown later, the nature of recovery bears on the profile of lawsuits filed by plaintiff attorneys.

The relationship between breach of duty, causation, and damages may be exemplified by the following situation. A patient who undergoes a screening mammogram on which a spiculated mass is overlooked, but who recognized a lump that she brings to clinical attention within a week and that is shown to represent cancer, may be able to show a breach of duty on the part of the radiologist. However, the resolution of the clinical problem defeats both the claim of causation (there is no demonstrable relationship of the misinterpretation to delay in diagnosis because the delay is not clinically significant) and damages. Thus, although a breach of duty may have occurred, there is no legal negligence.

A lawsuit will often set out many issues regarding negligence, otherwise known as "causes of action." Each cause of action may be viewed as a separate claim of negligence, wherein all elements must be satisfied for recovery.[13] In the preceding paradigm, one might raise issues about mental distress. Usually, claims of distress are derivative to ones of negligence, so that without a showing of negligence, the court will not hear claims of mental distress. Some states permit legal action for the intentional infliction of mental distress and others for the negligent infliction of mental distress, but these circumstances are uncommon. Sometimes, such claims arise with respect to the pain associated with mammograms but rarely, if ever, succeed, except in extraordinary circumstances. In addition, claims may apply to women who have disagreed with the manner in which mammography has been performed on their breast implants; as of this writing, I am not aware of anything but defendant verdicts at trial for the few cases that have been brought to legal attention.

Most cases reviewed by appellate courts involve the clinical management of breast signs and symptoms that preceded the diagnosis of breast cancer. The standards of care applicable to clinical examination are beyond the scope of this discussion, although the radiologist must recognize two issues.[14-19] First, not all clinical examinations are reasonable, although the radiologist probably may rely on a directed clinical breast examination. Thus, for equivocal clinical circumstances, the potential suboptimal nature of a clinical examination may be considered. Second, for practices accepting self-referred patients and performing clinical breast examination, such cases and circumstances may require closer review.

STANDARD OF CARE

As a matter of first course, mammographic studies should be documented as screening or diagnostic, according to criteria for potential signs or symptoms of breast cancer and other conditions distinguishing the two examinations. An intake sheet or history form will serve as a record to validate the triaging of patients in this respect. Because different standards of care may be assigned the different goals of respective screening and diagnostic studies, such validation is important.[20] It also serves as a basis for proper billing, as the issues of false claims and fraud and abuse have been applied to such situations.

The standard of care derives directly from the concept of duty. As mentioned, duty for imaging involves obtaining reasonable images, rendering a reasonable interpretation, and effectively communicating the interpretation.

Many efforts have been made to investigate the feasibility of screening with a form of imaging other than mammography. Historically, ultrasonography, thermography, and light transmission have proved unsuccessful. Interest in screening ultrasonography has emerged with published reports suggesting possible reconsideration, for which some of the issues are discussed later. In addition, screening with magnetic resonance imaging (MRI) has been considered, with commercial availability of one unit with a low-field-strength magnet dedicated to breast evaluation. At present, however, screening mammography remains virtually synonymous with screening breast imaging, fulfilling the public health–related criterion of being oriented toward high volume, low cost, and easily accessible implementation.

In this context, however, it should be noted that screening for breast cancer is not synonymous with screening mammography. The Breast Cancer Detection Demonstration Project (BCDDP) demonstrated that although many malignant lesions that are clinically occult may be detected by means of mammography, a finite percentage of palpable cancers is not seen radiographically.[21] Current clinical practice often prompts directed ultrasonography under such circumstances, a method that usually detects the cancer. Thus, acceptance of a patient for screening mammography is predicated on a physical examination that demonstrates no signs or symptoms of breast cancer—that is, the patient is asymptomatic. Generalized pain or multiple bilateral lumps ("lumpy bumpy disease") is considered a normal variant and also qualifies the patient for screening.[22] Because the purpose of screening mammography is to identify a small percentage of the population that requires additional (diagnostic) evaluation, cost-efficient approaches are not only desirable but also legally sound. For example, "on-line" review of films is not necessary, so long as a recall system is established.[23] For institutions in which radiologists contract with facilities or institutions, and screening films are "batch read," it may be advisable to establish, in a policy and procedure manual, the importance of having facility personnel reconcile the patient's history with the type of examination performed, as such records may not be routinely reviewed on a screening reading station. This approach also affords the facility the opportunity to identify patients who have been improperly scheduled for screening and for whom more problem-oriented or diagnostic evaluation is indicated.

Quality control, which applies to both screening and diagnostic imaging, is both mandated and prescribed by federal law (MQSA). Emerging protocols for digital mammography will likely fall under similar auspices, both of which may be supplemented by state requirement. As indicated earlier, violation of such standards may be prima facie evidence of breach of the standard of care. If an image is suboptimal but might otherwise be argued by a reviewing expert as reasonable, noncompliance with quality control standards for that day may undermine the defense of the image in question.

Many breasts do not lend themselves to optimal imaging, in which all of the breast tissue is visible in both of the universally prescribed craniocaudal and mediolateral oblique projections. However, it is incumbent upon facility personnel and the reviewing radiologist to be persuaded that a reasonable attempt has been made to image all breast tissue. This issue may be judged in part from prior films, if available. Issues regarding technique, such as lack of compression or motion blurriness, do not depend on prior films. Because MQSA charges the interpreting radiologist with the functional duty of approving films, unsatisfactory images must be repeated, either before the patient leaves the facility or at a later date.

Screening is concerned primarily with detection, but not necessarily characterization, of potentially significant abnormalities. Reasonable interpretation in the screening setting thus translates to reasonable detection. The issue of *foreseeability*, a concept central to a legal analysis of duty, emerges in identifying potentially significant abnormalities. Reviews, for example, of prior mammograms in which cancer has subsequently been diagnosed often demonstrate abnormalities that are not sufficiently foreseeable to necessitate recall of the patient for a second evaluation, even though the cancer was associated with the anatomic site.[24] In like manner, computer-aided detection studies may show evidence of otherwise benign-looking calcifications that the computer detects but for which the patients were not recalled.[25] In such studies, it is difficult to ascertain whether or not recall would have been prompted even with the highlighting of such areas by a computer model. Thus, expert opinion is often focused not only on whether a mammographic focus was seen but also on whether the patient should have been recalled for further evaluation. The application of an indeterminate impression for a screening mammogram is not only valid (e.g., American College of Radiology [ACR] Breast Imaging Reporting and Data System [BI-RADS] category 0) but also frequently preferred, pending further evaluation.

The final assessment of a diagnostic study, however, cannot be "indeterminate" or BI-RADS category 0. Some facilities prefer to use this term, pending more sophisticated technology or even retrieval of old films. Such practice should be discouraged—except in extraordinary circumstances—because the ambiguity after diagnostic evaluation invites mismanagement. Final impressions may be conditioned prospectively, that is, they may be expressed as subject to revision following additional studies or examination of prior films. In the case of mismanagement and consequent delay, the failure to assign a BI-RADS category 2, 3, 4, or 5 and its equivalent written explanation may represent a statutory breach in the standard of care, requiring no expert opinion.

Final evaluation and reasonable interpretation in the diagnostic setting are assessed on a case-by-case basis. Criteria for benign, probably benign, and suspicious abnormalities are reviewed extensively in this text. As has been mentioned, the law does not require a warranty of certainty but rather a reasonable interpretation. The interrelationship between reasonable interpretation and film quality is highlighted by a retrospective review of claims made against radiologists by the PIAA in association with the ACR.[26] Cases in which additional films were not obtained were linked to incorrect diagnostic impressions. Review of conventional films may afford sufficient confidence with respect to certain lesions (e.g., a spiculated mass seen in two orthogonal projections is virtually always suspicious, absent a history of trauma [including surgery] or infection). More often than not, potentially significant abnormalities are better evaluated with additional images, including but not limited to spot compression views with or without magnification, rolled or altered angled views, and ultrasonography. The reasonableness of the interpretation is thus assessed both by the image obtained and by the analysis of the abnormality. This approach is exemplified by cases for which BI-RADS category 3, "probably benign, short-term follow-up suggested," is employed. Usually, but not invariably, such a recommendation is issued pending evaluation of an abnormality for which no features inconsistent with a benign diagnosis are found.

Because most benign abnormalities lack pathognomonic features to ensure that they are benign (e.g., lipoid cyst of fat necrosis), a probably benign diagnosis is often rendered to afford the option of surveillance instead of biopsy, an approach that has been shown to be cost effective.[27] Note that an improperly obtained spot compression view—either blurry because of prolonged imaging time or misplaced over the wrong anatomic site—will lead to an erroneous interpretation. Radiologists, charged with reasonable interpretation, must be satisfied that the images obtained provide a reasonable basis for interpretation or indicate conditions that compromise this goal; for example, some patients decline adequate compression or a second set of films, and this limitation should be noted in the report.[28]

The issue of foreseeability applies to diagnostic impressions. Recall the current interest in screening ultrasonography or even MRI studies, often suggested for high-risk patients or patients with complicated mammographic patterns (a nebulous category, in that this definition may extend to most women undergoing screening).[29,30] When abnormalities are identified and considered probably benign, surveillance requires both validation of the technique and compliance. Compliance is an issue in any surveillance program, and if there is reason to suspect lack of follow-up, this approach may not be a viable option. This issue may also complicate MRI surveillance, for which the cost of follow-up studies must be considered. Validation trials for ultrasonographic or MRI surveillance are relatively lacking in current published literature. Although surveillance schedules have been advocated, personal audit validation may be important for issues for which there are no published reports.

Retention of films and reports by any radiology facility is generally governed by state statute.[31] MQSA requires that original films be released on request, although many facilities release copy films if originals are not requested. Exposure of the facility to potential legal problems arises when such films are lost, complicating either current management efforts or future comparisons. Signed releases should be obtained from the patient and kept when films are removed from the facility. Facilities accepting old films may find it advisable to keep logs or records of incoming and outgoing films. These records are almost universally admitted as evidence (over usual hearsay objections) when the issue requires judicial review. In like manner, state and federal law prescribes the length of time for retention of films and records, requirements that may be different from those for other kinds of radiologic studies.

Recovery of old films for comparison is problematic because of both the induced costs associated with the effort and the recognition that prior films often cannot be found. Because otherwise nonspecific neodensities cannot be recognized without old films, some lesions may go undetected without comparison of current and previous films. Likewise, biopsy of many abnormalities that are probably benign may be avoided if they can be shown to be stable through comparison. Attempting to retrieve films in a systematic manner may be evidence of reasonableness, given the lack of uniform success of retrieval that has been documented in the literature.[28]

Communication of results has in part been standardized by federal requirements that patients receive letters written in lay language about their mammographic studies. This directive applies to both screening and diagnostic examinations as well as to supplementary comparison studies. Historically, results have been communicated in writing to referring physicians. Results may be reported in a variety of methods, the primary directive for screening reports being the identification of abnormalities that require recall and further evaluation, and that for diagnostic reports a specific assessment. Screening studies in particular lend themselves to systematic methods such as computer-generated reports. The diagnostic study for a patient being evaluated for a specific sign or symptom should report a pertinent positive or negative finding in the area of clinical concern. These comments should be distinguished from general disclaimers such as "mammography is not a substitute for biopsy" and "malignancy cannot be excluded," historical phrases that neither relieve the radiologist of a reasonable interpretation nor assist the clinician in evaluation of a focal clinical abnormality. Frequently, the breast imaging report offers a likely etiologic factor for a clinical finding (e.g., cyst, suspicious lesion), so that when there is no imaging finding associated with the area of concern, clinical management becomes obligatory.

The ACR lexicon contains a number of descriptors that help characterize lesions, serving as a basis for commonly used terminology. Although the use of such descriptors is not mandatory, familiarity with them gives the mammographer the opportunity to consider their implementation. Tantamount in importance to the actual terminology of the lexicon, if not paramount in importance, is the notion that deliberate description of a lesion not only increases the likelihood of reaching a deductive, correct diagnostic impression but also validates the rationale for reaching that conclusion. In other words, even if the diagnosis is incorrect, a proper description of the lesion in question should form the basis for reasonable interpretation. From a risk management perspective, a conclusion that is incorrect without a reasoned description is more difficult to reconcile than one in which the findings are accurately described and reasonably, albeit incorrectly, assessed. On occasion, the radiologist indicates that a lesion is probably benign and even assigns a BI-RADS 3 category but includes a statement that biopsy is required.

Such discrepancies reflect the inability of the radiologist to recognize that a "benign" imaging diagnosis cannot be sufficiently sustained, so tissue diagnosis is required. When tissue diagnosis is required, the lesion is considered by definition to be suspicious enough for malignancy that surveillance is no longer a recommended option. Such inconsistencies may at first appear to protect the radiologist from legal redress but instead may subject him or her to greater legal exposure because, as mentioned, ambiguity invites mismanagement.

Because it is foreseeable that mailed letters do not always reach their intended parties, situations requiring proximal intervention (i.e., lesions requiring biopsy) generally necessitate direct communication. This proposition is supported by both legal cases and the ACR "Standard on Communication."[32] As an Ohio court expressly stated, "the communication of the diagnosis so that it may be beneficially utilized may be altogether as important as the diagnosis itself."[33] Direct communication requires either personal discussion or telephone conversation with the intended party. Facsimile transmission and e-mail communication are unlikely to satisfy this requirement for the same reason that posted letters may fail; namely, they may not reach the intended party. In other words, the duty of the radiologist is not static but dynamic and is raised to a level of direct communication when a lesion is considered suspicious for malignancy. If the referring physician is unavailable for a prolonged period, the information can be communicated to another physician covering the clinical practice. Certain offices may have office managers or other personnel so integral to the referring physician's practice that they may be designated as surrogates. However, this situation should be specifically identified, sometimes in a policy and procedure manual, because the regular communication of the need for biopsy to general office personnel may not satisfy the communication requirement.

Communication of less urgent results may be facilitated through more customary methods. Recommendations for short-term follow-up are assisted by reminder letters from the radiology facility, the clinician, or both. On the other hand, recommendations for recall may be facilitated by direct patient communication, often in concert with the referring physician. This method serves two purposes. First, the patient may seek additional imaging elsewhere and may not inform the screening facility; direct attempts at recall identify this situation. Second, patients may not appreciate the importance of recall, even with a letter sent to them. Tickler files or systems approaches developed by the facility help encourage additional imaging or identify those patients who are informed and decline. Such circumstances should be documented in the medical record. The test of all of these forms of communication is, again, reasonableness.

The relative duties of the referring physician and imaging facility to achieve the patient's compliance with suggested evaluation or follow-up are evolving. Different states may define the role of the radiologist in different manners. For example, the California Appellate Court has suggested that the radiologist, as consultant, subordinate his or her activities to the referring physician.[34] Other states hold different perspectives. Federal law as prescribed by MQSA preempts state law to the extent that state law can add to but not lessen the impact of federal statutory guidelines. The requirement for lay language communication of results to patients incorporates a legislative history that imposes responsibilities on the woman also to act reasonably once informed. In any given case, recommendations that are not successfully completed will be evaluated in the context of all of these considerations.

THE SELF-REFERRED PATIENT

The preceding discussion identifies the relative roles of the radiologist and referring physician, which may vary according to both state jurisdiction and actual circumstances. These roles merge for the patient who not only makes her own appointment for a mammogram prior to seeing her referring physician—a "self-initiated examination"—but in fact also has no ongoing relationship with a treating physician. Complex issues regarding whether or not clinicians are referring physicians in this context arise, such as the doctrine of continuous care, but are beyond the scope of this discussion.

Perhaps no other aspect of breast imaging distinguishes this field from other fields of current radiologic practice than does the issue of the self-referred patient.[35] Usually, imaging procedures are ordered by referring physicians consequent to clinical problems or ongoing surveillance. Even emerging trends of screening for lung or bowel cancer are unlikely to evolve without an intermediary clinician caring for the patient. However, many asymptomatic women seek to avail themselves of screening mammography services even though they are not under the direct care of a clinician. This may in part be due to the widespread publicity that attends breast cancer screening and the high prevalence of the disorder among women, especially younger women. Many facilities have adapted their referral base to include self-referred women, often helping to maximize the benefit of large-volume screening schedules that lend themselves to lower costs of service as well as the subsequent procedures derivative of such activities.

Facilities accepting self-referred women need to recognize certain aspects of the practice that may not pertain to traditional physician-referred practices. First, criteria should be established to identify and designate women who are considered self-referred. Specific time frames have not been established, but because most women have seen a physician during their lifetimes, simply naming a referring physician who may not be a currently bona fide treating physician invites problems when follow-up recommendations or referrals are made. Thus, the facility should specify a time of last contact with a referring physician beyond which the patient is properly considered self-referred. Conversely, facilities not accepting self-referred patients should establish similar guidelines in defining who they will accept.

Because screening for breast cancer is not, as discussed earlier, synonymous with mammographic screening, a physical examination is an important component of the evaluation. Facilities accepting self-referred women should either provide for a clinical examination or arrange for such an examination to be done. Triaging women for screening or diagnostic studies is important for both physician-referral and self-referral facilities in order to identify circumstances requiring ultrasonography or knowledge of palpable areas that convert otherwise subthreshold mammographic findings into areas of greater radiographic concern.[28] Recall the issue of foreseeability in helping to determine whether or not care rendered the patient was reasonable. Because it is foreseeable that some cancers may not be detected on mammograms but are palpable and can often be identified on focused ultrasonography, clinical examination is required for breast care. The self-referral facility assumes the role of primary care for the breast unless the patient is referred elsewhere for such care. The standard of care for clinical examination, as noted earlier, is beyond the scope of the current discussion. In this context, it might be noted that mammographers performing limited breast clinical examination for correlative purposes may need to indicate to the patient the limited nature of such examination and remind her that it does not substitute for or obviate a full clinical examination by her treating physician. For self-referred patients, this limited role is less applicable.

Communication of results for self-referred women has become similar to the method used for physician-referred women, following the MQSA requirement of result letters. Safeguards to ensure proper identifying demographic information may have to be more exacting. When physician-referred facilities err in such information gathering, they can often apply to the primary care physician to correct the data; this step may not be possible for self-referred women. One method of avoiding misinformation, especially when data are entered into a computer system or other printed record, is to have the woman verify that the information is accurate before she leaves the facility. Direct communication after a diagnostic evaluation, given the absence of an intermediary clinician, is accomplished by speaking to the patient, much the same as a primary care physician would do. All of the issues discussed previously for the situation in which the radiology facility works in concert with the clinician's office are reduced for self-referral facilities to the role of the imaging facility.

COLLATERAL ISSUES

Law of Agency

Personnel who work for the benefit and under the supervision of an individual or entity are considered agents of that person or entity. Errors and omissions of agents are attributed to the individual or entity under the law of agency by legal doctrines of vicarious liability, or respondeat superior. This issue arises for mammography facilities in several contexts.

First, as noted for self-referral facilities, the obtaining of incorrect demographic data, which may interfere with recall or other efforts, both places the health of the patient at risk and creates legal exposure for the facility. Second, technologists working according to policies and procedures of the facility are generally covered under this doctrine. More often than not, the nature of the employment helps determine what has historically been referred to as a master-servant relationship. Thus, in a free-standing facility owned by the radiologist, the radiologists and facility have an identity of interest. Where this is not the case, the facility is responsible for the agent, except to the extent that the "supervising radiologist" is responsible for approving the quality of the images obtained. Technologists or other personnel working on an interim basis (e.g., registry) should be familiar with protocol, because errors in procedure are more likely to be attributed to the facility that has not oriented such personnel.

Duty to Refer, Abandonment, and Negligent Referral

Imagers evaluating patients in physician-referral practices must directly notify the referring clinician of the need for biopsy when required. Most often, the clinician refers the patient to an appropriate facility or individual, commensurate with a legal duty. Sometimes the facility is that of the radiologist when image-guided tissue sampling is desired; other times, the patient is referred to a surgeon or oncologist. For self-referral practices, this *duty to refer* is assumed by the radiologist.

In like manner, the radiologist who performed an image-guided procedure such as core biopsy and has received the results may have to further confer with the referring physician or directly with the patient (for self-referred women) if additional surgery is required. The failure to do so, or to attend to any exigent circumstance that requires proximal action, is called *abandonment* and is legally actionable if an untoward consequence occurs.[36] For example, after a core biopsy showing florid atypical ductal hyperplasia, the radiologist is aware of the need for excisional biopsy because of anticipated tissue sampling error, but the referring clinician may not be familiar with such circumstances, which have been primarily addressed in the surgical and radiology literature.

If the radiologist knows or has reason to know that the person or facility to which he or she is referring the patients will not adequately care for the patient, and if an untoward event occurs, then the referring radiologist may be subject to the claim of *negligent referral*. For example, if surgery is required, and the physician to whom the patient is referred is not familiar with breast surgery for nonpalpable lesions, then failed surgery may implicate the referring radiologist.[36]

SECOND CONSULTATIVE OPINIONS

Although second opinions are commonly sought on an informal basis for imaging examinations, it behooves the interpreting radiologist to recall the definition of duty cited earlier in this chapter.[12] Specifically, whether rendered for a charge and formalized or given "gratuitously," the radiologist's interpretation is held to the same standard of care.

Because breast care litigation is common, the radiologist offering second opinions may wish to commit such opinions to a hard-copy formal report, whether or not there is a charge (an issue related to fraud and abuse claims, beyond the scope of this discussion). This may be especially important when the consultation involves a recommendation for either additional evaluation or biopsy. An alternative approach is to make a contemporaneous entry into a log book of some sort and to retain such records for several years. Contemporaneous entries may be admissible as evidence of the substance of the consultation as an exception to standard hearsay rules. Such evidence may refute inaccurate entries or recollections of the clinician who sought opinion without formal report. Recall that the purpose of the interpretative report is to commit to reproducible form the impression of the radiologist. Informal recollections defeat this purpose, so that in a field of high legal exposure such as breast imaging, additional efforts may prevent unnecessary consequences.

Double Reading and Computer-Aided Detection

The use of second opinions has been advocated in terms of double reading to improve both the sensitivity and specificity of mammographic abnormality detection. Although such efforts are laudable in an effort to provide excellence in mammographic services, the establishment of such a standard is problematic, for several reasons. Reimbursement for public health–oriented screening, in which double reading has been advocated to have the greatest impact, is limited, and the additional cost may prove to be a disincentive. Although cost considerations do not relieve a facility or radiologist from legal liability in the law of negligence,[37] the overall financial viability of a facility in helping women access mammography should be considered. Moreover, improved detection of lesions has also been studied for lung nodules, polyp detection during colon studies, and even evaluation by computed tomography of the pancreas for cancer. It may be that more than one physical examination would improve detection of breast cancer. One of the main issues in feasibility studies of double reading is the types of pairings of readers that are made during review. Claims of increased sensitivity without compromise in specificity are unacceptably difficult to reconcile.[38] Different pairs of readers (κ values) show different patterns of improved detection.[39] Double reading may be more useful for some individuals than others, and various approaches, such as technologist prereading and selective double reading, have been advocated. Double reading has not, for these and other reasons, evolved into a standard of care.

Computer-aided detection (CAD) is another approach to detect lesions that might be missed, in much the same manner as double reading. Current efforts to assign probabilities of malignancy to such lesions are investigational. Current published reports are based on cancers for which prior mammograms were reviewed by computer detector technology, showing a large majority of calcifications and a lesser but large number of masses being identified. This effort, like double reading, is afforded only by the identification of many abnormalities (false positive) that are of little clinical or radiographic concern.[25]

One of the problems in assessing the impact of CAD is that it is not possible to identify which lesions the radiologist saw in the past and considered below the threshold for recall or biopsy recommendation and which he or she did not see that might have modified interpretative recommendations if denoted by the computer. As was noted earlier, retrospective evaluation is sufficiently biased to complicate the issue.[24] If, indeed, areas of concern identified by the computer on prior occasions truly meet generally accepted threshold criteria, the assumption may be made that these were "missed" rather than seen and not recalled, as has been inferred in a recent report.[24] As with double reading, issues of cost, reimbursement, and overall efficacy apply to CAD. Ongoing evaluation will provide a better basis for the role of both CAD and assisted diagnosis.

Performing Interventional Procedures and Obtaining Consent

Those involved with interventional procedures after evaluation of nonpalpable breast lesions must consider two aspects of potential liability.[40] The first is consent. Implied consent is not considered valid beyond the obtaining of images, and invasive procedures raise the issue of the intentional tort (not usually covered by liability insurance policies) of battery (the unlawful touching of others). Consent is a complete defense to the charge of battery, but consents must be reasonably obtained or else they expose the interventionist to the charge of negligent consent. In a survey of those performing simple interventional procedures (not core biopsies), a large percentage of respondents indicated that they did not obtain consent before performing, for example, needle localizations for surgery.[41] Because there is a foreseeable miss rate during surgery, and because the radiologist is intimately involved in the success or failure of the excision, consent should be obtained by the person performing the intervention, and not by others, and the person should not rely on generalized hospital consent forms.

Material risks (those that may be severe) or risks of high frequency of occurrence need to be disclosed to the patient. Alternatives should also be discussed. This discussion can often be conducted by other personnel as a preliminary effort, but the interventionist must discuss the issue with the patient before performing an elective procedure. Written consent forms are evidence of the discussion and as such are important, but they are not substitutes for the substantive discussion.[42]

When a radiologist accepts an interventional procedure in a case that has been evaluated by another institution, the interventionist is responsible for reasonably ensuring that a lesion is present and can be approached (although re-evaluation of malignant potential is not necessarily required). Reports for both preoperative needle localization and core biopsy procedures demonstrate that many procedures are recommended when, in fact, there is no lesion.[43,44] Performing an intervention under such circumstances subjects the interventionist to legal exposure. In other words, the interventionist has a duty to act reasonably in the performance of the procedure, which includes validation of a bona fide target for intervention.

FACING A LAWSUIT

Most states have laws concerning the time frame within which a lawsuit may be filed, known as the *statute of limitations*. The purpose of such statutes, in part, is to avoid unending legal exposure of the defendant for circumstances tenuously related to the initial conduct that may prompt a plaintiff to seek legal regress. Given the time lag between the filing of a complaint and trial, more extended periods may invite confusion and loss of evidence as well as credible testimony with regard to the initial episode. The specific conditions and length of time for statutory limits vary with the jurisdiction, but the fundamental issue regards when a patient knows or should know that the defendant's act was potentially negligent ("the Discovery Rule"). This period is usually 1 to 2 years after the incident. After this time, actions against the defendant are barred.

Concealment or misrepresentation of information constitutes a form of civil fraud that will toll or extend the statute of limitations indefinitely. Often radiologists are asked (1) whether a lesion was present on a prior mammogram and (2) whether it should have been subject to further investigation. In an attempt to mitigate the patient's anxiety, and in recognition of both the bias of retrospective review and the need to avoid the charge of fraud, the radiologist under such circumstances may elect to disqualify himself of herself from such a determination and invite the patient to seek independent opinion if desired.

The receipt of a summons and complaint—a lawsuit—is often conditioned on either the filing of an affidavit of merit (e.g., Florida) or a pre-filing notice (e.g., California). The filing usually triggers serious emotional responses in the defendant, the nature of which are beyond the limits of this discussion. Nonetheless, certain guidelines should be employed after receipt of such notice. Frequently, the radiologist may attempt to retrieve the case in question and, hoping to validate the initial diagnostic impression, discuss it with a colleague. Any discussions after the filing of a lawsuit may be subject to discovery procedures, in which participants are under oath and required to disclose the nature of such discussions. If the colleague does not in fact agree with the initial interpretation, such testimony may be further damaging to the defendant.

Temptations to alter or add to records, even with bona fide intentions of making the record more complete, must be resisted. Plaintiff consultants include handwriting experts who may impugn the integrity of the radiologist on discovery that a record has been altered.

Radiologists are advised, therefore, upon learning of a lawsuit against them, to "freeze the episode in time and place."[36] Appropriate medical records and films should be sequestered if the facility maintains custody, because lost records are often viewed in an unfavorable manner. The risk manager of the case, often assigned by the insurance liability carrier, should be contacted immediately, and the carrier will assign an attorney to the case. The radiologist may wish to interview the attorney, determine the attorney's familiarity with issues of breast imaging, and direct the attorney when necessary to consultants or information to offer background education with respect to these issues. The attorney often contacts a potential expert to review the case, which may also serve to educate the attorney regarding not only the issues of the particular case but also the larger context in which the case arises. Indeed, the ACR is involved with preparing background materials for attorneys desiring more information.

The complaint is answered by the defendant attorney, and any conversations that the attorney has with the client are considered privileged and not subject to discovery by the other side. An objective determination will be sought as to whether the case is indeed defensible or whether it may be preferable to settle the case and avoid a formal trial. If the defendant identifies a potential conflict of interest in such a determination, other legal opinions may be sought.

In discovery procedures, attorneys for both sides seek to determine the facts of the case. Expert consultants are often used in the process. They are most useful when no advocacy is implied in their opinions, but rather they are asked to make a strict determination whether or not the applicable standard of care was met. Questions or "interrogatories" are often issued and should be answered by the defendant with the assistance of the attorney. Depositions may be taken, wherein testimony is given under oath, to help determine the prior course of events in assessing the conduct of the defendant. Preparation for such depositions is essential, because conflicting statements may be used to impeach the defendant's credibility if the case goes to trial.

The time course for this legal process may be short, depending on the status of the plaintiff, or it may extend for years. Often, mandatory settlement conferences are held to reassess the positions of the respective parties. Again, the law seeks to afford restitution to a plaintiff not for an unfortunate result but for negligent conduct. Both the substance of the conduct and the credibility of the defendant and witness play integrated roles in how a jury determines whether the standard of care has been met and whether there is sufficient evidence of damages caused by negligent conduct. Different juries may respond differently, so a trial verdict carries no legal precedent.

Table 10–1. Physical Findings on Examination in Malpractice Lawsuits for Failure to Detect Breast Cancer

Finding	No. Claims	Percentage of Claimants
Palpable mass	265	58.9
Pain in breast	73	16.2
Skin dimpling	53	11.8
Breast examination not done	41	9.1
Pain with palpation	31	6.9
Nipple retraction	29	6.4
Nipple bleeding/discharge	23	5.1
Palpable nodes	22	4.9
Asymmetrical breasts	21	4.7
Skin discoloration	12	2.7

Adapted from Physician Insurers Association of America: PIAA Breast Cancer Study, 3rd ed. Rockville, MD, PIAA, 2002.

CLAIMS DATA AND VERDICTS

The 1995 PIAA study referred to at the beginning of this chapter attempted to identify aspects of breast care that were associated with the filing of malpractice lawsuits.[3] Most of the data reflect the clinical practice of medicine, with implications for imagers (Table 10–1). However, radiologists were the most commonly named defendants in this study, in part because so many cases involve patients who have undergone mammography (Table 10–2). The average indemnity payment for imagers was $182,000, but this number has risen substantially. Although the incidence of breast cancer rises with age, 62% of the claimants in the PIAA study and 71% of the total reported that indemnity payments were for women younger than 50 years. Indeed, the trend of verdicts was the mirror image of the incidence of breast cancer, decreasing with age. Women younger than 40 years composed 31% of claimants and accounted for 37% of indemnity payments. The reasons for this observation likely relate to (1) faster cancer growth rates in younger women with the potential for higher stage of presentation after delay, (2) higher monetary damage assessment based on potential years of life loss and larger losses of income-generating years, and (3) case selection bias secondary to the contingency fee basis for attorney compensation in most malpractice cases. To encourage plaintiffs to find restitution for medical malpractice, attorneys usually accept cases on a contingency fee basis; that is, remuneration is in the form of a percentage of the recovered damages (subject to state-specific limitations) instead of hourly fees. The rationale is beyond the scope of this discussion, but the business of litigation introduces a natural and even necessary bias in the election of cases pursued.

Table 10–2. Domestic Malpractice Claims in the PIAA Breast Cancer Study

Specialty	No. of Claims	No. of Paid Claims	Average Indemnity	Total Indemnity
Radiology	242	184	$346,247	$63,709,403
Obstetrics/gynecology	167	133	$368,798	$49,050,183
Corporation	87	37	$264,518	$9,787,161
Surgical specialties	78	62	$334,393	$20,732,367
Family practice/General practice	62	52	$308,692	$16,051,984
Internal medicine	46	36	$246,538	$8,875,382
Other	22	12	$235,711	$2,828,528
Hospital	20	8	$144,063	$1,152,500
Pathology	9	7	$375,442	$2,628,091
Total	733	531	$329,220	$174,815,599

Adapted from Physician Insurers Association of America: PIAA Breast Cancer Study, 3rd ed. Rockville, MD, PIAA, 2002.

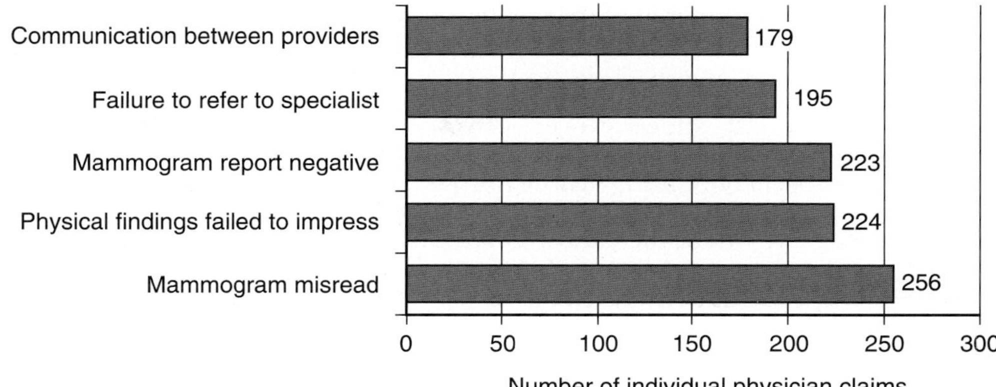

Figure 10–1. Physician-associated issues in legal claims brought for failure to detect breast cancer. (From Physician Insurers Association of America: PIAA Breast Cancer Study, 3rd ed. Rockville, MD, Physician Insurers Association of America, 2002.)

A majority of cases reviewed by PIAA indicated that the patient presented to the clinician with a lesion that was eventually diagnosed as cancer (Fig. 10–1). Delay in diagnosis suggests either that such signs and symptoms were not adequately evaluated at the time or that timely dynamic follow-up was not pursued. Pain was a presenting symptoms in 9% of cases, but this fact is difficult to evaluate because of the overwhelmingly large number of patients who have pain and no cancer.

A subsequent review of 199 cases from this study focusing on imaging aspects (100 screening examinations, 99 diagnostic examinations) indicated that the same kinds of issues discussed in this chapter were associated with radiologists' culpability.[26] Poor image quality affected outcome in 10% of screening cases and 17% of diagnostic cases, and the supervising radiologist was held accountable. The failure to obtain additional views applied to nearly half of the screening cases and nearly three fourths of the diagnostic cases. Errors in reporting occurred in almost one third of patients receiving indemnity payments. Sometimes these errors were due to clerical mistakes, and other times to misdiagnosis. Of significance in this context, in 82% of the diagnostic cases coming to legal attention, the radiologist made no direct communication of results to the referring physician (Table 10–3).

Although primary care physicians such as those practicing obstetrics and gynecology are most likely to be named in lawsuits, radiologists were the most commonly named defendants. This result is probably secondary to the fact that mammography is performed frequently and is referred by multiple different specialties as well as that lawsuits usually include either all potential defendants or those directly involved in the care of the woman.

FUTURE ISSUES

The development of digital mammography, reviewed in other sections of this text, reflects a variety of imaging and electronic strategies. Not only are there substantive differences in spatial and contrast resolution among different products, but also work stations processing such information vary. Whereas prior mammographic units and film-screen combinations varied somewhat (e.g., faster films with slower screens, and vice versa), the resulting hard copy images could be analyzed using a common reference scheme with respect to physical and imaging parameters. A review of such images for satisfactory quality thus employs a common denominator.

Because the specifications of different digital units are different, that common denominator for image review may vary. Reasonable specifications are likely to be supported by clinical trials necessary for approval by the U.S. Food and Drug Administration (FDA) as well as for commercial availability.

However, because mammographic interpretation is based on a variable and somewhat subjective

Table 10–3. Reasons for Liability of Radiologists Regarding Both Screening and Diagnostic Examinations in PIAA–American College of Radiology Breast Cancer Study

Reason	Percentage of Screening Exams (100 cases)	Percentage of Diagnostic Studies (99 cases)
Image quality problem	13	16
Outcome affected	86	92
Interpreting radiologist responsible	100	100
Impact on diagnosis	75	67
Errors in diagnosis	62	54
Omission of additional views	50	75
Poor image quality	10	20
No abnormality suggested	100	87
Errors in communication		
No direct contact to referring physician	71	82
No policy re: communication	35	35
Error in report	27	35
Patient misidentified	9	7
Typographical error	8	14
Errors in omission affecting cases	≈100	≈100
Consequent inadequate follow-up	75	60

Adapted from Physician Insurers Association of America: PIAA/ACR Practice Standards Study. Washington, DC, PIAA, 1996.

post-processing manipulation of data, review of such data may afford the opportunity to re-manipulate the data with different post-processing techniques. Consider a soft tissue mass that is considered suspicious and for which biopsy shows cancer. Retrospective review, commented on earlier, may demonstrate otherwise nonspecific findings.[24] Those prospectively viewed nonspecific findings may be reprocessed—with knowledge of where the cancer developed—to produce a more suspicious image if evaluated after the presence of cancer is known. The reprocessed image may be used as evidence to impugn the initial interpretation.

Review of images during expert assessment for potential liability should be a prospective exercise, more easily performed when hard copy film images are available. Proper review of digital images raises two issues. Hard copy images may need to be made of the post-processed images as they were interpreted, inviting criticism that the interpretation was made from the imaging monitor but is being reviewed in a different manner. This approach challenges the fundamental definition of reasonable conduct, wherein the measure is directed toward *similar circumstances*.[7] Alternatively, "soft copy" digital images may have to be reviewed, inviting a more deliberate attempt to window and level different areas in question, given the conditions under which such a review is requested. Again, the issue of *similar circumstances*[7] from a foreseeable perspective is challenged. There may be no way to avoid the greater bias introduced into such a review, and the resolution of these new issues may require future consensus-based guidelines.

Issues regarding CAD have already been discussed. Future concerns will likely emerge as diagnostic algorithms are developed appropriating likelihoods of suspicion to lesions detected by the computer. Given the relative sensitivities and specificities of such probability determinations, final interpretation not only will remain in the purview of the radiologist but also will be subject to the reasonableness standards already discussed. It is difficult to predict the influence of an external probability determination as might be generated by a computer readout, and most likely the issue would be resolved with the assistance of expert testimony, which would be directed not only to the lesion but also to the importance or reliability of the computer-generated probability.

References

1. Brenner RJ, Rothman B: Detection of primary breast cancer in women with known adenocarcinoma metastatic to the axilla: Use of magnetic resonance imaging following negative clinical and mammographic examination. J Magn Reson Imaging 1997;7:1153-1158.
2. Physician Insurers Association of America: Breast Cancer Study. Washington, DC, Physician Insurers Association of America, 1990.
3. Physician Insurers Association of America: Breast Cancer Study, 2nd ed. Rockville, MD, Physician Insurers Association of America, 1995.

3a. Physician Insurers Association of America: PIAA Breast Cancer Study, 3rd ed. Rockville, MD, Physician Insurers Association of America, 2002.

4. Beninger PR, Beninger ES, Fitzgerald FT: Survey on views and knowledge of house officers on medical legal issues. J Med Educ 1985;60:481-483.
5. Todd v Eitel Hospital, 237 NW2d 357 (Minn 1975).
6. Brenner RJ: Breast cancer and malpractice: A guide to the clinician. Semin Breast Dis 1998;1:3-14.
7. Sheffington v Bradley, 266 Mich 552, 115 NW 2d 303 (1962).
8. MQSRA (Mammography Quality Standards Re-authorization Act of 1998), Pub L No 105-248.
9. Francisco v Parchment Medical Clinic. 88 Mich App 583, 272 N.W.2d 736, 1978, modified 407 Mich 325, 1979.
10. French v Sinkford, 132 W Va 66, 54 SE 2d 38 (1948) as recited in Livengood v Kerr 391 SE 2d 371 at 375 (W Va 1990).
11. Kohn LT, Corrigan JM, Donaldson MS: To Err Is Human: Building a Safer Health System. Washington, DC, The National Academies Press, 1999.
12. Restatement of torts (second). Section 323 (a).
13. Brenner RJ: Medicolegal aspects of breast imaging. Radiol Clin North Am 1992;30:227-286.
14. Barton MB, Harris R, Fletcher SW: Does this patient have breast cancer? The screening clinical breast examination: Should it be done? How? JAMA 1999;282:1270-1280.
15. Goodson WH: Clinical breast examination. West J Med 1996; 164:355-358.
16. Foster R: Limitations of physical examination on early diagnosis of breast cancer. Surg Oncol Clin North Am 1994;3:55-66.
17. Donegan WL: Evaluation of a palpable breast mass. N Engl J Med 1992;327:937-941,
18. Amsler v Verilli, 119 App Div 2d 786, 506 NYS 2d 411 (NY, 2nd Div 1986).
19. Dettman v Flanary, 86 Wis 2d 728 (1979).
20. Brenner RJ: Medical legal aspects of breast imaging: Variable standards or care relating to different types of practices. AJR Am J Roentgenol 1991;156:719-723.
21. The breast cancer detection demonstration project: End results. CA Cancer J Clinic 1987;35:258-290.
22. Grady D, Hodgkins ML, Goodson WH 3d: The lumpy breast. West J Med 1988;149:226-9
23. Sickles EA, Weber WN, Galvin HB: Mammography screening: How to operate successfully at low cost. Radiology 1986;160: 95-101.
24. Harvey JA, Fajardo LL, Innis CA: Previous mammograms in patients with impalpable breast carcinomas: Retrospective versus blinded interpretation. AJR Am J Roentgenol 1993;161: 1167-1172.
25. Birdwell RL, Ikeda DM, O'Shaughnessy KF, et al: Mammographic characteristics of 115 missed cancers later detected with screening mammography and the potential utility of computer-aided detection. Radiology 2001;219:192-202.
26. Brenner RJ, Lucey LL, Smith JJ, et al: Radiology and medical malpractice claims: A report on the Practice Standards Survey of the Physicians Insurers Association of America and the American College of Radiology. AJR Am J Roentgenol 1998; 171:19-22.
27. Brenner RJ, Sickles EA: Surveillance mammography versus stereotactic core biopsy for probably benign breast lesions: A cost-comparison analysis. Acad Radiol 1997;4:419-425.
28. Brenner RJ: False negative mammograms: Medical legal, and risk management considerations. Radiol Clin North Am 2000; 38:741-757.
29. Kolb TM, Lichy J, Newhouse JH: Occult cancer in women with dense breasts: Detection with screening US—diagnostic yield and tumor characteristics. Radiology 1998;207:191-199.
30. Buchberger W, DeKoekkoek-doll P, Springer P, et al: Incidental findings on sonography of the breast: Clinical significance and diagnostic workup. AJR Am J Roentgenol 1999;173;921-927
31. Brenner RJ, Westenberg L: Film management and custody: Current and future medicolegal concerns. AJR Am J Roentgenol 1996;167:1371-1375.
32. American College of Radiology: ACR Standards 2000-2001. Reston, VA, American College of Radiology, 2001.

33. Phillips v Good Samaritan Hospital, 416 NE 2d 646 (Ohio, 1979).
34. Townsend v Turk, 218 Cal App 3d 278, 266 Cal Rptr 821 (1990).
35. Monsees B, Destouet JM, Evens RG: The self-referred mammography patient: A new responsibility for radiologists. Radiology 1988;166:69-73
36. Brenner RJ: Mammography and malpractice litigation: Current status, lessons, and admonitions. AJR Am J Roentgenol 1993; 161:931-935.
37. Wickline v State of California, 183 Cal App 1064, 118 Cal Rptr 661 (1986).
38. Beam CA, Sullivan DC: What are the issues in double reading of mammograms? Radiology 1994;193:582.
39. Taplin SH, Rutter CM, Elmore JG, et al: Accuracy of screening mammography using single versus independent double reading interpretation. AJR Am J Roentgenol 2000;174:1257-1262.
40. Brenner RJ: Interventional procedures of the breast: Medical legal considerations. Radiology 1995;195:611-615.
41. Reynolds HE, Jackson VP, Musick BS: A survey of interventional mammography practices. Radiology 1993;187:71-73.
42. Reuter SR: An overview of informed consent for radiologists. AJR Am J Roentgenol 1987;148:219-227.
43. Meyer JE, Sonnenfeld MR, Greenes RA, et al: Cancellation of preoperative breast localization procedures: Analysis of 53 cases. Radiology 1988;169:629-630.
44. Philpotts LE, Lee CH, Horvath LJ: Canceled stereotactic core-needle biopsy of the breast: Analysis of 89 cases. Radiology 1997;205:423-428.

Section III

OTHER DIAGNOSTIC TOOLS

Clinical Examination of the Breast

Malcolm M. Bilimoria and David P. Winchester

Clinical examination of the breast is an integral part of the three-tiered approach to well breast care (the other two parts being yearly mammograms and monthly breast self-examinations). If one considers that 10% to 15% of the approximately 180,000 new breast cancers this year in the United States will not be detected by conventional imaging, one realizes that at least 18,000 breast cancers have to be detected early by physical examination alone (be it by the physician or the patient).[1] That is, of course, if one assumes that all women 40 years or older comply with the recommendation of yearly mammograms.

Before physical examination of the breast, a thorough medical history is needed to set the groundwork. For example, the date of the last menstrual period and the regularity of the menstrual cycles are important considerations in the evaluation of nodularity, pain, or cysts in a premenopausal woman. Similarly, postmenopausal women should be carefully questioned about hormone replacement therapy, knowledge of which is important if the examination reveals a breast mass. Benign breast masses are uncommon in postmenopausal women who are not currently taking hormone replacement.[2] Important components of the medical history for breast patients are highlighted in Table 11–1.

TECHNIQUE OF BREAST EXAMINATION

A robe should be provided for all patients undergoing breast examination, along with instructions to undress completely from the waist up. Attention to modesty is important, because if an examination is uncomfortable for the patient, she may be deterred from following through with subsequent clinical examinations. First, a visual examination is performed. Both breasts are viewed with the patient in a sitting position with her hands on her hips. Attention to asymmetry, retraction of the skin or nipple, and any breast erythema is important. A comparison of breast size and shape is noted, with particular attention to the chronicity of the differences. It is not unusual for a woman's breasts to differ slightly in size, but recent changes in either size or shape should be noted because they may be manifestations of underlying disease.

Superficial tumors may be evident as bulges in the natural contour of the breast. More often, however, a visual examination in a woman with a malignancy shows retraction of the overlying skin. This can be seen when tumors deep in the breast cause shortening of fibrous septa within the breast or when more superficial tumors cause direct puckering of the skin. Not all skin retraction necessarily results from cancer. Mondor disease or superficial thrombophlebitis of the thoracoepigastric veins can cause skin retraction of the lateral aspect of the breast.[3] Fat necrosis and the associated fibrosis is also a rare cause of skin retraction.

Edema of the breast skin, also referred to as peau d'orange, is another important visual finding of breast examination. It is usually the result of dermal lymphatic obstruction secondary to an underlying malignancy. Another cause, however, is previous axillary lymph node dissections resulting in skin edema along the lateral aspect of the breast. Localized radiation therapy can also cause edema of the skin overlying the irradiated breast which, at times, is confused with tumor recurrence.[4]

Visual inspection is also important in identifying erythema of the breast. Erythema may be secondary to cellulitis, recent breast irradiation, or an inflammatory carcinoma. Inflammatory carcinoma is distinguished from cellulitis by the absence of tenderness and fever.

Examination of the nipples should be initiated with attention to symmetry, retraction, and the presence of eczematous changes. Eczematous changes or ulceration of the nipple may be indicative of Paget disease of the nipple, signifying an underlying malignancy. Ashikari and colleagues[5] reported that of 214 patients presenting with Paget disease, only 6 (2.8%) had no evidence of either invasive cancer or ductal carcinoma in situ.

The physician should inspect the breast with the patient's hands on her hips and with her arms raised. These maneuvers allow for thorough evaluation for even subtle areas of skin retraction.

Next, the physician initiates examination for palpable masses. Examination is started with the patient in an upright position with her hands on her hips. The examiner should use the pads of the middle three fingers, rather than the fingertips or any portion of the hand, to perform the examination. Each physician must develop his or her own systematic, consistent method of examination. Common methods are examination of the breast in a concentric manner and in the direction of spokes on a wheel. It is important to avoid pinching breast tissue between two fingers, which often leads to a false appreciation of a mass.

The physician then examines the breasts while the patient assumes the supine position with the ipsilateral arm raised above her head. Examination

Table 11–1. Important Components of the Medical History in Patients Undergoing Breast Examination

All women	Age at menarche and menopause Last menstrual period and regularity of cycles Breast changes noted with menstrual period (pain, nodularity) History of nipple discharge (frequency, color, bilateral or unilateral discharge) Number of pregnancies and age at first pregnancy History of oral contraceptive use (age at start, duration, dose) History of hormone replacement therapy (age at start, duration, dose) Previous breast biopsies and corresponding diagnoses Family history of breast cancer, including affected relatives and ages Family history of other cancers: ovarian or primary peritoneal cancer (*BRCA1* gene), pancreatic cancer (*BRCA2* gene), sarcomas or adrenocortical tumors (Li-Fraumeni gene)
Woman presenting with a breast mass	How and when it was first noticed Previous mass at this location Trauma at this location Changes in the mass (size, shape, consistency) Changes in surrounding skin

of the breast should include palpation from the clavicles to the inferior rib cage and from sternal border to midaxillary line. Any masses should be evaluated for size, tenderness, firmness, location, and fixation to underlying or surrounding tissue. If there is a question of a nonsuspicious mass in a premenopausal woman, a second examination at a different time during the menstrual cycle may be helpful.

If the patient has a history of nipple discharge or if nipple discharge is elicited during the examination, the examiner should try to discern which quadrant of the breast is responsible by initiating palpation away from the nipple and traveling toward the nipple. The discharge should be examined for amount, consistency, and color. If the discharge is not obviously bloody, a test for occult blood may be performed. The characteristics of nipple discharge that should raise the index of suspicion for malignancy are spontaneous and unilateral discharge that is bloody, serosanguineous, or watery in consistency and is associated with an underlying mass.

Evaluations of the supraclavicular, infraclavicular, and axillary nodal basins are also key elements of the breast examination. Each nodal basin should be examined with the patient in the upright and supine positions. Nodal masses are evaluated for size, tenderness, location, and fixation or being matted. Lymph nodes that are smaller than 1 cm, mobile, and bilateral are of low suspicion and can often be felt in thin women.

If the breast physical examination yields findings suspicious for carcinoma, the American Joint Committee on Cancer (AJCC) clinical stage should be included in the medical record.

Another important aspect of the clinical breast examination is teaching the patient how to examine her own breasts, which serves as reinforcement of breast self-examination. Such teaching helps the patients feel more comfortable with breast self-examination. This issue is particularly important in light of studies showing that women who perform breast self-examination are less likely to die from breast cancer. In the Canadian National Breast Screening Study, 45,000 women were taught three key elements of the breast self-examination.[6] They were then subsequently evaluated according to whether they performed each of the three key components. The odds ratio for death from breast cancer was 1.82 for women omitting one component of the examination, whereas women who did not perform self-examinations at all were almost three times more likely to die from breast cancer (odds ratio, 2.95). Other, smaller studies have similarly confirmed the benefits of breast self-examination.[7,8] A thorough clinical breast examination is important not only as a method of physician-based breast cancer detection but also as a tool to teach breast self-examination to patients.

References

1. Greenlee RT, Murray T, Bolden S, Wingo PA: Cancer Statistics 2000. CA Cancer J Clin 2000;50:7.
2. Haagensen CD: Diseases of the Breast. Philadelphia, WB Saunders, 1986, p 502.
3. Tabar L, Dean P: Mondor's disease: clinical, mammographic, and pathologic features. Breast 1981;7:17.
4. Morrow M: Clinical evaluation. In Harris JR, Lippman ME, Morrow M, Hellman S (eds): Diseases of the Breast. Philadelphia, Lippincott-Raven, 1996, p 67.
5. Ashikari R, Park K, Huvos AG, et al: Paget's disease of the breast. Cancer 1970;26:680.
6. Baines CJ: The Canadian National Breast Screening Study. Ann Intern Med 1994;120:326.
7. Gastrin G, Miller AB, To T, et al: Incidence and mortality from breast cancer in the Mama Program for Breast Screening in Finland, 1973-1986. Cancer 1994;73:2168.
8. Newcomb PA, Weiss NS, Storer BE, et al: Breast examination in relation to the occurrence of advanced breast cancer. J Natl Cancer Inst 1991;83:260.

Chapter

12 Breast Ultrasonography

Valerie P. Jackson and Victoria J. Edmond

Wild and Neal first described the use of ultrasound (US) to examine the breast in 1951.[1] Since that time, US has undergone major technological improvements, and it is now the most widely used and effective adjunctive technique to mammography.

TECHNICAL ASPECTS

Breast ultrasonography should be performed with high-resolution real-time US equipment. Mechanical sector transducers are no longer acceptable for breast ultrasonography. Although 7 MHz is the *minimum* frequency that can be used, 10- to 13-MHz transducers are preferable to get optimal benefit from ultrasonography of the breast. Ten- to 13-MHz transducers have higher spatial and contrast resolution while maintaining sufficient depth of penetration to image back to the chest wall in the vast majority of patients (Fig. 12–1). Newer developments such as panoramic imaging[2,3] (Fig. 12–2) and real-time compound imaging[4-6] (Figs. 12–3 and 12–4) have also improved the ability of US to depict masses and aid in diagnosis. Linear array transducers should be used because they have a relatively wide field of view and can be used to guide interventional procedures. Currently available linear array transducers have focal zones that can be varied in number and depth so that the region of best focus can be placed at the appropriate depth for optimal image quality.

Accurate breast ultrasonography requires high-quality equipment that is properly calibrated and maintained. Unfortunately, the breast imaging section may receive the "castoffs" of the general ultrasonography division of the radiology department, or it may have such a limited budget that only inexpensive equipment can be purchased. There are wide variances in the prices and quality of US equipment marketed for breast imaging. Image quality, rather than price, should be the major element in the decision regarding the purchase of new equipment. Substandard equipment, technique, or interpretation will diminish the potential benefit of US in breast imaging.

The operator should have a thorough knowledge of breast anatomy and pathology as well as the technical aspects of both mammography and US. Whenever possible, breast ultrasonography should be performed in the mammography facility by the same radiologists or technologists who perform or interpret mammography. The mammogram must be available when ultrasonography is performed so that the proper area is examined. When a palpable abnormality is examined, clinical examination must be performed to ensure that the ultrasonographic findings correspond to the palpable lesion. After US gel is applied, the operator may be able to feel masses that are not otherwise palpable. For nonpalpable, mammographically detected masses, the operator must determine the proper area to scan from the mammogram and correlate the size and location of the ultrasonographically visualized lesion with the mammographic findings. For example, if the mammogram demonstrated a 2-cm mass and the ultrasonographer found a 5-mm cyst, the ultrasonographic findings would not correlate with the mammogram.

In most cases, ultrasonography is performed with the patient supine on an examination table, with her ipsilateral arm abducted over her head. The operator should strive to minimize the thickness of the breast, maintain a normal angle of incidence of the US beam to the breast parenchyma, and use the chest wall as a means of posterior compression. Thus, for lateral lesions, the patient should be placed in the contralateral posterior oblique position with the aid of a pillow or sponge wedge. For medial lesions, the woman should be flat on her back. Appropriate compression with the transducer minimizes the breast thickness and improves image quality.

Proper placement of the focal zone(s) is critical to the ultrasonographic examination. Accurate depiction of the margin characteristics requires the use of a high-resolution transducer, with the focal zone(s) placed at the level of the mass (Fig. 12–5). If the lesion is superficial and the focal zone cannot be moved electronically, a standoff pad should be used to physically move the transducer away from the breast, thus placing the focal zone in the superficial region of the breast.

The time-compensated gain (TCG) or depth-compensated gain (DCG) must be set appropriately for accurate assessment of the internal matrix of the lesion. As shown in Figures 12–6 and 12–7, if the gain is set too low, a hypoechoic solid mass may appear to be anechoic, whereas if the gain is too high, a simple cyst fills in with low-level internal echoes, leading to the erroneous diagnosis of a solid mass. Posterior enhancement is an inconsistent finding, and its prominence depends on the type of equipment used, the size and location of the cyst, and the amount or type of fluid within it. It is important to remember that posterior enhancement can occur behind solid masses as well as cysts.

It may be difficult to correlate the location of a lesion seen on mammography with its location in a

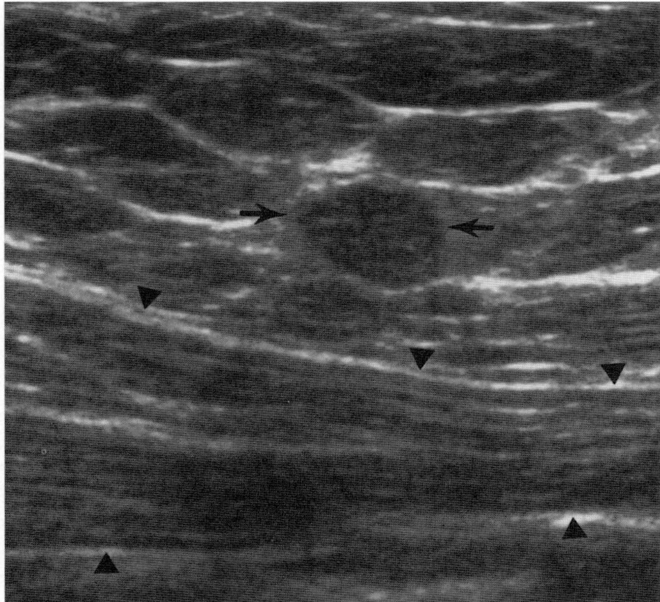

Figure 12–1. Radial 12-MHz ultrasonogram of oval circumscribed mass (*arrows*) that is slightly hypoechoic relative to fat. The breast tissue would be classified as "homogeneous background echotexture—fat." The breast is well penetrated by the sound beam, with visualization through the pectoralis muscle (*arrowheads*).

woman in the supine position. If a question exists regarding the correlation between the mammographic and ultrasonographic findings for a nonpalpable lesion, US can be performed through the "window" of a fenestrated mammographic compression paddle used for needle localization procedures. The patient's breast remains compressed in the mammographic unit while a film is obtained. The coordinates of the lesion on the film are used to guide the placement of the transducer in the window of the paddle for ultrasonography (Fig. 12–8).[7-9]

We perform breast ultrasonography as a tailored examination of an area of mammographic or palpable abnormality, rather than as a complete survey of one or both breasts. The role of US as a screening technique is controversial because ultrasonography has a high false-positive rate and is very operator dependent. Scans should be obtained in the area of interest in at least two orthogonal planes. Many ultrasonographers scan longitudinally and transversely, although radial and antiradial planes may be more effective.[10] The operator should sweep through the entire lesion and obtain hard copy images of representative sections of the lesion or of the area if no ultrasonographic abnormality is seen. These should be clearly labeled with the location and plane of the scan. Masses should be measured on the hard copy images with electronic calipers in three dimensions. Additional images of each mass should be obtained without calipers because the caliper marks may obscure the borders of small lesions.

Given the small field of view with US, it is important to properly label the images. The American College of Radiology (ACR) Practice Guideline for Breast Ultrasound recommends the elements shown in Table 12–1.[11]

Artifacts

Artifacts are commonly encountered in ultrasonography and can cause confusion and misdiagnosis if not correctly interpreted.[12-16] Most are easily

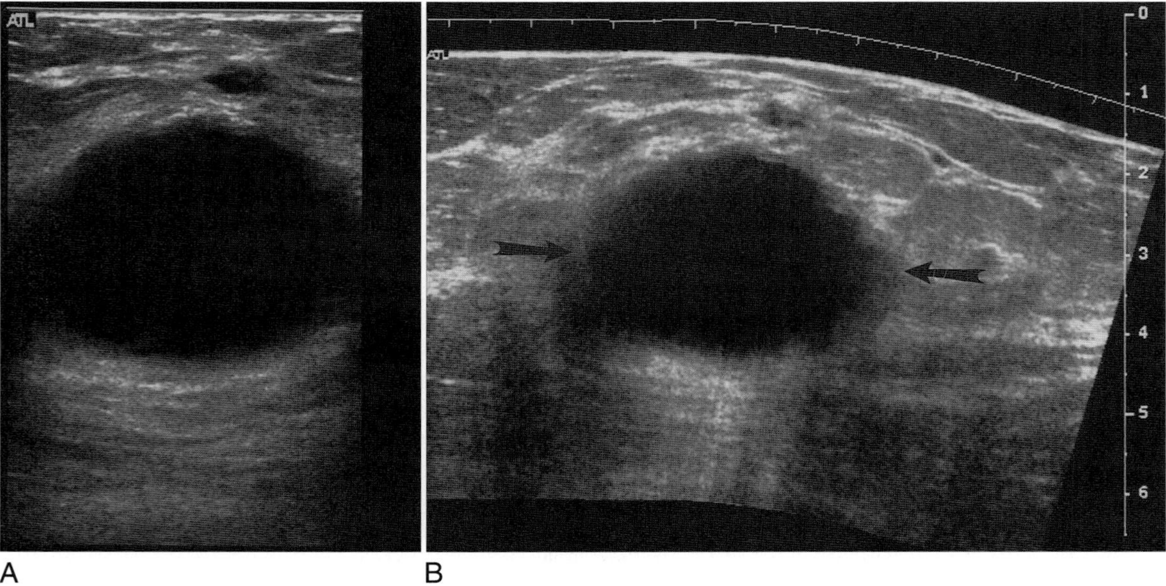

Figure 12–2. Conventional 12-MHz ultrasonogram (**A**) and extended field-of-view ultrasonogram (**B**) of a 3.5-cm invasive ductal carcinoma. The size of the lesion and surrounding tissue are better seen on the extended field-of-view image. Note that the mass is hypoechoic to fat, appearing nearly anechoic. The margins are indistinct.

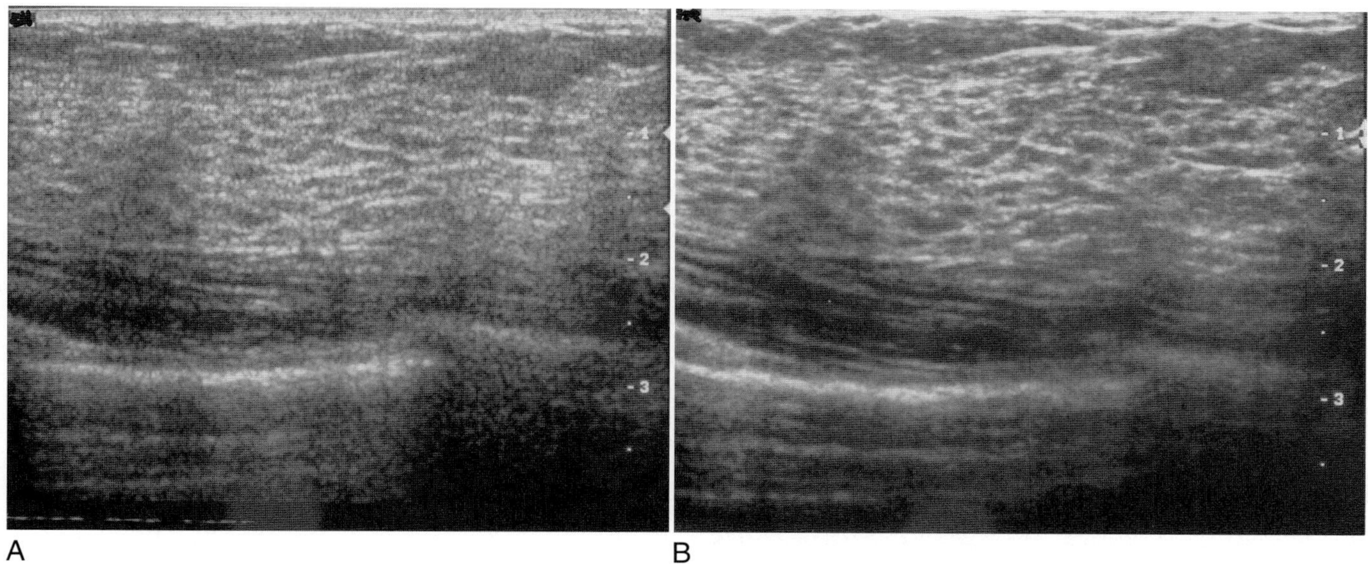

Figure 12–3. Conventional 12-MHz (**A**) versus 12-MHz real-time compound imaging scan (**B**). Note that the resolution is improved and the image appears "smoother" on the compound imaging scan of this area of normal fibroglandular tissue ("homogeneous background echotexture—fibroglandular").

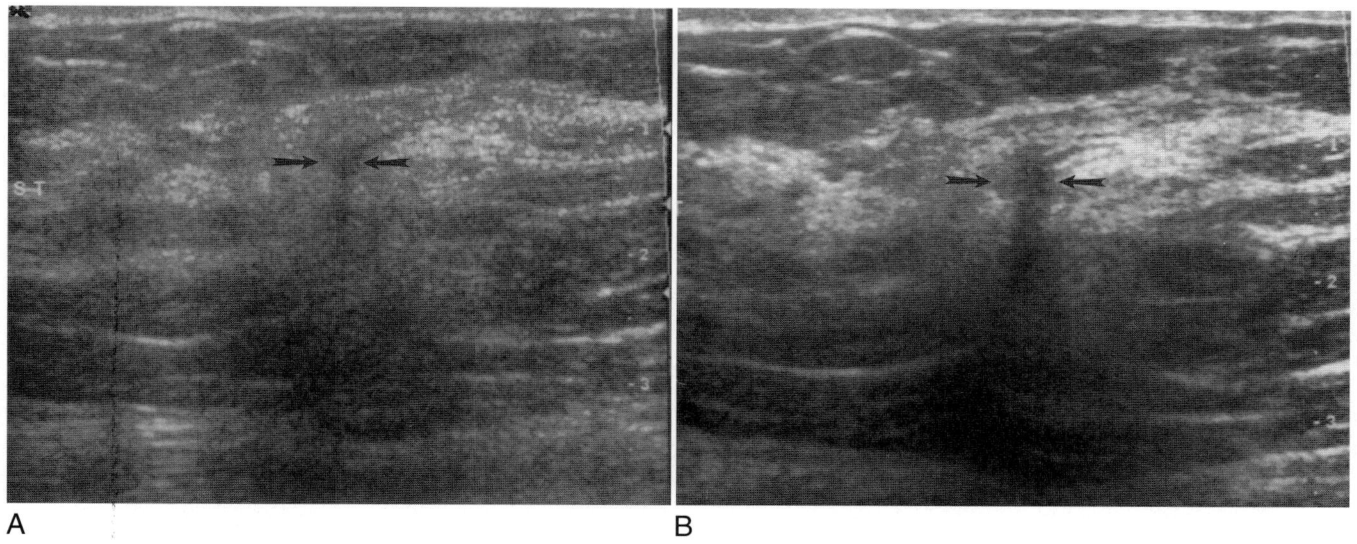

Figure 12–4. Conventional 12-MHz (**A**) versus 12-MHz real-time compound imaging scan (**B**) of a 4-mm invasive ductal carcinoma (*arrows*). Note that the tumor is more visible on the compound imaging study because of improved spatial and contrast resolution.

Table 12–1. Recommended Labeling for Breast Ultrasound

Permanent identification label with:
Facility name and location
Examination date
Patient's first and last name
Patient's identification number or date of birth
Anatomic location using quadrant, clock face, or labeled diagram of breast
Indication of distance from nipple (may be helpful)
Sonographer's or sonologist's identification number, initials, or other symbol

Adapted from ACR Practice Guideline for the Performance of a Breast Ultrasound Examination.[11]

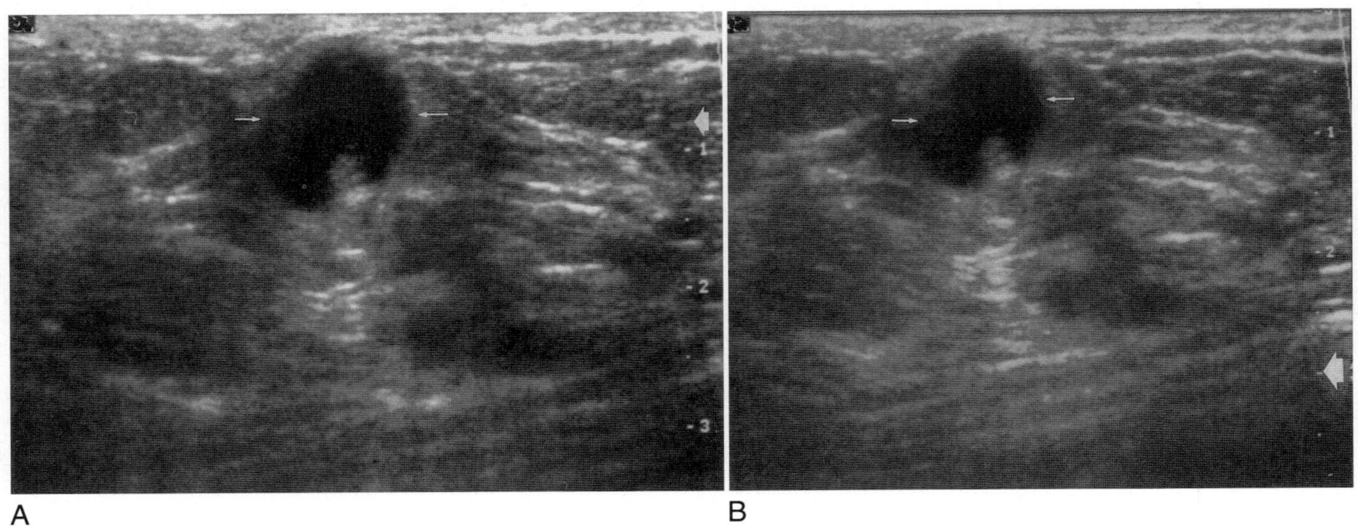

Figure 12–5. Effect of focal zone placement. The 9-mm complex mass (*small arrows*) is better seen when the focal zone is placed in the region of the mass (**A,** *large arrow*) than when the focal zone is placed in the region of the pectoralis muscle (**B,** *large arrow*).

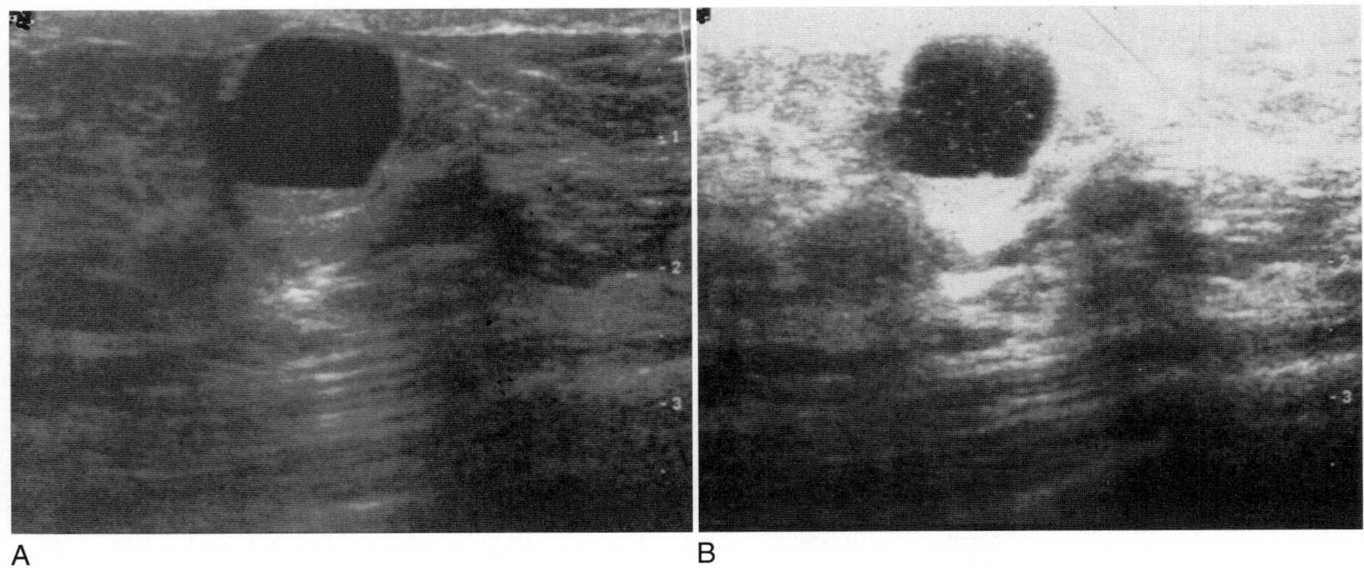

Figure 12–6. Effect of gain setting. This 1-cm cyst appears anechoic when the gain is appropriately set (**A**). When the gain is set too high (**B**), multiple echoes are seen within the cyst, simulating a complicated cyst or solid mass. At aspiration, clear yellow fluid was aspirated.

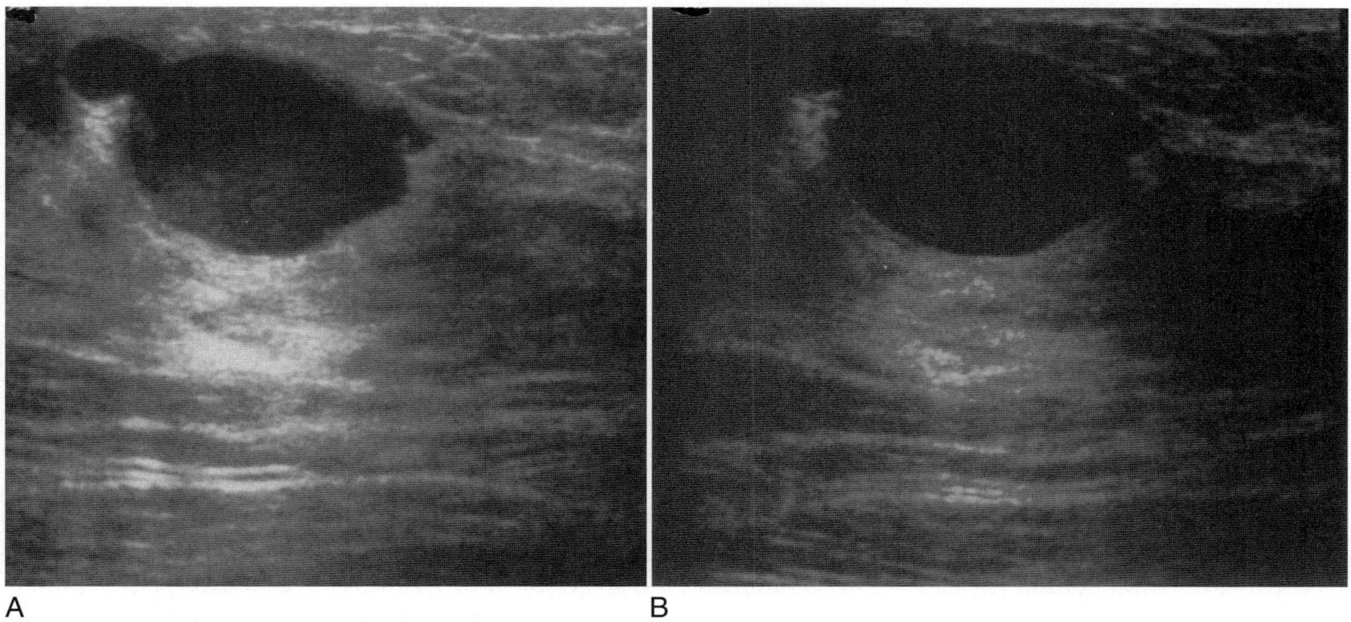

Figure 12–7. Effect of gain setting. When the gain is appropriately set, debris is clearly visible within this complicated cyst (**A**). When the gain is set too low (**B**), the cyst, as well as most of the surrounding fat, appears anechoic.

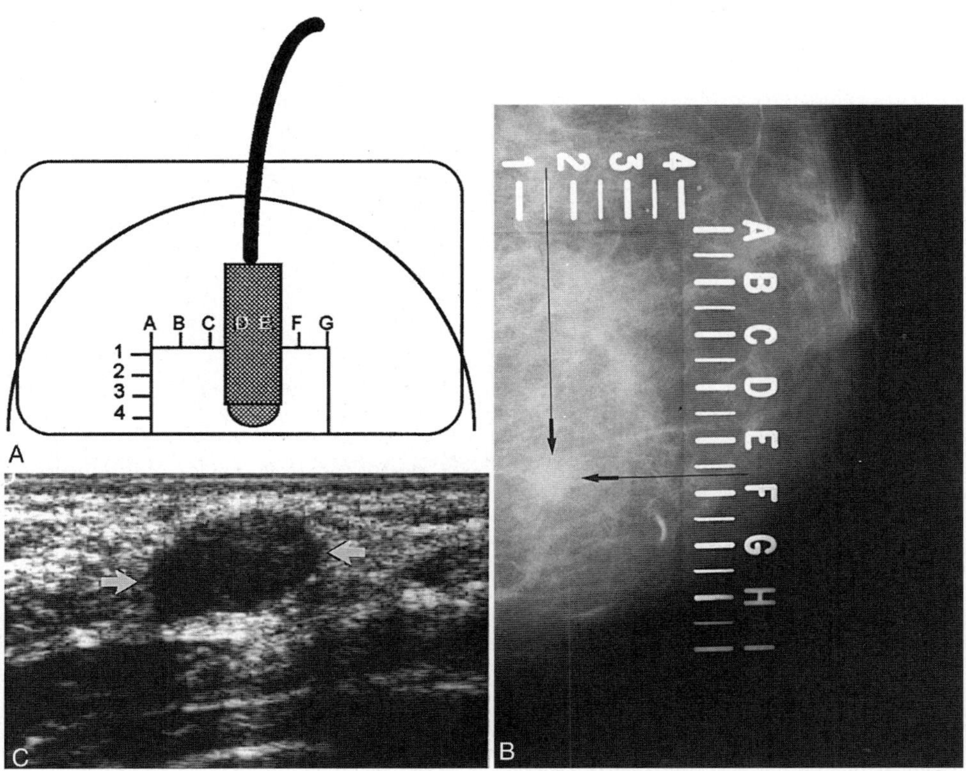

Figure 12–8. Ultrasonography can be performed in a fenestrated mammographic compression paddle to ensure that the proper lesion is evaluated with US. The breast is compressed within the mammography unit, and the film is processed. The coordinates of the lesion on the mammogram are used to guide placement of the US transducer (**A**). An example of a small, partly circumscribed, partly obscured mass found on mammography (**B,** *arrows*), with US of the lesion (**C,** *arrows*) in the fenestrated compression paddle, demonstrating its solid internal matrix. At biopsy, this was a fibroadenoma.

recognized by experienced operators and interpreters. Some "artifacts," such as posterior enhancement and shadowing, serve as signs that aid in the ultrasonographic diagnosis of lesions. Many, however, make interpretation difficult if not recognized as artifacts. An experienced operator works to minimize their effects, realizing that artifacts cannot be totally eliminated. As stated by Dr. George Kossoff, "Skilled interpreters of ultrasonic images follow three golden rules: never make an interpretation on a single image; just because a feature is displayed do not consider that it is necessarily real; and just because a feature is not displayed do not consider that it is necessarily not there."[14]

BASIC INTERPRETATION

The ACR recently published a lexicon for breast US as part of the fourth edition of the Breast Imaging Reporting and Data System (BI-RADS).[17] The descriptors follow those used for mammography BI-RADS as closely as possible, with additional descriptors for the features unique to US. Table 12–2 lists the features in the US BI-RADS lexicon, and examples of each are shown in Figures 12–9 to 12–31.

Cysts

Ultrasonography depicts the internal matrix of masses, and it is 96% to 100% accurate in the diagnosis of cysts.[18-21] To achieve such accuracy, one must use strict criteria for the diagnosis of cysts. Most simple cysts have circumscribed margins and sharp anterior and posterior borders, are anechoic, and usually have posterior enhancement (see Fig. 12–11). When cysts are multiple, clustered, or surrounded by

Text continued on p. 186

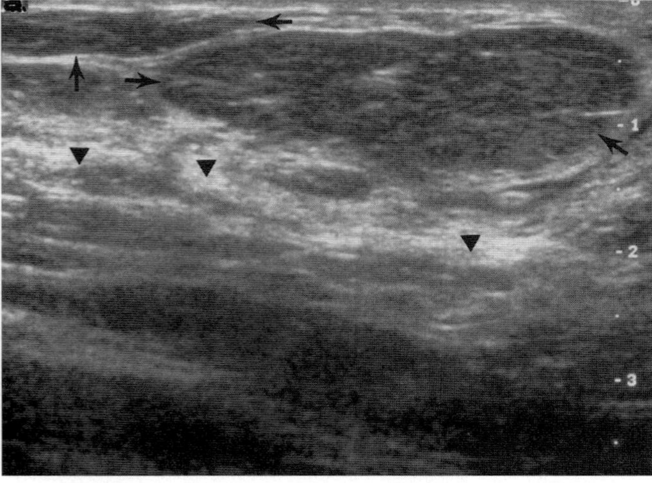

Figure 12–9. Heterogeneous background echotexture. The fibroglandular tissue (*arrowheads*) is hyperechoic, whereas the fat lobules (*arrows*) are hypoechoic.

Table 12–2. American College of Radiology BI-RADS Breast Ultrasonography Lexicon

Feature	Figure(s)
Background Echotexture	
Homogeneous background echotexture—fat	12–1
Homogeneous background echotexture—fibroglandular	12–3
Heterogeneous background	12–9
Shape	
Oval	12–10
Round	12–11
Irregular	12–12
Orientation	
Parallel to skin	12–10
Not parallel to skin	12–11, 12–12
Margin	
Circumscribed	12–10, 12–11
Not circumscribed	
Indistinct	12–13
Angular	12–14
Microlobulated	12–12
Spiculated	12–15
Lesion Boundary	
Abrupt interface	12–10, 12–11
Echogenic halo	12–12, 12–14, 12–16
Echo Pattern	
Anechoic	12–11, 12–17
Hyperechoic	12–18
Complex	12–19, 12–20
Hypoechoic	12–12 to 12–16
Isoechoic	12–21, 12–22
Posterior Acoustic Features	
No posterior acoustic features	12–12, 12–21
Enhancement	12–11, 12–17
Shadowing	12–14 to 12–16
Combined pattern	
Effect on Surrounding Tissue	
None	12–17
Duct changes (abnormal caliber and/or arborization)	12–14
Cooper's ligament changes (straightening or thickening)	12–15, 12–23
Edema	12–12
Architectural distortion	12–14
Skin thickening	12–16, 12–20
Skin retraction/irregularity	12–24
Calcifications	
None seen	
Macrocalcifications	12–25, 12–26
Microcalcifications out of a mass	
Microcalcifications in a mass	12–27
Special Cases	
Clustered microcysts	12–28
Complicated cysts	12–29
Mass in or on skin	12–30
Foreign body	
Lymph nodes—intramammary	12–31
Lymph nodes—axillary	
Vascularity	
Color or power Doppler findings compared with normal tissue	
Present or not present	
Present immediately adjacent to lesion	
Diffusely increased vascularity in surrounding tissue	

Adapted from ACR BI-RADS, 4th ed.[17]

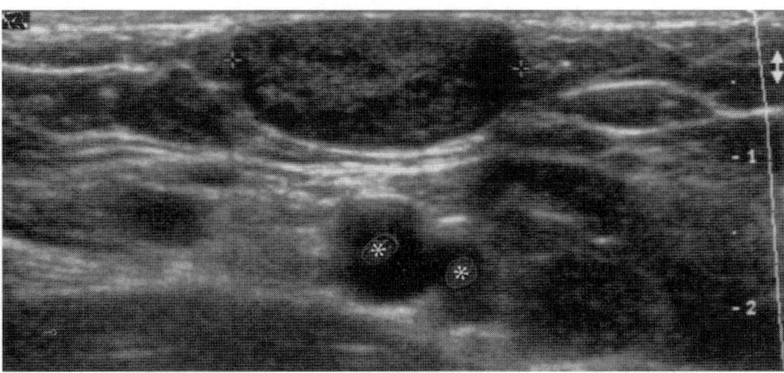

Figure 12–10. Oval circumscribed hypoechoic mass (*calipers*). The orientation of the mass is parallel to the skin. This is a sebaceous cyst located in the axilla. There is an abrupt interface with the surrounding breast tissue. The anechoic structures located posteriorly (*asterisks*) are the axillary artery and vein.

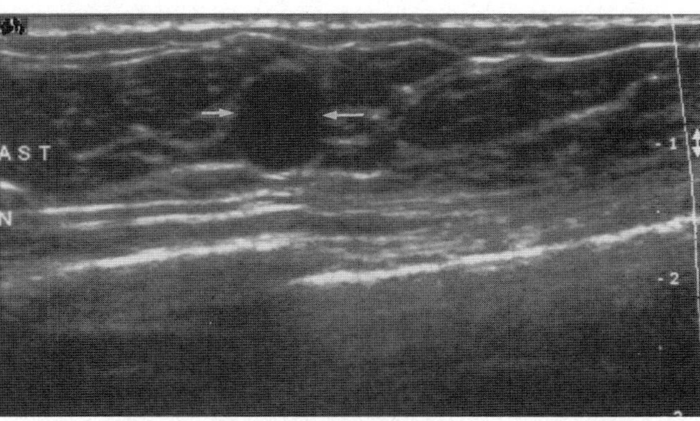

Figure 12–11. Round circumscribed anechoic mass (*arrows*). This is a benign simple cyst. The orientation of the mass is not parallel to the skin. There is an abrupt interface with the surrounding breast tissue.

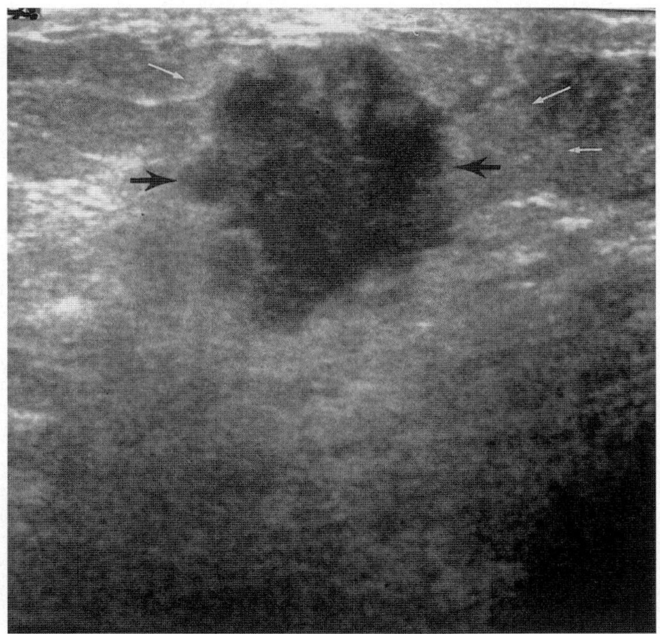

Figure 12–12. Irregular hypoechoic mass with microlobulated and indistinct margins (*black arrows*). The orientation of the mass is not parallel to the skin. There is an echogenic halo (*white arrows*) of edema or desmoplastic reaction around this invasive ductal carcinoma. This vague band of increased echogenicity is generally seen only with malignancy or an inflammatory process such as an abscess. There are no posterior acoustic changes.

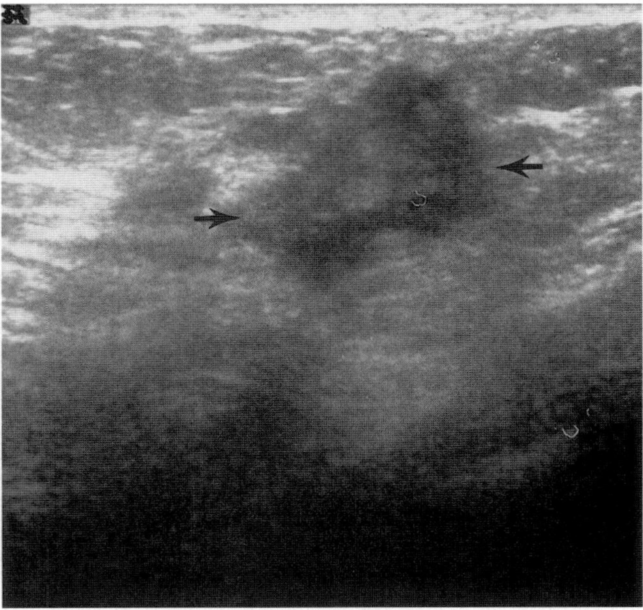

Figure 12–13. Irregular hypoechoic invasive ductal carcinoma (*arrows*) with indistinct margins.

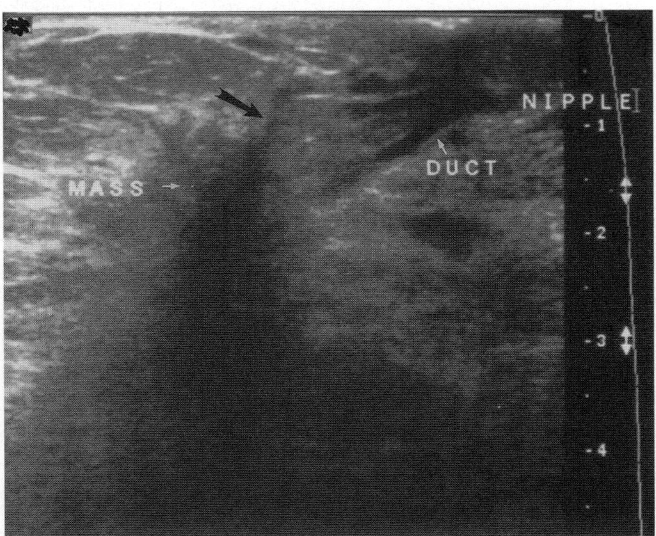

Figure 12–14. Carcinoma with surrounding architectural distortion. Irregular hypoechoic invasive ductal carcinoma with an angular margin (*black arrow*) and duct changes (dilatation and cutoff). There is a surrounding echogenic halo and intense posterior acoustic shadowing.

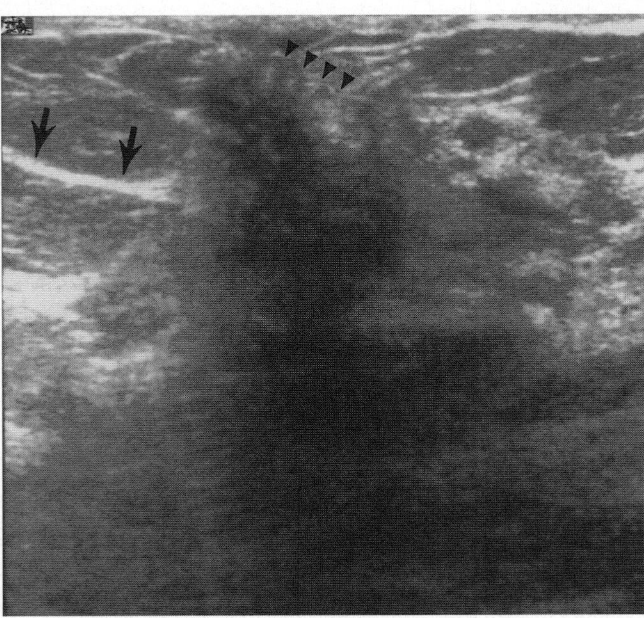

Figure 12–15. Irregular hypoechoic invasive ductal carcinoma with spiculated margins (*arrowheads*) and associated thickening of Cooper's ligaments (*arrows*). There is posterior acoustic shadowing.

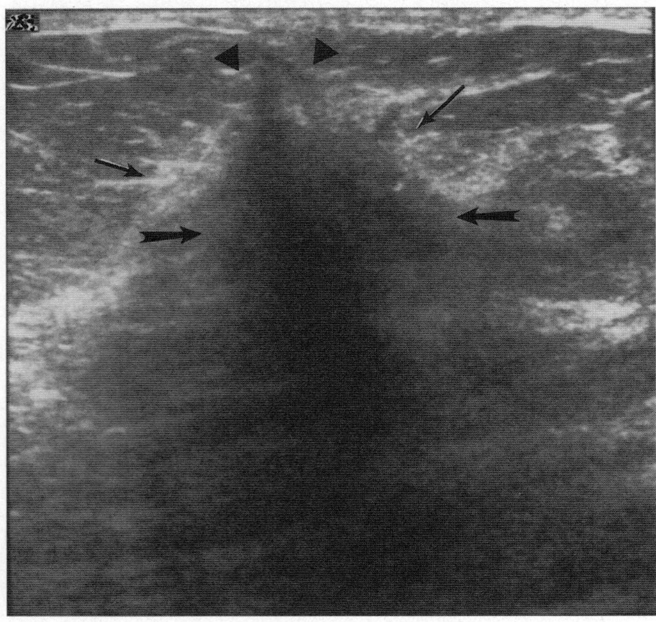

Figure 12–16. Irregular hypoechoic invasive ductal carcinoma (*large arrows*) with indistinct margins, a surrounding echogenic halo (*small arrows*), and associated skin thickening (*arrowheads*). There is posterior acoustic shadowing.

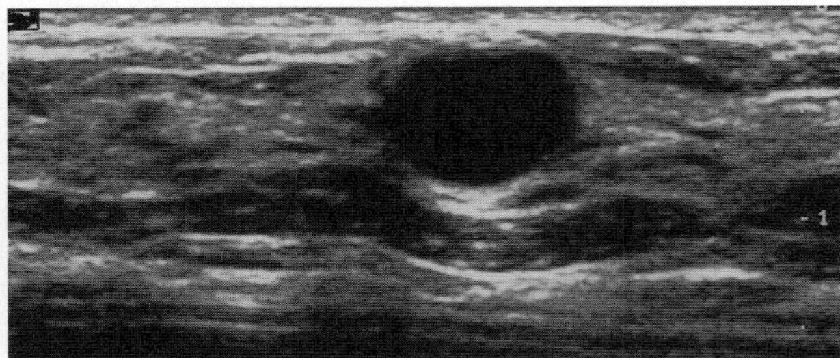

Figure 12–17. Anechoic circumscribed mass (benign simple cyst). The mass is oriented parallel to the skin. There is posterior acoustic enhancement. The surrounding tissue is normal.

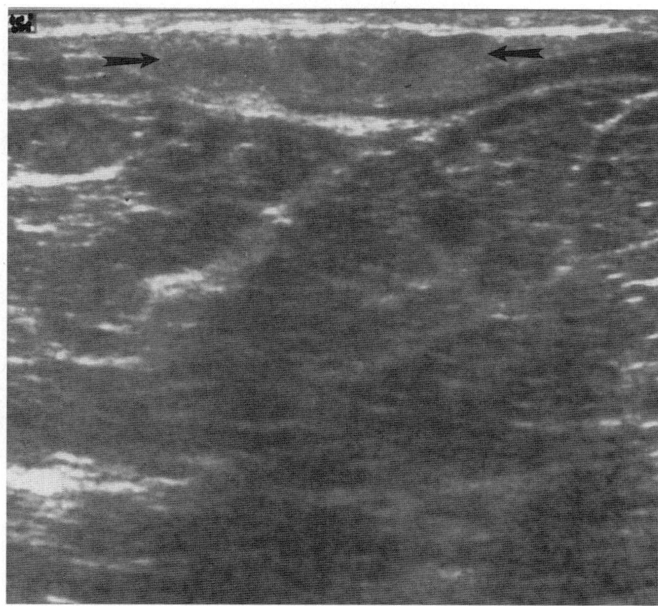

Figure 12–18. Hyperechoic mass (*arrows*). The patient had a history of trauma to the area. This was an area of fat necrosis that resolved on follow-up.

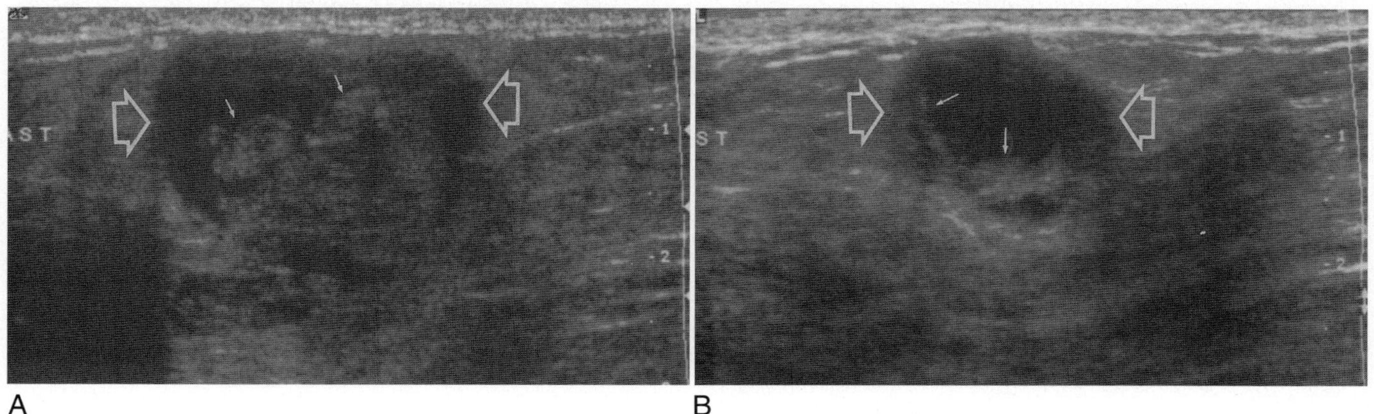

A B

Figure 12–19. Complex mass. Radial (**A**) and antiradial (**B**) ultrasonograms of an intracystic papillary carcinoma (*open arrows*) demonstrate solid material (*small arrows*) within the fluid of the mass.

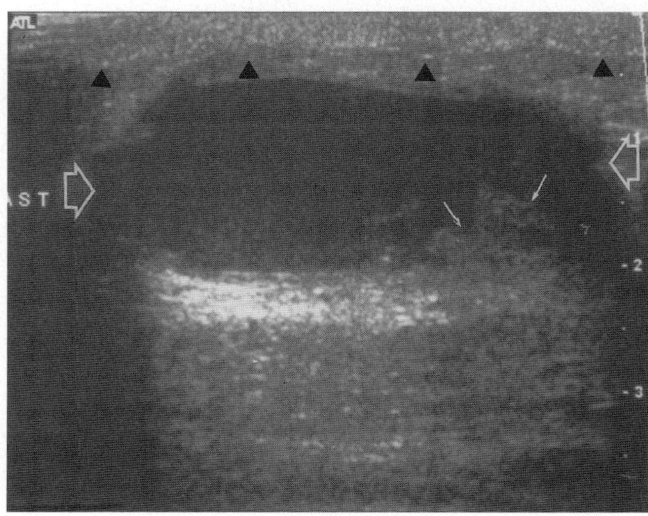

Figure 12–20. Complex mass. This oval mass (*open arrows*) has indistinct margins and both cystic and solid (*small arrows*) components. Note the associated skin thickening (*arrowheads*). This was invasive ductal carcinoma, but an abscess could have an identical ultrasonographic appearance.

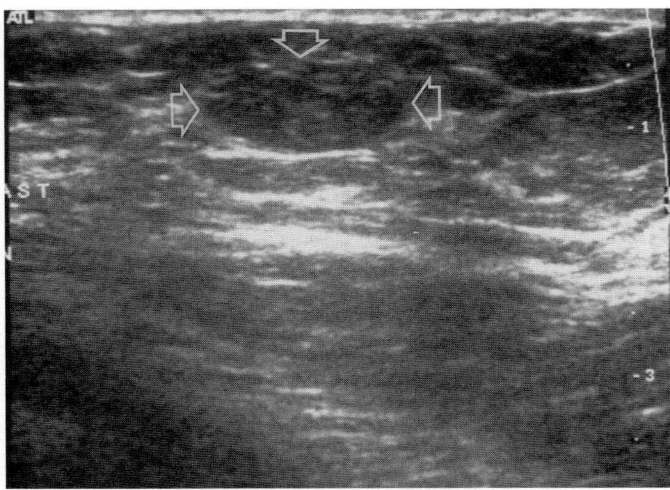

Figure 12–21. Isoechoic mass. This circumscribed, oval fibroadenoma (*arrows*) has an internal echo texture identical to fat. There are no posterior acoustic changes.

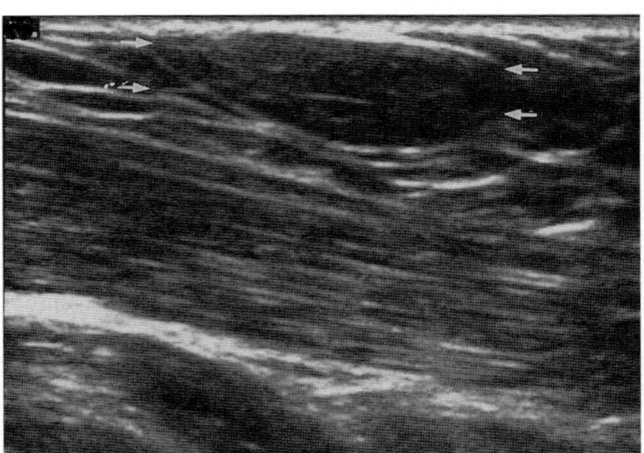

Figure 12–22. Isoechoic mass. This circumscribed, oval lipoma (*arrows*) has an internal echo texture identical to fat. There is no specific ultrasonographic appearance for a lipoma. Some are hyperechoic relative to fat, whereas others are isoechoic.

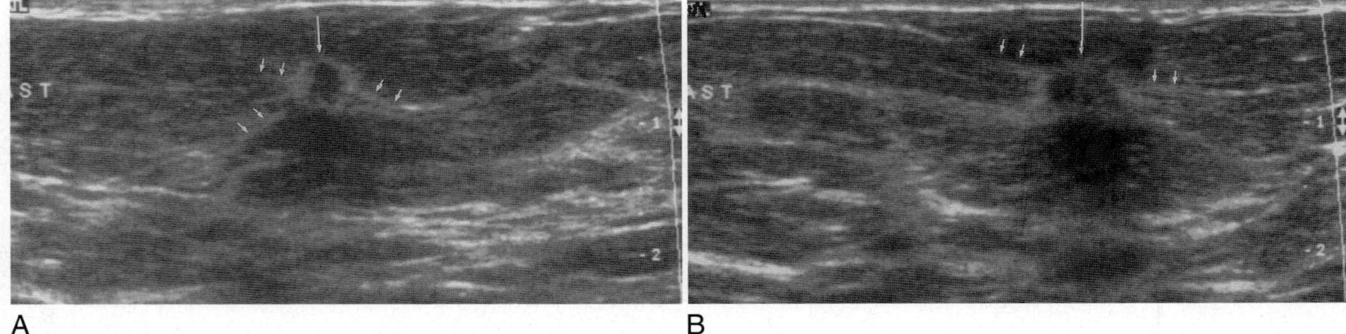

Figure 12–23. Cooper's ligament changes. Longitudinal (**A**) and transverse (**B**) ultrasonograms of a 5-mm invasive ductal carcinoma (*long arrows*). The mass is hypoechoic and has indistinct margins. There is an echogenic halo around the mass. There is associated thickening and straightening of Cooper's ligaments (*small arrows*).

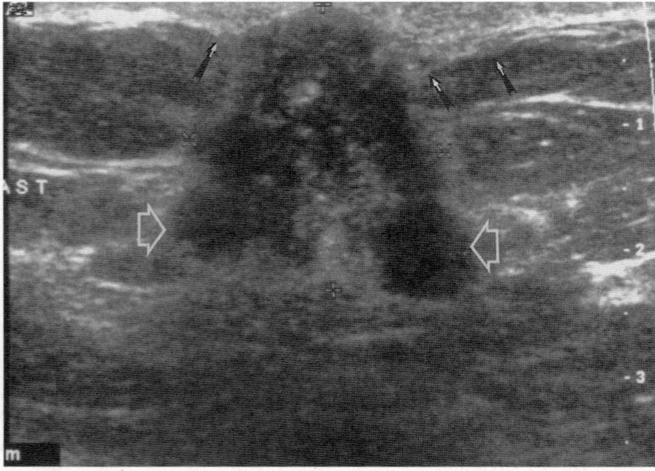

Figure 12–24. Skin retraction and irregularity. This 2-cm, irregular, hypoechoic invasive ductal carcinoma (*open arrows*) has an orientation that is not parallel to the skin. There is associated irregular skin thickening (*small arrows*). The clinically apparent skin retraction is not visible on the ultrasonogram because of the compression from the transducer.

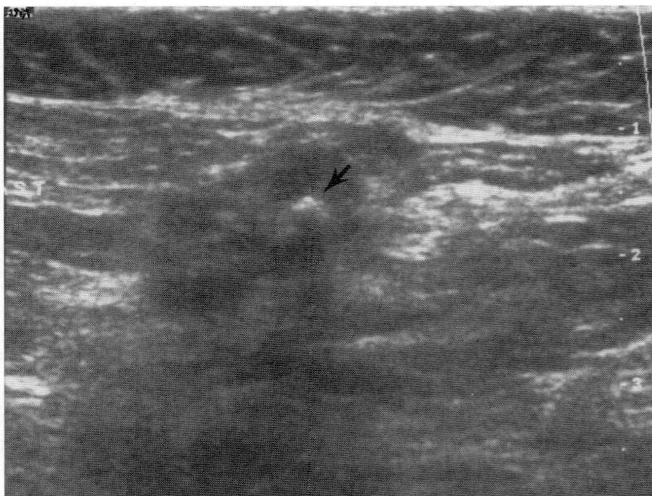

Figure 12–25. Macrocalcification (*arrow*) in an axillary lymph node.

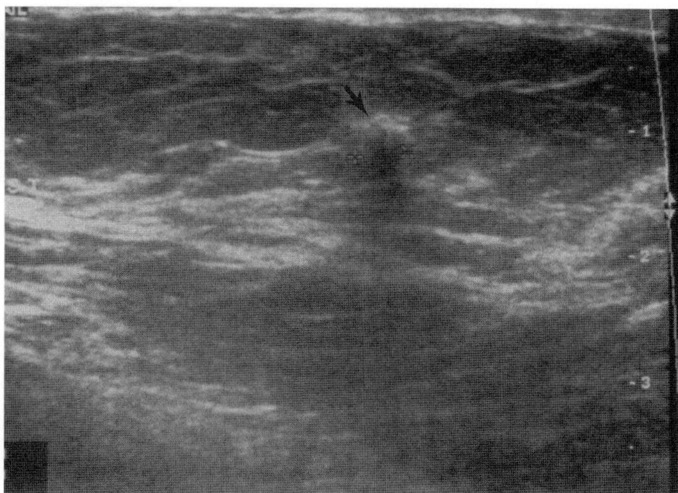

Figure 12–26. Macrocalcification (*arrow*) in an involuting fibroadenoma (*calipers*). The diagnosis was obvious on the mammogram, but the ultrasonographic appearance mimics a small invasive ductal carcinoma with posterior acoustic shadowing.

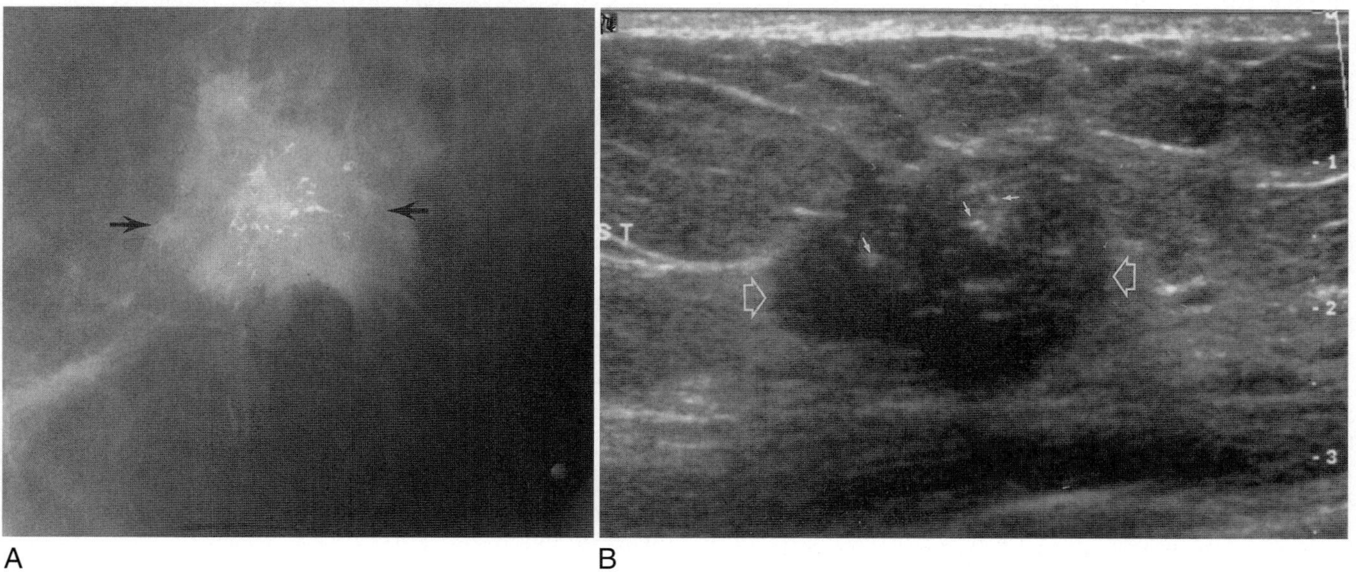

Figure 12–27. Microcalcifications within a mass. Mammogram (**A**) of an invasive ductal carcinoma (*arrows*) with internal microcalcifications. The ultrasonogram (**B**) demonstrates an irregular hypoechoic mass (*open arrows*) with internal bright reflectors (*small arrows*), which represent the microcalcifications.

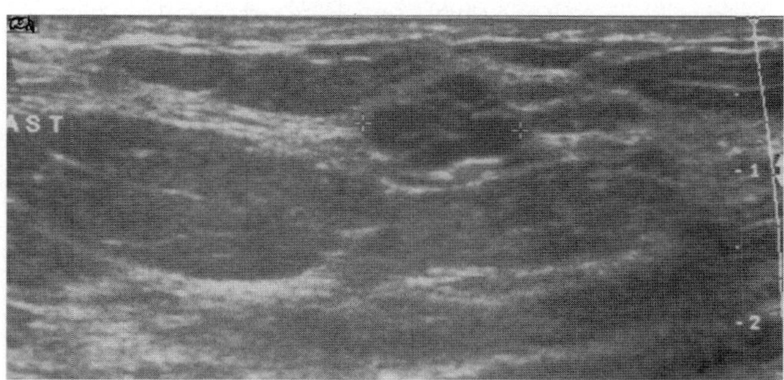

Figure 12–28. Clustered microcysts. This appearance is suggestive of apocrine metaplasia.

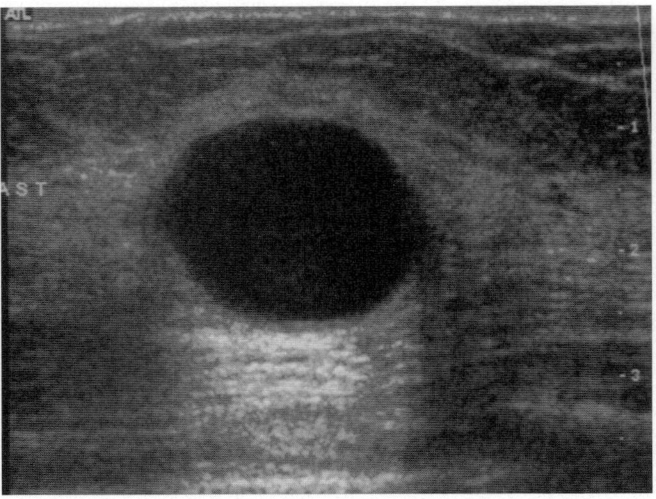

Figure 12–29. Complicated cyst. This round mass has slightly indistinct margins and low-level internal echoes. There is marked posterior acoustic enhancement. Clear greenish fluid was aspirated, and the lesion has not recurred.

fibrous tissue, they may have angulated margins. Not all simple benign cysts display the classic features described previously. When internal echoes are seen within a cyst, the most common causes are artifactual from improper gain or power adjustment, reverberation (Fig. 12–32), or other artifacts. When "real" echoes are found within a cyst, they are usually attributed to proteinaceous material, cellular debris, hemorrhage, infection, or cholesterol crystals within the cyst (Fig. 12–33).

There is continued controversy regarding the smallest size of circumscribed mass for which US should be attempted. This varies with the lesion location, breast size and composition, and type of equipment used. Using good-quality, high-frequency equipment, one can diagnose cysts as small as 2 to 3 mm in diameter in many breasts. Conversely, a 2-cm cyst may be difficult to diagnose when located deep within a large fatty breast. For many small cysts, differentiation is not possible because of "partial voluming" or "side lobe artifacts." It is difficult to predict how often this will occur; therefore, no hard and fast rule exists regarding the smallest lesion that can be evaluated with US.

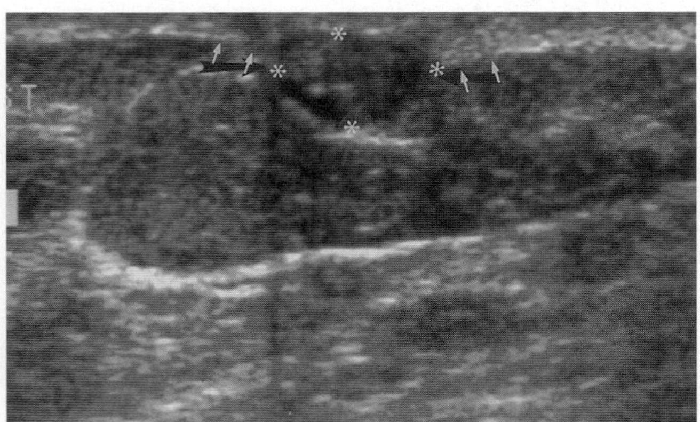

Figure 12–30. Mass in skin. The posterior aspect of the skin (*arrows*) forms a "claw" around this 1-cm sebaceous cyst (*asterisks*).

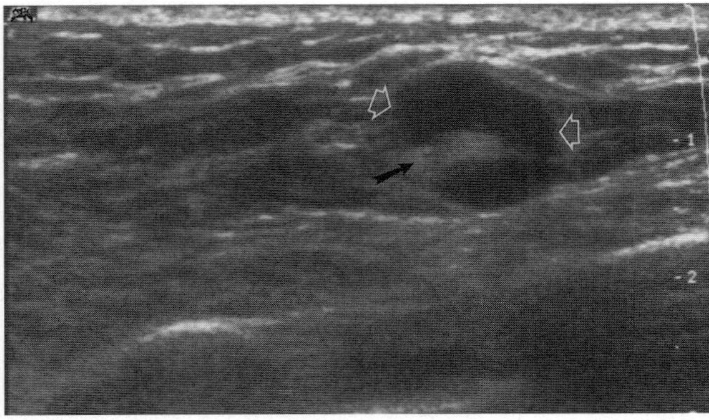

Figure 12–31. Intramammary lymph node. This enlarged lymph node (*open arrows*) maintains its fatty hilum (*black arrow*). This is a reactive node in a patient with psoriasis.

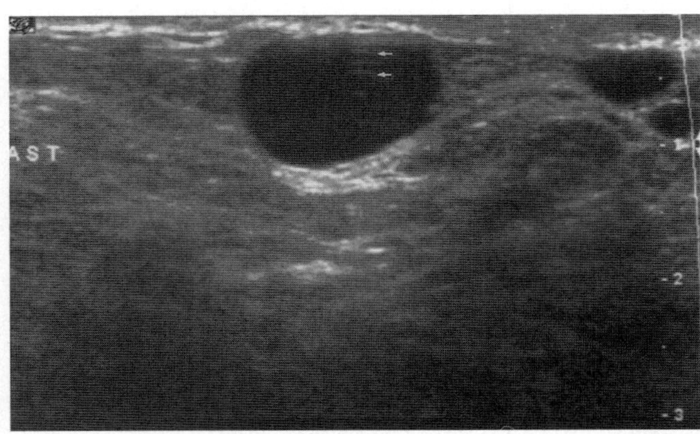

Figure 12–32. Reverberation artifact (*arrows*) in a cyst.

It is important to carefully scan in two orthogonal planes, looking for wall irregularity or solid projections into the cyst, which may indicate an intracystic tumor (see Figs. 12–5, 12–19, and 12–20). Intracystic benign and malignant tumors are unusual, and several studies have described the ultrasonographic features.[22-25]

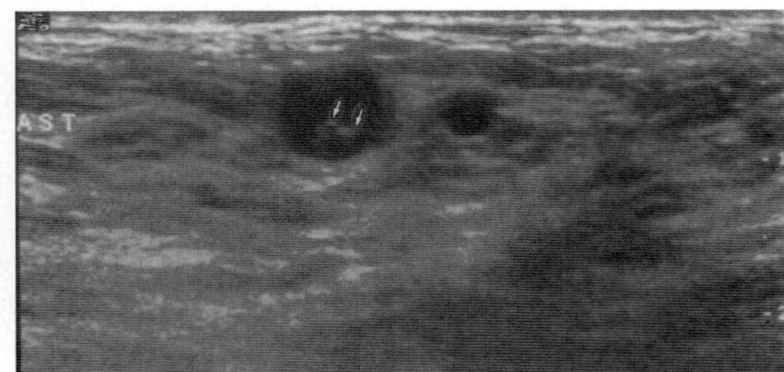

Figure 12–33. Cellular debris (*arrows*) within a benign cyst.

The use of ultrasonography for the diagnosis of cysts is clinically important because simple cysts, particularly those that are not palpable, do not require aspiration or biopsy. This saves patients the expense, anxiety, and discomfort associated with surgery or percutaneous needle placement. Aspiration, rather than US, has been advocated for the evaluation of palpable masses,[26] because this is less expensive at many centers and often therapeutic. Over the years, however, US has become the dominant method for the determination of whether a mass is a cyst. At most institutions, if a palpable mass is documented to be a simple cyst, aspiration is not performed unless the patient has pain or anxiety associated with the palpable lump.

US is most commonly performed for evaluation of noncalcified masses with circumscribed, indistinct, or obscured margins for which cysts are in the differential diagnosis. Masses with spiculated margins and circumscribed masses containing microcalcifications do not require US examination for determination of the internal matrix. If calcifications (macro- or micro-) are in the central portion of the mass, the lesion is solid. Calcifications layered within the dependent portion of a mass, documented by both horizontal and vertical beam mammograms, are diagnostic of milk of calcium within a cyst, and US is not required for confirmation. When spiculated margins or suspicious microcalcifications are seen within a mass on mammography, the lesion requires biopsy, even if a simple cyst is found with US. When a mass is completely or predominantly obscured by adjacent fibroglandular tissue on mammography, the character of the margins is unknown, and US is useful for determination of the margin characteristics as well as the internal matrix. In all of these situations, even if US is not necessary for evaluation of the internal matrix of the lesion, ultrasonography is very useful to determine if the lesion can be targeted with US for subsequent intervention, such as needle biopsy.

Solid Masses

"Typical" ultrasonographic features of benign and malignant solid breast masses have been described.[27-29] Most ultrasonographically visible infiltrating carcinomas are irregular hypoechoic masses with posterior acoustical shadowing (Fig. 12–34). Many fibroadenomas are oval, smooth, hypoechoic masses (Fig. 12–35). Many solid masses do not display a "typical" ultrasonographic appearance. Some carcinomas are circumscribed (Fig. 12–36), and some fibroadenomas are irregular or have indistinct margins (Fig. 12–37). In addition, many small solid masses are not visible with US. If a discrete cystic or solid lesion is *not* visualized with US, one must assume that the mass is solid, rather than that no abnormality exists. In such cases, one should base the need for biopsy or follow-up on the mammographic appearance or clinical findings.

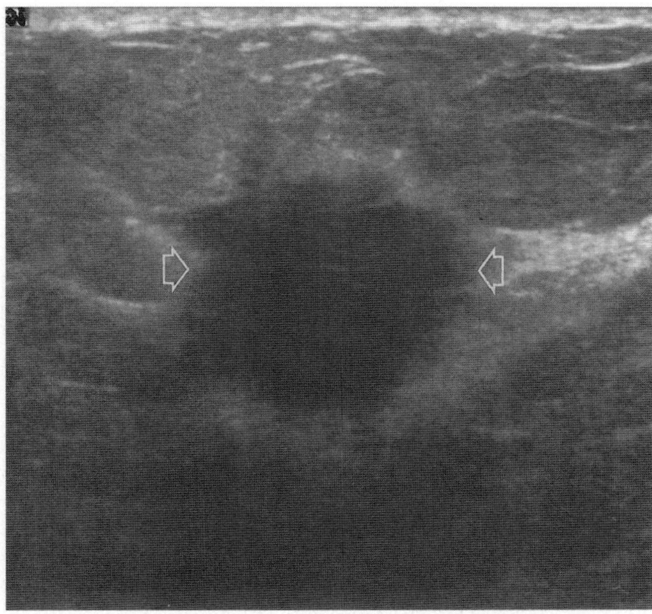

Figure 12–34. Typical ultrasonogram of invasive ductal carcinoma (*arrows*). The mass has an irregular shape and indistinct margins, and its orientation is not parallel to the skin. The mass is hypoechoic relative to fat, and there is a surrounding echogenic halo. There is mild posterior acoustic shadowing.

Indications for Breast Ultrasound
(Table 12–3)

Differentiation of Cysts from Solid Masses

As stated previously, one of the most important roles for US is the determination of the cystic or solid nature of circumscribed noncalcified masses seen on

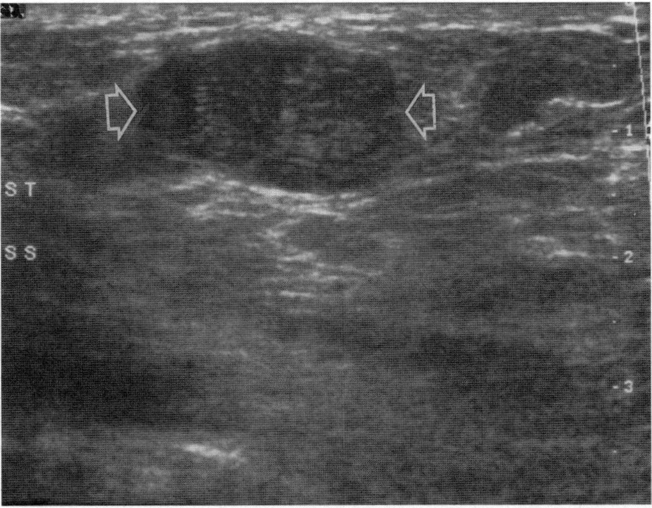

Figure 12–35. Typical ultrasonogram of a fibroadenoma (*arrows*). The circumscribed oval mass is oriented parallel to the skin. There are no surrounding architectural changes other than displacement of adjacent breast tissue. The mass is hypoechoic relative to fat, and in this case there is mild posterior acoustic enhancement.

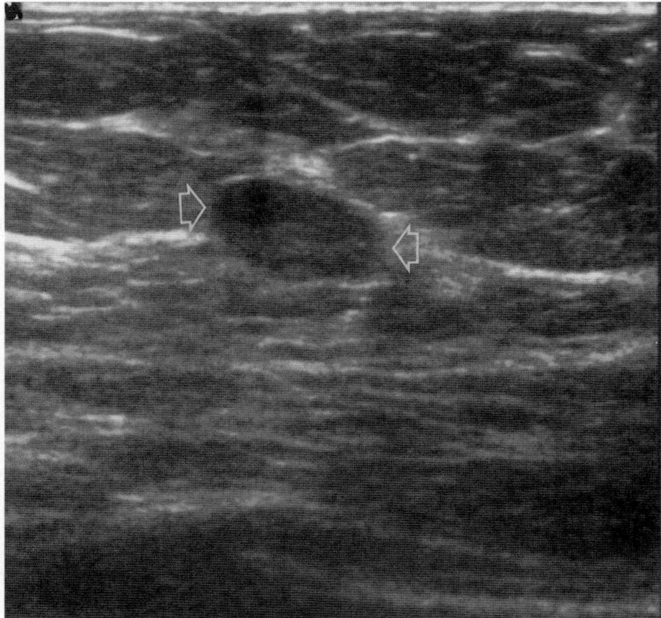

Figure 12–36. Circumscribed carcinoma. This 1-cm invasive ductal carcinoma (*arrows*) has circumscribed margins, an oval shape, and orientation parallel to the skin and is isoechoic to fat.

mammography or found on palpation. When typical ultrasonographic features are present, US is virtually 100% accurate in the diagnosis of a cyst.

Evaluation of a Palpable Mass Not Visible in a Radiographically Dense Breast

Normal fibroglandular tissue may partly or completely obscure masses on mammography. When a palpable mass is not mammographically visible and sufficient radiographic density is present so that the lesion could be hidden, the role of US is primarily to determine if the mass is cystic or solid. Many investigators have found cases in which US demonstrated palpable breast cancers not seen on mammography.[18,30-41] US does not display all solid masses, however, even in dense breasts.[38,42] Although the negative predictive value for a negative mammogram and ultrasonogram has been reported to be as high as 99% to 100%,[43-45] biopsy should still be considered if the clinical findings are suspicious.[39,46a]

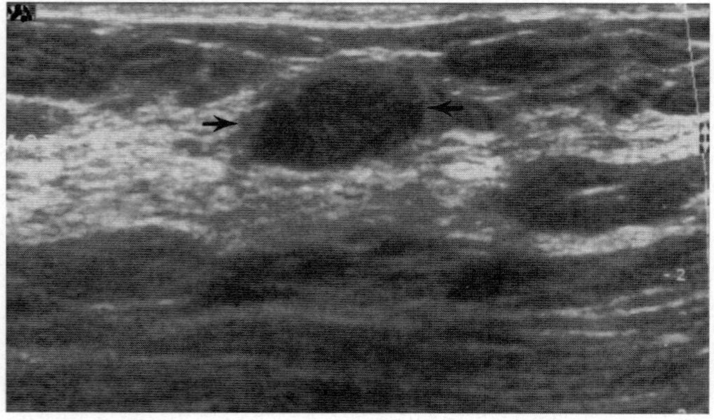

Figure 12–37. Fibroadenoma with indistinct margins. The mass (*arrows*) is oval and oriented parallel to the skin, but the margins are indistinct.

Table 12–3. Indications for Breast Ultrasonography

Differentiation of cysts from solid masses
Evaluation of a palpable mass not visible in a radiographically dense breast
Evaluation of a partially obscured nonpalpable mass found on mammography
Assessment of a mass that cannot be completely evaluated with mammography because of location
Evaluation of a woman younger than 30 years with a palpable mass
Evaluation of an infected breast for an abscess
Evaluation of an area of asymmetrical density
Guidance for interventional procedures

Assessment of a Mass that Cannot Be Completely Evaluated with Mammography because of Location

With creative positioning, the technologist can place almost all palpable breast masses on the mammogram. Rarely, for extremely peripheral masses in very thin women, the technologist may find it difficult or impossible to place the lesion on the film. In these unusual cases, US is indicated for determination of the cystic or solid nature of the lesion. It is important to remember that US should not be used to compensate for poor positioning, and negative ultrasonographic findings do not rule out carcinoma.

Evaluation of a Young Patient with a Palpable Mass

Ultrasound is generally the primary method for evaluation of a woman younger than the age of 30 with a palpable mass.[47-51] The breasts of these women are more sensitive to radiation than are those of older women, and breast cancer in this age group is relatively rare. Thus, it is desirable to limit the radiation exposure in young women. In our practices, we usually perform US as the initial imaging study. If a suspicious solid mass is found on ultrasonography, mammography should be considered to evaluate for additional lesions. For women older than 30 years, we begin with mammography and supplement with US when necessary. Imaging is not justified if a focal clinical abnormality is not present, unless the woman has a personal or unusually strong family history of breast cancer.[47,49]

Evaluation of an Infected Breast for an Abscess

Diffuse mastitis is usually diagnosed and treated clinically. Occasionally, mastitis does not respond appropriately to antibiotics, or focal clinical findings may suggest abscess formation. In these cases, mammography may be difficult to perform because of pain and edema of the breast. Mammography usually does not demonstrate a discrete abscess cavity within an area of increased density from inflammation unless a gas-forming organism is involved. US is an excellent method for detection of an abscess cavity (Fig. 12–38) within an area of mastitis, and it can guide surgical or percutaneous drainage, if necessary.

Evaluation of an Area of Asymmetrical Density

Asymmetrical density is a common mammographic finding, and the cause is usually asymmetrical fibroglandular tissue. This is generally readily apparent from the mammogram alone. If there is any question after mammographic workup, US is useful to distinguish between fibroglandular tissue and a mass or architectural distortion.[52]

Guidance for Interventional Procedures

Ultrasound has been successfully used to guide cyst aspiration, fine-needle aspiration biopsy of solid masses, and preoperative needle or wire localization.[53-63] A variety of methods may be used, and, with experience, US localization is rapid and accurate.

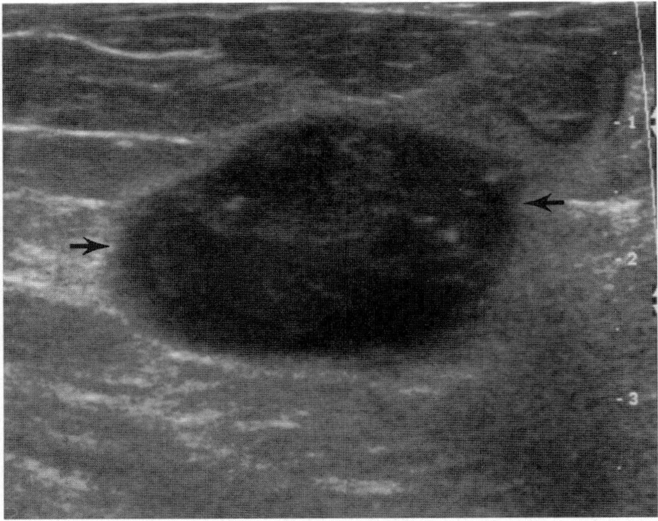

Figure 12–38. Abscess. This 3-cm mass (*arrows*) has indistinct margins and a heterogeneous hypoechoic internal echo texture indistinguishable from a carcinoma.

These techniques are described in Chapters 16, 17, and 20.

Controversial Uses of Breast Ultrasound

There are two major areas of continued controversy regarding indications for US of the breast: differentiating benign from malignant solid masses and the use of US for screening for breast cancer. The cost of ultrasonography and lack of scientifically demonstrated benefit for the patient make the usefulness of US in these situations unclear. Further research is necessary before we can determine the true benefit (or potential harm) that may derive from the use of ultrasonography in these situations.

Differentiation of Benign from Malignant Solid Masses

Considerable overlap occurs between the US appearances of fibroadenomas and carcinomas using current US imaging techniques and criteria.[19,27,28,64-66,66a,67] In addition, there is lack of uniformity in observers' use of terminology to describe ultrasonographic features, which reduces the accuracy of ultrasound in distinguishing between benign and malignant masses.[67-79] The use of a standardized lexicon, such as ACR BI-RADS,[17] should help to reduce the variability in the terminology. The configuration or shape of the tumor,[70-72] ultrasonic tissue characterization,[73] and pulsed[74-79] or color[80-82] Doppler findings show potential as methods to differentiate between benign and malignant solid masses. Further research with large sample sizes is necessary to determine whether these are any more reliable than the "classic" findings described in the early 1980s.

Screening of the Asymptomatic Radiographically Dense Breast

For value as a single screening modality, US must detect all cancers that would be visible mammographically, as well as a substantial number of nonpalpable cancers that are not mammographically visible. US does not adequately perform either of these tasks. Ultrasonography's sensitivity is reduced in the detection of small solid masses in fatty or mixed breast tissue, and US usually does not detect microcalcifications.

There has been renewed interest in the use of US for screening for breast cancer in women with radiographically dense breasts. Early studies showed that US had unacceptably high false-negative rates, ranging from 0.3% to 47% (mean = 20.7%).[18,28,30,32,33,38,40,76,83-85] Most of the carcinomas reported in these series were palpable. The false-negative rates would be expected to be higher for smaller, clinically occult cancers. Most important, US failed to detect a significant number of *nonpalpable* carcinomas in women with good-quality negative mammograms.[42] Ultrasound was also shown to have a substantial false-positive rate in asymptomatic women. In other words, many "lesions" were found on breast ultrasonograms, but these were rarely clinically significant. Kopans et al.[38] followed 94 cases with abnormal US but normal mammographic and physical examinations for 3 to 4 years; none of these lesions was malignant. Sickles et al.[21] found 80 solid masses in 587 asymptomatic women with dense breasts, but none was found to be carcinoma. In 1990, Fung and Jackson[86] reported biopsy of 62 lesions found only by US in radiographically dense breasts of asymptomatic women. All were benign.

More recent studies have demonstrated that current state-of-the-art, high-frequency, real-time equipment (with 10- to 12-MHz transducers) can be used to find small, nonpalpable cancers.[87-95] The studies published to date, however, have not been blinded (i.e., the US operator knew the results of the clinical breast examination and mammogram at the time of ultrasonography, which leads to bias).[96] Cilotti et al.[89] compared the results of breast ultrasonography performed by two independent, equally experienced operators—one was aware of the mammographic findings, and the other was not. The sensitivity of US for detection of breast cancer by the operator who knew the mammographic findings was 85%, whereas the sensitivity for the "blinded" operator was only 35%. The ACR Imaging Network (ACRIN) Trial 6666, currently in progress, will evaluate the use of screening US in a high-risk population. The ultrasonograms will be performed in a systematic fashion by trained, experienced radiologists who are blinded to the results of other imaging studies. This large, multicenter trial should help answer the remaining questions regarding the efficacy and cost-effectiveness of US for screening for breast cancer.[97]

References

1. Wild JJ, Neal D: Use of high frequency ultrasonic waves for detecting changes of texture in living tissues. Lancet 1951;1: 655-657.
2. Fornage BD, Atkinson EN, Nock LF, Jones PH: US with extended field of view: Phantom-tested accuracy of distance measurements. Radiology 2000;214:579-584.
3. Weng L, Tirumalai AP, Lowery CM, et al: US extended-field-of-view imaging technology. Radiology 1997;203:877-880.
4. Huber S, Wagner M, Medl M, Czerbirek H: Real-time spatial compound imaging in breast ultrasound. Ultrasound Med Biol 2002;28:155-163.
5. Kwak JY, Kim E-K, You JK, Oh KK: Variable breast conditions: Comparison of conventional and real-time compound ultrasonography. J Ultrasound Med 2004;23:85-96.
6. Malich A, Marx C, Sauner D: Assessment of conventional versus real-time spatial compound imaging in breast ultrasonography: Preliminary results. J Clin Ultrasound 2003;31: 59-60.
7. Brem RF, Gatewood OMB: Template-guided breast US. Radiology 1992;184:872-874.
8. Conway WF, Hayes CW, Brewer WH: Occult breast masses: Use of mammographic localizing grid for US evaluation. Radiology 1991;181:143-146.
9. Lunt LG, Peakman DJ, Young JR: Mammographically guided ultrasound: A new technique for assessment of impalpable breast lesions. Clin Radiol 1991;44:85-88.
10. Stavros AT, Dennis MA: The ultrasound of breast pathology. In Parker SH, Jobe WE (eds): Percutaneous Breast Biopsy. New York, Raven Press, 1993, pp 111-127.
11. American College of Radiology: Practice Guideline for the Performance of a Breast Ultrasound Examination. Reston, VA, American College of Radiology, 2002.
12. Baker JA, Soo MS, Rosen EL: Artifacts and pitfalls in ultrasonographic imaging of the breast. AJR Am J Roentgenol 2001;176:1261-1266.
13. Bassett LW, Kimme-Smith C: Breast ultrasonography. AJR Am J Roentgenol 1991;156:449-455.
14. Kossoff G: Basic physics and imaging characteristics of ultrasound. World J Surg 2000;24:134-142.
15. Kremkau FW: Diagnostic Ultrasound: Principles, Instruments, and Exercises, 3rd ed. Philadelphia, WB Saunders, 1989, pp 147-174.
16. Scanlon KA: Ultrasonographic artifacts and their origins. AJR Am J Roentgenol 1991;156:1267-1272.
17. American College of Radiology: Breast Imaging Reporting and Data System (BI-RADS), 4th ed. Reston, VA, American College of Radiology, 2003.
18. Egan RL, Egan KL: Detection of breast carcinoma: Comparison of automated water-path whole-breast ultrasonography, mammography, and physical examination. AJR Am J Roentgenol 1984;143:493-497.
19. Hilton SV, Leopold GR, Olson LK, Willson SA: Real-time breast ultrasonography: Application in 300 consecutive patients. AJR Am J Roentgenol 1986;147:479-486.
20. Jellins J, Kossoff G, Reeve TS: Detection and classification of liquid-filled masses in the breast by gray scale echography. Radiology 1977;125:205-212.
21. Sickles EA, Filly RA, Callen PW: Benign breast lesions: Ultrasound detection and diagnosis. Radiology 1984;151:467-470.
22. Berg WA, Campassi CI, Ioffe OB: Cystic lesions of the breast: Ultrasonographic-pathologic correlation. Radiology 2003;227: 183-191
23. Kasumi F, Tanaka H: Diagnosis of intracystic tumors by ultrasound. In Jellins J, Kobayashi T (eds): Ultrasonic Examination of the Breast. New York, John Wiley & Sons, 1983, pp 283-291.
24. Omori LM, Hisa N, Ohkuma K, et al: Breast masses with mixed cystic-solid ultrasonographic appearance. J Clin Ultrasound 1993;21:489-495.
25. Reuter K, D'Orsi CJ, Reale F: Intracystic carcinoma of the breast: The role of ultrasonography. Radiology 1984;153:233, 234.
26. Kopans DB: What is a useful adjunct to mammography? Radiology 1986;161:560, 561.
27. Cole-Beuglet C, Soriano RZ, Kurtz AB, Goldberg BB: Fibroadenoma of the breast: Ultrasonomammography correlated with pathology in 122 patients. AJR Am J Roentgenol 1983;140: 369-375.
28. Cole-Beuglet C, Soriano RZ, Kurtz AB, Goldberg BB: Ultrasound analysis of 104 primary breast carcinomas classified according to histopathologic type. Radiology 1983;147:191-196.
29. Egan RL, Egan KL: Automated water-path full-breast ultrasonography: Correlation with histology in 176 solid lesions. AJR Am J Roentgenol 1984;143:499-507.
30. Bassett LW, Kimme-Smith C, Sutherland LK, et al: Automated and hand-held breast US: Effect on patient management. Radiology 1987;165:103-108.
31. Cosmacini P, Veronesi P, Galimberti V, et al: Ultrasonographic evaluation of palpable breast masses: Analysis of 134 cases. Tumori 1990;76:495-498.
32. Croll J, Kotevich J, Tabrett M: The diagnosis of benign disease and the exclusion of malignancy in patients with breast symptoms. Semin Ultrasound CT MR 1982;3:38-50.
33. Dempsey PJ: The importance of resolution in the clinical application of breast ultrasonography. Ultrasound Med Biol 1988;14(suppl 1):43-48.

34. Dempsey PJ, Moskowitz M: Is there a role for breast ultrasonography? In McGahan JP (ed): Controversies in Ultrasound. New York, Churchill Livingstone, 1987, pp 17-36.
35. Durfee SM, Selland D-L, Smith DN, et al: Ultrasonographic evaluation of clinically palpable breast cancers invisible on mammography. Breast J 2000;6:247-251.
36. Frazier TG, Cole-Beuglet C, Kurtz AB, et al: Further evaluation by ultrasound of mammographically determined breast dysplasia. J Surg Oncol 1982;19:69, 70.
37. Guyer PB: Direct-contact B-scan ultrasonomammography—an aid to x-ray mammography. Ultrasound Med Biol 1988;14:49-52.
38. Kopans DB, Meyer JE, Lindfors KK: Whole-breast US imaging: Four-year follow-up. Radiology 1985;157:505-507.
39. Moy L, Slanetz PJ, Moore R, et al: Specificity of mammography and ultrasound in the evaluation of a palpable abnormality: Retrospective review. Radiology 2002;225:176-181.
40. Sickles EA, Filly RA, Callen PW: Breast cancer detection with ultrasonography and mammography: Comparison using state-of-the-art equipment. AJR AM J Roentgenol 1983;140:843-845.
41. Vilaro MM, Kurtz AB, Needleman L, et al: Hand-held and automated ultrasonomammography: Clinical role relative to x-ray mammography. J Ultrasound Med 1989; 8:95-100.
42. Pamilo M, Soiva M, Anttinen I, et al: Ultrasonography of breast lesions detected in mammography screening. Acta Radiol 1991;32:220-225.
43. Dennis MA, Parker SH, Klaus AJ, et al: Breast biopsy avoidance: The value of normal mammograms and normal ultrasonograms in the setting of a palpable lump. Radiology 2001;219: 186-191.
44. Soo MS, Rosen EL, Baker JA, et al: Negative predictive value of ultrasonography with mammography in patients with palpable breast lesions. AJR Am J Roentgenol 2001;177:1167-1170.
45. Shetty MK, Shah YP: Prospective evaluation of the value of negative ultrasonographic and mammographic findings in patients with palpable abnormalities of the breast. J Ultrasound Med 2002;21:1211-1216.
46. Kopans DB: Pathologic, mammographic, and ultrasonographic correlation. In Kopans DB: Breast Imaging, 2nd ed. Philadelphia, Lippincott-Raven, 1997, pp 511-615.
46a. Kopans DB: Negative mammographic and US findings do not help exclude breast cancer. Radiology 2002;222:857-858.
47. Bassett LW, Ysrael M, Gold RH, Ysrael C: Usefulness of mammography and ultrasonography in women less than 35 years of age. Radiology 1991;180:831-835.
48. Feig SA: The role of ultrasound in a breast imaging center. Semin Ultrasound CT MR 1989;10:90-105.
49. Harris VJ, Jackson VP: Indications for breast imaging in women under age 35 years. Radiology 1989;172:445-448.
50. Shaw de Paredes E, Marsteller LP, Eden BV: Breast cancers in women 35 years of age and younger: Mammographic findings. Radiology 1991;177:117-119.
51. Williams SM, Kaplan PA, Petersen JC, Lieberman RP: Mammography in women under age 30: Is there clinical benefit? Radiology 1986;161:49-51.
52. Shetty MK, Watson AB: Ultrasonographic evaluation of focal asymmetric density of the breast. Ultrasound Q 2002;18:115-121.
53. Ciatto S, Catarzi S, Morrone D, Del Turco MR: Fine-needle aspiration cytology of nonpalpable breast lesions: US versus stereotaxic guidance. Radiology 1993;188:195-198.
54. D'Orsi CJ, Mendelson EB: Interventional breast ultrasonography. Semin Ultrasound CT MR 1989;10:132-138.
55. Fornage BD: Percutaneous biopsies of the breast: State of the art. Cardiovasc Intervent Radiol 1991;14:29-39.
56. Fornage BD, Coan JD, David SL: Ultrasound-guided needle biopsy of the breast and other interventional procedures. Radiol Clin North Am 1992;30:167-185.
57. Fornage BD, Faroux MJ, Simatos A: Breast masses: US-guided fine-needle aspiration biopsy. Radiology 1987;162:409-414.
58. Fornage BD, Sneige N, Faroux MJ, Andry E: Ultrasonographic appearance and ultrasound guided fine-needle aspiration biopsy of breast carcinomas smaller than 1 cm^3. J Ultrasound Med 1990;9:559-568.
59. Gordon PB, Goldenberg SL, Chan NHL: Solid breast lesions: Diagnosis with US-guided fine-needle aspiration biopsy. Radiology 1993;189:573-580.
60. Kopans DB, Meyer JE, Lindfors KK, Bucchianeri SS: Breast ultrasonography to guide cyst aspiration and wire localization of occult solid lesions. AJR Am J Roentgenol 1984;143:489-492.
61. Parker SH, Jobe WE, Dennis MA, et al: US-guided automated large-core breast biopsy. Radiology 1993;187:507-511.
62. Rifkin MD, Schwartz GF, Pasto ME, et al: Ultrasound for guidance of breast mass removal. J Ultrasound Med 1988;7:261-263.
63. Rissanen TJ, Makarainen HP, Kiviniemi HO, Suramo II: Ultrasonographically guided wire localization of nonpalpable breast lesions. J Ultrasound Med 1994;13:183-188.
64. Heywang SH, Dunner PS, Lipsit ER, Glassman LM: Advantages and pitfalls of ultrasound in the diagnosis of breast cancer. J Clin Ultrasound 1985;13:525-532.
65. Heywang SH, Lipsit ER, Glassman LM, Thomas MA: Specificity of ultrasonography in the diagnosis of benign breast masses. J Ultrasound Med 1984;3:453-461.
66. Jackson VP, Rothschild PA, Kreipke DL, et al: The spectrum of ultrasonographic findings of fibroadenoma of the breast. Invest Radiol 1986;21:34-40.
66a. Kopans DB, Meyer JE, Steinbock RT: Breast cancer: The appearance as delineated by whole breast water-path ultrasound scanning. J Clin Ultrasound 1982;10:313-322.
67. Rahbar G, Sie AC, Hansen GC, et al: Benign versus malignant solid breast masses: US differentiation. Radiology 1999;213: 889-894.
68. Arger PH, Sehgal CM, Conant EF, et al: Interreader variability and predictive value of US descriptions of solid breast masses: Pilot study. Acad Radiol 2001;8:335-342.
69. Baker JA, Kornguth PJ, Soo MS, et al: Ultrasonography of solid breast lesions: Observer variability of lesion description and assessment. AJR Am J Roentgenol 1999;172:1621-1625.
70. Adler DD, Hyde DL, Ikeda DM: Quantitative ultrasonographic parameters as a means of distinguishing breast cancers from benign solid masses. J Ultrasound Med 1991;10:505-508.
71. Fornage BD, Lorigan JG, Andry E: Fibroadenoma of the breast: Ultrasonographic appearance. Radiology 1989;172:671-675.
72. Nishimura S, Matsusue S, Koizumi S, Kashihara S: Size of breast cancer on ultrasonography, cut surface of resected specimen, and palpation. Ultrasound Med Biol 1988;14(suppl 1):139-142.
73. Golub RM, Parsons RE, Sigel B, et al: Differentiation of breast tumors by ultrasonic tissue characterization. J Ultrasound Med 1993;12:601-608.
74. Burns PN, Halliwell M, Wells PNT, Webb AJ: Ultrasonic Doppler studies of the breast. Ultrasound Med Biol 1982;8: 127-143.
75. Halliwell M, Burns PN, Wells PNT: An ultrasonic duplex breast scanner. Ultrasound Med Biol 1982; 8(Suppl 1):72.
76. Jellins J, Kossoff G, Gill RW, Reeve TS: Combined B-mode and Doppler examination of the breast. Ultrasound Med Biol 1982; 8(Suppl 1):89.
76a. Jellins J, Reeve TS, Croll J, Kossoff G: Results of breast echographic examinations in Sydney, Australia, 1972-1979. Semin Ultrasound CT MR 1982;3:58-62.
77. Minasian H, Bamber JC: A preliminary assessment of an ultrasonic Doppler method for the study of blood flow in human breast cancer. Ultrasound Med Biol 1982;8:357-364.
78. Wells PNT, Halliwell M, Skidmore R, et al: Tumour detection by ultrasonic Doppler blood-flow signals. Ultrasonics 1977;15: 231, 232.
79. White DN, Cledgett PR: Breast carcinoma detection by ultrasonic Doppler signals. Ultrasound Med Biol 1978;4:329-335.
80. Cosgrove DO, Bamber JC, Davey JB, et al: Color Doppler signals from breast tumors. Work in progress. Radiology 1990; 176:175-180.
81. Cosgrove DO, Kedar BP, Bamber JC, et al: Breast diseases: Color Doppler US in differential diagnosis. Radiology 1993;189:99-104.
82. McNicholas MMJ, Mercer PM, Miller JC, et al: Color Doppler ultrasonography in the evaluation of palpable breast masses. AJR Am J Roentgenol 1993; 61:765-771.

83. Giuseppetti GM, Rizzatto G, Gozzi G, Ercolani P: Ruolo dell'ectomografia nella diagnosi del carcinoma infraclinico della mammella. Radiol Med 1989;78:339-342.
84. Smallwood JA, Guyer P, Dewbury K, et al: The accuracy of ultrasound in the diagnosis of breast disease. Ann R Coll Surg Engl 1986;68:19-22.
85. van Dam PA, Van Goethem MLA, Kersschot E, et al: Palpable solid breast masses: Retrospective single- and multimodality evaluation of 201 lesions. Radiology 1988;166:435-439.
86. Fung HM, Jackson FI: Clinically and mammographically occult breast lesions demonstrated by ultrasound. J R Soc Med 1990;83:696-698.
87. Berg WA, Gilbreath PL: Multicentric and multifocal cancer: Whole-breast US in preoperative evaluation. Radiology 2000; 214:59-66.
88. Buchberger W, DeKoekkoek-Doll P, Springer P, et al: Incidental findings on ultrasonography of the breast: Clinical significance and diagnostic workup. AJR Am J Roentgenol 1999;173: 921-927.
89. Cilotti A, Bagnolesi P, Moretti M, et al: Comparison of the diagnostic performance of high-frequency ultrasound as a first- or second-line diagnostic tool in non-palpable lesions of the breast. Eur Radiol 1997;7:1240-1244.
90. Gordon PB, Goldenberg SL: Malignant breast masses detected only by ultrasound. A retrospective review. Cancer 1995;76: 626-630.
91. Kaplan SS: Clinical utility of bilateral whole-breast US in the evaluation of women with dense breast tissue. Radiology 2001;221:641-649.
92. Kolb TM, Lichy J, Newhouse JH: Occult cancer in women with dense breasts: Detection with screening US—diagnostic yield and tumor characteristics. Radiology 1998;207:191-199.
93. Kolb TM, Lichy J, Newhouse JH: Comparison of the performance of screening mammography, physical examination, and breast US and evaluation of factors that influence them: An analysis of 27,825 patient evaluations. Radiology 2002;225: 165-175.
94. Leconte I, Feger C, Galant C, et al: Mammography and subsequent whole-breast ultrasonography of nonpalpable breast cancers: The importance of radiologic breast density. AJR Am J Roentgenol 2003;180:1675-1679.
95. Moon WK, Noh D-Y, Im J-G: Multifocal, multicentric, and contralateral breast cancers: Bilateral whole-breast US in the preoperative evaluation of patients. Radiology 2002;224:569-576.
96. Kopans DB: Effectiveness of US breast cancer screening remains to be demonstrated. Radiology 2003;227:606.
97. Berg WA: Rationale for a trial of screening breast ultrasound: American College of Radiology Imaging Network (ACRIN) 6666. AJR Am J Roentgenol 2003;180:1225-1228.

Chapter 13 Digital Mammography, CAD, and Other Digital Applications

Stephen A. Feig and Martin J. Yaffe

Film-screen mammography is an effective tool for the detection and diagnosis of breast cancer. Several limitations of current mammographic technology have been identified, and good evidence now exists that improved image quality and reduced radiation dose can be achieved if mammograms are acquired directly in digital form. In this chapter, the rationale for digital mammography is presented, and various approaches to the design of a digital mammography system are described. Current challenges in achieving a practical, clinically acceptable digital mammography system are discussed, and applications of digital mammography to computer-aided detection, telemammography, and quantitative imaging are suggested.

There is good evidence that early detection of breast cancer can reduce mortality from the disease (see Chapter 23). Film-screen x-ray mammography has been shown to have greater sensitivity and specificity for detection of breast tumors than any other noninvasive diagnostic technique currently available. Over the past few decades, many improvements have been made in the mammographic x-ray unit, the film-screen image receptor, film processing, and the radiographic technique used for mammography (see also Chapters 1-3).[1] Nevertheless, several technical factors limit the ability of mammography to display the finest or most subtle details while at the same time producing images with the most efficient use of the radiation dose to the patient.[2,3] A mammographic imaging system that acquires mammograms directly in digital form effectively overcomes these limitations and may improve the performance of mammography.

LIMITATIONS OF CONVENTIONAL MAMMOGRAPHY

In film-screen mammography, the film must act as an image acquisition detector as well as a storage and display device. It performs very well in providing excellent spatial resolution of high-contrast structures and is an efficient medium for long-term storage of image data. However, as in any situation in which several jobs must be done simultaneously, certain compromises result; they are discussed here.

Contrast and Latitude

Breast tumors, microcalcifications, and architectural distortions are visualized in the mammogram because of differences in x-ray attenuation between these structures and normal breast tissue. The overall displayed contrast of structures on the mammogram results as a combination of this "attenuation contrast" and the photographic (optical density) gradient of the mammographic film.

Figure 13–1 shows measured x-ray attenuation coefficients of fibroglandular breast tissue, fat, and breast carcinoma versus x-ray energy.[4] The very small differences between these curves illustrate why mammography is such a challenging imaging task, particularly when the tumor is surrounded by fibroglandular tissue.[5] As shown in Figure 13–2, attenuation contrast decreases rapidly with increasing x-ray energy. To maximize attenuation contrast, mammography is conventionally carried out with low-energy x-ray spectra, typically with the use of a molybdenum anode x-ray tube operated at a potential of approximately 26 kilovolt peak (kVp), with additional molybdenum beam filtration. The breast attenuates x-rays very strongly at these energies; therefore, so that adequate signal is obtained from the image receptor at a relatively high dose compared with that for general radiography, 1 to 2.5 milligray mean glandular dose per image is received by the breast.

The display contrast properties of the radiographic film are described by the slope or gradient of its characteristic curve (Fig. 13–3). Because of the sigmoidal shape of the characteristic curve, the range of x-ray exposures over which the film display gradient is significant, or the *image latitude*, is limited to a factor of about 25. This may be a problem, because the maximum range of transmitted exposures can be 100:1 or more, depending on the thickness and composition of the breast. For a tumor located in either a relatively radiolucent or a relatively opaque region of the breast, even though adequate attenuation contrast is provided by the x-ray beam, the final contrast displayed to the radiologist may be severely reduced because of the limited gradient of the film. This is particularly a concern in patients with dense breasts.

Noise

All radiologic images contain random fluctuation or noise owing to the statistics of x-ray quantum absorption. This noise can limit the reliability of detection of small or subtle structures. In addition, other sources of noise, such as those resulting from the structure of the fluorescent screen and the granularity of the film emulsion used to record the image, compound this problem.[2] An ideal imaging system

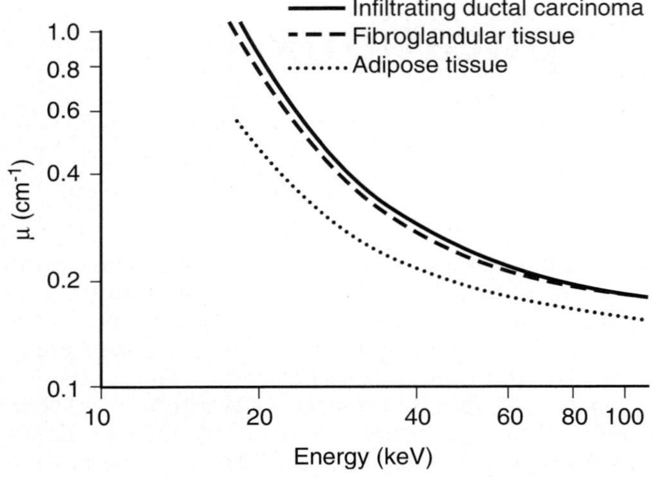

Figure 13–1. Measured x-ray linear attenuation coefficients of unfixed samples of fibroglandular and adipose breast tissue and infiltrating ductal carcinoma of the breast, plotted versus x-ray energy in kiloelectron volts.

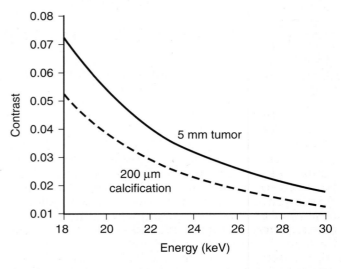

Figure 13–2. Dependence of attenuation contrast on x-ray energy. Calculation is for a 5-millimeter-diameter infiltrating ductal carcinoma and a 0.2-mm calcification in a 5-cm-thick breast composed of 50% adipose and 50% fibroglandular tissue.

would be "quantum-limited," meaning that x-ray quantum noise is the dominant source of random fluctuation. Generally, existing mammographic film-screen systems are not quantum limited, and particularly for fine structures, noise in the imaging system is dominated by fluctuation associated with the imaging system.

An imaging system can be made quantum limited through reduction of intrinsic noise sources and the use of more x-rays to form the image. For a fixed-system speed, the latter is best accomplished through an increase in the x-ray interaction efficiency of the screen, which is typically only 60%. When a system is quantum limited, further reduction in noise requires an increase in the number of x-rays incident on the imaging system—that is, an increase in patient dose. With film, such an increase could cause diagnostically important information to be shifted

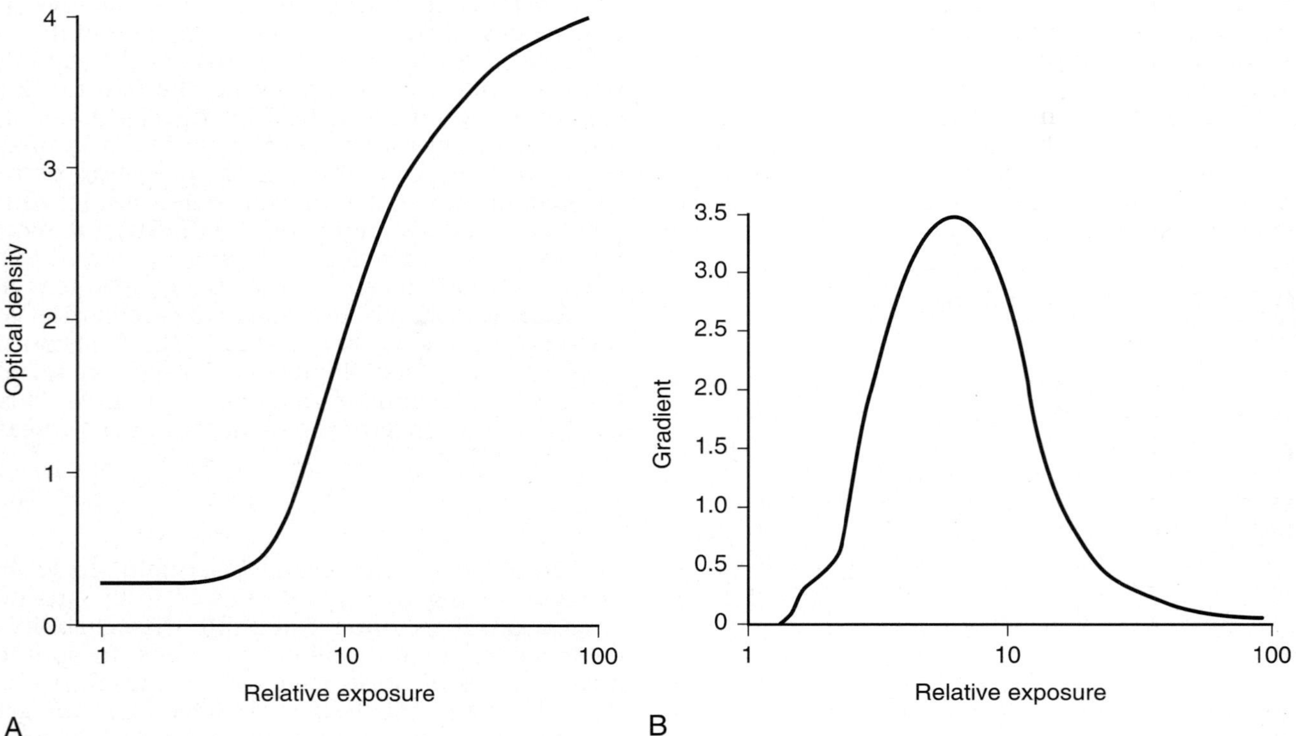

Figure 13–3. **A,** Characteristic (Hurter and Driffield [H & D]) curve of a mammographic film-screen image receptor. **B,** Slope of the characteristic curve gives the gradient, which describes the amount of contrast amplification (or attenuation) provided by the film.

to a region of the characteristic curve where the gradient is less (see Fig. 13–3B), thereby diminishing contrast. To avoid such a loss of contrast, it might be necessary to accompany the exposure increase with the use of a less sensitive film.

Compromise between Resolution and Efficiency

Another key limitation of film-screen mammography is the tradeoff between spatial resolution and detector x-ray interaction (detection) efficiency. When a fluorescent screen is used with film, spatial resolution is limited by blur due to diffusion of light in the screen. Screen blur worsens as the thickness of the screen is increased. For high resolution, mammographic screens must be kept relatively thin, resulting in suboptimal x-ray detection efficiency and higher radiation dose.

Inefficiency of Scatter Rejection

Even at the low x-ray energies used in mammography, Compton x-ray scattering is an important process of interaction between the x-ray beam and the breast. The magnitude of singly and multiply scattered x-ray quanta impinging on the imaging system is generally comparable to the intensity of directly transmitted primary radiation.[6] By adding a "uniform," noisy background to the image, detection of scattered quanta reduces image contrast, signal-to-noise ratio (SNR), and the dynamic range available for recording useful information.

Modern mammography is performed with a specially designed radiographic grid that discriminates geometrically against scattered radiation. Although the scattered radiation does not carry useful information, it does contribute to achieving the required optical density on the film. The loss of this scattered radiation and inefficiencies of the grid in transmitting the desired primary radiation to the screen necessitate a higher radiation dose to the patient. Typically, this increase is a factor of 2 to 3 compared with the dose from imaging without a grid.[6]

BINARY NUMBERS

Imaging systems such as digital mammography that depend on computers to process and store images use binary numbers rather than decimal numbers (Table 13–1). Digits in a decimal system can assume 1 of 10 values. However, when a computer fills in a position in a binary number (bit), it has a choice of only two values, 0 and 1. A bit may be considered similar to a light switch, which can be either on or off. Functionally, a bit may represent a transistor in a computer memory or the state of magnetization of a microscopic portion on a magnetic disk or tape.

Digits in a decimal system express multiples of the base 10. Thus, the value in each successive place in a digital number increases by a factor of 10 (i.e., 1, 10, 100, 1000). Because bits in a binary system express multiples of the base 2, the value of each successive place to the left increases by a factor of 2 (i.e., 1, 2, 4, 8, 16).

Table 13–1. Comparison of Decimal and Binary Numbers and Values

Decimal System				
Place number	3	2	1	0
10 possible decimal digit entries (0–9) for each place	9	9	9	9
	8	8	8	8
	7	7	7	7
	6	6	6	6
	5	5	5	5
	4	4	4	4
	3	3	3	3
	2	2	2	2
	1	1	1	1
	0	0	0	0
Decimal digit value = decimal digit entry ×	10^3	10^2	10^1	10^0
	maximum value for four-place decimal number = 9999			
Binary System				
Place number	3	2	1	0
Two possible binary digit (bit) entries (0 or 1) for each place	1	1	1	1
	0	0	0	0
Binary digit values = binary digit ×	2^3	2^2	2^1	2^0
	8 +	4 +	2 +	1 = 15
	or	or	or	or
	0 +	0 +	0 +	0 = 0
	maximum value for a four-place binary number = 15			

Because binary numbers can represent many fewer values than decimal numbers of the same number of digits, and because computers must process and store vast amounts of information, the capacity of a computer memory or storage device is usually described in terms of kilobytes (KB), megabytes (MB), gigabytes (GB), and terabytes (TB) (Table 13–2). Examples of the first nine corresponding decimal and binary numbers along with their bit values are shown in Table 13–3.

DIGITAL VERSUS ANALOG IMAGES

The limitations of film mammography discussed here arise from the film and screen (e.g., restricted latitude and display contrast, low quantum detection efficiency, and noise) and from the image acquisition geometry (e.g., inefficiency of scatter rejection). Many of these limitations can be effectively

Table 13–2. Binary Storage Capacity Units

Kilobyte = 2^{10} bytes = 1024 bytes or approximately 1000 bytes
Megabyte = 2^{20} bytes = 1024 kilobytes or approximately 1 million bytes
Gigabyte = 2^{30} bytes = 1024 megabytes or approximately 1 billion bytes
Byte = 8 bits

Table 13–3. Representation of Numbers in Decimal and Binary Systems and Bit Value

Decimal	Binary	Bit Value
0	0	0
1	1	1
2	10	0 + 2 + 0
3	11	0 + 2 + 1
4	100	4 + 0 + 0
5	101	4 + 0 + 1
6	110	4 + 2 + 0
7	111	4 + 2 + 1
8	1000	8 + 0 + 0 + 0

overcome with a digital mammography imaging system in which image acquisition, display, and storage are performed independently, allowing optimization of each.

The major differences between digital and analog images are illustrated in Figure 13–4. The analog image is a more or less continuous representation of the spatial and intensity variations of the x-ray pattern transmitted by the patient (Fig. 13–4A), whereas the digital image is obtained by "sampling" of the x-ray pattern at discrete increments of spatial position and image signal intensity (Fig. 13–4B). Spatially, the digital image is formed as a two-dimensional matrix of (usually) square picture elements (pixels) of a fixed size (Fig. 13–4C), typically 0.05 to 0.1 mm on a side. Within each pixel, the image takes on a single value representing the signal strength or "brightness" of the image, averaged over the area represented by that pixel.

Both pixel size and the potential spatial resolution supported by that pixel size can be easily calculated if the dimensions of the image field and the number of pixels across the image are known: pixel size dimension of image field divided by number of pixels along that dimension. For example, the pixel size of the digital image shown in Fig. 13–4C is:

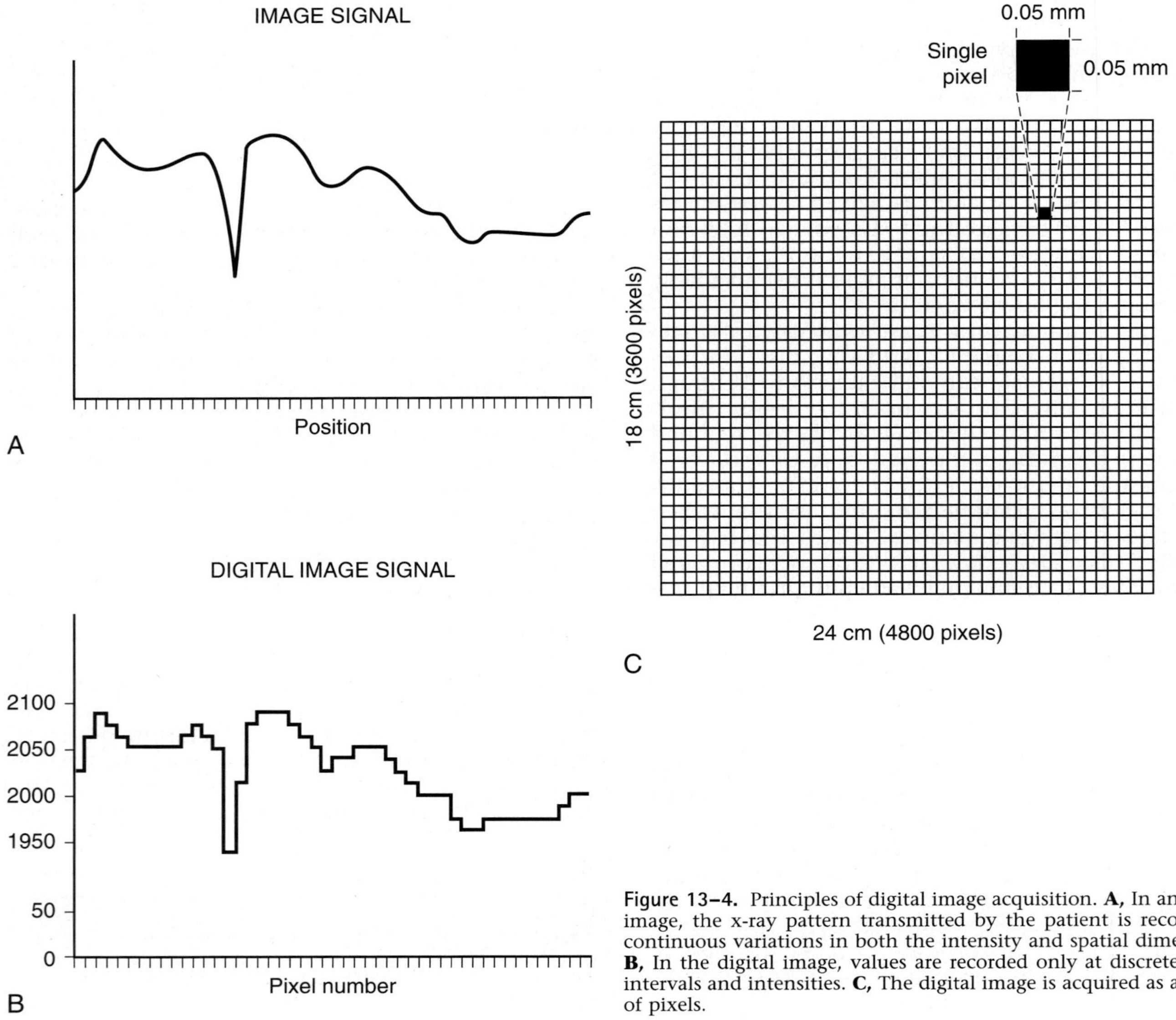

Figure 13–4. Principles of digital image acquisition. **A,** In an analog image, the x-ray pattern transmitted by the patient is recorded as continuous variations in both the intensity and spatial dimensions. **B,** In the digital image, values are recorded only at discrete spatial intervals and intensities. **C,** The digital image is acquired as a matrix of pixels.

$$\frac{18 \text{ cm}}{3600} \text{ or } \frac{24 \text{ cm}}{4800} = 0.05$$

Spatial resolution of an imaging system may be measured in terms of line-pairs per millimeter (lp/mm). A line-pair target consists of a series of progressively narrower lines (highly attenuating, such as provided by lead) and spaces (radiolucent). Within each member of a series, the line and space have equal width. For example, 10 lp/mm means that there are 10 lead strips per millimeter, each 0.05 mm wide, and 10 spaces per millimeter, each 0.05 mm wide. The spatial resolution of an imaging system can be evaluated from the number of line-pairs per millimeter that can be clearly seen on a radiograph. Because a line and a space must be represented by at least two pixels, then the number of line-pairs per millimeter that an imaging system can provide can be no greater than the number of pixel pairs/mm (i.e., 1 divided by pixel size × 2). For the digital image shown in Figure 13–4C, the maximum spatial resolution in line-pairs/mm can be no greater than $1/(0.05 \times 2) = 1/0.1 = 10$ lp/mm. It should be noted that other factors, such as the size of the x-ray focal spot, light blur in phosphors, and patient motion, may reduce the spatial resolution below this level.

The term *matrix size* refers to the number of pixels in a matrix rather than the physical dimensions of a matrix. For an image field of a given size, a larger matrix field provides a less "blocky" image with higher resolution. The numeric value of each pixel determines its shade of gray (Fig. 13–5). The number of bits available to describe the gray level of a pixel is referred to as the *bit depth*. Matrices with a greater bit depth are capable of displaying more shades of gray. The total number of bytes required to store an image depends on matrix size and bit depth. For example, a 1024 × 1024 digital image with a bit depth of 8 (1 byte) requires 1024 × 1024 × 8 = 8,388,608 bits, or 8 Mbit (1 MB). Because of the way computers are designed, numbers are represented by an integral number of bytes. One byte provides only 256 signal levels, which is inadequate for digital mammography; typically between 10 and 14 bits of digitization are used. In each case, however, the resultant number for each pixel occupies 2 bytes in computer memory. For an image with matrix size 1900 × 2300, there are 4,370,000 pixels, occupying 8.74 MB.

Because the number of shades of gray that can be displayed in a single pixel represents an exponential function of bit depth, doubling the bit depth much more than doubles the largest number of shades of gray that can be displayed. For example, if 4 bits can display 15 ($2^4 - 1$) shades of gray, then 8 bits can display 255 ($2^8 - 1$) shades of gray.

In a digital imager (Fig. 13–6), a detector absorbs the x-rays and produces an electronic signal for each pixel, which is translated into a digital value by a solid-state device known as an analog-to-digital converter (ADC). These numbers are then transmitted to a memory buffer. The intensity representing the x-ray pattern is measured as one of a finite set of "gray levels" (see Fig. 13–5B).

Once the digital image is stored in computer memory, it can be displayed with contrast independent of the detector properties and can be defined by the needs of the radiologist. This feature allows considerable flexibility and is one of the main benefits of digital mammography.

REQUIREMENTS FOR A DIGITAL MAMMOGRAPHY SYSTEM

Spatial Considerations

The pixel size must be adequately small if fine detail in the breast is to be depicted accurately. If the pixels are too large, then the borders of structures will be jagged and poorly defined. Under these circumstances, although the *presence* of microcalcifications might be evident, *details* of their shapes and edge structures might be inadequate. An example of the effect of pixel size on image quality is given in Figure 13–7.

The limiting resolution of the film-screen image receptor for mammography is on the order of 20 lp/mm. To provide this level of resolution, a digital system would have pixels spaced no further apart than 25 μm. This implies, for the large image receptor, a matrix of 9600 × 12000 pixels! It is not currently feasible to acquire or display digital images

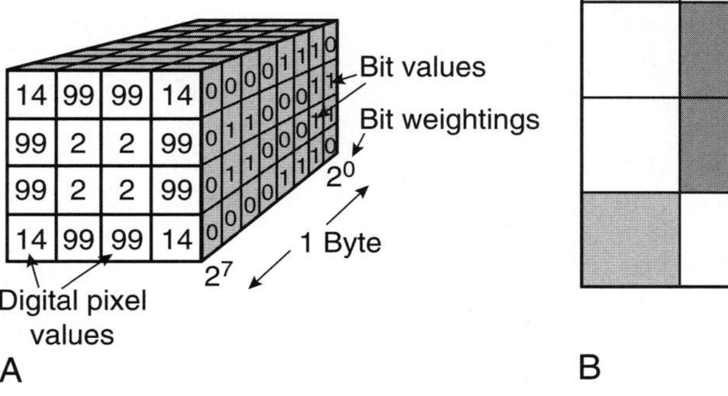

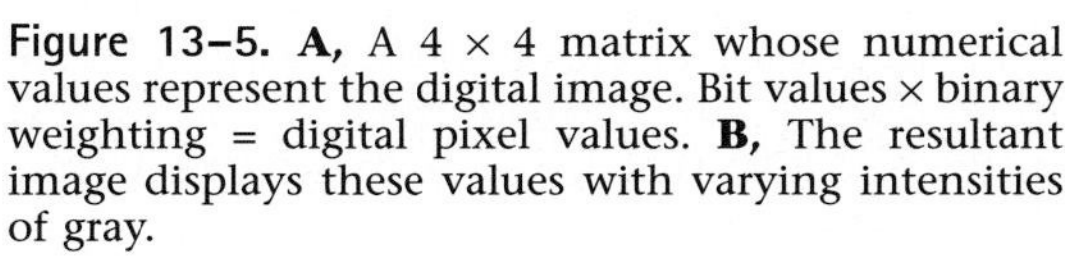
Figure 13–5. A, A 4 × 4 matrix whose numerical values represent the digital image. Bit values × binary weighting = digital pixel values. **B,** The resultant image displays these values with varying intensities of gray.

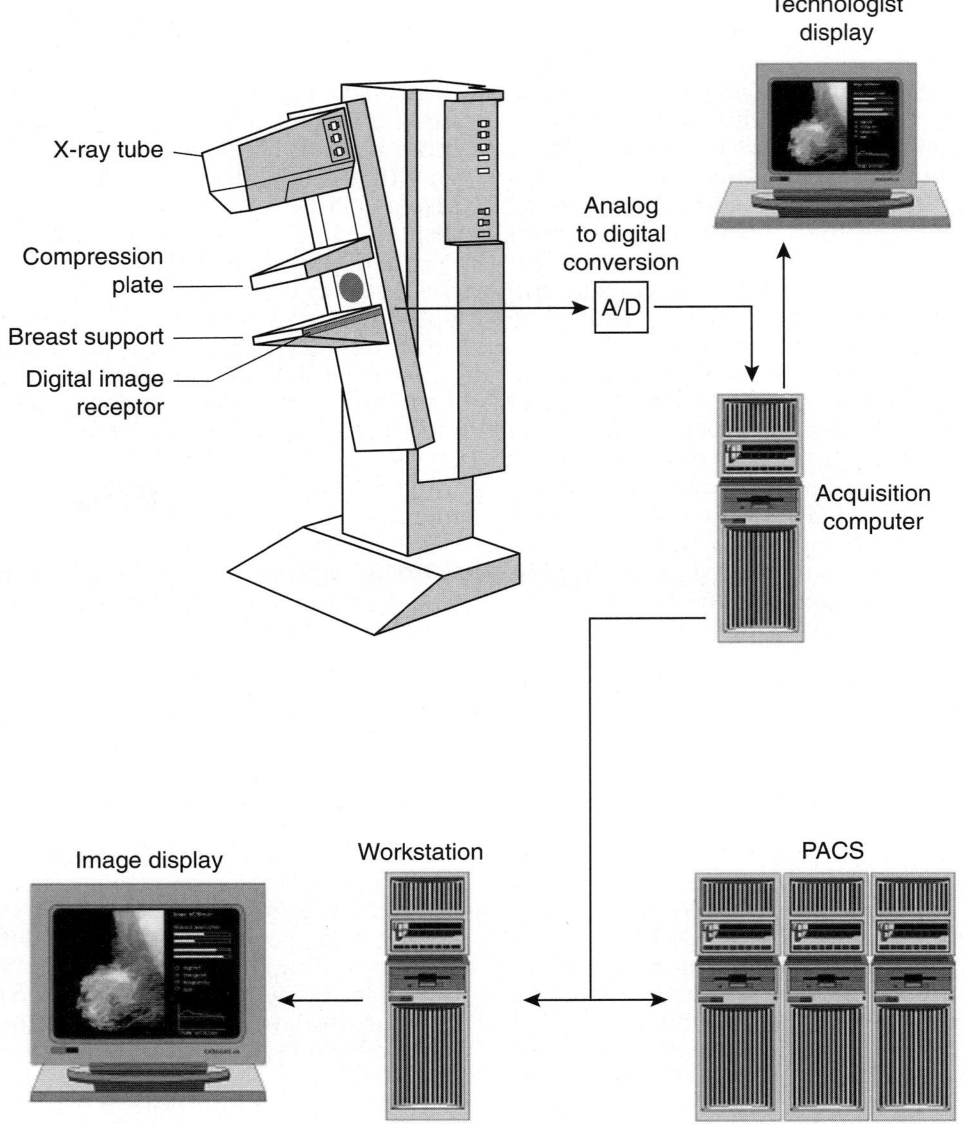

Figure 13–6. Schematic diagram of a digital mammography system. PACS, picture archiving and communications system.

of the entire breast with such resolution. To determine whether digital mammography with larger pixel sizes, say 50 μm, would be suitable for breast imaging, one must consider the issue of resolution more closely and link it to considerations of contrast and noise. Limiting spatial resolution is measured using test objects of nearly 100% contrast, objects that do not exist in the breast. For the low-contrast objects found in the breast, detectability may be limited not by spatial resolution but also by lack of displayed contrast or by insufficient SNR; therefore the limiting spatial resolution is certainly not the only parameter determining image quality and, in many cases, may not be the most important parameter.

Evidence that digital mammography, even with a modest limiting resolution of less than 10 lp/mm, may improve lesion detectability is illustrated in Figure 13–8, which compares images of a contrast-detail test pattern containing disks of varying diameter and subject contrast. The images were obtained on a digital mammography system with 100-μm pixels and on a state-of-the-art mammography film-screen system. Even though the digital system has a lower limiting resolution, it can provide superior detectability, not only of large, low-contrast disks but also of submillimeter disks of moderate contrast. The pixel size, matrix size, and limiting spatial resolution of the digital mammography systems that either are in routine clinical use or are being evaluated are shown in Table 13–4. It has been suggested that although adequate detection of structures may be achieved at 100 μm, smaller pixel sizes are probably required for the determination of the shape of these structures, often an important feature in the diagnosis of microcalcifications.[7] The actual spatial resolution requirements for digital mammography are still not known definitively and will be determined only in careful future experimental studies or possibly through comparison of the

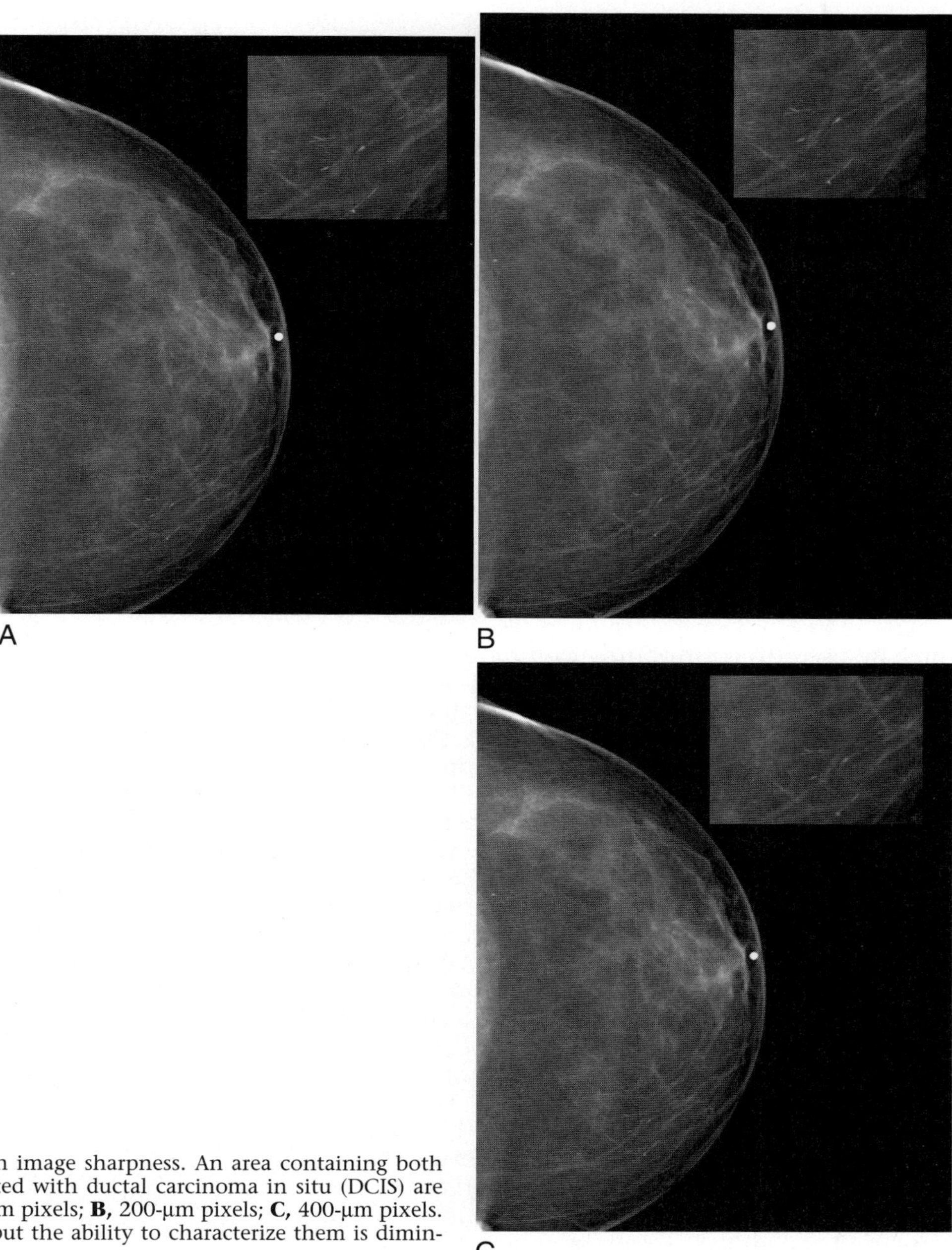

Figure 13–7. The effect of pixel size on image sharpness. An area containing both benign calcifications and those associated with ductal carcinoma in situ (DCIS) are shown magnified in the *insets*. **A,** 100-μm pixels; **B,** 200-μm pixels; **C,** 400-μm pixels. Calcifications can be seen in all cases, but the ability to characterize them is diminished with increased pixel size.

clinical performance of commercial systems that provide different levels of spatial resolution.

Number of Bits of Digitization

In Figure 13–4B, the number of levels required to represent signal intensity relates to the subtlety of changes in x-ray transmission that must be displayed and to the range of x-ray transmission that is present behind different regions (highly dense versus lucent) in the breast. In turn, to justify use of a certain number of bits of digitization, both the intrinsic x-ray noise in the image and the noise associated with the detector and circuitry must be appropriately low. These requirements dictate the radiation dose that

Table 13–4. Basic Design Parameters of Current Digital Mammography Systems

Manufacturer	Detector Element Size (μm)	Matrix	Bit Depth	Technology	Grid?
GE	100	1.9K × 2.3K	14	CsI phosphor/a-Si	Yes
Fischer	50 (25)	4K × 5.6K	12	CsI phosphor/charged-coupled device	No
Fuji	50	4.7K × 6K	10 (log)	Photostimulable phosphor	Yes
Lorad/Hologic	70	3K × 4K	14	Amorphous selenium	Yes

a-Si, amorphous silicon; CsI, cesium iodide.

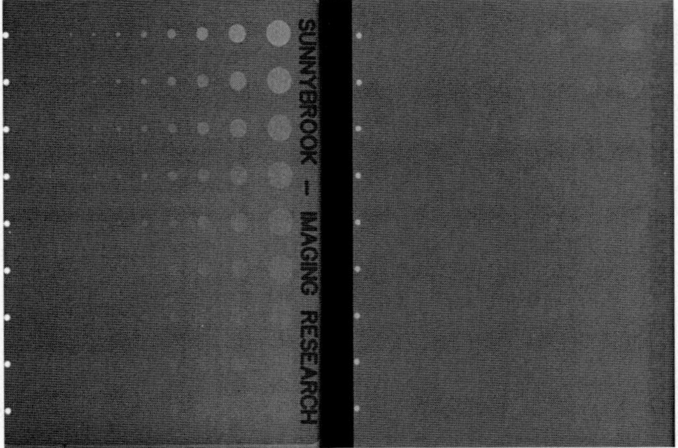

Figure 13–8. Comparison of contrast-detail performance of film-screen versus that of a prototype digital mammography system. **A,** Film image was obtained under standard conditions of 26 kVp with a molybdenum/molybdenum (Mo/Mo) spectrum. **B,** The digital image was acquired at 45 kVp with a tungsten target x-ray tube.

must be used (to control quantum mottle) as well as the quality of the system components. Use of too few gray levels causes information to be lost and gives the image a "terraced" appearance with artificial contrasts that may be disturbing to the radiologist (Fig. 13–9).

The number of gray levels with which transmission data should be digitized can be estimated by considering the exposure range that must be accommodated and the precision of digitization needed at the low end of that range. For a 5-cm-thick, compressed breast of average fat and fibroglandular composition, the attenuation factor at 25 kiloelectron volts (keV) is approximately 7.5. For a dense breast 8 cm in thickness, the attenuation factor is about 75. Assuming that a high enough radiation exposure is used to overcome quantum noise, detection of a lesion representing a 1% decrease in transmitted radiation (e.g., a 0.5-cm tumor) would require a detector whose exposure range capability was 750 for the average breast and 7500 for the dense breast. This calculation implies that digitization to between 12 and 13 bits is required if linear digitization is employed. If, alternatively, the logarithm of the image is calculated before digitization, the number of bits required may be able to be reduced to 10; however, logarithmic processing makes "flat-fielding" operations (discussed later) more difficult. For comparison, in computed tomography (CT) images, the raw data are usually stored to 16 bits (65,536 gray levels); in digital subtraction angiography (DSA), 10 bits, or 1024 levels, are used.

DIGITAL MAMMOGRAPHY SYSTEM DESIGNS

Detectors for digital mammography should have the following characteristics:

1. Efficient absorption of the incident radiation beam.
2. Linear (or logarithmic) response over a wide range of incident radiation intensity.
3. Low intrinsic noise.
4. Adequate spatial resolution (sample spacing at 50 to 100 μm).
5. Ability to accommodate a field size of *at least* 18 × 24 cm (and an approach to allow imaging of larger breasts).
6. Image receptor configuration that allows proper breast positioning technique.
7. Acceptable imaging time to avoid problems with patient motion and discomfort and excessive heat loading of the x-ray tube.

Acquisition of digital mammograms can be point-by point, line-by-line, multi-line, slot, or full-area. The first two approaches almost certainly require too long an image acquisition time to be practical. Systems of the other types have been developed and either are currently being used clinically or are under evaluation.

Area Detectors: Full Field

Conventional film-screen mammography images are obtained with a single, brief radiation exposure of an area detector. This approach is attractive for digital mammography, in that it is convenient, allows good throughput, and makes efficient use of the heat loading applied to the x-ray tube. To be acceptable for digital mammography, an area detector must possess an appropriate combination of spatial resolution, field coverage, and signal-to-noise performance. Some approaches to area detection and their strengths and weaknesses are described here.

Demagnification Cameras

A high-resolution x-ray detector can be produced by coupling an x-ray–absorbing phosphor with a smaller-area photodetector, such as a charge-coupled device (CCD) array via demagnifying lenses or fiberoptic tapers (Fig. 13–10). These CCDs are built on single silicon chips and typically cover only a field of less than 3 × 3 cm. The CCD output is then digitized to produce a high-resolution digital image.

This configuration has been used since 1992 for producing small-area (5 × 5-cm) digital images for guiding stereotactic breast biopsy. Such systems typically provide 1024 × 1024–pixel images with a pixel size of 50 or 100 μm.

It is not practical to extend this approach to full breast imaging by employing a larger phosphor surface and simply increasing the amount of optical demagnification, to a factor of about 8. Unfortunately, the collection of light then becomes very inefficient and causes image noise to be increased to unacceptable levels. One commercial system produced by Trex Medical (Danbury, Connecticut) was constructed as a mosaic of 12 (3 rows of 4)

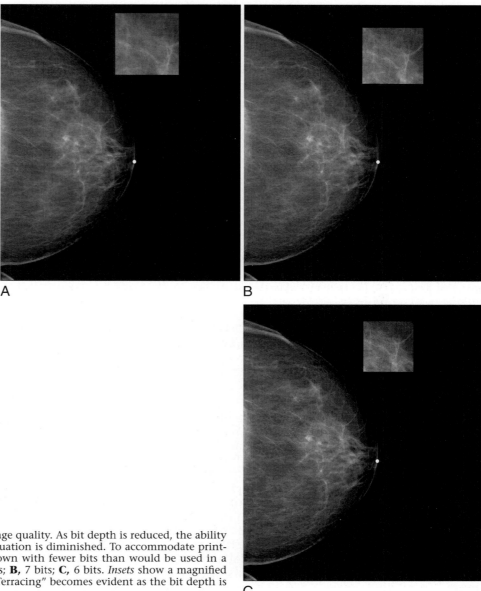

Figure 13–9. Effect of bit depth on image quality. As bit depth is reduced, the ability to depict subtle changes in tissue attenuation is diminished. To accommodate printing limitations, all images here are shown with fewer bits than would be used in a digital mammography system. **A,** 8 bits; **B,** 7 bits; **C,** 6 bits. *Insets* show a magnified area containing benign calcification. "Terracing" becomes evident as the bit depth is decreased.

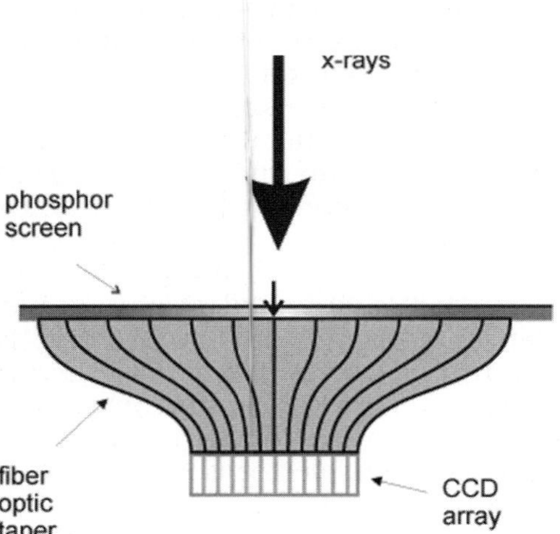

Figure 13–10. A small-format digital camera, in which an x-ray image produced by a phosphor is optically demagnified and coupled to a photodetector. Coupling can be by lenses or fiberoptics. These detectors are typically used in stereotactic biopsy guidance systems. CCD, charge-coupled device.

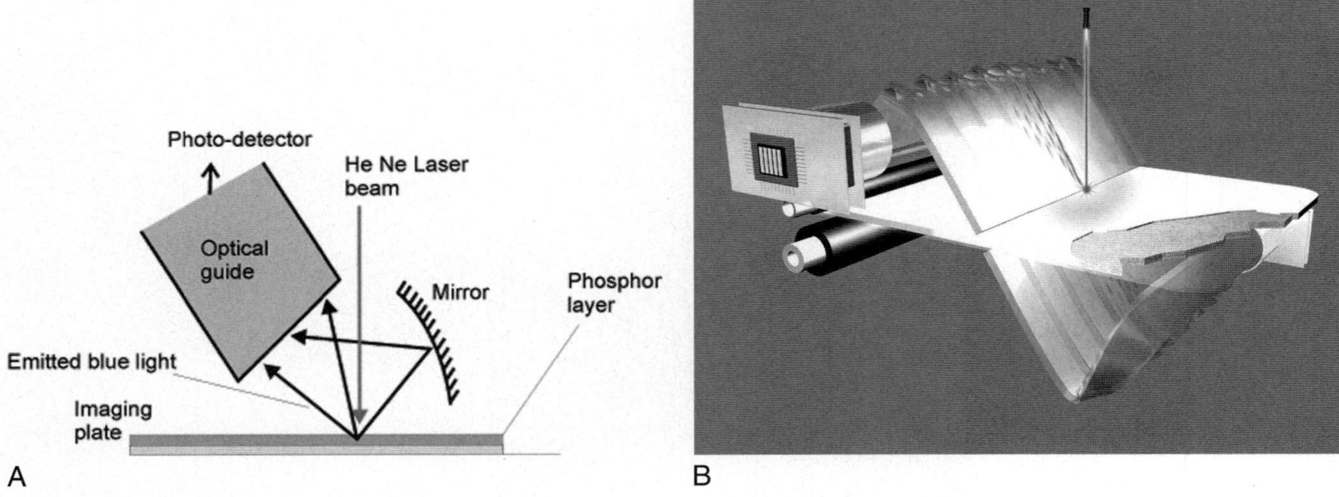

Figure 13–11. **A,** Photostimulable phosphor readout system. The emitted light is collected from the upper surface of the plate, measured, and digitized. **B,** Photostimulable phosphor plate in a dual-sided reader. (Courtesy Fuji Medical Systems.)

small-format detectors to cover the full breast. This system is no longer commercially available.

Photostimulable Phosphors

Photostimulable or storage phosphors have been successfully developed as an imaging system for general radiography, and it is possible to extract the information from such devices in digital form. Energy from absorbed x-rays causes electrons in the phosphor to be excited. Rather than decaying immediately to give off light, as would be the case in a normal phosphor, some of the electrons are captured and stored in "traps" in the phosphor crystals. The number of traps filled is proportional to the exposure received by the phosphor, and the spatial arrangement of these trapped electrons forms the latent image. The digital image is created in a reader by scanning of the phosphor plate with a finely focused red laser beam. This stimulation releases electrons from the traps, giving rise to emission of light of a shorter wavelength (blue), which is collected point by point as the laser scans over the plate.

The original version of this system provided a sampling element of 100 μm, limiting the theoretical spatial resolution to 5 lp/mm.[8] In this system, the light given off was collected by an optical system located above the plate (Fig. 13–11A). The resolution in this design is limited in part by the laser light scattering within the volume of the phosphor and stimulating a larger region of the material than the initial width of the laser beam. A second important factor is that the collection of stimulated light is inefficient, resulting in a loss of SNR because of a secondary quantum sink in the system.[9] More recently, a more efficient design was introduced in which the light is collected from the bottom surface of the plate as well (Fig. 13–11B). In addition, the phosphor plate has been improved, allowing the sampling interval to be decreased to 50 μm.

Flat-Plate Phosphor Systems

As illustrated in Figure 13–12A, an array of light-sensitive diodes can be deposited on a plate of amorphous silicon[10] such that each element provides the signal for one pixel of the image. The diodes are covered by a suitable x-ray–absorbing phosphor, such as thallium-activated cesium iodide (CsI), and the electric charge stored on each diode after x-ray exposure can be read out through a network of thin-film transistor (TFT) switches. These switches are located in the corner of each detector element. They are activated by signals sent along lines that run between the columns of the array. When a line is activated, the TFTs for elements on every row down that column connect the respective photodiodes to lines that run along each row. Each of these is connected to an output amplifier and an ADC. In this way, the entire array is read, with the use of a number of external connections equal to the sum of the number of rows and columns of the detector ($r + c$) instead of the total number of elements ($r \times c$).

The system produced by General Electric Medical Systems (Waukasha, Wisconsin), illustrated in Figure 13–12B, has detector dimensions of 19 × 23 cm with detector elements 100 μm on a side and 14-bit digitization. Although it is possible to produce smaller detector elements, doing so would impose major engineering challenges. As the detector element is reduced in size, proportionately more of its area is occupied with the readout switches and lines, and less is actually sensitive to the incident x-rays. The geometric efficiency of the detector is thus reduced. In addition, with the higher number of elements that would result, the complexity in connecting readout

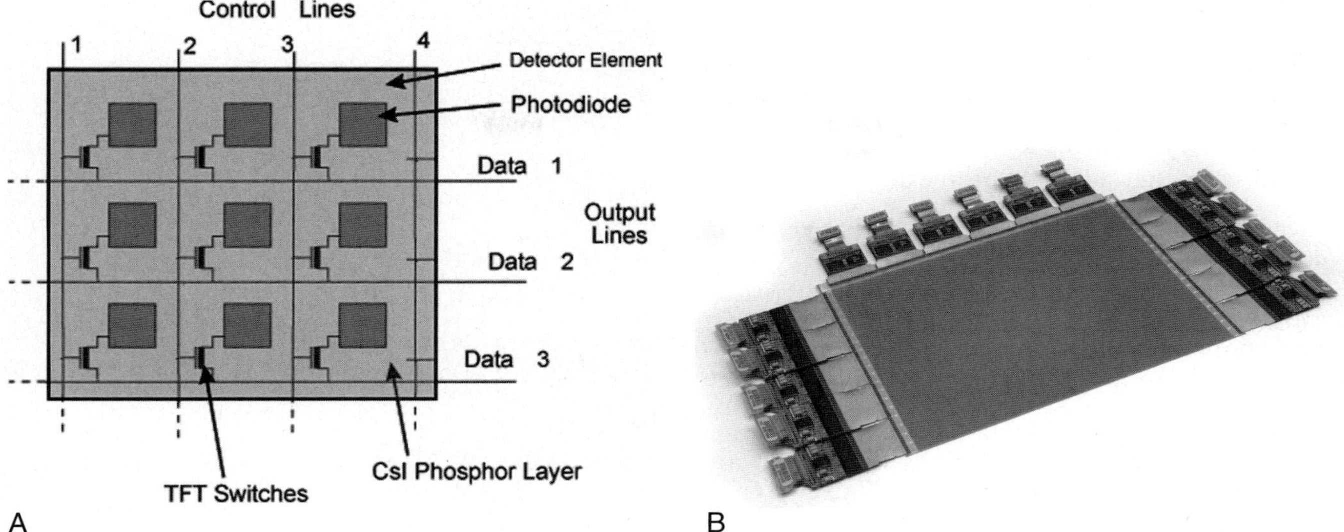

Figure 13–12. Area detector based on amorphous silicon. **A**, Schematic diagram of detector elements. **B**, Photograph of detector plate. CsI, cesium iodide; TFT, thin-film transistor.

wires to all of the rows and columns of the matrix while maintaining minimal loss of coverage at the chest wall side of the imaging system becomes progressively greater.

Direct-Conversion X-ray Detectors

In phosphor-based detectors, at least two energy conversion stages occur: x-ray to light and light to electronic charge. Because of inefficiencies in energy conversion and signal collection, these systems can be limited in sensitivity and suffer from increased noise.[11] Several detector technologies in which x-ray energy is directly and efficiently converted to charge have been considered. They include crystalline silicon detectors or zinc cadmium telluride detectors hybridized directly to CCDs, amorphous selenium, lead iodide, or mercuric iodide deposited on a flat-plate TFT readout, and high-pressure gas ionization detectors. In these detectors, the direct conversion process generally provides a much greater electronic charge signal than is available when phosphors are employed.

Amorphous Selenium

In phosphor-based detectors, when x-rays are absorbed, they produce light. The light spreads as it travels to the photodetector, which in turn is used as the readout device. This arrangement results in a loss of spatial resolution. As the detector is made thicker to improve quantum interaction efficiency, the resolution gets worse. Direct-conversion detectors like selenium have some important advantages over phosphor-based detectors for imaging. Because it is a photoconductor, the electrical charge produced in selenium can be propelled by an electrostatic field placed across the detector, so that the charge spreading is minimal, even for a thick, efficient detector (Fig. 13–13).[12] Rowlands and colleagues,[13] Zhao and coworkers,[14] and Lee and associates[15] have investigated amorphous selenium as a detector for digital mammography.

In current implementations by two companies, Lorad (Danbury, CT) and Analogic (Peabody, MA), the selenium is deposited on a plate containing a matrix of electrode pads, which define the detector elements (*dels*). The charge produced in the selenium is collected by means of an electric field and stored on these electrodes. Readout is accomplished in the same manner as used for the phosphor, flat-panel system, by TFT switches on each del connected to activation lines and data lines.

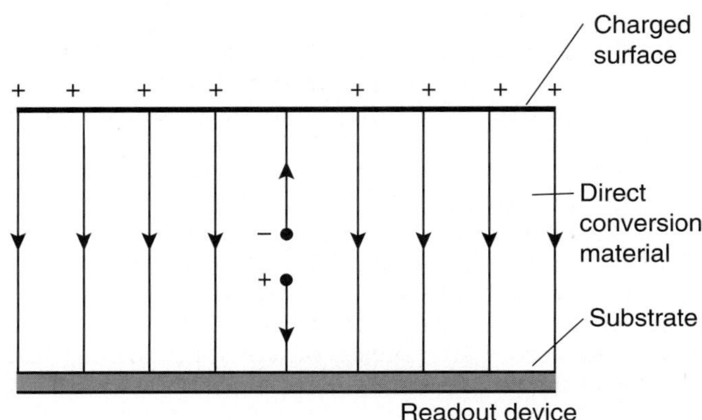

Figure 13–13. In a direct-conversion x-ray detector, an electric field across the detector causes the liberated charge to drift quickly to a collection electrode, minimizing loss of spatial resolution due to lateral spreading.

Scanned-Beam Detectors

An alternative approach for acquisition of digital mammograms is to use a long, narrow detector that covers only part of the breast at one time. To build up a full image, the detector is scanned, in conjunction with the radiation beam, across the entire breast.

Because the image is acquired sequentially in a scanning system, the total acquisition time is longer than with an area detector. A major offsetting advantage of scanned-beam systems, however, is that because only part of the volume of the breast is irradiated at any one time, it is much easier and more efficient than in an area system to control the detrimental effects of scattered radiation at the image receptor. Less scattered radiation is created during the acquisition of each subimage. Furthermore, it is easier to interpose antiscatter collimators between the breast and the detector without the need for attenuating interspace material, as in the grids used for area detectors. The result is far more dose-efficient rejection of scatter than in an area system.

A slot-beam system for digital mammography was originally proposed by Nelson and coworkers[16] in 1987; our group at the University of Toronto has also worked on the design.[17] A commercial system, developed by Fischer Imaging Corp (Denver, CO), uses a detector that is approximately 10 mm in width and 22 cm long. The x-ray beam, which is collimated to match the detector dimensions, is scanned across the breast parallel to the chest wall in synchrony with the detector. After transmission through the breast, x-rays are absorbed by a cesium iodide phosphor, and the emitted light is conveyed via a fiberoptic coupling plate to several CCD arrays whose electrical signals are then digitized. Fiberoptic coupling overcomes, in part, the problem of reduced resolution caused by diffusion of light in the screen. The restricted angular acceptance of the optical fibers causes each fiber to collimate the light incident from the screen, thereby increasing the effective resolution. In addition, the high optical coupling efficiency attainable with fiberoptics minimizes signal losses, thereby facilitating an x-ray quantum-limited system. The fiberoptic glass acts as an attenuator to keep direct radiation from reaching the CCD. This would cause unwanted signal and could also damage the CCD.

To allow a smooth mechanical motion, the images are acquired through use of a time-delay integration (TDI) technique.[18] The CCD is designed so that charge accumulated in an element of the device can be shifted in a controlled manner from element to element down columns of the CCD. As the detector is moved across the breast at constant speed, the charge collected in each element of the CCD is shifted down its column at the same speed as the scan but in the opposite direction. When the charge packet reaches the last element in the CCD, the charge signals in the columns are read out at high speed. In this way, the signal corresponding to a given pixel in the image is acquired by integration down columns of the detector. Depending on the slot width, a scanning system can acquire a mammogram in 3 to 6 seconds. Figure 13–14 is a photograph of the Fischer system, illustrating the similarity of the appearance of such a system to a conventional mammography unit.

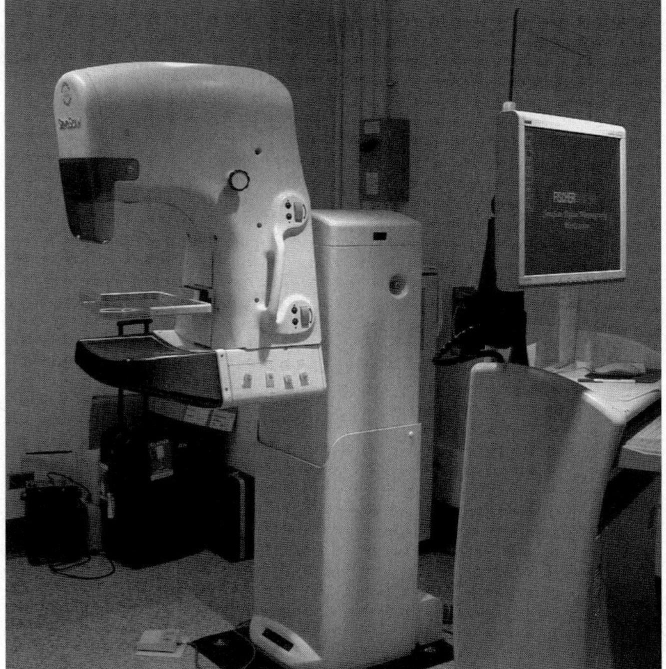

Figure 13–14. Photograph of the Fischer digital mammography system.

EXPOSURE TECHNIQUE

The technique (e.g., kilovoltage, filtration) for film-screen mammography has been established largely by trial and error over several decades of the practice of mammography. For digital systems, in which contrast can be freely manipulated, the optimal spectra may be different from those for film. In a digital imaging system, the operating kilovoltage and the amount of radiation used to form an image should be defined strictly by signal-to-noise considerations rather than by contrast or film "blackening" requirements. Fahrig and associates[19] have shown, in computer models of scanning digital mammography, that compared with film-screen technique, increased kilovoltage improves efficiency and output of the x-ray tube, resulting in images with a high SNR while allowing lower radiation dose and scan time.

IMAGE STORAGE

Although the technology for digital mammography will continue to improve, current systems have reached a level of performance at which they rival screen-film mammography. For these systems to be truly practical, however, they must be effectively integrated with radiology picture archiving and communications systems (PACSs). Digital mammograms require vast amounts of digital storage; however, this should not be a major problem because the capacity of both random access memory and short- and long-term digital storage is steadily growing, with a concurrent reduction in the cost per megabyte. More challenging problems relate to image processing and display.

IMAGE PROCESSING

Flat-Field Correction

On most systems, certain basic operations are performed on the digital image before it is presented for viewing. The first of these is referred to as *flat-field correction*. Frequently, there are spatial variations in sensitivity in the detector. In a film-screen system, nothing can be done about this problem, and the manufacturer goes to great lengths to minimize this type of "structural noise." In a digital detector, it is possible to correct for such variation, often by making two measurements. The first step is to record the response of all detector elements in the absence of x-ray exposure. This is a measurement of the so-called dark signal, and because this value can vary with time and temperature, such measurements may be carried out quite frequently. The value of the dark signal can be subtracted from the measured digital values produced by the detector during imaging of the breast. The second measurement is of the detector elements' response to a uniform field of x-rays. This is done by placing either nothing or a uniform attenuator in the x-ray beam and acquiring an image. This measurement should be made with many x-rays (e.g., by averaging a number of such acquired images together) to ensure that the noise in the measurement is low. This set of data is then used to match the sensitivity of all the detector elements. The result is an image that is essentially free of structural variations. It should be noted that such a simple correction works well only if the detector response is linear. If the response is nonlinear or if transformations such as a logarithm are intentionally performed before flat-field correction, correction is much more difficult.

For display of a digital image, mapping from pixel value to video intensity on a soft-copy display or optical density on a printed laser film must take place. Various types of image processing, such as contrast enhancement, can be employed to improve the conspicuity of relevant anatomic information before display. Several methods of contrast enhancement can be used. The simplest, and perhaps most useful, operations are "look-up table" (LUT) or translation table modifications. As discussed earlier, the image is recorded on a numerical scale, typically from 0 to 4095 (12 bits) or 0 to 16,383 (14 bits). This exceeds the sensitivity capability of the eye for contrast perception and also the capability of both film and most electronic display devices. Typically, on a cathode ray tube (CRT), it is considered feasible to display the image in terms of 8 bits or 256 shades of brightness at any one time. An LUT is used by the digital mammography computer to map the original image data from the original acquired range down to the 256 levels available for display. For every pixel value, the table contains a number representing the video display intensity or printed optical density to which that pixel value is mapped. A digital-to-analog converter converts this number to an analog voltage signal. The use of the Barten model[20,21] has been incorporated in the digital imaging and communications in medicine (DICOM) display standard for optimization of display lookup tables. In this model, each level in the table represents the same "perceptual" increment. This means that an object with 5% subject contrast will be seen equally well in the brightest and darkest areas.

A method of contrast enhancement known as *linear scaling and clipping* or *windowing and leveling* is illustrated in Figure 13–15.[22] In this type of LUT modification, the viewer makes selections on window and level controls to enhance image features. A window level (L) is set, which describes the image value that is displayed as the midvalue of display intensity, and a window (W) or range of original image values to be displayed is also chosen. Image values below L – W/2 are displayed as black and are visible on the monitor, and those above L + W/2 are displayed at the maximum intensity of white. Intermediate values are displayed on a linear range of gray values between black and white so that the entire range of display values is used. The sloped portion of the graph is termed the *ramp*. The width of the ramp is the W setting, and the midportion of the ramp is the L setting. This allows the user to ensure that the anatomy of interest is viewed in the optimum part of the display brightness and to adjust contrast as desired. For example, if the user wishes to enhance contrast differences in the brightest portions of the

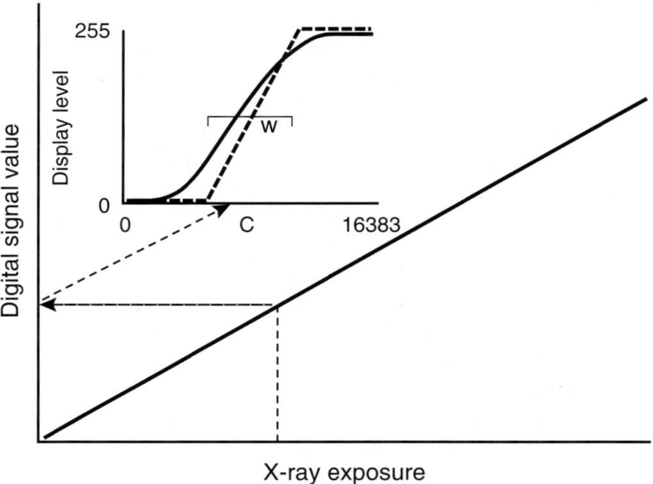

Figure 13–15. In digital imaging, a wide range of intensity information is acquired by the detector. Intensities of interest can be enhanced in the display process, for example by manipulation of L (window level) and W (window range) controls. *Inset* shows how contrast may be increased by reducing W.

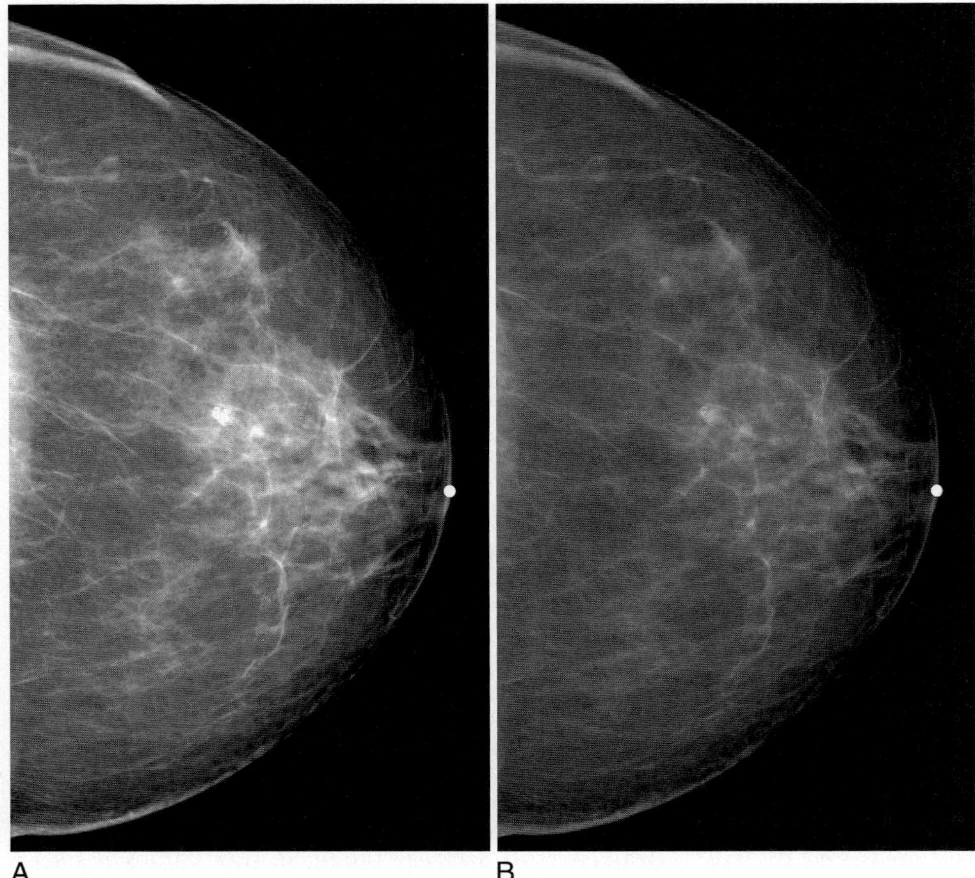

Figure 13–16. Display contrast adjustment. Contrast has been increased from A to B.

image, the W and L can be increased to encompass higher pixel values. Controlling W and L allows one to use the display window to inspect regions of the breast that vary greatly in density. The user can increase the degree of contrast with which the image is displayed (without the necessity to reimage the breast) by reducing W so that the ramp is made steeper (curve slope is increased), because the entire range of gray-scale values must be obtained from a narrower range of pixel values. This is illustrated in the *inset* in Figure 13–15. An example of display contrast adjustment of a mammogram is shown in Figure 13–16.

The value of W can be reduced until the appearance of noise in the displayed image becomes unacceptable. This is determined by the intrinsic noise of the image acquisition, which in turn can be controlled by the use of very-low-noise x-ray detection systems and by the dose to the breast. The dose can be chosen according to the required SNR for a particular imaging situation rather than by the need to produce an image of a given "brightness."

More generally, it may be found that other, nonlinear mappings (e.g., logarithmic) from image intensity to display brightness may be more suitable. These may be found to better compensate for deficiencies in the display device or for the perceptual characteristics of the observer. For example, if the curve in Figure 13–15 were concave upward (exponential), contrast in the brighter portions of the image would be enhanced. If the curve were concave downward (reverse exponential), contrast in the darker portions of the image would be enhanced. An optimal LUT modification remains to be determined.

Another means of enhancing the display is through modification of the histogram of image display values. If the histogram is calculated, it is frequently found that certain display values are not used or are infrequently used. Histogram equalization is a technique of remapping the image display values so that all gray levels in the display are used with more-or-less equal frequency. This can help make better use of the capability of the display; however, care must be taken to control the amplification of display contrast to avoid excessive appearance of noise. Modifications of equalization, such as contrast-limited adaptive histogram equalization (CLAHE), have been tested on digital mammograms by Pisano and associates[22,23] at the University of North Carolina.

It is also possible to improve the sharpness of display with various edge-enhancement techniques. Those familiar with xeromammography will recall the high edge contrast that tended to enhance the visibility of structures by outlining their borders. One convenient technique for edge enhancement that can be used to advantage is "unsharp masking." A blurred version of the original mammogram is made by filtering the image in the computer with a convolution kernel. The nature of this function determines the degree of blurring. When this blurred mask is subtracted from the original image, the resulting difference image is composed mainly of the sharp features of the mammogram without the broad area structures. This edge map can be added to the original image to provide enhancement of the edges of microcalcifications, fine fibers, and blood vessels. The amount of edge enhancement is controlled by a weighting constant by which the edge image is multiplied before the addition takes place. One of the important advantages of digital imaging is that these image-processing features can be turned on and off instantly to allow the radiologist to view the images under different enhancement conditions. This can facilitate the determination of whether suspicious structures are real or artifactual. Although very sophisticated image processing is possible, it is likely that the main benefit of image enhancement will derive from relatively simple operations that improve contrast in dense regions or that sharpen subtle structures. The optimal manner in which to display image contrast scales, the possible value of equalization, and the role of edge enhancement and other image sharpening techniques in digital mammography must be carefully investigated in terms of their efficacy.

IMAGE DISPLAY

In screen-film mammography, images of the entire breast are recorded on either 18 × 24–cm or 24 × 30–cm film, depending on breast size. With digital mammography, display of the full breast on a monitor having the same 18 to 20 lp/mm resolution as screen-film mammography is not currently feasible, because it would require 9600 × 12,000 pixels (picture elements). Even the display of a full breast at 10 lp/mm resolution would require 4000 × 5000 pixels. At present, the highest-resolution monochrome displays that are commercially available have formats of 2048 × 2560 pixels. Newer flat-panel displays of 3840 × 2400 pixels are available but have not been evaluated in commercial mammography systems. From Table 13–4, it can be seen that only a single 19 × 23–cm format image at 100-μm sampling can be displayed on this flat-panel monitor. An examination generally consists of four views, and it is often desirable to display a previous examination for comparison. Therefore, if one attempts to emulate the method of viewing film mammograms, up to eight monitors would be required. However, for larger image formats and images with pixels smaller than 100 μm, even this expensive solution would not be workable, because it would not be possible to display an entire single image on a monitor at full spatial resolution.

A solution to this problem is to temporarily reduce the number of pixels in the image by averaging, so that the whole image can be displayed on the monitor. Of course, averaging will blur the image slightly. Then, when a suspicious region of interest is identified, the image can be "zoomed" to display that region at full, acquired spatial resolution (Fig. 13–17). This image can then be panned, so that a larger area or the entire breast is sequentially visualized at full resolution. One of the challenges with this approach to display is to allow the radiologist to maintain orientation with respect to the overall image of the breast.

In current digital mammography systems, two display monitors are typically used. The radiologist can easily format the display to present one or several mammograms per monitor. If the system is well designed, the radiologist can quickly navigate among these images and can zoom any image to regain full spatial resolution and pan over the zoomed image to scrutinize adjacent tissue structures. When a radiologist zooms the image beyond the point where one acquired image point is displayed per pixel on the monitor, it will continue to be enlarged, but the resolution will not increase. This type of zooming is similar in nature to using a loupe to magnify the image.

After digital images are manipulated on the monitor to optimize demonstration of anatomic and pathologic features, hard-copy films can be produced by means of a laser film printer. Existing laser printers can provide an adequate number of pixels and a sufficiently small pixel size to record a mammogram without loss of spatial resolution.

To record x-ray transmission through the breast with sufficient precision, intensity data from the x-ray detector are typically digitized to 4096 or 16,384 possible levels, requiring 12 to 16 bits or 2 bytes of computer memory for storage.[17] This is a much wider range of signal intensities than can adequately be displayed either with a single LUT setting on a monitor or with a single set of printing conditions on laser film. In soft-copy display on the monitor, interactive adjustment of the LUT can be used to ensure that all relevant parts of the signal scale are presented with appropriate display brightness and contrast. However, this process can be very time consuming. In the case of hard-copy display on film, once the display printing parameters are set, the characteristics of the printed image are fixed, and if one wants to explore the signal domain with other parameters, additional images must be printed. Again, this is time consuming and expensive.

The range of signal intensity that must be displayed can be reduced considerably without sacrificing diagnostic quality through the use of a type of image processing called *peripheral equalization*.[24,25] This process seeks to suppress the largest signal variations in the image, which are associated with changes in thickness from one part of the breast to another, especially at the edges. If it is done properly, peripheral equalization can be accomplished while maintaining the information associated with

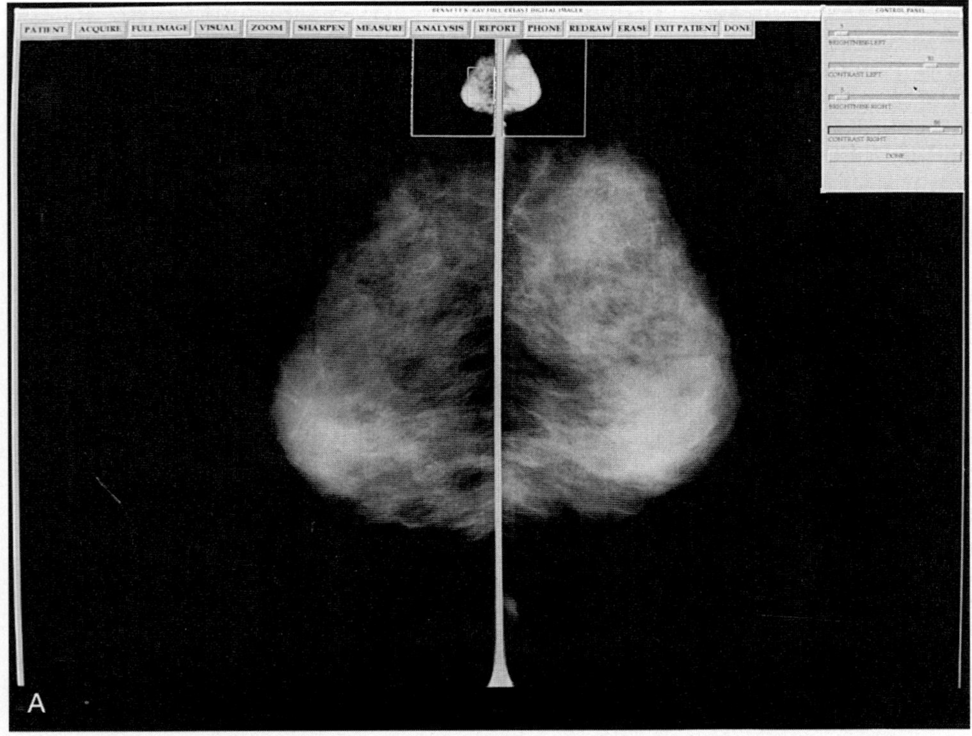

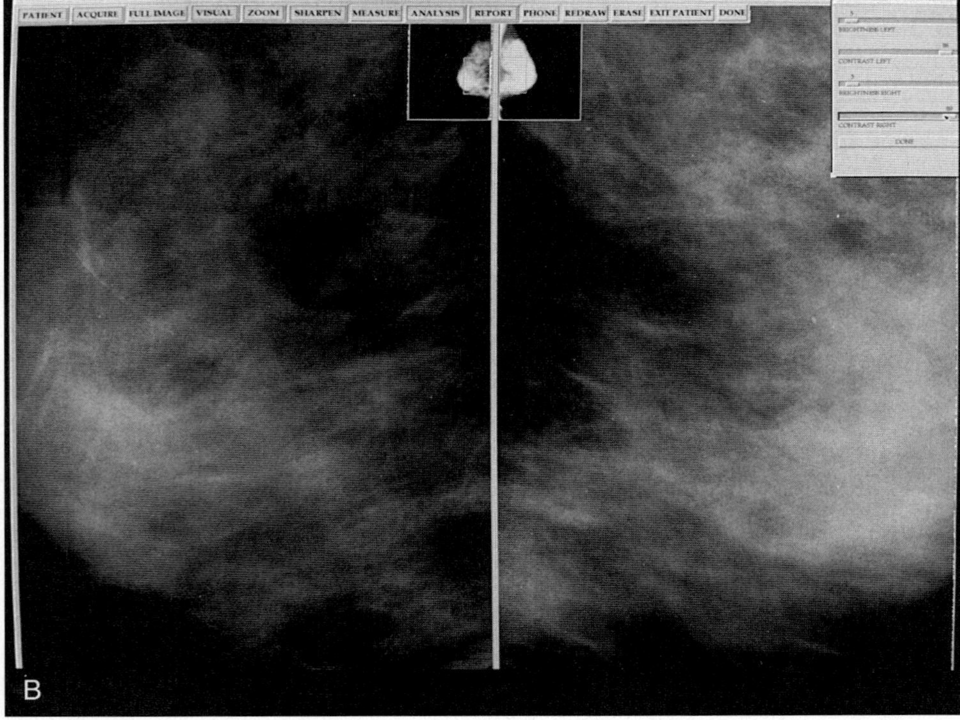

Figure 13–17. Display design for digital mammography. In this design scheme, identical views of both breasts are shown side by side on the same monitor. **A,** Full images. **B,** Full-resolution "magnified" zooms of comparable regions of each breast. Note the control panel for brightness (level) and contrast (window width). (Courtesy of Bennett X-ray Corp, Copiague, NY.)

changes in tissue composition, related to the normal and possibly abnormal structures in the breast.

In the long run, soft-copy display will probably be the method of choice for viewing digital mammograms, because it is more flexible with respect to manipulating the image and does not require the use of film. Until digital mammography workstations are widely available, however, hard-copy images may provide the most easily transferable record of the examination to another facility.

Another challenge presented by digital mammography is that of comparison of a patient's digital mammogram with previous screen-film images. This could be accomplished in one of three ways: (1) films printed from the digital system could be compared with previous films, (2) older studies could be digitized and displayed on the digital workstation, or (3) images on the CRT monitor could be compared with preexisting screen-film studies. Each of these options has advantages and disadvantages in terms of effort, cost, and, possibly, diagnostic accuracy.

The advantage of digital mammography comes largely from decoupling of the image acquisition, storage, and display operations and using improved detector technology to obtain information from the breast more precisely. The use of soft-copy display is attractive, but at present, several practical problems must be solved, and a new learning curve must be formulated for the radiologist in interpreting such images.

For hard-copy display of digital mammograms on film, the image can be displayed briefly on a computer monitor at less than full resolution to allow image processing to be performed. The image is then printed on film with a laser printer. The disadvantage of this approach is that the radiologist is reviewing a fixed image, placing the responsibility for proper image display either on the technologist or on an automatic display algorithm in the digital mammography system.

To provide a preferable alternative to film, the digital display should duplicate several practices that are performed in film interpretation. Just as a radiologist is able to mark and circle film features with a wax pencil, he or she should be able to mark (annotate) digital images during soft-copy viewing on the monitor. The monitor should also be able to mask areas around selected features to enhance visual perception. To help the technologist position patients for special views, hard-copy images with the lesion circled should be available, or there should be a monitor in the examination room. The latter arrangement is essential if needle localization procedures are to be performed with the digital mammography system.

COMPUTER-AIDED DETECTION

Rationale

Digital mammography greatly facilitates the use of *computer-aided detection* (CAD), which may be defined as detection by a radiologist who takes into account images and analysis from a computer. These serve as a "second opinion" that the radiologist can take into consideration in making the final interpretation. In the absence of digital mammography, performance of CAD requires the initial cumbersome and time-consuming step of digitization of film images to provide suitable input for the computer.

Even with high-quality modern mammography, some breast cancers may be missed on initial interpretation yet are visible in retrospect (Table 13–5). Reading of screening mammograms by a second radiologist has been shown to improve the cancer detection rate by 10% to 15%.[26-28] Presumably, CAD could have the same type of effect.

Table 13–5. Image Storage Requirements for Digital Mammography

	Image Dimensions (cm)	Pixel size (μm) 100	50	40
Single image	18 × 24	8.6	34.6	54.0
(megabytes)	24 × 30	14.4	57.6	90.0
Annual workload	18 × 24	0.6	2.5	3.9
(terabytes)	24 × 30	1.0	4.2	6.5

CAD might have some advantages over human observers. Because computers are not subject to fatigue or distraction, CAD results should be reproducible as long as the same computer program is used. The computer should show no intraobserver variation. As Vyborny[29] has observed, "One does not need a radiograph to demonstrate limitations in human search performance; a bottle of catsup and any crowded refrigerator will do."

Detection refers to finding an abnormality on screening of women without any possible sign or symptom of breast cancer, whereas *diagnosis* is the evaluation of a known mammographic or clinical abnormality. The term *computer-aided diagnosis* has been used more generally in reference to either detection or diagnosis of mammographic lesions. In this chapter, however, we assess these functions separately.

Detection Methods for Microcalcifications and Mass Lesions

Microcalcifications are an especially important sign of early breast cancer. Of nonpalpable cancers detected on screening, 30% to 50% are visible on the basis of microcalcifications alone.[30] Among nonpalpable minimal carcinomas (noninfiltrating cancers and cancers smaller than 0.5 cm), about 70% are detected on the basis of microcalcifications alone.[31] Calcifications are the dominant abnormality in 95% of in-situ carcinomas.[30] Thus, as earlier-stage cancers are considered, the proportion of lesions detected on the basis of microcalcifications becomes increasingly greater.

Because histologic examination shows that 80% of breast cancers contain microcalcifications,[32] any means that improves the mammographic demonstration or radiologist's perception of microcalcifications should improve detection. Microcalcifications are suitable objects for CAD because of their easily definable difference in density, size, and shape from normal anatomic structures and their potential subtlety.

The computer vision process developed by the University of Chicago group consists of five steps (Fig. 13–18).[33] The first step is segmentation, by which the breast area is extracted (segmented) from the previously digitized mammogram so that image processing can subsequently be performed.[34] The second step, spatial (linear) filtration, is designed to enhance

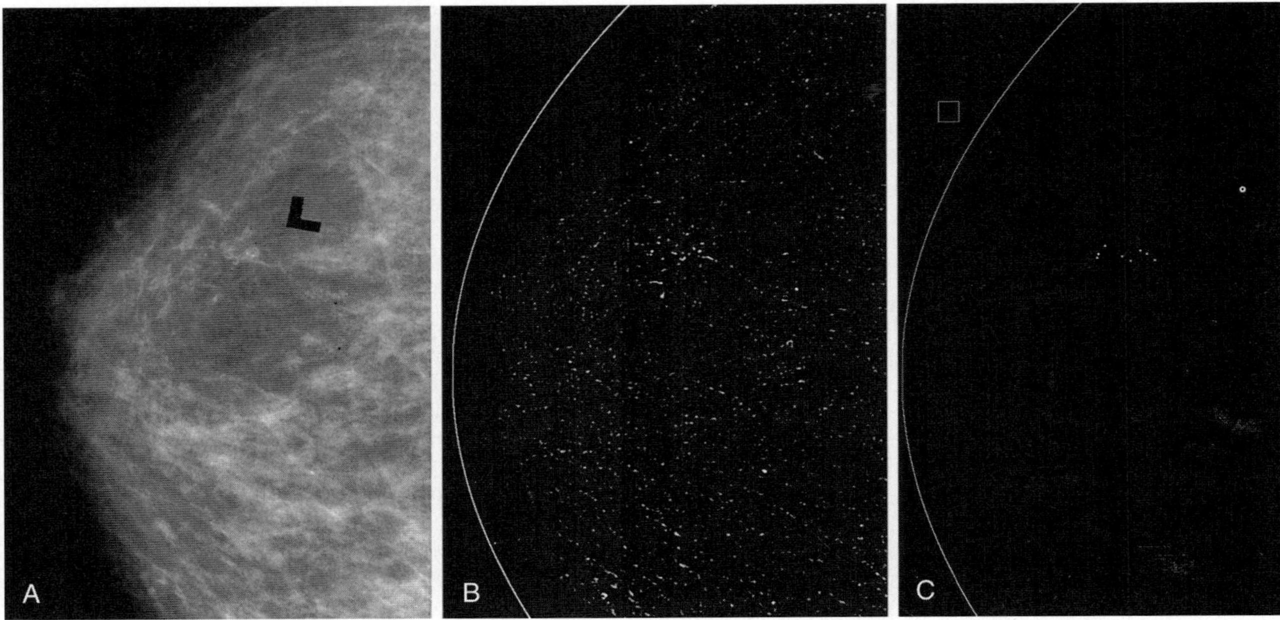

Figure 13–18. Illustration of the steps involved in the automated detection of clustered microcalcifications. **A,** Original mammogram with a cluster of microcalcifications (*arrowhead*). **B,** The mammogram is filtered to enhance microcalcifications by suppression of the normal background structure of the breast, and then this filtered image is subjected to a gray-level thresholding. **C,** Next, feature analysis, in which the size, contrast, texture, and spatial distribution of potential microcalcifications are used to eliminate false computer detections. The computer detected the true cluster. (Courtesy of Robert Nishikawa, PhD, University of Chicago, Chicago, IL.)

microcalcifications and to deemphasize background structures. The digitized image is spatially filtered twice, first to increase the SNR of the calcifications and then to suppress them. The two images are then subtracted to produce a "difference image" containing the calcifications but largely devoid of background density.

The third step, signal extraction (Fig. 13–18B), segments microcalcifications from the difference image by means of global gray-level thresholding and local gray-level thresholding technique.[35,36] Global gray-level thresholding eliminates a very high preselected percentage of pixels (e.g., 98%), whose values are lower than those of a much lower preselected percentage of pixels (e.g., 2%) that are retained. Local thresholding eliminates those pixels whose values are lower than a preselected absolute threshold value. The fourth step, feature analysis (feature extraction) (Fig. 13–18C), removes signals that are likely to arise from structures other than microcalcifications. Features used to distinguish calcifications from noncalcifications include signal area, concentration, spatial distribution, texture, and contrast.[37,38] Finally, a computer tool known as an *artificial neural network* can use input from the first four steps to further reduce the numbers of false-positive clusters.[39-41] Its use can classify unknown cases on the basis of learning from experience with known cases. The computer then indicates the location of the calcifications by means of circles, arrows, or text.

During the past several years, numerous other investigators have entered the field and have reported other approaches to CAD of microcalcifications.[33] The growing interest in this field may be attributed to the greater use of screening mammography and development of full-field digital mammographic units. Although all previous studies of CAD have used digitized mammograms, direct input of data from a full-field digital unit will facilitate the use of CAD by eliminating the need for preprocessing digitization.

Because mammographic differences in optical density and morphology between mass lesions and surrounding breast tissues are less than those for calcifications, computerized detection of mass lesions is considerably more difficult than detection of microcalcifications. Initial attempts at CAD were based on differences in optical density among different areas of the same breast and between the corresponding areas of the right and left breasts as well as differences between the directions of the breast densities.[42-44]

A later computer vision scheme developed by Giger[33] and Yin and coworkers[45-47] is also based on differences between the normal bilateral symmetry of the breasts. Gray-level thresholding is performed before subtraction. Feature extraction techniques—morphologic filtering, size, shape, and distance from the borders of the breast—are then used to reduce the number of false-positive findings. Several different approaches to CAD of breast masses have been pursued by other investigators.[46-50]

The relative efficacy of different CAD schemes cannot be reliably compared unless they are tested on identical series of cases and interpreted by the same set of radiologists. Even then, the relative advantages and disadvantages of different systems may vary according to the overall composition of the case material and overall ability of the radiologist.

If CAD is used as a second opinion rather than as a substitute for the radiologist, it need not be better than or even as good as the radiologist. Even if CAD does not detect all lesions found by the radiologist, it might still find other lesions missed by the radiologist. Moreover, because the final decision comes from the radiologist rather than from the computer, false-positive diagnoses from the computer may be tolerable, so long as they do not lead to unnecessary biopsies or even to excessive additional mammographic exposures. These possible consequences of CAD must be monitored. Obviously, any increase in the sensitivity of CAD is desirable. An improvement in CAD's specificity also may be desirable as long as no concomitant decrease in sensitivity occurs.

False-positive detections by the computer may prolong the subsequent review by the radiologist. When sensitivity and specificity levels are set for the computer, this drawback must be weighed against improved detection. However, several studies have reported that the higher false-positive rate of the computer did not significantly slow the reading speed of radiologists.[49]

A future objective of CAD could be to detect changes on sequential mammograms, such as increase in the size of a mass or number of microcalcifications, change in breast architecture, and presence of a new mass or calcifications. This application, however, would require compensation for differences in positioning between mammographic studies.

Need for CAD in Detection of Missed Cancers

There is evidence that some potentially detectable breast cancers may not always be detected, even when high-quality images are interpreted by experienced radiologists. Double reading of screening mammograms has been shown to improve breast cancer detection rates by 10% to 15%.[26-28,51-55] Additionally, a number of studies have found that many cancers can be identified in retrospect on mammograms that were performed before the one on which they were detected (Table 13–6).

Missed cancers are cancers that are potentially detectable at screening but were not detected by the radiologist. Birdwell and associates[56] used the term "missed cancers" for those that were appreciated by the majority of radiologists on blinded retrospective review of previous mammograms. Among the missed cancers in their study, 51% were in breasts that were fatty or contained scattered fibroglandular densities, 30% were seen as calcifications alone, 21% were seen as masses with calcifications, and 47% were seen as noncalcified masses. Sixty-four percent of the masses were 11 mm or larger, and 57% of the calcification cases were in areas larger than 11 mm. These characteristics suggest that many missed cancers could have been detected by improved interpretation or the use of CAD.

Several studies have sought to determine how frequently nonpalpable cancers detected at screening mammography can be identified in retrospect on a previous mammogram. Martin and colleagues[57] evaluated 48 malignancies that surfaced clinically between annual screening intervals at four Breast Cancer Detection Demonstration Project (BCDDP) Centers. Of these interval cancers, 29% (14/48) were missed through obvious oversights, and 38% (18/48) went undetected because of less obvious errors that were noted in retrospect by experienced examiners. In only 33% of cases (16/48) were no diagnostic radiographic signs found on review.

Bird and coworkers[58] identified 77 cancers that were "missed" at screening mammography among 320 cancers found in a screened population between 1985 and 1990. Double reading had been performed in all cases. Forty-seven (61%) of the "missed" cancers were visible in retrospect on a previous mammogram that had been interpreted as being normal. Eleven (14%) of the missed cancers were evaluated as normal by the first reader but underwent biopsy by virtue of being suspicious to the second reader. Only 25% (19/77) of the "missed" cancers had no mammographic findings.

Harvey and colleagues[59] evaluated previous mammograms in 73 patients in whom nonpalpable breast cancers were detected on subsequent mammograms. Reviews were performed two ways: (1) blinded (without knowledge that cancer had been detected on a later examination) and (2) nonblinded (side-by-side comparison of earlier and later studies). Findings of blinded reviews were categorized as "positive" if biopsy was recommended or additional views were requested of the area where the cancer was finally detected. On such reviews, Harvey and colleagues[59] found that the interpretation was positive in 41% (30/73) of patients. Because it is unknown whether additional views would have led to a biopsy recommendation, it is possible that this classification may have overestimated the number of cancers that were missed as a result of reader error. Additionally, when blinded reviews do not mix cancer cases with enough normal and benign cases, observers may be more suspicious about mammographic findings than they would be under everyday circumstances.[60] A subsequent nonblinded retrospective review found evidence of cancer in 25 of the 43 patients for whom blinded review had normal findings. Because nonblinded reviews give observers the advantage of hindsight, such studies may overestimate the number of cancers that are identifiable even by the best readers. Nevertheless, Harvey and colleagues[59] found that findings in 75% (55/73) of cancers were positive on either blinded or nonblinded review of previous mammograms.

A similar nonblinded review by Van Dijck and associates[61] found that 57% (25/44) of screen-detected breast cancers and 46% (18/40) of interval cancers from a program in Holland could be identified retrospectively on a previous mammogram. Jones and coworkers[62] reviewed previous mammograms of 133 patients in whom cancer was detected 3 years later at the first incident screen. Of these cancers, mammographic results in 22.6% (30/133) could be classified as false-negative or missed at the prevalent screen 3 years earlier.

Daly and colleagues[63] reviewed first-round screening films of 100 women in whom cancer was detected in the second round of the United Kingdom National Health Service Breast Screening Programme. On initial blind review of the first screening mammograms, a lesion later proven histologically to be the cancer was correctly identified in 25% (25/100) of women. Review with knowledge of the site of the lesion at second round identified an additional 19 false-negative lesions, for a total false-negative rate of 44% (44/100) on nonblinded retrospective review. Similar results were obtained in a blinded retrospective study conducted by Vitak and coworkers[64] in Sweden, in which two external reviewers identified 25% of missed cancers for further evaluation.

Retrospective reviews in which readers are blinded and cancer cases are mixed with an adequate number of normal and benign cases provide more realistic estimates. One such review was conducted by Warren-Burhenne and associates.[65] Among 427 breast cancers detected by screening mammography at 13 facilities in the United States, 67% (286/427) were visible at nonblinded retrospective review of previous mammograms. At blinded retrospective assessment of these previous mammograms, panels of five radiologists independently reviewing these cases enriched with normal cases found that 27% (115/427) would have required biopsy or additional imaging.

Another "enriched" review of breast cancers missed during routine screening in North Carolina was conducted by Yankaskas and colleagues.[66] Four community-based radiologists experienced in mammography performed independent, blinded, retrospective reviews of the screening mammograms of 339 asymptomatic women. These included 93 women who were diagnosed with breast cancer within 1 year of a normal screening mammogram and 246 women in whom no breast cancer developed during that year. Using the majority interpretation of the four radiologists, the researchers found that 42% of the 93 false-negative mammograms would have been further evaluated but that the average rate of further evaluation for the 246 true-negative mammograms was 13%. Yankaskas and colleagues[66] subtracted the true-negative rate from the false-negative rate to estimate that abnormalities on 29% of false-negative mammograms could have been detected at screening.

Two further studies of missed cancers have been neither blinded nor enriched. Taft and Taylor[67] in Australia found that 38% (19/50) of screen-detected cancers could be seen retrospectively on previous mammograms that had been interpreted as normal. In a study of screen-detected invasive lobular carcinoma, a type of cancer known to be difficult to detect, Evans and associates[68] found that 77% (31/40) of cases were seen on nonblinded retrospective review of previous mammograms by expert radiologists.

Table 13–6. Evaluation of Screening Mammograms Interpreted as Normal and Breast Cancer Subsequently Developed: How Often Can Breast Cancer be Seen on Second Reading?

Study*	Type of Study	Detection of Cancer on Re-review (%)
Martin et al (1979)[57]	Nonblinded	67
Bird et al (1992)[58]	Nonblinded	75
Harvey et al (1993)[59]	Blinded	41
	Nonblinded	75
Van Dijck et al (1993)[61]	Nonblinded	57
Jones et al (1996)[62]	Nonblinded	23
Daly et al (1998)[63]	Blinded	25
	Nonblinded	44
Vitak (1998)[64]	Blinded	25
Warren-Burhenne et al (2000)[65]	Blinded	27
	Nonblinded	67
Yankaskas et al (2001)[66]	Blinded	29
Taft and Taylor (2001)[67]	Nonblinded	38
Evans et al (2002)[68]	Nonblinded	77
Brem et al (2003)[69]	Blinded	33

*Superscript numbers indicate chapter references.

Brem and coworkers[69] reviewed 377 screening mammograms interpreted as showing normal or benign findings 9 to 24 months before cancer diagnosis. Each study was reviewed independently and in blinded fashion by three radiologists. Additional views were requested by at least two of three reviewers in 33% (123/377) of cases.

In summary, six separate studies involving blinded retrospective reviews of screening mammograms in women in whom breast cancer subsequently developed found lesions requiring evaluation or biopsy in 25% to 41% of cases. The two of the blinded studies that were enriched with normal cases found that 27% to 29% of cancers could be seen in retrospect. Nine nonblinded retrospective reviews identified 23% to 77% of missed cases (see Table 13–6).

Cancers Missed by Radiologists: Retrospective Reviews Using CAD

The ability of CAD to identify malignant masses that had been missed by radiologists was first demonstrated by te Brake and colleagues[70] in 1998. Their research system found 34% (22/65) of these cancers.

Warren-Burhenne and associates[65] used missed cancer cases to evaluate the potential of CAD to improve mammographic detection rates. Among 115 breast cancers identified on a blinded retrospective review of mammograms that had been performed at least 9 months before the actual date of detection, these investigators found that CAD detected 77% (89/115). Their study also illustrates that the sensitivity of CAD depends on how *missed cancers* are defined. When Warren-Burhenne and associates[65] expanded their database to include missed cancers identified on nonblinded retrospective review of the previous studies, they evaluated a larger number of missed cancers (286 versus 115), included more subtle lesions, and found that CAD had a lower detection sensitivity, 60% (171/286).

Garvican and colleagues[71] found that CAD (R-2 Image Checker V 2.0) could detect 52% (15/29) of interval cancers from the National Health Service Breast Screening Programme (NHSBSP) in East Kent, United Kingdom, that had been missed by screening readers but had been seen on retrospective non-blinded review by expert radiologists.

In Sweden, Moberg and coworkers[72] evaluated the mammograms of 59 women in whom interval cancers surfaced clinically after a screening that had been originally interpreted as normal. Retrospective reviews by experienced radiologists found 26 of the cancers. CAD flagged 13 of these 26 cancers, yielding a CAD sensitivity of 50% (13/26) for interval cancers identified by one or more radiologists on retrospective review. The relatively lower sensitivity of CAD can be explained by the appearance of interval cancers, which are more likely to appear as subtly asymmetrical. Identification of such lesions often depends on comparison between current and previous studies, subtle asymmetry between the two breasts, or both. CAD sensitivity is lower for interval cancers, in which spiculation and microcalcifications are often absent.

Taft and Taylor[67] in Australia found that CAD retrospectively detected 88% (88/100) of screen-detected cancers and 63% (12/19) of cancers that had been missed at screening and found on retrospective review by expert radiologists. CAD actually performed better than either of two nonexpert readers, who each found 42% (8/19), and better than the two nonexpert readers together, who found 53% (10/19) of missed cancers that were identified in retrospect by the experts. Among 31 cases of invasive lobular carcinoma that had been missed by radiologists and were identified in retrospect on previous films by expert radiologists, Evans and colleagues[68] reported that CAD marked 77% (24/31).

How Does the Mammographic Appearance of Masses and Calcifications Affect the Sensitivity of CAD?

The relative ability of CAD to identify breast calcifications and masses has been evaluated in multiple clinical studies (Table 13–7). Most of these clinical studies have been performed on the R-2 Image Checker (Fig. 13–19). Landmark studies such as those of Warren-Burhenne and colleagues[65] and Birdwell and associates[56] demonstrated that the sensitivity of CAD is better for calcifications than for masses. Additionally, Birdwell and associates[56] found that CAD had a higher sensitivity for masses containing calcifications than for noncalcified masses—83% (20/24) and 67% (36/54), respectively—yielding an average 71% (56/78) sensitivity for all masses. Castellino and associates[73] demonstrated the effect of an updated algorithm (V2.2) on mass detection. Using the same set of cancers detected at screening as used by Warren-Burhenne and colleagues,[65] Castellino and associates[73] found a detection rate for masses of 86% (580/677), compared with 75% (506/677) detected with the V1.2 algorithm used by the earlier researchers.

Table 13–7. Sensitivity of Computer-Aided Detection (CAD) for Breast Cancer Screening: Calcifications versus Masses

Study*	CAD System†	Case Material	Study Design	All Cancers‡	Sensitivity	
					Calcifications	Masses
te Brake et al (1998)[70]	Research	MC	R			34% (22/65)
Nakahara et al (1998)[74]	V1.0	DC	R	86% (56/65)	100% (22/22)	79% (34/43)
Thurfjell et al (1998)[79]	V1.0	DC + MC	R	50% (37/74)		
Warren-Burhenne et al (2000)[65]	V1.2	DC	R	84% (906/1083)	99% (400/406)	75% (506/677)
		MC		77% (89/115)		
		MC		60% (171/286)	79% (87/110)	48% (84/176)
Vyborny et al (2000)[75]	V2.0	DC	R			76% (513/677)
Castellino et al (2000)[73]	V2.2	DC	R	90% (979/1083)	98% (399/406)	86% (580/677)
Garvican and Field (2001)[71]	V2.0	MC	R	52% (15/29)		
Moberg et al (2001)[72]	V1.2	MC	R	50% (13/26)		
Taft and Taylor (2001)[67]	CADx	DC	R	88% (88/100)		
		MC		63% (12/19)		
Birdwell et al (2001)[56]	V2.0	MC	R	76% (86/113)	86% (30/35)	72% (56/78)
Freer and Ulissey (2001)[80]	V2.0	DC + MC	P	82% (40/49)	100% (22/22)	67% (18/27)
Evans et al (2002)[68]	V2.2	DC	R	91% (86/94)	100% (10/10)	95% (53/56)
		MC		77% (24/31)	83% (5/6)	93% (13/14)
Brem et al (2003)[69]	CADx V3.4	MC	R	65% (80/123)		
Baker et al (2003)[76]	V2.5	DC	R	48% (13/27)		
	CADx 4.0	DC	R	19% (5/27)		

DC, detected cancers; MC, missed cancers; P, prospective; R, retrospective.
*Superscript numbers indicate chapter references.
†These studies used the Image Checker (R2 Technology, Inc., Los Altos, CA) version 1.0 (V1.0), 1.2 (V1.2), 2.0 (V2.0), or 2.2 (V2.2) or Second Look (CADx Systems, Beaverhook, OH) version 3.4 (V3.4) or 4.0 (V4.0).
‡Total cancers include calcifications, masses, architectural distortion, and focal asymmetrical densities.

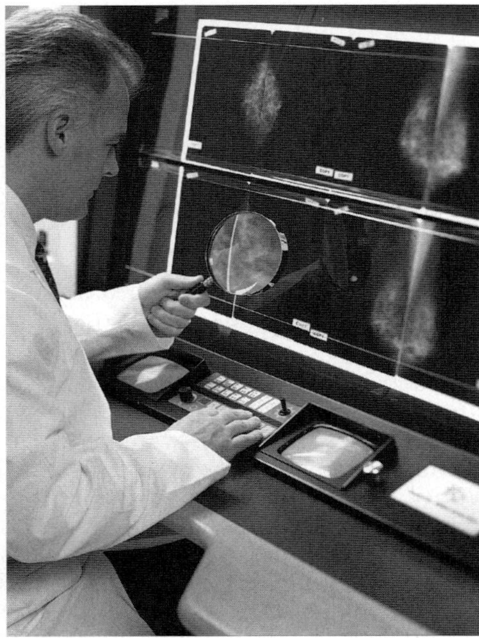

Figure 13–19. Mammography interpretation at the viewbox with computer-aided detection. (Courtesy of R-2 Technology Inc., Sunnyvale, CA.)

Nakahara and coworkers[74] found that CAD could identify 86% (55/65) of cancers that were detected by his group of radiologists in Japan, including 100% (22/22) of malignant calcifications and 79% (34/43) of malignant masses. Among 94 cases of invasive lobular carcinoma detected at screening mammography, Evans and associates[68] found that retrospective evaluation by CAD marked 95% (53/56) of masses, 85% (17/20) of architectural distortions, 75% (6/8) of asymmetrical densities, and 100% (10/10) of calcifications that represented the tumors. Among invasive lobular carcinomas identified in retrospect on previous mammograms that had been interpreted as normal, these investigators found that CAD identified 93% (13/14) of masses, 50% (3/6) of architectural distortions, 60% (3/5) of asymmetrical densities, and 83% (3/8) of calcifications that represented tumor.

A study by Vyborny and associates[75] assessed the effect of spiculation on CAD. Malignant masses were labeled as either nonspiculated or spiculated by three radiologists on separate reviews. Masses considered spiculated were termed "possibly spiculated," "spiculated," or "clearly spiculated." Among 677 malignant masses, 14% (92/677) were considered not spiculated, 13% (87/677) were possibly spiculated, 18% (123/677) were spiculated, and 55% (375/677) were clearly spiculated. CAD results were then compared with radiologist ratings for spiculation. The CAD system marked 86% (322/375) of clearly spiculated masses, 72% (89/123) of spiculated masses, 61% (53/87) of possibly spiculated masses, and 53% (49/92) of masses that were not spiculated. When similar categories were combined, 74% (498/677) of breast masses were considered spiculated or clearly spiculated and 26% (179/677) were considered not spiculated or possibly spiculated by at least two of the three radiologists. When these groupings were used, CAD marked 83% (411/498) of masses in the combined spiculated and highly spiculated categories and 57% (102/179) of masses classified as either possibly spiculated or nonspiculated.

Vyborny and associates[75] also assessed these malignant masses for their subtlety apart from the presence or absence of spiculation. Among the malignant masses, 13% (88/677) were considered subtle, 23% (154/677) were moderately well visualized, and 64% (435/677) were obvious. In these three groups, CAD marked 45% (40/88), 61% (94/154), and 87% (379/435), respectively. Thus, sensitivity of CAD was highest for masses that were obvious and lowest for masses that were subtle. The investigators also evaluated the effect of breast density on CAD, finding that CAD performance appeared to be independent of density.

Brem and colleagues[69] found that CAD identified 65% (80/123) of missed cancers (masses and calcifications combined) that were seen by experts on retrospective review of previous mammograms. Using spiculated cancers that were detected by radiologists on screening mammograms, Baker and associates[76] compared the performance of two commercially available CAD systems. One CAD system detected distortion in 48% (13/27) of cases. The other CAD system identified distortion in 19% (5/27) of cases in the same set. When the sample set was expanded to include both malignant and benign cases with distortion, the detection rates of the two systems were 49% (22/45) and 33% (15/45), respectively.

In summary, detection sensitivity of CAD is higher for calcifications than for masses. Masses that do not contain calcifications or spiculation that is not prominent are less likely to be identified by CAD. Cancers in which the mass appears subtle to radiologists or also looks like an architectural distortion or asymmetrical density rather than a mass are also less likely to be flagged by CAD.

How Well Does CAD Improve Cancer Detection Rates for Expert versus Nonexpert Readers?

Several studies also suggest that the additive value of CAD depends on the experience of the radiologist. Nawano and colleagues[77] had five doctors who did not specialize in mammography perform retrospective readings on mammograms of 43 women with palpable breast cancer and 43 normal women. Images were also evaluated by a research CAD software system. When the radiologists interpreted studies with the use of CAD, there were significant ($P < 0.02$) increases (0.92 vs 0.84) in the area under the receiver operating characteristic (ROC) curve, which plots true-positive fraction as a function of false-positive fraction.

Using a research CAD system, Kegelmeyer and associates[78] had four radiologists perform a blinded retrospective review both with and without the assistance of CAD on mammograms of 36 spiculated cancers that had been detected at screening mixed with 49 normal mammograms. The computer reports increased the average radiologist sensitivity by 9.7% (range 3% to 14%), moving from 80.6% to 90.3% with no decrease in average specificity. The radiologists ranged in experience from a third-year resident to the head of the radiology department. The amount of improvement resulting from CAD was generally inversely proportional to the radiologist's level of experience.

A study by Thurfjell and coworkers[79] suggested that even some experienced radiologists may benefit from CAD. Three radiologists interpreted 120 mammographic examinations from a first screening round in Uppsala, Sweden. Among these 120 cases, 32 cancers had been detected at the first screening round, 10 cancers surfaced clinically during the subsequent interval between screens, and 32 cancers were not detected until the second round; 46 mammograms were normal at both screening rounds. Thus, the material contained a wide range from obvious cases to those that were very subtle and had escaped detection at the first screening round. The CAD system correctly marked 37 cancers, 30 of the 32 cancers that had been detected in the first screening round and 7 of the 32 cancers that were not detected until the second screening round. On retrospective review of these 120 cases, one radiologist, an expert screener with 30 years of experience in mammography including 15 years in mass screening, detected 44 cancers without the aid of CAD. These included all 37 cancers that were marked by CAD. The second radiologist, with 5 years of experience in mammography including 2 years performing mass screening, detected 42 cancers alone and 43 cases when aided by CAD. The third radiologist had 7 years of experience in mammography; she detected 35 cases without CAD and 38 cancers with CAD prompting. Thus, the additive value of CAD seemed to vary among radiologists and to depend on their experience and skill.

Encouraged by results from retrospective studies such as those of Warren-Burhenne and associates[65] and Birdwell and colleagues,[56] Freer and Ulissey[80] performed prospective interpretation of 12,860 mammograms over a 2-year period using the Image Checker M1000 version 2.0 (R2 Technology, Inc., Los Angeles, CA) at their private practice office in Texas. Among these screening studies, 3437 (27%) represented a baseline evaluation, and the remaining 9423 (73%) had previous mammograms available for comparison. Each mammogram was read twice by a radiologist, first without CAD and then after CAD input. With CAD, the detection rate increased from 3.2% (41/12,860) to 3.8% (49/12,860). There was a 19.5% increase in the number of cancers detected, and the proportion of detected malignancies that were early stage (0 and 1) rose from 73% to 78%. CAD located all 22 cancers seen as calcifications; radiologists had initially detected 15, finding the other 7 after CAD prompting. Among 27 cancers that appeared to be masses, the radiologists originally detected 26 without help from CAD and corroborated an additional case after CAD review. CAD located 18 malignant masses and missed 9. Although CAD led to improved cancer detection rates, prospective CAD sensitivity was 67% for masses versus 100% for malignant calcifications.

These encouraging results are at variance with those from two other studies. Brem and colleagues[81] challenged an R-2 CAD system by using dedicated mammographers who were given 42 mammograms with malignant microcalcifications, 40 with benign microcalcifications, and 24 normal mammograms. Ninety-eight percent (41/42) of malignant calcifications and 80% (32/40) of benign microcalcifications were flagged by the CAD system. The mean sensitivity for malignant microcalcification detection was 89.6% (±6.3 SD) for the radiologists alone and 91.8% (±3.9 SD) for the radiologists with the CAD system. The mean difference without and with the CAD system was 2.2% (range 0 to 7%). The major reason that CAD did not increase the radiologists' detection rate more in this study was not that CAD did not flag enough malignant calcifications but that the radiologists were not sufficiently suspicious of the 98% of malignant microcalcifications that were marked by CAD.

In a retrospective study, Moberg and coworkers[72] found that the addition of CAD (R-2 Image Checker V1.2) did not improve the detection rates for interval cancers found by expert reviewers subsequent to normal screening examinations. Readers had 2 to 8 years of experience in screening and 5 to 10 years of experience in reading clinical mammograms.

Gur and associates[82] assessed changes in cancer detection rates among 24 radiologists in a clinical practice in Pittsburgh after the introduction of a computer-aided R-2 detection system. The investigators found no statistically significant change (3.49% before vs. 3.55% after) in breast cancer detection rates for the entire group of radiologists or for the subset of radiologists who interpreted high volumes of mammograms. On reanalysis of the data, Feig and coworkers[83] pointed out that the low-volume readers had a 19.7% (3.64 versus 3.05) increase in cancer detection rate that was not statistically significant ($P = 0.37$). Additionally, the study had a weakness inherent in any longitudinal study that compares detection rates for mammograms performed during two different time periods.

Nevertheless, similar results were obtained in a retrospective review of interval and screen-detected cancers interpreted without and with CAD (R-2 Image Checker 1,000) in Great Britain. Taylor and associates[84] found no difference in cancer detection sensitivity (0.78 vs. 0.78). No difference due to CAD was found for either well or poorly performing film readers.

How Does CAD Affect Interpretation Time, Screening Recall Rates, Recommendations for Short-Term Follow-Up, and False-Positive Biopsy Rates?

Successful clinical application of CAD to screening mammography requires higher detection rates without any excessive increase in interpretation time, recall rates, and false-positive biopsies. Current detection algorithms are heavily weighted toward sensitivity, thereby sacrificing the specificity of any computer-generated mark on the mammogram. On the basis of observational-judgment skills that no computer can yet duplicate, the radiologists can act on or ignore any marks that the computer has made to indicate possible masses or calcifications.

In their separate studies of CAD, Freer and Ulissey[80] and Birdwell and colleagues[56] found that the computer made 2.8 and 2.9 marks, respectively, per four-view screening mammogram on locations that were not cancer. Of the marks made by the computer in the Freer and Ulissey study,[80] 97% were dismissed without the need for additional mammographic views. Although no study has yet addressed the potential effect of CAD on interpretation time, it would seem that any increase would be relatively small.

Recall rates refer to the percentage of patients asked to return immediately for additional imaging evaluation after batch interpretation of their screening mammograms. Recall rates that are too high lead to patient inconvenience and anxiety as well as higher cost and greater inefficiency of the screening process. Excessive recall rates represent a disincentive for clinicians to advise screening, for patients to undergo screening, for radiologists to perform screening, and for medical care payers to support screening. If, however, recall rates are too low, some subtle cancers may be missed, and benign lesions may undergo unnecessary biopsy when supplementary views and ultrasonography are not performed to provide more definitive evaluation of findings detected at screening.

The American College of Radiology (ACR)[85] recommends that the screening recall rate be 10% or less. Because of the availability of previous films for comparison, recall rates for periodic screenings can be lower than those for initial screenings.[86] Yankaskas and coworkers[87] estimated that a recall rate of 4.9% to 5.5% represents the best tradeoff between sensitivity and positive predictive value.

Most clinical studies suggest that the effect of CAD on recall rates is very slight. Warren-Burhenne and colleagues[65] calculated the recall rates of 14 radiologists at five facilities over a 4-month period before CAD was available. Their average recall rate for screening studies was 8.3% (1961/23,682). With the aid of CAD, the same radiologists had a recall rate of 7.6% (1126/14,817). Several of the studies suggest that CAD does not reduce specificity or increase recall rates for highly experienced readers but does raise recall rates for less experienced readers.[71,72]

In the study by Freer and Ulissey,[80] each of 12,860 screening mammograms was first interpreted without CAD and then immediately after CAD. Average recall rates for these readings were 6.5% (830/12,860) and 7.7% (986/12,860), respectively. Gur and associates[82] found that CAD had no effect on recall rates, which they found to be 11.39% (6430/56,532) without CAD and 11.40% (6,741/59,139) with CAD. Data from a study by Garvican and coworkers[71] suggest that for less experienced readers, CAD may result in a greater increase in recall rates.

Freer and Ulissey[80] also found a slight increase in the number of lesions assigned to the probably benign (ACR Breast Imaging Reporting and Data System [BI-RADS] 3) category: 1.9% (257/12,860) before CAD and 2.3% (298/12,860) when studies were interpreted with CAD. Probably benign lesions have an extremely low likelihood of malignancy (usually less than 1%).[88] Immediate biopsy of such lesions is not recommended.[85] Rather, short-interval mammographic follow-up, usually 6 months after the screening examination, is recommended. Biopsy is then advised only for the few lesions (usually less than 4%) that have changed in size or appearance.

The *positive predictive value* (PPV) is commonly defined as the percentage of biopsies performed as a result of a "positive" mammographic finding that resulted in a diagnosis of cancer. A PPV that is too low indicates an excessive rate of false-positive biopsies. A PPV that is too high suggests that some cancers having an atypical appearance for malignancy are being missed. An appropriate value for PPV depends on factors such as age, breast cancer risk, and clinical signs and symptoms, which vary from one practice population to another. Therefore, the ACR[85] recommends a PPV in the range of 25% to 40%. In their study, Freer and Ulissey[80] found that CAD had no effect on the PPV of 38% at their center.

Computer-Aided Diagnosis

Computerized methods are also being developed to help the radiologist assess the likelihood of malignancy for a given lesion. The input into such schemes may come directly from computer vision or from the radiologist. These artificial intelligence techniques include discriminant analysis methods, rule-based expert systems, and artificial neural networks. The aim of such systems is to reduce the number of false-positive biopsies with virtually no loss in biopsies of malignant lesions.

The computer vision characterization scheme used by Giger and associates[33] to distinguish benign from potentially malignant masses is based on the presence or absence and degree of spiculation of the mass margins. Characteristics used to classify calcifications by other computer-extracted feature schemes used have included the number of calcifications in a cluster, spatial relationship among the calcifications in a cluster, length and width of clusters, and shape and border characteristics of individual particles. Thus far, no artificial intelligence system that derives its input directly from a mammographic image has been shown to improve accuracy of diagnosis beyond that of the unaided radiologist.

Computer classification schemes that derive their input from subjective identification and interpretation of mammographic features by a radiologist have been based on discriminant analysis,[89-91] rule-based expert systems, and artificial neural networks.[39] Input from the radiologist may come in the form of a checklist entry system. Both radiographs and clinical information may be included.[92,93] Although systems based on input from the radiologist do seem to be of value to radiologists who are not proficient in breast imaging, even these systems have not been shown to help radiologists who are more expert.[49,94]

The potential ability of computers to distinguish benign from malignant masses and calcifications could be limited by the reliability and applicability of mammographic signs that compose the database input. The intelligence of the computer depends on how well it is taught. Over the years, radiologists have found many features to differentiate benign from malignant masses[95] and calcifications.[96] Better determination of the reliability of these signs as well as identification of new signs should be a high-priority goal.

Computer Assessment of Breast Density and Breast Cancer Risk

Following pioneering work by Wolfe,[97] Boyd and Yaffe have been assessing whether quantitative analysis of density data and textures of digitized film mammograms of asymptomatic women can allow prediction of future risk of breast cancer.[98,99] Good evidence now exists that this is the case,[98] and a relative risk factor of 4 to 6 has been associated with high-density versus low-density mammographic patterns. Density scores and other relevant information could be automatically extracted from digital mammograms to help, for example, in defining the optimal screening interval for different risk groups or to monitor whether risk can be reduced by dietary or drug interventions.[99]

TELEMAMMOGRAPHY

Telemammography is the transmission of mammographic images from one location to another in digital format. These locations can be within a particular facility—for example, the mammography clinic and the operating room. Alternatively, the images can be sent over much longer distances, such as between a mammography unit in a remote facility lacking a qualified interpreting physician and a center of expertise where interpretation or consultation would be provided.[100-102]

Although teleradiology is commonly used in many areas of radiology,[103] telemammography is currently only used to a very limited extent.[104,105] A number of different technologies are available for digital image data transmission (Table 13–8). Many health care facilities are now equipped with fiberoptic communications infrastructures and network backbones allowing multiple users to communicate at 100 Mbit/second or 1Gbit/second transmission rates. At 100 Mbit/second, an image composed of 100-μm pixels can be sent from one location to another in about 1 second, and a 50-μm pixel image in about 4 seconds. With the higher speed connection, the transmission times are truly negligible, although it must be remembered that generally, the communication lines are shared with other digital image traffic. PACSs have very-high-speed servers designed to cope with many connections at a time. At these transmission speeds, it is doubtful that image compression is worthwhile, and compression may slow down transmission if the workstation is underpowered.

For transmission between facilities, there are a number of possibilities. Standard Internet connections such as "high-speed" or ADSL (asynchronous digital subscriber line) are likely to be much too slow, especially for high-volume situations, although they might be acceptable for occasional consultations between radiologists or with surgeons. T1 or higher-speed Internet connections may be practical. It is also possible to use wireless links between facilities if the distances involved are sufficiently short. In all cases, if public communications channels are to be used, appropriate attention must be given to security of medical data. This involves establishing Virtual Private Networks (VPNs) or encryption of data. Authentication of users and control over the use of the images must be handled in a way that meets legal and regulatory standards (e.g., Health Insurance Portability and Accountability Act [HIPAA]). Medical images are currently stored and transmitted within a facility using DICOM standards. This method works within a local secure

Table 13–8. Transmission of Digital Images with Various Currently Available Technologies*

Transmission Method	ISDN 56K	TCP/IP T1 Native NT-4	TCP/IP T1 NT-5	TCP/IP 100BT
Effective Mbits/sec	0.057	0.126	1.544	100
Time for 1 image	2.3 hr	35 min	190 sec	3 sec
Time for patient	9.3 hr	140 min	12.7 min	12 sec
Patients/day	1	3	38	2400

*Times are based on images composed of 50-μm pixels.

environment, but security considerations and the overhead involved with DICOM "handshaking" (authentication of each transmission) suggest that another protocol should be used between facilities or over the public media.

A common method for sending digital data through a network involves the division of information into "packets." Each packet has a label so that when information is sent it can be reassembled at the receiving end even though the individual packets may not arrive in the order that they were sent. In the most familiar protocol, known as TCP/IP (transmission control protocol/Internet protocol), the receipt of each packet is acknowledged, and if a packet is not received within a predefined period, it is resent. In this way, TCP/IP provides error-free service. In addition, because the cost of the communication link may be based on the amount of information transmitted, image compression may be desirable under these conditions.[106]

Technically, one can separate the telemammography system into two levels, (1) the basic network hardware and software and (2) a "user application" with which the operator/radiologist interacts. Because the technology of image communication is likely to undergo rapid change and improvement, it is important to provide this separation so that the system will appear more or less the same to the user even though drastic modifications may be made at the basic network level to enhance performance as technology develops.

The telemammography system must not degrade the diagnostic quality of the mammograms. Therefore, any data coding, compression, and display strategies must maintain the high intrinsic quality of the images and must introduce no unacceptable artifacts. Image compression might have to be performed to reduce transmission costs and increase speed. It can be either loss-less (no information is deleted from the image) or "lossy." A popular type of loss-less compression is the LempelZivWelch (LZW) algorithm, which is used in most modems and in GIF images. Although lossy compression such as wavelet compression can provide greater compression ratios—reduction of the amount of data in an image by a factor of 10 or more—the more moderate gains (a factor of 2 to 3) obtained with loss-less compression may be preferable for legal reasons and may be completely satisfactory with high-speed transmission.

The transmission speed (and cost) depends on the type of network technology that is employed. The requirements for speed depend on the total number of images to be sent. Another consideration is whether the images are to be sent as a batch, perhaps overnight, or sent and interpreted in real time. For batch transmission, even networks of modest speed may be acceptable, if the images can be sent during times when the network is not heavily loaded. For real-time applications, even slight delays of several seconds may be disturbing to the radiologist, and if the utilization approaches the rated bandwidth, the packet error rate will rise and the throughput will be seriously degraded because the network is occupied with resending packets.

Depending on needs and budget, image transmission could be carried out over standard T1 telephone links (1.544 Mbit/sec) or higher-speed asynchronous transfer mode (ATM) links. For more remote locations where the infrastructure for these links may not exist, satellite communication may be more appropriate, despite the higher initial setup cost, because it can provide arbitrarily high speed (based on price and size of antenna) and can be operated virtually anywhere, including mobile vans.

Several possible applications of telemammography can be anticipated. At present, when diagnostic mammography is performed in the absence of an on-site expert radiologist, patients may need to make a second appointment to receive supplementary views so that their breast problem can be adequately evaluated. Telemammography would allow radiologists to monitor and interpret problem-solving mammography on line from a nearby or even distant location. Screening studies could also be read remotely, eliminating the need to transport films from the remote fixed site or mobile van to the main facility. Clinical images could be remotely monitored for technical quality as they are performed so that patients would not have to return for second exposures. Telemammography could also facilitate second-opinion interpretation by nationally recognized experts. Radiologists at different locations could see and discuss the same case simultaneously. Interactive teaching conferences could be conducted between different sites. Finally, mammographic images could be transmitted to the offices of referring physicians, expediting patient care and eliminating the need for patients to transport and possibly misplace their mammograms.

DUAL-ENERGY MAMMOGRAPHY, TOMOSYNTHESIS, AND CONTRAST-ENHANCED DIGITAL MAMMOGRAPHY

It has been suggested that even if the contrast limitations of film-screen mammography were overcome with digital mammography, some lesions would still be missed, particularly in dense breasts, because of the complexity of overlying fibroglandular structures. Unwanted contrasts caused by these structures form "clutter" noise, which masks the structures of greatest interest. The availability of digital imaging facilitates the implementation of techniques to increase lesion conspicuity. One technique is dual-energy mammography.[107] If digital images with two substantially different x-ray spectra are combined, they produce hybrid images in which the contrast of relevant structures is preserved while the unwanted masking contrasts are largely removed. This process could be done at the viewing station so that various structures within the image can be surveyed dynamically.

Another way to reduce image clutter is to provide tomographic images of the breast. While dedicated breast CT systems are under investigation, possibly a simpler way to remove out-of-plane information is to perform a variant of blurring tomography called tomosynthesis.[108] Tomosynthesis can be built as a modification to a digital mammography system, primarily by allowing the x-ray tube support to be rotated about a pivot point located near the breast as in Figure 13–20. In tomosynthesis, a number of exposures are produced with the x-ray beam incident upon the breast at different angles ranging over approximately ±20 degrees from the normal. After each exposure, the digital image is read out and recorded. Shifting the images with respect to one another and adding them appropriately allows "reconstruction" of different planes in the breast, providing good isolation of the anatomy and three-dimensional information about the location of structures within the breast.

Still another way of simplifying the image and increasing the conspicuity of relevant structures is by digital subtraction imaging.[109,110] In this technique, the breast is compressed lightly to avoid disrupting blood flow and then is imaged at high kilovoltage to suppress soft tissue contrast and allow a low radiation dose to be used. Then, an intravenous injection of non-ionic iodine contrast medium is administered, and a series of low-dose digital images is obtained. If logarithms of the mask and post-injection images are taken and the mask is subtracted from each subsequent image, the breast anatomy is largely eliminated except where iodine has accumulated (Fig. 13–21). This accumulation generally occurs in areas of angiogenesis, a process that frequently accompanies the development of a lesion. From the series of images, which might be acquired every 2 minutes out to 10 minutes, kinetic data on uptake and washout in a focal area of interest can also be computed. The combination of morphology of the area of uptake and the rates of uptake and washout may be helpful in characterizing lesions. The fact that the image is based on functional rather than simply anatomic changes associated with cancer may help the radiologist better identify the extent of disease for the surgeon.

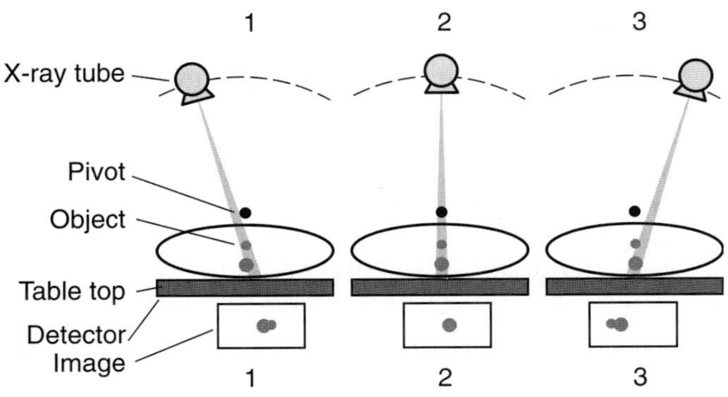

Figure 13–20. Schematic of tomosynthesis imaging system based on digital mammography.

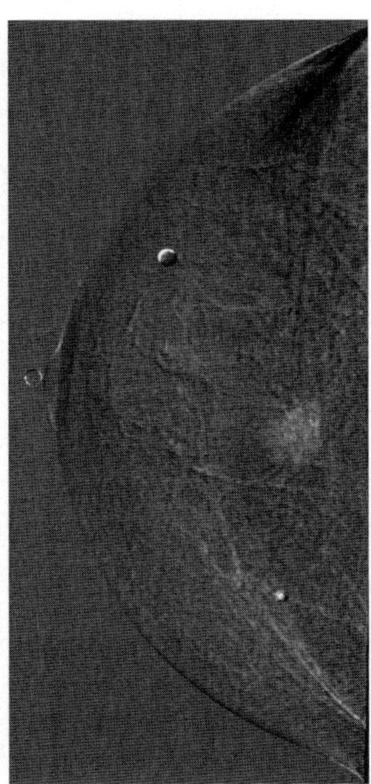

Figure 13–21. Contrast subtraction digital mammogram illustrating angiogenesis in the location of an infiltrating ductal carcinoma.

CLINICAL SCREENING TRIALS

Several studies have compared digital mammography with screen-film mammography for cancer detection and specificity among screened women. Lewin and associates[111,112] screened 4945 women at two institutions in Colorado and Massachusetts. Each woman underwent both conventional and digital mammography, performed on General Electric units. All images were interpreted independently. Thirty-five cancers were detected, 22 with screen-film mammography and 21 with digital mammography. Digital mammography had a slightly but statistically significant lower recall rate (11.5% versus 13.8%, $P < 0.03$).

In a similarly designed trial performed on 3683 women in Norway, Skaane and colleagues[113] found that screen-film mammography depicted 28 malignancies and that digital mammography performed using a General Electric unit depicted 23 malignancies. The difference between cancer detection rates was not significant ($P = 0.23$). The recall rate for digital mammography was slightly higher than that for conventional mammography (4.6% versus 3.5%). The investigators attributed this difference to a learning curve effect.

The Digital Mammographic Imaging Screening Trial (D-MIST), supported by the American College of Radiology Imaging Network (ACRIN) and the National Cancer Institute (NCI), has completed accrual of 49,528 women at 34 centers in the United States and Canada.[114,115] Each woman underwent both conventional and digital mammography with independent interpretation. Digital images were acquired on five different types of units—General Electric, Fischer, Fuji, Hologic, and Trex. Accrual of subjects was completed in March 2004. Follow-up will continue through January 2005. Analysis and presentation of data are expected in early 2005 with publication in late 2005.

CONCLUSIONS

The rationale for digital mammography and several approaches to design of digital mammography systems have been described. Problems still remaining to be solved in development of a practical digital mammography system have been discussed, and some of the applications that can be attempted with digital mammography and computer-aided detection (CAD) have been considered.

Although digital mammography has many potential advantages, not least of which may be the ability to provide better images of dense tissue owing to contrast enhancement, it has several potential disadvantages (Table 13–9). Undoubtedly, many of these drawbacks can be minimized through technical progress. However, clinical trials are necessary to reassess the relative advantages and disadvantages of digital mammography at each stage in its technologic progress.

Table 13–9. Potential Advantages and Disadvantages of Digital Mammography Compared with Conventional Film-Screen Mammography

Potential advantages	
Primary	Increased image contrast
	Wider display latitude
	Ability to alter contrast and latitude of selected areas or entire image after exposure
	Lower detector noise
Secondary	Picture archiving and retrieval
	Computer-aided detection
	Computer-aided diagnosis
	Telemammography
	Computer assessment of breast density and breast cancer risk
	Dual-energy mammography
	Tomosynthesis
	Contrast-enhanced digital mammography
Potential disadvantages and technical challenges	Lower detection resolution
	Limited resolution of display monitors
	Design of efficient workstation
	More costly system
	Extremely large data storage requirement
	Raster noise of monitor

One major question relates to the degree of resolution necessary for digital mammography to image fine detail of microcalcifications and mass margins. Current screen-film systems have a resolution equivalent to approximately 0.025-mm pixels. It is not known whether a digital system with a pixel size of 0.1 mm will be adequate because of its higher contrast and lower noise. A prospective clinical study involving large numbers of subtle lesions may be necessary to resolve this question, especially because other factors, such as relative exposure times, also affect resolution.

Another problem is that digital mammography requires a display monitor of at least 4000 × 4000 pixels. Currently available medical monitors can display only 2048 × 2560 pixels; however, improvement is expected in the next 5 years. Laser cameras are capable of producing a 0.05-mm pixel hard-copy image. Moreover, hard-copy laser camera images have less inherent noise than display monitors.

The ability of digital mammography to include as much posterior tissue as screen-film mammography on the mediolateral oblique view is another potential concern because of the larger size and shape of many digital mammography image receptors. The effect of the relatively longer exposure times of digital mammography on motion unsharpness of clinical images also must be assessed.

The cost of a digital mammography unit is in the range $300,000 to $400,000, compared with about $90,000 for a top-of-the-line screen-film unit. Additional equipment for digital image processing, display, and storage will add further substantial costs. These costs must be weighed against potential advantages of digital mammography for better detection and diagnosis and possible improvements in efficiency.

One final challenge will be development of an interpretation setup that is as efficient as when the radiologist places old and new routine and supplementary film-screen mammographic views side by side on a viewbox. It is not yet certain whether digital mammography, after contrast enhancement on the monitor, will be interpreted from an ergonomically efficient workstation composed of banks of monitors or from hard-copy films.

Substantial numbers of cancers are missed at screening mammography interpretation, and many of these may be retrospectively identified on either blinded or nonblinded review. CAD has been able to identify a portion of missed cancers. Performance of CAD is better for calcifications than for masses. CAD can more easily identify masses that are strongly speculated or contain calcifications than subtle masses, architectural distortions, and asymmetrical densities. The incremental value of CAD may vary inversely according to the interpretive skill of the radiologist.

Although many more studies are needed for confirmation, initial investigations indicate that for some radiologists, CAD can improve screening detection rates with no undue effect on rates for additional imaging, short-term follow-up or false-positive biopsies.

References

1. Haus AG: Dedicated mammographic x-ray equipment, screen-film-processing systems, and viewing conditions for mammography. Semin Breast Dis 1999;2:30-54.
2. Haus AG, Yaffe MJ: Screen-film and digital mammography: Image quality and radiation dose considerations. Radiol Clin North Am 2000;38:871-898.
3. Rothenberg LH, Feig SA, Haus AG, et al: A guide to mammography and other breast imaging procedures. (NCRP Report No. 72.) Bethesda, MD, National Council on Radiation Protection and Measurements, 2004.
4. Johns PC, Yaffe MJ: X-ray characterization of normal and neoplastic breast tissues. Phys Med Biol 1987;32:675-695.
5. Feig SA, Shaber GS, Patchefsky A: Analysis of clinically occult and mammographically occult breast tumors. AJR Am J Roentgenol 1977;128:403-408.
6. Wagner AJ: Contrast and grid performance in mammography. In Barnes GT, Frey GD (eds): Screen-Film Mammography Imaging Considerations and Medical Physics Responsibilities. Madison, WI, Medical Physics Publishing, 1991, pp 115-134.
7. Freedman MT, Steler DE, Jafroudi H, et al: Digital mammography: Tradeoffs between 50 and 100 micron pixel size. Proc SPIE 1995;2432:114-125.
8. Kato H: Photostimulable phosphor radiology design considerations. In Seibert JA, Barnes GT, Gould RG (eds): Specification, Acceptance Testing and Quality Control of Diagnostic X-ray Imaging Equipment. (AAPM Monograph No. 20.) Woodbury, NY, American Institute of Physics, 1994, pp 303-357.
9. Nishikawa RM, Mawdsley GE, Fenster A, et al: Scanned projection digital mammography. Med Phys 1987;14:717-727.
10. Street RA: Hydrogenated Amorphous Silicon. New York, Cambridge University Press, 1991, p 391.
11. Rougeot H: Direct x-ray photoconversion processes. In Hendee WR, Trueblood JH (eds): Digital Imaging. Madison, WI, Medical Physics Publishing, 1993, pp 49-96.
12. Feig SA: Xeromammography. In Bassett LW, Gold RH (eds): Breast Cancer Detection: Mammography and Other Methods in Breast Imaging, 2nd ed. Orlando, FL, Grune & Stratton, 1987, pp 89-109.
13. Rowlands JA, Hunter DM, Araj N: X-ray imaging using amorphous selenium: A photoinduced discharge readout method for digital mammography. Med Phys 1991;18:421-431.
14. Zhao W, Rowlands JA, German S: Digital radiology using self-scanned readout of amorphous selenium: Design considerations for mammography. Proc SPIE 1995;2432:250-259.
15. Lee DL, Cheung LK, Jeromin LS: New digital detector for projection radiography. Proc SPIE 1995;2432:237-249.
16. Nelson RS, Barbaric Z, Bassett LW: Digital slot scan mammography using CCD's. Proc SPIE 1987;767:102-108.
17. Maidment AD, Fahrig R, Yaffe MJ: Dynamic range requirements in digital mammography. Med Phys 1993;20:1621-1633.
18. Holdsworth DW, Nishikawa RM, Mawdsley GE, et al: Slot beam digital mammography using a time-delay integration (TDI) CCD. Proc SPIE 1989;1090:306-313.
19. Fahrig R, Maidment AD, Yaffe MJ: Optimization of peak kilovoltage and spectral shape for digital mammography. Proc SPIE 1992;1651:74-83.
20. Barten PGJ: Physical model for the contrast sensitivity of the human eye. Proc SPIE 1992;1666:57-72.
21. Barten PGJ: Contrast Sensitivity of the Human Eye and its Effects on Image Quality. Bellingham, WA, SPIE Press, 1999.
22. Pisano ED, Cole EB, Major S, et al: Radiologist preference for imaging processing algorithm for different clinical tasks for digital mammography display. Radiology 2000;216:820-830.
23. Pisano ED, Cole EB, Hemminger BM, et al: Image processing algorithms for digital mammography—a pictorial essay. Radiographics 2000;20:1479-1491.
24. Bick U, Giger ML, Schmidt RA, et al: Peripheral density correction of digital mammographs. Radiographics 1996;16:1403-1411.
25. Byng JW, Critten JP, Yaffe MJ: Thickness equalization processing for mammographic images. Radiology 1997;203:564-568.
26. Anderson ED, Muir BB, Walsh JS, et al: The efficacy of double reading mammograms in breast screening. Clin Radiol 1994;49:248-251.
27. Thurfjell EL, Lernevall KA, Taube AAS: Benefit of independent double reading in a population-based mammography screening program. Radiology 1994;191:241-244.
28. Harvey SC, Geller B, Oppenheimer RG, et al: Increase in cancer detection and recall rates with independent double interpretation of screening mammography. AJR Am J Roentgenol 2003;180:1461-1467.
29. Vyborny CL: Can computers help radiologists read mammograms? Radiology 1994;191:315-317.
30. Feig SA, Galkin BM, Muir HD: Evaluation of breast microcalcifications by means of optically magnified tissue specimen radiographs. Recent Results Cancer Res 1987;105:111-123.
31. Moskowitz M: The predictive value of certain mammographic signs in screening for breast cancer. Cancer 1983;51:1007-1011.
32. Fisher ER, Gregorio RM, Fisher B, et al: The pathology of invasive breast cancer. Cancer 1975;36:1-85.
33. Giger ML: Computer-aided diagnosis. In Haus AG, Yaffe MJ (eds): Syllabus: A Categorical Course in Physics—Technical Aspects of Breast Imaging. Oak Brook, IL, Radiological Society of North America, 1999, pp 249-272.
34. Bick U, Giger ML, Schmidt RA, et al: Automated segmentation of digitized mammograms. Acad Radiol 1995;2:1-9.
35. Chan HP, Doi K, Galhotra S, et al: Image feature analysis and computer-aided diagnosis in digital radiography. I: Automated detection of microcalcifications in mammography. Med Phys 1987;14:538-548.
36. Nishikawa RM, Giger ML, Doi K, et al: Computer-aided detection of clustered microcalcifications on digital mammograms. Med Biol Eng Comput 1995;33:174-178.
37. Chan HP, Doi K, Vyborny CJ, et al: Improvement in radiologists' detection of clustered microcalcifications on mammograms: The potential of computer-aided diagnosis. Invest Radiol 1990;25:1102-1110.
38. Nishikawa RM, Giger ML, Doi K, et al: Computer-aided detection of clustered microcalcifications: An improved method for grouping detected signals. Med Phys 1993;20:1661-1666.
39. Wu Y, Doi K, Giger ML, et al: Computerized detection of clustered microcalcifications in digital mammograms: Applications of artificial neural networks. Med Phys 1992;19:555-560.
40. Wu Y, Giger ML, Doi K, et al: Artificial neural networks in mammography: Application to decision making in the diagnosis of breast cancer. Radiology 1993;187:81-87.
41. Zhang W, Doi K, Giger ML, et al: Computerized detection of clustered microcalcifications in digital mammograms using a shift-invariant-artificial neural network. Med Phys 1994;21:517-524.
42. Giger ML, Yin FF, Doi K, et al: Investigation of methods for the computerized detection and analysis of mammographic masses. Proc SPIE 1990;1233:183-184.
43. Kimme C, O'Loughlin BJ, Sklansky J: Automatic detection of suspicious abnormalities in breast radiographs. In Klinger A, Fu KS, Kunii TL (eds): Data Structures, Computer Graphics and Pattern Recognition. New York, Academic Press, 1975, pp 427-447.
44. Winsberg F, Elkin M, Macy J: Detection of radiographic abnormalities in mammograms by means of optical scanning and computer analysis. Radiology 1967;89:211-215.
45. Yin FF, Giger ML, Doi K, et al: Computerized detection of masses in digital mammograms: Analysis of bilateral subtraction images. Med Phys 1991;18:955-963.

46. Yin FF, Giger ML, Doi K, et al: Computerized detection of masses in digital mammograms: Investigation of feature-analysis techniques. J Digit Imaging 1994;7:18-26.
47. Yin FF, Giger ML, Vyborny CJ, et al: Comparison of bilateral-subtraction and single-image processing techniques in the computerized detection of masses. Invest Radiol 1993;28:473-481.
48. Brzakovic D, Luo XM, Brzakovic P: An approach to automated detection of tumors in mammograms. IEEE Trans Med Imaging 1990;9:233-241.
49. Kegelmeyer WP Jr, Pruneda JM, Bourland PD, et al: Computer-aided mammographic screening for spiculated lesions. Radiology 1994;191:331-337.
50. Lai SM, Li X, Bischof WF: On techniques for detecting circumscribed masses in mammograms. IEEE Trans Med Imaging 1989;8:377-386.
51. Attinen I, Pamilio M, Soiva M, et al: Double reading of mammography screening films: One radiologist or two? Clin Radiol 1993;48:414-421.
52. Anderson ED, Muir B, Walsh JS, et al: The efficacy of double reading mammograms in breast screening. Clin Radiol 1994;49:248-251.
53. Ciatto S, Turco MRD, Morrone D, et al: Independent double reading of screening mammograms. J Med Screening 1995;2:99-101.
54. Warren RM, Duffy SW: Comparison of single reading with double reading of mammograms and change in effectiveness with experience. Br J Radiol 1995;69:958-962.
55. Deans HE, Everington D, Cordiner C, et al: Scottish experience of double reading in the National Breast Screening Programme. The Breast 1998;7:75-79.
56. Birdwell RL, Ikeda DM, O'Shaughnessy KF, et al: Mammographic characteristics of 115 missed carcinomas later detected with screening mammography and the potential utility of computer-aided detection. Radiology 2001;219:192-202.
57. Martin JE, Moskowitz M, Milbrath JR: Breast cancer missed by mammography. AJR Am J Roentgenol 1979;132:737-739.
58. Bird RE, Wallace TW, Yankaskas BC: Analysis of cancers missed at screening mammography. Radiology 1992;184:613-617.
59. Harvey JA, Fajardo LL, Innis CA: Previous mammograms in patients with impalpable carcinoma: Retrospective vs blinded interpretation. AJR Am J Roentgenol 1993;161:1167-1172.
60. Moberg K, Grundstrom H, Tornberg S, et al: Two models for radiological reviewing of interval cancers. J Med Screen 1999;6:35-39.
61. Van Dijck J, Verbeek A, Hendriks J, Holland R: The current delectability of breast cancer in a mammographic screening program: A review of the previous mammograms of interval and screen-detected cancers. Cancer 1993;72:1933-1938.
62. Jones RD, McLean L, Young JR, et al: Proportion of cancers detected at the first incident screen which were false negative at the prevalent screen. The Breast 1996;5:339-343.
63. Daly CA, Apthorp L, Field S: Second round cancers: How many were visible on the first round of the UK National Breast Screening Programme, three years earlier? Clin Radiol 1998;53:25-28.
64. Vitak B: Invasive interval cancers in the Ostergotland Mammographic Programme: Radiological analysis. Eur Radiol 1998;8:639-646.
65. Warren-Burhenne LS, Wood SA, D'Orsi CJ, et al: Potential contribution of computer-aided detection to the sensitivity of screening mammography. Radiology 2000;215:554-562.
66. Yankaskas BC, Schell MJ, Bird RE, Desrochers DA: Reassessment of breast cancers missed during routine screening mammography: A community-based study. AJR Am J Roentgenol 2001;177:535-541.
67. Taft R, Taylor A: Potential improvement in breast cancer detection with a novel computer-aided detection system. Applied Radiol Dec 2001;25-28.
68. Evans WP, Warren-Burhenne LJ, Laurie L, et al: Invasive lobular carcinoma of the breast: Mammographic characteristics and computer-aided detection. Radiology 2002;225:182-189.
69. Brem RF, Baum J, Lechner M, et al: Improvement in sensitivity of screening mammography with computer-aided detection: A multiinstitutional trial. AJR Am J Roentgenol 2003;181:687-693.
70. te Brake GM, Karssemeijer N, Hendriks JH: Automated detection of breast carcinomas not detected in a screening program. Radiology 1998;207:465-471.
71. Garvican L, Field S: A pilot evaluation of the R-2 Image Checker System and user's response in the detection of interval breast cancers on previous screening films. Clin Radiol 2001;56:833-837.
72. Moberg K, Bjurstam N, Wilczek B, et al: Computer-assisted detection of interval breast cancers. Eur J Radiol 2001;139:104-110.
73. Castellino RA, Roehrig, J, Zhang W: Improved computer-aided detection (CAD) algorithms for screening mammography [abstract]. Radiology 2000;217(P):400.
74. Nakahara H, Namba K, Fukami A, et al: Computer-aided diagnosis (CAD) for mammography: Preliminary results. Breast Cancer 1998;5:401-405.
75. Vyborny CJ, Doi T, O'Shaughnessy KF, et al: Breast cancer: Importance of spiculation in computer-aided detection. Radiology 2000;215:703-707.
76. Baker JA, Rosen EL, Lo JY, et al: Computer-aided detection (CAD) in screening mammography: Sensitivity of commercial CAD systems for detecting architectural distortion. AJR Am J Roentgenol 2003;181:1083-1088.
77. Nawano S, Murakami K, Moriyama N, et al: Computer-aided diagnosis in full digital mammography. Invest Radiol 1999;34:310-316.
78. Kegelmeyer WP Jr, Pruneda JM, Bourland PD: Computer-aided mammographic screening for spiculated lesions. Radiology 1994;191:331-337.
79. Thurfjell E, Thurfjell MG, Egge E, Bjurstam N: Sensitivity and specificity of computer-assisted breast cancer detection in mammography screening. Acta Radiol 1998;39:384-388.
80. Freer TW, Ulissey MJ: Screening mammography with computer-aided detection: Prospective study of 12,860 patients in a community breast center. Radiology 2001;220:781-786.
81. Brem RF, Schoonjans JM: Radiologist detection of microcalcifications with and without computer-aided detection: A comparative study. Clin Radiol 2001;56:150-154.
82. Gur D, Sumkin JH, Rockette HE, et al: Changes in breast cancer detection and recall rates after the introduction of a computer-aided detection system. J Natl Cancer Inst 2004;96:185-190.
83. Feig SA, Sickles EA, Evans WP, et al: Changes in breast cancer detection rates (letter to the editor). J Natl Cancer Inst 2004;96:1260-1261.
84. Taylor PM, Champness J, Given-Wilson RM, et al: An evaluation of the impact of computer-based prompts on screen readers' interpretation of mammograms. Brit J Radiol 2004;77:21-27.
85. American College of Radiology (ACR): Breast Imaging Reporting and Data System (BI-RADS™), 4th ed. Reston, VA, American College of Radiology, 2003.
86. Hunt KA, Rosen EL, Sickles EA: Outcome analysis for women undergoing annual versus biennial screening mammography: A review of 24,211 examinations. AJR Am J Roentgenol 1999;173:285-289.
87. Yankaskas BC, Cleveland RJ, Schell MJ, et al: Association of recall rates with sensitivity and positive predictive values of screening mammography. AJR Am J Roentgenol 2001;177:543-549.
88. Sickles EA: Management of probably benign lesions. Radiol Clin North Am 1995;33:1123-1130.
89. Gale AB, Roebuck EJ, Riley P, et al: Computer aids to mammographic diagnosis. Br J Radiol 1987;60:887-891.
90. Getty DJ, Pickett RM, D'Orsi CJ, et al: Enhanced interpretation of diagnostic images. Invest Radiol 1988;23:240-252.
91. Swets JA, Getty DJ, Pickett RM, et al: Enhancing and evaluating diagnostic accuracy. Med Decis Making 1991;11:9-18.
92. Swett HA, Fisher PA, Cohn AI, et al: Expert system controlled image display. Radiology 1989;172:487-493.

93. Swett HA, Miller PA: ICON: A computer based approach to differential diagnosis in radiology. Radiology 1987;163:555-558.
94. Vyborny CJ, Giger ML: Computer vision and artificial intelligence in mammography. AJR Am J Roentgenol 1994;162:699-708.
95. Feig SA: Breast masses: Mammographic and sonographic evaluation. Radiol Clin North Am 1992;30:67-92.
96. Feig SA: Mammographic evaluation of calcifications. In Kopans DB, Mendelson EB (eds): Syllabus: Categorical Course in Breast Imaging. Oak Brook, IL, RSNA Publications, 1995, pp 93-105.
97. Wolfe JN: Risk for breast cancer development determined by mammographic parenchymal pattern. Cancer 1976;37:2486-2492.
98. Boyd NF, Byng JW, Jong RA, et al: Quantitative classification of mammographic densities and breast cancer risk: Results from the Canadian National Breast Screening Study. J Natl Cancer Inst 1995;87:670-675.
99. Yaffe MJ, Boyd NF: Mammographic image analysis of breast cancer risk assessment. Semin Breast Dis 2002;5:238-246.
100. Abdel-Malek A: Experience with a proposed teleradiology system for digital mammography. Proc SPIE 1995;2435:200-209.
101. Mattheus RA, Temmerman Y, Verhellen P, et al: Management system for a PACS network in a hospital environment. Proc SPIE 1991;1446:341-351.
102. Viitanen J, Sund T, Rinde E, et al: Nordic teleradiology development. Comp Methods Programs Biomed 1992;37:273-277.
103. Bidgood WD Jr, Staab EV: Understanding and using teleradiology. Semin Ultrasound CT MR 1992;13:102-112.
104. Sickles EA: Computer-aided diagnosis and telemammography: Clinical perspective. In Haus AG, Yaffe MJ (eds): Physical Aspects of Breast Imaging—Current and Future Considerations. Oak Brook, IL, RSNA Publications, 1999, pp 283-285.
105. Fajardo LL, Yoshino MT, Seeley GW, et al: Detection of breast abnormalities on teleradiology transmitted mammograms. Invest Radiol 1990;25:1111-1115.
106. Batnitzky S, Rosenthal SJ, Siegal EL, et al: Teleradiology: An assessment. Radiology 1990;177:11-17.
107. Johns PC, Yaffe MJ: Theoretical optimization of dual-energy x-ray imaging with application of mammography. Med Phys 1985;12:289-296.
108. Niklason LT, Christian BT, Niklason LE, et al: Digital tomosynthesis in breast imaging. Radiology 1997;205:399-406.
109. Lewin JM, Isaacs PK, Vance V, et al: Dual energy contrast-enhanced digital subtraction mammography—feasibility. Radiology 2003;229:261-268.
110. Jong RA, Yaffe MJ, Skarpathiotakis M, et al: Contrast digital mammography: Initial clinical experience. Radiology 2003;228:842-850.
111. Lewin JM, Hendrick RE, D'Orsi CJ, et al: Comparison of full-field digital mammography to screen-film mammography for cancer detection: results of 4945 paired examinations. Radiology 2001;218:873-880.
112. Lewin JM, D'Orsi CJ, Hendrick RE, et al: Clinical comparison of full-field digital mammography to screen-film mammography for breast cancer detection. AJR Am J Roentgenol 2002;179:671-677.
113. Skaane P, Young K, Skjennald: Population-based mammography screening: Comparison of screen-film and full-field digital mammography with soft-copy—Oslo I Study. Radiology 2003;229:877-884.
114. Pisano ED, Yaffe MJ, Hemminger BM, et al: Current status of full-field digital mammography. Acad Radiol 2000;7:266-280.
115. Pisano ED: Digital Mammographic Imaging Screening Trial: D-MIST. Syllabus, 31st National Conference on Breast Cancer. Reston, VA, American College of Radiology 2004, pp 191-204.

Magnetic Resonance Imaging of Breast Tumors

Nanette D. DeBruhl, Dawn Michael, and Lawrence W. Bassett

Magnetic resonance imaging (MRI) has rapidly progressed over the past several years to being a valuable modality for evaluating breast diseases. The first MRI studies for the evaluation of breast cancer were conducted in the mid-1980s and were based primarily on breast tissue characterization using T1-weighted and T2-weighted images.[1-6] These early investigations, without the benefit of MRI contrast agents, attempted to use calculated T1- and T2-weighted values and MRI signal intensities on various MRI sequences to differentiate malignant from benign breast tumors. The investigators theorized that malignant tumors would have specific cellular MRI characteristics that could be used to differentiate them from benign lesions. However, it became evident that the signal intensity of both benign and malignant lesions is predominantly determined by the water content as well as the cellular content of the breast tumors.[7] Malignant and benign lesions have high water content, and many malignant and benign tumors consist of extensive fibrosis. Therefore, the MRI signal intensities would not be sufficient to reliably differentiate malignant from benign breast lesions.

In 1986, Heywang and associates[8] first applied the use of an MRI contrast agent to determine whether this would improve differentiation of benign from malignant lesions. This technique involved obtaining one image before administration of the contrast agent (precontrast image) and two images obtained after administration of the agent (postcontrast images) with the use of limited temporal resolution, relatively high spatial resolution, and three-dimensional (3D) gradient echo, which revealed strong contrast enhancement of breast cancers relative to normal breast parenchyma. The results were encouraging, with most malignant tumors showing enhancement and most benign breast lesions not enhancing. Many investigators confirmed the initial experience with MRI contrast agents in breast lesions and further contributed their experience and expertise to MRI of the breast.[2,7-23]

A common obstacle of breast MRI research was technical restrictions. The early technology was limited in its ability to yield images with high spatial resolution and high temporal resolution simultaneously. Because of this limitation, researchers chose to explore only one of the two imaging techniques.

Temporal imaging, also referred to as *dynamic imaging*, primarily reported by the European investigators, focused on contrast uptake based on time using short (10- to 90-second), repetitive scans. They used dynamic, two-dimensional (2D) and 3D temporal imaging during gadolinium enhancement. Researchers using this methodology believed that the most useful information about breast lesions is the time course of gadolinium enhancement, also referred to as *kinetics* (Figs. 14–1 and 14–2).[2,7,8,11-18] Investigators initially believed that malignant tumors enhanced more quickly and more intensely than benign tumors.

As researchers continued investigating the characteristics of the uptake of contrast agent in lesions, the aspects of kinetic analysis further developed to include percentage enhancement, rate of enhancement, intensity of enhancement, time to peak enhancement (steepest slope), and time–signal intensity profiles. Kaiser and colleagues[17] initially investigated the percentage enhancement and tracked the rapid signal intensity changes that occur in the early postcontrast period. They focused on interpreting signal intensity relative to the baseline lesion signal intensity, instead of fatty tissue, according to the following equation:

$$[(SI_{post} - SI_{pre})/SI_{pre}] \times 100$$

where SI_{pre} represents signal intensity before contrast agent administration, and SI_{post} represents signal intensity after contrast agent administration.[17]

The theories presented by Gilles and associates[24] were based on the timing of lesion enhancement relative to arterial enhancement. These researchers proposed that any enhancement within the first postcontrast image should be considered malignant. Heywang and coworkers[11] assessed signal intensity of lesion enhancement in relation to the signal of fatty tissue using a normalization factor and units to allow for adjustments of MRI parameters that may have been used in different patients. The imaging was performed on 0.35-tesla (T) and 1-T magnets. On the basis of these criteria, results showed a sensitivity of 100% and a specificity of 27%.

Buadu and colleagues[25] described the steepest slope calculation that helped determine the time to peak enhancement, defined as the time between administration of contrast agent and maximum signal intensity value. Szabo and associates[26] determined the best diagnostic predictors for malignancy by using the following calculation:

$$Slope_i = E\ peak / T\ peak$$

where $Slope_i$ is the initial slope, *E peak* is maximum percent enhancement, and *T peak* is time to peak.

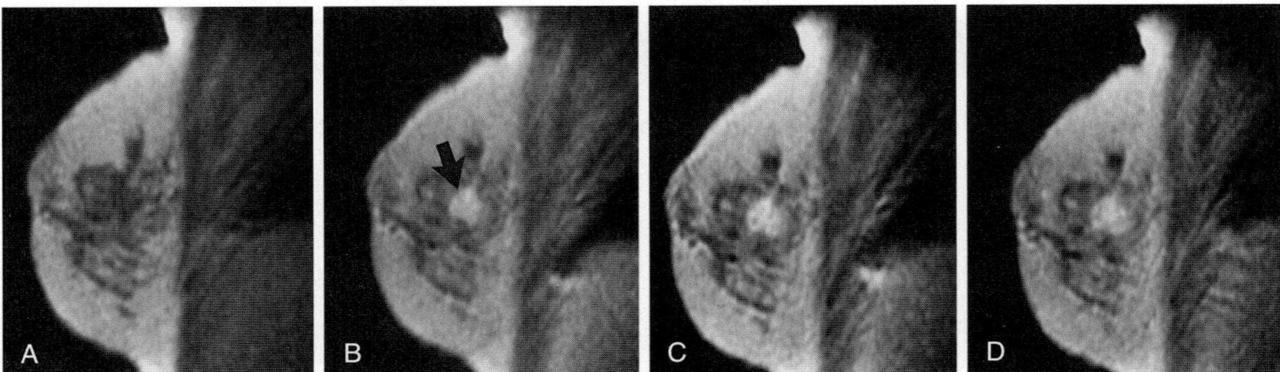

Figure 14–1. Two-dimensional dynamic sagittal (non–fat-suppressed) magnetic resonance images of an infiltrating ductal carcinoma (*arrow*). Images were obtained at 0 seconds (**A**), 60 seconds (**B**), 120 seconds (**C**), and 180 seconds (**D**) after administration of contrast agent. The irregular, heterogeneous, focal mass (*arrow*) enhanced rapidly, reaching peak intensity between 90 and 180 seconds.

Time–signal intensity curves described by Fischer and coworkers[27] and Kuhl and associates[28] expanded the postcontrast analysis period to include not only an early analysis but also intermediate and late postcontrast phases. They realized that valuable information could be ascertained from the time–signal intensity curve of any given lesion. This classification scheme was as follows (Fig. 14–3):

- *Type 1a:* Lesion continues to enhance over entire acquisition period.
- *Type 1b:* Lesion signal gain begins to slow down in the late postcontrast period, thus creating a bowing of the signal curve.
- *Type 2:* Lesion signal plateaus after the early increase.
- *Type 3:* Lesion loses signal intensity due to washout of contrast agent immediately after signal intensity peak.

Additional interpretations of the time–signal intensity curves proved that benign lesions and malignant intensity curves were significantly different. The distribution of curve types for benign lesions were as follows: type 1 = 83%, type 2 = 11.5%, and type 3 = 5.5 %. Conversely, malignant lesions showed the following distribution: type 1 = 8.9%, type 2 = 33.6%, and type 3 = 57.4%.[29] It appeared that benign lesions

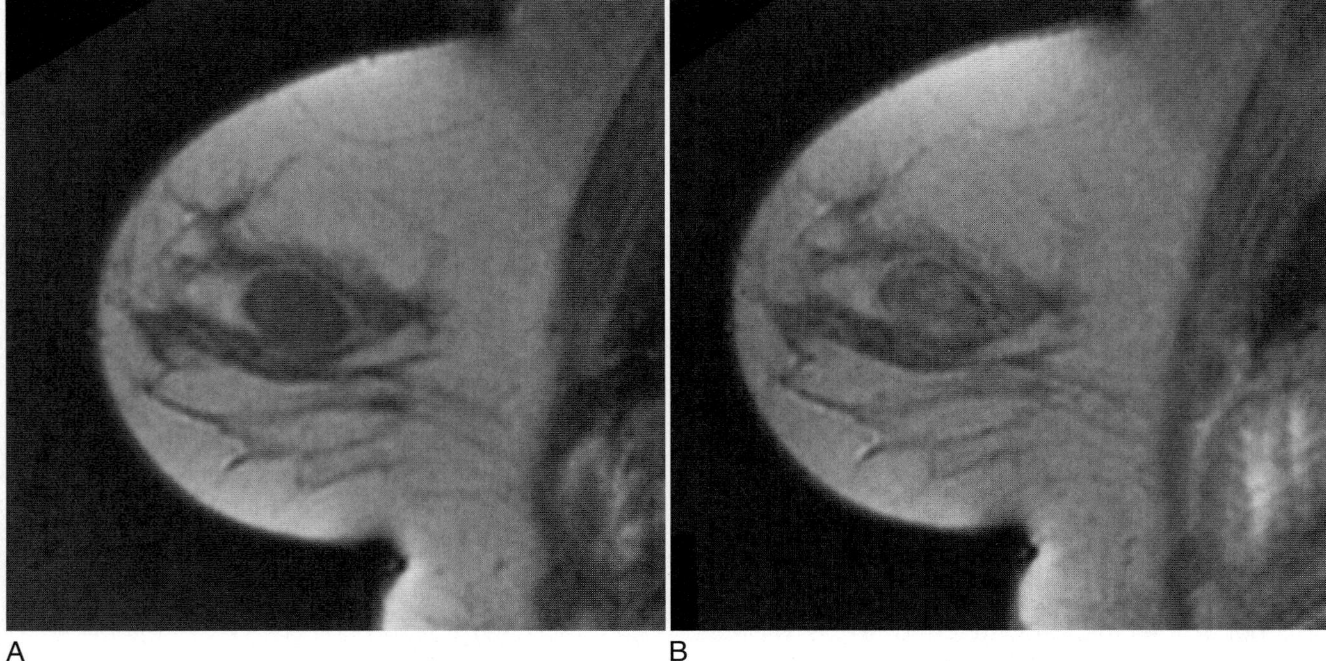

Figure 14–2. Two-dimensional dynamic sagittal (non–fat-suppressed) magnetic resonance images of an oval, smooth, heterogeneous, focal mass. Images were obtained at 0 seconds (**A**), 90 seconds, 180 seconds, and 270 seconds (**B**) after administration of contrast agent. The oval circumscribed 2.5-cm mass enhanced slowly.

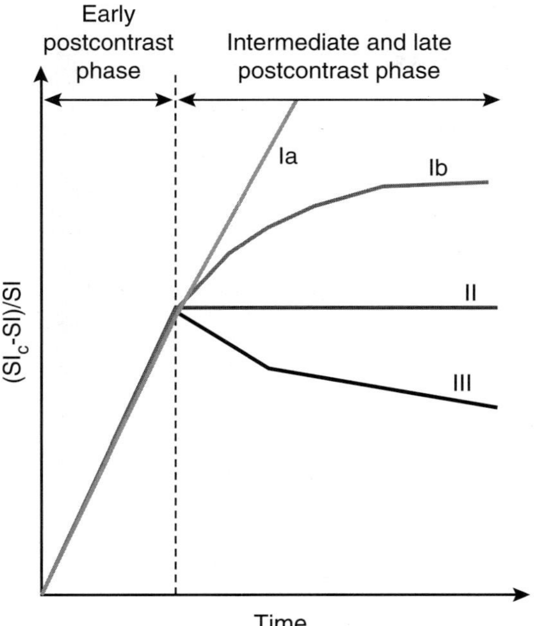

Figure 14–3. Schematic drawing of the time–signal intensity curve types. Type I corresponds to a straight (Ia) or curved (Ib) line; enhancement continues over the entire dynamic study. Type II is a plateau curve with a sharp bend after the initial upstroke. Type III is a washout time course ([SI_c – SI]/SI). (From Kuhl CK, et al: Dynamic breast MRI: Are signal intensity time course data useful for differential diagnosis of enhancing lesions? Radiology 1999; 211:101-110.)

tended to demonstrate a type 1 curve, whereas malignant lesions tended to demonstrate type 2 or 3 curves.[28] This method showed a sensitivity of 91%, a specificity of 83%, and a diagnostic accuracy of 86%.[28,29]

Other investigators advocated spatial imaging, also referred to as static imaging. Spatial imaging focused on the morphology, based on architectural characteristics that were better visualized with a longer imaging acquisition time (2.5 to 4 minutes). Those who advocated spatial imaging believed that the better architectural detail obtained through the use of delayed 3D imaging after gadolinium enhancement improved the detection of lesions.[4,9,20-23] Harms and colleagues[10] initially focused on the spatial aspect of breast imaging to improve analysis of subtle morphologic details. Their approach was based on the well-known fact that malignant lesions exhibit characteristic MRI features similar to those seen on mammography. Nunes and associates[30,31] designed a morphologic model using shape, margins, enhancement pattern, and lesion distribution to distinguish benign from malignant lesions and thus improve specificity. A follow-up study for reproducibility successfully confirmed that diagnostic performance characteristics remained highly predictive for determining outcome.[30,31]

Advancements in technology have allowed the union of optimal temporal and spatial resolution with each breast MRI performed. As evident from the history of the "dynamic" method and "static" evaluations, each method can provide valuable information necessary to characterize lesions. Furthermore, no method has proved to be 100% effective standing alone because of the occasional superimposed presentation of benign and malignant lesions. Benign lesions tend to favor the type 1 curve and smooth edges, and malignant lesions tend to demonstrate a washout curve and nonsmooth or spiculated borders. However, overlap among these lesion features remains.

In an effort to overcome the obstacle of lesion feature overlap, novel approaches to interpretation were taken. Currently, the most acceptable method is a combined approach using morphologic features and kinetic analyses to evaluate and diagnose lesions. This combined approach has been shown to yield higher sensitivity and specificity than either method alone.

Kinkel and coworkers[32] assessed the reproducibility of diagnosing suspicious breast lesions through the use of dynamic and morphologic parameters. They evaluated 57 patients with either palpable findings or suspicious mammographic findings and prospectively analyzed each lesion with contrast-enhanced MRI preoperatively, on the basis of a predetermined classification and regression tree.[32] Histopathologic specimens were used as the standard of reference. Results showed that the washout enhancement pattern combined with lesion margin assessment (spiculated or "non-smooth") with dynamic contrast-enhanced high-resolution MRI of the breast allowed reproducible lesion characterization. This study yielded a sensitivity and positive predictive value (PPV) of 97% and a specificity and negative predictive value (NPV) of 96%.[32]

Schnall and colleagues[33] also examined the advantage of combining architectural (morphologic) features interpretation with kinetic analysis in 100 cases (50 benign and 50 malignant lesions). They concluded that addition of qualitative classification of the time–signal intensity curve to an architectural interpretation significantly improves performance. These researchers found that qualitative classification of enhancement curves was the most predictive of the kinetic features. They agreed with previous studies that reported the washout feature as a moderate predictor of malignancy when used alone, and they realized that the washout feature was the key to further evaluating equivocal architectural findings.[33] The combined method has proved to be the superior method with the highest reproducible sensitivity and specificity (Fig. 14–4). Table 14–1 shows the sensitivities and specificities from various studies for MRI of the breast.

PATHOPHYSIOLOGY OF ENHANCEMENT

The interpretation of breast MRI has been a challenge because of the shared characteristics of benign and malignant lesions with regard to contrast enhancement and morphologic features as well as within

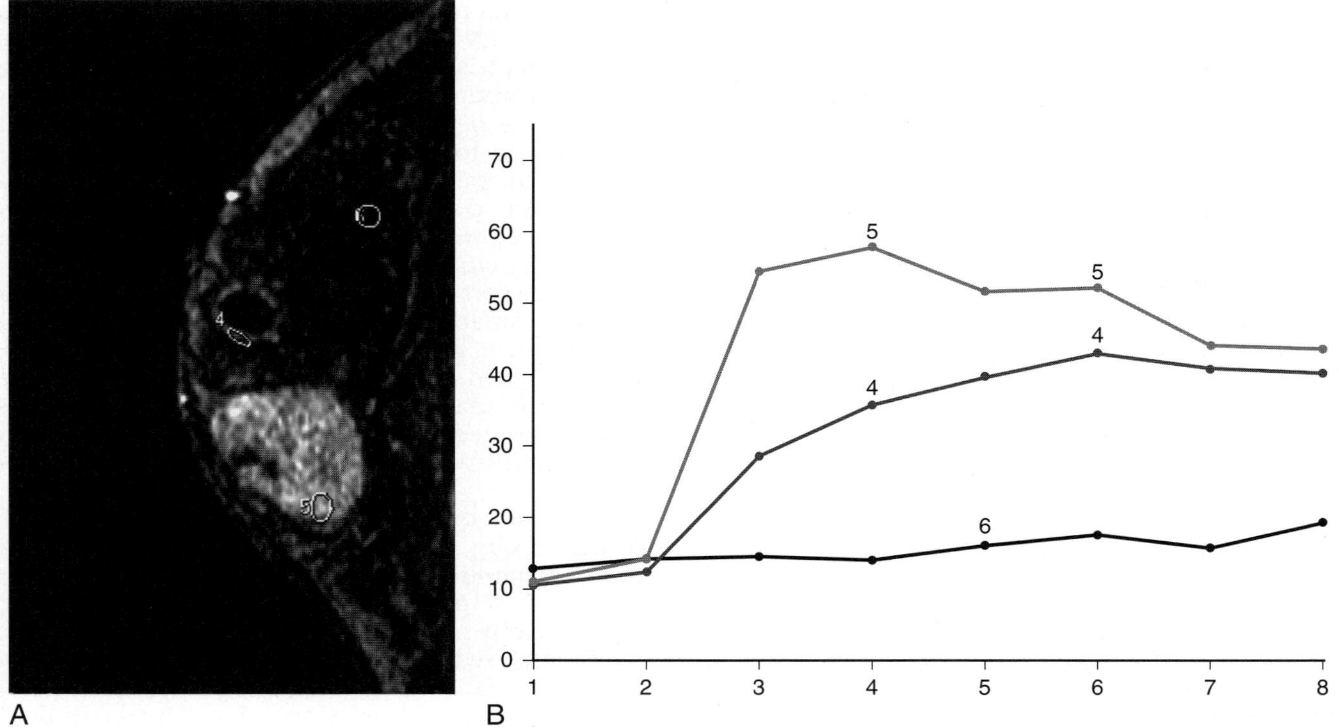

Figure 14–4. **A** and **B,** Contrast-enhanced, T1-weighted, dynamic fat-saturated sagittal spoiled gradient-recalled (SPGR) image, status postprocessing with subtraction. The patient had a history of infiltrating ductal carcinoma, and imaging was performed for further evaluation of extent of disease. **A** depicts large enhancing mass in the lower quadrant with a suspicious time–signal intensity curve, number 5 (**B** 5). The more superior round mass is a known cyst that has a smooth rim with a benign enhancement pattern number 4 (**B** 4). Time–signal intensity curve number 6 (**B** 6) is the baseline pattern of enhancement within fatty tissue.

kinetic curve analyses. The biggest overlap lies within the features of contrast enhancement. Many have wondered why benign lesions can enhance in a pattern similar to that of malignant lesions. The pathophysiology behind this enhancement has been examined and has not yet been fully clarified. Studies investigating the potential causes of rate enhancement, rate enhancement decline, and no enhancement have been carried out so that the strengths and weaknesses of contrast agent–enhanced breast MRI and differential diagnosis can be better understood.[34-37] A fundamental understanding was developed from these studies.

Research has shown that malignant lesions possess and release substances called *angiogenic factors*.[38-44]

Table 14–1. Sensitivity and Specificity of Various Studies for Magnetic Resonance Imaging of the Breast*

Study*	% Sensitivity	% Specificity
Kaiser[16]	97	97
Heywang-Kobrunner[12]	99	28
Harms et al[10]	94	37
Giles et al[24]	95	53
Nunes et al[69]	96	79
Kuhl[29]	91	83

*Superscript numbers indicate chapter references.

The factor most commonly reported is vascular endothelial growth factor (VEGF), also known as vascular permeability factor (VPF). VEGF/VPF is actually a family of proteins that stimulate the growth of preexisting capillaries as well as new capillaries. When viewed histologically, however, the de novo vessels exhibit pathologic vessel wall architecture with leaky endothelial linings.[39,40,45] Invasive ductal carcinoma and high-grade ductal carcinoma in situ (DCIS) have been associated with high VEGF/VPF expression with receptors, but infiltrating lobular carcinoma has low VEGF/VPF expression. There is no significant difference in vascular density between these two types of invasive cancers. This finding suggests that other factors are stimulating vessel density in infiltrating lobular carcinoma.[40,44]

As a result of the increase in vascular density and permeability, the influx and efflux of contrast material are significantly affected in these focal areas within a lesion. Additionally, arteriovenous shunts due to the reformed architecture in the already existing capillaries have been discovered. Unfortunately, vessel density is not specific for malignancy. Benign lesions can also have prominent vascularity related to their growth. For example, benign lesions have displayed unexpected vessel density with locally increased permeability. Up to 10 % of cancers, usually the true lobular invasive and scirrhotic or desmoplastic invasive ductal cancers, can show shallow enhancement related to low vessel density.[28,44] Extensive research studies have examined the correlation among vessel density, signal intensity, and patterns of enhancement in the postcontrast image, with conflicting results. It is clear that there is a correlation between the percentage of maximal signal increase after contrast administration and high vessel density in known cancers.[41-43,46,47] Variations in biologic presentation are reflected in the differences in contrast enhancement patterns. This has been a source of frustration for radiologists and is reason enough to support the belief that interpretation based on contrast enhancement alone is not sufficient. With all the issues involved, dynamic contrast enhancement patterns are accurate and extremely useful in differential diagnosis. The number of vessels is just one of the factors that affect imaging. Tissue relaxation times, vessel architecture, permeability, and interstitial pressure gradients are also important in determining contrast enhancement.[28,48]

BENEFITS AND DISADVANTAGES OF BREAST MAGNETIC RESONANCE IMAGING

Magnetic resonance imaging has been reported to have several important benefits in evaluating the breast. The fact that the modality does not use ionizing radiation eliminates the potential for radiation-induced cancers.[49,50] To date, MRI has not been linked to breast cancer induction. Actually, this benefit of MRI is not convincing because the incidence of mammography-induced breast cancer is unknown, if it does exist. Modern mammography technology and federal regulation of mammography have ensured safe radiation doses. Furthermore, if a risk exists, it is probably related to a small, high-risk population. Furthermore, mammography is still indicated in these high-risk patients for correlation with MRI examinations.

One benefit of MRI is the ability to use variable pulse sequences, including tissue suppression techniques and postprocessing, which aids in the detection and characterization of breast lesions.[4,10,21,23,24,51] This feature has been useful in differentiating benign and malignant lesions.[20,26,30,33] MRI provides a 3D evaluation of the extent of lesions, including multiple foci of carcinoma in the same breast, to provide further information for staging and treatment options.[27,52] MRI has been used in the surveillance of women with a history of breast conservation surgery for malignancy, to differentiate recurrence or residual disease from postoperative or postirradiation changes when results of other methods have been inconclusive.[15,18,53,54] Others report the ability of MRI to assist in the analysis of problematic mammography findings.[55]

MRI also has a number of potential disadvantages, including cost, time, limited availability, poor depiction of microcalcifications, lack of standardized methods, injection requirement, and medical constraints. MRI examinations are expensive, usually costing $1000 to more than $4000. Furthermore, in our experience, individual payers may not reimburse for breast MRI examinations. Therefore, the information derived must be clinically useful and must not have been obtainable by less expensive means. In addition to cost, MRI may take up to 30 minutes per patient. Contraindications to MRI can be due to implantable devices that are not MRI compatible, such as pacemakers, metallic aneurysm clips, brain stimulators, and indwelling delivery pumps. Another potential disadvantage is the injection of contrast agent, which is necessary to delineate tumor from normal parenchyma. Medical constraints, such as claustrophobia, make it difficult for some patients to complete an MRI procedure. Another potential limitation is unreliable depiction of calcifications that can be associated with DCIS.[28,56] Calcifications are best seen on mammography; with MRI, however, the surrounding tissue can markedly enhance and can reveal a larger area of involvement than what was identified on mammography (Fig. 14–5). It is important to integrate the MRI findings with the mammographic findings. All of the potential benefits and limitations must be evaluated and compared with those of the standard breast imaging modalities, mammography and ultrasonography.

MRI sequences and methodologies used to image breast tumors are not yet standardized. Imaging results cannot always be clearly reproduced or interpreted from one facility to another because of varied initial scanning plane (i.e., sagittal, coronal, or axial), slab thickness, imaging time, and strength of MRI units/superconducting magnets. MRI units can vary from 0.5 to 3.0 T, although most imaging is currently performed with 1.5-T magnets. In addition, most imaging interpretation is performed on monitors or with software packages that will allow for 3D viewing of the breast. An intense focus can be immediately evaluated with time–signal intensity curves and with manipulation of the images so the location can be confirmed. When films or compact discs (CDs) are sent to another facility for a second opinion or interpretation, the receiving facility's radiologist has to rely on the submitted format and is currently unable to reorient the images. Thus, he or she is neither able to evaluate a potentially suspicious finding in all three planes nor able to generate time–signal intensity curves for analysis.

Although it is unlikely that MRI will ever be a standalone modality for breast cancer detection, many studies suggest that the modality will continue to have an important role as an adjunct to mammography and ultrasonography.

TECHNIQUES OF BREAST MAGNETIC RESONANCE IMAGING

MRI techniques vary widely from center to center across the world. As a general rule, most MRI im-

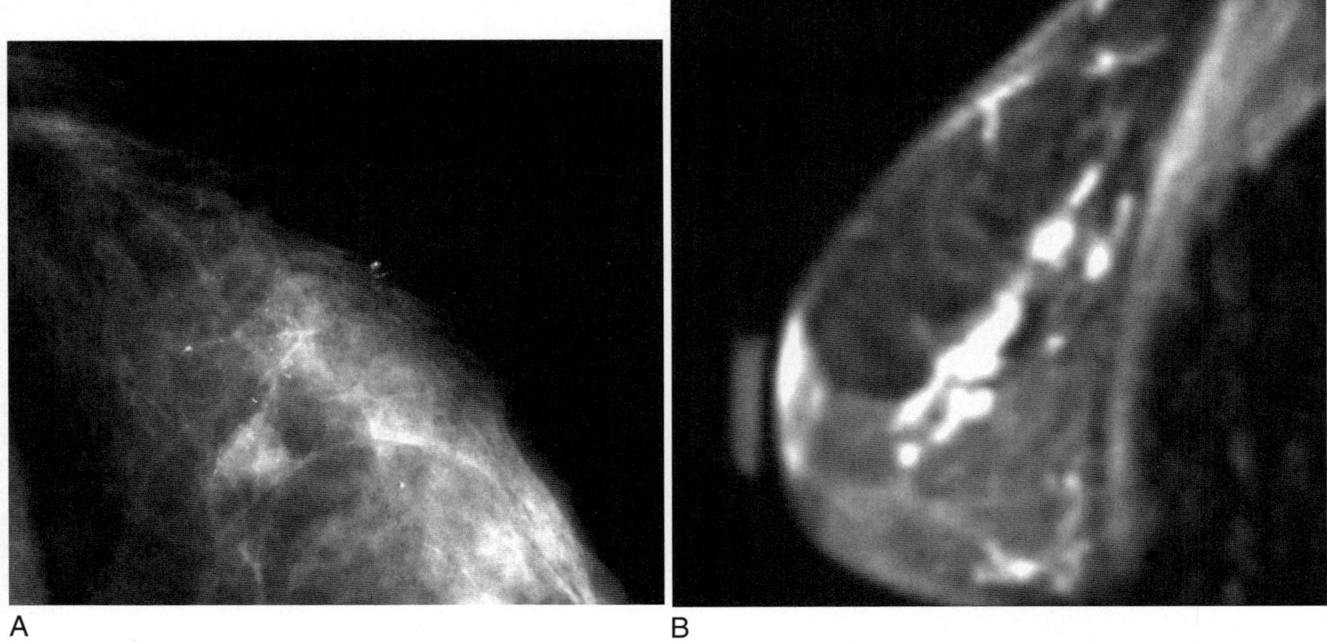

Figure 14–5. Malignant calcifications. **A,** Craniocaudal mammogram shows extensive pleomorphic calcifications in the upper hemisphere of the left breast. **B,** Three-dimensional volume contrast-enhanced, fat-suppressed sagittal magnetic resonance images show intense segmental, homogenous contrast enhancement with clumping that corresponds to the location of suspicious calcifications (*arrow*). Biopsy demonstrated ductal carcinoma in situ.

agers follow the same fundamentals. Variations in techniques do not affect image quality or data acquisition. Most imagers use a 1.5-T magnet with a dedicated dual breast coil for either bilateral or unilateral imaging. Dedicated breast coils are needed to obtain adequate resolution and to improve signal-to-noise ratios. Of note, high-quality images and data have been obtained with MRI units with magnets less than 1.5 T.

Imaging is best performed with the patient in the prone position with the breasts suspended or slightly compressed in a dedicated breast coil. Image acquisition planes are usually in the sagittal or axial position. These planes correlate to a lateral and craniocaudal view on the mammogram. However, some radiologists also have protocols that image in the coronal plane. Regardless, volume acquisition allows for reconstruction of images in any of the three planes. The radiologist must choose the initial scan plane he or she is most comfortable with in the evaluation, because there is some loss of information with reconstruction. Finally, it is very important that a complete evaluation of a breast MRI study includes monitor reading. This step allows the reader to manipulate the images in the sagittal, coronal, and axial planes to determine whether a lesion exists or a finding is normal breast vascularity or tissue. If there is a lesion, correlation of size, location, and rate of enhancement can be performed for further evaluation.

Imaging is usually obtained with the patient in the prone position because it decreases the respiratory motion artifact and has helped alleviate the effects of claustrophobia. Newer coils allow for feet-first entrance into the scanner, further reducing claustrophobia. In our practice, we have found that playing music through headphones worn by the patient can be helpful and that conscious sedation, if necessary, can be achieved with oral or sublingual short-acting hypnotics or antianxiety medications to diminish symptoms. For more severe symptoms, intravenous sedation has been helpful. The tools needed to perform MRI are universal. On the other hand, the methodologies used to interpret breast MRI reflect significant divergence.

As previously stated, two different MRI methodologies in assessing breast disease with gadolinium enhancement emerged: (1) dynamic 2D and 3D imaging during gadolinium enhancement and (2) delayed 3D imaging after gadolinium enhancement. A combination of dynamic and high-resolution MRI has been introduced in clinical as well as research protocols nationally and internationally. The goal of this combination is to achieve the highest sensitivity and specificity possible. Imaging protocols have been developed, and as MRI technology advances, guidelines are constantly revised to optimize image quality and interpretation. Protocols are changing, and the software sequences will evolve as the hardware advances. It is important to achieve high temporal and spatial imaging simultaneously with higher signal-to-noise ratios for the best resolution while making dynamic information readily available.

IMAGING APPEARANCE OF TYPICAL MALIGNANT BREAST TUMORS

Malignant breast tumors have been extensively evaluated with contrast-enhanced MRI and reported on in the literature. Two major aspects of the evaluation of all breast tumors with contrast-enhanced MRI must be considered. First, one must determine whether the breast tumor demonstrates contrast enhancement. Second, one must evaluate the morphology of the enhancement, which is similar to evaluating the morphology of a lesion on mammography.[21]

Malignant breast tumors typically have irregular or spiculated margins on contrast-enhanced MRI, as they do on mammography. Studies have reported a PPV of 91% for a spiculated margin (Fig. 14–6).[30] It also has been reported that tumors with rim enhancement on MRI are highly suspicious for malignancy, with a PPV of 86% (Fig. 14–7).[32,46,48] Ductal enhancement is another architectural feature that has displayed a PPV of 85%.[30] However, a number of breast cancers have circumscribed, smooth borders on MRI, just as they do on mammography (Fig. 14–8).[30]

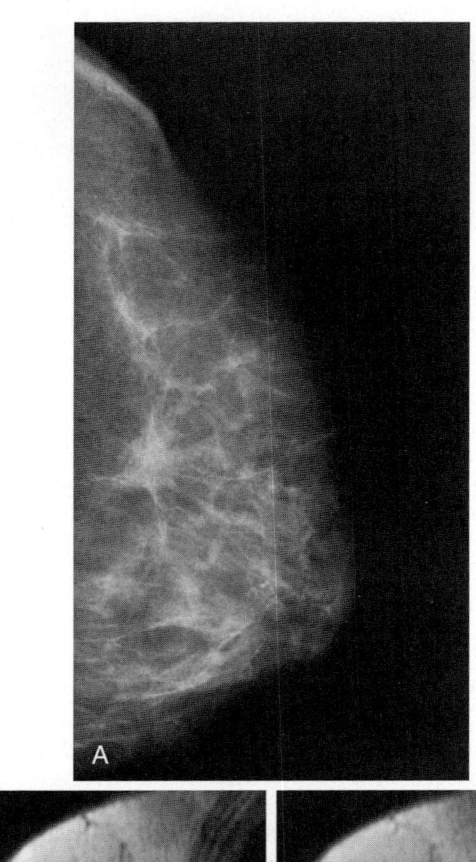

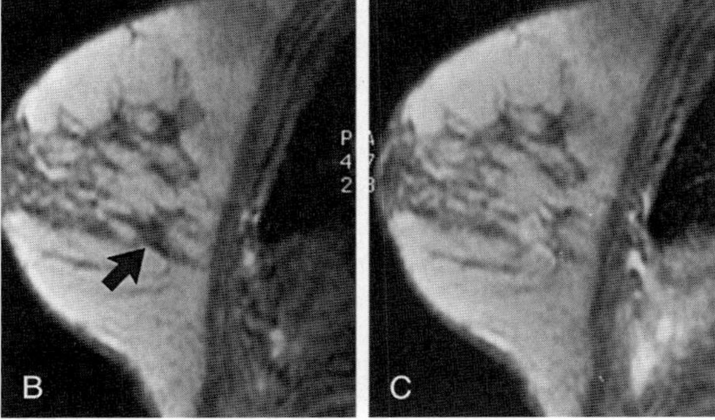

Figure 14–6. Infiltrating ductal carcinoma. **A,** Exaggerated craniocaudal mammogram shows a spiculated mass in the left breast. Two-dimensional dynamic sagittal precontrast (**B**) and postcontrast (**C**) magnetic resonance images show an irregular rapidly enhancing mass (*arrow*).

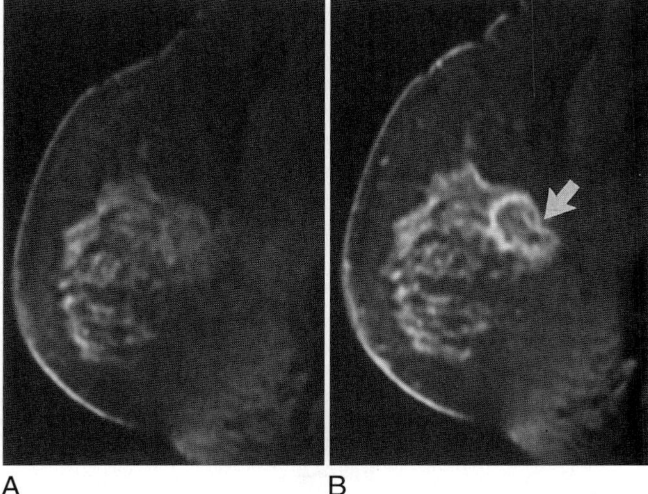

Figure 14–7. Invasive ductal carcinoma with ring enhancement. Three-dimensional volume precontrast (**A**) and postcontrast (**B**) fat-suppressed sagittal magnetic resonance images show striking ring enhancement of a lobulated, irregular, heterogeneous mass (*arrow*).

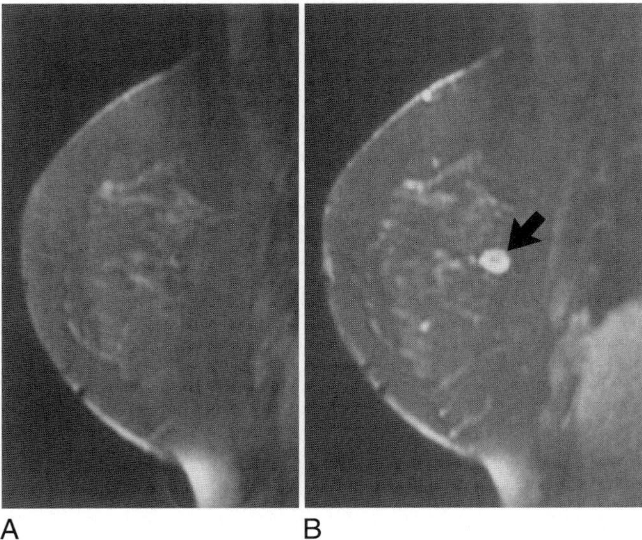

Figure 14–8. Circumscribed infiltrating ductal carcinoma in a patient with a history of right breast cancer who presented with a new right breast lump. Sagittal three-dimensional, spoiled gradient-recalled (SPGR) precontrast (**A**) and postcontrast (**B**) magnetic resonance images show a round, smooth, heterogeneous rim-enhancing mass (*arrow*) on the postcontrast images.

Malignant breast tumors can appear as rapidly enhancing lesions that have an initial rate of increase of the time–signal intensity curve to levels three times the initial start point within 90 to 120 seconds of injection. They can either maintain high signal intensities for 10 to 15 minutes after intravenous injection of gadolinium or demonstrate rapid washout of contrast agent, which is a marked descent of the time–signal intensity curve, often after 3 to 5 minutes (see Fig. 14–4). Invasive ductal and lobular carcinomas as well as DCIS can demonstrate these MRI enhancement patterns. There is evidence of differences in enhancement characteristics between non–high-grade DCIS and high-grade DCIS. Research has been performed to determine sensitivity and specificity of contrast-enhanced MRI in patients with DCIS.[56-58] The high-grade lesions reported were larger. Very small lesions or distant foci of non–high-grade DCIS may be missed on MRI, either because of slice thickness or limitations of resolution, or because they do not enhance. A negative MRI finding seems to exclude high-grade DCIS (see Figs 14–5 and 14–21).[58] The washout pattern has a high PPV for malignancy but is not pathognomonic. In our experience, lymph nodes and some fibroadenomas commonly demonstrate this pattern.

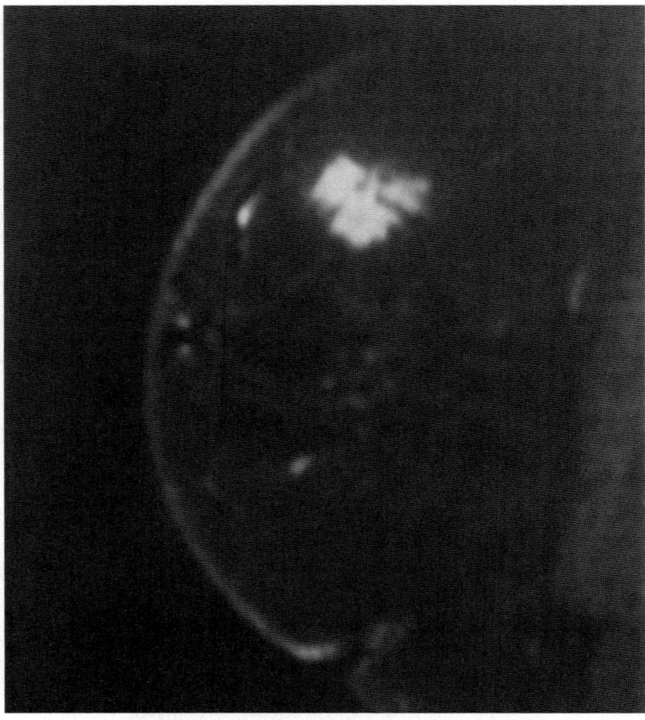

Figure 14–9. Subtraction image of a sagittal T1-weighted, contrast-enhanced spoiled gradient-recalled (SPGR) sequence. Intensely enhancing irregular mass with nonenhancing internal septations. Biopsy demonstrated infiltrating ductal carcinoma.

IMAGING APPEARANCE OF TYPICAL BENIGN BREAST TUMORS

Contrast-enhanced MRI of benign breast tumors has also been reported in the literature.[1-5,7-23] As with all breast tumors, two major MRI features must be evaluated. First, one must determine whether the breast tumor demonstrates contrast enhancement. The classic appearance of benign breast tumors with contrast-enhanced MRI is a nonenhancing or slowly enhancing breast lesion (see Fig. 14–2).

Second, one must evaluate the morphology of the breast tumor. As with their morphology on mammography, benign breast tumors are typically circumscribed on MRI (see Fig. 14–2). Other architectural features with significant NPVs are no visible lesion on MRI (96%), mild regional enhancement (92%), smooth borders (95%), lobulated borders (90%), internal septations (95%), no or minimal enhancement (92%), no enhancement (95%), and minimal enhancement (89%).[30] Fibroadenomas in postmenopausal women typically show either slow enhancement or no enhancement and circumscribed margins.[59] Some fibroadenomas may also demonstrate nonenhancing internal septations; in a study of 57 patients, a 95% NPV for malignancy was reported in lesions with such septations.[30] Conversely, the appearance of nonenhancing septations in an irregular, spiculated mass is not suggestive of a benign abnormality (Fig. 14–9). Modifiers that assist in evaluating lesions are not stronger predictors than morphologic features alone. Furthermore, a significant proportion of benign tumors demonstrate rapid, intense contrast enhancement and could potentially be mistaken for malignant tumors (Fig. 14–10). In our experience, some fibroadenomas—especially those in younger women, lymph nodes, some cases of sclerosing adenosis, and most phyllodes tumors—have demonstrated rapid, intense uptake of contrast agent (Fig. 14–11).

IMAGE ANALYSIS AND ASSESSMENT

In an effort to standardize breast MRI description, interpretation, and assessment, a core group of radiologists, who are known nationally and internationally and have extensive breast MRI experience, developed a dictionary with a vocabulary of the words or phrases used to describe the MRI findings and then refined it into a lexicon.[60,61] The lexicon followed the format of the American College of Radiology Breast Imaging Reporting and Data System (ACR BI-RADS) for mammography and applied it to breast MRI. It comprises terminology, imaging techniques, evaluation of kinetic and morphologic contrast-enhancement patterns, breast composition, impressions, recommendations, and treatment (Table 14–2).[62]

The breast MRI lexicon has been a work in progress for several years while being tested by experienced breast MRI radiologists for interobserver agreement on interpretation of images.[32,63,64] The goal of the

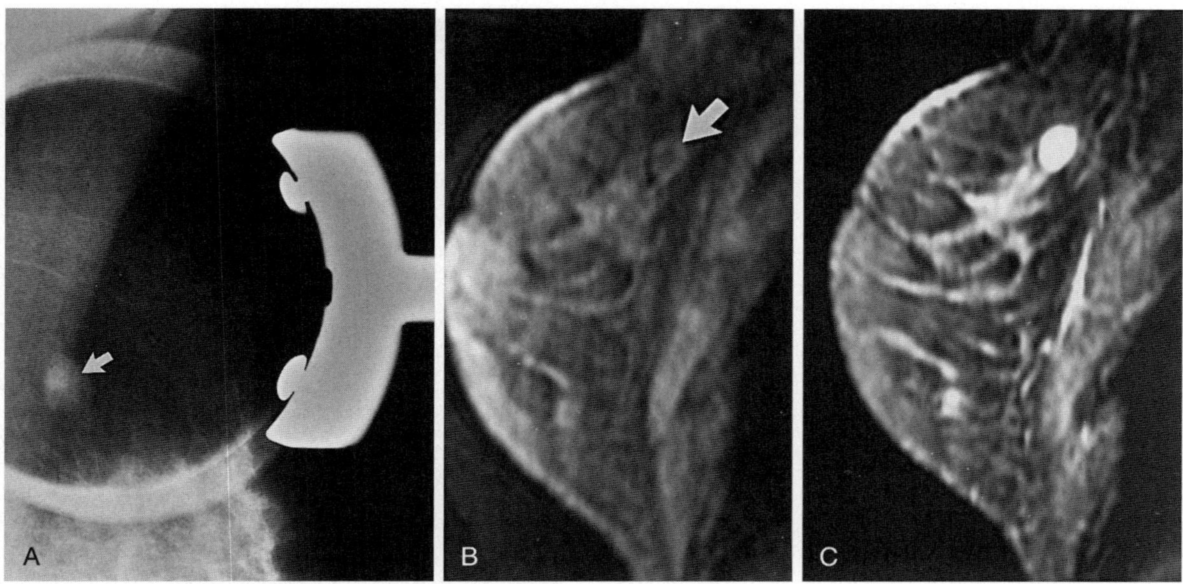

Figure 14–10. Fibroadenoma. **A,** Close-up of spot compression mammographic view shows an oval circumscribed mass (*arrow*) anterior to the pectoralis major muscle. Three-dimensional volume precontrast (**B**) and postcontrast (**C**) fat-suppressed sagittal magnetic resonance images are shown. The mass (*arrow*) demonstrates intense contrast enhancement.

lexicon was to accurately describe imaging findings to facilitate communication between radiologist and referring physicians as well as to allow retrospective analysis for validation of patient management.[65]

Lexicon testing for morphology reproducibility among readers of 85 contrast-enhanced MRI studies showed substantial agreement about breast density; moderate agreement about lesion type, mass margins, and shape; and fair agreement about interpretation of internal enhancement. Although there was a positive outcome for reproducibility of breast density and lesion type, all categories of the lexicon must be reproducible for breast MRI language and reporting to be uniform.[60] On the basis of this study, further testing and refinement led to a final version published in the ACR BI-RADS *Breast Imaging Atlas* in 2003.[62] Ongoing studies continue to evaluate the efficacy of image evaluation using the breast MRI lexicon, with temporal and spatial imaging.[66,67]

As discussed previously, one of the challenges of breast MRI was the lack of standardized medical terminology. The MRI lexicon has provided

Table 14–2. Lesion Classification Form for American College of Radiology Breast Imaging Reporting and Data System (BI-RADS): Magnetic Resonance Imaging*

Lesion Type (select one)	
A. Focus/Foci (tiny spot of enhancement, <5 mm); if only finding, *GO TO SECTION E*	
B. Mass (three-dimensional space-occupying lesion that is one process, usually round, oval, or irregular in shape)	
Shape *(select one)*	Description
❑ Round	Spherical or ball-shaped
❑ Oval	Elliptical or egg-shaped
❑ Lobular	Undulating contour
❑ Irregular	Uneven shape (not round, oval, or lobulated)
Margin *(select one)*	Description
❑ Smooth	Well-circumscribed and well-defined margin
❑ Irregular	Uneven margin can be round or jagged (not smooth or spiculated)
❑ Spiculated	Characterized by radiating lines
Mass Enhancement *(select one)*	Description
❑ Homogeneous	Confluent uniform enhancement
❑ Heterogeneous	Nonspecific mixed enhancement
❑ Rim enhancement	Enhancement more pronounced at the periphery of mass
❑ Dark internal septation	Dark nonenhancing lines within a mass
❑ Enhancing internal septation	Enhancing lines within a mass
❑ Central enhancement	Enhancement more pronounced at center of mass

Continued

Table 14–2. Lesion Classification Form for American College of Radiology Breast Imaging Reporting and Data System (BI-RADS): Magnetic Resonance Imaging*—*cont'd*

Lesion Type (select one)

C. Non–Mass-like Enhancement (in an area that is not a mass)

Distribution Modifiers *(select one)*	Description
❑ Focal area	Enhancement in a confined area, less than 25% of quadrant
❑ Linear	Enhancement in a line that may not conform to a duct
❑ Ductal	Enhancement in a line that may have branching, conforming to a duct
❑ Segmental	Triangular region of enhancement, apex pointing to nipple, suggesting a duct or its branches
❑ Regional	Enhancement in a large volume of tissue not conforming to a ductal distribution, geographic
❑ Multiple regions	Enhancement in at least two large volumes of tissue not conforming to a ductal distribution, multiple geographic areas, patchy areas of enhancement
❑ Diffuse	Enhancement distributed uniformly throughout the breast

Internal Enhancement *(select one)*	Description
❑ Homogeneous	Confluent uniform enhancement
❑ Heterogeneous	Nonuniform enhancement in a random pattern
❑ Stippled, punctate	Punctate, similar-appearing enhancing foci, sand-like or dot-like
❑ Clumped	Cobblestone-like enhancement, with occasional confluent areas
❑ Reticular, dendritic	Enhancement with finger-like projections extending toward nipple, especially seen on axial or sagittal images, in women with partly fatty–involuted breasts

D. Symmetrical or Asymmetrical (bilateral scans only)

Symmetrical or Asymmetrical *(select one)*	Description
❑ Symmetrical	Mirror-image enhancement
❑ Asymmetrical	More in one breast than in the other

E. Other Findings *(select all that apply)*

❑ None apply	❑ Edema
❑ Nipple retraction	❑ Lymphadenopathy
❑ Nipple invasion	❑ Pectoralis muscle invasion
❑ Pre-contrast high ductal signal	❑ Chest wall invasion
❑ Skin thickening (focal)	❑ Hematoma/blood
❑ Skin thickening (diffuse)	❑ Abnormal signal void
❑ Skin invasion	❑ Cysts

F. Kinetic Curve Assessment

Kinetic Curve Assessment *(select one)*	Description
❑ Initial rise	Slow, medium, rapid
❑ Delayed phase	Persistent, plateau, washout

G. Assessment Category

Assessment Category *(select one)*	Description
❑ **Category 0**—Incomplete: Need additional imaging evaluation	Finding for which additional evaluation is needed
Final Assessment	
❑ **Category 1**—Negative	No abnormal enhancement, no lesion found (routine follow-up)
❑ **Category 2**—Benign finding	Benign, no malignant features; i.e., cyst (routine follow-up)
❑ **Category 3**—Probably benign finding	Probably benign finding (short interval follow-up)
❑ **Category 4**—Suspicious abnormality	Low to moderate suspicion for malignancy (biopsy should be considered)
❑ **Category 5**—Highly suggestive of malignancy	High probability of malignancy (appropriate action should be taken)
❑ **Category 6**—Known cancer	Biopsy-proven malignancy diagnosis on the imaged finding prior to definitive therapy (appropriate action should be taken)

*Instructions to user: For each of the following categories, select the term that best describes the dominant lesion feature. Wherever possible, definitions and descriptions used in BI-RADS for mammography will be applied to MRI of the breast. This form is for data collection and does not constitute a written MRI report.

From American College of Radiology: ACR BI-RADS—Magnetic Resonance Imaging. In ACR Breast Imaging Reporting and Data System, Breast Imaging Atlas. Reston VA, American College of Radiology, 2003, pp 111-113.

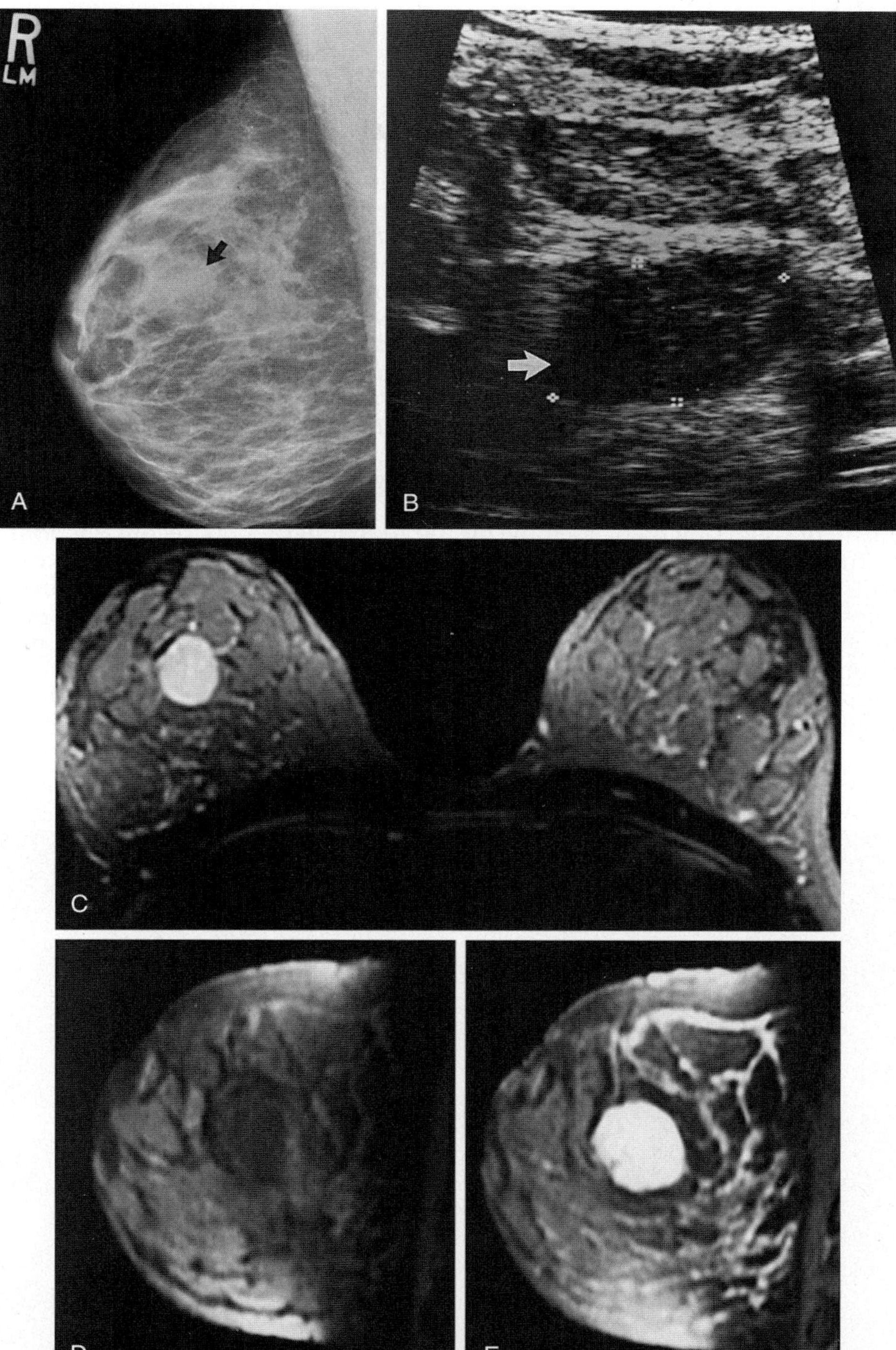

Figure 14–11. Benign mass with rapid contrast enhancement on magnetic resonance imaging. **A,** 90-degree lateral mammogram shows a round, isodense mass (*arrow*) that appeared solid on ultrasonography (**B**). **C,** Axial T2-weighted, fast spin-echo, fat-suppressed magnetic resonance images show a round, circumscribed, homogeneous mass with increased signal intensity. Three-dimensional volume precontrast (**D**) and postcontrast (**E**) fat-suppressed sagittal images show intense contrast enhancement of the mass. Excisional biopsy demonstrated benign phyllodes tumor.

standardized interpretation; however, some variability still exists between the interpreting radiologist's technique and analysis.

Additional benefits of breast MRI remain to be acquired and are contingent on the success of this unified lexicon for interpreting and reporting breast MRI. The lexicon would potentially solve the problems of suboptimal medical communication, fragmented online information resources, lack of standard formats for online teaching files, and irreconcilable research results.[68] Development of this unified lexicon has allowed the field of breast MRI to advance in all areas—diagnosis, staging, treatment, and, possibly, screening trials in the future. More important, investigators will be equipped with a system that will enable similar data collection methods to facilitate prospective and retrospective research on an individual or combined basis.[68]

Assessment and Reporting

Breast imaging analysis involves many steps and usually follows a multidisciplinary approach. It is imperative to have an accurate history and physical findings, recent mammograms, and ultrasonographic or other pertinent imaging studies available for comparison. The nipples can be marked for orientation as well as scars or other areas of interest. The first step in image analysis requires a gestalt view of the breast before injection of contrast agent through a review of the precontrast T1- and T2-weighted images. Retroareolar ductal fluid, fluid collections, biopsy sites, and benign cystic or solid masses can have varying levels of intensity on the T1- and T2-weighted images. Image analysis is further improved with postprocessing through subtraction of the precontrast images from the postcontrast images (Fig. 14–12) and the use of maximum-intensity projections (Fig. 14–13), which assemble all the individual millimeter slices or slab images into one 3D model. Most of the precontrast imaging findings are removed from the postcontrast images if there is relatively no change in the appearance after injection of contrast agent. However, there may be incomplete removal or slight uptake of contrast imaging, and the finding will appear on the postcontrast images. That is why it is important to review the images before postprocessing to avoid potential misinterpretations.

If there is enhancement, the imager must determine whether it signifies a real mass, vascularity, or normal breast tissue. The tools necessary to complete this analysis are kinetics and morphology. To obtain optimal interpretation of the architectural features of the breast image, at least one postcontrast image should be obtained and interpreted between 90 and 270 seconds.[69] Studies have shown that contrast enhancement of malignant lesions usually peaks by 2 minutes and curve analyses are usually done over approximately a 7-minute period (400 seconds).[16,29]

Computer-aided diagnosis and detection programs have been commercially available for mammographic analysis for several years. The same technology has now become available for MRI. This technology may prove to provide a comprehensive program in evaluating MRI breast images, to include 3D reconstructions in all three planes, angiogenic mapping based on variations in uptake of contrast, and dynamic time–signal intensity curves, all within minutes of completion of the examination.

A significant amount of time and effort has been devoted to improving and unifying breast MRI reporting. On the basis of retrospective and prospective studies evaluating dynamic and static imaging,

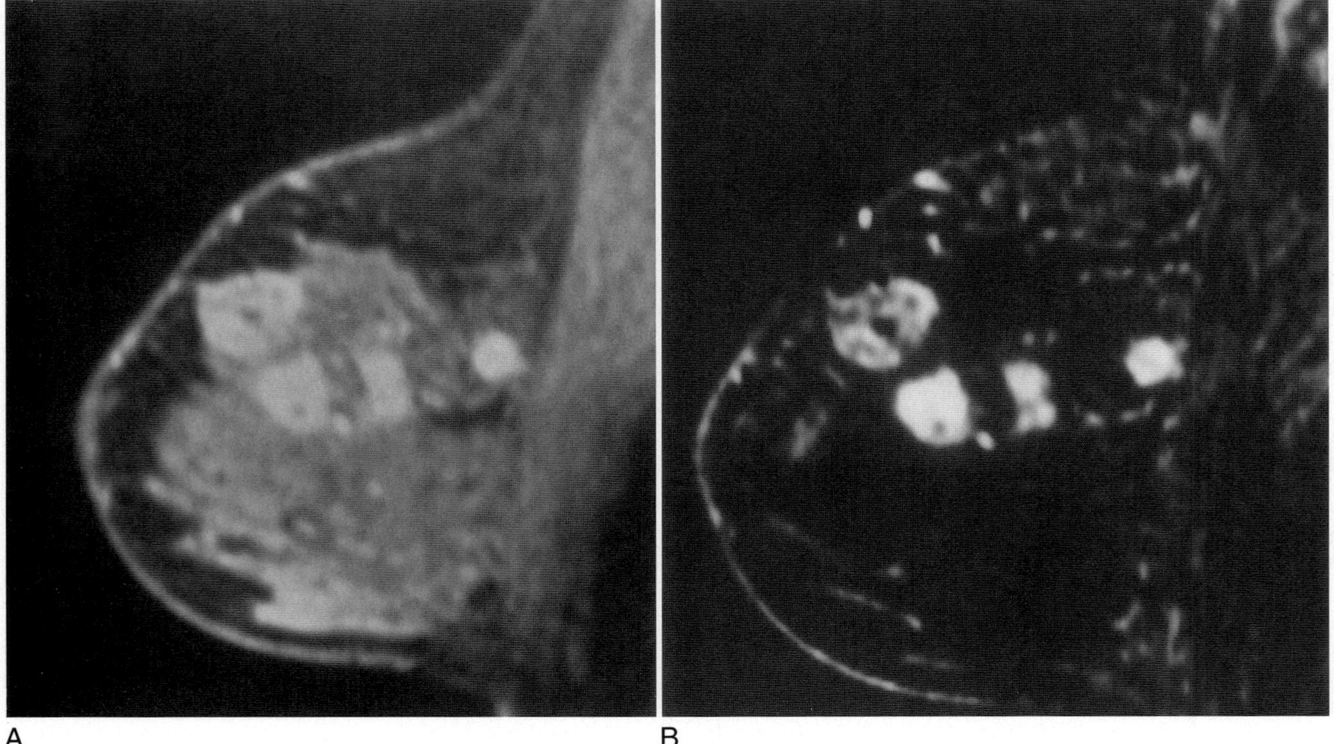

Figure 14–12. A 35-year-old woman with dense breasts presented with a palpable right breast mass. Mammography and ultrasonography identified a 40-mm mass. Clinically the mass was greater than 50 mm. Magnetic resonance imaging was performed for further evaluation. **A,** Contrast-enhanced sagittal T1-weighted three-dimensional spoiled gradient-recalled (SPGR) magnetic resonance image showed multiple large, round, irregular, heterogeneous masses in a linear, segmental distribution extending to the chest wall. **B,** Subtraction image improves conspicuity of the multifocal mass. Imaging findings are now concordant with the clinical findings.

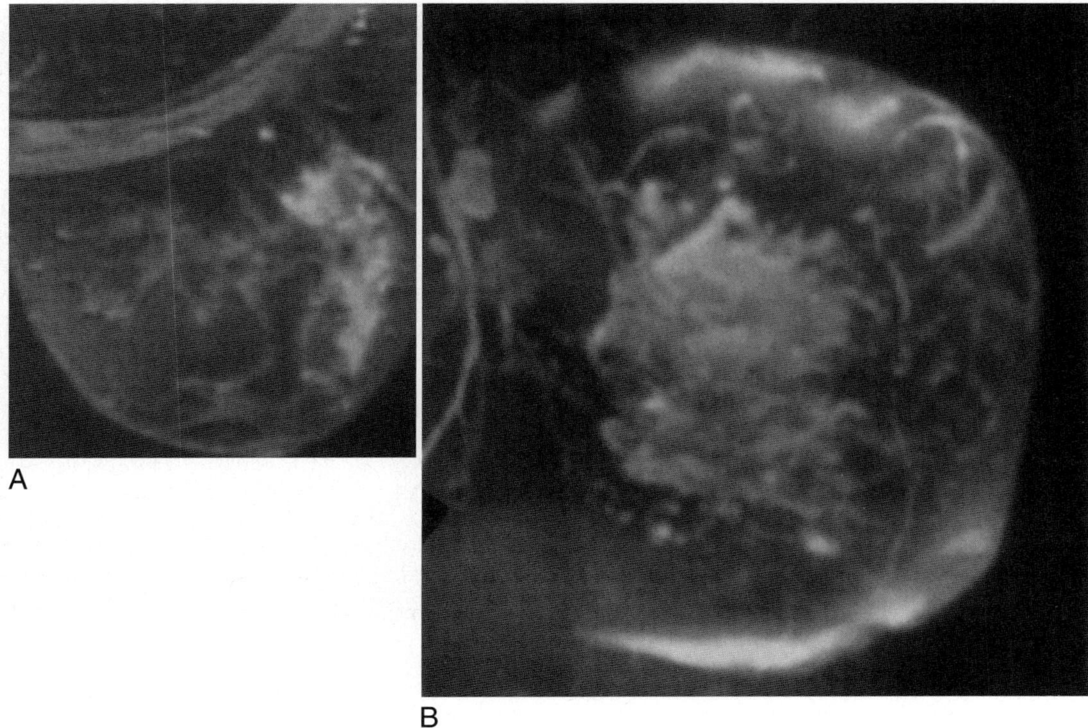

Figure 14–13. A 45-year-old woman had a large palpable mass that was not visualized on mammography and was ill defined on ultrasonography. Biopsy demonstrated lobular cancer. Magnetic resonance imaging was performed to determine extent of disease. **A,** An axial single-slice (slab) contrast-enhanced spoiled gradient-recalled (SPGR) subtraction image of the right outer hemisphere in the area of the palpable mass. **B,** Contrast-enhanced, sagittal, maximum-intensity projection (MIP) shows the full extent of the tumor and adenopathy in the axilla.

alone and combined, recommendations have been made regarding what standard reporting should include. The components are divided into the five categories: (1) lesion type, (2) other findings, (3) kinetic curve analyses, (4) assessment/impression, and (5) recommendations.[62,65]

Lesion type is a broad category that has many subsets, including focus/foci, mass enhancement, and non-mass enhancement. Using the lexicon, the reader should then further describe mass shape, mass margin, mass enhancement distribution, and non-mass enhancement description and distribution.

Additionally, some images may have noteworthy findings, such as diffuse or regional enhancement (Fig.14–14), cysts (Fig.14–15), nipple retraction (Fig. 14–16), and lymphadenopathy (Fig. 14–17). These findings should be reported as well because they contribute significantly to the final assessment and treatment recommendations.

Kinetic curve analyses, previously described as types 1, 2, and 3 (see Fig. 14–3), should be used to further evaluate regions of interest (ROIs) to differentiate benign from malignant. Essentially, the reader should evaluate the shape of the curve, the initial rise, and the time course. For example, if a lesion with indeterminate morphology is identified and the reader evaluates the shape of the curve as a steady rise with plateau, this lesion would be classified as probably benign. A sharp rise and steady decline defines a washout pattern more suspicious for malignancy. Evidence has shown that benign lesions such as young fibroadenomas and some lymph node views can occasionally display a washout pattern. A washout pattern does not occur in every malignant tumor. It is beneficial when a washout curve is present because it increases the level of suspicion for malignancy.

Harms and associates[70] developed an algorithmic approach to the evaluation of a mammographic finding and MRI enhancement patterns. The lesion type, significant findings, and kinetic curve analysis should be considered to arrive at the final assessment. This assessment should include the reader's impression and final diagnosis along with recommendations. MRI BI-RADS final assessment categories should be determined and reported like those for mammography, as follows (see Table 14–2):

0. Incomplete: need additional imaging evaluation.
1. Negative.
2. Benign finding.
3. Probably benign finding—short-interval follow-up.
4. Suspicious abnormality—biopsy should be considered.
5. Highly suggestive of malignancy—appropriate action should be taken.
6. Known cancer—appropriate action should be taken.

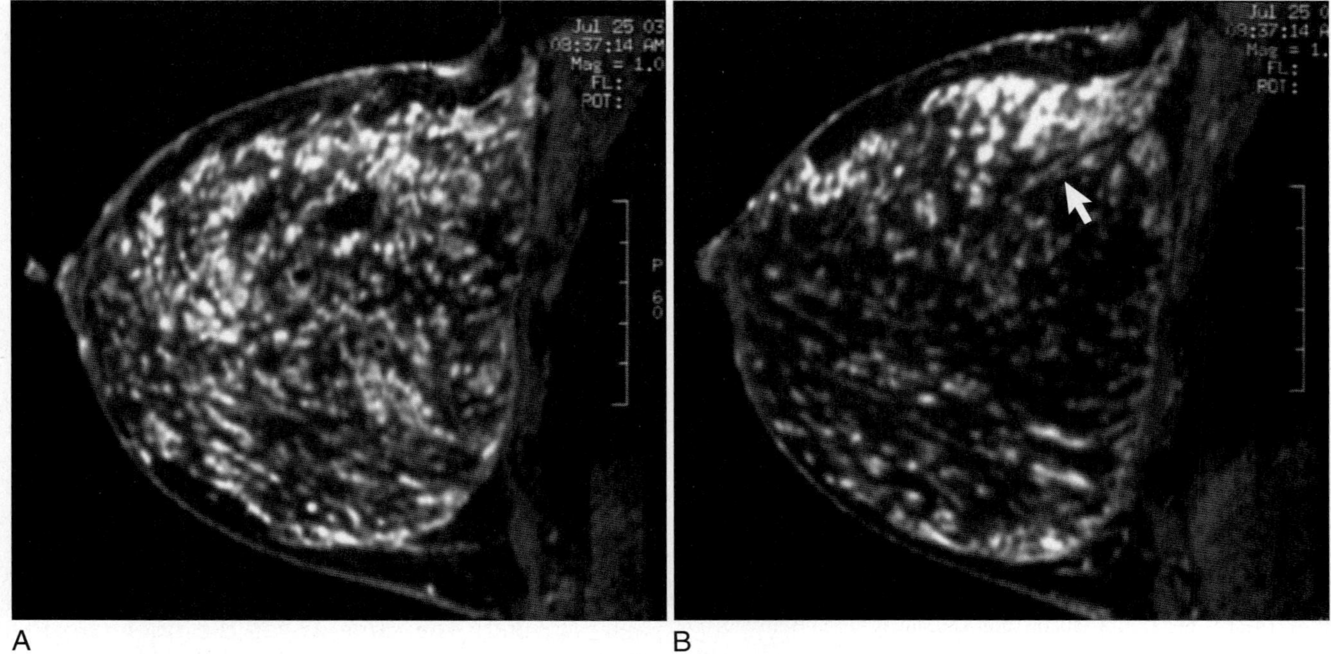

Figure 14–14. A 38-year-old woman with dense breasts and a high risk for breast cancer underwent screening with magnetic resonance imaging using research protocol. **A,** Contrast-enhanced subtraction sagittal image of the right breast shows a diffuse benign nonspecific enhancement pattern. **B,** Subtraction image of the contrast-enhanced sagittal image demonstrates regional benign enhancement in the same breast (*arrow*).

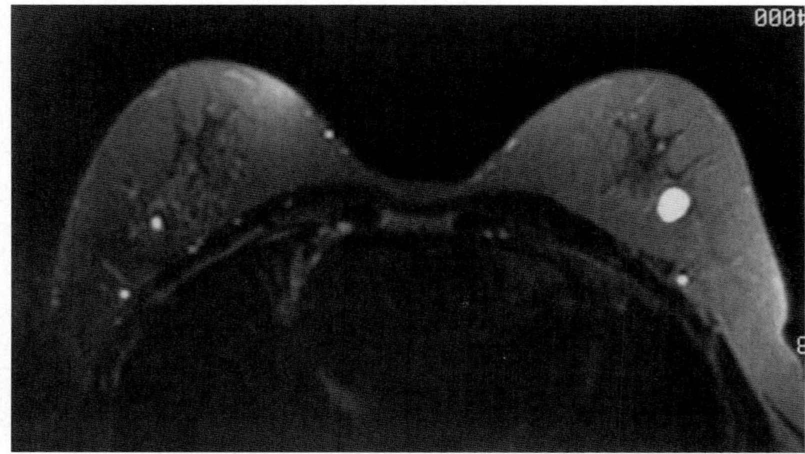

Figure 14–15. T2-weighted axial fat-suppressed magnetic resonance image shows a round high-signal-intensity mass that did not enhance on the T1-weighted postcontrast images (*not shown*). This finding is consistent with a simple cyst.

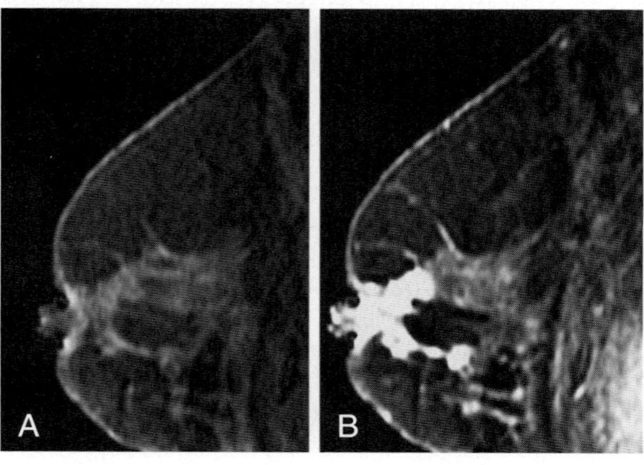

Figure 14–16. Magnetic resonance imaging in surveillance of the conservatively treated breast. The patient had a long history of left breast deformity and nipple retraction after undergoing lumpectomy. Mammographic findings were inconclusive, showing a dense retroareolar region that could have been secondary to previous surgery and irradiation and that was not significantly changed from its appearance on previous mammograms. Three-dimensional spoiled gradient-recalled (SPGR) precontrast (**A**) and postcontrast (**B**) fat-suppressed sagittal images show postcontrast segmental enhancement Clumped areas of enhancement are seen in the retroareolar breast tissue. Surgery demonstrated recurrent infiltrating ductal carcinoma.

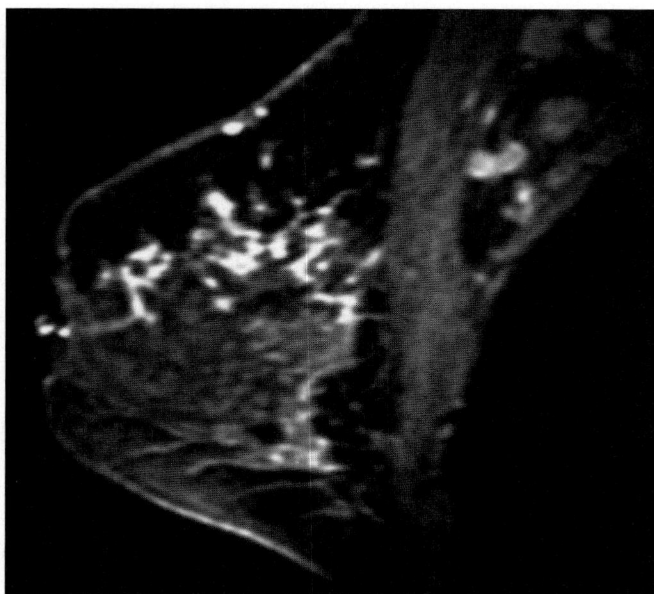

Figure 14–17. Segmental suspicious calcifications and irregular masses were observed on mammography and ultrasonography in a 65-year-old woman. Abnormal lymph nodes were also palpated. A contrast-enhanced postsubtraction single magnetic resonance image shows segmental irregular enhancement extending from the nipple to the chest wall. Adenopathy appears in the axilla with multiple enhancing masses.

CURRENT CLINICAL PRACTICE FOR IMAGING THE BREAST

Current clinical practices for MRI of the breast include (1) imaging of the augmented breast; (2) preoperative evaluation for extent of tumor, size, and additional lesions; (3) postoperative evaluation, that is, surveillance after breast conservation surgery and radiotherapy for residual or recurrent disease; (4) evaluation of malignant axillary adenopathy to search for the unknown primary; (5) further evaluation for inconclusive findings of mammography, ultrasonography, or positron emission tomography (PET) or for suspicious clinical findings with negative imaging findings; (6) analysis of chest wall invasion; and (7) evaluation of tumor response to neoadjuvant chemotherapy.[61,71]

These practices are constantly under evaluation, challenge, and refinement by researchers and investigators. MRI interpretation must be accompanied by mammography, ultrasonography, and other pertinent clinical or imaging information. MRI is best as an adjunct study, and therefore integration of MRI findings with those of the other modalities is essential for accurate diagnosis and interpretation.

Imaging the Augmented Breast

Magnetic resonance imaging is the most effective method for the detection of either intracapsular or extracapsular rupture of a breast implant.[72] More information concerning MRI of breast implants can be found in Chapter 32.

Standard mammographic views are limited in the detection of breast cancer in women with implants. Although special methods have been developed to improve the mammographic evaluation of the breast with implants, such as implant-displaced views, cancers may still be excluded from these views. Ultrasonography of palpable areas and breast physical examination in conjunction with mammography will offer additional benefit in detection of breast cancer.[73] Later studies have shown that the risk of development of breast cancer is not higher in women with augmented breasts. In addition, the stage and prognosis of tumors were not influenced by breast implants, despite the lower accuracy of mammography.[74,75] When these methods are inconclusive, MRI has proved useful in tumor detection, because the implant does not obscure breast tissue on MRI (Fig. 14–18).[14] Protocols for imaging the augmented breast for the breast parenchyma and tumor analysis are essentially the same as for the nonaugmented breast. At our facility, we add an inversion recovery sequence with water suppression to assess implant integrity in addition to the tumor protocols.

Evaluation of the Extent of Breast Cancer

Investigators have found MRI to be more reliable than mammography or clinical breast examination in determining the extent of tumor involvement or multifocal lesions.[27,55,76,77] Chest wall invasion can also be depicted well on MRI images when tumors are located in the posterior aspect of the breast.[78] It has been noted that mammography may underestimate the extent of tumor involvement compared with MRI (Fig. 14–19). Studies have shown that MRI has detected multifocal disease in many patients in whom mammography shows only focal disease (see Figs. 14–12 and 14–19).[52,63] As a result of these findings, MRI has been used as an aid in preoperative treatment planning (lumpectomy vs. mastectomy). Lee and coworkers[79] reported an overlap in the appearances of benign and malignant lesions that limited the efficacy of breast MRI in detection of postoperative residual disease. They also found that MRI can show additional suspicious lesions that are likely to be multicentric or multifocal disease. The MRI findings changed the original treatment plan for approximately 30% of the affected breasts in this study.[79]

Controversy surrounds MRI and its role in preoperative planning. It has been argued that the current clinical practice of evaluating with MRI before breast surgery may actually be increasing the number of mastectomies. Breast cancer is often multifocal, but treatment with lumpectomy and irradiation has been associated with low rates of local recurrence. However, once MRI fully delineates the tumor size

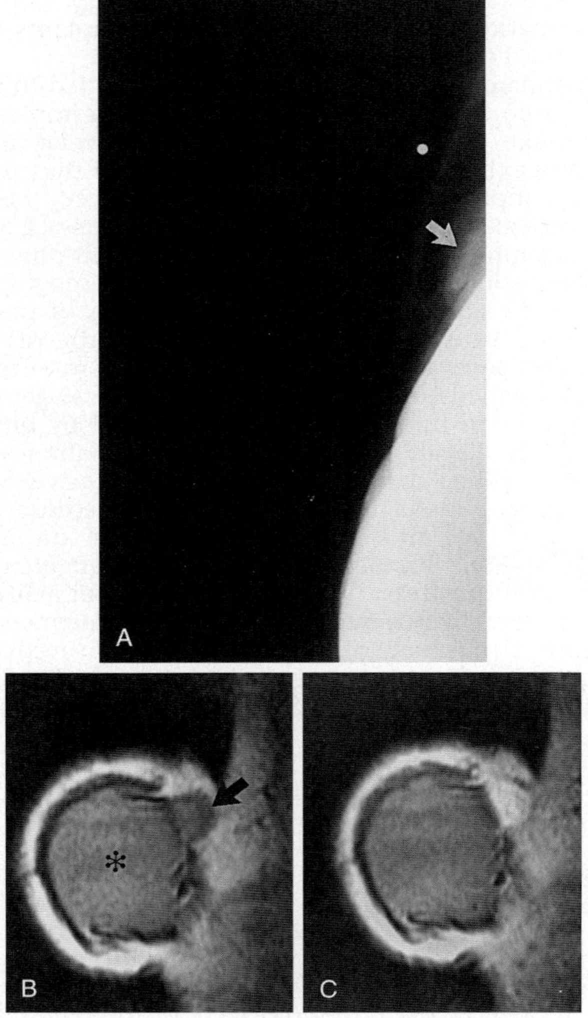

Figure 14–18. Invasive lobular carcinoma in a woman with silicone breast implants. The patient presented with a lump in her right breast. **A,** Tangential mammogram image of the palpable abnormality shows the anterior boundary of a round, smooth mass (*arrow*) just posterior to the lead marker (BB). **B** and **C,** Two-dimensional dynamic sagittal magnetic resonance images show a round, smooth, heterogeneous, rapidly enhancing mass (*arrow*) adjacent to the implant (*asterisk*).

and identifies multicentric lesions, a mastectomy becomes a more viable option than lumpectomy and irradiation.[80] MRI may reveal a large tumor that is amenable to neoadjuvant chemotherapy, with the possibility of reducing tumor size and providing the option of lumpectomy, which might not have been considered. It is important to realize that all lesions within the breast that enhance with contrast agent are not necessarily additional foci of malignancy. The incidentally enhancing lesion (IEL) has been reported as a focus of enhancement of 5 mm or less and should be considered benign if there is no evidence of malignancy.[62,81] However, if a malignancy is present, such lesions become more suspicious and increase the reporting of additional lesions. On the basis of the findings, histologic confirmation of suspected multicentric disease should be obtained before decision-making for treatment is undertaken.[52] Research is currently under way to answer these questions and to achieve an understanding of the clinical significance of detecting additional lesions and how it would affect treatment and outcome.

Surveillance after Breast-Conserving Surgery and Radiotherapy for Breast Cancer

Another potential use of MRI of the breast is the ongoing evaluation of women who are undergoing breast conservation therapy for cancer. Mammography and clinical breast examination are limited in the evaluation of the conservatively treated breast because of postoperative and post-irradiation changes.[14,15,18,53,82] Postoperative changes can result in contrast enhancement, and MRI is not effective for evaluation of the postoperative breast immediately after surgery. The timing can be important, especially for patients whose surgical specimens had positive margins and who are candidates for reexcision.[54] One study recommends waiting at least 28 days after surgery to search for the positive margin.[83] After approximately 12 to 18 months, the majority of postoperative changes are less active, and most scars do not enhance after 1 year. MRI has the potential to identify tumor recurrence, but fat necrosis and inflammation may have enhancement patterns that can be confusing.[52,84] Enhancement after 1 year is suggestive of residual or recurrent breast tumor, depending on the enhancement pattern, morphologic characteristics, and kinetics (see Fig. 14–16).

Evaluating Tumor Response to Neoadjuvant Chemotherapy

Preoperative neoadjuvant chemotherapy is defined as combined chemotherapy given to patients with breast cancer who have large tumor masses (stage T3 or T4), regional lymph node involvement, or both, before they undergo definitive surgical treatment.[63] Many of these patients tend to have distant micrometastases, and the goal of this therapy is to improve overall survival and postoperative cosmetic results. Response to therapy is usually followed by physical examination to detect residual tumor, but it may be difficult to differentiate tumor from fibrotic changes or to identify small nonpalpable disease clinically. Therefore, MRI has been the most useful modality as an adjunct in the assessment of the residual tumor burden.[85-88] In one series, the percentage reduction in the early contrast uptake after two cycles of neoadjuvant chemotherapy was predictive of the achievement of a pathologically complete response (Fig. 14–20).[89] In our experience, MRI is very accurate in the quantitative analysis of residual tumor; however, false-negative findings have occurred. They may be related to the effects of

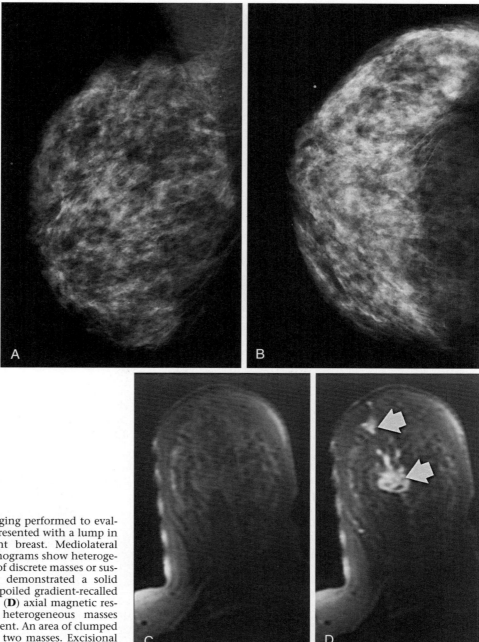

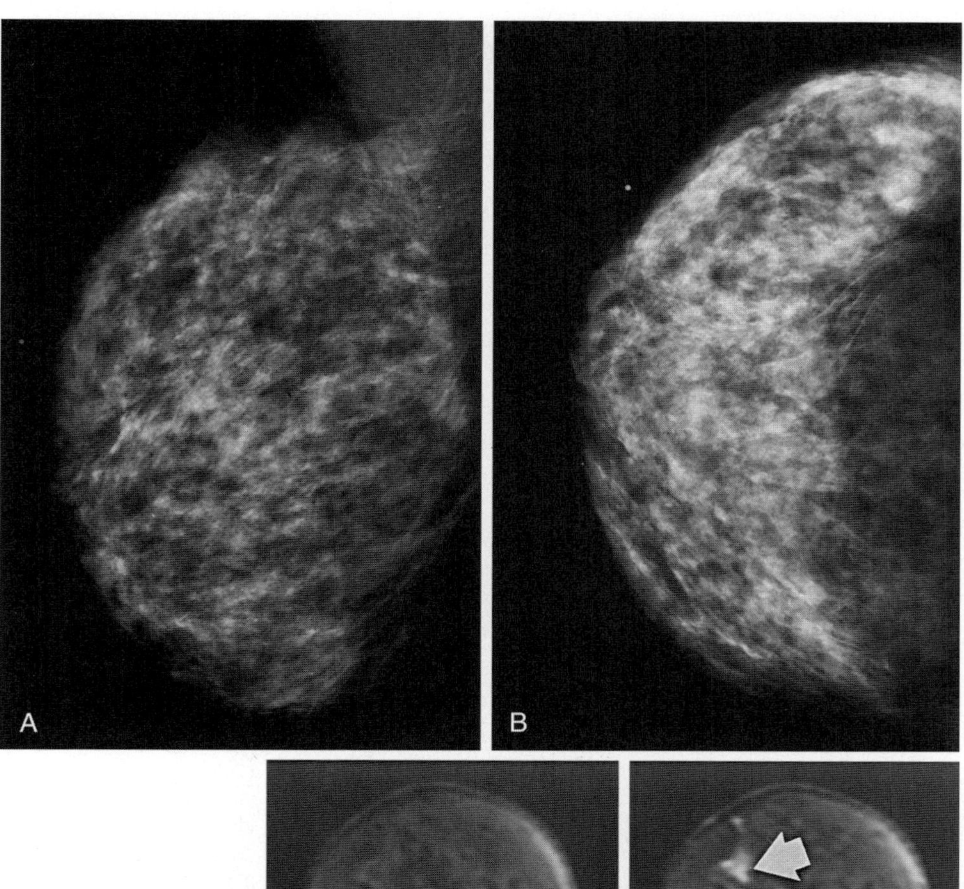

Figure 14–19. Magnetic resonance imaging performed to evaluate extent of carcinoma. The patient presented with a lump in the upper-outer quadrant of her right breast. Mediolateral oblique (**A**) and craniocaudal (**B**) mammograms show heterogeneously dense breasts without evidence of discrete masses or suspicious calcifications. Ultrasonography demonstrated a solid mass (not shown). Three-dimensional spoiled gradient-recalled (SPGR) precontrast (**C**) and postcontrast (**D**) axial magnetic resonance images show two irregular, heterogeneous masses (*arrows*) with intense contrast enhancement. An area of clumped enhancement can be seen between the two masses. Excisional biopsy demonstrated multifocal ductal carcinoma.

chemotherapy on the microvasculature, decreasing uptake of contrast agent within the tumor. Multicenter clinical trials are under way to evaluate the response of neoadjuvant chemotherapy with MRI, mammography, ultrasonography, and PET.

Evaluation of Axillary Adenopathy and the Unknown Primary

Breast cancer manifesting as axillary metastases without mammographic or clinical evidence of the primary tumor within the breast is an uncommon occurrence. The incidence is low; this finding accounts for 0.3% to 0.8% of all patients with breast cancer at the time of presentation.[90] Studies have shown that MRI is effective in imaging multifocal disease and finding unsuspected foci of breast cancer within a known affected breast. The use of MRI to search for the primary source of axillary metastases has shown promise. Several studies have shown that breast MRI is effective in identifying the primary in the ipsilateral breast in 75% to 86% of patients.[90-92] Treatment for women with positive axillary nodes and negative clinical and mammographic findings is usually mastectomy. With the high sensitivity of MRI and its accuracy in identifying a primary tumor, lumpectomy becomes an option that otherwise would have not been considered. Now that imaging of both breasts can be performed in a

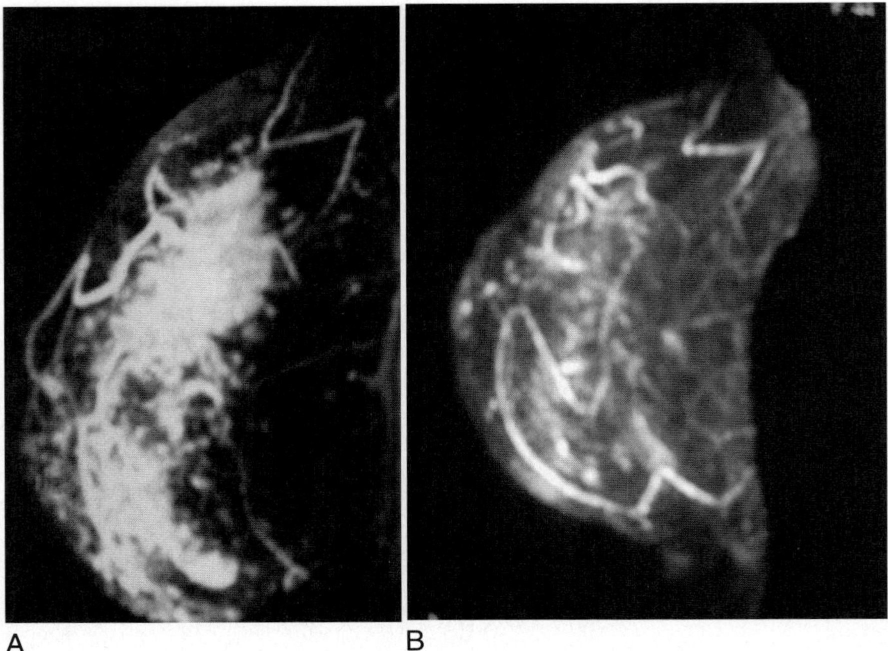

Figure 14–20. **A,** Contrast-enhanced sagittal maximum intensity projection (MIP) magnetic resonance image of an intensely enhancing mass of infiltrating ductal carcinoma involving the entire breast. **B,** Contrast-enhanced sagittal image obtained after neoadjuvant chemotherapy shows complete resolution of mass.

short time, synchronous cancers as well as the possibility of a contralateral primary cancer can also be evaluated.[91]

Evaluation of Nipple Discharge

Breast MRI has also been applied to the evaluation of nipple discharge. Nakahara and colleagues[93] imaged 55 women with galactography, ultrasonography, and MRI. The purpose of their study was to evaluate the efficacy of MRI with the imaging standards of mammography after the injection of contrast agent into a discharging duct and ultrasonography to identify dilated ducts with filling defects or focal masses. Their results were encouraging. MRI identified all the malignant lesions, including DCIS.[93] Orel and associates[94] had similar results, although the design of their study was different. The two studies suggested that there is a potential role for MRI as a noninvasive alternative to galactography.[93,94] We have evaluated only four women with MRI for bloody nipple discharge. One case was positive for DCIS, which was identified only on MRI (Fig. 14–21); galactography and ultrasonography in this case showed duct ectasia without filling defects, suggesting benign disease.

Evaluation with Positron Emission Tomography and Magnetic Resonance Imaging

Positron emission tomography is used to assess abnormal biochemical changes in the body. The modality has proved to be useful in detection of both primary tumor and metastases, cerebrovascular disease, and epilepsy. In some patients, an abnormal focus of activity is visualized in the breast on a PET study that was obtained for another clinical indication. Breast MRI as well as mammography and ultrasonography can be used to further evaluate this abnormal finding. Walter and coworkers[95] investi-

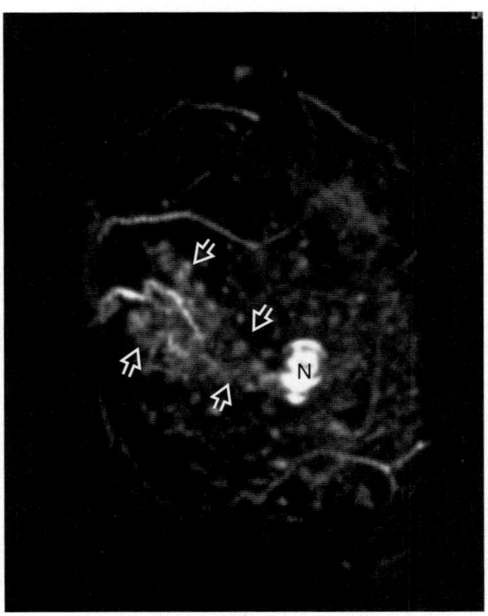

Figure 14–21. A 47-year-old woman presented with bloody discharge from her right nipple. Ductography and ultrasonography identified multiple nonspecific dilated ducts without filling defects. No suspicious findings. Magnetic resonance imaging showed a large, discrete, triangular enhancement (*open arrows*), an appearance consistent with a segmental distribution extending into the nipple. (N represents the nipple marker.) Pathologic diagnosis was ductal carcinoma in situ.

gated the diagnostic value of MRI and PET as single diagnostic tools and in combination for differentiation between malignant and benign disease. Nineteen malignant and 23 benign breast lesions (of 42 lesions in 40 patients) were proven histologically. The combination of the two imaging methods reduced the need for biopsy from 55% to 17%. Only one false-negative finding, in a patient pretreated with chemotherapy, was observed with the use of both methods. The combination of breast MRI and PET using fluorodeoxyglucose (FDG) can help decrease the number of biopsies performed on benign breast lesions. Walter and coworkers[95] suggested that because of their high cost, these technologies be limited to use in problematic cases to rule out or demonstrate malignancy. The best diagnostic strategy is achieved if breast MRI is used first; if the diagnosis is still questionable, FDG-PET can be performed.[95]

In a study by Rieber and associates,[96] MRI and PET were superior to conventional methods in nearly all areas studied—diagnosis, extent of disease, and contralateral malignancies. The findings of one or both of the methods positively affected patients' surgical treatment in 12.5% to 15% of cases. PET is also used to monitor patients after breast reconstruction and to gauge the response to neoadjuvant chemotherapy. It suffers the same pitfalls as MRI, with false-negative findings secondary to chemotherapy and false-positive findings in the reconstructed breast due to inflammation and fat necrosis.

POTENTIAL ROLES FOR BREAST MAGNETIC RESONANCE IMAGING

Research has provided tremendous insight into the genetics of breast cancer and its pathogenesis. Each year sees an expansion of our understanding of the basic mechanisms of breast cancer initiation and progression as well as clinical applications of this knowledge. Within radiology and nuclear medicine, there is also an evolution of technical advances that continue to give researchers the tools necessary to answer the clinical questions as they develop.

Potential roles in the future include screening women at high risk of breast cancer in comparison with members of the general population who also have heterogeneously dense or extremely dense breast tissue. Breast MRI screening for the general population is too costly, and the specificity is varied. The information needed to support the screening may come from multicenter clinical trials, or a specific trial may have to be performed to answer these questions.

Clinical trials are currently being carried out to determine the efficacy and long-term benefits of screening. However, for MRI to be viable as a screening tool, MRI-guided biopsy and localization must be perfected to allow for tissue diagnosis of lesions that are not depicted by other means.[97]

Screening High-Risk Women and Dense Breast Tissue

MRI for the detection of breast cancer is not limited by breast density. Thus, breast MRI may play an important role in the evaluation of women who have dense breast tissue, who have undergone breast augmentation with silicone injections, or who are at high risk for breast cancer. The standard methods for the assessment of dense breast tissues are clinical breast examination, mammography, and ultrasonography. Many women with dense breast tissue have palpable nodules. In our practice, many women with dense breast tissue and palpable nodularity are imaged frequently with mammography and ultrasonography. Usually the clinical findings are due to physiologic nodularity, and the mammograms and ultrasonography findings are normal. If conventional imaging findings are inconclusive and the clinical findings are suspicious or the woman is at high risk for breast cancer, breast MRI may be requested (Fig. 14–22).

Mammography and ultrasonography are limited in evaluating women with silicone injections. The silicone granulomas are poorly penetrated with mammography, and therefore the mammograms are extremely dense with limited visualization of breast tissue. Ultrasound beams are scattered in the presence of silicone, and the underlying tissue cannot be visualized. However, breast MRI can adequately visualize the breast tissue once a contrast agent is given (Fig. 14–23). We are currently monitoring several women who have silicone injections, and to date their examinations have been negative for breast cancer.

High-risk applies to women who have tested positive for the gene mutations *BRCA1* and *BRCA2* or who have biopsy-proven atypical ductal hyperplasia (ADH) or lobular carcinoma in situ (LCIS), at least one first-degree relative with a history of breast cancer or ovarian cancer, or a personal history of breast cancer. Female carriers of *BRCA1* mutations can have a lifetime risk of breast cancer of 80% or higher and of ovarian cancer of almost 60%. Carriers of *BRCA2* mutants have a similar risk of breast cancer and a more moderately increased risk of ovarian cancer.[98,99] Other rare syndromes that have been reported to increase the risk of breast cancer are Li-Fraumeni syndrome, a hereditary cancer syndrome that predisposes people to develop early-onset breast cancer and sarcomas and other early-onset cancers; Cowden syndrome, an autosomal dominant disorder associated with skin lesions and multiple hamartomas; and Peutz-Jeghers syndrome, a disorder or pigmentation and gastrointestinal hamartoma. Ataxia-telangiectasia, a progressive cerebellar ataxia with ocular apraxia and telangiectasia, has also been implicated but not yet proven in increasing cancer risk.[100] Approximately 80% to 90% of hereditary breast cancer cases are caused by mutations in the *BRCA1* and *BRCA2* genes.[101] However, only 5% to 10% of breast cancers are associated with genetic

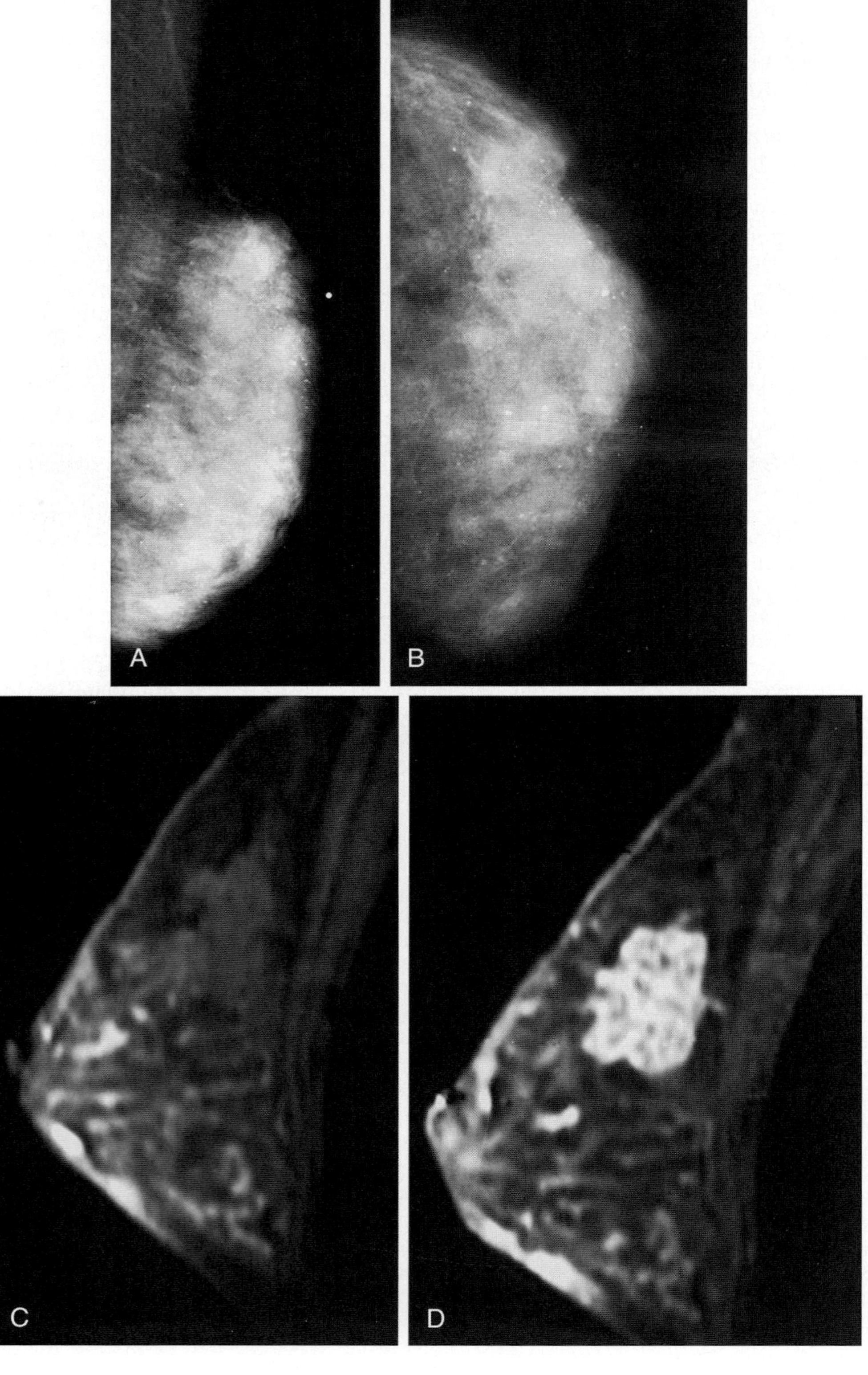

Figure 14–22. Carcinoma obscured by dense tissue on mammography. A woman presented with a lump in her left breast. Mediolateral oblique (**A**) and craniocaudal (**B**) mammograms show heterogeneously dense breasts with diffuse, benign-appearing calcifications. The lead marker (BB) seen in **A** is at the site of the palpable mass. Three-dimensional spoiled gradient-recalled (SPGR) precontrast (**C**) and postcontrast (**D**) fat-suppressed sagittal magnetic resonance images show a large, irregular, heterogeneous, contrast-enhancing mass with enhancing internal septations. Excisional biopsy demonstrated infiltrating ductal carcinoma.

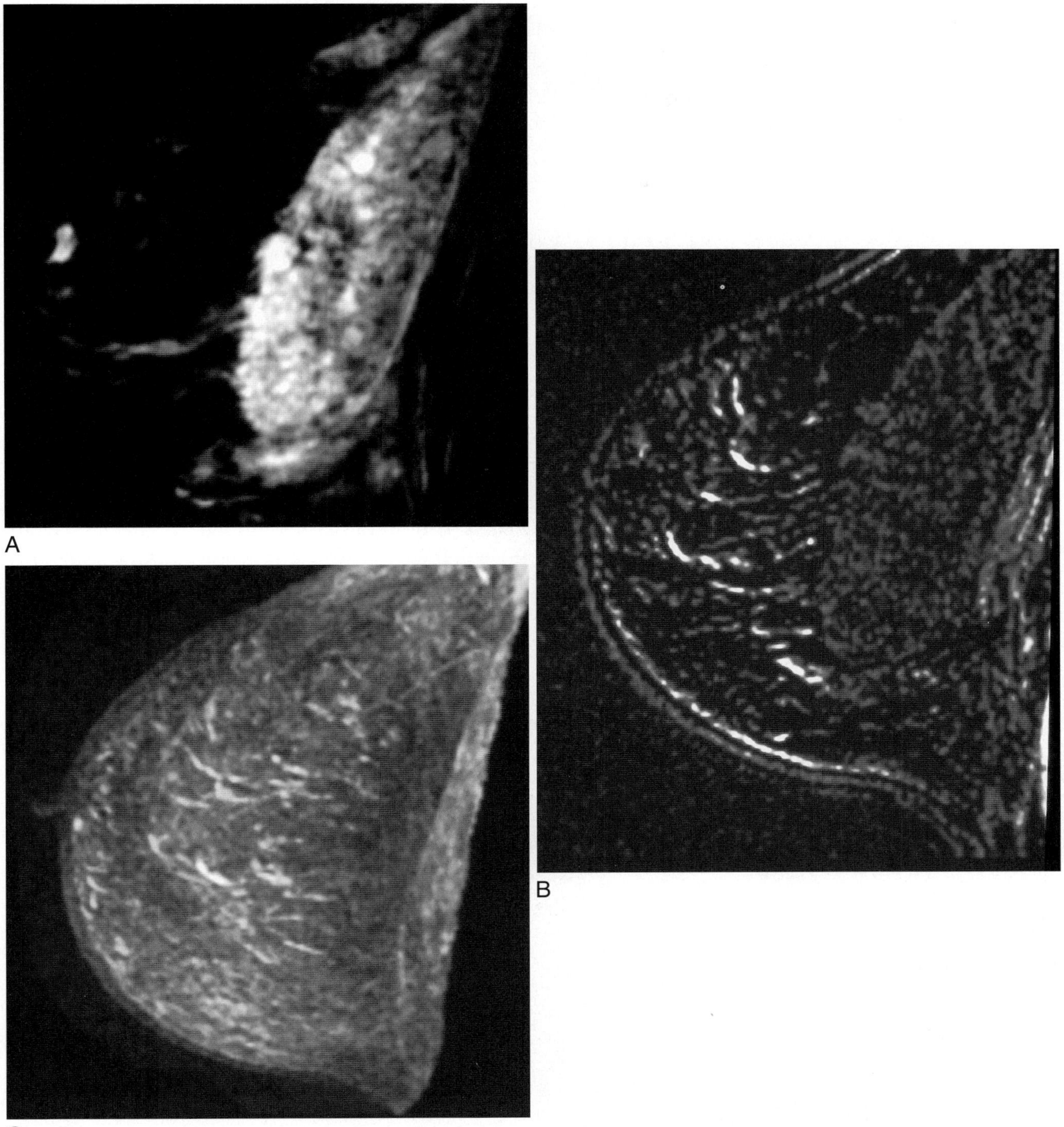

Figure 14–23. Evaluation of breasts with silicone injections. **A,** Non–contrast-enhanced, short-tau inversion recovery (STIR) magnetic resonance image shows diffuse silicone injections primarily involving the posterior aspect of the breast. **B,** Contrast-enhanced subtraction image demonstrates no evidence of suspicious enhancement. **C,** Maximum intensity projection (MIP) image with subtraction combines all the single-slice images into one to provide a three-dimensional projection of the breast tissue. Note that the silicone granulomas are not seen on this image because of subtraction.

predisposition. The key to identifying women who are at risk for a hereditary breast cancer lies in obtaining an adequate, three-generation family history, including ethnic background.[101] Absolute risk factors are added values that can be incorporated in the breast cancer risk assessment models that are commonly used, known as the Gail or Claus models. These models look at age, age at menarche, age at first live birth, nulliparity, presence or absence of a first-degree relative (mother or sister) with breast cancer, and a personal history of benign biopsy findings.[102] An association between low-dose diagnostic x-ray exposure or therapeutic radiation treatment and breast cancer risk has not been established.

Several studies have been conducted to compare MRI with conventional imaging (mammography and ultrasonography) in screening high-risk women.[49,50,103] The results have confirmed that breast MRI is superior to mammography and ultrasonography. Breast MRI can find occult primaries not seen with the other modalities.

MRI-GUIDED BIOPSY AND WIRE LOCALIZATION

MRI of the breast is very sensitive in detecting breast cancers as well as benign breast lesions. When a suspicious abnormality is detected only on MRI, a method must be available to localize the finding for preoperative wire localization or image-guided percutaneous core needle biopsy.[71,97,104,105] Heywang-Köbrunner and associates[106] and Fischer and colleagues[97] were the first to report successful MRI-guided needle localizations using prototype biopsy devices. Freehand methods have also been reported (Fig. 14–24).[107-109]

MRI-guided interventional procedures have been modified from the standard methods used in mammography. Many of the required features are similar—access to the breast, immobilization of the breast, image localization of the lesion, needle placement, and image confirmation of needle placement. Many prototypes have developed over the years, most based on the system developed by Heywang-Köbrunner.[107,110-112] With the help of manufacturers, the investigators' efforts were realized, because the best features of their devices were incorporated and ultimately became commercially available. MRI-guided localization using a dedicated breast biopsy device with the patient in the prone position has been performed for more than 10 years.[97,106,107,110,113] Access is still primarily limited to the lateral approach with commercially available biopsy devices, but improvements to allow medial access are in progress.

The magnetic field creates challenges for needle localizations and biopsies by means of MRI. The material used to manufacture the localization device,

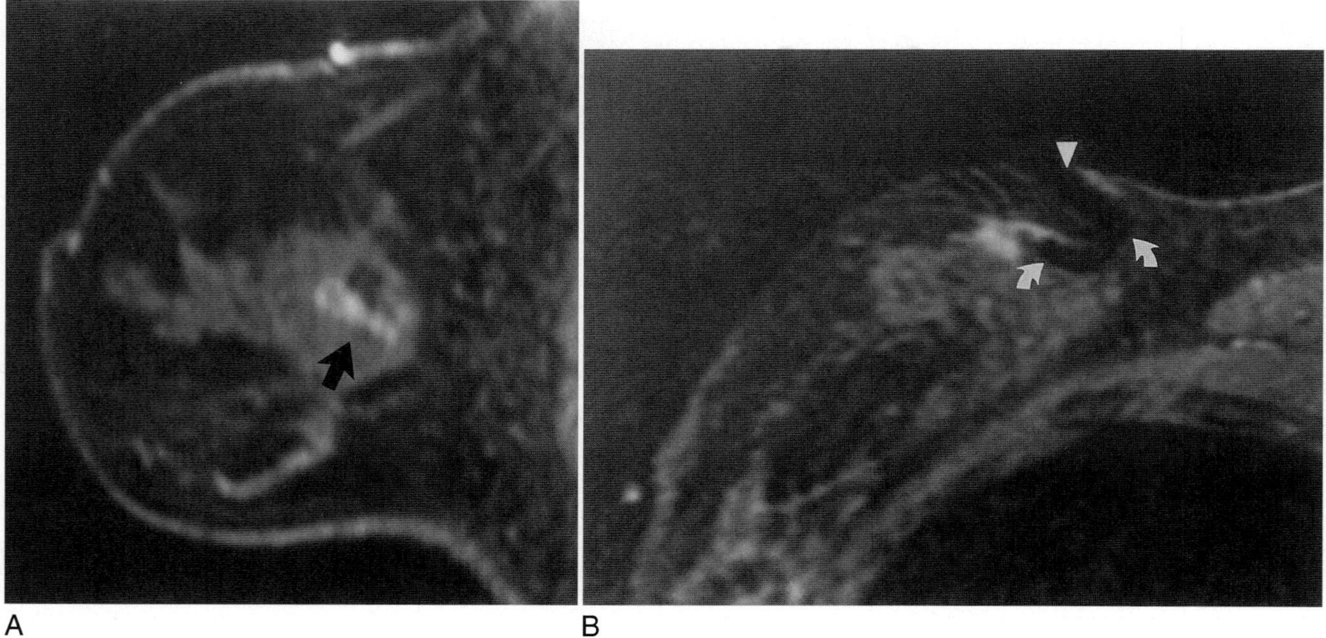

Figure 14–24. Preoperative needle wire localization with magnetic resonance imaging (MRI) guidance in a 58-year-old woman with ductal carcinoma in situ who had undergone core needle biopsy. Post–core biopsy ultrasonography was negative, and the mass was no longer visualized or palpable. MRI was performed to evaluate for potential areas of residual disease. **A,** Contrast-enhanced three-dimensional, T1-weighted, spoiled gradient-recalled (SPGR) image with fat suppression identifies an 8-mm ductal enhancement in the area of the prior biopsy (*arrow*). **B,** MRI–guided needle placement was performed with an MRI-compatible needle and wire. The *arrowhead* identifies the entry site of the needle-wire system. The hook of the J wire (*curved arrows*) is within the focus of enhancement.

including the compression plate, must be compatible with a strong magnetic field. In the commercially available dedicated MRI biopsy systems, the grids are plastic and MRI compatible. Efforts have been made to find magnetic field–compatible needles that do not compromise the quality and effectiveness of breast biopsy. Nonferrous needles have been acceptable because they can remain in the breast during imaging for localization of the lesion before biopsy. Technical innovations have allowed the combination of nonferrous with ferrous needles through the use of a new MRI-compatible coaxial needle for localization of the lesion, followed by biopsy with a standard stainless steel 14-gauge core biopsy needle.[105,107] The accuracy rate for mammography-guided stereotactic core needle biopsy (SCNB) is within the 95th percentile.[114] MRI-guided core needle biopsy has been reported as accurate and is gaining interest because of the minimal complications, compared with the perioperative risk and scarring associated with surgical biopsy after wire localization.

As our experience grows, MRI-guided core needle biopsies will be performed to obtain a diagnosis before or in lieu of a lumpectomy or excisional biopsy for diagnosis.[107] Vacuum-assisted MRI-guided core biopsies are also increasing in use.[107] A substitute needle is placed and its position confirmed with the contrast-enhanced MRI. This needle is then removed and the large-bore vacuum-assisted core system needle is placed to the appropriate depth. Postprocedure marker clips can be placed in the biopsy cavity via the biopsy instrument.[107] These large-bore core needle biopsy systems used with MRI have the same risks and complications as those used with mammography and ultrasonography.

Despite advancements in equipment and pulse sequences, the role of MRI of the breast will remain limited until MRI-guided breast biopsy and prebiopsy needle localization become reliable and widely available. One of the major limitations of wire localization or core needle biopsy of lesions detected solely on MRI is the inability to document the removal of these lesions with specimen radiography. A method to reliably verify that the breast lesion was actually removed remains a challenge. Further limitations include limited access to areas of interest in the medial aspect of the breast or near the chest wall.

At our institution, if a lesion is found on MRI, directed ultrasonography is recommended. We commonly identify the abnormality ultrasonographically. If the lesion is deemed suspicious, a biopsy is performed under ultrasonographic guidance. When there is a question of concordance between ultrasonographic and MRI findings, we place an MRI-compatible needle within the lesion under ultrasonographic guidance and confirm the location with a contrast-enhanced MRI. Therefore, percutaneous MRI-guided interventional procedures are limited to the few cases in which other imaging modalities are unable to visualize the suspicious lesion detected on MRI. Reports in the literature support our findings.[111,115]

We have used both freehand and dedicated biopsy devices successfully in localizing MRI-detected lesions (see Fig. 14–23). The MRI-guided localization or core biopsy procedures require approximately 60 to 90 minutes (from setup, intravenous access, and breast positioning to lesion localization). After one injection of gadolinium, the breast lesion(s) can be clearly visualized. The lesion conspicuity usually remains throughout the procedure without the need for a second injection. However, additional injections of gadolinium might be required to ensure adequate visualization of some lesions during the entire localization procedure. The development of contrast agents that provide prolonged lesion enhancement may eliminate the need for multiple injections.

Future innovations may include new MRI-compatible contrast agents (e.g., antibody-specific, non-ionic gadolinium) that may be more effective in differentiating malignant from benign tumors. Minimally invasive procedures such as MRI-guided tumor ablation and MRI-guided lumpectomies have the potential to precisely localize the margins of a tumor to ensure complete removal.[71,111]

SUMMARY

Breast MRI began in the early 1980s but was not successful for tumor evaluation until the development of contrast-enhanced breast MRI in 1986. MRI has been used in multiple research and academic institutions and now in the clinical arena throughout the world in patients who have symptoms or positive findings on conventional imaging. Advances in both spatial and temporal resolution, imaging sequences, pharmacokinetics of contrast agent uptake, use of dedicated and phased-array breast coils, and gadolinium-based contrast agents have played a role in the evolution of breast MRI.

Current clinical indications for breast MRI include the evaluation of implant integrity and tumors, inconclusive conventional imaging findings, preoperative evaluation (extent and multifocality), postoperative evaluation (residual or recurrent, axillary adenopathy/unknown primary, neoadjuvant chemotherapy), and pre- and post-treatment evaluations. Breast MRI's role in screening remains unresolved, especially in patients who have augmented breasts and those at high risk for breast cancer. Additional research is needed to determine the clinical role of breast MRI and the optimal pulse sequences. Furthermore, MRI-guided biopsy must be refined to expedite the biopsy of lesions depicted only on MRI. Additional benefits of breast MRI remain to be determined.

Standardized guidelines for reporting breast MRI results have improved significantly since contrast-enhanced agents were introduced in 1986. Multiple approaches to the interpretation of breast MRI have been examined because of the overlap in presentation of benign and malignant lesions. The ACR BI-RADS lexicon for breast MRI has provided the capacity for better reporting, communication, and collection of data from multiple studies.

References

1. Alcorn FS, et al: Magnetic resonance imaging in the study of the breast. Radiographics 1985;5:631-652.
2. Heywang SH, et al: MR of the breast: Histopathologic correlation. Eur J Radiol 1987;3:175-183.
3. Murphy WA, Gohagan JK: Breast. In Stark DD, Bradley WG Jr (eds): Magnetic Resonance Imaging. St. Louis: CV Mosby, 1987, pp 861-886.
4. Partain CL, et al: Magnetic resonance imaging of the breast: Functional T1 and three-dimensional imaging. Cardiovasc Intervent Radiol 1986;8:292-299.
5. Stelling CB, et al: Prototype coil for magnetic resonance imaging of the female breast. Radiology 1985;154:457-462.
6. Wiener JI, et al: Breast and axillary tissue MRI: Correlations of signal intensities and relaxation times with pathologic findings. Radiology 1986;160:299-305.
7. Heywang-Köbrunner SH: Contrast-enhanced magnetic resonance imaging of the breast. Invest Radiol 1994;29:94-104.
8. Heywang SH, et al: MRI of the breast using gadolinium-DTPA. J Comput Assist Tomogr 1986;10:199-204.
9. Harms SE, et al: Fat-suppressed three-dimensional MRI of the breast. Radiographics 1993;13:247-267.
10. Harms SE, et al: MRI of the breast with rotating delivery of excitation off resonance: Clinical experience with pathologic correlation. Radiology 1993;186:493-501.
11. Heywang SH, et al: MRI of the breast with Gd-DTPA: Use and limitations. Radiology 1989;171:9.
12. Heywang-Köbrunner SH: Contrast-enhanced MRI of the breast-overview after 1250 patient examinations. Electromedica 1993;2:43-52.
13. Heywang-Köbrunner SH: Non-mammographic breast imaging techniques. Curr Opin Radiol 1992;4:146-154.
14. Heywang-Köbrunner SH, et al: Contrast-material enhanced MRI of the breast in patients with postoperative scarring and silicon implants. J Comput Assist Tomogr 1990;14:348-356.
15. Heywang-Köbrunner SH, et al: Contrast-enhanced MRI of the breast after limited surgery and radiation therapy. J Comput Assist Tomogr 1993;17:891-900.
16. Kaiser WA: MRM promises earlier breast cancer diagnosis. Diagn Imaging Int 1992;11:44-50.
17. Kaiser WA, Zeitler E: MRI of the breast: Fast imaging sequences with and without Gd-DTPA. Radiology 1989;170: 681-686.
18. Lewis-Jones HG, Whitehouse GH, Leinster SJ: The role of MRI in the assessment of local recurrent breast carcinoma. Clin Radiol 1991;43:197-204.
19. Merchant TE, et al: Clinical magnetic resonance spectroscopy of human breast disease. Invest Radiol 1991;26:1053-1059.
20. Orel S, et al: Suspicious breast lesions: MRI with radiologic-pathologic correlation. Radiology 1994;190:485-493.
21. Pierce WB, et al: Three-dimensional gadolinium-enhanced MRI of the breast: Pulse sequence with fat suppression and magnetization transfer contrast. Radiology 1991;181:757-763.
22. Revel D, et al: Gd-DTPA contrast enhancement and tissue differentiation in MRI of experimental breast carcinoma. Radiology 1986;158:319-323.
23. Rubens D, et al: Gadopentetate dimeglumine-enhanced chemical-shift MRI of the breast. AJR Am J Roentgenol 1991;157:267-270.
24. Gilles R, et al: Nonpalpable breast tumors: Diagnosis with contrast-enhanced subtraction dynamic MRI. Radiology 1994;191:625-631.
25. Buadu LD, et al: Breast lesions: Correlation of contrast medium enhancement patterns on MR images with histopathologic findings and tumor angiogenesis. Radiology 1996;200:639-649.
26. Szabo BK, et al: Dynamic MRI of the breast. Acta Radiol 2003;44:379-386.
27. Fischer U, Kopka L, Grabbe E: Breast carcinoma: Effect of preoperative contrast-enhanced MRI on the therapeutic approach. Radiology 1999;213:881-888.
28. Kuhl CK, Schild HH: Dynamic image interpretation of MRI of the breast. J Magn Reson Imaging 2000;12:965-974.
29. Kuhl CK, et al: Dynamic breast MRI: Are signal intensity time course data useful for differential diagnosis of enhancing lesions? Radiology 1999;211:101-110.
30. Nunes LW, Schnall MD, Orel SG: Update of breast MRI architectural interpretation model. Radiology 2001;219:484-494.
31. Nunes LW, Schnall MD, Orel SG, et al: Correlation of lesion appearance and histologic findings for the nodes of a breast MRI interpretation model. Radiographics 1999;19:79-92.
32. Kinkel K, et al: Dynamic high-spatial resolution MRI of suspicious breast lesions: Diagnostic criteria and interobserver variability. AJR Am J Roentgenol 2000;175:35-43.
33. Schnall MD, et al: A combined architectural and kinetic interpretation model for breast MR images. Acad Radiol 2001;8:591-597.
34. Bone B, et al: Mechanism of contrast enhancement in breast lesions at MRI. Acta Radiol 1998;39:494-500.
35. Degani H., et al: Mapping pathophysiological features of breast tumors by MRI at high spatial resolution. Nat Med 1997;3:780-782.
36. Frouge C, et al: Correlation between contrast enhancement in breast lesions at MRI. Invest Radiol 1994;29:1043-1049.
37. Buckley DL, et al: Microvessel density of invasive breast cancer assessed by dynamic Gd-DTPA enhanced MRI. J Magn Reson Imaging 1997;7:461-464.
38. Folkman J, Klagsbrun M: Angiogenic factors. Science 1987; 235:442-447.
39. Dvorak HF, Brown LF, Detmar M, Dvorak AM: Vascular permeability factor/vascular endothelial growth factor, microvascular hyperpermeability, and angiogenesis. Am J Pathol 1995;146:1029-1039.
40. Brown LF, et al: Expression of vascular permeability factor (vascular endothelial growth factor) and its receptors in breast cancer. Hum Pathol 1995;26:86-91.
41. Stomper PC, Winston JS, Herman S, et al: Angiogenesis and dynamic MRI gadolinium enhancement of malignant and benign breast lesions. Breast Cancer Res Treat 1997;45:39-46.
42. Tuncbilek N, Unlu E, Karakas H, et al: Evaluation of tumor angiogenesis with contrast-enhanced dynamic magnetic resonance mammography. Breast J 2003;9:403-408.
43. Buadu LD, et al: Patterns of peripheral enhancement in breast masses: Correlation of findings on contrast medium enhanced MRI with histologic features and tumor angiogenesis. J Comput Assist Tomogr 1997;21:421-430.
44. Lee AH, Dublin EA, Bobrow LG, Poulsom R: Invasive lobular and invasive ductal carcinoma of the breast show distinct patterns of vascular endothelial growth factor expression and angiogenesis. J Pathol 1998;185:394-401.
45. Giavazzi R, Albini A, Bussolino F, et al: The biological basis for antiangiogenic therapy. Eur J Cancer 2000;36:1913-1918.
46. Matsubayashi R, Matsuo Y, Edakuni G, et al: Breast masses with peripheral rim enhancement on dynamic contrast-enhanced MR images: Correlation of MR findings with histologic features and expression of growth factors. Radiology 2000;217:841-848.
47. Esserman L, et al: Contrast-enhanced magnetic resonance imaging to assess tumor histopathology and angiogenesis in breast carcinoma. Breast J 1999;5:13-21.
48. Sherif H, Mahfouz AE, Oellinger H, et al: Peripheral washout sign on contrast-enhanced MR images of the breast. Radiology 1997;205:209-213.
49. Den-Otter W, Merchant TE, Beijerinck D, Koten JW: Breast cancer induction due to mammography screening in hereditarily affected women. Anticancer Res 1996;16:3173-3175.
50. Kuhl CH, Schmutzler RK, Leutner CC, et al: Breast MRI screening in 192 women proved or suspected to be carriers of a breast cancer susceptibility gene: Preliminary results. Radiology 2000;215:267-279.
51. Boetes C, et al: MR characterization of suspicious breast lesions with a gadolinium-enhanced Turbo FLASH subtraction technique. Radiology 1994;193:777-781.

52. Orel SG, Schnall MD: MRI of the breast for the detection, diagnosis, and staging of breast cancer. Radiology 2001;220: 13-30.
53. Dao TH, et al: Tumor recurrence versus fibrosis in the irradiated breast: Differentiation with dynamic gadolinium-enhanced MRI. Radiology 1993;187:751-755.
54. Orel SG, et al: Breast carcinoma: MRI before re-excisional biopsy. Radiology 1997;205: 429-436.
55. Lee CH, et al: Clinical usefulness of MRI of the breast in the evaluation of the problematic mammogram. AJR Am J Roentgenol 1999;173:1323-1329.
56. Orel SG, Mendonca MH, Reynolds C et al: MRI of ductal carcinoma in situ. Radiology 1997;202:413-420.
57. Soderstrom CE, Harms SE, Copit DS, et al: Three-dimensional RODEO breast MRI of lesions containing ductal carcinoma in situ. Radiology 1996;201:427-432.
58. Neubauer H, Li M, Kuehne-heid R, et al: High grade and non-high grade ductal carcinoma in situ on dynamic MR mammography: Characteristic findings for signal increase and morphological pattern of enhancement. Br J Radiol 2003;76: 3-12.
59. Hochman, MG, et al: Fibroadenomas: MRI appearances with radiologic-histopathologic correlation. Radiology 1997;204: 123-129.
60. Ikeda DM, et al: Development, standardization, and testing of a lexicon for reporting contrast-enhanced breast magnetic resonance imaging studies. J of Magn Reson Imaging 2001; 13:889-895.
61. Harms SE, et al: Technical report of the International Working Group on Breast MRI. J Magn Reson Imaging 1999; 10:979-1015.
62. American College of Radiology (ACR): ACR BI-RADS®—Magnetic Resonance Imaging. In: ACR Breast Imaging Reporting and Data System, Breast Imaging Atlas. Reston, VA: American College of Radiology, 2003.
63. Ikeda DM, Baker DR, Daniel BL: Magnetic resonance imaging of breast cancer: Clinical indications and breast MRI reporting system. J Magn Reson Imaging 2000;12:975-983.
64. Liberman L, et al: The breast imaging reporting and data system-positive predictive value of mammographic features and final assessment. AJR Am J Roentgenol 1998;171:35-40.
65. Morris EA: Illustrated breast MR lexicon. Semin Roentgenol 2001;36:238-249.
66. Liberman L, et al: Breast lesions detected on MRI: Features and positive predictive value. AJR Am J Roentgenol 2002; 179:171-178.
67. Kim SJ, Morris EA, Liberman L: Observer variability and applicability of BI-RADS® terminology for breast MRI: Invasive carcinomas as focal Masses. AJR Am J Roentgenol 2001; 177:551-557.
68. Langlotz CP, Caldwell SA: The completeness of existing lexicons for representing radiology report information. J Digit Imaging 2002;15:201-205.
69. Nunes LW, Englander SA, Charafeddine R, et al: Optimal post-contrast timing of breast MR image acquisition for architectural feature analysis. J Magn Resonance Imaging 2002;16:42-50.
70. Harms SE, Flamig DP: Breast MRI. J Clin Imaging 2001;25: 227-246.
71. Kneeshaw PJ, Turnbull LW, Drew PJ: Current applications and future direction of MR mammography. Br J Cancer 2003;88:4-10.
72. Gorczyca DP: MRI of breast implants. Magn Reson Imaging Clin North Am 1994;2:659-672.
73. Fajardo LL, Harvey JA, McAleese KA, et al: Breast cancer diagnosis in women with subglandular silicone gel-filled augmentation implants. Radiology 1995;194:859-862.
74. Miglioretti DL, Rutter CM, Geller BM, et al: Effect of breast augmentation on the accuracy of mammography and cancer characteristics. JAMA 2004;291:442-450.
75. Pukkala E, Boice JD Jr, Hovi SL, et al: Incidence of breast and other cancers among Finnish women with cosmetic breast implants, 1970-1999. J Long Term Eff Med Implants 2002; 12:271-279.
76. Boetes C, et al: Breast tumors: Comparative accuracy of MRI relative to mammography and US for demonstrating extent. Radiology 1995;197:743-747.
77. Weinstein SP, et al: MRI of the breast in patients with invasive lobular carcinoma. AJR Am J Roentgenol 2001;176:399-406.
78. Morris EA, et al: Evaluation of pectoralis major muscle in patients with posterior breast tumors on breast MR images: Early experience. Radiology 2000;214:67-72.
79. Lee JM, et al: MRI before reexcision surgery in patients with breast cancer. AJR Am J Roentgenol 2004;182:473-480.
80. Tillman GF, et al: Effect of breast magnetic resonance imaging on the clinical management of women with early-stage breast carcinoma. J Clin Oncol 2002;16:3413-3423.
81. Brown J, Smith RC, Lee CH: Incidental enhancing lesions found on MRI of the breast. Am J Roentgenol 2001;176:1249-1254.
82. Gilles R, et al: Assessment of breast cancer recurrence with contrast-enhanced subtraction MRI: Preliminary results in 26 patients. Radiology 1993;188:473-478.
83. Frei KA, et al: MRI of the breast in patients with positive margins after lumpectomy. AJR Am J Roentgenol 2000;175: 1577-1584.
84. Solomon B, et al: Delayed development of enhancement in fat necrosis after breast conservation therapy: A potential pitfall of MRI of the breast. AJR Am J Roentgenol 1998;170: 966.
85. Gilles R, Guinebretiere, JM, Toussaint C, et al: Locally advanced breast cancer: Contrast-enhanced subtraction MRI of response to preoperative chemotherapy. Radiology 1994; 191:633-638.
86. Delille JP, Slanetz PJ, Yeh ED, et al: Invasive ductal breast carcinoma response to neoadjuvant chemotherapy: Noninvasive monitoring with functional MRI pilot study. Radiology 2003;228:63-69.
87. Rosen EL, Blackwell KL, Baker JA, et al: Accuracy of MRI in the detection of residual breast cancer after neoadjuvant chemotherapy. AJR Am J Roentgenol 2003;181:1275-1282.
88. Londero V, Bazzocchi M, Del Frate C, et al: Locally advanced breast cancer: comparison of mammography, sonography and MR imaging in evaluation of residual disease in women receiving neoadjuvant chemotherapy. Eur Radiol 2004;14: 1371-1379.
89. Martincich L, et al: Role of magnetic resonance imaging in the prediction of tumor response in patients with locally advanced breast cancer receiving neoadjuvant chemotherapy. Radiol Med (Torino) 2003;106:51-58.
90. Fourquet A, De La Rochefordiere A, Campana F: Occult primary cancer with axillary metastases. In Harris JR, Lippman ME, Morrow M, Hellman S (eds): Diseases of the Breast. Philadelphia: Lippincott-Raven, 1996, pp 892-896.
91. Morris EA, et al: MRI of the breast in patients with occult primary breast carcinoma. Radiology 1997;205:437-440.
92. Orel SG, et al: Breast MRI in patients with axillary node metastases and unknown primary malignancy. Radiology 1999;212:543-549.
93. Nakahara H, et al: A comparison of MRI, galactography and ultrasonography in patients with nipple discharge. Breast Cancer 2003;10:320-329.
94. Orel SG, et al: MRI in patients with nipple discharge: Initial experience. Radiology 2000;216:248-254.
95. Walter C, et al: Clinical and diagnostic value of preoperative MR mammography and FDG-PET in suspicious breast lesions. Eur Radiol 2003;13:1651-1656.
96. Rieber A, et al: Pre-operative staging of invasive breast cancer with MR mammography and/or PET: Boon or bunk? Br J Radiol 2002;75:789-798.
97. Fischer U, et al: MR-guided biopsy of suspect breast lesions with a simple stereotaxic add-on device for surface coils. Radiology 1994;192:272-273.
98. Lancaster JM, Carney ME, Futreal PA: BRCA 1 and 2—a genetic link to familial breast and ovarian cancer. Medscape Womens Health 1997;2:7.
99. Ford D, et al: Genetic heterogeneity and penetrance analysis of the BRCA1 and BRCA2 genes in breast cancer families. The Breast Cancer Linkage Consortium. Am J Hum Genet 1998;62:676-689.

100. Thull DL, Vogel VG: Recognition and management of hereditary breast cancer syndromes. Oncologist 2004;9:13-24.
101. Greene MH: Genetics of breast cancer. Mayo Clin Proc 1997;72:54-65.
102. McTiernan A, et al: Comparisons of two breast cancer risk estimates in women with a family history of breast cancer. Cancer Epidemiol Biomarkers Prev 2001;10:333-338.
103. Warner E, et al: Comparison of breast magnetic resonance imaging, mammography, and ultrasound for surveillance of women at high risk for hereditary breast cancer. J Clin Oncol 2001;19:3524-3531.
104. Heywang-Köbrunner SH, et al: Interventional MRI of the breast: Lesion localization and biopsy. Eur Radiol 2000;10:36-45.
105. Lehman CD, et al: MRI-guided breast biopsy using a coaxial technique with a 14-gauge stainless steel core biopsy needle and a titanium sheath. AJR Am J Roentgenol 2003;181:183-185.
106. Heywang-Köbrunner SH, et al: Prototype breast coil for MR-guided needle localization. J Comput Assist Tomogr 1994;18:876-881.
107. Viehweg P, et al: MR-guided interventional breast procedures considering vacuum biopsy in particular. Eur J Radiol 2002; 42:32-39.
108. Brenner RJ, et al: Technical note: Magnetic resonance imaging-guided pre-operative breast localization using "freehand technique." Br J Radiol 1995;68:1095-1098.
109. Daniel BL, et al: Freehand MRI-guided large gauge core needle biopsy: A new minimally invasive technique for diagnosis of enhancing breast lesions. J Magn Reson Imaging 2001;13:896-902
110. Kuhl CK, Morakkabati N, Leutner CC, et al: MRI-guided large-core (14-gauge) needle biopsy of small lesions visible at breast MRI alone. Radiology 2001;220:31-39.
111. Helbich TH: Localization and biopsy of breast lesions by the magnetic resonance imaging guidance. J Magn Reson Imaging 2001;13:903-911.
112. Doler W, et al: Stereotaxic add-on device for MR-guided biopsy of breast lesions. Radiology 1996;200:863-864.
113. Orel SG, et al: MRI-guided localization and biopsy of breast lesions: Initial experience. Radiology 1994;193:97-102.
114. Parker SH, et al: Percutaneous large-core breast biopsy: A multi-institutional study. Radiology. 1994;193:359-64.
115. LaTrenta LR, et al: Breast lesions detected with MRI: Utility and histopathologic importance of identification with US. Radiology 2003;227:856-861.

Chapter 15

Nuclear Medicine Applications in Breast Imaging

Juanita Yun, Bao To, Mohan Ramaswamy, and Randall A. Hawkins

A variety of nuclear medicine imaging techniques and radiopharmaceuticals have been evaluated and actively used in the detection and staging of breast cancer. These techniques include planar and single photon emission computed tomography (SPECT) (using perfusion agents, monoclonal antibodies, peptides, and nonspecific agents), positron emission tomography (PET), most commonly with fluorodeoxyglucose (FDG) but also with other radiopharmaceuticals, and lymphoscintigraphy for identification and localization of sentinel lymph nodes (see later). These nuclear medicine modalities are used currently as adjuncts to mammography, primarily in the post-biopsy tumor staging process and differ from other radiographic imaging techniques in that they focus on biochemical and physiologic characteristics of tumors and metastases.

Depending on the particular radiotracer injected, nuclear medicine techniques can take advantage of the specific uptake characteristics of that tracer by a breast tumor, often resulting in a high ratio of tumor to background, enabling differentiation of tumor from functionally different tissue, such as scar or fat. These methods can be useful (1) in the evaluation of a palpable lesion in the absence of a mammographic abnormality, (2) for detection of lesions in patients whose mammograms are difficult to interpret, (3) as complementary procedures used to add specificity in differentiating between benign and malignant lesions, and (4) as minimally invasive modalities for the staging of breast cancers. An emerging role for PET is the evaluation of tumor response to chemotherapy.

One of the earliest examples of nuclear medicine in the detection of breast cancer was in the use of phosphorous 32 (^{32}P) in 1942.[1] Since then, a variety of radiopharmaceuticals have been investigated. The more commonly used radiopharmaceuticals in planar and SPECT scintimammography are technetium Tc 99m (^{99m}Tc) sestamibi and ^{99m}Tc tetrofosmin, both commonly used in myocardial perfusion agents, and methylene diphosphonate (MDP), also a bone imaging agent. The clinical use of FDG, a structural analogue of glucose, in PET is widespread. Other positron-emitting agents that have been used for breast cancer imaging are radioactive carbon (^{11}C)–labeled methionine, ^{11}C tyrosine, radioactive oxygen (^{15}O)–labeled tracers, and radioactive fluoride (^{18}F)–labeled estradiol (FES). ^{99m}Tc sulfur colloid, which is used in lymphoscintigraphy and for mapping of sentinel lymph nodes (see later), has had favorable results.

TECHNETIUM Tc 99M SESTAMIBI AND Tc 99M TETROFOSMIN

^{99m}Tc sestamibi has been investigated as an imaging agent in a variety of tumors. The first cases of breast cancer detection with ^{99m}Tc sestamibi were described by Aktolun and colleagues[2] in 1992; these researchers imaged 4 breast cancer patients of 34 cancer patients with both ^{99m}Tc sestamibi and thallium. Subsequent investigations have examined the use of both planar and SPECT in breast cancer detection.[3-6] Technetium Tc 99m customarily distributes homogeneously in normal breast tissue regardless of density and concentrates in malignant breast tumors, so that uptake by tumors is six times higher than that by adjacent, normal breast or fat tissue. A positive study result consists of focal increased activity within the breast or axilla compared with the surrounding breast tissue (Figs. 15–1 and 15–2). In more than 2600 cases reported (including a large multicenter clinical trial involving 42 institutions in North America), the sensitivity of ^{99m}Tc sestamibi scintimammography ranges from 80% to 90%, with an average of 85%.[7] Although criteria defining a positive scan result have not been clearly established and can be somewhat reader dependent, reported specificities are in a similar range as those for sensitivity, averaging about 89%.[8,9] Lesions that can cause false-positive uptake of sestamibi include fibroadenomas, fibrocystic change, inflammation, sclerosing adenosis, and epithelial hyperplasia. The experience with a second myocardial perfusion agent, ^{99m}Tc tetrofosmin, is still limited, initial studies suggesting sensitivity and specificity similar to those for ^{99m}Tc sestamibi.[10] Khalkhali and associates[11] examined scintimammography in 558 patients with dense and fatty breasts as classified by mammography and found that the diagnostic accuracy of scintimammography was unchanged by breast tissue density.

The exact mechanism of sestamibi concentration within tumor cells is not completely understood. ^{99m}Tc sestamibi is lipophilic, allowing passive transport through tumor cell membranes. Ninety percent of ^{99m}Tc sestamibi localizes to the cell mitochondria.[12] Cells with increased mitochondrial content demonstrate greater sestamibi uptake. Interestingly it has also been observed that ^{99m}Tc sestamibi is a substrate of the P-glycoprotein (Pgp-170), which is present in cells expressing the multidrug resistance gene (MDR1). Efflux of sestamibi in patients with high

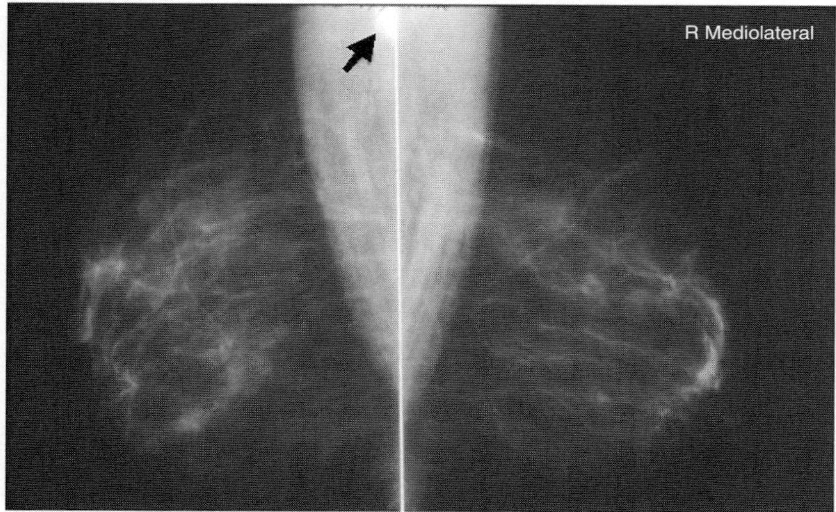

A

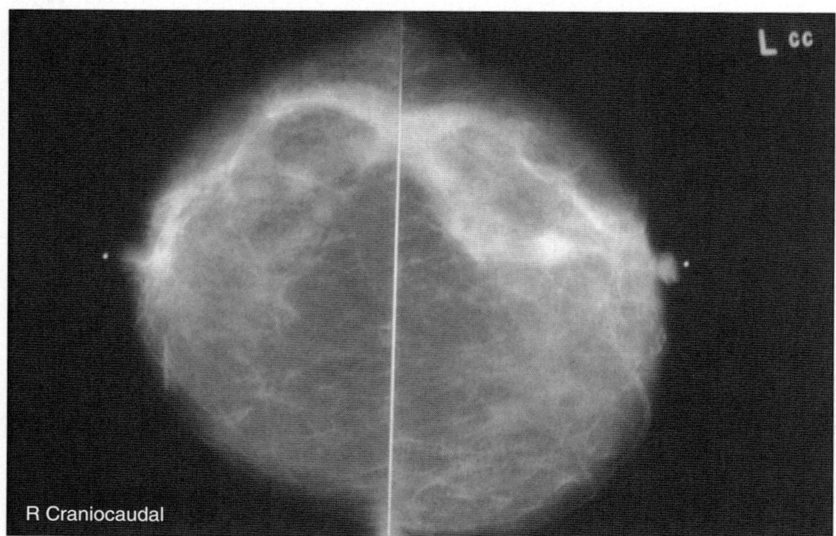

B

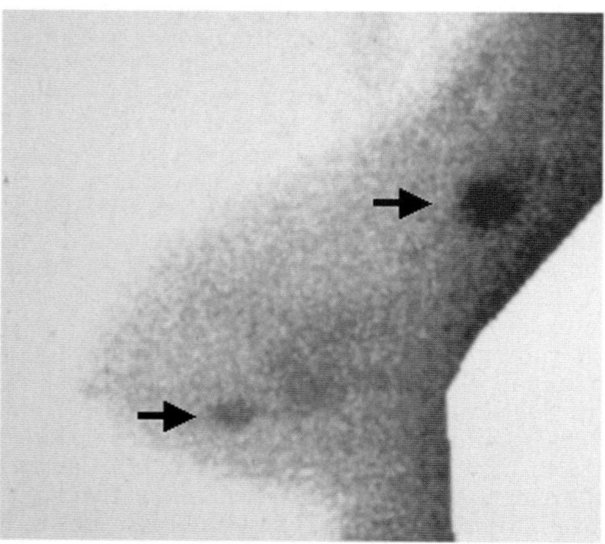

C

Figure 15–1. **A,** Mediolateral projection mammogram of a 47-year-old woman who presented with a palpable left axillary 1.5-cm lymph node. The mammogram shows a small left axillary lymph node (*arrow*). No primary tumor was noted. **B,** Craniocaudal projection mammogram with no primary tumor noted. **C,** Scintimammograms of the same patient demonstrating a focus of intense uptake in the left axilla (*top arrow*) and a focal region of uptake in the lower portion of the left breast (*bottom arrow*). Fine-needle aspiration of the left axillary mass demonstrated infiltrating breast carcinoma. A focus of 1.3-cm invasive ductal carcinoma was found in the mastectomy specimen in the lower and inner portion of this breast. (Courtesy of Dr. Iraj Khalkhali, Harbor-UCLA Medical Center.)

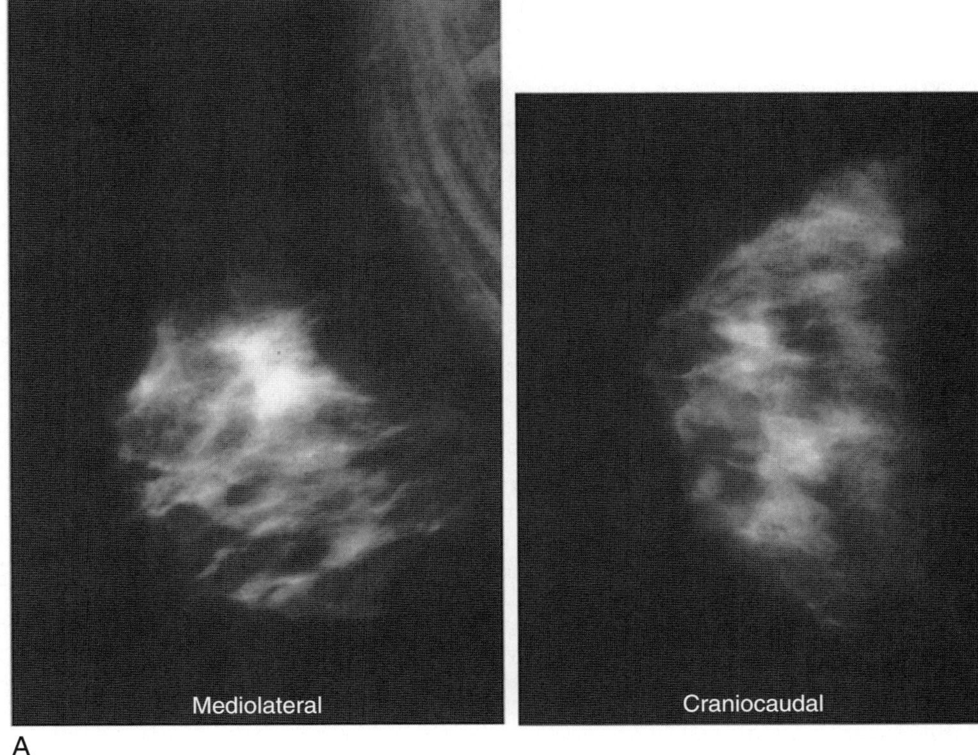

A

B

Figure 15–2. **A,** Mediolateral and craniocaudal projection mammogram of the right breast demonstrating asymmetrical density in the upper outer quadrant. The patient is a 64-year-old woman who presented with a questionable mass in the same region. Biopsy result was benign at that time. **B,** Scintimammogram of the right breast approximately 4 months after mammography and biopsy, demonstrating intense focal uptake in the retroareolar region (*arrow*). A second mammogram and ultrasonogram did not show any abnormality in this area. Localization using a guide wire with nuclear medicine techniques followed by excisional biopsy demonstrated a 1.8-cm invasive ductal carcinoma. The patient then underwent radical mastectomy. (Courtesy of Dr. Iraj Khalkhali, Harbor-UCLA Medical Center.)

level of P-glycoprotein is increased, a feature that may allow for functional imaging at the level of MDR1 expression and detection of the induction of multidrug resistance in patients undergoing chemotherapy.[13-16] Tetrofosmin is also a substrate for P-glycoprotein.

Protocol for ^{99m}Tc Sestamibi Breast Imaging

No specific patient preparation is necessary. To exclude the possibility of nonspecific ^{99m}Tc sestamibi uptake, scintimammography should not be performed before or 7 to 10 days after a fine-needle aspiration, 2 weeks after core biopsy, 4 to 6 weeks after a breast biopsy, or 2 to 3 months after breast surgery or radiotherapy. A standard dose of ^{99m}Tc sestamibi of about 20 mCi (740 Mbq) is injected intravenously into the arm opposite the side of the suspected breast lesion, to avoid nonspecific uptake in the ipsilateral axillary lymph nodes. If involvement of both breasts or axillae is suspected, a foot injection may be used.

To obtain the best possible study, the patient is imaged in both the prone and supine positions. Prone imaging, with either a special table with lateral cutouts or a foam cushion (with semicircular lateral cutouts), results in better visualization of breast tissue, allowing separation from the liver and myocardium (both of which demonstrate normal sestamibi uptake) and from the other breast. Prone imaging also minimizes the distance between the breast and the camera, enabling deeper breast tissue to be evaluated. Supine images better visualize the axilla and can also provide better tumor localization. Images are acquired over 10 minutes and are obtained 5 to 15 minutes after radiotracer injection. Additional anterior or posterior oblique images can be obtained if needed. Although the role of the routine use of SPECT has not been established, this modality may better characterize a lesion or may detect the presence of axillary metastases. However, SPECT alone is not recommended.[7,8]

Potential Roles for Scintimammography

Because ^{99m}Tc sestamibi has a lower sensitivity in small lesions (less than 10 mm), it is not considered useful in general screening for breast cancer. However, because the sensitivity of ^{99m}Tc sestamibi is not affected by the density of breast tissue, it can be useful in detecting disease or recurrence in women who have dense breasts, small breasts, prior breast surgery, radiotherapy, or breast implants, in whom lesion detection by radiographic mammography may be more difficult.

Magnetic resonance imaging (MRI) has been shown to have slightly higher sensitivity than ^{99m}Tc sestamibi scintimammography (91% and 88%, respectively). The specificity, however, of MRI both before and after contrast enhancement may be lower than for ^{99m}Tc scintimammography (52% and 83%, respectively), particularly in those patients with indeterminate mammographic findings,[17] although Helbich and associates[18] demonstrated MR to be more sensitive and as specific as scintimammography.

Scintimammography can also be potentially useful for selection of a lesion for biopsy in patients with multiple mammographic abnormalities. Sestamibi uptake can also provide helpful information regarding metastatic axillary lymph node involvement, although it may not be sensitive or specific enough for the use as a basis of treatment decisions. Finally, scintimammography can be offered as a possible alternative for those women who, for various reasons, may refuse recommended mammography.

ANTIBODY TUMOR IMAGING

The use of antibody imaging with radiolabeled monoclonal antibody and antibody fragments in breast cancer is under active investigation, with the clinical role of these agents yet to be determined. Radiopharmaceuticals include a ^{99m}Tc-radiolabeled anti-carcinoembryonic antigen (CEA) antibody Fab′ fragment, CEA Scan (Immunomedicis, Inc, Morris Plains NJ), radioactive yttrium 90 or I 131 linked monoclonal MUC-1 antibody, which targets epithelial glycoprotein mucin on the cell surfaces of 90% of breast cancers, and growth factor receptors EGF-R and HER-2/Neu.

Immunohistochemical methods have demonstrated the expression of oncofetal CEA in approximately 60% to 80% of breast cancers.[19] Numerous studies have examined the use and localization of a variety of CEA antibodies in primary and axillary breast cancer.[20] Goldenberg and colleagues[21] demonstrated a specificity of 91% and a sensitivity of 61% for scintigraphic images obtained with ^{99m}Tc-labeled anti-CEA Fab′ in 104 patients scheduled for biopsy confirmation of mammographic and physical findings. Tumor size less than or equal to stage T1 tumors significantly affected the sensitivity of the radioantibody images in the majority of missed lesions, and a proliferative histology significantly affected the specificity.[21] CEA scanning may prove to be especially useful in those patients with palpable and nonpalpable breast lesions found to be indeterminate on mammography (American College of Radiology Breast Imaging Reporting and Data System [BI-RADS] category IV), necessitating further follow-up or biopsy.[22]

An area of great interest is the possible therapeutic use of radiolabeled antibodies. Radioimmuno-guided breast surgery using a handheld probe during surgery after a preoperative injection of radiolabeled monoclonal antibodies is a technique being explored for the intraoperative diagnosis and staging of breast cancer as a guide to conservative surgery. There is also growing interest in radioimmunotherapy (RAIT), in which the combination of a high-energy, β-emitting radioactive isotope with a monoclonal antibody can provide targeted treatment to a variety of tumors, including breast cancer.[23]

POSITRON EMISSION TOMOGRAPHY IN BREAST CANCER

PET has been used in several centers for the evaluation of breast carcinoma. FDG is the PET agent most commonly used in clinical situations. FDG is transported from plasma to tissue via glucose transporter carrier–facilitated diffusion and is then phosphorylated by hexokinase to FDG-6-PO_4, analogous to glucose phosphorylation. Rather than being further metabolized like glucose-6-PO_4, however, FDG-6-PO_4 remains trapped intracellularly. Subsequent decay

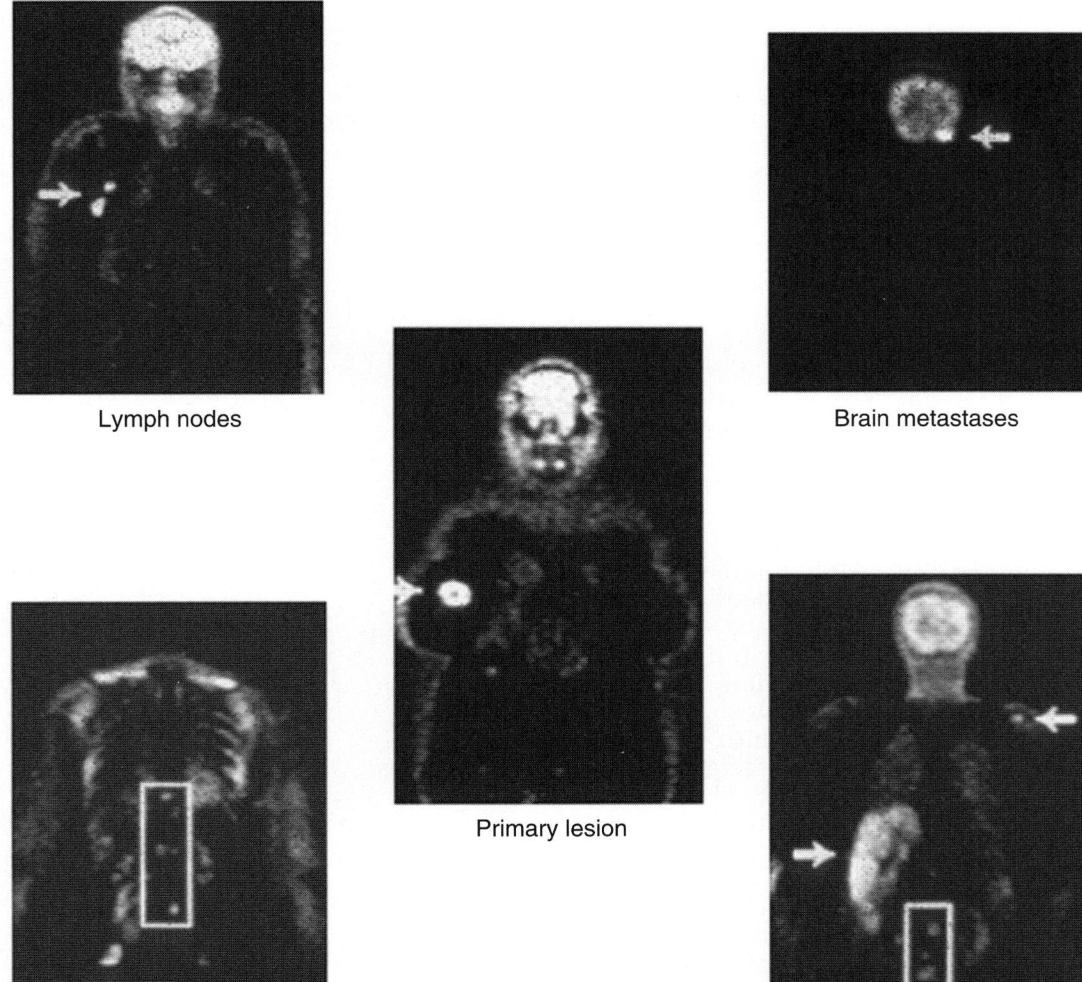

Figure 15–3. Whole-body fluorodeoxyglucose (FDG) imaging for multiple–organ system evaluation of breast carcinoma. The *middle image* shows primary breast carcinoma with high focal FDG uptake compared with normal breast tissue (*arrow*). Other views demonstrate metastases involving lymph nodes, bone, brain, and liver (*arrows*).

results in the emission of positrons that can be detected and imaged after annihilation with electrons. Primary breast carcinomas demonstrate high focal FDG uptake compared with normal breast tissue, resulting in images with a very high tumor-to-background ratio (Fig. 15–3). In contrast, benign cystic and solid lesions consistently demonstrate absence or low levels of FDG uptake, making FDG PET useful in differentiating benign lesions from tumor.

Evaluation of Breast Masses with FDG PET

The reported sensitivity of PET with FDG ranges from 80% to 100%, with reported specificities also in a similar range. The differences in these study findings result from differences in imaging techniques, patient populations, scanner resolutions, and primary lesion sizes.[24] Lesions as small as 0.4 cm have been detected in the breast with FDG PET. FDG uptake by in situ cancer has been found to be less intense than that by invasive ductal cancer. Importantly, PET is able to identify unsuspected multifocal carcinoma in the breast. This modality can also unequivocally identify primary breast cancers in women who have breast implants or dense breasts, in whom accurate mammographic imaging can be difficult.[25-27]

Protocol

Patients should be fasting for at least 4 hours before PET to reduce myocardial uptake and other background soft tissue uptake that could interfere with lesion detection. A dose of FDG of about 10 mCi (370 Mbq) is injected intravenously into the arm opposite the side of the suspected breast lesion, to avoid nonspecific uptake in the ipsilateral axillary lymph nodes. A whole-body PET scanner is used. Because the whole-body imaging mode will limit the scan duration at each bed, a dedicated emission scan of the breast acquired with the patient in a prone position can be used to optimize visualization of breast tissue. Whole-body images to detect metastases are usually acquired with the patient in the supine position.

Other PET Agents

Tumor aggressiveness and prognosis are governed by the estrogen receptor status. Dehdashti and colleagues[28] compared in vitro assays for estrogen receptors with PET scans performed with FDG and FES. These investigators found positive correlations between the estrogen receptor assays and FES PET but did not find a similar relationship between estrogen receptor status and FDG uptake. ^{11}C methionine is an amino acid used in protein synthesis. This agent, which can be used for tumor detection with PET, demonstrates increased accumulation in breast tumors.[28] Studies with ^{11}C methionine imaging of breast masses demonstrate a strong correlation between uptake of tracer and the proliferative rate of the tumor, with a standardized uptake value (SUV) of 8.5 ± 3.3 in a small series of 7 patients. ^{11}C methionine PET has also been demonstrated to be efficacious in the identification of distant metastases and may provide a better tumor-to-background ratio than FDG.[29] However, given the short half-life of ^{11}C, which makes an on-site cyclotron necessary, the possible clinical use of this agent is limited.

STAGING AND EVALUATION OF BREAST CANCERS

In the staging of breast cancer, the presence or absence of axillary lymph node metastases is a key prognostic indicator. A noninvasive method to determine axillary node involvement could reduce the number of women who undergo axillary node dissection, the associated costs, including those of hospitalization, and possible complications, including lymphedema. Several studies have demonstrated the effective use of FDG in the detection of axillary lymph node involvement of breast cancers. One of the largest, conducted by Utech and colleagues,[30] involved 124 patients with known breast cancer who were evaluated for the involvement of axillary lymph nodes with FDG PET. The study found this modality to demonstrate a sensitivity of 100% with no false-negative results and 20 false-positive results. Wahl and associates,[31] evaluating the efficacy of FDG PET for staging of breast cancer, found that PET was not only useful for imaging axillary node metastases but also able to detect unexpected internal mammary node involvement.

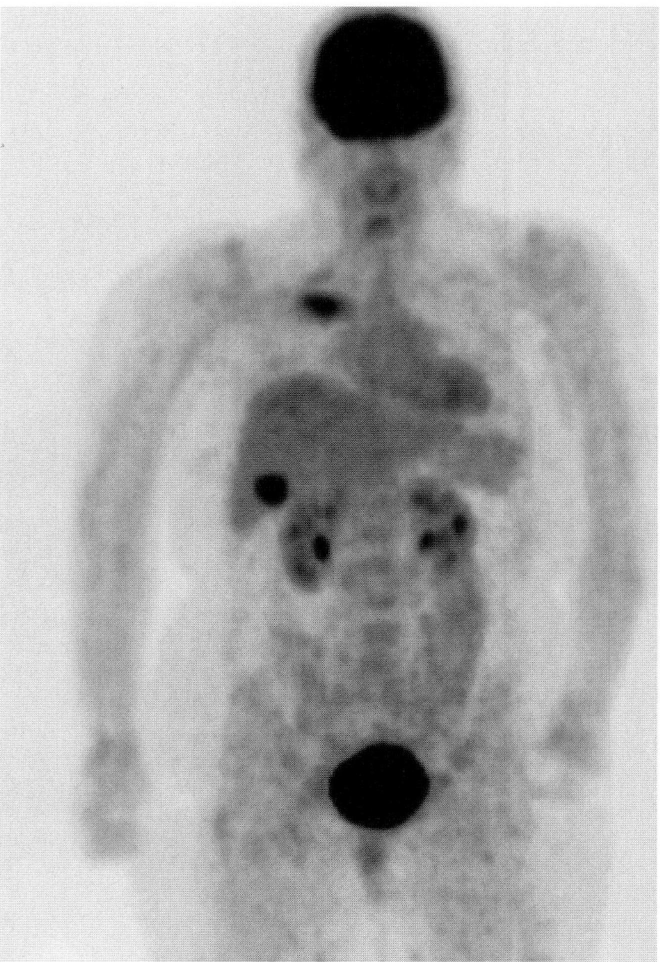

Figure 15–4. Whole-body fluorodeoxyglucose–positron emission tomography (FDG PET) image, frontal view. The patient is a 47-year-old woman with breast carcinoma who underwent right mastectomy, radiation therapy, and chemotherapy several years before this image was obtained. She presented for an FDG PET study because of new right chest wall thickening. FDG PET showed evidence of right chest wall tumor involvement with an unsuspected metastatic focus in the right lobe of the liver.

PET can help identify axillary node involvement and aid in the identification of women who would benefit from axillary node dissection. PET also has the advantage of providing whole-body imaging. This allows not only primary tumor detection but also metastatic evaluation of axillary lymph nodes and of distant lesions, including those in the brain, the liver, bone, and bone marrow, to help assign patients to various treatment categories (Figs. 15–3 and 15–4). Whole-body PET can also enable the evaluation and staging of recurrent disease.[30,31]

EVALUATION OF RESPONSE TO THERAPY

PET with FDG and ^{11}C methionine can be used in the assessment of the response of primary cancer and metastases to therapy. The specific usefulness of PET lies in the fact that it can serve as an earlier predictor of response to therapy than other available clinical parameters and anatomic end points. Using serial PET scans, Jansson and colleagues[32] demonstrated that 6 to 13 days after the first chemotherapy course, a decrease in the uptake of FDG, equivalent to a reduction greater than 10%, in the primary breast mass after therapy was a significant predictor of adequate response.[32] They found a median interval of 8 days after the initiation of chemohormonal therapy to be the optimum time for assessing tumor response. Several other studies have demonstrated similar findings; tumors that responded to the first course of chemotherapy—the response confirmed by subsequent histopathology—showed a significant decrease in FDG uptake compared with a baseline PET.[33,34] This emerging role for PET may provide early data regarding tumor response that can be used in determining the role and timing of the variety of surgical and chemotherapeutic alternatives available.

BREAST LYMPHOSCINTIGRAPHY AND THE SENTINEL LYMPH NODE

The lymph node status in patients with early breast cancer remains a powerful predictor of recurrence and survival. Lymphoscintigraphy involves the evaluation of the regional lymph node drainage from a malignancy after the injection of a small amount of radiocolloid at the tumor site. Imaging the movement of radiocolloid through the lymphatic channels allows identification of channels associated with the tumor site and, in particular, of the sentinel node. The *sentinel node* is the first lymph node to receive regional lymphatic flow from the tumor. Performing this procedure preoperatively followed by the use of a handheld gamma survey probe during surgery enables further localization of the sentinel or nodes for biopsy and subsequent evaluation for the presence or absence of tumor metastases. Sentinel node evaluation can spare the patient a more extensive axillary dissection and the associated morbidity and mortality.

Liberman and coworkers[35] reviewed results of sentinel node biopsy and compared them with results of axillary dissection in women with breast carcinoma. Reviewing a total of more than 2000 published sentinel node procedures, these investigators found that in the 90% of patients in whom a sentinel node was identified, the status of the sentinel node accurately predicted the status of the axilla in 98% of all patients and in 94% of patients in whom nodes were "positive" for carcinoma. The highest accuracy of sentinel node biopsy is in women with small (T1) infiltrating carcinomas. Given that less than half of the patients presenting with small tumors have evidence of axillary tumor involvement, sentinel lymph node biopsy is currently an alternative to axillary dissection in women with small infiltrating breast carcinomas and no clinical evidence of axillary involvement. Sentinel node biopsy can also permit a more focused pathologic examination, by the application of multiple sections or immunohistochemical analysis to the nodes of potentially highest yield, and can detect micrometastases more frequently than routine axillary dissection.[36] In this regard, sentinel lymph node biopsy may prove to be valuable in the future, in addition to axillary dissection, resulting in improved tumor staging.

Technique of Lymphoscintigraphy

Technical protocols for sentinel lymph node biopsy have not been standardized. It is clear from multiple studies that the technique is challenging, with success dependent on the multidisciplinary team performing the procedure and on patient characteristics, such as age and location of the primary tumor. Success rate improves with experience. Thus, it is important to stress the need for each institution and individual to establish a successful method until further technical standards are established and approved for widespread use in clinical practice.

Sentinel lymph node biopsy without imaging can be performed with blue dye. Several studies have demonstrated best results with concomitant use of radiocolloid and blue dye, enabling radiolocalization and visual identification of the lymph node during surgery. Both filtered and unfiltered ^{99m}Tc sulfur colloids have been used, with movement of the particle inversely related to its size. Smaller particles have shorter migration times to sentinel nodes but may cause visualization of multiple nodes or may pass through sentinel nodes, resulting in more diffuse axillary activity. The optimal radiopharmaceutical, therefore, may vary according to the timing of the imaging and the surgical procedure.[37] The volume injected and the site of injection also may affect success. Using radiotracer and blue dye, Linehan and associates[37] found that intradermal and parenchymal lymphatics of the breast drain to the same sentinel lymph node in most patients. The intradermal injection also simplified the technique and was more effective in successful localization of the sentinel lymph nodes. In a study of 68 patients, a single subareolar parenchymal injection of ^{99m}Tc sulfur colloid was as accurate in locating the sentinel lymph node as a peritumoral injection of blue dye, regardless of tumor location.[38]

A Lymphoscintigraphy Protocol

A single intradermal injection of 0.1 mCi of ^{99m}Tc sulfur colloid, filtered through a 0.22-μm sieve, in 0.1 mL normal saline is injected intradermally directly over the tumor site or cephalad to the biopsy scar or localization needle. At our institution, the injection site is first infiltrated with a single injection of 1% buffered lidocaine, which, in addition to acting as an analgesic, may facilitate the migration of sulfur colloid by increasing the volume injected at the site. The patient is positioned with the ipsilateral arm above her head, and images are obtained on a gamma camera with high-resolution collimation.

Our imaging protocol involves a dynamic set of images collected for 10 minutes. If no movement of tracer is identified after the first 10 minutes, a second injection is performed with subsequent imaging. After the dynamic image acquisition, frames are summed for further evaluation of channel activity. Static images in the anterior, lateral, and lateral anterior oblique positions are obtained for 2 to 3 minutes. The skin overlying the regions corresponding to lymph node activity are identified and marked with gentian violet in the anterior and 45-degree projections. Data corresponding to the number of channels, basins, and nodes marked as well as any specific problems encountered during lymphoscintigraphy are recorded, and the documentation is forwarded to the operating room. To avoid any confusion, a verbal detailed report of the lymphoscintigraphy is also given to the surgeon.

In the operating room, a handheld gamma probe is used to scan the marked regions and to locate the region of the radioactive nodes within the axilla before incision. If necessary, a collimator can be placed on the probe to reduce background noise, thereby facilitating detection of the sentinel nodes. If blue dye is used, it is injected either around the tumor site or superolateral to the tumor. Approximately 5 to 10 minutes later, a skin incision is made, and the probe is used to further survey the incision site to identify each lymph node, with probe counts obtained in vivo and ex vivo. After localization, isolation, and removal of the radioactive nodes, the bed is further surveyed until the dissection area is free of or has minimal radioactivity.

Given the small amount of radiation dose, strict radiation guidelines for patients, surgical personnel, and pathologists handling the node biopsy specimens are not required. Nevertheless, the usual delay in processing specimens, 2 to3 days after surgery, would further reduce any minimal radiation exposure for pathology personnel.[38,39]

FUTURE TECHNOLOGY

The clinical role of nuclear medicine imaging in the detection and diagnosis of breast cancer has been limited by the poor detection of small lesions. The development of dedicated gamma cameras and PET cameras specifically for breast and axillary imaging and the use of better gamma crystal technology can result in higher resolution and improved sensitivity, which are especially important for the detection of these smaller lesions.[40,41] The ongoing development of a combined imaging scanner unit that provides accurate co-registration of either PET or gamma emission nuclear medicine images with conventional mammography or other available radiographic technique may produce a technique that can provide both metabolic and anatomic information for diagnosis and localization of breast and axillary lesions.[42] Continued development of production methods and radiolabeling techniques for nuclides, which can be used for imaging, dose planning, and optimization of targeted tumor radioimmunotherapy, may play an important role in future cancer treatment.[43]

CONCLUSION

Nuclear medicine imaging methods are useful adjuncts in detection of breast cancer. Widely utilized techniques now include sentinel node detection with ^{99m}Tc sulfur colloid, breast cancer staging, and monitoring with FDG PET and, in some centers, scintimammography.

References

1. Low-Beer BVA, Bell HG, McCorkle HJ: Measurement of radioactive phosphorus in breast tumors in situ: A possible diagnostic procedure. Radiology 1946;47:492-493.
2. Aktolun C, Bayhan H, Kir M: Clinical experience with 99mTc MIBI imaging in patients with malignant tumors: Preliminary results and comparison with Tl-201. Clin Nucl Med 1992; 17:171-176.
3. Taillefer R, Robidoux A, Turpin S, et al: Metastatic axillary lymph node 99mTc MIBI imaging in primary breast cancer. J Nucl Med 1998;39:459-464.
4. Khalkhali I, Cutrone J, Mena I, et al: Technetium-99m-sestamibi scintimammography of breast lesions: Clinical and pathological follow-up. J Nucl Med 1995;36:1784-1789.
5. Kao CH, Wang SJ, Liu TJ: The use of technetium-99m methoxyisobutylisonitrile breast scintigraphy to evaluate palpable breast masses. Eur J Nucl Med 1994;21:432-436.
6. Palmedo H, Schomburg A, Grunwald F, et al: Technetium-99m-MIBI scintimammography for suspicious breast lesions. J Nucl Med 1996;37:626-630.
7. Khalkhali I, Vargas HI: The role of nuclear medicine in breast cancer detection: Functional breast imaging. Radiol Clin North Am 2001;39:1053-1068.
8. Taillefer R: The role of 99mTc sestamibi and other conventional radiopharmaceuticals in breast cancer diagnosis. Semin Nucl Med 1999;29:16-40.
9. Khalkhali I, Villanueva-Meyer J, Edell SL, et al: Diagnostic accuracy of 99mTc sestamibi breast imaging: Multicenter trial results. J Nucl Med 2000;41:1973-1979.
10. Obwegeser R, Berghammer P, Rodrigues M, et al: A head-to-head comparison between technetium-99m-tetrofosmin and technetium-99m-MIBI scintigraphy to evaluate suspicious breast lesions. Eur J Nucl Med 1999;26:1553-1559.
11. Khalkhali I, Baum JK, Villanueva-Meyer J, et al: (99m)Tc sestamibi breast imaging for the examination of patients with dense and fatty breasts: Multicenter study. Radiology 2002; 222:149-155.
12. Carvalho PA, Chiu ML, Kronauge JF, et al: Subcellular distribution and analysis of technetium-99m-MIBI in isolated perfused rat hearts. J Nucl Med 1992;33:1516-1522.
13. Piwnica-Worms D, Chiu ML, Budding M, et al: Functional imaging of multidrug-resistant P-glycoprotein with an organotechnetium complex. Cancer Res 1993;53:977-984.
14. Cordobes MD, Strazec A, Delmon-Moingeon L, et al: Technetium-99m sestamibi uptake by human benign and malignant breast tumor cells: Correlation with mdr gene expression. J Nucl Med 1996;37:286-289.

15. Cwikla JB, Buscombe JR, Barlow RV, et al: The effect of chemotherapy on the uptake of technetium-99m sestamibi in breast cancer. Eur J Nucl Med 1997;24:1175-1178.
16. Del Vecchio S, Ciarmiello A, Pace L, et al: Fractional retention of technetium-99m-sestamibi as an index of P-glycoprotein expression in untreated breast cancer patients. J Nucl Med 1997;38:1348-1351.
17. Tiling R, Sommer H, Pechmann M, et al: Comparison of technetium-99m sestamibi scintimammography with contrast-enhanced MRI for diagnosis of breast lesions. J Nucl Med 1997;38:58-62.
18. Helbich TH, Becherer A, Trattnig S, et al: Differentiation of benign and malignant breast lesions: MR imaging versus 99mTc sestamibi scintimammography. Radiology. 1997;202(2): 421-429.
19. Reynoso G, Chu TM, Holyoke D, et al: Carcinoembryonic antigen in patients with different cancers. JAMA 1972;220(3): 361-365.
20. Nabi HA: Antibody imaging in breast cancer. Semin Nucl Med 1997;27:30-39.
21. Goldenberg DM, Abdel-Nabi H, Sullivan CL, et al: Carcinoembryonic antigen immunoscintigraphy complements mammography in the diagnosis of breast carcinoma. Cancer 2000;89:104-115.
22. Goldenberg DM, Nabi HA: Breast cancer imaging with radiolabeled antibodies. Semin Nucl Med 1999;29:41-48.
23. Goldenberg DM: Targeted therapy of cancer with radiolabeled antibodies. J Nucl Med 2000;43:693-713.
24. Hoh CK, Schiepers C: 18-FDG imaging in breast cancer. Semin Nucl Med 1999;29:49-56. Review.
25. Wahl RL, Helvie MA, Chang AE, Anderson I: Detection of breast cancer in women after augmentation mammoplasty using fluorine-18-fluorodeoxyglucose-PET. J Nucl Med 1994; 35:872-875.
26. Hoh CK, Hawkins RA, Dahlbom M, et al: Cancer detection with whole body PET with 2-[F-18]fluoro-2-deoxy-D-glucose (FDG). J Comput Assist Tomogr 1993;17:582-589.
27. Tse N, Hoh CK, Hawkins RA, et al: Application of positron emission tomography with 2-[F-18]fluoro-2-deoxy-D-glucose (FDG) to the evaluation of breast disease. Ann Surg 1992; 216:27-34.
28. Dehdashti F, Mortimer JE, Siegel BA, et al: Positron tomographic assessment of estrogen receptors in breast cancer: comparison with FDG-PET and in vitro receptor assays. J Nucl Med 199;36:1766-1774.
29. Leskinen-Kallio S, Nagren K, Lehikoinen P, et al: Uptake of 11C-methionine in breast cancer studied by PET: An association with the size of S-phase fraction. Br J Cancer 1991;64: 1121-1124.
30. Utech CI, Young CS, Winter PF: Prospective evaluation of fluorine-18 fluorodeoxyglucose positron emission tomography in breast cancer for staging of the axilla related to surgery and immunocytochemistry. Eur J Nucl Med 1996;23:1588-1593.
31. Wahl RL, Cody RL, Hutchins GD, Mudgett EE: Primary and metastatic breast carcinoma: Initial clinical evaluation with PET with the radiolabeled glucose analogue 2-(F-18)-fluoro-2-deoxy-D-glucose. Radiology 1991;179:765-770.
32. Jansson T, Wetlin JE, Ahlstom H, et al: Positron emission tomography studies in patients with locally advanced and/or metastatic breast cancer: A method for early therapy evaluation? J Clin Oncol 1995;13:1470-1477.
33. Schelling M, Avril N, Nahrig J, et al: Positron emission tomography using [(18)F]-fluorodeoxyglucose for monitoring primary chemotherapy in breast cancer. J Clin Oncol 2000; 18:1689-1695.
34. Smith IC, Welch AE, Hutcheon AW, et al: Positron emission tomography using [(18)F]-fluorodeoxy-D-glucose to predict the pathologic response of breast cancer to primary chemotherapy. J Clin Oncol 2000;18:1676-1688.
35. Liberman L, Cody HS 3rd, Hill AD, et al: Sentinel lymph node biopsy after percutaneous diagnosis of nonpalpable breast cancer. Radiology 1999;211:835-844.
36. Turner RR, Ollila DW, Stern S, Giuliano AE: Optimal histopathologic examination of the sentinel lymph node for breast carcinoma staging. Am J Surg Pathol 1999;23:263-267.
37. Linehan DC, Hill AD, Akhurst T, et al: Intradermal radiocolloid and intraparenchymal blue dye injection optimize sentinel node identification in breast cancer patients. Ann Surg Oncol 1999;6:450-454.
38. Glass E, Essner R, Giuliano A: Sentinel node localization in breast cancer. Semin Nucl Med 1999;24:57-68.
39. Klimberg VS, Rubio IT, Henry R, et al: Subareolar versus peritumoral injection for location of the sentinel lymph node. Ann Surg 1999;229:860-865.
40. Doshi NK, Shao Y, Silverman RW, Cherry SR: Design and evaluation of an LSO PET detector for breast cancer imaging. Med Phys 2000;27:1535-1543.
41. Williams MB, Goode AR, Galbis-Reig V, et al: Performance of a PSPMT based detector for scintimammography. Phys Med Biol 2000;45:781-800.
42. Bergman AM, Thompson CJ, Murthy K, et al: Technique to obtain positron emission mammography images in registration with x-ray mammograms. Med Phys 1998;25:2119-2129.
43. Lundqvist H, Lubberink M, Tolmachev V, et al: Positron emission tomography and radioimmunotargeting—general aspects. Acta Oncol 1999;38:335-341.

Section IV

Interventional Breast Imaging Procedures

Chapter

16 Presurgical Needle Localization

Valerie P. Jackson

PROCEDURE

If a nonpalpable breast lesion is to undergo surgical excision, a preoperative localization procedure is necessary to maximize the chance that the proper area is removed. Many devices are available to aid in mammographic localization, including special fenestrated compression paddles and a multitude of needles, needle-wire assemblies, and localizing dyes.[1-4] Ultrasonography can also be used to guide localization of ultrasonographically visible lesions, and magnetic resonance imaging (MRI) can be used to localize lesions visible only on that modality. Localization with ultrasonography and MRI are discussed in Chapters 14 and 20. The appropriate choice of guidance method and localizing device depends on the location of the lesion, the available equipment, and the experience and preferences of the radiologist and surgeon.

Teamwork is essential for proper evaluation of nonpalpable suspicious breast lesions. The "team" consists of patient, mammography technologist, radiologist, surgeon, and pathologist. Only with good communication and close follow-up by all members of the team can accurate and safe results be achieved.

The needle or hook-wire system for presurgical localization should be chosen jointly by the radiologist and the surgeon. Some surgeons prefer to have a rigid needle left in place, allowing an incision in the periareolar region or another location distant from the wire entry site. In these cases, the needle or a stiffener serves as a palpable localizer for the surgeon. Other surgeons prefer to make the incision at the site of the localizing device. This requires a stable anchor, such as a strong barb-type hook-wire, rather than a curved J-wire or straight needle.

Some surgeons and radiologists prefer to use a blue dye as a localizing marker. In such cases, close coordination between the localization and operating room schedules is needed, because the dye diffuses with time, producing an unsatisfactory marker and leading to removal of an unnecessarily large specimen. Because methylene blue may interfere with estrogen-receptor protein-binding capacity assay,[5] isosulfan blue has been suggested as an alternative.[6] Toluidine blue has been suggested as a marker that diffuses less than methylene blue.[7] Nonetheless, although dye is often used for sentinel lymph node mapping and biopsy, it is seldom used alone today for presurgical needle localization procedures. Some radiologists use both dye and a needle or wire in case the metal localizer accidentally moves. Promising alternatives include the use of nondiffusing carbon particles for localization[8-11] and the placement of a radioactive seed at the site of the abnormality.[12,13] Both of these techniques allow the localization procedure to be done one or more days before surgery or at the time of percutaneous needle biopsy, reducing scheduling pressures on the day of surgery.

Before any localization procedure, the radiologist must review the imaging studies to be sure that the lesion has been appropriately evaluated and to plan an approach. Proper mammographic evaluation is needed to ensure that the lesion is "real" and that biopsy is appropriate.[14] Next, the radiologist must know the exact location of the lesion so as to plan a suitable approach. Although suspicious lesions are occasionally seen in only one mammographic projection, this is an unusual occurrence when appropriate evaluation has been performed.[15-17]

My colleagues and I routinely obtain written informed consent from the patient before all needle localization procedures.[18] We do so partly for medical-legal reasons and also to improve the patient's cooperation during the procedure. When patients are accurately and calmly informed about the procedure, they have less anxiety, are more cooperative, and tolerate the procedure better.

The technique for mammographic localization with a fenestrated mammography compression plate is simple and accurate. The original mammograms are reviewed to determine the appropriate needle length and the skin surface closest to the lesion (Fig. 16–1A through C). Although the approach is usually from the superior, inferior, lateral, or medial aspect of the breast,[19] any degree of angulation is possible.[20] The Mammography Quality Standards Act (MQSA) requires that the x-ray tube and image receptor be able to rotate 180 degrees, allowing localization from the inferior aspect of the breast for lesions in that region. Occasionally, the patient's body habitus precludes a from below (FB) approach. In these cases, the breast can sometimes be rolled enough to bring the lesion close to the fenestration of the compression paddle (Fig.16–2), or an inferior approach can be used with the patient in the recumbent position.[21,22]

The patient is positioned with the fenestrated paddle against the proposed skin entry surface. Small ink marks may be placed on the skin at the corners of the window of the compression paddle to allow rapid detection of any patient motion and to facilitate repositioning of the paddle if the lesion is not

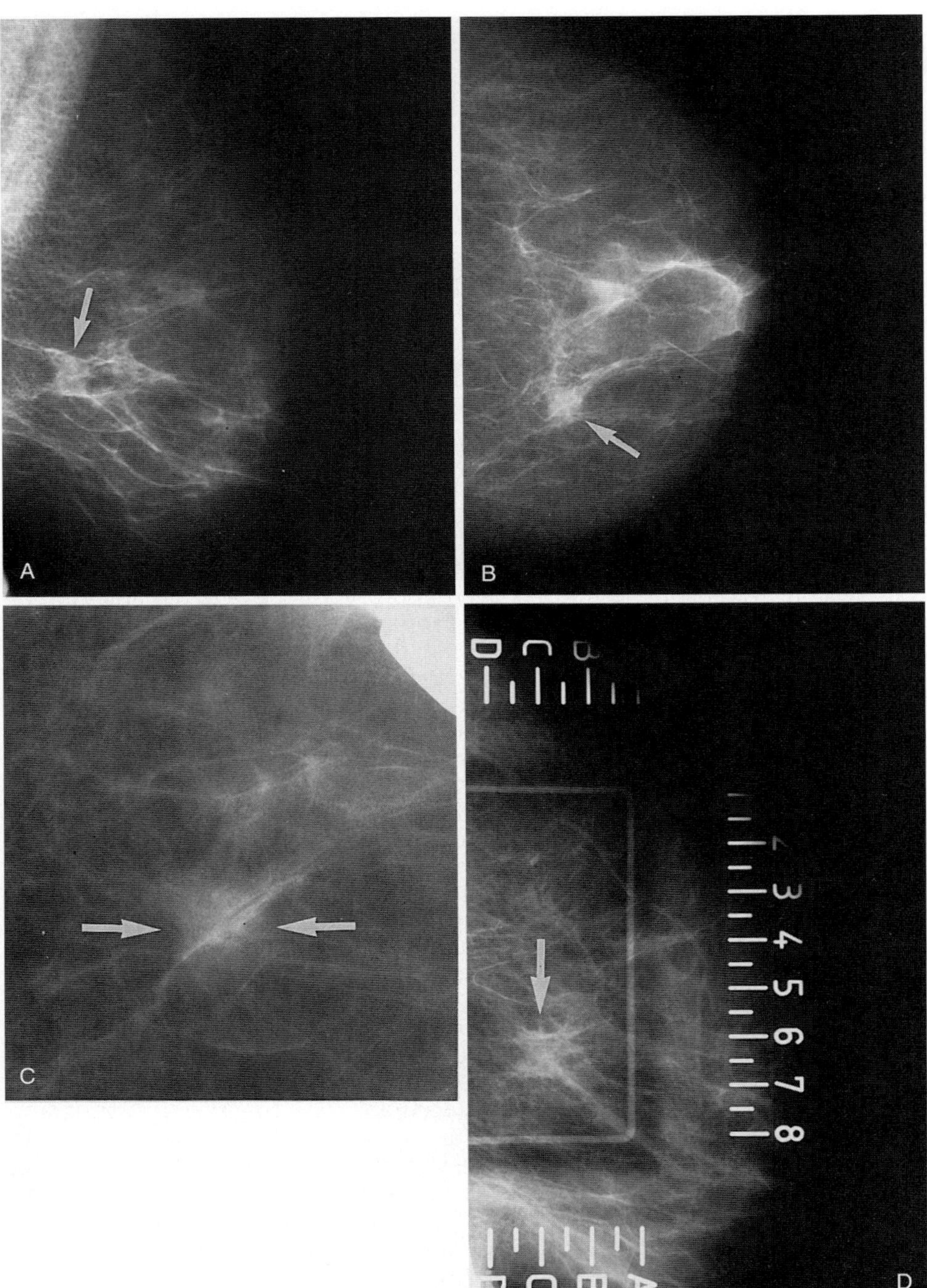

Figure 16–1. Sixty-year-old female with a 1.2-cm spiculated mass in the left breast (*arrows*). The lateromedial (**A**), craniocaudal (CC) (**B**), and spot compression magnification CC (**C**) views show the mass located at the 9-o'clock region of the medial aspect of the breast. **D,** The fenestrated compression paddle has been placed against the medial aspect of the breast, which is the skin surface closest to the lesion (*arrow*). The breast remains compressed while the film is processed and reviewed.

present within the window. A scout film is obtained (see Fig. 16–1D), and the breast is left compressed in the unit while this film is processed and reviewed to ensure that the lesion is under an open area. If it is not, the breast is appropriately repositioned until the lesion is accessible. The coordinates of the lesion are then determined from the scout film, and the skin is cleansed with sterile soap. Local anesthesia is optional,[23] but many women prefer to have it. Usually, 1 mL of 1% lidocaine, administered into the skin and subcutaneous tissue, is enough anesthetic for this procedure.

The breast is immobilized in the mammography unit, so that passage of the needle through the lesion is usually quick and the compression leads to some degree of numbness of the breast. The needle path must replicate the x-ray beam in order for the needle to pass through the lesion, so it is important to use the field-localizing light of the mammography unit to ensure that the shadow of the hub of the needle remains superimposed on the skin entry site.[24] No attempt should be made to gauge the distance to the lesion in this position; rather, the needle should be passed as far as possible into the breast. A radiograph

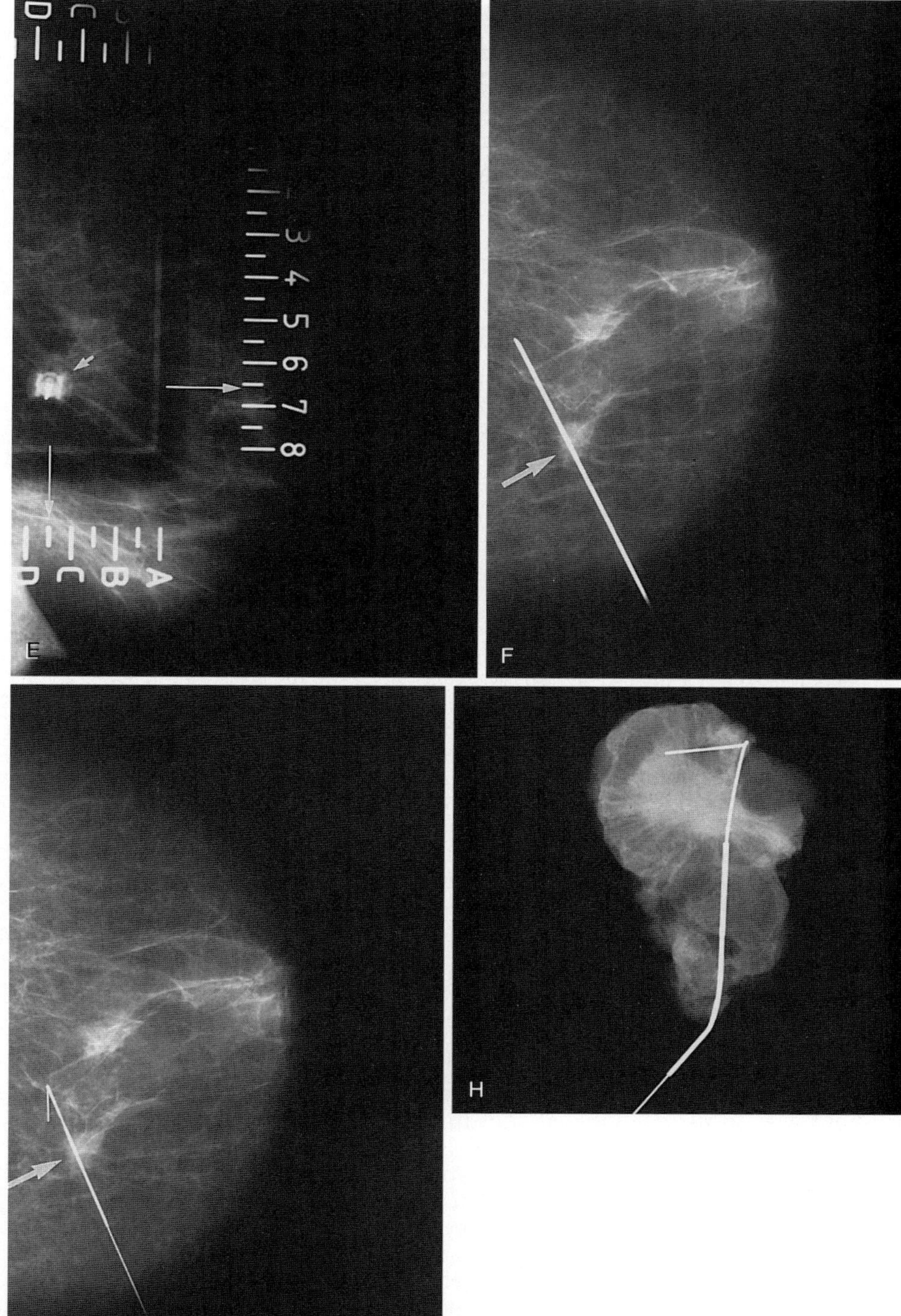

Figure 16–1, cont'd. **E,** The needle (*short arrow*) has been inserted into the mass at the coordinates shown by the *long arrows*. **F,** Craniocaudal view shows the needle entering the medial aspect of the breast and coursing through the mass (*arrow*). The distance from the mass to the end of the needle was measured and the needle was pulled back 2 cm, to the level of the far edge of the mass. If there is any doubt as to the position of the needle, another film should be obtained before the wire is after-loaded. **G,** CC view demonstrating the mass (*arrow*) at the thick part of the wire. The hook is approximately 1 cm beyond the mass. **H,** Specimen radiograph with localizing wire. This specimen film was obtained with a dedicated specimen x-ray machine at 20 kVp. Histologic analysis showed the lesions to be invasive ductal carcinoma. Note that the spiculations of the tumor extend to the surface of the specimen. The wire has been pulled back slightly, either during the surgery or after the removal of the specimen from the breast.

is then obtained in this first projection to verify that the needle is superimposed on the lesion (see Fig. 16–1E). While the radiologist maintains control of the needle (and keeps it advanced into the tissue), the compression paddle is carefully removed, and the patient is positioned for the orthogonal projection. Depending on the size of the breast, this view may be done with either a standard compression paddle or a small spot-compression device. The needle should have traveled beyond the lesion (see Fig. 16–1F) and then should be pulled back an appropriate distance before the hook-wire is after-loaded. The goal is to have the hook approximately 1 cm beyond the lesion. If the needle tip is at the lesion on the initial orthogonal view, no needle movement is necessary. However, if the needle is *short* of the lesion,

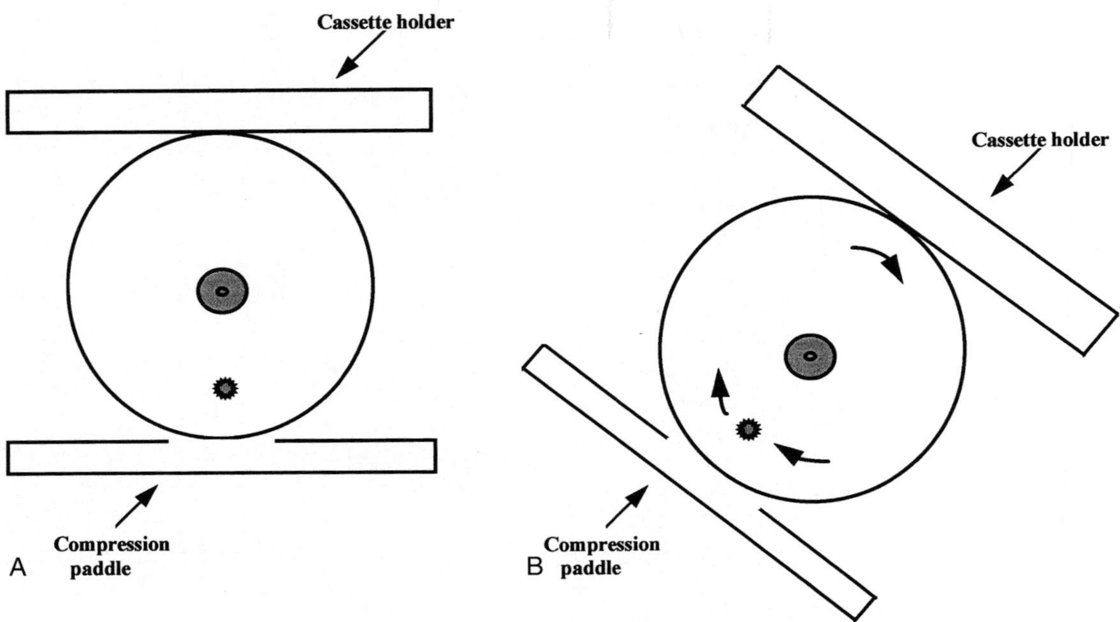

Figure 16–2. Localization of a lesion in the inferior aspect of the breast. When a nonpalpable, suspicious mammographic abnormality is present in the 6-o'clock region of the breast, the best method for localization uses a caudocranial (from below [FB]) approach (**A**), with the fenestrated compression paddle against the inferior skin surface. If the patient has a large abdomen, the image receptor should be maximally rotated given the patient's physical constraints, and the breast can be rolled before it is placed in compression, in order to bring the undersurface of the breast to the fenestration of the compression paddle (**B**). Taut compression is needed to prevent motion from the breast unrolling during the procedure.

advancement is difficult because the needle often deviates away from the lesion and one can no longer confirm its exact position until the wire is placed.

A final full-field mammogram is obtained showing the final wire position (see Fig. 16–1G). A metallic marker (BB) is placed at the skin entry site to allow measurement of the distance between the skin and the lesion. This film, together with that showing the needle passing through the lesion with the fenestrated compression paddle, should be adequate for demonstration of the position of the wire for the surgeon. However, some surgeons request orthogonal full-field wire films to review at the time of surgery. In this situation, only minimal compression should be used to obtain the full-field view done in the projection used for the initial needle placement, so as not to push the wire farther into the breast. The wire is coiled on the patient's skin surface, covered with gauze, and then bandaged. The patient is sent to surgery with her films appropriately marked for the surgeon.

The entire localization procedure is usually completed in 20 to 30 minutes. If digital mammography equipment is used for localization, the process is the same except that digital images, rather than radiographic films, are obtained and the entire process takes considerably less time. Dershaw and associates[25] found that the use of a digital image receptor on a mammography unit reduced the time required for needle localization by 50%.

When faint microcalcifications or vague masses are localized, they are sometimes difficult to visualize on the scout film obtained with the fenestrated compression paddle. The reason is the relative lack of compression of the breast tissue in the area within the window. Additional compression can be achieved within the window by placement of a sterile plastic surgical adhesive draping sheet on the undersurface of the compression paddle, against the skin surface.[26] The patient's skin must be cleaned with sterile soap before the sterile plastic sheet is placed. In some cases, the localization procedure must be done with a magnification technique to adequately visualize suspicious microcalcifications.[27]

When multiple suspicious abnormalities are present, multiple wires should be used to mark each lesion individually. In some cases, the needles and wires can be placed through the fenestrated compression paddle at the same time. More often, after one lesion is localized, the fenestrated compression paddle must be moved to a new location to provide appropriate localization of additional lesions. When a large abnormality, such as extensive microcalcifications, is localized, multiple wires are often used to "bracket" the boundaries of the lesion to help the surgeon remove the entire area at the initial excision (Fig. 16–3). This is particularly helpful before lumpectomy for a known carcinoma that has been previously diagnosed with imaging-guided needle biopsy.

Some surgeons and radiologists prefer to approach breast lesions from the anterior aspect of the breast, using a "freehand" method. This approach may be accurate in some mammographers' hands, but for most it is not as fast or as precise as the use of a

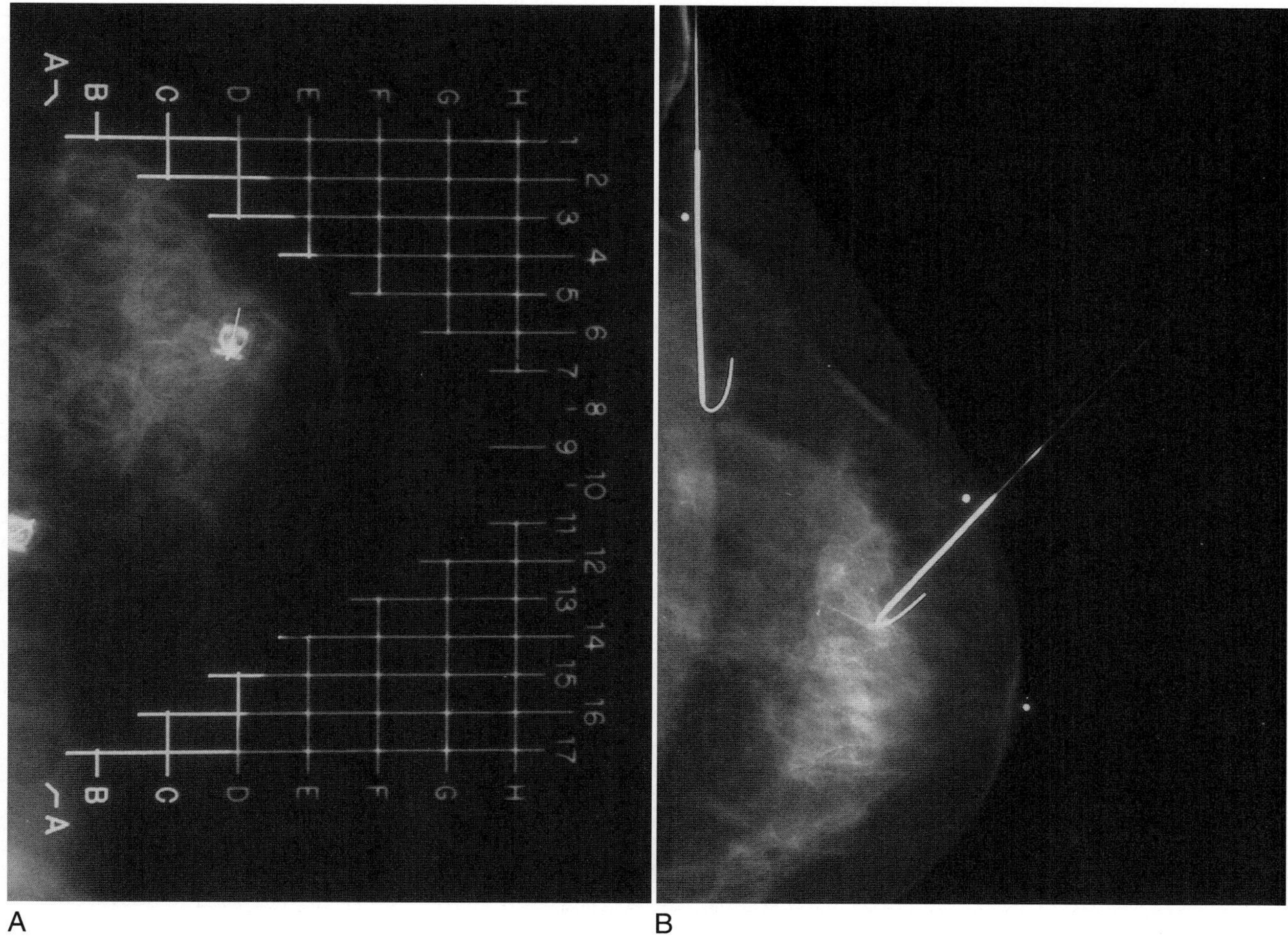

Figure 16–3. Bracketing localization of a large lesion before lumpectomy for breast carcinoma. There is a large area of very faint microcalcifications in the left breast. With digital mammography and the craniocaudal projection, needles were placed at the anterior and posterior margins of the region of calcifications (**A**). The mediolateral view (**B**) shows the needles and wires marking the extent of the calcifications.

fenestrated compression plate. The freehand technique commonly requires multiple repositionings of the needle to achieve adequate localization, and each movement of the needle requires two orthogonal mammograms to determine the needle's position. This method involves more time and radiation exposure and is usually less accurate than the use of a fenestrated compression paddle. Therefore, it is rarely, if ever, used. An anterior approach is sometimes advocated for lesions that are in the subareolar region, deep to the nipple and not close to any one skin surface. However, by rolling the breast during positioning in the fenestrated compression paddle, one can bring a more anterior skin surface over the lesion to reduce the distance between the skin entry site and the lesion, providing the surgeon with a quick and accurate "pseudoanterior approach" (Fig. 16–4).

Stereotactic devices are accurate for placement of needles for various types of needle biopsy but almost always require more time and are often less accurate for depth determination for presurgical needle localization than a fenestrated compression paddle. Digital image receptors on stereotactic units significantly reduce the time required for the procedure, but the fact that the entire procedure is performed with the breast compressed in a single direction leads to unpredictable final depth of wire placement (Fig. 16–5). Thus, stereotactic units are not recommended for routine preoperative needle localization of breast lesions.[28]

When a nonpalpable suspicious abnormality is ultrasonographically visible, it may be localized with ultrasonography quickly and accurately.[29] A "freehand" technique, whereby the length of the needle is directly visualized during real-time ultrasonography, should be used for needle and subsequent wire placement (see Chapter 20). It is important to plan the approach so that the needle path is as short as possible. When ultrasonographic localization is used for mammographically visible lesions, final wire-placement mammograms are always obtained and sent with the patient to the operating room.

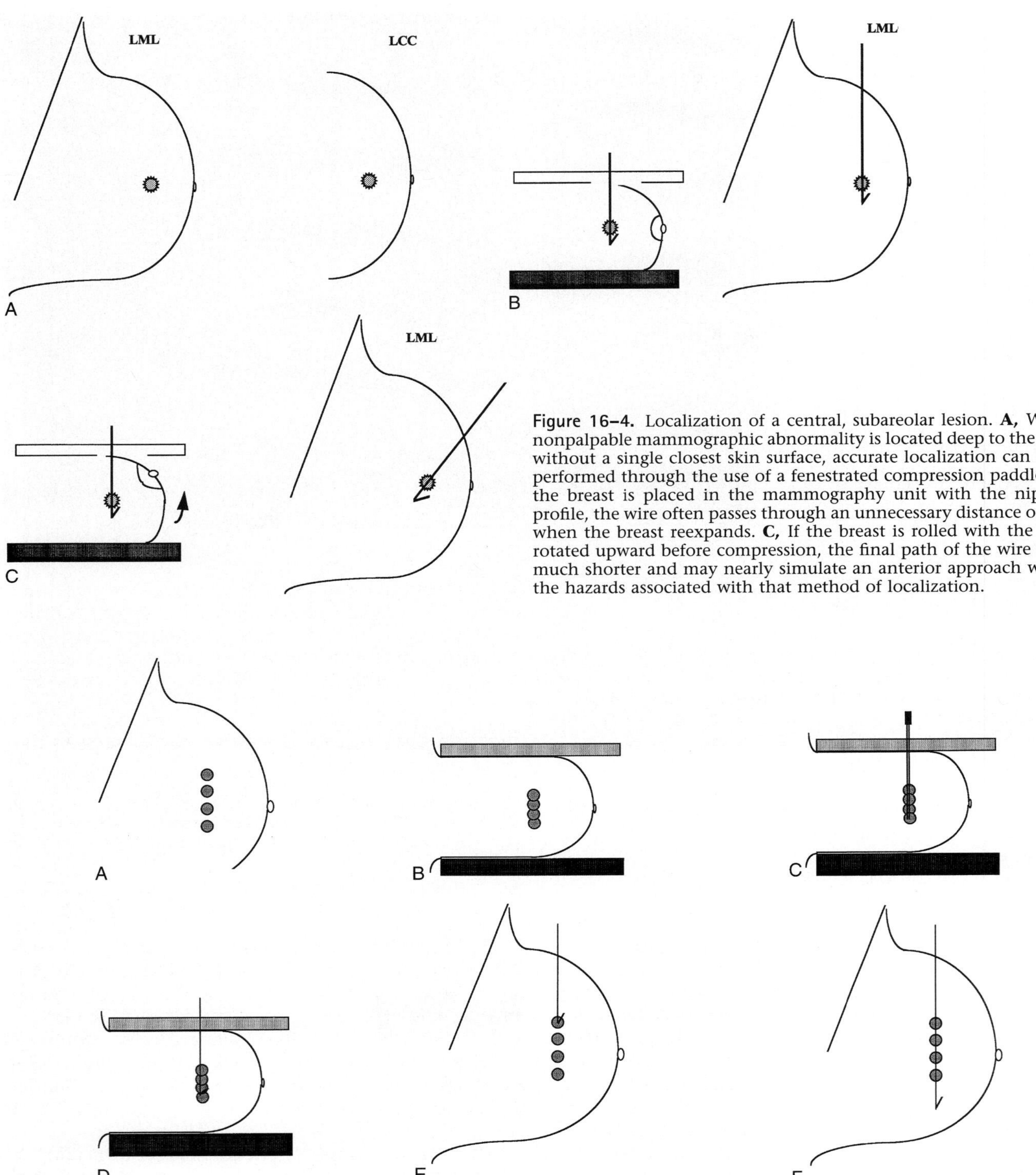

Figure 16–4. Localization of a central, subareolar lesion. **A,** When a nonpalpable mammographic abnormality is located deep to the nipple without a single closest skin surface, accurate localization can still be performed through the use of a fenestrated compression paddle. **B,** If the breast is placed in the mammography unit with the nipple in profile, the wire often passes through an unnecessary distance of tissue when the breast reexpands. **C,** If the breast is rolled with the nipple rotated upward before compression, the final path of the wire will be much shorter and may nearly simulate an anterior approach without the hazards associated with that method of localization.

Figure 16–5. Stereotactic needle localization. The final depth of the hook is unpredictable because the entire procedure is performed with the breast compressed in a single direction. A hypothetical model is used to demonstrate this concept. **A,** Mediolateral mammogram with four lesions at different depths (but the same *x* and *y* coordinates) within the breast. **B,** With compression for needle localization or needle biopsy, the lesions compact together, as do all other structures within the breast. **C,** Needle placement is accurate for needle biopsy in this position. **D,** Wire placement. If the hook is engaged while the breast is still compressed in one direction, the four lesions remain compacted together. **E,** When the breast reexpands after removal of compression, the final wire location may be unpredictable. In this case, the wire placement would be fine for the lesion in the most superior location but unsatisfactory for the most caudally located lesion. **F,** Some stereotactic equipment manufacturers recommend that the hook of the wire be deployed 1 to 2 cm deep to the lesion, so that the wire is more likely to remain through the lesion when the breast reexpands. However, this practice can lead to suboptimal placement of the hook beyond the lesion. In this example, the position of the hook-wire would be fine for the deepest lesion but suboptimally beyond the other three locations.

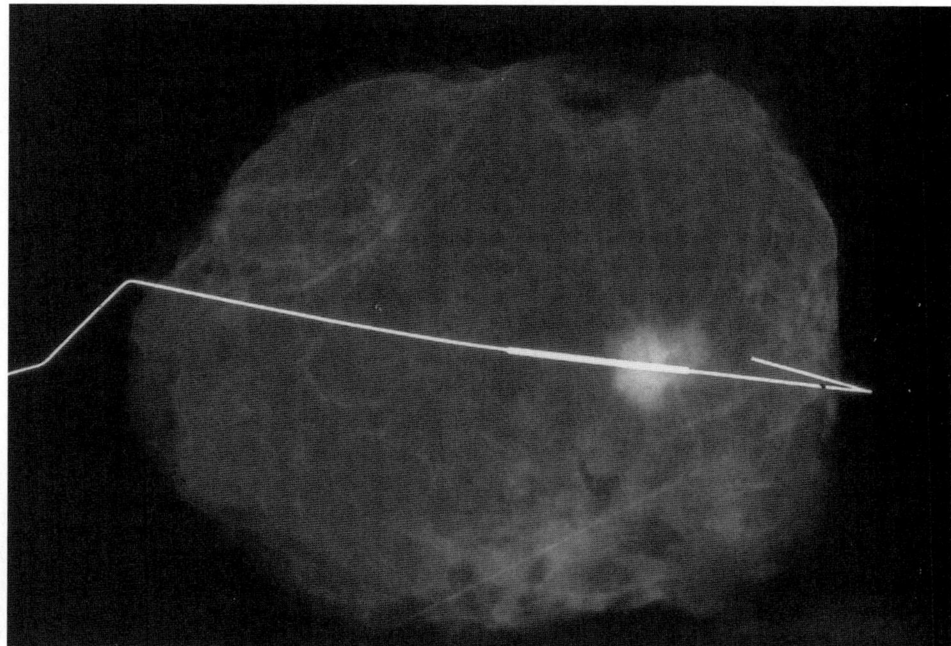

Figure 16–6. Specimen radiography. An 8-mm spiculated mass (invasive ductal carcinoma) is surrounded by a wide rim of normal-looking breast tissue.

SPECIMEN RADIOGRAPHY

Specimen radiography is an important part of the localization and surgical biopsy procedure for all types of nonpalpable breast lesions. It allows documentation that the lesion has been at least partially removed and demonstrates the location of the abnormality for the pathologist. A radiograph must be taken of the biopsy specimen (for calcified *and* noncalcified lesions) to ensure that the lesion and the localizing device have been removed.[30-32] Figures 16–1H and 16–6 through 16–9 demonstrate various specimen radiographs. Magnification and compression are usually used for specimen radiographs, particularly for noncalcified lesions.[33] There has been some speculation that the use of compression for specimen radiography may lead to inaccurate assessment of histologic margin status.[34] Nonetheless, most radiologists use compression because it makes the lesion more conspicuous on the radiograph.

Specimen radiography can be done with either a mammography unit or a dedicated specimen x-ray machine with low-kVp technique (20 to 23 kVp). Ideally, the specimen radiograph should be reviewed while the patient is still in the operating room by the radiologist who actually performed the localization. In any event, the patient's mammograms must be available for review at the time of specimen radiography. If the lesion is not seen in the specimen, the surgeon should be notified so that he or she can consider removing more tissue. Any additional tissue removed should be submitted for specimen radiography. The radiologist should also notify the surgeon if the entire localizing device or the entire lesion does not appear to be within the specimen.

For some vague noncalcified masses, the specimen radiograph may be equivocal. Turning the specimen 90 degrees and taking another radiograph may allow visualization of the lesion.[35] In addition, specimen radiographs obtained in orthogonal planes give

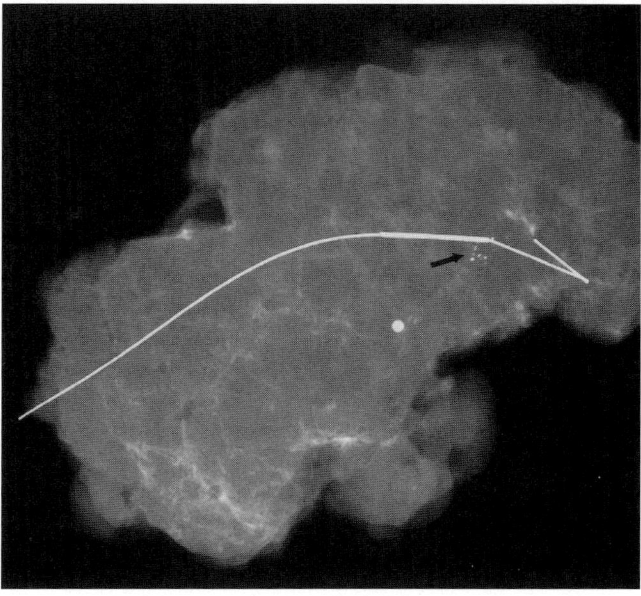

Figure 16–7. Specimen radiography. A 5-mm cluster of microcalcifications (*arrow*) that has been completely removed in a relatively large specimen. When all of the calcific particles that were previously visible on magnification mammography are present within the specimen, surrounded by a wide margin of radiographically normal breast tissue, one can be relatively sure that the lesion visible on imaging has been removed. However, such an appearance does not ensure histologically negative margins, because there may be a noncalcified component to the lesion. The lesion in this case was a fibroadenoma with focal calcification.

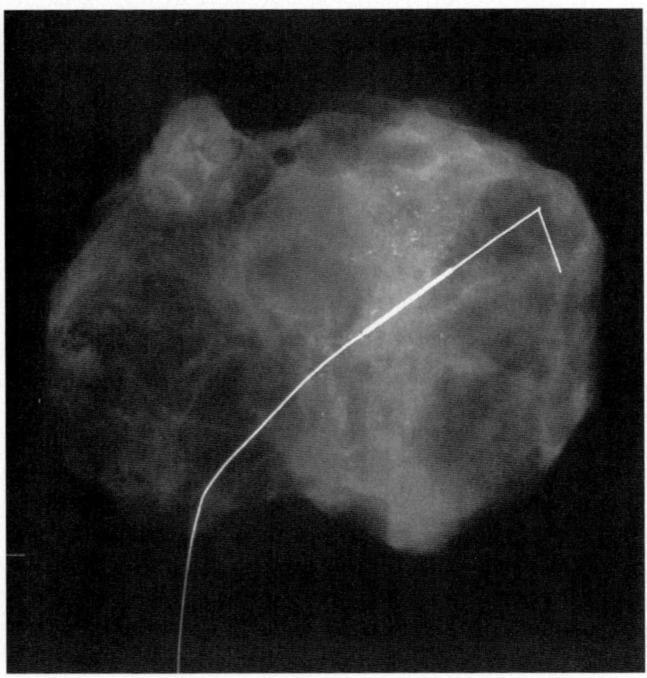

Figure 16–8. Specimen radiography. Large area of microcalcifications, with calcifications extending to the edge of the specimen (*arrows*). The margins are likely to be positive for malignancy in this situation. The surgeon should be notified immediately that the calcifications extend to the edge of the specimen. This lesion was ductal carcinoma in situ.

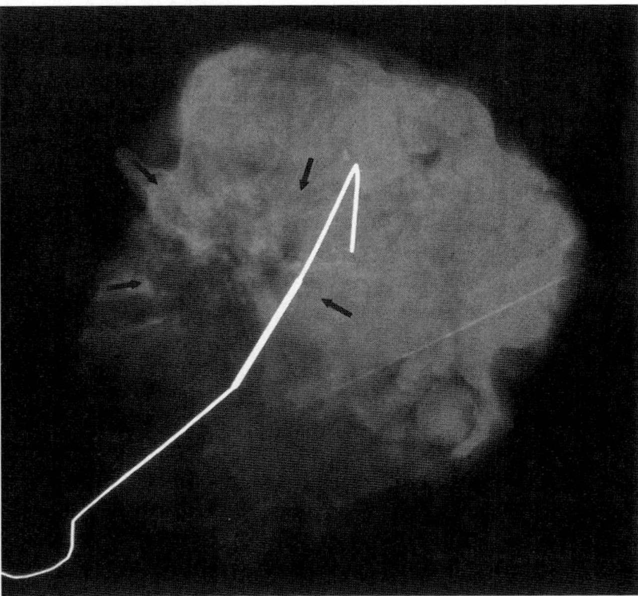

Figure 16–9. Specimen radiography. A 2-cm area of architectural distortion (invasive ductal carcinoma, *arrows*) that extends to the edge of the specimen. It is likely that the histologic margins will be positive for malignancy in this sort of situation. The surgeon should be notified immediately that the architectural distortion is at the edge of the specimen.

the surgeon and pathologist a better indication of whether the entire lesion has been removed.

The American College of Radiology Standard for the Management of Invasive Breast Carcinoma[36] recommends that specimen radiography preferably be performed in two directions. Even though specimen radiography is poor for predicting the margin status of resection of carcinomas,[37,38] it remains an important part of the procedure to document removal of at least a portion of the lesion. If the specimen radiograph and pathology report remain equivocal, repeat mammography should be performed within 2 to 3 months of surgery to see whether the lesion was actually removed.

The lesion should be marked within the specimen so that the pathologist knows the correct area to section for histologic analysis. The marking can be easily done with a variety of commercially available specimen-handling systems. Many of these systems have an alphanumeric coordinate system embedded within an immobilizing device, so that the coordinates of the lesion can be marked on the specimen radiograph that is submitted to the pathologist. Other devices have small holes to allow placement of a needle into the suspicious area of the tissue. However, in some states, it is illegal to submit material bearing needles for pathology. It is occasionally necessary to radiograph the specimen blocks or the sliced specimen to precisely localize the lesion within the tissue for the pathologist.[39,40]

When ultrasonographic localization is used for mammographically visible lesions, specimen radiography should be performed in the usual manner to document that the lesion has been removed. In the unusual instance of a mammographically invisible but ultrasonographically detected nonpalpable lesion, the specimen can be immersed in saline solution and specimen ultrasonography performed.[30,40] Unfortunately, for lesions that have been detected and localized with MRI, there is no way to do specimen evaluation at this time.

POTENTIAL COMPLICATIONS

All localization procedures carry the same potential risks: bleeding, infection, and vasovagal reaction.[41] Bleeding is rarely, if ever, a problem for needle localization procedures because the needle used is so small. Sterile technique should be used to minimize the chance of infection. Vagal reaction is the most dramatic and severe complication of presurgical needle localization procedures. After the needle has been placed, the patient should *never* be left alone in the room. A cart and basic resuscitation equipment should be nearby. The patient must be alert and able to cooperate with the procedure; therefore, no preoperative sedative medication should be given before the localization procedure. Anterior localization procedures carry the additional risk of pneumothorax, which is not a problem with approaches that are parallel to the chest wall.

Potential surgical complications include migration of the wire and cutting of the wire during dissection.[42,43] The surgeon should be aware that the wire should not be cut during preparation of the breast for surgery. The use of sufficiently sturdy wires or the placement of a needle or cannula over the wire helps minimize the risk of cutting the wire during surgery.

References

1. Homer MJ: Localization of nonpalpable breast lesions with the curved-end, retractable wire: Leaving the needle in vivo. AJR Am J Roentgenol 1988;151:919-920.
2. Homer MJ, Pile-Spellman ER: Needle localization of occult breast lesions with a curved-end retractable wire: Technique and pitfalls. Radiology 1986;161:547-548.
3. Kopans DB, Lindfors K, McCarthy KA, Meyer JE: Spring hookwire breast lesion localizer: Use with rigid-compression mammographic systems. Radiology 1985;157:537-538.
4. Kwasnik EM, Sadowsky NL, Vollman RW: An improved system for surgical excision of needle-localized nonpalpable breast lesions. Am J Surg 1987;154:476-477.
5. Hirsch JI, Banks WL, Sullivan JS, Horsley JS: Effect of methylene blue on estrogen-receptor activity. Radiology 1989;171: 105-107.
6. Hirsch JI, Banks WL, Sullivan JS, Horsley JS: Noninterference of isosulfan blue on estrogen-receptor activity. Radiology 1989;171:109-110.
7. Czarnecki DJ, Feider HK, Splittgerber GF: Toluidine blue dye as a breast localization marker. AJR Am J Roentgenol 1989; 153:261-263.
8. Canavese G, Catturich A, Vecchio C, et al: Pre-operative localization of non-palpable lesions in breast cancer by charcoal suspension. Eur J Surg Oncol 1995;21:47-49.
9. Langlois SLP, Carter ML: Carbon localisation of impalpable mammographic abnormalities. Australas Radiol 1991;35:237-241.
10. Moss HA, Barter SJ, Nayagam M, et al: The use of carbon suspension as an adjunct to wire localization of impalpable breast lesions. Clin Radiol 2002;57:937-944.
11. Mullen DJ, Eisen RN, Newman RD, et al: The use of carbon marking after stereotactic large-core-needle breast biopsy. Radiology 2001;218:255-260.
12. Gray RJ, Giuliano R, Dauway EL, et al: Radioguidance for nonpalpable primary lesions and sentinel lymph nodes(s). Am J Surg 2001;182:404-406.
13. Gray RJ, Salud C, Nguyen K, et al: Randomized prospective evaluation of a novel technique for biopsy or lumpectomy of nonpalpable breast lesions: Radioactive seed versus wire localization. Ann Surg Onc 2001;8:711-175.
14. Meyer JE, Sonnenfeld MR, Greenes RA, Stomper PC: Cancellation of preoperative breast localization procedures: Analysis of 53 cases. Radiology 1988;169:629-630.
15. Kopans DB, Waitzkin ED, Linetsky L, et al: Localization of breast lesions identified on only one mammographic view. AJR Am J Roentgenol 1987;149:39-41.
16. Sickles EA: Practical solutions to common mammographic problems: Tailoring the examination. AJR Am J Roentgenol 1988;151:31-39.
17. Swann CA, Kopans DB, McCarthy KA, et al: Localization of occult breast lesions: Practical solutions to problems of triangulation. Radiology 1987;163:577-579.
18. Reynolds HE, Jackson VP, Musick BS: A survey of interventional mammography practices. Radiology 1993;187:71-73.
19. Kopans DB: Preoperative imaging-guided needle placement and localization of clinically occult lesions. In Kopans DB (ed): Breast Imaging. Philadelphia, JB Lippincott, 1989, pp 320-341.
20. Vyborny CJ, Merrill TN, Geurkink RE: Difficult mammographic needle localizations: Use of alternate orthogonal projections. Radiology 1986;161:839-841.

21. Homer MJ: Preoperative needle localization of lesions in the lower half of the breast: Needle entry from below. AJR Am J Roentgenol 1987;149:43-45.
22. Pisano ED, Hall FM: Preoperative localization of inferior breast lesions. AJR Am J Roentgenol 1989;153:272.
23. Reynolds HE, Jackson VP, Musick BS: Preoperative needle localization in the breast: Utility of local anesthesia. Radiology 1993;187:503-505.
24. Caldarelli J, Cronan JJ, Scola FH, Schepps B: Shadow technique: A method for accurate and quick mammographic needle localization. Breast Dis 1987;1:29-31.
25. Dershaw DD, Fleischman RC, Liberman L, et al: Use of digital mammography in needle localization procedures. AJR Am J Roentgenol 1993;161:559-562.
26. Bates BF, Gaskin H: A modified technique for breast compression during needle localization. AJR Am J Roentgenol 1992; 159:1189-1190.
27. Berkowitz JE, Horan PM: Preoperative needle localization of subtle breast calcifications: Magnification technique. Radiology 1992;185:277.
28. Jackson VP, Bassett LW: Stereotactic fine-needle aspiration biopsy for nonpalpable breast lesions. AJR Am J Roentgenol 1990;154:1196-1197.
29. Fornage BD, Coan JD, David CL: Ultrasound-guided needle biopsy of the breast and other interventional procedures. Radiol Clin North Am 1992;30:167-185.
30. D'Orsi CJ: Management of the breast specimen. Radiology 1995;194:297-302.
31. Homer MJ, Berlin L: Radiography of the surgical breast biopsy specimen. AJR Am J Roentgenol 1998;171:1197-1199.
32. Stomper PC, Davis SP, Sonnenfeld MR, et al: Efficacy of specimen radiography of clinically occult noncalcified breast lesions. AJR Am J Roentgenol 1988;151:43-47.
33. Lee MJ, Birdwell RL, Dirbas F, et al: Does intraoperative radiography of breast tissue specimens require compression? J Women's Imaging 2002;4:156-164.
34. Graham RA, Homer MJ, Katz J, et al: The pancake phenomenon contributes to the inaccuracy of margin assessment in patients with breast cancer. Am J Surg 2002;184:89-93.
35. Rebner M, Pennes DR, Baker DE, et al: Two-view specimen radiography in surgical biopsy of nonpalpable breast masses. AJR Am J Roentgenol 1987;149:283-285.
36. American College of Radiology: Standard for breast conservation therapy in the management of invasive breast carcinoma. In: Standards. Reston, VA, American College of Radiology, 2001, pp 231-248.
37. Graham RA, Homer MJ, Sigler CJ, et al: The efficacy of specimen radiography in evaluating the surgical margins of impalpable breast carcinoma. AJR Am J Roentgenol 1994;162:33-36.
38. Lee C, Carter D: Detecting residual tumor after excisional biopsy of impalpable breast carcinoma: Efficacy of comparing preoperative mammograms with radiographs of the biopsy specimen. AJR Am J Roentgenol 1995;164:81-86.
39. Cardenosa G, Eklund GW: Paraffin block radiography following breast biopsies: Use of orthogonal views. Radiology 1991; 180:873-874.
40. Frenna TH, Meyer JE, Sonnenfeld MR: US of breast biopsy specimens. Radiology 1994;190:573.
41. Helvie MA, Ikeda DM, Adler DD: Localization and needle aspiration of breast lesions: Complications in 370 cases. AJR Am J Roentgenol 1991;157:711-714.
42. Davis PS, Wechsler RJ, Feig SA, March DE: Migration of breast biopsy localization wire. AJR Am J Roentgenol 1988;150:787-788.
43. Homer MJ: Transection of the localization hooked wire during breast biopsy. AJR Am J Roentgenol 1983;141:929-930.

Imaging-Guided Core Needle Biopsy of the Breast

Christine H. Kim and Lawrence W. Bassett

Large core needle biopsy (CNB) has become the preferred method of tissue diagnosis for lesions in the breast that are apparent on imaging. The main reasons are that large CNB is less invasive than open surgical biopsy as well as more cost-effective[1-6] because it eliminates the need for surgery to establish a diagnosis. The majority of benign lesions can be identified and managed with surveillance protocols. Malignant lesions can be diagnosed and characterized histologically before definitive surgery, eliminating the need for two operations (one to establish a diagnosis and another for definitive treatment). Automated large CNB can also differentiate between invasive and noninvasive cancers, a distinction that determines whether lymph node sampling should be performed at the time of surgery. In addition, some investigators have reported a lower rate of positive (cancerous) margins after lumpectomy in patients diagnosed with CNB than in patients diagnosed with needle-localized excisional biopsy.[7-10] The accuracy of large CNB has been reported to be comparable to that of surgical biopsy,[11-13] with rates of 92% to 99% for sensitivity and 94% to 100% for specificity.[11-15]

The two methods of imaging guidance widely used with CNB are mammography (stereotaxis) and ultrasonography. CNB guided by magnetic resonance imaging (MRI) is just beginning to be performed at some institutions.[16,17] The imaging modality used is generally the one that best depicts the abnormality (Fig. 17–1). For example, most microcalcifications are best seen on mammography and most often undergo biopsy with stereotactic guidance. For lesions that are apparent on both modalities, other factors may be considered, such as patient comfort (the patient lies supine during ultrasound-guided procedures and is either prone, decubitus, or upright for stereotactic procedures) and anatomic limitations (lesions in small or thin breasts or lesions that are extremely close to the chest wall may be difficult or impossible to sample with stereotactically guided biopsy). Ultrasound-guided core biopsies with an automated biopsy gun can also be less time-consuming and more cost effective[6] than stereotactic procedures. Other methods that are or have been used for diagnostic tissue sampling are fine-needle aspiration (FNA) biopsy and sampling with the Advanced Breast Biopsy Instrumentation (ABBI) device.

STEREOTACTIC CORE NEEDLE BIOPSY

Stereotactic imaging was first used in interventional breast procedures in Sweden in 1977 to guide FNA biopsy. In 1986, the first stereotactic unit was installed in the United States at the University of Chicago. In 1990, Parker and colleagues[18] introduced stereotactic (mammographically guided) CNB, also known as stereotactic mammotomy, after a short trial in the late 1980s in which the stereotactic method was used for preoperative needle localization.[19,20] Today, stereotactic breast biopsies can be performed using either (1) a dedicated stereotactic biopsy unit (LORAD, Danbury, CT, and Fischer Imaging, Denver, CO), which consists of a combined digital mammography unit, prone biopsy table, and an 11-gauge, vacuum-assisted directional cutting device (Mammotome Biopsy System, Biopsys Medical, Inc., Irvine, CA) (Fig. 17–2), or (2) a smaller "add-on" stereotactic unit that attaches to a conventional mammography unit (Fig. 17–3). An add-on unit can be used with either the vacuum-assisted device (VAD) or a spring-loaded automated large-core (ALC) biopsy gun.[21] The dedicated biopsy unit requires a large open space and is much more expensive than the add-on unit but enables faster image acquisition. Prone positioning on the dedicated stereotactic tables also allows for greater patient comfort while making it easier for the patient to remain still. The standard add-on unit is less expensive and can be used in a much smaller space with the patient in either an upright or decubitus position, but image acquisition takes longer and there is a greater chance of patient movement, especially in the upright position. In addition, the potential effect of vasovagal reactions becomes more significant when the patient is positioned upright. The add-on unit may be upgraded to employ digital mammography for faster image acquisition, but this process can be very expensive.

Mammographic Abnormalities Selected for Stereotactic Core Needle Biopsy

The majority of mammographic abnormalities that are sampled using stereotactic guidance can be divided into the following two basic categories:

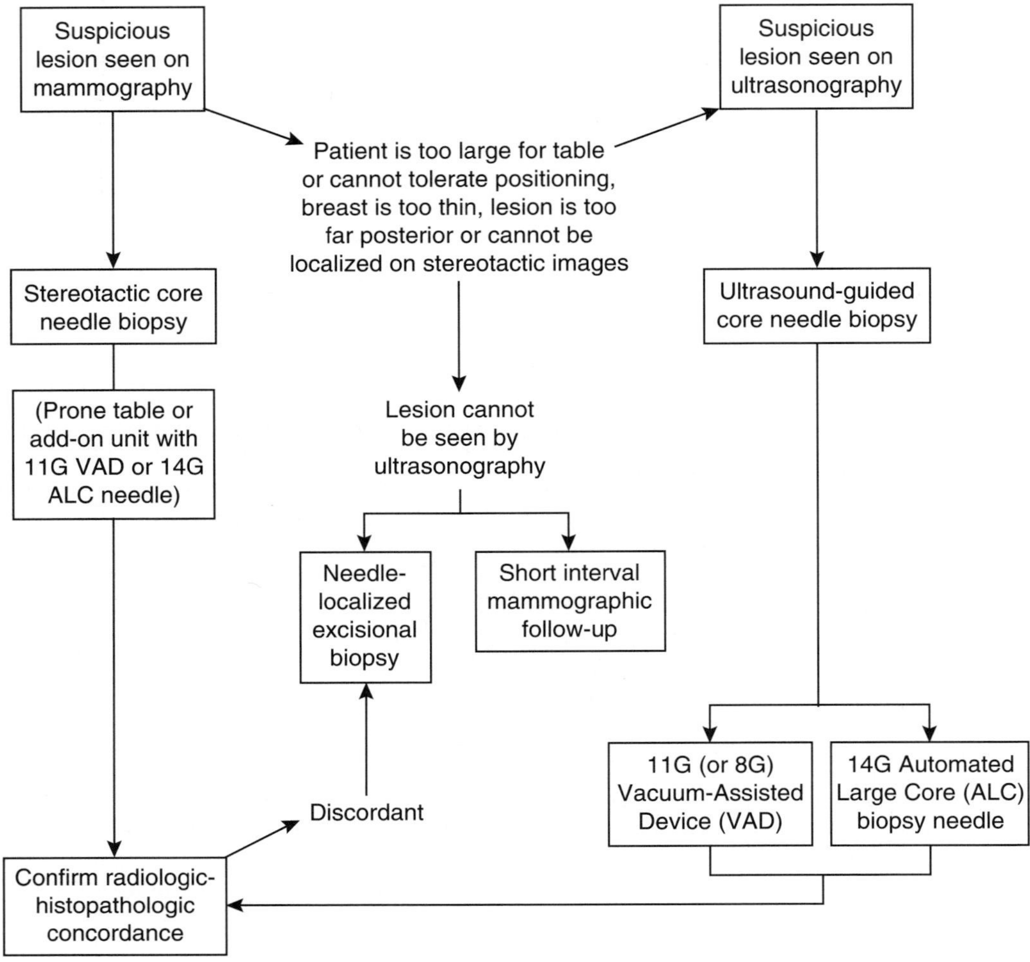

Figure 17–1. Algorithm for imaging-guided core needle biopsy of the breast.

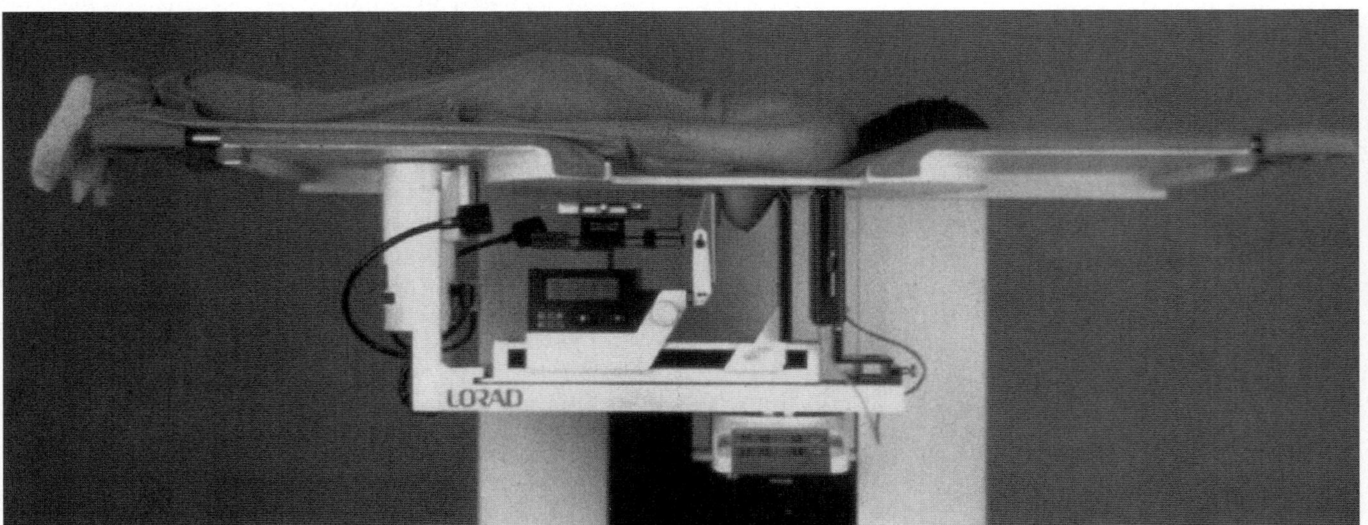

Figure 17–2. Patient lying prone on dedicated stereotactic biopsy table with breast suspended through an opening in the table.

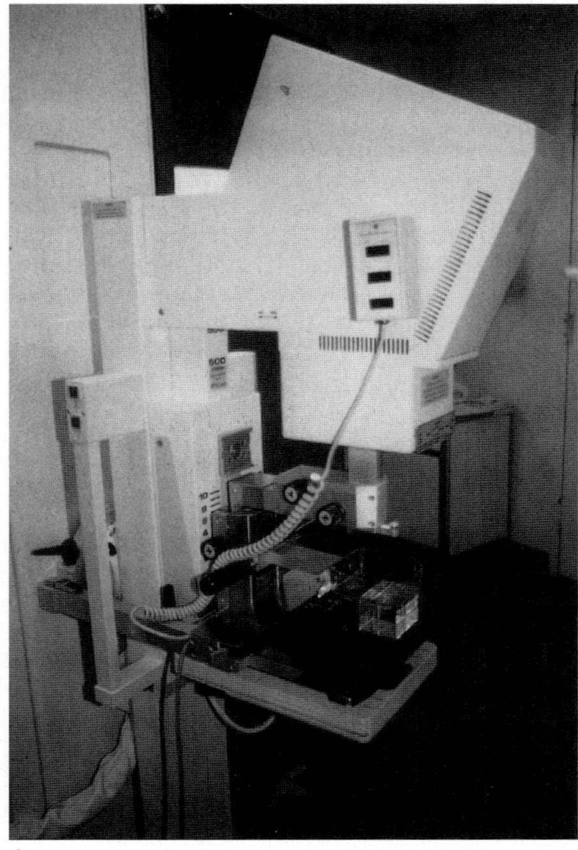

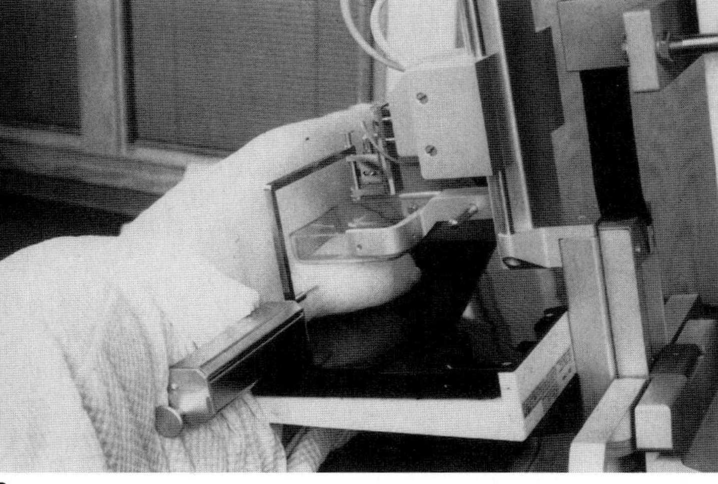

A B

Figure 17–3. **A,** "Add-on" device (in upright position) attached to a conventional mammography unit. **B,** Patient in lateral decubitus position during stereotactic biopsy using add-on device attached to a conventional mammography unit.

- Suspicious abnormalities, classified by the American College of Radiology's Breast Imaging Reporting and Data System (BI-RADS) as category 4
- Abnormalities that are highly suggestive of malignancy (BI-RADS category 5)

These abnormalities include masses, microcalcifications, and architectural distortion with suspicious or changing features (Table 17–1). For patients with mammographic findings that are probably benign (BI-RADS 3), a 6-month follow-up evaluation is the usual recommendation. Occasionally, CNB may be

Table 17–1. Breast Imaging Reporting and Data System (BI-RADS) Final Assessment Categories for Mammography

Category	Assessment	Description	Recommendation
0	Incomplete	Needs additional imaging evaluation and/or prior films for comparison	Additional imaging workup and/or comparison with prior studies
1	Negative	Nothing to comment on	Routine screening
2	Benign findings	Negative mammogram, but interpreter chooses to describe a benign finding	Routine screening
3	Probably benign	Very high probability of benignity (less than 2% risk of malignancy)	Short interval follow-up to establish stability
4	Suspicious	Finding without the classic appearance of malignancy but with a reasonable probability of being malignant	Biopsy should be considered
5	Highly suggestive of malignancy	High probability (>95%) of being malignant	Appropriate action should be taken
6	Known malignancy	Cancer that is biopsy proven	Appropriate action should be taken

Adapted with permission from the American College of Radiology (ACR): ACR Breast Imaging Reporting and Data System (BI-RADS), 4th ed. Reston, VA, American College of Radiology, 2003, pp 193-197. No other representation of these documents is authorized without express, written permission from the American College of Radiology.

performed on probably benign lesions for patients who have a personal or family history of breast cancer or who are extremely anxious; however, the cost-to-benefit ratio of these lesions can be quite high.[22]

Risks and Complications of Stereotactic Core Needle Biopsy and Informed Consent

Once the decision to perform stereotactic CNB is made, the findings, recommendations, and procedure, including the potential risks and alternatives, are explained to the patient. The main complications are discussed; they are infection, bleeding, ecchymosis or hematoma formation, the possibility of not obtaining a diagnostic tissue sample, and the possible complication of implant rupture. Placement of a localizing marker clip, if applicable, is also explained. Once the patient understands and accepts the risks and complications and agrees to proceed, she is asked to sign an informed consent form (Fig. 17–4). The patient is then advised to discontinue anticoagulation therapy in advance, if possible, and, at some institutions, may be offered a short-acting sedative on the day of the biopsy to reduce anxiety. Patients should also be advised that in a small percentage of cases, surgical biopsy may still be necessary if there is any question about the pathologic diagnosis after CNB.

Technique

At the time of the biopsy, the patient is asked to lie prone on the biopsy table with the breast suspended through an opening in the table (Fig. 17–5). The breast is positioned against the image receptor plate, and compression is applied with an open biopsy compression paddle so that the lesion lies in the center of the field of view (Figs. 17–6 and 17–7). Two mammographic images are taken at +15-degree and −15-degree angles from the plane perpendicular to the image receptor; these images are then viewed at either a digital monitor or a special viewbox that is electronically integrated with the biopsy equipment. The location of the lesion is marked on each of the stereotactic images on the monitor or on the viewbox, and numerical coordinates are automatically calculated to localize the lesion in the x, y, and z planes (Fig. 17–8). The needle position is calibrated to assign a zero starting position. The calculated biopsy coordinates are transmitted to the biopsy gun. It is important for the physician to confirm that the spatial orientation of x, y, and z coordinates within the breast is appropriate, because targeting errors can occur (Fig. 17–9). The skin in the biopsy field is thoroughly cleansed with povidone-iodine solution, and local anesthetic is injected from the skin down to the breast tissue surrounding the lesion. Sterile technique is maintained throughout the procedure.

The VAD is a hollow 11-gauge beveled needle with an aperture on the side of the needle shaft for sample retrieval (Fig. 17–10). The functions of the needle are controlled by a computer touch screen or handheld remote. An inner cutting sheath closes the window of the sample chamber before the needle is positioned within the breast. A small (2- to 3-mm) incision is made in the skin, and the tip of the biopsy needle is inserted through the dermis and positioned just in front of the lesion (Fig. 17–11). When the spatial coordinates are deemed acceptable, the needle is "fired" into the lesion. Once the sample chamber is situated next to the lesion, the window is opened, and a vacuum is applied to draw the adjacent tissue into the chamber. The cutting sheath then severs the tissue as it closes the window, and the vacuum continues to draw the specimen backwards through the hollow needle (which remains in position), from which it can be retrieved outside the breast. The window is rotated to sample areas of the surrounding tissue 360 degrees around the needle shaft. At our institution, an average of 12 to 16 samples are obtained.

If an ALC biopsy gun is used, the needle is also fired directly into the lesion. However, because the caliber of the samples is smaller, the needle position should be readjusted slightly for each pass to ensure that representative samples are taken from different areas of the lesion.

After sampling is determined to be sufficient, a stainless steel or titanium microclip is often placed at the biopsy site via the hollow biopsy needle (Fig. 17–12), especially if it is thought that the lesion will no longer be radiographically apparent after biopsy. If any further intervention is required, the microclip can later serve as a target for needle localization before surgery. No side effects or risks have been associated with the presence of the microclip, even in patients undergoing MRI.[23] The only drawback is that the clip can occasionally migrate from the biopsy site either initially or some time later.[24,25] For this reason, immediately post-biopsy orthogonal-view mammograms are recommended to document the location of the clip relative to the biopsy site.

Mammographic Findings after Stereotactic Biopsy

There are several reasons to obtain orthogonal-view mammographic images (usually craniocaudal [CC] and 90-degree lateral) immediately after stereotactic CNB. The first, as mentioned previously, is to confirm appropriate positioning of the microclip. A second reason (especially if a clip is not used) is to see how much of the targeted lesion remains. If the pathology results are discordant and the targeted lesion appears unchanged on the post-biopsy mammograms, one may question whether the lesion was actually sampled. Other inconsequential findings that may be apparent on immediate post-biopsy

Text continued on p. 283

INFORMED CONSENT INFORMATION

IMAGING-GUIDED CORE NEEDLE BIOPSY

You have decided to have an important breast biopsy procedure and we appreciate your selecting UCLA Healthcare to meet your needs. It is important to you and to us that you fully understand the risks, benefits and alternatives to the breast core needle biopsy you have planned. The purpose of this document is to provide written information regarding the risks, benefits and alternatives to imaging-guided breast core needle biopsy. The information provided here is a supplement to the discussions you have had with our physicians in preparation for the procedure. You should read this material and ask your doctors any questions you have before giving your consent.

The Procedure: Abnormalities shown in mammograms or ultrasound that are determined to require biopsy are usually not cancer. Approximately 70% of breast biopsies result in a benign (not cancer) diagnosis. Surgical or "open" biopsy is the conventional method for performing the biopsy. Breast core needle biopsy guided by stereotactic mammography or ultrasound is considered a less invasive alternative to surgical biopsy. At UCLA we have performed over 1,000 core needle biopsies guided by stereotactic mammography or ultrasound since 1992. Core needle biopsy offers some advantages over surgical biopsy but also has risk and limitations. These are explained below.

Benefits

If your core needle biopsy is successful and is complemented by compliance with follow-up recommendations after the biopsy, you may receive the benefits explained below. The doctors cannot guarantee you will receive any of these benefits. Only you can decide if the potential benefits are worth the risks. The potential benefits are:

1. If successful, core needle biopsy does not leave any permanent scar on the breast.
2. If successful, core needle biopsy can be accomplished in approximately 1 hour. This is less than the overall surgical biopsy procedure, which involves needle localization first to guide the surgeon and then the actual surgical biopsy.
3. If successful, core needle biopsy can provide a definitive benign (not cancer) or cancer diagnosis. If benign and consistent with the mammography and ultrasound findings an open (surgical) biopsy could be avoided.
4. Core needle biopsy does not leave any significant changes (scars) within the breast that could change the appearance future mammograms and potentially be confusing.

Risks

There are risks associated with undergoing one of these procedures, and it is essential to understand the associated risks. The following risks are well recognized, but there may also be risks not included in this list that are unforeseen by your doctors.

1. The procedure may not be successful for the following technical reasons:
   - The abnormality does not show up well enough on the stereotactic mammography or ultrasound to guide the core biopsy needle properly.
   - The abnormality is in a difficult location (too close to the skin surface or too deep in the breast) so that the core biopsy needle cannot be safely performed.
   - For stereotactic mammography guided core needle biopsy you will have to lie prone (stomach down) on the biopsy table for about 30 minutes. The breast to be biopsied will be suspended through a hole in the table and will have to be compressed. If you have problems lying this way the procedure cannot be done.
2. If the core needle biopsy results are not definitive an open (surgical) biopsy may have to be performed a few weeks later. Overall, a surgical biopsy is required in about 15% of patients after the core needle biopsy. This can happen in the following circumstances:
   - When the core needle biopsy results do not adequately explain the mammography or ultrasound findings
   - The core needle biopsy results show a difficult diagnosis that requires more tissue be removed to be sure that an associated cancer was not missed. An example would be a diagnosis of "atypical ductal hyperplasia". A diagnosis of atypical ductal hyperplasia does not mean that you have cancer but it means that a surgical biopsy is necessary because some of the tissue removed is not typical and there could be cancer nearby. Again, this does not mean that there is cancer but it does mean that a surgical biopsy should be done to examine more tissue in the same area.
   - The core needle biopsy does not provide sufficient tissue to give a diagnosis.

Figure 17–4. Example of consent form used for core needle biopsy.

Continued

3. Cancer may be present but not diagnosed on the core needle biopsy despite a benign (not cancer) diagnosis. This is reported to occur in about 2% of cases. For this reason, if the results of the core needle biopsy are benign you will be asked to comply with a follow-up surveillance protocol including a 6-month follow-up mammography and/or ultrasound examination. It is important to comply with the follow-up recommendations. If you cannot return for follow-up mammography or ultrasound, core needle biopsy may not be the appropriate method for your biopsy.
4. Some patients experience bleeding after the core needle biopsy and this would require application of compression over the area for 10 minutes or longer. Prolonged bleeding is uncommon and has not occurred in our experience but this is a potential complication of having a needle biopsy or surgery.
5. A hematoma may occur. This is a collection of blood at the biopsy site which can feel like a breast lump. If you felt a lump before it may feel bigger because of the hematoma. This should get smaller or completely go away in a few weeks.
6. Bruising around the needle biopsy entry site on the skin frequently occurs. This usually resolves within a few weeks.
7. Infection is a potential complication of needle biopsy. Although we have not encountered this complication, it is a potential risk when a needle is placed in the breast.
8. If the procedure is done with ultrasound guidance and the needle entered the chest wall behind the breast it could result in a pneumothorax (puncture of the lung lining or "pleura"). This is a rare complication since the ultrasound-guided procedure is done in such a way as to avoid this complication. However, if pneumothorax occurred it would require that a chest x-ray examination be performed. The chest x-ray would determine whether any treatment of the pneumothorax, such as placing a chest tube to remove air or fluid, was necessary.

If you have breast silicone or saline implants, the needle could potentially puncture the implant. This could result in implant leakage or collapse. This is a rare complication since the procedure is done in such a way as to avoid this complication.

Alternatives

The abnormality could also be removed by a surgical procedure. Surgical biopsy would require mammography-guided or ultrasound-guided presurgery needle localization if the abnormality cannot be felt by the surgeon or is difficult to feel.

Patient Initials:____________

Date:________________

Figure 17–4—Cont'd.

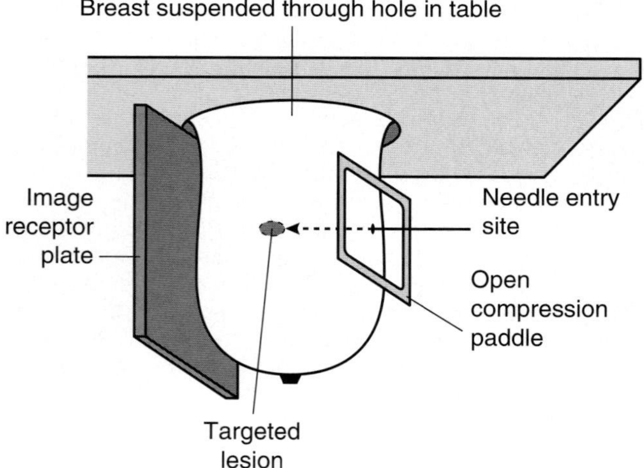

Figure 17–5. Side view of breast suspended through opening in prone biopsy table and in compression beneath the table.

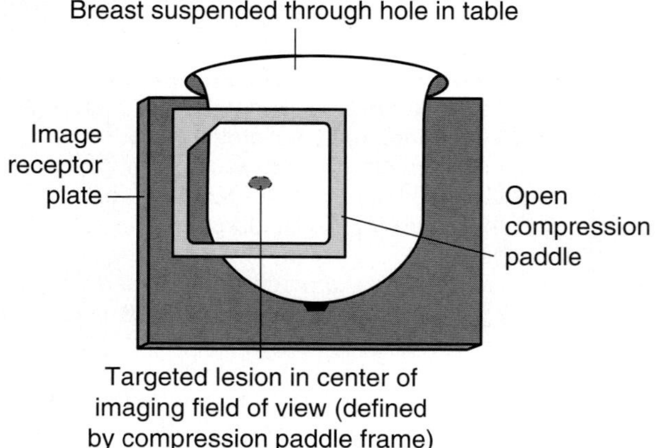

Figure 17–6. Frontal view of breast in compression with targeted entry site in center of compression paddle frame.

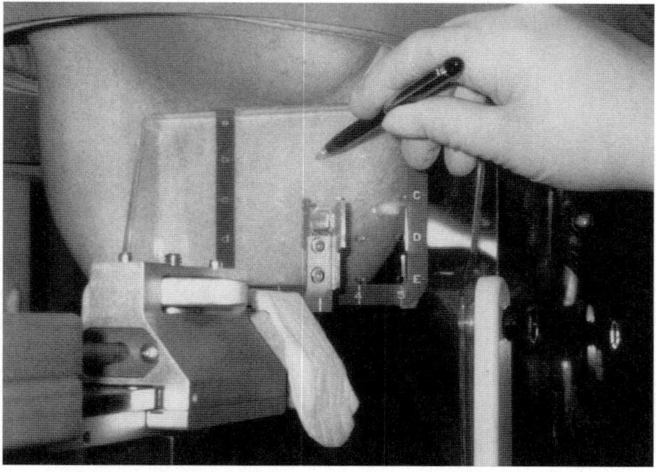

Figure 17–7. Breast in compression with targeted skin entry site within the center of imaging field of view (defined by compression paddle frame).

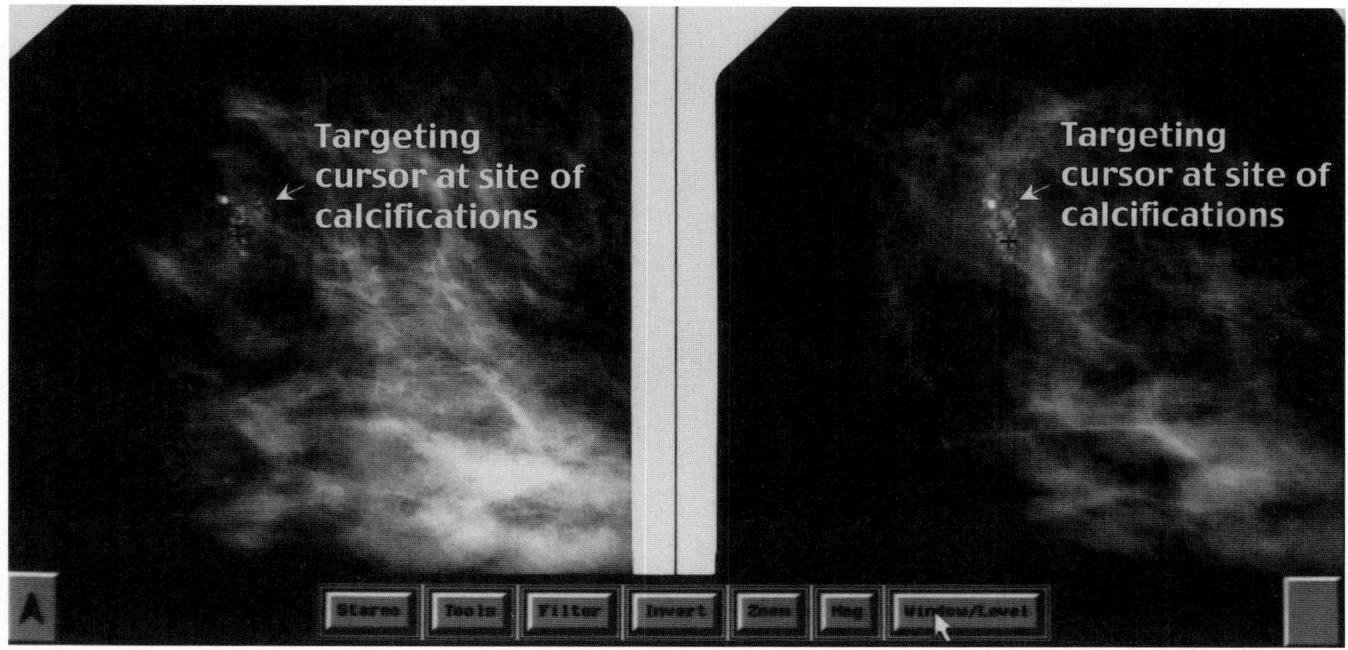

Figure 17–8. Stereotactic images after targeting a cluster of microcalcifications for biopsy.

Proper Targeting

−15° view +15° view

Pre-fire stereotactic images
Needle tip just in front of the lesion

−15° view +15° view

Post-fire stereotactic images
Needle tip and sample chamber in desired position within the lesion

A

−Z Error: Needle Not In Far Enough

−15° view +15° view

Pre-fire stereotactic images
Needle tip not close enough to lesion

−15° view +15° view

Post-fire stereotactic images
Needle tip and sample chamber not in far enough

B

+X Error: Needle Too Far Lateral

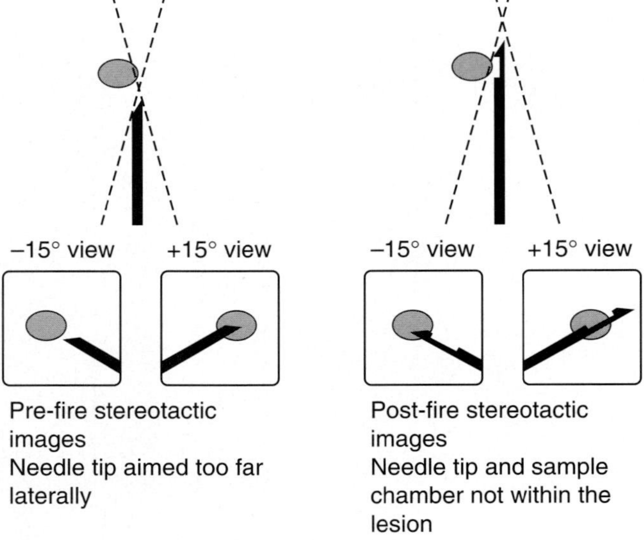

C

Figure 17–9. A, Example of proper stereotactic targeting. **B,** Example of –Z error: Needle is not advanced deep enough into the breast. **C,** Example of +X error: Needle is positioned too far lateral with respect to the lesion.

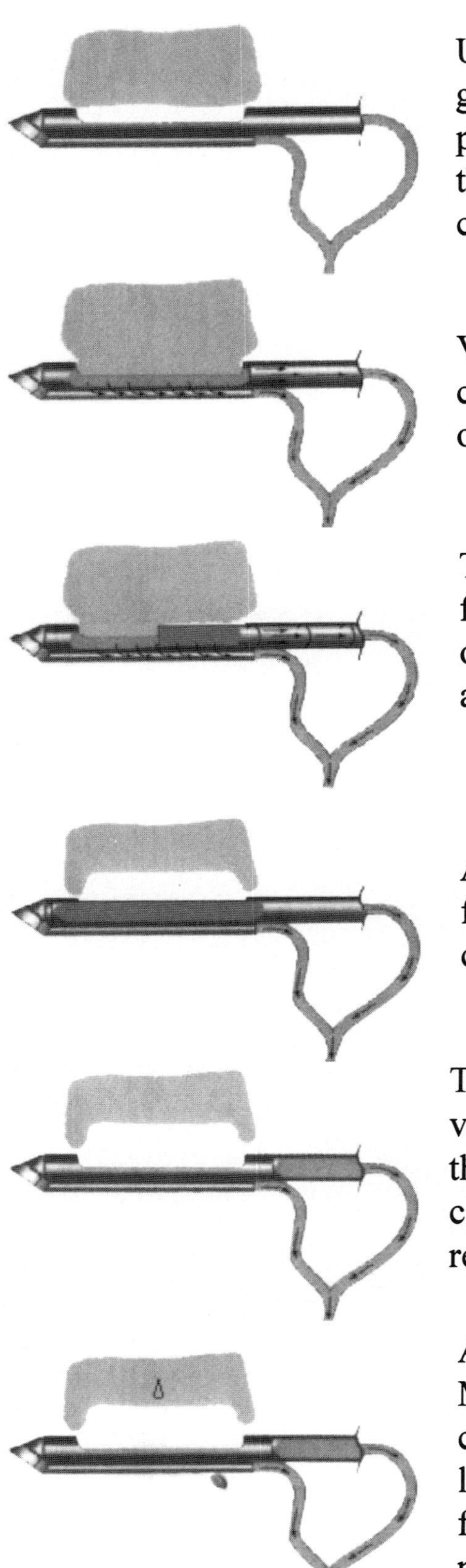

Under stereotactic or ultrasound guidance, the probe is positioned in the breast to align the center of aperture with the center of the lesion.
Vacuum aspiration gently captures the specimen in the open aperture.
The rotating cutter is advanced forward, capturing a specimen of the tissue that is in the aperture of the probe.
After the cutter has reached its full forward position, rotation ceases.
The cutter is withdrawn, and the vacuum system helps transport the specimen to the tissue collection chamber to be retrieved.
After the biopsy is complete, a MicroMark™ II Tissue Marker can be permanently placed to locate the site in the event of further surgical or mammographic follow-up.

Figure 17–10. Cutting mechanism of a vacuum-assisted device biopsy needle. (Illustrations courtesy of Ethicon Endo-surgery, Inc.)

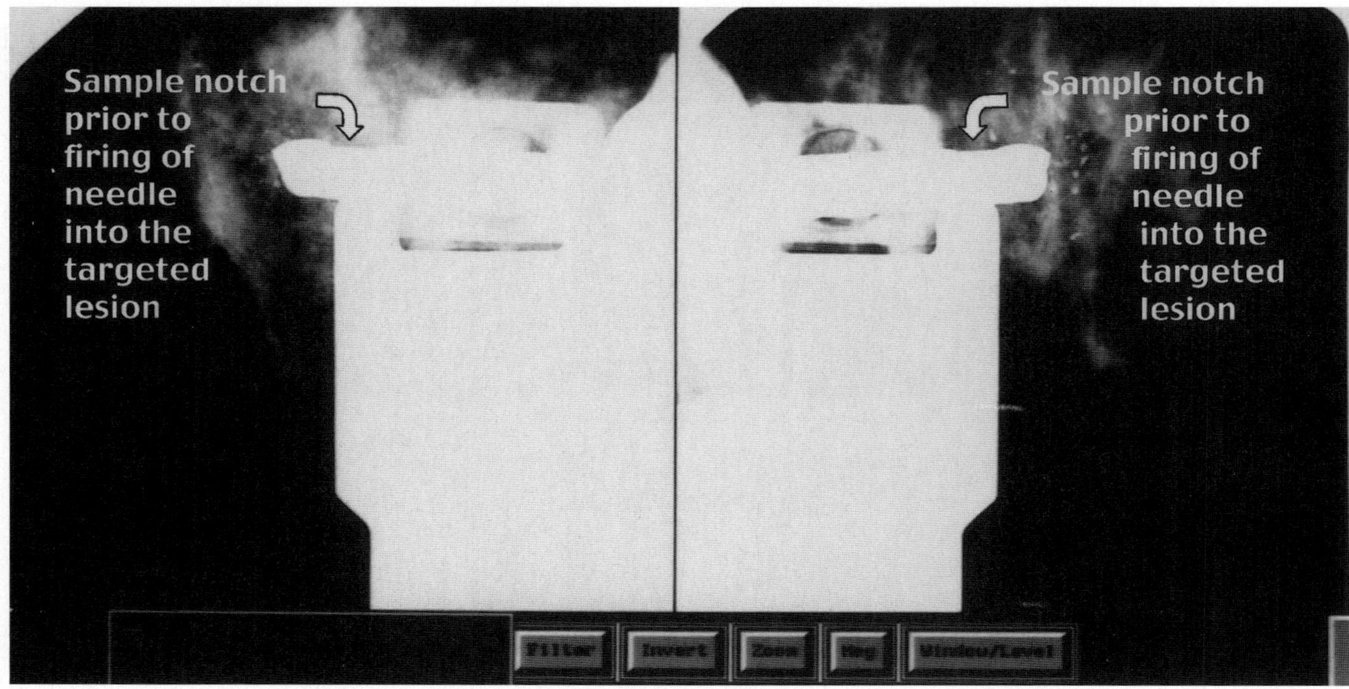

Figure 17–11. Stereotactic images prior to firing of needle, showing the sample notch positioned just in front of a targeted cluster of microcalcifications.

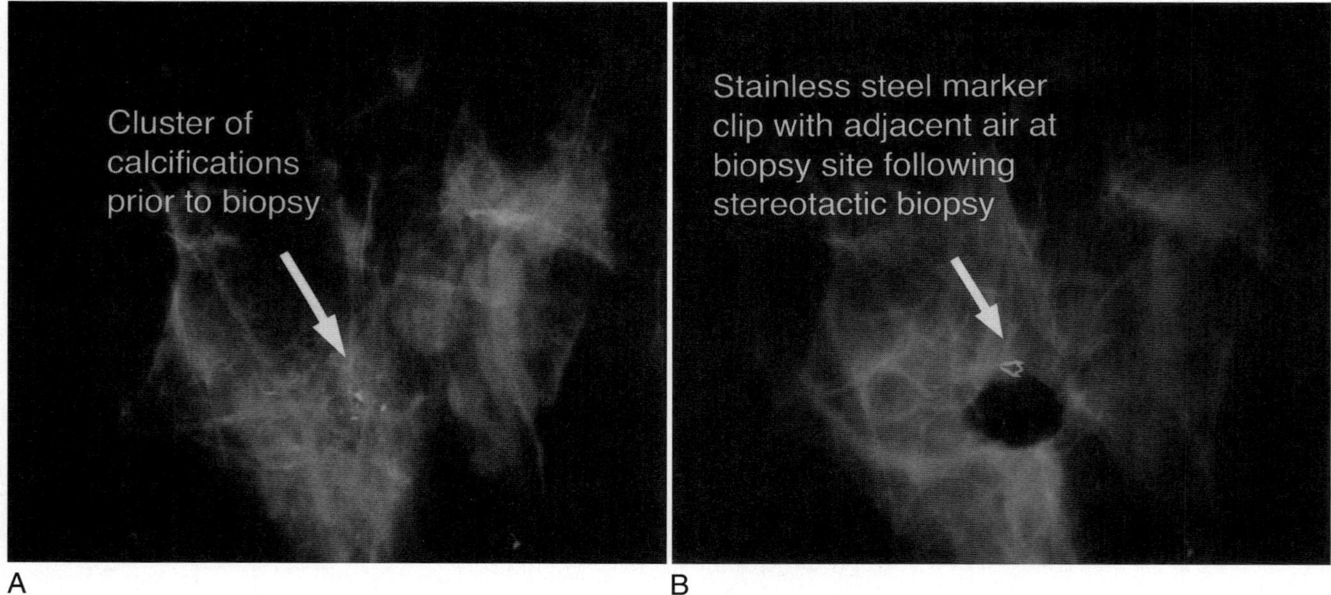

Figure 17–12. **A** and **B,** Stereotactic images showing a cluster of microcalcifications before biopsy and a biopsy marker clip with air in the biopsy cavity immediately after sampling.

images are air at the biopsy site or along the biopsy track (Figs. 17–12B and 17–13) and increased density, either focally at the biopsy site secondary to hematoma formation or diffusely around the biopsy site secondary to lidocaine infiltration. In a small percentage of patients, a small focal density may be seen on mammography 6 months or more after stereotactic biopsy with the 11-gauge VAD.[26] This density, thought to represent a post-biopsy needle scar, is reportedly seen best on a single mammographic view in the same projection in which the biopsy was performed (Fig. 17–14). Another finding that can appear after stereotactic biopsy, although less common, is fat necrosis (Fig. 17–15).

ULTRASOUND-GUIDED CORE NEEDLE BIOPSY

The first ALC biopsy gun was introduced in 1982 by Lindgren in Sweden. In 1993, ultrasound-guided CNB of the breast using a 14-gauge needle with an automated biopsy gun was reported by Parker and colleagues.[27] Now, two different types of biopsy needles are available for sampling lesions that are visible on ultrasonography. The first and more commonly used device is the spring-loaded ALC biopsy gun, available from several different manufacturers; it can be used with 14-, 16- or 18-gauge needles, although the 14-gauge needle has been shown to be most accurate for CNB diagnoses.[28] In our practice, the ALC biopsy gun is used in conjunction with a hollow introducer needle to facilitate multiple entries. The second is the handheld VAD (Fig. 17–16), which can be used with either an 11- or 8-G needle and does not require an introducer.[29]

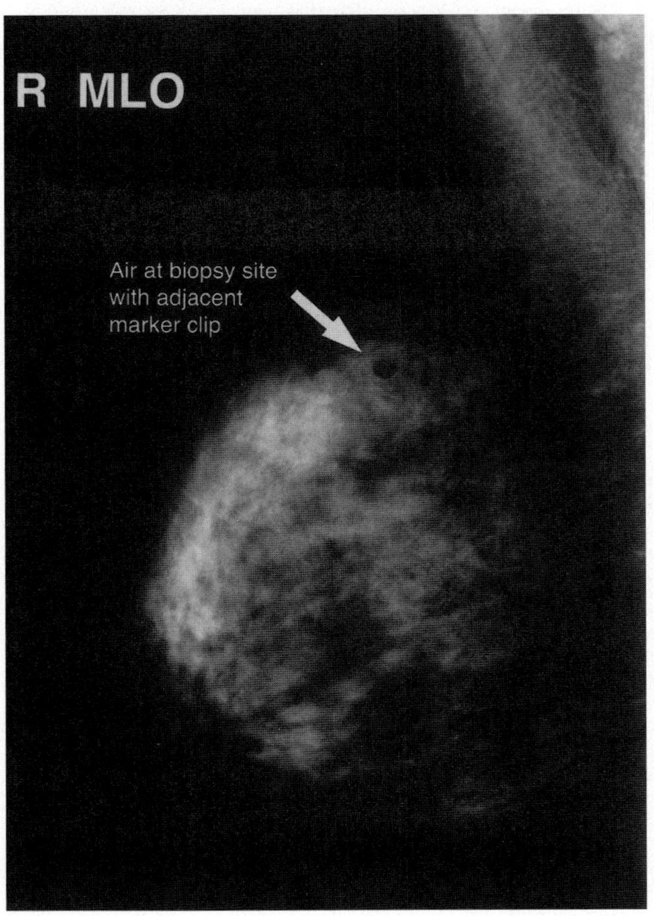

Figure 17–13. Mediolateral oblique view of the right breast immediately after stereotactic biopsy showing the biopsy marker clip with air at the biopsy site.

Ultrasonographic Abnormalities Selected for Ultrasound-Guided Core Needle Biopsy

Like the mammographic abnormalities selected for biopsy, the majority of ultrasonographically apparent abnormalities selected for biopsy are BI-RADS category 4 (suspicious) or 5 (highly suggestive of malignancy) lesions. They include any lesion with ultrasonographic features of malignancy, whether or not it is visible on mammography. Some of the features that have been used to differentiate malignant from benign lesions are irregular or angular shape, microlobulated or spiculated margins, taller-than-wide dimensions (orientation within the breast is not parallel to the skin surface), and posterior acoustic shadowing.[30] Other findings that may prompt the decision to perform core needle biopsy are complex cysts with eccentric wall thickening, mural nodules, and benign-appearing lesions that undergo rapid unexpected growth. Under special circumstances, ultrasound-guided CNB, like stereotactic CNB, may be performed on BI-RADS 3 (probably benign) lesions.

Risks and Complications of Ultrasound-Guided Core Needle Biopsy and Informed Consent

Once the decision to perform ultrasound-guided CNB is made, the findings, recommendations, and procedure, including the risks and alternatives, are explained to the patient. The main complications, although rare, are discussed; they are bleeding, ecchymosis, hematoma formation, infection, pneumothorax, implant rupture, and the possibility of not obtaining a diagnostic tissue sample. Placement of a localizing marker clip, if applicable, is also explained. Once the patient understands and acknowledges the risks and complications and agrees to proceed, she is asked to sign an informed consent form. The patient is advised to discontinue anticoagulation therapy in advance, if possible, and, at some institutions, may be offered a short-acting sedative on the day of the biopsy to reduce anxiety.

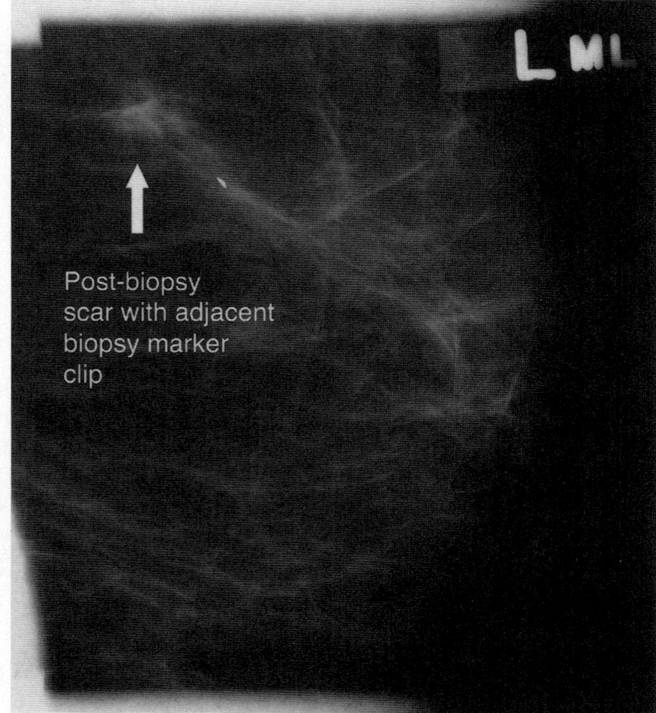

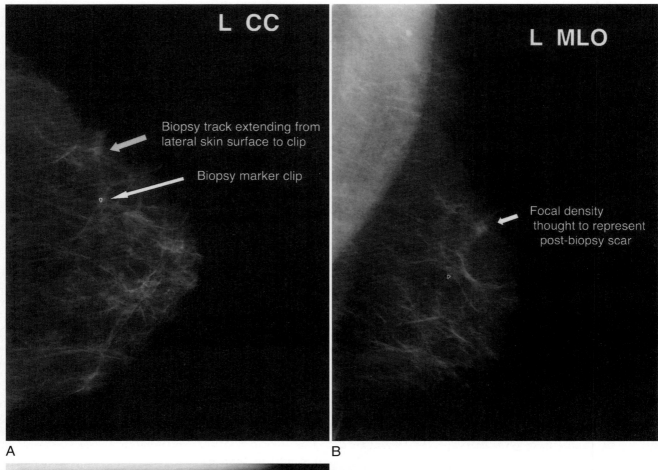

Figure 17–14. A, Craniocaudal view of left breast 6 months after a stereotactic biopsy with benign findings, showing a linear density extending from the lateral skin surface centrally, thought to represent the biopsy track. **B,** Mediolateral oblique view of the left breast 6 months after biopsy showing a focal irregular density in the vicinity of the biopsy track, consistent with biopsy scar. **C,** 90-degree mediolateral spot magnification view of the left breast showing the focal density with adjacent biopsy marker clip.

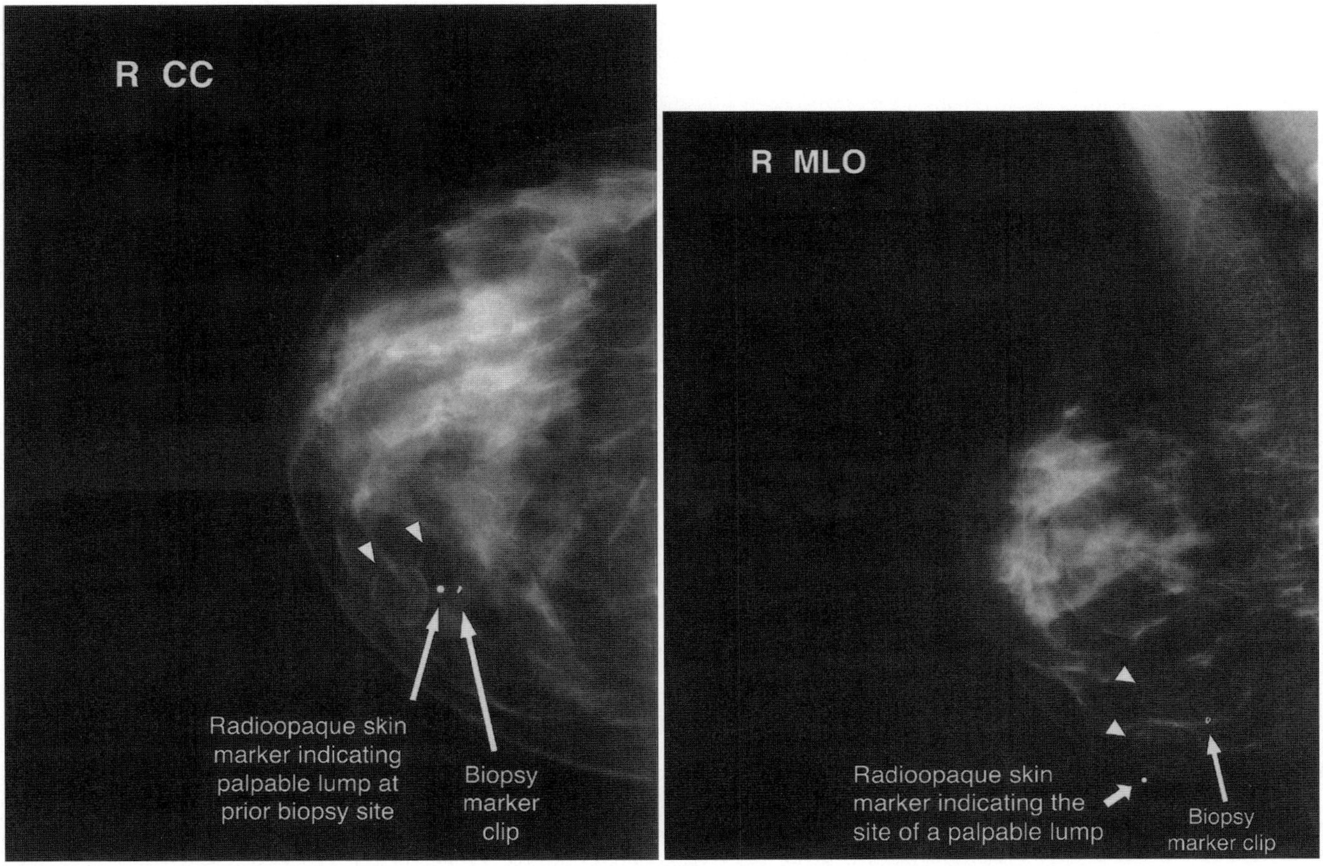

Figure 17–15. A, Craniocaudal view of the right breast 1 year after a benign stereotactic biopsy with a stainless steel marker clip at the biopsy site. A radiopaque lead marker (BB) indicates a palpable lump at the biopsy site where at least 2 oil cysts of fat necrosis are seen (*arrowheads*). **B,** Mediolateral oblique view of the right breast 1 year after stereotactic biopsy. A radiopaque BB indicates a palpable lump at the biopsy site where at least two oil cysts of fat necrosis can be seen (*arrowheads*).

Technique

The decision as to which biopsy instrument to use depends on a number of different factors, many of which are related to the size of the needle. Lesions that have a higher probability of sampling error (for example, very small or obscure lesions or complex cystic lesions) should probably be sampled with the larger-caliber VAD rather than the smaller-caliber ALC gun. For complex cystic lesions, a portion of the fluid can be aspirated beforehand with a fine-gauge needle and syringe to maximize the amount of solid tissue obtained with the VAD. The VAD has also been used to completely remove benign lesions smaller than 2 or 3 cm (such as fibroadenomas) that are palpable and would have otherwise been removed surgically. A biopsy marker clip should always be placed when the lesion is no longer present or is

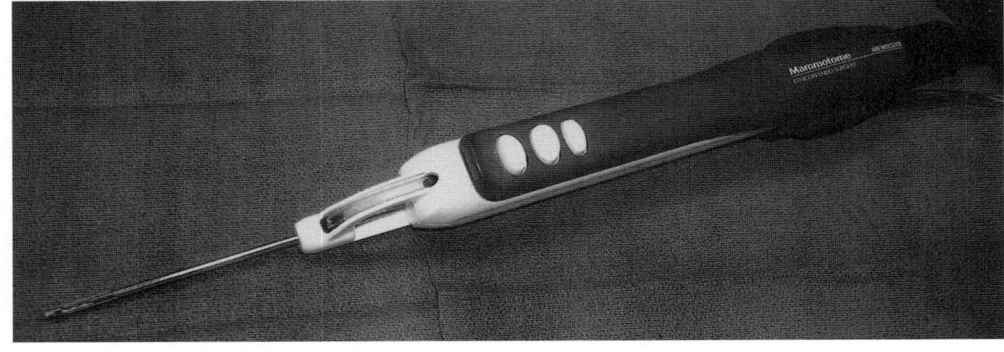

Figure 17–16. Example of a handheld vacuum-assisted device used for ultrasound-guided breast biopsies (Mammotome, Ethicon Endosurgery).

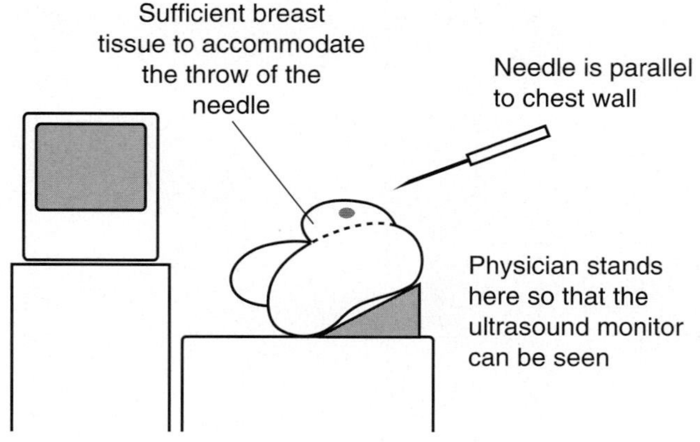

Figure 17–17. Proper patient positioning for ultrasound-guided core biopsy.

more difficult to visualize after biopsy. There are instances, however, in which a smaller needle is desirable because of anticipated bleeding problems; for example, the patient may have a bleeding diathesis that cannot be completely corrected or the lesion to be sampled is highly vascular. The ALC gun is also much less expensive than the VAD.

Once the lesion is identified, the patient is appropriately positioned to enable percutaneous access by the shortest route with the needle parallel to the chest wall throughout the procedure (Fig. 17–17). For example, if a lesion is in the upper outer quadrant of the left breast, the patient should be placed in the right posterior oblique position with the arm raised to facilitate lateromedial entry.

Sterile technique is used (Fig. 17–18), and local anesthetic is injected into the surrounding skin and breast tissue. A linear-array ultrasonography transducer with a frequency of at least 7 MHz or greater is used to visualize the needle and the lesion throughout the procedure.

If a VAD is used, a small incision is made in the skin. Using ultrasound guidance, the needle is inserted to the appropriate depth and is advanced parallel to the chest wall, either through or directly subjacent to the lesion; it remains in place throughout the procedure (Figs. 17–19A and 17–20A). The needle depth is maintained but the needle itself is manually rotated to sample adjacent areas of tissue with vacuum assistance (see Fig. 17–20B to C). The functions of the needle can be controlled manually by buttons on the holster or with a foot pedal, depending on operator preference.

If an ALC gun is used with an introducer, a skin incision is usually not necessary. With ultrasound guidance, a 13-gauge introducer is inserted to the appropriate depth and is advanced parallel to the chest wall, just proximal to the lesion. The sharp inner cannula of the introducer is removed, leaving the hollow outer sheath in position. A 14-gauge ALC biopsy needle is then inserted through the introducer sheath (see Fig. 17–19B), and the gun is fired into the lesion, automatically cutting a small core sample. The biopsy needle is removed, leaving the introducer in place, and the specimen is exposed for retrieval. The biopsy needle is then re-inserted, and another sample is obtained. This process is repeated several times until different areas of the lesion are sampled. Usually, between three and six samples are taken with either the ALC or VAD technique. Some authors recommend that at least four nonfragmented samples be obtained for optimal diagnostic yield.[31]

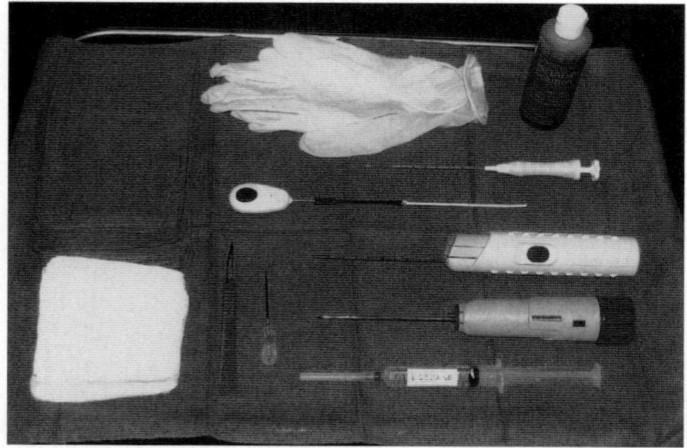

Figure 17–18. Sterile equipment setup tray for ultrasound-guided core needle biopsy, showing just a few of the different types of automated large-core biopsy guns and marker clips that are available.

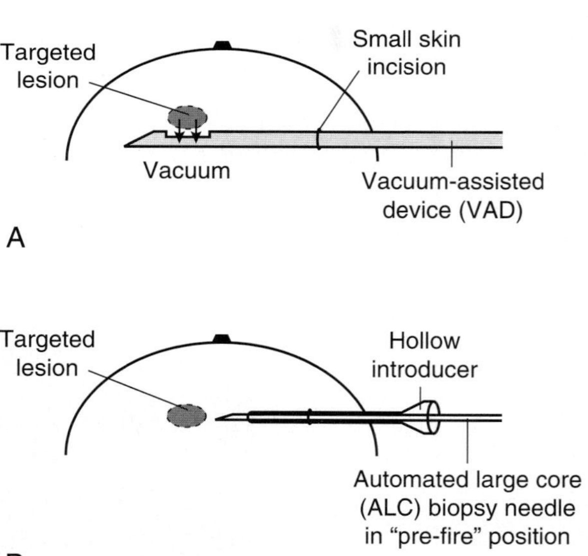

Figure 17–19. A and **B,** Schematic diagram showing some of the differences in needle positioning and sampling between ultrasound-guided biopsy using an automated large core (ALC) needle versus a vacuum-assisted device (VAD).

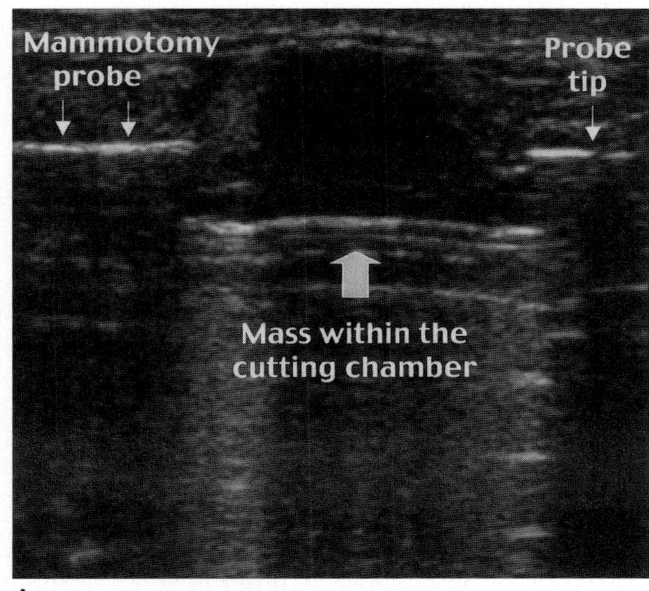

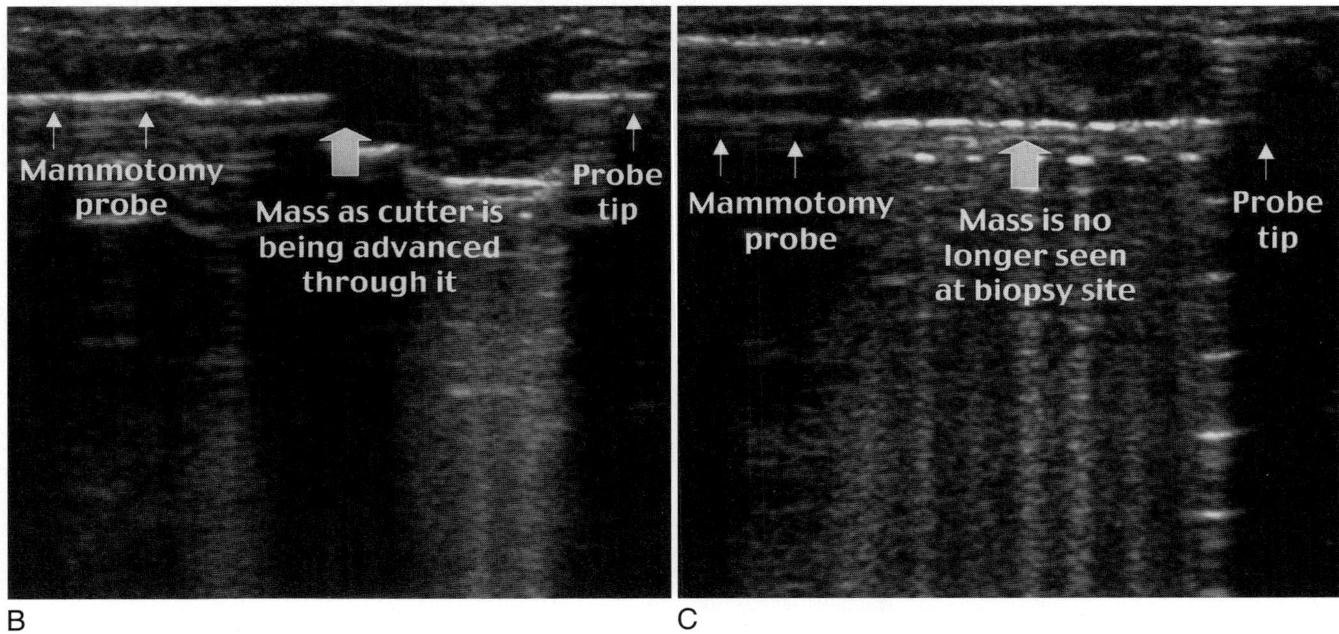

Figure 17–20. **A,** Ultrasonographic image of targeted mass situated within the open sample notch (cutting chamber) of a vacuum-assisted device. **B,** Ultrasonographic image of targeted mass as a sample is being cut. **C,** Ultrasonographic image of the biopsy site after sampling. No visible remnant of the mass is left, and a marker clip was placed to identify the biopsy site.

As for stereotactic biopsy, placement of a biopsy marker clip can often be useful after ultrasound-guided core biopsy. The handheld VAD is designed to accommodate the same biopsy marker clips that are used with stereotactic biopsy. Stainless steel microclips have also been used with the 14-gauge ALC biopsy gun; the microclip is deposited at the biopsy site via the introducer.[32]

ADVANCED BREAST BIOPSY INSTRUMENTATION

The ABBI device was first introduced in 1995 as an alternative to the existing CNB and excisional biopsy techniques. This system uses a large-bore cutting device (up to 2 cm in diameter) to remove breast tissue under stereotactic guidance. The goal is to obtain an accurate histologic diagnosis and possible definitive treatment as well. For example, if a cancer is completely removed and margins of the specimen are "negative" for malignancy, no additional surgical procedure is necessary.

Although the ABBI device is still available, it has not been widely accepted, largely because of the relatively high rate of complications and low rate of complete lesion retrieval reported for its use. Complications (including significant hematoma, infection, and vasovagal reactions), rates of which have ranged from 2% to 17%,[33-35] are likely due to the large size of the incision (2 to 3 cm) as well as the amount of tissue removed, which usually measures approximately 5 cm in length by 1 to 2 cm wide (although the width may vary with the size of the cutting instrument). In addition, a study investigating the size of the lesion with respect to overall specimen size obtained with the ABBI device found that less than 10% of the specimen was occupied by the lesion and more than 90% of the specimen included uninvolved surrounding breast tissue.[36] Nevertheless, positive margins on ABBI specimens are found in as many as 57% to 86% of lesions,[33,37] necessitating further surgery for complete extirpation. Furthermore, 72% to 88% of lesions excised with the ABBI device have turned out to be noncancerous, benign lesions,[33,35] for which a smaller, less invasive core needle biopsy would have been sufficient for diagnosis. Although the sensitivity and specificity of this method have been reported to be comparable to those of excisional biopsy and CNB,[38] ABBI does not appear to have a significant advantage over CNB, and its use involves a larger incision and removal of a larger volume of normal breast tissue.

FINE-NEEDLE ASPIRATION CYTOLOGY

Fine-needle aspiration (FNA) of the breast first gained popularity in the 1970s as an alternative to open surgical biopsy. The sensitivity and specificity of this procedure have been reported to range from 75% to 99% and 56% to 99%, respectively.[39-41] Although it is still a widely used method of tissue diagnosis, fine-needle aspiration has fallen out of favor in this country, and CNB has become the preferred method for biopsy of the breast. One of the reasons is that CNB is believed to have a greater specificity than fine needle aspiration cytology (FNAC).[42] In addition, there can be a high rate of insufficient or nondiagnostic samples with FNAC, ranging from 0 to 50%,[39] whereas the insufficiency rates for CNB have been reported to be between 3% and 7%.[43,44] Part of the wide variability in reported performance of FNAC has been attributed to differences in operator experience or training; however, other factors that may be involved are differences in the number of passes taken and in needle size.[45] Further reasons that CNB is often preferred over FNAC are that CNB provides more tissue upon which additional tests, such as hormone receptor assays, may be performed and that CNB can distinguish between in situ and invasive cancers, whereas FNAC cannot.

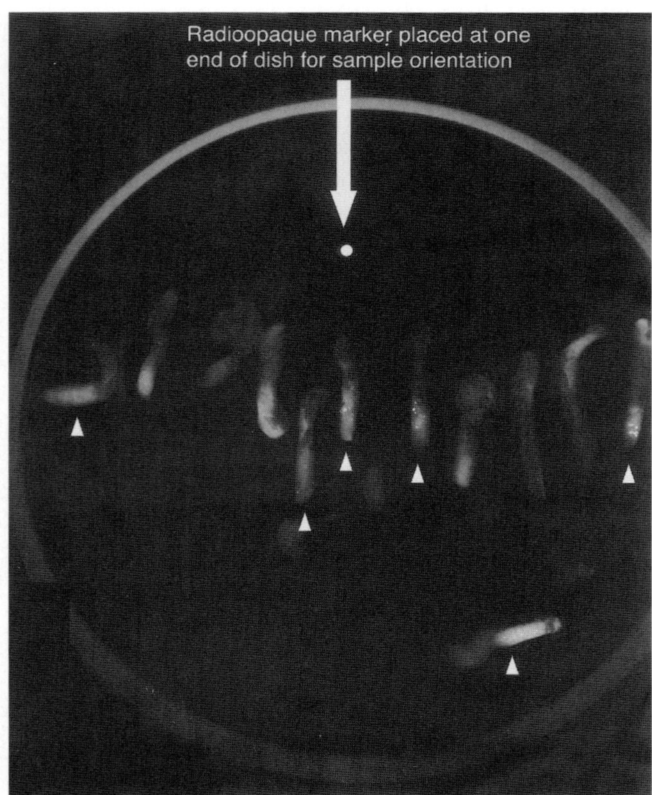

Figure 17–21. Specimen radiograph of core biopsy samples containing calcifications (indicated by *arrowheads*).

PATHOLOGY

Specimen Handling

Once the samples are obtained, specimen radiography is often performed to confirm the presence of a lesion if it has been seen on mammography. Microcalcifications should be radiographically visible within the samples if they are the targeted lesion (Fig. 17–21). Specimen radiography can be useful even when noncalcified lesions are sampled. Samples showing dense material on specimen radiography can confirm the presence of a targeted nodule, especially in patients with predominantly fatty breast tissue (Fig. 17–22).[46] A radiopaque lead marker (BB) may be placed at one end of the collection plate for orientation. If the lesion in question includes calcifications, the samples may be sorted and placed into separate cassettes labeled "with" and "without" calcifications to further assist the pathologist. All specimens from the biopsy are placed into a jar of formalin that has been carefully labeled with the patient's name and medical record number, the date of the biopsy, and the exact anatomic location of the

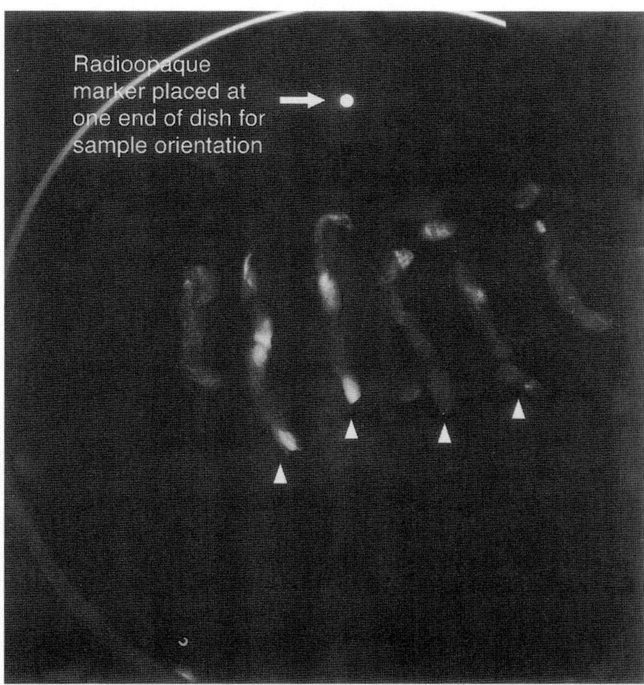

Figure 17–22. Specimen radiograph of core biopsy samples containing dense tissue from a nodule (indicated by *arrowheads*).

biopsy site (Fig. 17–23). A standard pathology requisition form is also carefully filled out to include the patient's name, medical record number, date and anatomic location of the biopsy, radiologic findings, and BI-RADS assessment as well as any other pertinent clinical information that may be useful to the pathologist (Fig. 17–24).

Radiologic-Histopathologic Concordance

Once a lesion has been sampled, it is extremely important that the pathology results correlate with the radiologic findings. If the results are not concordant, one must consider the possibility of negative sampling error. With lesions containing calcifications, specimen radiography can help confirm adequate sampling. The presence of calcium within the tissue samples (or absence of calcium on post-biopsy stereotactic images of the breast) can verify that the appropriate area was sampled. With noncalcified lesions, the presence of dense tissue within the samples can be reassuring, although it is more difficult to be certain that the target lesion has been sampled. Even ultrasound-guided core biopsies with real-time imaging are subject to the possibility of sampling error. Therefore, the pathologist should confirm the presence of calcifications that are radiographically visible within the samples, and discrete lesions seen on imaging should be explained by a focal pathologic process. For example, if a discrete mass is seen, fibroadenoma, papilloma, lymph node, cyst, fat necrosis, sclerosing adenosis, or even focal fibrosis would be an acceptable diagnosis. Normal fatty breast tissue without a discrete mass, however, would be a discordant finding, and a second core or excisional biopsy may be needed. Close collaboration among the radiologists, pathologists, and surgeons is necessary to ensure radiologic-histopathologic concordance and to reduce the likelihood of a missed diagnosis.

CONTRAINDICATIONS TO CORE NEEDLE BIOPSY

Some of the circumstances that may hinder successful stereotactic core biopsy are the following:

- Patient weight is greater than 300 lb
- Patient is unable to tolerate prone, immobile positioning for duration of biopsy
- Breast is too thin under compression to accommodate the needle

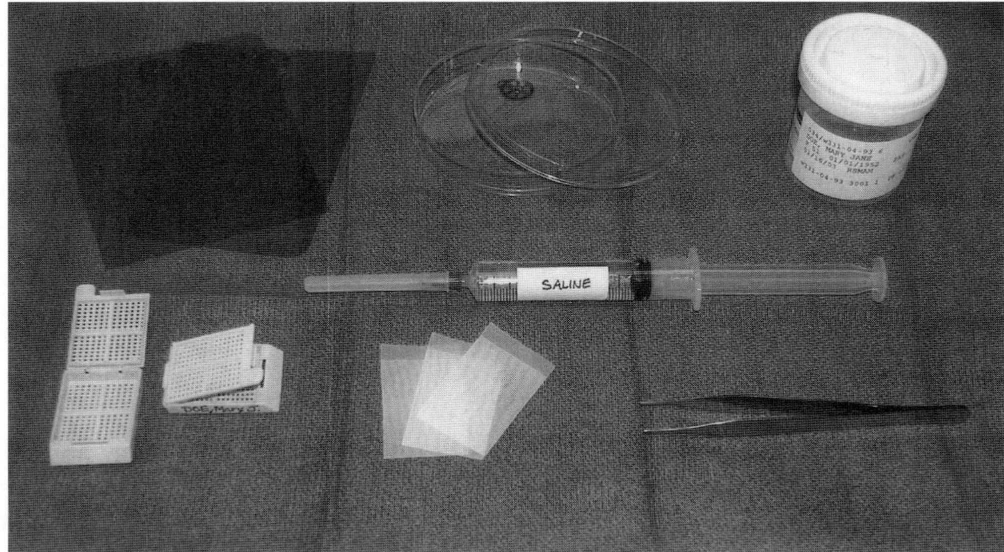

Figure 17–23. Specimen collection equipment with properly labeled tissue cassettes and jars.

Pathology Requisition

Patient ID Number: ______________________ Date: ______________

Last Name: ______________________ First: ____________________ Age: _____________

Ordering Physician: _______________________________________ ID: ____________________

Attending Physician: _______________________________________ ID: ____________________

Attending Address: _______________________________________ Phone: _________________

Location

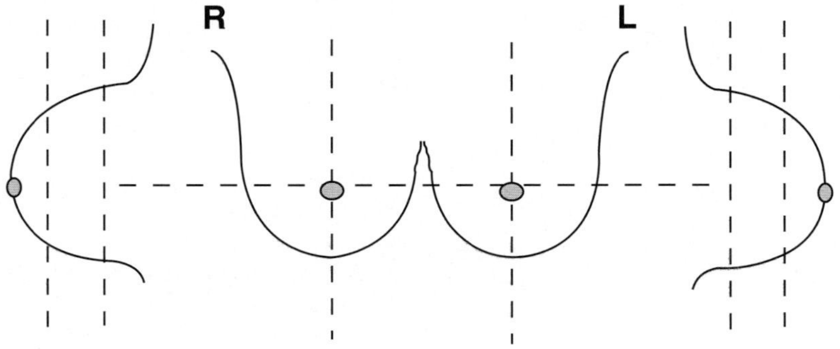

R L

Abnormality: Mass ☐ **Calcifications** ☐ **Other** ☐

Impression: Likely benign ☐ **Suspicious** ☐

Imaging final assessment: 2 3 4A 4B 4C 5

Biopsy specimens contain calcifications ☐
(Placed in bag in specimen container)

Comments:

____

Figure 17–24. Example of pathology requisition slip to be submitted with core needle biopsy specimens.

- Lesion is too far posterior to be positioned within the imaging field of view
- Lesion cannot be seen clearly on both stereotactic images

Relative Contraindications to Core Needle Biopsy

The circumstances under which stereotactic biopsy may be performed with caution are the following:

- Implants—biopsy can be performed only if the lesion can be clearly visualized on both stereotactic images with the implant edge fully displaced from the target site on both images
- Coagulopathy—permission should be obtained from the patient's primary care physician, and appropriate blood products, if necessary, should be given in advance

COMPLICATIONS OF CORE NEEDLE BIOPSY

The potential complications of CNB are few and infrequent, with rates ranging from 0 to 3.9%.[47,48] Complications that have been reported in the immediate post-biopsy period include hematoma (mostly self-limited but in extremely rare cases requiring surgical intervention), infection, pneumothorax (more common with ultrasound-guided procedures), implant rupture, and vasovagal reactions (more common with the upright positioning used for stereotactic units).

Other secondary outcomes associated with core needle biopsy pertain to displacement of tumor or epithelial cells (or both) along the needle track. This question was first addressed in the 1950s when various articles began to suggest the occurrence of malignant seeding after various diagnostic needle procedures.[49-52] Since then, the incidence of tumor cell displacement after needle procedures (including FNA, needle localization, and large CNB) has been studied in greater depth. Although the incidence of tumor cell displacement has been reported in up to 32% of CNB cases,[53] it has not been found to contribute to an increased incidence of local tumor recurrence after appropriate treatment.[54] This finding is believed to be due to the fact that the isolated tumor cells do not survive outside the primary tumor site, possibly because of host immune response, the effects of local radiation therapy, or both. The hypothetical risk of tumor seeding along the needle track can be avoided through the use of a VAD or introducer with an ALC biopsy gun.

One potential pitfall related to tumor cell displacement, however, can occur as a result of CNB when ductal carcinoma in situ (DCIS) is present without invasion. Rarely, the displacement of nests of DCIS outside the main biopsy site can mimic stromal invasion and therefore lead to the false diagnosis of invasive cancer.[53,55] This pitfall can be avoided if the pathologist is provided with a detailed patient history, including anatomic location of prior needle procedures.

POST-BIOPSY PATIENT INSTRUCTIONS

Immediately after CNB, manual pressure is applied directly over the biopsy site for at least 10 to 15 minutes or until all bleeding has subsided. The skin opening is then reapproximated with sterile tapes (Fig. 17–25), and the patient is instructed not to shower for 24 to 48 hours. A pressure dressing may

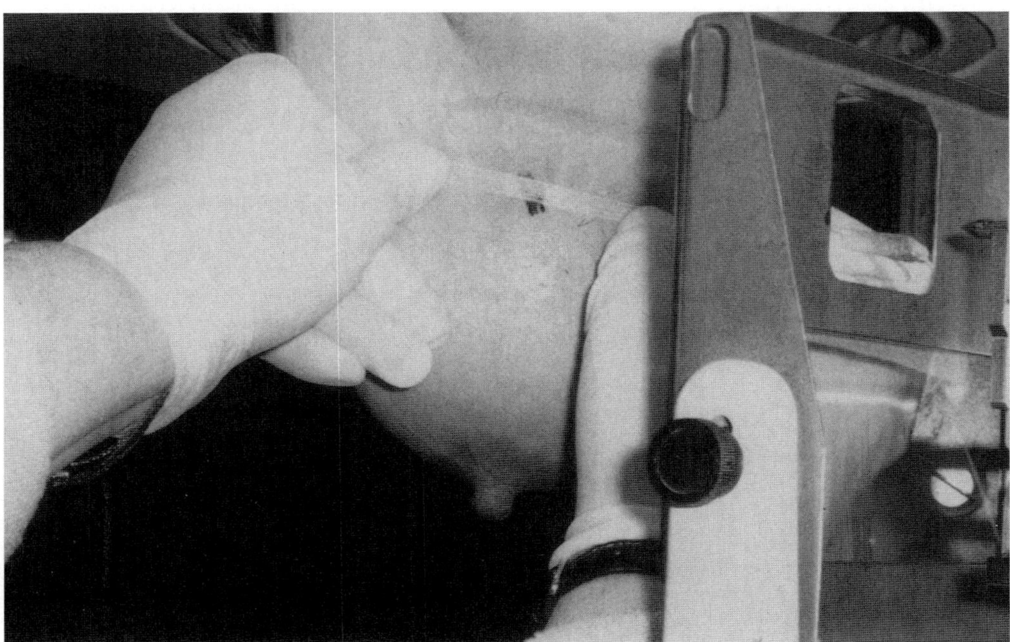

Figure 17–25. Sterile tapes are used to close the skin incision after stereotactic core needle biopsy.

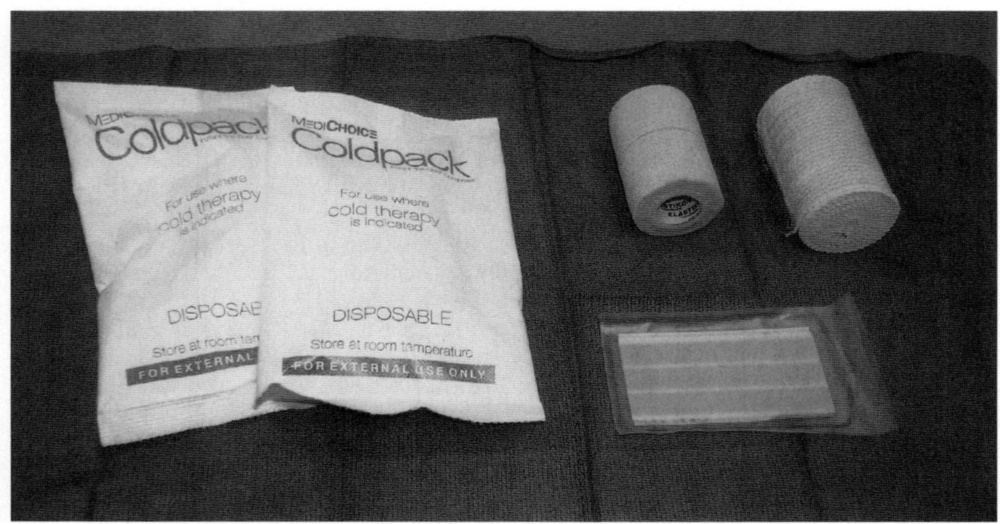

Figure 17–26. Sterile dressings and ice packs for post-biopsy wound care.

be helpful if significant bleeding has occurred (Fig. 17–26). The patient may sponge-bathe, being careful to keep the biopsy area dry, and ice packs should be applied for several hours after the procedure to reduce swelling and discomfort. Acetaminophen may be taken for persistent pain, but to avoid rebleeding, the patient should not take aspirin or other products containing salicylic acid for at least 2 to 3 days after the biopsy.

The patient is told that if she experiences any signs of infection (erythema, purulent discharge, swelling, fever, increased warmth of the sampled breast), she should go to the breast center, to her referring physician, or to an emergency room for reevaluation and possible antibiotic therapy.

POST-BIOPSY IMAGING FOLLOW-UP

For benign diagnoses that are concordant with imaging findings and do not require surgical excision, imaging follow-up is recommended. Although the percentage of false-negative diagnoses from core needle biopsy is small, they do occur, and suspected missed cancers have been discovered at benign biopsy sites more than 1 year later.[56] The recommended intervals for initial and subsequent post-biopsy follow-up evaluations vary from institution to institution, but most authorities recommend an initial 6-month follow-up imaging study (some may tailor this interval to the pathology diagnosis, recommending an initial follow-up at 6 months for a nonspecific benign diagnosis or at 1 year for a specific benign diagnosis), with continued annual surveillance for at least 2 years thereafter.[57-59]

AMERICAN COLLEGE OF RADIOLOGY ACCREDITATION

For a facility to be accredited by the American College of Radiology to perform breast biopsy, it

Table 17–2. Clinical Image Requirements for Stereotactic Breast Biopsy

For masses	Two-view mammogram (orthogonal views) with the mass to be sampled marked on each film Stereo images: For "true-cut" gun-needle biopsy system: Stereo pair images clearly labeled "Pre-fire" and "Post-fire" demonstrating needle positioning before and after biopsy of the lesion For vacuum-assisted cutting needle biopsy system: A post-fire stereo pair showing the side hole in the cutting needle positioned at the lesion to be sampled
For calcifications	Two-view mammogram (orthogonal views) with the calcifications to be sampled marked on each film Stereo images: For "true-cut" gun-needle biopsy system: Stereo pair images clearly labeled "Pre-fire" and "Post-fire" demonstrating needle positioning before and after biopsy of the lesion For vacuum-assisted cutting needle biopsy system: A pre-fire stereo pair showing the side-hole in the cutting needle positioned at the lesion to be sampled Specimen radiograph demonstrating calcium
For fine-needle aspiration cytology (FNAC)	Two-view mammogram (orthogonal views) with the mass to be sampled marked on each film Pre-FNAC stereo image pair demonstrating the needle within the lesion

Adapted from American College of Radiology: Stereotactic Breast Biopsy Accreditation Program Requirements, p 14. Available online in printer-downloadable format at www.acr.org/dyna/?doc=mammography/index.html

Table 17–3. Clinical Image Requirements for Ultrasound-Guided Breast Biopsy

For core needle biopsy	Two-view mammogram—craniocaudal (CC) and mediolateral oblique (MLO)—with the mass to be sampled marked on each film. The mammogram should be submitted even if the mass is not visible mammographically Pre-biopsy ultrasonogram demonstrating the mass in two orthogonal views with the mass to be sampled clearly labeled Ultrasonograms clearly labeled "Pre-fire" and "Post-fire" demonstrating needle positioning before and after biopsy of the lesion
For fine-needle aspiration cytology	Two-view mammogram (CC, MLO) with the mass to be sampled marked on each film. The mammogram should be submitted even if the mass is not visible mammographically. Pre-biopsy ultrasonogram demonstrating the mass in two orthogonal views with the mass to be sampled clearly labeled Ultrasonogram during the procedure demonstrating the long axis of the needle tip positioned within the lesion

Adapted from American College of Radiology: Breast Ultrasound Accreditation Program (Including Ultrasound-Guided Breast Biopsy) Requirements, p 10. Available online in printer-downloadable format at www.acr.org/dyna/?doc=mammography/index.html

must satisfy certain requirements. Separate guidelines have been established for stereotactic and ultrasound-guided breast biopsy, including personnel qualifications (for physician, radiologic technologist, and, in some cases, medical physicist) as well as requirements pertaining to equipment, quality control, quality assurance, and clinical images. For stereotactic biopsies, there are additional guidelines regarding phantom images and radiation dose. The guidelines are summarized in Tables 17–2 and 17–3.

References

1. Burkhardt JH, Sunshine JH: Core-needle and surgical breast biopsy: Comparison of three methods of assessing cost. Radiology 1999;212:181-188.
2. Liberman L, Sama MP: Cost-effectiveness of stereotactic 11-gauge directional vacuum-assisted breast biopsy. AJR Am J Roentgenol 2000;175:53-58.
3. Logan-Young W, Dawson AE, Wilbur DC, et al: The cost-effectiveness of fine-needle aspiration cytology and 14-gauge core needle biopsy compared with open surgical biopsy in the diagnosis of breast carcinoma. Cancer 1998;82:1867-1873.
4. Lee CH, Egglin TK, Philpotts L, et al: Cost-effectiveness of stereotactic core needle biopsy: Analysis by means of mammographic findings. Radiology 1997;202:849-854.
5. Liberman L, Goodstine SL, Dershaw DD, et al: One operation after percutaneous diagnosis of nonpalpable breast cancer: Frequency and associated factors. AJR Am J Roentgenol 2002;178:673-679
6. Liberman L, Feng TL, Dershaw DD, et al: US-guided core breast biopsy: Use and cost-effectiveness. Radiology 1998;208:717-723.
7. Verkooijen HM, Peeters PHM, Buskens E, et al: Diagnostic accuracy of large-core needle biopsy for nonpalpable breast disease: A meta-analysis. Br J Cancer 2000;82:1017-1021.
8. Elvecrog EL, Lechner MC, Nelson MT: Nonpalpable breast lesions: Correlation of stereotaxic large-core needle biopsy and surgical biopsy results. Radiology 1993;188:453-455.
9. Gisvold JJ, Goellner JR, Grant CS, et al: Breast biopsy: A comparative study of stereotaxically guided core and excisional techniques. AJR Am J Roentgenol 1994;162:815-820.
10. Kaufman CS, Delbecq R, Jacobson L, et al: Excising the reexcision: Stereotactic core-needle biopsy decreases need for reexcision of breast cancer. World J Surg 1998;22:1023-1027.
11. Verkooijen HM: Diagnostic accuracy of stereotactic large-core needle biopsy for nonpalpable breast disease: Results of a multicenter prospective study with 95% surgical confirmation. Int J Cancer 2002;99:853-859.
12. White RR, Halperin TJ, Olson JA, et al: Impact of core-needle breast biopsy on the surgical management of mammographic abnormalities. Ann Surg 2001;33:769-777.
13. Brenner RJ, Bassett LW, Fajardo LL, et al: Stereotactic core-needle breast biopsy: A multi-institutional prospective trial. Radiology 2001;218:866-872.
14. Fuhrman GM, Cederbom GJ, Bolton JS, et al: Image-guided core-needle breast biopsy is an accurate technique to evaluate patients with nonpalpable imaging abnormalities. Ann Surg 1998;227:932-939.
15. Nguyen M, McCombs MM, Ghandehari S, et al: An update on core needle biopsy for radiologically detected breast lesions. Cancer 1996;78:2340-2345.
16. Smith LF, Henry-Tillman R, Mancino AT, et al: Magnetic resonance imaging-guided core needle biopsy and needle localized excision of occult breast lesions. Am J Surg 2001;182:414-418.
17. Kuhl CK, Morakkabati N, Leutner CC: MR imaging-guided large-core (14-gauge) needle biopsy of small lesions visible at breast MR imaging alone. Radiology 2001;220:31-39.
18. Parker SH, Lovin JD, Jobe WE, et al: Stereotactic breast biopsy with a biopsy gun. Radiology 1990;176:741-747.
19. Dowlatshahi K, Gent HJ, Schmidt R, et al: Nonpalpable breast tumors: Diagnosis with stereotaxic localization and fine-needle aspiration. Radiology 1989;170:427-433.
20. Hendrick RE, Parker SH: Stereotaxic imaging. In Haus AG, Yaffe MJ (eds): Syllabus: A Categorical Course in Physics—Technical Aspects of Breast Imaging. Oakbrook, IL, RSNA, 1994, pp 263-274.
21. Georgian-Smith D, D'Orsi C, Morris E, et al: Stereotactic biopsy of the breast using an upright unit, a vacuum-suction needle, and a lateral arm-support system. AJR Am J Roentgenol 2002; 178:1017-1024.
22. Bassett LB, Winchester DP, Caplan RB, et al: Stereotactic core-needle biopsy of the breast: A report of the Joint Task Force of the American College of Radiology, American College of Surgeons, and College of American Pathologists. CA Cancer J Clin 1997;47:171-190.
23. Shellock FG: Metallic marking clips used after stereotactic breast biopsy: Ex vivo testing of ferromagnetism, heating and artifacts associated with MR imaging. AJR Am J Roentgenol 1999;172:1417-1419.
24. Rosen EL, Vo TT: Metallic clip deployment during stereotactic breast biopsy: retrospective analysis. Radiology 2001;218:510-516.
25. Philpotts LE, Lee CH: Clip migration after 11-gauge vacuum-assisted stereotactic biopsy: Case report. Radiology 2002; 222:794-796.
26. Lamm RL, Jackman RJ: Mammographic abnormalities caused by percutaneous stereotactic biopsy of histologically benign lesions evident on follow-up mammograms. AJR Am J Roentgenol 2000;174:753-756.
27. Parker SH, Jobe WE, Dennis MA: US-guided automated large-core breast biopsy. Radiology 1993;187:507-511.

28. Helbich TH, Rudas M, Haitel A, et al: Evaluation of needle size for breast biopsy: comparison of 14-, 16- and 18-gauge biopsy needles. AJR Am J Roentgenol 1998;171:59-63.
29. Parker SH, Klaus AJ, McWey PJ, et al: Sonographically guided directional vacuum-assisted breast biopsy using a handheld device. AJR Am J Roentgenol 2001;177:405-408.
30. Rahbar G, Sie AC, Hansen GC, et al: Benign versus malignant solid breast masses: US differentiation. Radiology 1999;213: 889-894.
31. Fishman JE, Milikowski C, Ramsinhani R, et al: US-guided core needle biopsy of the breast: How many specimens are necessary? Radiology 2003;226:779-782.
32. Phillips SW, Gabriel H, Comstock CE, et al: Sonographically guided metallic clip placement after core needle biopsy of the breast. AJR Am J Roentgenol 2000;175:1353-1355.
33. Insausti LP, Alberro JA, Regueira FM, et al: An experience with the Advanced Breast Biopsy Instrumentation (ABBI) system in the management of non-palpable breast lesions. Eur Radiol 2002;12:1703-1710.
34. Marti WR, Zuber M, Oertli D, et al: Advanced breast biopsy instrumentation for the evaluation of impalpable lesions: A reliable diagnostic tool with little therapeutic potential. Eur J Surg 2001;167:15-18.
35. Rebner M, Chesebrough R, Gregory N: Initial experience with the advanced breast biopsy instrumentation device. AJR Am J Roentgenol 1999;173:221-226.
36. Smathers RL: Advanced breast biopsy instrumentation device: Percentages of the lesion and surrounding tissue removed. AJR Am J Roentgenol 2000;175:801-803.
37. Leibman AJ, Frager D, Choi P: Experience with breast biopsies using the Advanced Breast Biopsy Instrumentation system. AJR Am J Roentgenol 1999;172:1409-1412.
38. Schwartzberg BS, Goates JJ, Keeler SA, et al: Use of advanced breast biopsy instrumentation while performing stereotactic breast biopsies: Review of 150 consecutive biopsies. J Am Coll Surg 2000,191:9-15.
39. Ljung BM, Drejet A, Chiampi N, et al: Diagnostic accuracy of fine-needle aspiration biopsy is determined by physician training in sampling technique. Cancer 2001;93:263-268.
40. Ariga R, Bloom K, Reddy VB, et al: Fine-needle aspiration of clinically suspicious palpable breast masses with histopathologic correlation. Am J Surg 2002;184:410-413.
41. Pisano ED, Fajardo LL, Caudry DJ, et al: Fine-needle aspiration biopsy of nonpalpable breast lesions in a multicenter clinical trial: Results from the Radiologic Diagnostic Oncology Group V. Radiology 2001;219:785-792.
42. Westenend PJ, Sever AR, Beekman-de Volder HJ, et al: A comparison of aspiration cytology and core needle biopsy in the evaluation of breast lesions. Cancer 2001;93:146-150.
43. Dronkers DJ: Stereotaxic core biopsy of breast lesions. Radiology 1992;183:631-634.
44. Liberman L, Dershaw DD, Rosen PP, et al: Stereotaxic 14-gauge breast biopsy: How many core biopsy specimens are needed? Radiology 1994;192:793-795.
45. The uniform approach to breast fine needle aspiration biopsy: A synopsis. Breast J 1996;2:357-363.
46. Berg WA, Jaeger B, Campassi C, et al: predictive value of specimen radiography for core needle biopsy of noncalcified breast masses. AJR Am J Roentgenol 1998;171:1671-1678.
47. Margolin FR, Leung JW, Jacobs RP, et al: percutaneous imaging-guided core breast biopsy: 5 years' experience in a community hospital. AJR Am J Roentgenol 2001;177:559-564.
48. Lai JT, Burrowes P, MacGregor JH: Vacuum-assisted large-core breast biopsy: Complications and their incidence. Can Assoc Radiol J 2000;51:232-236.
49. Robbins GF, Brothers JH, Eberhart WF, et al: Is aspiration biopsy of breast cancer dangerous to the patient? Cancer 1954;7:774-778.
50. Harter LP, Curtis JS, Ponto G, et al: Malignant seeding of the needle track during stereotaxic core needle breast biopsy. Radiology 1992;185:713-714.
51. Youngson BJ, Liberman L, Rosen PP: Displacement of carcinomatous epithelium in surgical breast specimens following stereotaxic core biopsy. Am J Clin Pathol 1995;103:598-602.
52. Chao C, Torosian MH, Boraas MC, et al: Local recurrence of breast cancer in the stereotactic core needle biopsy site: Case reports and review of the literature. Breast J 2001;7:124-127.
53. Diaz LK, Wiley EL, Venta LA: Are malignant cells displaced by large-gauge needle core biopsy of the breast? AJR Am J Roentgenol 1999;173:1301-1313.
54. Chen AM, Haffty BG, Lee CH: Local recurrence of breast cancer after breast conservation therapy in patients examined by means of stereotactic core-needle biopsy. Radiology 2002;225: 707-712.
55. Liberman L, Vuolo M, Dershaw DD, et al: Epithelial displacement after stereotactic 11-G directional vacuum-assisted breast biopsy. AJR Am J Roentgenol 1999;172:677-681.
56. Parker SH, Burbank F, Jackman R, et al: Response to "Caution on core." Radiology 1994;193:326-327.
57. Lee CH, Philpotts LE, Horvath LJ, et al: Follow-up of breast lesions diagnosed as benign with stereotactic core-needle biopsy: Frequency of mammographic change and false-negative rate. Radiology 1999;212:189-194.
58. Jackman RJ, Nowels KW, Rodriguez-Soto J, et al: Stereotactic, automated, large-core needle biopsy of nonpalpable breast lesions: False-negative and histologic underestimation rates after long-term follow-up. Radiology 1999;210:799-805.
59. Maganini RO, Klem DA, Huston BJ, et al: Upgrade rate of core biopsy-determined atypical ductal hyperplasia by open excisional biopsy. Am J Surg 2001; 182:355-358.

Chapter 18 After the Imaging-Guided Needle Biopsy

Anne C. Hoyt and Lawrence W. Bassett

Over the past decade, imaging-guided breast core needle biopsy (CNB) has become the most common biopsy performed at our facility for nonpalpable and many palpable breast lesions. It is now a widely used and widely accepted, cost-effective alternative to open surgical biopsy.[1,2] The use of needle biopsy to obtain a histologic diagnosis of breast lesions requires that the physician performing the procedure have a good understanding of postprocedural responsibilities and management. After the biopsy, the physician must evaluate the results for concordance between imaging and pathology findings, carry out appropriate patient follow-up, develop a management plan, and communicate results to the referring health care provider, the patient, or both.

Once the technical component of the examination is completed, important patient management and follow-up issues must be addressed. In our experience, patients rarely have significant physical problems after the procedure, other than temporary discomfort and bruising at the site of the biopsy. However, they do experience considerable anxiety about the biopsy findings, so results should be obtained in a reasonable time and communicated to them. Usually this goal can be accomplished in 2 to 3 days without compromising accuracy. We avoid asking for and communicating "wet" or "stat" readings from the pathologist, because changing a diagnosis from a benign ("negative") wet reading to a malignant ("positive") final reading can be devastating for the patient.

ASSESSING FOR CONCORDANCE

The process of assessing concordance involves comparison of the imaging findings that led to the biopsy with the pathology results. Success of an imaging-guided needle biopsy program requires a good working relationship between radiologist and pathologist. To optimize the process, the pathologist must have adequate clinical information.

To assist the pathologist with this process, we have devised a modified pathology requisition for needle biopsy cases (Fig.18–1). The requisition includes the following information:

- Location of the lesion.
- The most relevant imaging findings (e.g., mass versus calcifications).
- The probability of malignancy; we use a modified American College of Radiology Breast Imaging Reporting and Data System (BI-RADS) numbering system, wherein the Suspicious Category is subdivided into 4A (mild suspicion), 4B (moderate suspicion), and 4C (high suspicion).

When a high likelihood of malignancy is communicated in the pathology requisition (e.g., 4C or 5), the pathologist frequently telephones us if he or she does not find a cancer. When calcifications are present in the biopsy specimen, the specimens that contain the calcifications are placed in a separate bag ("tea bag") within the specimen jar. The pathologist recuts the specimen if imaging demonstrated calcifications but none were identified in the initial histologic slides.

After the biopsy is performed and interpreted, the next step is to assess the pathology results for concordance with the imaging findings that led to the biopsy and with any relevant clinical findings. The concept of concordance has origins in the fine-needle aspiration biopsy "triple test" protocol, which compares clinical findings, imaging findings, and pathology results.[3] If the results are "benign triplets" (clinical, imaging, and pathology findings are benign), the patient is followed clinically or with further imaging in 6 months. If the results are "malignant triplets" (all three types of findings indicate malignancy), definitive surgery can be planned. When pathology findings are malignant, definitive surgery would follow pathologic confirmation (permanent or frozen section). "Mixed triplets" or "inconclusive triplets" mandate an open biopsy. These basic principles for correlating clinical, imaging, and pathology findings can be applied to CNB. Of course, there are usually no clinical findings, but the imaging and pathology findings can be compared with the biopsy findings.

The assessment for concordance can be done in a number of ways:

1. A case-by-case or regularly scheduled meeting with the pathologist (Fig. 18–2).
2. Viewbox review of mammographic images alongside the written pathology reports.
3. Comparison of written imaging reports and pathology reports for concordance.

The correlation process involves determining whether pathology results adequately explain imaging findings. The imaging documentation of the procedure is reviewed to verify that the lesion was accurately targeted (e.g., in ultrasonography-guided biopsies, the needle traversed the lesion) and that post-biopsy images confirm that the lesion was sampled. For stereotactically guided biopsies of calcifications, the specimen radiograph is reviewed to verify that the specimens contained adequate

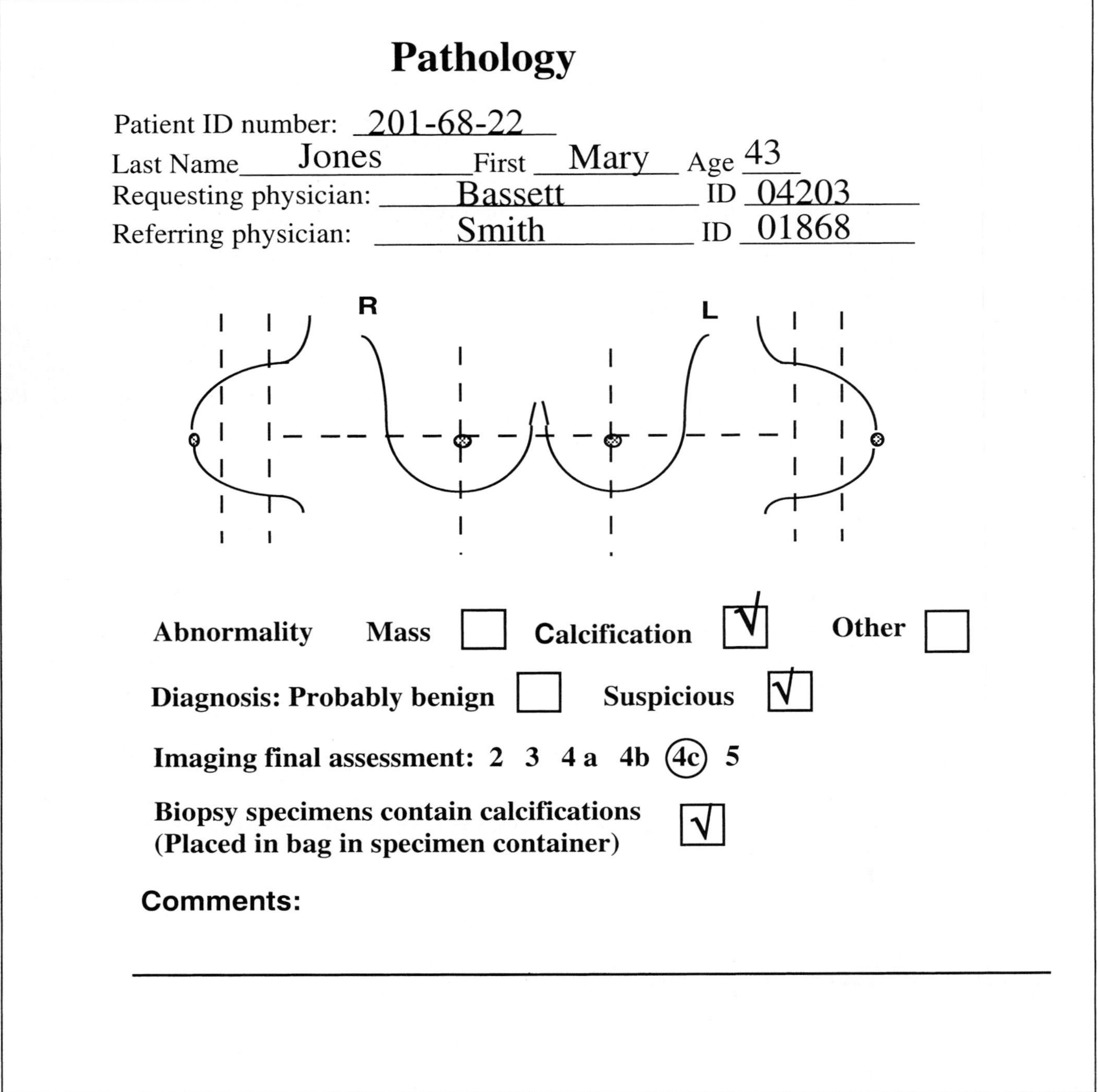
Pathology

Patient ID number: 201-68-22
Last Name Jones First Mary Age 43
Requesting physician: Bassett ID 04203
Referring physician: Smith ID 01868

Abnormality **Mass** ☐ **Calcification** ☑ **Other** ☐

Diagnosis: Probably benign ☐ **Suspicious** ☑

Imaging final assessment: 2 3 4 a 4b (4c) 5

Biopsy specimens contain calcifications (Placed in bag in specimen container) ☑

Comments:

Figure 18–1. Pathology requisition for breast core needle biopsy.

numbers of calcifications. *Concordance* means that the imaging findings of concern are adequately explained by the pathology results. *Discordance* indicates that the imaging findings are not consistent with or are not adequately explained by the pathology results.

Once concordance or discordance between imaging and pathology findings has been established, a post-CNB management plan is devised. In our practice, patients with discordant findings and patients in whom accurate targeting or limited sampling is a concern are referred for open surgical biopsy. Patients with "positive" results, in which cancer is diagnosed, are referred to a surgeon for definitive treatment.

For most patients with benign concordant imaging-biopsy findings, a 6-month follow-up is recommended in order to identify any false-negative

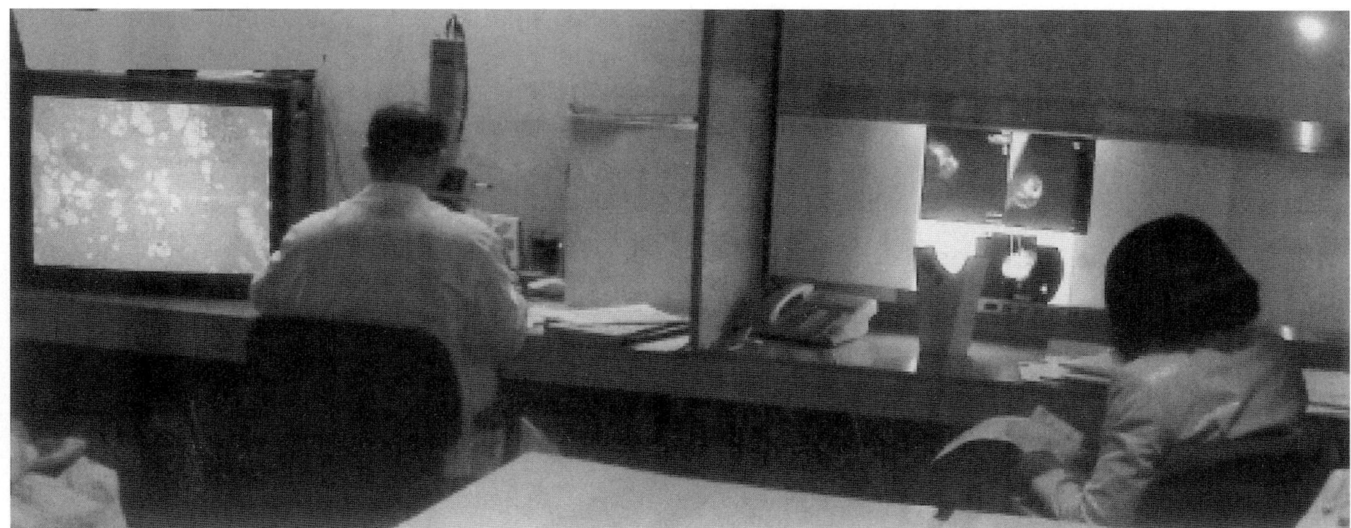

Figure 18–2. Radiology-pathology correlation conference. The radiologist presents the history and imaging findings. The pathologist shows the histologic findings. Concordance or discordance is determined, and a management plan is developed.

results as soon as possible. Some investigators believe that a 1-year follow-up is adequate for "definite" benign cases, such as a typical fibroadenoma identified at imaging with a CNB diagnosis of fibroadenoma (Fig. 18–3). We, however, apply the 6-month follow-up protocol in all cases. Our uniform 6-month follow-up protocol simplifies the patient follow-up tracking process and also reflects our experience with two phyllodes tumors that were diagnosed as fibroadenomas on CNB. The modality used for follow-up imaging (mammography or ultrasonography) should be the modality that better demonstrates the lesion.

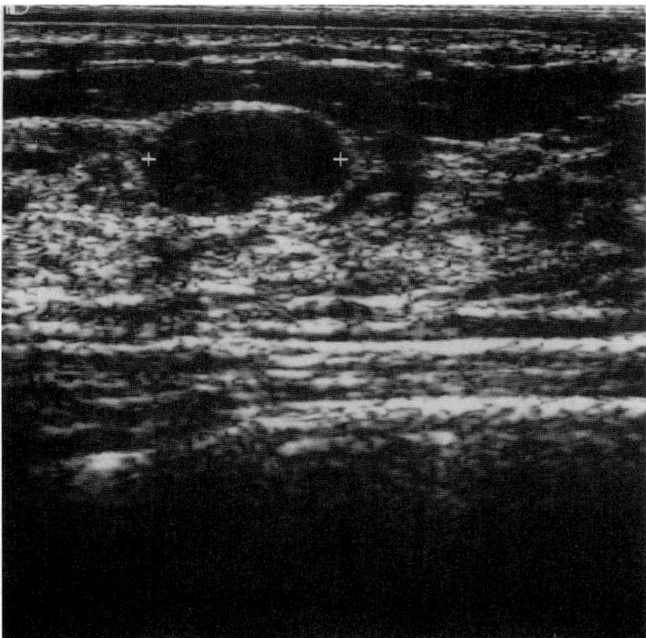

Figure 18–3. "Definite benign." A 35-year-old woman presented with a palpable breast mass. Ultrasonography shows an oval solid mass that is wider than it is tall (parallel to the skin surface), with circumscribed margins and a thin echogenic pseudocapsule, considered typical of fibroadenoma. Histologic examination of a core needle biopsy specimen showed fibroadenoma.

A *false-negative CNB result* is defined as a benign CNB finding in a patient in whom cancer is detected at the biopsy site within 2 years after the biopsy (Fig. 18–4). Reports in the literature indicate that the false-negative rate for breast CNB is approximately 2%.[4] However, this rate may be lower when the physician performing the biopsy is experienced.[5]

Understanding the limitations of CNB is important. Several uncommon "benign" and "high-risk" pathology diagnoses have been linked to "underestimation" of disease, because adjacent carcinoma was missed as a result of sampling error. When there is the possibility of underestimation of disease, open biopsy should be performed. There is universal agreement that after a CNB diagnosis of atypical ductal hyperplasia (ADH), open biopsy should be performed to rule out underestimation of disease. The need for open biopsy is controversial for the following conditions: radial scar, papillary lesions, lobular carcinoma in situ (LCIS), atypical lobular hyperplasia (ALH), and columnar cell lesions. In addition, approximately 20% of cases with CNB diagnosis of ductal carcinoma in situ (DCIS) show evidence of invasive carcinoma at surgical excision, another example of underestimation of disease.

ATYPICAL DUCTAL HYPERPLASIA

ADH is the classic high-risk lesion in terms of possible underestimation of disease. Surgical excision after a CNB diagnosis of ADH can yield in situ or invasive carcinoma in a significant number of cases.

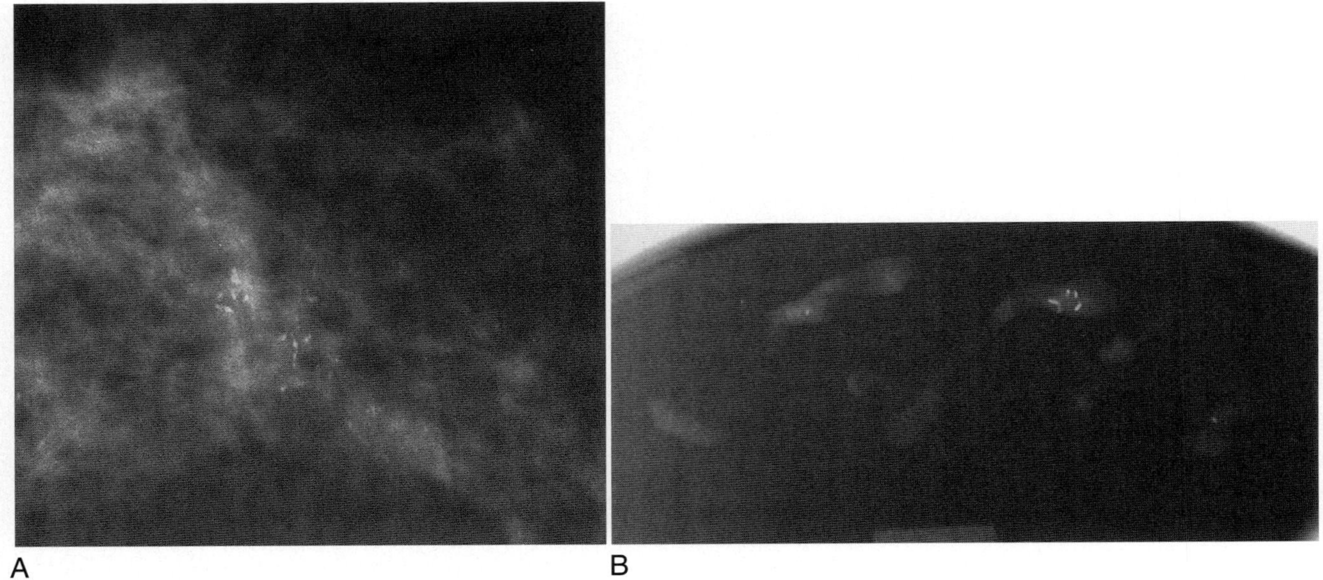

Figure 18–4. False-negative result of core needle biopsy (CNB) in a 54-year-old woman. **A,** Screening mammogram showed numerous heterogeneous, linear and branching calcifications. **B,** Breast CNB specimen radiograph verifies calcifications in three of the specimens. Histology found benign calcifications of sclerosing adenosis. Because the calcifications appeared suspicious, follow-up was recommended at 6-month intervals. Six-month follow-up mammograms showed an increase in calcifications, and excisional biopsy revealed high-grade ductal carcinoma in situ. The false-negative CNB result was attributed to sampling error.

For this lesion, underestimation is defined as a diagnosis of ADH on CNB with identification of DCIS or invasive ductal carcinoma in the subsequent surgically excised specimen. Underestimation rates for ADH vary with the type of biopsy device used. Underestimation of in situ or invasive carcinoma has been reported in 20% to 25% of CNB diagnoses of ADH, even with the use of an 11-gauge vacuum-assisted device.[6,7] Use of 14-gauge automated (spring-loaded) biopsy devices has underestimation rates of up to 58%.[8-11]

The post-biopsy management of this entity is universally agreed upon. When ADH is identified after CNB, surgical excision is indicated. Even complete removal of the mammographic lesion during CNB does not ensure benign findings at subsequent surgical excision.[12-14] Both histologic and mammographic factors make accurate diagnosis difficult. Some cases of ADH have a similar histologic appearance to that of DCIS, making differentiation difficult. Individual pathologists may disagree on whether borderline cases are ADH or DCIS. Furthermore, the two entities frequently coexist and may manifest as mammographically identical microcalcifications (Fig. 18–5). Increasing the number of CNB specimens obtained can reduce the frequency of ADH diagnoses and the rates of ADH underestimation.[10]

RADIAL SCAR

Management of radial scars is controversial. For the patient in whom mammographic findings suggest radial scar, many investigators suggest that open biopsy rather than CNB should be performed.[15-17] Typically, radial scars manifest as an area of architectural distortion with a lucent center (Fig. 18–6). However, confident imaging diagnosis of radial scar is difficult because the architectural distortion may look identical to invasive ductal carcinoma. Furthermore, an unexpected histologic diagnosis of radial scar is not uncommon, because lesions can manifest as a mass or calcifications. Other

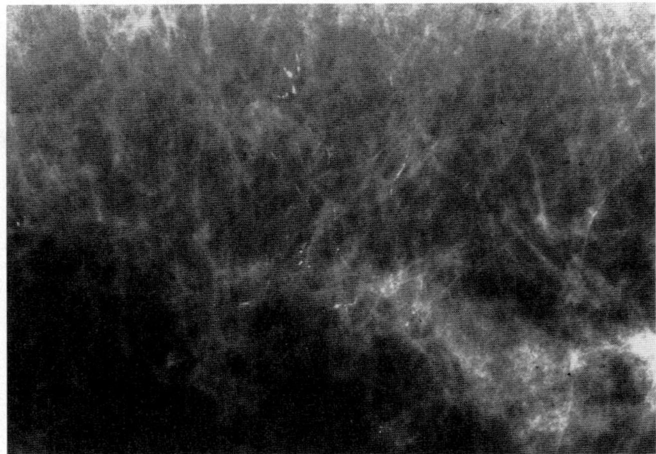

Figure 18–5. Atypical ductal hyperplasia (ADH) versus ductal carcinoma in situ (DCIS). In a 60-year-old woman, the mammogram showed linear, branching calcifications throughout the lower breast, which were considered suspicious for DCIS. Breast core needle biopsy revealed ADH. To rule out underestimation of disease, an excisional biopsy was performed to remove the remaining calcifications. The histologic diagnosis of the surgical specimen was extensive ADH.

Figure 18–6. Radial scar in a 52-year-old woman with an abnormal mammogram. **A,** The right mediolateral oblique mammogram showed an architectural distortion in the upper hemisphere (*arrow*). **B,** Spot compression mammogram showed an architectural distortion (spicules with no central mass). Differential diagnosis was radial scar versus carcinoma. **C,** Excisional biopsy was performed because of concern about coexistent radial scar and carcinoma. Histologic diagnosis was radial scar.

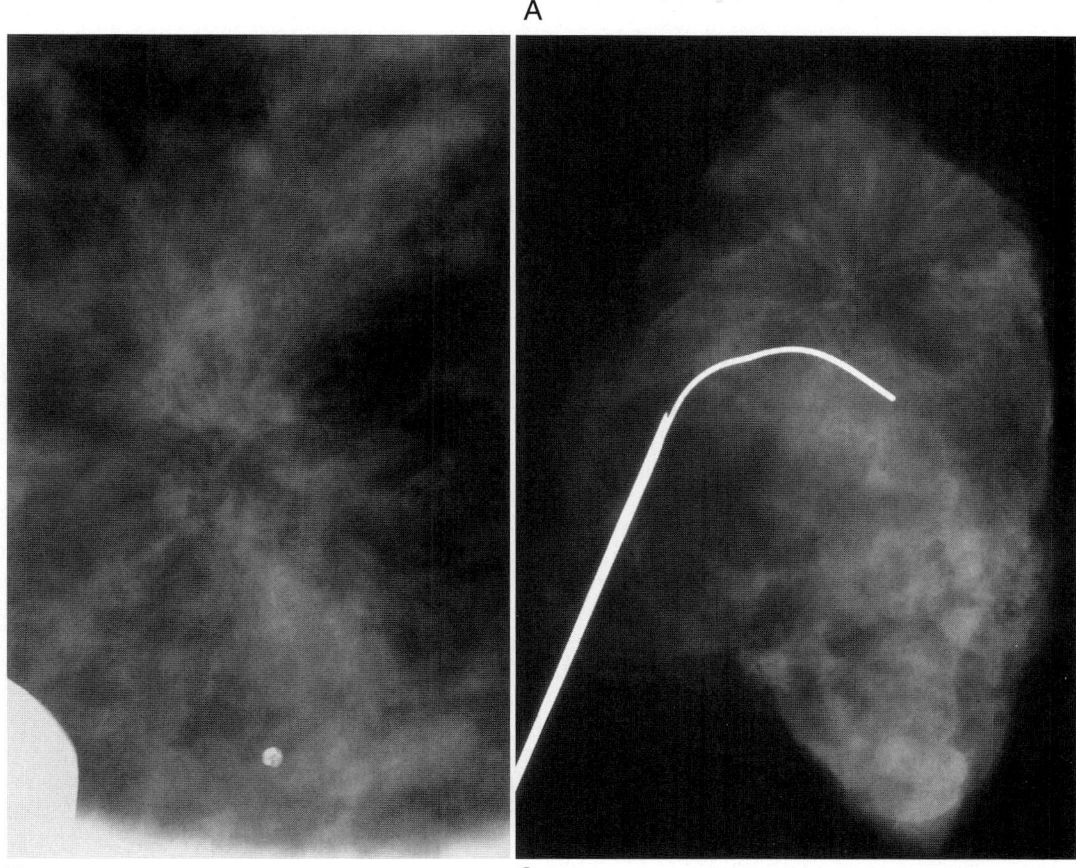

radial scars are small, microscopically visible lesions, incidentally identified in a pathologic specimen.

Experts no longer believe that radial scar itself is a high-risk lesion or precursor of tubular carcinoma, but it may coexist with DCIS or invasive carcinoma.[18] Histologically, radial scars harbor an array of proliferative elements. The ducts within a radial scar are often distorted by a central fibroelastic core but maintain both epithelial and myoepithelial cell layers with a surrounding basement membrane. This two-cell layer and basement membrane differentiates radial scar from tubular carcinoma, which has only a single cell layer and no basement membrane.

Reported rates of carcinoma found at excision of radial scars vary from 0 to 40%; however, the total number of cases is small.[2,9,19] A large multi-institutional study of 157 cases of radial scar diagnosed at CNB found carcinoma in 8% at surgical excision.[6] The risk was 28% if the radial scar was associated with atypia (ADH, ALH, LCIS) but was 4% if no atypia was present. Furthermore, the cancer miss rate was 0 in cases in which 12 or more CNB specimens were obtained. Our current policy is to recommend excisional biopsy for imaging-expected radial scars, for CNB-diagnosed radial scars associated with atypia, and for imaging-pathology discordance.

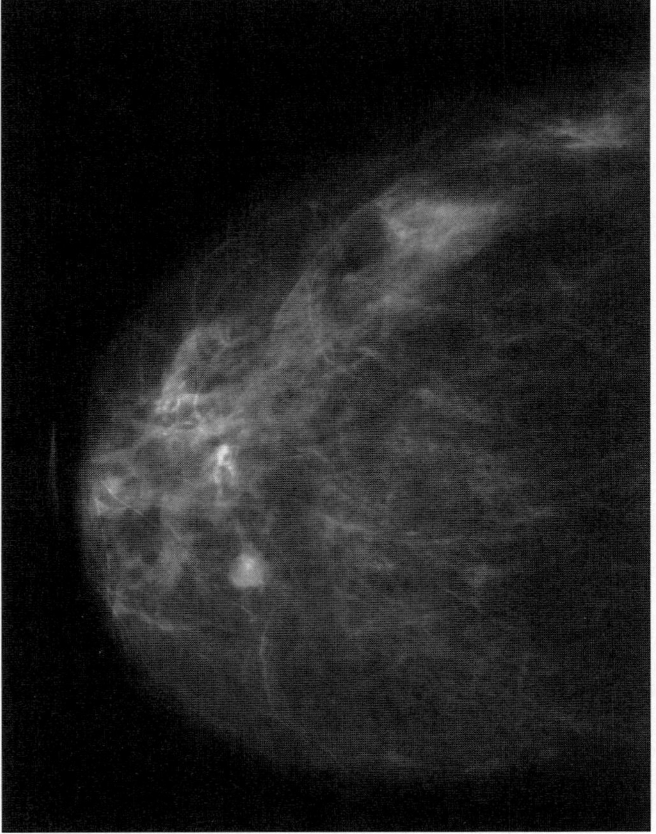

Figure 18–7. Papilloma. In a 51-year-old woman, the mammogram showed a round mass with partially obscured margin. Breast core needle biopsy revealed a papilloma. Excisional biopsy performed to rule out coexistent carcinoma showed only papilloma.

PAPILLARY LESIONS

Papillomas are a diverse group of lesions ranging from a typically solitary, large central duct papilloma to multiple peripheral papillomas. A papilloma is composed of arborescent fronds of fibrovascular stroma with a stalk that arises from the duct lumen. The fronds are usually covered with a benign two-cell epithelial layer; however, this lining may undergo hyperplasia and evolve into ADH, DCIS, or invasive papillary carcinoma. The appearance of this epithelial lining determines whether the papilloma is benign, high-risk, or malignant. As with ADH, there is variability among pathologists in differentiating borderline benign from malignant lesions.

Mammographically, a papilloma may appear as a circumscribed mass or a group of microcalcifications (Fig. 18–7). Clinical features of central large duct papillomas include bloody or clear nipple discharge, whereas peripheral papillomas are more likely to be asymptomatic. It used to be thought that multiple peripheral papillomas raised a woman's risk of breast cancer but central solitary papillomas did not. However, a study by Page and colleagues[21] documented that increased risk from papilloma was related to the presence or absence of ADH in a papilloma rather than the papilloma's location.

A papilloma diagnosed at CNB warrants open biopsy if ADH is found in its epithelium. However, routine performance of open biopsy after a CNB diagnosis of papilloma without atypia is controversial. Many investigators believe that 11-gauge vacuum-assisted devices adequately sample papillomas and that open biopsy is not necessary unless atypia is identified or there is imaging-pathology discordance.[19,22,23] A large study of 46 papillary lesions subjected to biopsy with either 14-gauge, automated, large core, or 11- or 14-gauge, vacuum-assisted devices further support the latter recommendation.[24]

LOBULAR NEOPLASIA

Our knowledge of lobular neoplasia is evolving. It used to be believed that lobular neoplasia was not a precursor to malignancy but, rather, a marker that identified an increased risk of development of invasive breast cancer in either breast. These concepts are in evolution. Page and associates found that the relative risk of development of breast cancer after a benign biopsy showing ALH was 3.1.[25] Furthermore, subsequent breast cancers were approximately three times more likely to develop in the ipsilateral breast than in the contralateral breast of women with such biopsy findings. These investigators therefore suggest that ALH may be a lesion intermediate between a local precursor and a generalized bilateral risk factor for breast cancer.

Lobular neoplasia does not have any clinical or mammographic features. Lobular neoplasia comprises a spectrum of lesions, from LCIS to ALH to ductal involvement with cells of ALH. Histologically, LCIS is characterized by a lobule distended by small, uniform cells. When the same small uniform cells proliferate but do not distend the lobule, ALH is diagnosed. Cancerization of the lobules occurs when DCIS grows retrograde into the lobules from the involved ducts, and this condition can mimic LCIS. Because cancerization of the lobules requires lumpectomy and radiation treatment, the pathologist must be able to differentiate these two conditions.

The necessity for open biopsy after a CNB diagnosis of lobular neoplasia (LCIS, ALH) remains controversial. This is in part due to the fact that these lesions are relatively uncommon, with an incidence of <2% in most core needle biopsy studies.[19,26,27] A paper by Liberman and associates suggests some potential guidelines.[27] In this paper, excisional biopsy was recommended only when there was overlap of the histologic features of LCIS and DCIS, when imaging-histologic discordance was identified, or when the LCIS co-existed with a high-risk lesion (radial scar, ADH). Different experienced radiologists use different approaches to manage lobular neoplasia when diagnosed at CNB. More investigation is necessary before there is a clear answer to this question.

COLUMNAR CELL LESIONS

Breast biopsy for microcalcifications may reveal a columnar cell lesion. Columnar cell lesions include a wide variety of pathologic lesions distinguished by the presence of columnar cells lining the terminal duct lobular unit.[28] These entities range from benign to atypical to DCIS with columnar cell features. Benign columnar changes of the terminal duct lobular unit are described by terms such as "blunt duct adenosis," "columnar alteration of the lobules," and "metaplasie cylindrique."[29,30] An entity known as "columnar alteration with prominent apical snouts and secretions" (CAPSS) may or may not be associated with atypia (Fig. 18–8). When associated with atypia, CAPSS lesions are two times more likely to show DCIS at surgical excision.[31] Until further large studies more conclusively delineate appropriate management of columnar cell lesions, surgical excision should be considered if a CNB specimen demonstrates a columnar cell lesion with associated atypia.

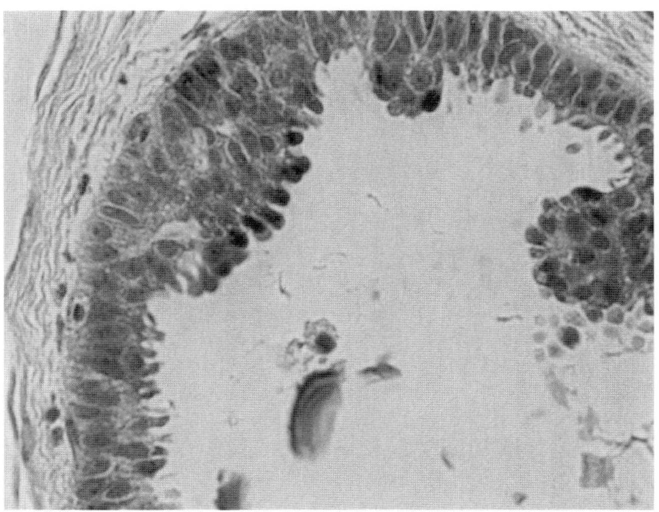

Figure 18–8. Columnar alteration with prominent apical snouts and secretions (CAPSS). The histologic specimen showed a lobular structure lined with epithelial cells with prominent apical cytoplasmic snouts. Some of the cells are in a single layer, and other areas show stratification and tufting.

SCLEROSING ADENOSIS

Sclerosing adenosis is a benign proliferative condition characterized by proliferation of the lobules (adenosis) and fibrous tissue. Occasionally, the associated fibrosis is so severe that the lobules are distorted enough to mimic invasive carcinoma. Mammographically, sclerosing adenosis is characterized by a cluster of microcalcifications that can range from uniform and round to pleomorphic or linear. Less commonly, it may manifest as a mass. Sclerosing adenosis does not carry a significantly increased risk of future malignancy, but it can lead to a false-positive CNB diagnosis of malignancy. A *false-positive CNB diagnosis* occurs when the CNB result is interpreted as malignant, but surgical excision reveals a benign condition and reevaluation of the original CNB pathology indicates that the diagnosis should have been sclerosing adenosis rather than invasive cancer. We have encountered only two false-positive CNB results. In both cases, sclerosing adenosis mimicked an invasive carcinoma. Subsequent review by an expert in breast pathology found that the correct diagnosis was sclerosing adenosis, not carcinoma. If there is doubt, special stains can be used on the pathologic specimen to identify the presence of myoepithelial cells, which are seen in sclerosing adenosis but are not seen in carcinoma (Fig. 18–9).

FALSE-POSITIVE RESULTS

As already mentioned, a false-positive CNB result consists of an original pathology interpretation of malignancy with subsequent decision that the original diagnosis should have been benign. If a false-positive CNB result is suspected because the surgical excision specimen does not demonstrate carcinoma, the original pathology specimen should be reviewed. If the review finds a benign lesion, the CNB result

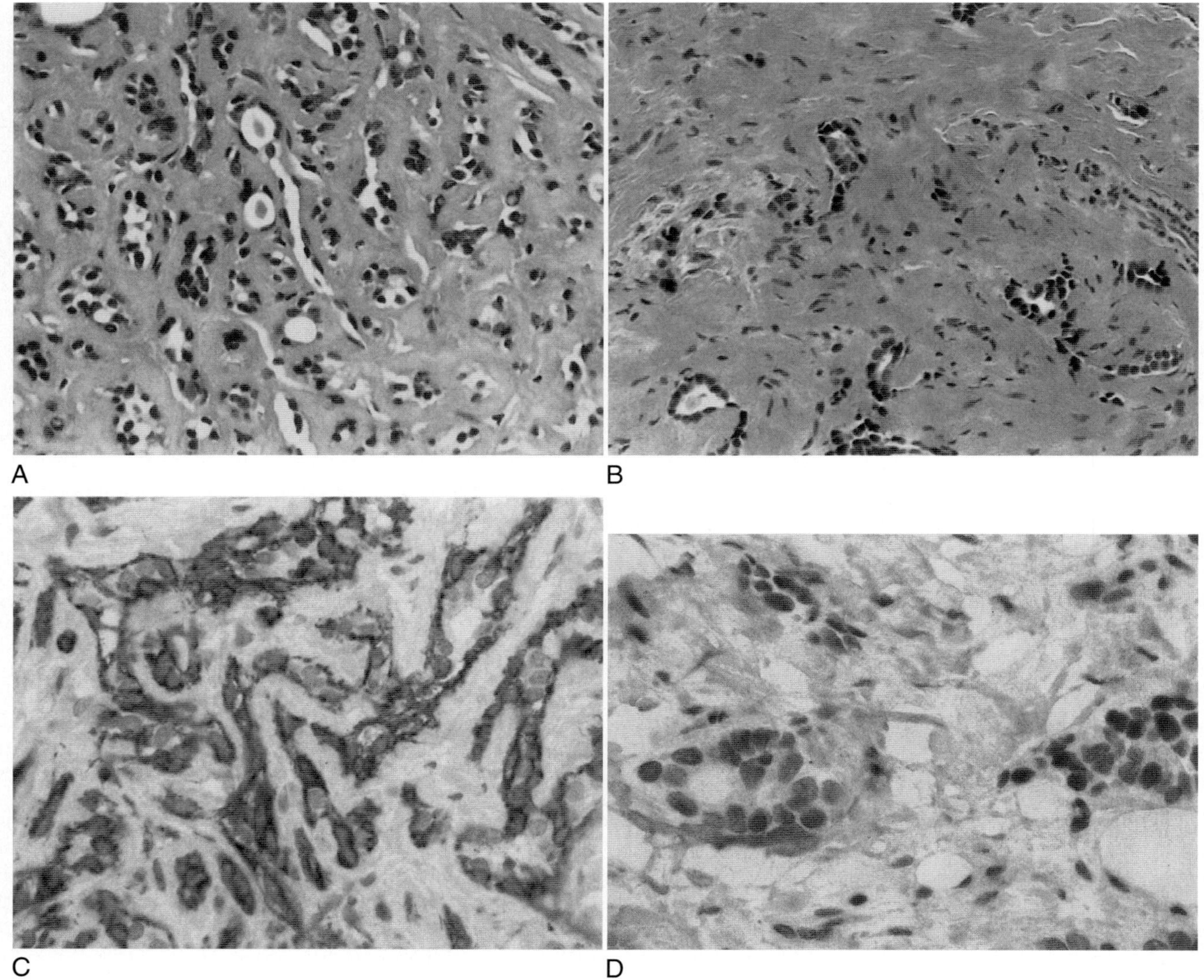

Figure 18–9. Sclerosing adenosis: a potential false-positive CNB result. **A** and **B,** Both histologic sections show disorganized ductal structures surrounded by fibrosis, suggesting invasive carcinoma. **C,** Anti–smooth muscle chain stain for histologic section **A** shows uptake of the stain by myoepithelial cells, indicating the diagnosis is sclerosing adenosis. **D,** Anti–smooth muscle chain stain for histologic section **B** shows no uptake of the stain, indicating absence of myoepithelial cells and a diagnosis of invasive carcinoma (tubular carcinoma).

was a false-positive. If review confirms a malignancy, then further imaging is performed to verify that the mammographic abnormality was removed at the surgical excision. If the postoperative imaging finding is negative and pathologic review confirmed a malignancy in the CNB specimen, it is likely that the original lesion was removed entirely during the CNB. Complete removal of lesions is more likely to occur with the more efficient sampling devices, such as the 8- and 11-gauge, vacuum-assisted devices.

COMMUNICATION RESPONSIBILITIES

Communicating post biopsy management recommendations to the referring health care provider is an important responsibility of the physician performing the CNB. A study from Stanford University found poor patient compliance with recommendations for CNB follow-up management; only 74% of patients acted on recommendations for open surgical biopsy, and only 54% returned for the recommended short-term follow-up imaging studies.[32]

Once a management plan is devised (6-month follow-up or surgical excision), the results are communicated to the referring clinician and the patient. In our practice, the referring clinician usually conveys the results and recommendations to the patient; however, we assume this role whenever this task is not easily or quickly accomplished by the referring clinician. We convey our recommendations to the health care provider in two ways. First, a phone call is made to the referring physician with the results and management recommendations. Second, an addendum to the original biopsy report is issued that summarizes the recommendations from the radiology-pathology correlation conference as well as our post-CNB management recommendations.

SUMMARY

Management of the patient undergoing breast CNB does not end with the performance of the biopsy. Follow-up management includes correlating pathology results and imaging findings for concordance, developing a patient management plan, communicating this plan to the referring health care provider, and monitoring compliance with the recommendations.

References

1. Bassett L, Winchester DP, Caplan RB, et al: Stereotactic core-needle biopsy of the breast: A report of the Joint Task Force of the American College of Radiology, American College of Surgeons, and College of American Pathologists. CA Cancer J Clin 1997;47:171-190.
2. Lee CH, Egglin TK, Philpotts L, et al: Cost-effectiveness of stereotactic core needle biopsy: Analysis by means of mammographic findings. Radiology 1997;202:849-854.
3. The Uniform Approach to Breast Fine Needle Aspiration Biopsy: A Synopsis. Developed and Approved at the National Cancer Institute–Sponsored Conference, Bethesda, Maryland, September 9-10, 1996. Breast J 1996;2:357-363.
4. Lee CH, Philpotts LE, Horvath LJ, Tocino I: Follow-up of breast lesions diagnosed as benign with stereotactic core-needle biopsy: Frequency of mammographic change and false-negative rate. Radiology 1999;212:189-194.
5. Pfarl G, Helbich TH, Riedl CC, et al: Stereotactic 11-gauge vacuum-assisted breast biopsy: A validation study. AJR Am J Roentgenol 2002;179:1503-1507.
6. Brem RF, Behrndt VS, Sanow L, Gatewood OM: Atypical ductal hyperplasia: Histologic underestimation of carcinoma in tissue harvested from impalpable breast lesions using 11-gauge stereotactically guided directional vacuum-assisted biopsy. AJR Am J Roentgenol 1999;172:1405-1407.
7. Philpotts LE, Shaheen NA, Carter D, et al: Comparison of re-biopsy rates after stereotactic core-needle biopsy of the breast with 11-gauge vacuum suction probe versus 14-gauge needle and automatic gun. AJR Am J Roentgenol 1999;172: 683-687.
8. Brenner RJ, Bassett LW, Fajardo LL, et al: Percutaneous core breast biopsy: A multiinstitutional prospective trial. Radiology 2001;218:866-872.
9. Jackman RJ, Nowels KW, Rodriquez-Soto J, et al: Stereotactic, automated, large-core needle biopsy of nonpalpable breast lesions: False-negative rates and histologic underestimation rates after long-term follow-up. Radiology 1999;210:799-805.
10. Jackman RJ, Nowels KW, Shepard MJ, et al: Stereotaxic large-core needle biopsy of 450 non-palpable breast lesions with surgical correlation in lesions with cancer or atypical hyperplasia. Radiology 1994;193:91-95.
11. Liberman L, Cohen MA, Dershaw DD, et al: Atypical ductal hyperplasia diagnosed at stereotaxic core biopsy of breast lesions: An indication for surgical biopsy. AJR Am J Roentgenol 1995;164:1111-1113.
12. Jackman RJ, Birdwell RL, Ikeda DM: Atypical ductal hyperplasia: Can some lesions be defined as probably benign after stereotactic 11-gauge vacuum-assisted biopsy, eliminating the recommendation for surgical excision? Radiology 2002;224: 548-554.
13. Liberman L, Dershaw DD, Rosen PP, et al: Percutaneous removal of malignant mammographic lesions at vacuum-assisted biopsy. Radiology 1998;206:711-715.
14. Liberman L, Kaplan JB, Morris EA, et al: To excise or to sample the mammographic target: What is the goal of stereotactic 11-gauge vacuum-assisted breast biopsy? AJR Am J Roentgenol 2002;179:679-683.
15. Ciatto S, Morrone D, Catarzi S, et al: Radial scars of the breast: Review of 38 consecutive mammographic diagnoses. Radiology 1993;187:757-760.
16. Frouge C, Tristant H, Guinebretiere JM, et al: Mammographic lesions suggestive of radial scars: Microscopic findings in 40 cases. Radiology 1995;195:623-625.
17. Kopans DB: Pathologic, mammographic, and sonographic correlation. In Breast Imaging, 2nd ed. Philadelphia, Lippincott-Raven, 1998, pp 551-615.
18. Anderson JA, Gram JB: Radial scar in the female breast: A long term follow-up of 32 cases. Cancer 1984;15:2557-2560.
19. Philpotts LE, Shaheen NA, Jain KS, et al: Uncommon high-risk lesions of the breast diagnosed at stereotactic core-needle biopsy: Clinical importance. Radiology 2000;216:831-837.
20. Brenner RJ, Jackman RJ, Parker SJ, et al: Percutaneous core needle biopsy of radial scars of the breast: When is excision necessary? AJR Am J Roentgenol 2002;179:1179-1184.
21. Page DL, Salhany KE, Jensen RA, et al: Subsequent breast carcinoma risk after biopsy with atypia in a breast papilloma. Cancer 1996;78:258-266.
22. Liberman L, Bracero N, Vuolo MA, et al: Percutaneous large-core biopsy of papillary breast lesions. AJR Am J Roentgenol 1999;172:331-337.
23. Mercado CL, Hamele-Bena D, Singer C, et al: Papillary lesions of the breast: Evaluation with stereotactic directional vacuum-assisted biopsy. Radiology 2001;221:650-655.
24. Rosen EL, Bentley RC, Baker JA, Soo MS: Imaging-guided core needle biopsy of papillary lesions of the breast. AJR Am J Roentgenol 2002;179:1185-1192.
25. Page DL, Schuyler PA, Dupont WD, et al: Atypical lobular hyperplasia as a unilateral predictor of breast cancer risk: A retrospective cohort study. Lancet 2002;361:125-129.
26. Berg WA, Mrose HE, Ioffe OB: Atypical lobular hyperplasia or lobular carcinoma in situ at core-needle breast biopsy. Radiology 2001;218:503-509.
27. Liberman L, Sama M, Susnik B, et al: Lobular carcinoma in situ at percutaneous breast biopsy: Surgical biopsy findings. AJR Am J Roentgenol 1999;173:291-299.
28. Jacobs TW, Connolly JL, Schnitt SJ: Nonmalignant lesions in breast core needle biopsies: To excise or not to excise? Am J Surg Pathol 2002;26:1095-1110.
29. Page DL, Anderson TJ: Diagnostic Histopathology of the Breast. Edinburgh, Churchill Livingstone, 1987, pp 86-88.
30. Trojani M: Atlas en couleurs d'histopathologie mammaire. Paris, Maloine, 1988, pp 38-43.
31. Fraser JL, Raza S, Chorny K, et al: Columnar alteration with prominent apical snouts and secretions: A spectrum of changes frequently present in breast biopsies performed for microcalcifications. Am J Surg Pathol 1998;22:1521-1527.
32. Goodman KA, Birdwell RL, Ikeda DM: Compliance with recommended follow-up after percutaneous breast biopsy. AJR Am J Roentgenol 1998;170:89-92.

Handling of Pathology Specimens

Karin L. Fu and Yao S. Fu

Earlier detection of earlier breast cancers gives the patients more options in treatment, including breast-conserving surgery and radiotherapy. In addition, more adjuvant therapies are available today. Important decisions for breast cancer management depend heavily on the pathologic findings.[1] The following discussion presents general recommendations for the handling of cytologic and histologic specimens.

FINE-NEEDLE ASPIRATION

Fine-needle aspiration cytology (FNAC) for the biopsy of a clinically palpable abnormality, when performed and interpreted by well-trained and qualified physicians, has proved to be accurate.[2] On the basis of a correlation of the FNAC and clinical findings, appropriate decisions can be made as to whether observation, biopsy, excision, or definitive treatment is needed. FNAC has been demonstrated to be cost-effective.[3,4] FNAC guided by mammography or ultrasonography can also be performed for nonpalpable, mammographically detected abnormalities, with good results.[5]

The material obtained through FNA is usually sufficient to prepare two types of smears and stains: air-dried smears for Giemsa or Quick-Diff stains, and smears fixed immediately in 95% alcohol for Papanicolaou or hematoxylin and eosin (H & E) stains. Each provides useful information. One limitation of FNAC is its difficulty distinguishing between in situ and invasive ductal carcinomas.

According to the review of literature by Bedard and Pollett,[6] the sensitivity and specificity of FNAC for both benign and malignant conditions are 74% to 97% and 82% to 100%, respectively. False-negative FNAC interpretation of specimens that are actually malignant tumors remain problematic, at a rate of about 10% or less (Fig. 19–1). The most common reason is failure to recognize hypocellular, inadequate specimens, which are caused by dense fibrous stroma, necrotic cystic tumor, and technical problems. Well-differentiated ductal carcinoma and lobular carcinoma can be challenging to interpret correctly.

False-positive FNAC interpretation occurs occasionally. Fibroadenoma with hyperplastic ducts, lactational changes, fat necrosis, granulation tissue, atypical hyperplasia, papillary lesions, and nuclear atypia secondary to treatment effects, such as surgery, radiotherapy, and chemotherapy, are pitfalls of "over-interpretation." The interpreter of FNAC specimens, especially if he or she has not personally performed the FNA procedure, should have adequate clinical and radiographic findings before making the diagnosis.

The liquid-based ThinPrep specimen has become available in many laboratories in the United States. The aspirated material in the syringe is rinsed, stored, and submitted in a transport solution for automated processing and Papanicolaou stain. Compared with conventional smears, the only advantage of ThinPrep smears is the lower rate of unsatisfactory specimens (28% versus 34%). The sensitivity and specificity of the conventional preparations and ThinPrep have been found to be similar.[6]

CORE NEEDLE BIOPSY OF THE BREAST

Core needle biopsy (CNB) of the breast can also be performed for palpable abnormalities and is gaining popularity for imaging-guided biopsy of nonpalpable lesions.[7] A satisfactory core biopsy specimen should measure more than 1 cm in length and at least 1 mm in thickness with intact contiguous tissue (Fig. 19–2). In benign conditions, the border between normal and abnormal tissue is circumscribed, whereas in most malignant conditions, the border is irregular. In the malignant specimen, the presence of tumor cells infiltrating into the adjacent fat is a helpful diagnostic feature (Fig. 19–3). Tissue less than 1 cm in length is often fragmented and is less likely to include borders between normal and abnormal areas, making interpretation more difficult (Fig. 19–4).

Ideally, when the fresh tissue is removed from the biopsy gun, it is laid on a piece of paper or index card to be flattened and straightened. After a few minutes, the tissue, along with the underlying paper, is placed in formalin for several hours. This simple maneuver helps minimize tissue distortion and eases retrieval of all tissue fragments for sectioning. The core biopsy specimens are received in the pathology laboratory in the formalin and submitted in entirety for sectioning. The specimens are sectioned at different levels to ensure inclusion of representative areas for histologic study. If biopsy is performed on more than one lesion, the specimens should be properly labeled and submitted separately.

The accuracy of 224 14-gauge needle biopsies, when compared with excisional specimens, had an overall concordance rate of 93.8% (60 of 64) for cancer specimens. Four discordant specimens included two cases each of ductal carcinoma in situ (DCIS) and invasive ductal carcinoma, which is underdiagnosed as atypical ductal hyperplasias

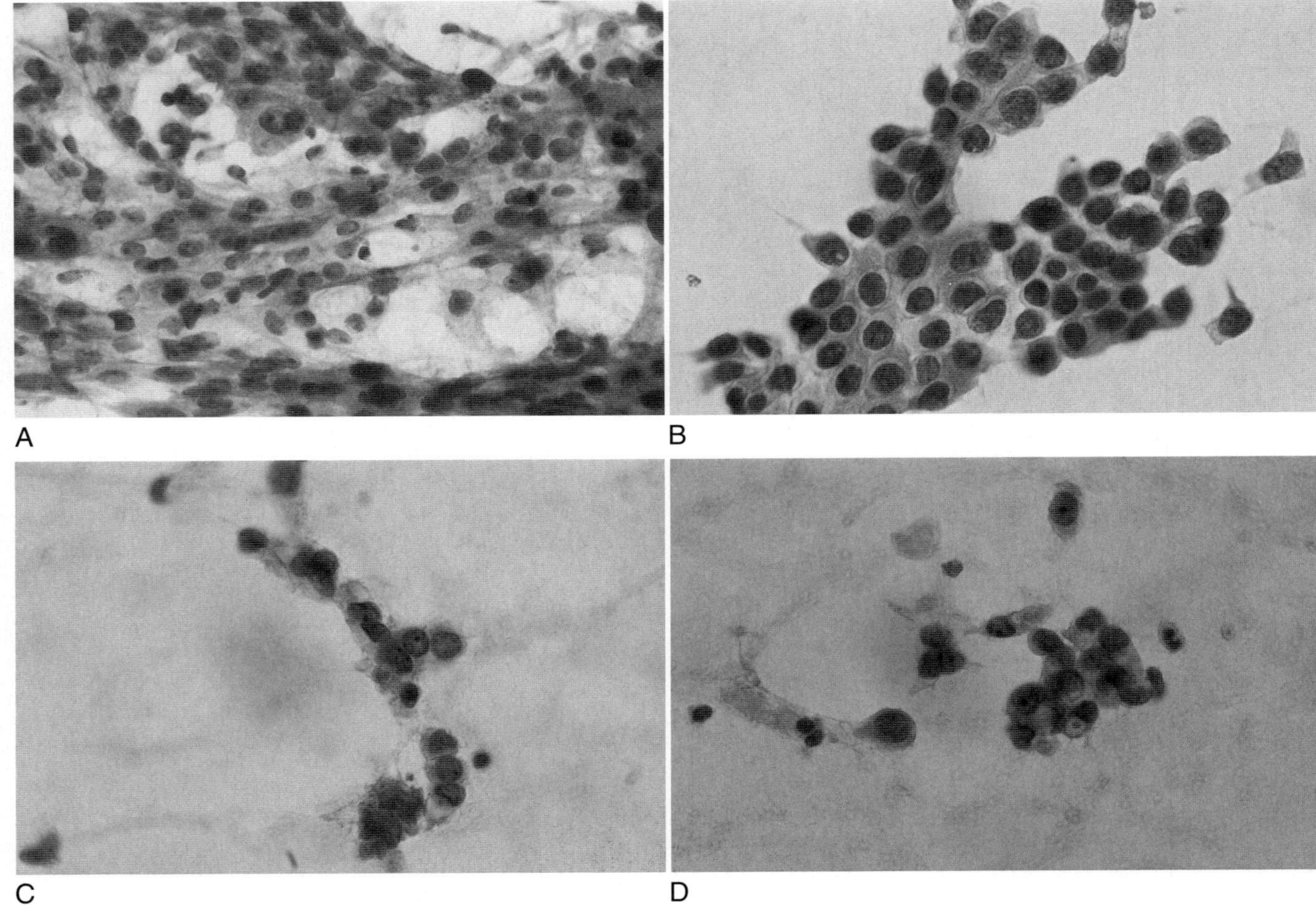

Figure 19–1. Fine-needle aspiration specimens of breast carcinomas. **A,** In poorly differentiated ductal carcinoma, the smear contains abundant malignant cells, which have large irregular hyperchromatic nuclei and prominent nucleoli. **B,** Aspiration specimen of a well-differentiated ductal carcinoma contains fewer tumor cells, which have uniformly round to oval nuclei and indistinct nucleoli. Some cells maintain cuboid shape, supporting a ductal origin. The lack of myoepithelial cells in a homogeneous population of cells favors the diagnosis of carcinoma. **C,** Aspiration specimen of an infiltrating lobular carcinoma usually provides a limited number of tumor cells, which are arranged in a single file. The nuclei are small and slightly irregular in shape. **D,** Cells of infiltrating lobular carcinoma contain vacuolated cytoplasm and intracytoplasmic lumens.

(ADH) in core biopsy specimens. The sensitivity of needle biopsy in this study was 96.9% and specificity 100%.[8]

In another comparative study of core needle biopsy specimens obtained with a 14-gauge needle and excisional specimens from invasive carcinomas, there was agreement on histologic type in 81% and on histologic grade in 75% of cases (higher than excision in 16%, lower in 9%). Vascular lymphatic space invasion was not evident in 21% of biopsy specimens. Invasive carcinomas with extensive in situ carcinoma were evident in only 29% of biopsy specimens.[9]

ADH is one of the most difficult diagnostic problems in CNB interpretation (see Fig. 19–4). Fifty percent of women in whom ADH was diagnosed from CNB were proved to have carcinoma, usually DCIS, in the subsequent excisional specimens.[10] In a review of literature, 52% to 75% of women with diagnosis of ADH from CNB were found to have carcinomas, the majority being DCIS and 19% to 25% of which were invasive.[8] These inherent limitations appear to be acceptable, because patient management is unlikely to be based on CNB results.[9]

EFFECTS OF FINE-NEEDLE ASPIRATION CYTOLOGY AND CORE BREAST BIOPSY

Information from previously performed FNAC and CNB should be given to the pathologist who handles the subsequent excisional specimens, because of artifacts caused by these procedures. In a study of 184 consecutive breast excisions performed after FNAC, Connolly and associates[1] found that 9.2% of specimens had hemorrhage with infarct, hemosiderin deposit, granulation tissue, and inflammatory reaction. Scar formation, hemorrhage, fat necrosis, and

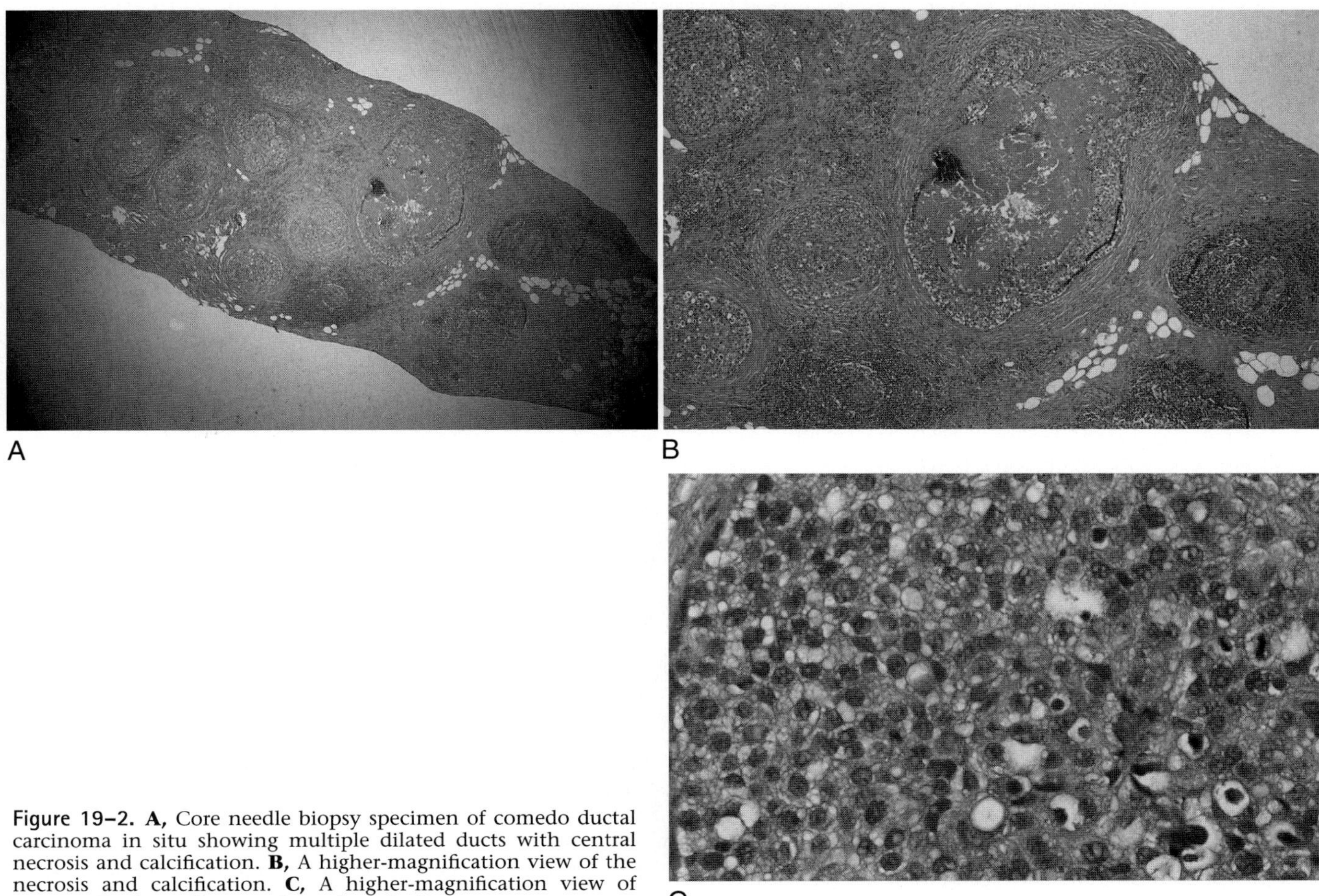

Figure 19–2. **A,** Core needle biopsy specimen of comedo ductal carcinoma in situ showing multiple dilated ducts with central necrosis and calcification. **B,** A higher-magnification view of the necrosis and calcification. **C,** A higher-magnification view of tumor cells shows large nuclei and nucleoli.

inflammatory reaction were the most common findings in excisional specimens that had previously undergone CNB (Figs. 19–5 and 19–6). Epithelial cells adjacent to the areas of prior FNAC or biopsy frequently appeared reactive and atypical, with nuclear hyperchromasia and prominent nucleoli. Less frequently, displacement of epithelial cells caused diagnostic difficulties in excisional specimens. In one case, fragments of intraductal papilloma embedded in the granulation tissue simulated invasive carcinoma. In a patient with DCIS, small aggregates of tumor cells were found in the granulation tissue, raising the possibility of invasive carcinoma.[11] Similar findings were reported by Youngson and colleagues,[12] who also found displaced epithelial cells in the vascular lymphatic space.

Carter and associates[13] reported a series of 15 cases in which axillary lymph nodes were removed 14 days to 4 months after initial CNB or excisional biopsy for invasive carcinoma or DCIS. In the subcapsular sinusoidal spaces were rare tiny clusters of epithelial cells. In 11 cases, these epithelial cells were judged to be malignant tumor cells. In 4 cases, however, the epithelial cells were considered to be benign, resembling papillary fragments and benign breast glands. These benign and malignant epithelial cells were accompanied by hemosiderin-laden macrophages, foreign body giant cells, and damaged red blood cells. The investigators concluded that CNB or excisional biopsy may cause mechanical transport of benign epithelial cells to the subcapsular region of lymph nodes and that this occurrence has no prognostic significance.

Perhaps most distressing is the failure to find carcinoma in the excision biopsy or mastectomy specimen after FNAC or CNB diagnosis of malignancy. In a study by Casey and associates,[14] 37 women underwent mastectomy for in situ or invasive carcinoma diagnosed by 14-gauge needle CNB. Carcinoma was found in 34 (92%) mastectomy specimens. However, no tumor could be found in the remaining three (8%) specimens. One of the 3 women had a 6- to 8-mm circumscribed colloid carcinoma, a second had a 6- to 9-mm, irregular nodule of tubular carcinoma, and the third had comedo DCIS and abnormal microcalcification on needle biopsy. These events may be explained by (1) the presence of a small lesion that was completely removed by previous biopsy, (2) biopsy-caused inflammatory reaction and tissue necrosis, (3) a false-positive interpretation of biopsy

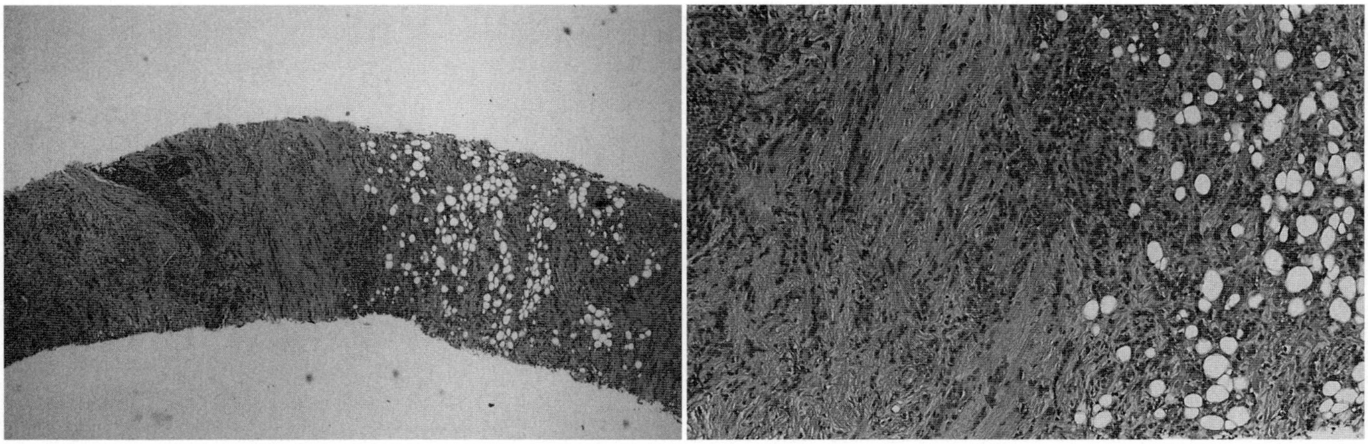

A

B

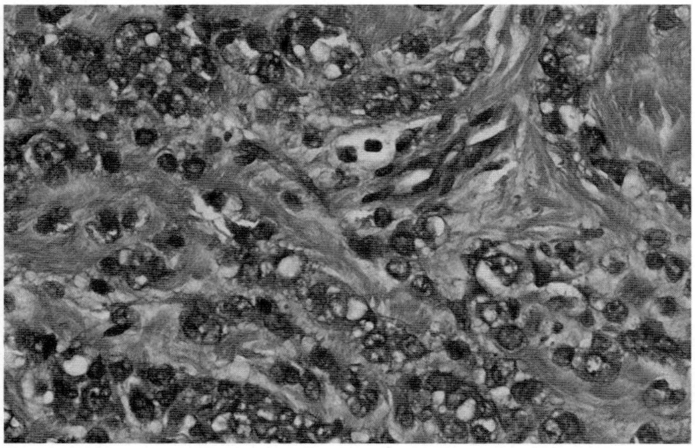

C

Figure 19–3. A, Core needle biopsy specimen of infiltrating ductal carcinoma with tumor cells infiltrating the fibrous breast tissue and adipose tissue. **B,** Higher-magnification view illustrates infiltration of the fat, a useful diagnostic feature for malignancy. **C,** Higher-magnification view shows poorly differentiated tumor cells.

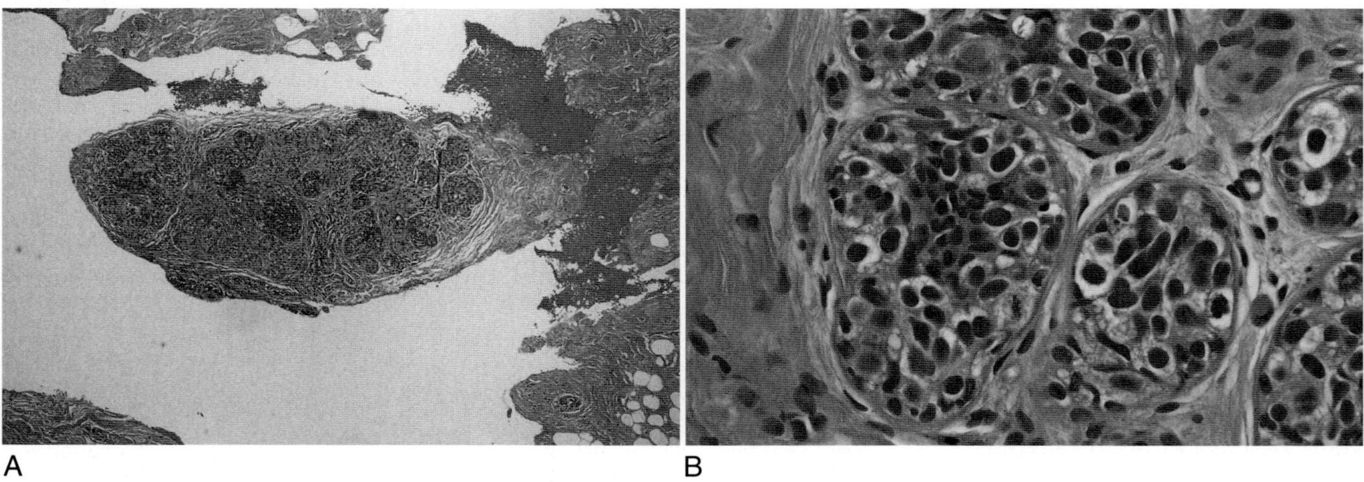

Figure 19–4. A, A fragmented core needle biopsy (CNB) specimen containing a lobule. **B,** Higher-magnification view reveals solid filling of the ductules by large atypical ductal cells and smaller, darker myoepithelial cells, which support the diagnosis of atypical ductal hyperplasia. Subsequent excision confirmed the diagnosis of ductal carcinoma in situ, which was not evident in the CNB specimen.

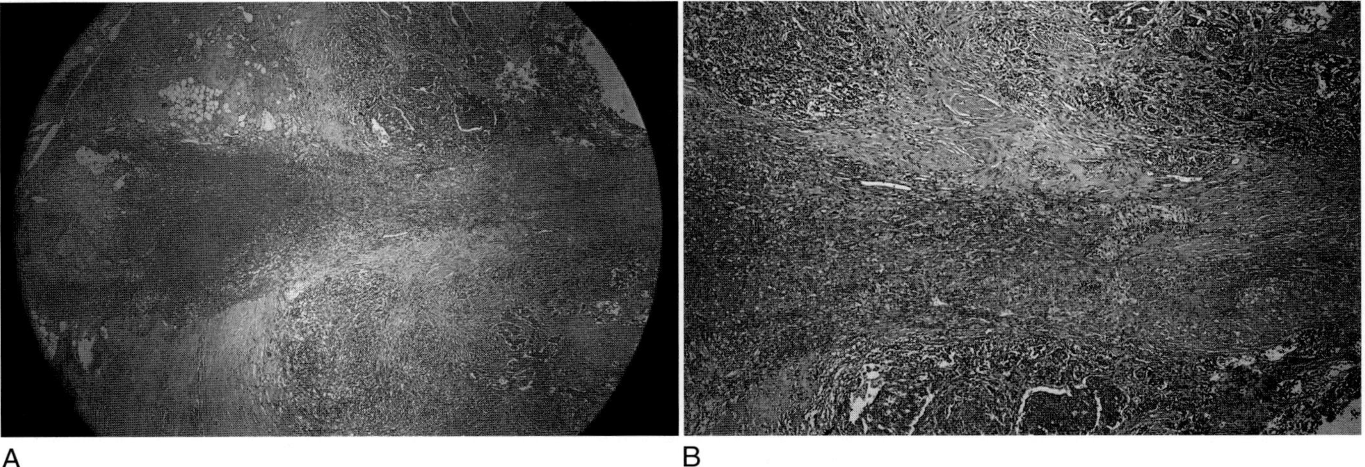

Figure 19–5. **A** and **B,** Needle track of previous core needle biopsy in excised infiltrating ductal carcinoma, showing hemorrhage and granulation tissue.

findings, (4) a mix-up of biopsy specimens in the procedure room, clinic, or laboratory, or (5) an inadequate sampling of mastectomy specimen.[14]

INCISIONAL BIOPSY

An incisional biopsy of the breast is most often performed for a breast mass associated with a skin lesion overlying the breast and nipple erosion. If an inflammatory breast carcinoma is suspected, multiple sections should be prepared. Special stains and immunohistochemical stains are performed as needed to rule out Paget disease.

Excisional Specimens

An excisional specimen should be submitted intact so that surgical borders can be accurately assessed. For best results, the original orientation of the tissues should be indicated by sutures or clips identifying the superior or inferior, medial or lateral, and superficial or deep borders. A J wire is sometimes placed in the area of mammographic abnormality.

Although there are some differences in the handling of excisional specimen for mammographic abnormality and palpable mass, the basic principles are similar. In the pathology laboratory, the specimen is properly oriented by the pathologist. The surface of the specimen is dried, painted with different-colored inks for specific margins, and placed briefly in a Bouin solution to coagulate the ink (Fig. 19–7). The entire specimen is then sectioned serially at 3- to 4-mm intervals. All slices are laid consecutively for inspection and palpation. When a mass or abnormality is identified, its dimensions, gross appearance, relationship with the adjacent tissue, and distance to each excision margin should be recorded. In addition, the lesion characteristics, such as the tumor

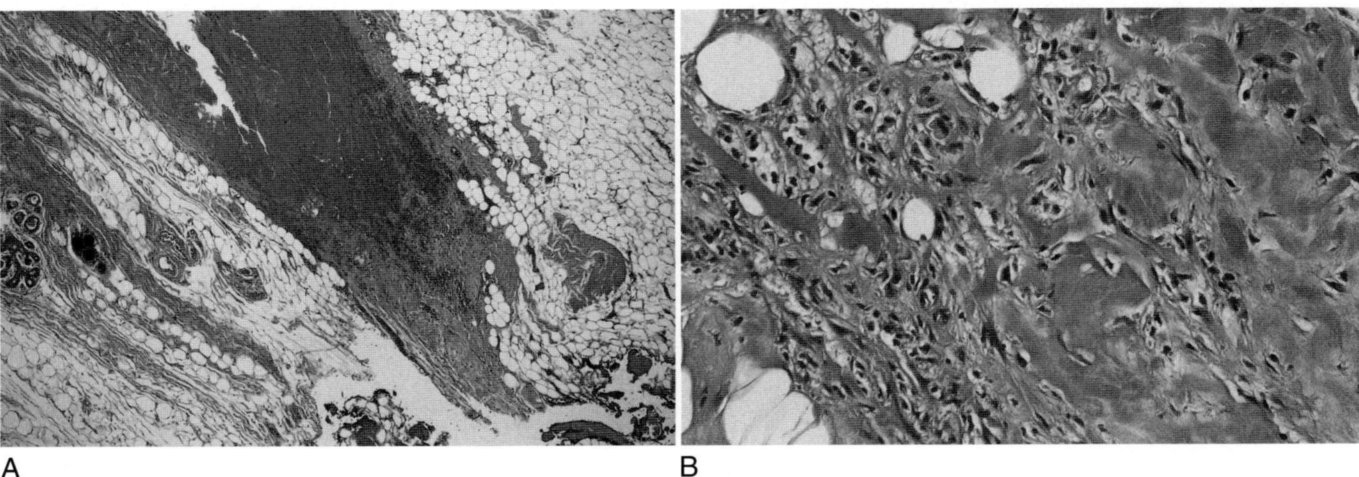

Figure 19–6. **A** and **B,** Excision performed 6 weeks after core needle biopsy reveals hemorrhage, fibroblastic proliferation, and scar tissue.

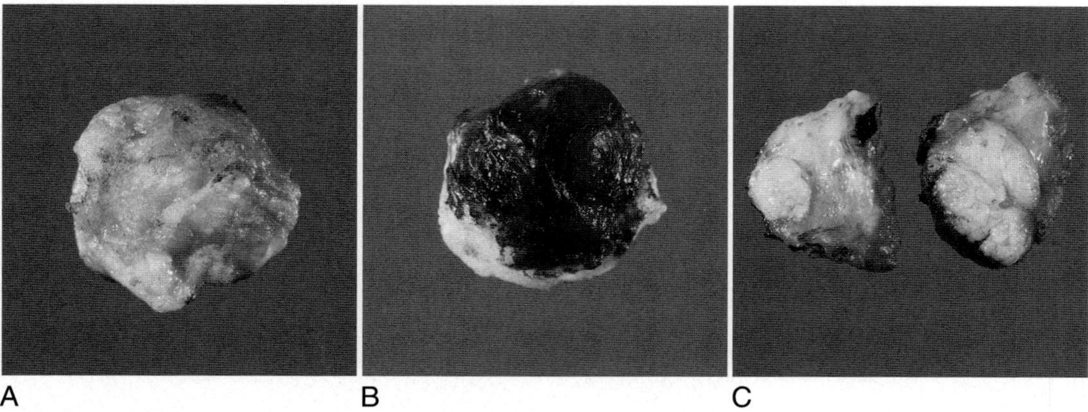

Figure 19–7. **A,** Excision of a palpable mass. **B,** The anterior surface is covered with blue ink, and the posterior margin with red ink (*top*). **C,** Cross-sections show a well-circumscribed fibroadenoma with fibrous stroma and cleftlike spaces.

borders (well-circumscribed, smooth, irregular, or infiltrative), consistency (soft, rubbery, firm, rock hard), and other features (e.g., cyst formation, necrosis, hemorrhage) should be described (Figs. 19–7 and 19–8). The tissue is then placed in paraffin blocks and submitted for histologic examination. The identity of the tissue placed in each cassette is also recorded.

Depending on the institutional policy and surgeon's preference, needle localization specimens are first sent to the radiology department for radiographs to confirm the presence of the lesion and also its completeness of excision. These radiographs are given to the pathologist to enable him or her to sample the abnormal area for histologic sections. Purple, laminated calcifications made up of calcium phosphate can be readily visualized in the section (Fig. 19–9). Calcium oxalate appearing as bright rectangular to irregular crystals is not stained with H & E and can be easily missed without polarized light (Fig. 19–10). These particles are most commonly found in the lumen of cysts and ducts, especially with apocrine metaplasia.[15] In the absence of calcium under polarized light, multiple deeper sections, radiograph of the remaining tissue block, or both become necessary to localize the calcification.

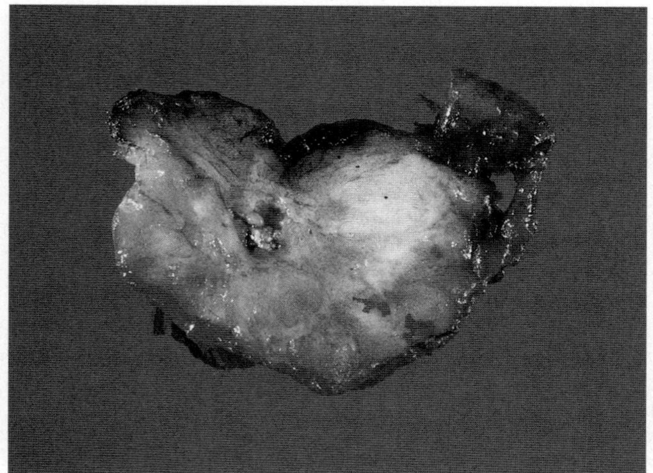

Figure 19–8. Gross appearance of cystic change (*left*) and an ill-defined mass extending to the margin (*blue ink, top*).

Some surgeons may request intraoperative consultation on excised specimen. For lesions smaller than 1 cm, frozen-section examination is not recommended,[16] because obtaining a frozen section may leave insufficient tissue for permanent-section diagnosis. In fact, 12% of cases with a discrepancy between the frozen-section and permanent-section diagnoses can be attributed to obtaining of a frozen section from a small lesion.[17] Furthermore, artifact caused by frozen section often precludes the ability to distinguish between in situ carcinoma and atypical ductal hyperplasia because of homogenization of the chromatin and poor preservation of cellular details.

In this age of cost containment, it is necessary to consider the extent of sampling that should be performed for histologic analysis. In one study, 157 consecutive specimens removed for mammographic abnormalities were studied by submission of the entire specimens for histologic study.[18] This group of cases consisted of 32% carcinomas, 12% atypical hyperplasias, and 56% benign changes without atypia. If only calcified areas were submitted for histologic study, 1 of 50 (2%) carcinomas and 5 of 19 (26%) atypical hyperplasias would have been missed. If areas of calcification and fibrous parenchyma were submitted for histologic analysis, all 50 carcinomas and 17 of 19 (89%) atypical hyperplasias would have been correctly identified. Thus, for specimens excised because of mammographic abnormalities, at least all calcified areas and fibrous parenchyma, with the exception of the surrounding fat tissue, should be submitted for histologic sections.

In another study, 384 specimens were removed because of palpable lesions, including carcinomas (6%) and atypical hyperplasias (0.8%).[19] When the

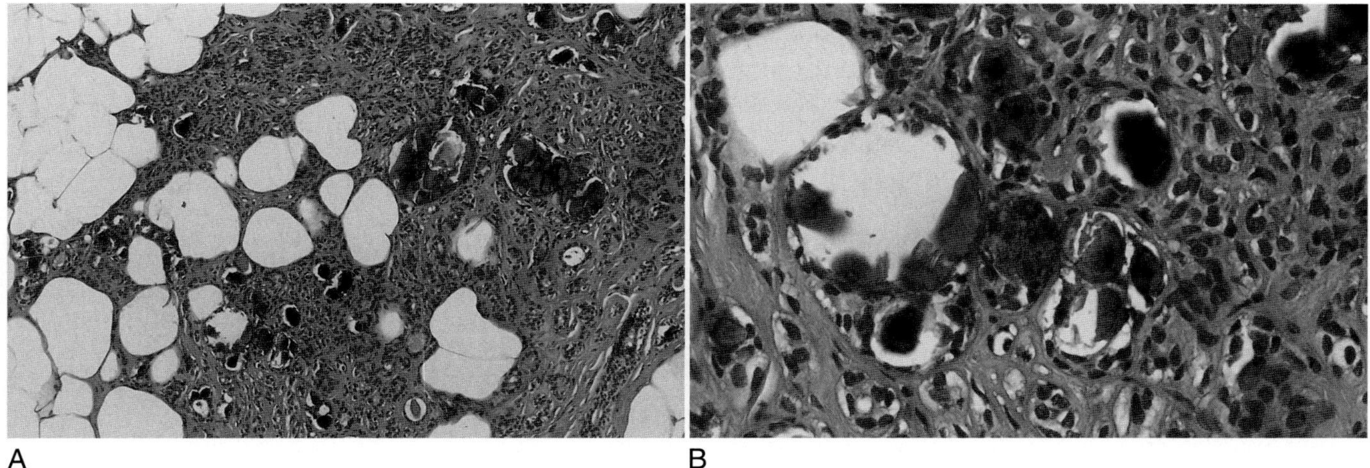

Figure 19–9. **A,** Sclerosing adenosis with multiple microcalcifications. **B,** Higher magnification reveals laminated, purple calcium phosphate.

number of paraffin blocks was limited to 5 per specimen, 23% of carcinomas or atypical hyperplasias were missed. When the number of blocks was increased to 10 per specimen, consisting primarily of fibroglandular tissue, 25 of 26 (96%) carcinomas and atypical hyperplasias were detected. The only tumor not detected was a lobular carcinoma in situ present only in the adipose tissue. The latter study confirmed the importance of submitting fibrous stroma of the breast. Only a small number of in situ carcinomas and atypical hyperplasias would not be detected if the adipose tissue were not examined. Thus, for the specimens excised because of mammographic abnormalities or palpable lesions, all areas with suspicious calcifications and fibroglandular tissue should be submitted for histologic study. Depending on the specimen size, either all or selective parts of the adipose tissue should be submitted.

Reexcision and Segmental Specimens

Segmental specimens and specimens obtained with reexcision are processed in the same manner as described earlier for excisional specimens. Orientation of the specimen with sutures is highly desirable. After the exterior surface is marked with India ink, the specimen is fixed and sectioned serially at 3- to 4-mm intervals. Frozen-section diagnosis may be performed for residual tumor and surgical margins. When residual tumor is identified, its dimensions and character are recorded. In addition, the relationship of residual tumor to the specimen margins, overlying skin, and nipple should be noted.

Abraham and coworkers[20] investigated the extent of sampling for histologic study in 97 consecutive reexcision specimens for in situ or invasive carcinoma. When totally embedded, 47 specimens contained in

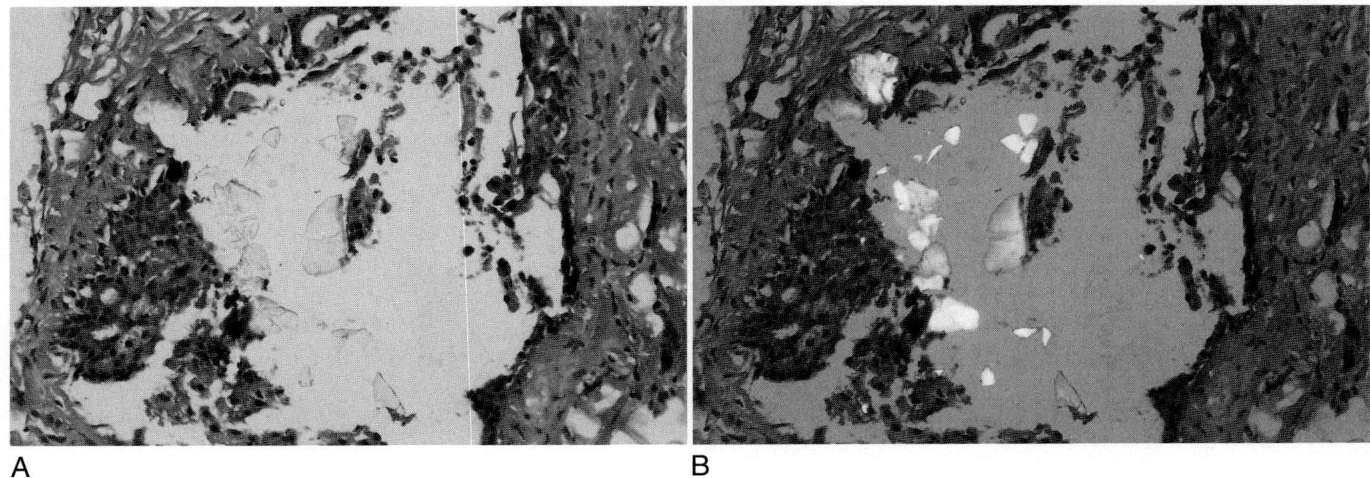

Figure 19–10. **A,** Calcium oxalate crystals in a cystic space do not react with hematoxylin and eosin stain. **B,** Under polarized light, crystals are readily detected.

situ or invasive carcinoma. The pathologic findings resulted in major changes in patient management (additional surgery) in 30 (64%) cases, minor modifications in radiation dose or chemotherapy regimen in 10 (21%) cases, and no change in management in 7 (15%) cases. When only one block per centimeter of specimen was submitted for histologic study, the results were 52% fewer paraffin blocks taken, detection of 88% of cases with major changes in therapy, and detection of 81% of all cases with major or minor changes. When two blocks were submitted per centimeter of specimen, 97% of cases with major changes in management and 95% of all cases with management changes were detected. This study reaffirms the importance of adequate sampling for histologic analysis.

Microscopic Evaluation of Surgical Margins on Excisional and Reexcision Specimens

The status of surgical margins in excisional and reexcision specimens is usually reported as positive, negative, or close to tumor. A *positive margin* indicates the presence of tumor cells at the inked margin. A *negative margin* indicates failure to find tumor cells at the inked margin (Fig. 19–11). When the tumor is close to the margin, its distance should be specified, such as less than 1 mm, 1 to 2 mm, and so on. In some instances, the margins cannot be determined with certainty because of cautery artifact (see Fig. 19–11). Unfortunately, multiple problems exist in reporting excision margins, as exemplified by the finding of residual carcinoma in reexcision specimens in 51% to 69% of cases with positive margins and in 26% to 33% with negative margins.[21-25]

Common problems include irregular, complex excision surfaces subject to sampling error and laboratory variation in handling specimens, submission of more than one fragment without orientation, and lack of uniform definition for terminology used. The effects of surgery, such as tissue necrosis and repair, may explain the finding of no residual tumor in a re-excision specimen with a previous positive margin. Complex three-dimensional ductal structures involved by multicentric or multifocal carcinoma in situ can also explain the false-negative results (Fig. 19–12).[26]

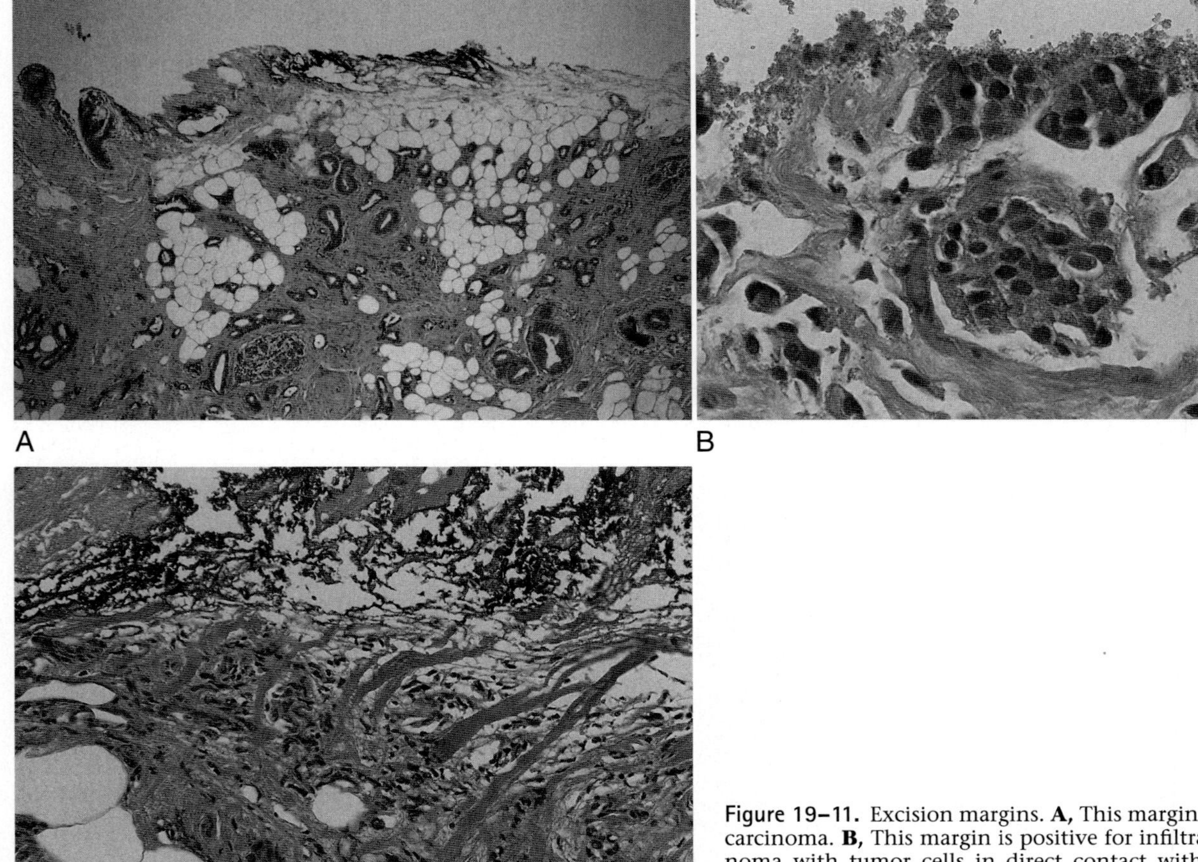

Figure 19–11. Excision margins. **A,** This margin is clear of tubular carcinoma. **B,** This margin is positive for infiltrating ductal carcinoma with tumor cells in direct contact with yellow ink (*top*; borders on white space). **C,** This margin is positive for infiltrating lobular carcinoma. Tumor cells with cautery artifact are in contact with blue ink (*top*; darker outlines).

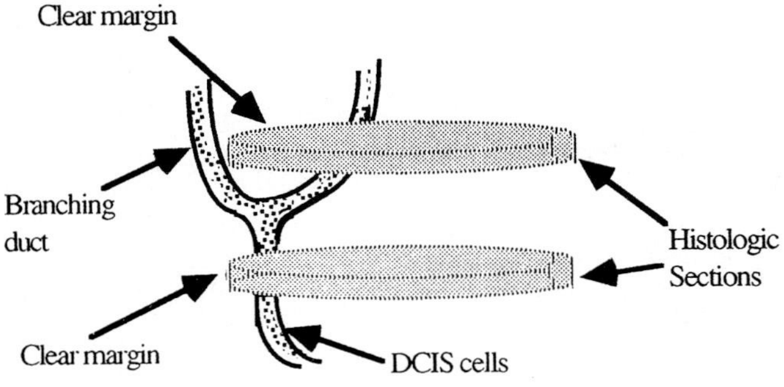

Figure 19–12. The complex branching of the duct system can lead to errors in histologic evaluation of the margins of intraductal cancers. For example, in this illustration of extensive ductal carcinoma in situ, the histologic sections would show a clear margin despite the presence of tumor in the branching duct beyond the surgical specimen.

Finally, ink flows from the surface to underlying tissue through defects on the surface caused by surgery, pathologic examination, or cysts. Thus, the presence of ink alone is not necessarily indicative of a positive margin.[27,28] This concept is particularly important for the pathologist at another institution who has not personally examined the original specimen. Any question or disagreement should be communicated to the original pathologist for clarification.

The surgeon can counteract the preceding limitations by submitting separate specimens from different margins.

MASTECTOMY SPECIMENS

All mastectomy specimens, especially those without axillary contents, must be marked for orientation by the surgeon. The descriptions before sectioning should include the dimensions of the breast and skin, changes in the nipple and skin, tissue on the deep margin, and axillary content. The breast tissue is sliced from the deep margin to the skin at 1- to 2-cm intervals. Previous biopsy site, surgical cavity, residual tumor, and any additional lesions are recorded and submitted for histologic confirmation. Routine sections should also include nipple, resection margins, and representative sections from each quadrant.

Axillary Lymph Node Dissection

The axillary lymph nodes are part of the modified radical mastectomy specimen or are received separately when breast-conserving surgery has been performed. In some cases, surgeons may isolate lymph nodes from a particular region, such as the apex, and submit them separately. After proper orientation, the lymph nodes are divided into proximal third, middle third, and distal third. The fat pad is sliced to identify lymph nodes by palpation and inspection. Small lymph nodes are submitted entirely with or without bisection. Larger lymph nodes are sliced at 2- to 3-mm intervals and submitted entirely or in representative sections, depending on institutional policy. When more than one lymph node is placed in a cassette, different lymph nodes can be distinguished with colored ink.

In the pathology report, the number of involved lymph nodes and the anatomic location and the maximal dimension of metastasis are described for the purpose of prognosis and staging of the tumor. Extracapsular involvement by the tumor, when present, should be described, defined, and reported; some investigators believe that extracapsular involvement adversely affects the prognosis.

Axillary Sentinel Lymph Node Sampling

Axillary sentinel lymph node sampling for breast carcinoma after the injection of blue dye or a radioactive substance at the primary site has gained popularity. These lymph nodes are frequently submitted at the time of surgery for detection of metastasis by frozen section, cytologic examination, or both.[29,30] If the sentinel node is negative for tumor, the probability of finding tumor in non-sentinel nodes is only 1%. If the sentinel node is positive for tumor, 18% to 38% of patients have additional metastases, thereby justifying axillary lymph node dissection (Fig. 19–13).[31] Questions remain about the accuracy of intraoperative diagnosis by frozen-section diagnosis and cytologic evaluations of sentinel nodes.

Turner and colleagues[32] reported using both frozen section and imprint cytology on the sentinel node at intraoperative pathologic consultation. The lymph node was bisected along the longitudinal plane. If the width of the sentinel node exceeded 6 to 8 mm, additional cuts were made at 2- to 3-mm intervals. Frozen sections were cut at two levels. The first was made after minimal trimming. Nine additional frozen sections were made for molecular studies. A second frozen section was then prepared. Permanent sections were cut at two to four levels, including immunohistochemical staining for keratin. The accuracy of frozen section and imprint cytology combined was 79%, compared with the final diagnosis based on immunohistochemical (IHC) staining for keratin. Thus, the false-negative rate for this combined approach was 21%.[32]

Immunohistochemical staining for keratin is routinely performed for sentinel lymph nodes to detect rare tumor cells that are not easily detectable on sections routinely stained with H & E. In a study of 278 women undergoing axillary sentinel node biopsies, metastasis was detected in 72 (25.9%) women through routine H & E staining of slides. Through immunohistochemical staining for keratin, an additional 14% of metastases were detected in 39

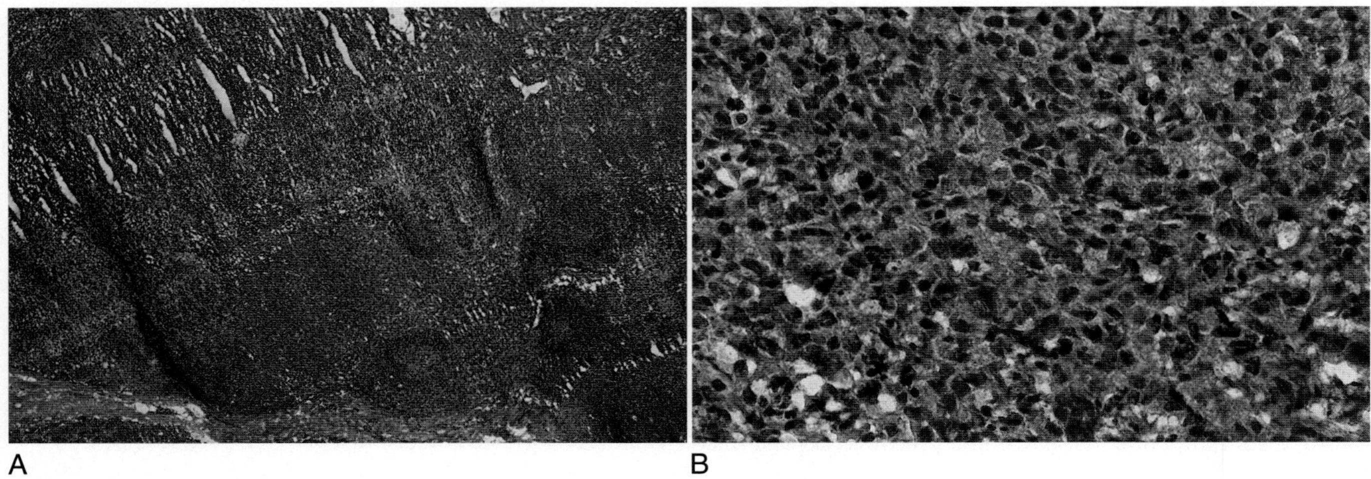

Figure 19–13. A, Frozen section of a sentinel lymph node with a metastasis beneath the capsule. **B,** Higher-magnification view demonstrates sheets of tumor cells with irregular nuclei.

women, making the total positive rate 39.9%. In other words, 35% of metastases in sentinel nodes would have been missed if immunohistochemical staining for keratin had not been performed (Fig. 19–14).[32]

Turner and colleagues[33] recommend that sentinel nodes submitted for permanent section be cut at two levels at 40-μm intervals for H & E staining and IHC staining for keratin. Additional cuts at 3 to 10 levels detected only two (4%) metastatic sentinel nodes from one patient (3%) and, thus, is not recommended.

It should be remembered that sentinel node biopsy requires surgical expertise. Ninety percent to 95% of sentinel nodes can be identified with training and experience. There are occasional skip metastases in about 1% of cases in which sentinel node biopsy is performed; in this situation, tumor cells may pass through the lymph node or in the vicinity of the sentinel node without being detected. Rare patients may have hematogenous spread of tumor without lymph node metastasis. Finally, there is no uniform handling of sentinel nodes among the pathologists, such as the number of sections and levels prepared, and the accuracy of interpretation varies. At least two levels of permanent sections for H & E stain and an immunohistochemical stain for keratin are recommended for all sentinel nodes.[33,34] Reverse transcriptase–polymerase chain reaction technique for messenger RNA of structural proteins and enzymes from tumor cells appears to be too sensitive for clinical use. Many cases were reported to be positive in studies evaluating the technique, but no tumor cells could be found on histologic examination.

Is it possible to use sentinel node sampling technique after neoadjuvant chemotherapy? To answer this question, Cohen and associates[35] conducted sentinel node mapping in 38 women with stage II or III breast cancer who had been treated with neoadjuvant chemotherapy. All lymph nodes were studied on three slides with H & E stain and one slide with IHC stain for keratin. In 82% (31 of 38) of patients, sentinel lymph nodes were identified. The accuracy of sentinel node sampling in predicting axillary lymph node status was 90% (28/31). The overall sensitivity was 83%, specificity 100%, positive predictive value 100%, and negative predictive value 81%. The researchers concluded that in breast cancer patients undergoing neoadjuvant therapy, sentinel node mapping can accurately determine status of axillary lymph nodes.[35]

When radioactive material is used for sentinel node sampling, 0.4 to 1.0 mCi of ^{99m}Tc sulfur colloid is typically used. The half-life is 6 hours, and radiation levels decrease to background levels after 60 hours. Because of very low radiation exposure for laboratory staff, it is not necessary to delay the handling of sentinel lymph nodes for intraoperative consultation and frozen-section examination. Whether there is a need for quarantine of the primary tumor excision specimen should be determined by the institutional radiation safety officer.[36]

IMMUNOHISTOCHEMISTRY AND SPECIALIZED TECHNIQUE

Immunohistochemical staining for breast diseases is used (1) to aid in pathologic diagnosis, (2) to improve prognostication and prediction of therapeutic responses, and (3) to investigate breast cancer. These staining procedures are routinely performed in pathology laboratories and are suitable for formalin-fixed, paraffin-embedded tissue sections as well as for

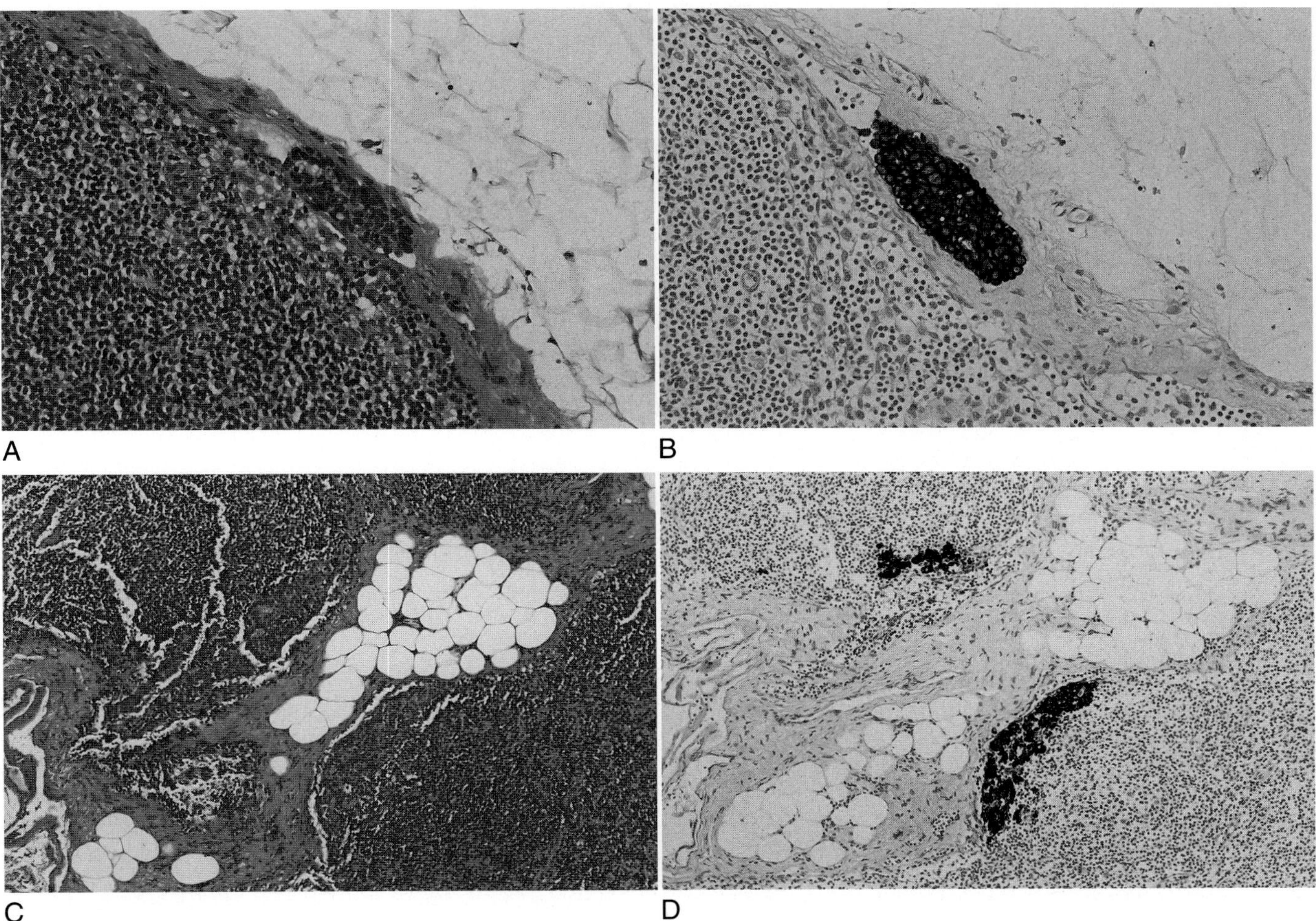

Figure 19–14. **A,** Permanent section stained with hematoxylin and eosin (H & E) reveals a cluster of tumor cells in the capsular lymphatic space. **B,** Immunohistochemical stain confirms keratin-positive tumor cells with brown immunoreactivity (appearing here as a *dark area*) in the cytoplasm. **C,** Two small foci of metastasis in the subcapsular region do not demonstrate any tissue reaction and can be easily missed on this H & E–stained section. **D,** Immunohistochemical stain for keratin confirms the presence of tumor cells with brown cytoplasm (appearing here as *dark areas*).

cells in FNA specimens and body fluids. Archival paraffin blocks prepared many years earlier are also suitable for IHC assay.

Pathologic Diagnosis

In the differential diagnoses of ADH versus DCIS and of atypical lobular hyperplasia (ALH) versus lobular carcinoma in situ (LCIS), immunohistochemical stains for S-100 protein and smooth muscle actin are valuable. These stains identify myoepithelial cells, which are found beneath the benign ductal and lobular epithelial cells, such as ductal hyperplasia and sclerosing adenosis. In ADH, myoepithelial cells are reduced in number but persist. In DCIS, the proliferating cells are homogeneous without myoepithelial cells. Myoepithelial cells are limited to the periphery of the ducts (Fig. 19–15). Similarly, myoepithelial cells remain in ALH but are largely absent in LCIS. In invasive ductal carcinoma as well, myoepithelial cells are absent, a finding useful to distinguish tubular carcinoma from sclerosing and microglandular adenosis (Fig. 19–16).

When there is difficulty in determining ductal or lobular carcinoma, immunohistochemical stain for E-cadherin is useful. The cell adhesion molecule E-cadherin regulates cell-to-cell adhesion, polarization, and interaction with adjacent stroma. In a study of E-cadherin reactivity of noninvasive ductal and lobular lesions, all 37 DCIS lesions had strong E-cadherin reactivity, compared with only 2 (9%) of 22 LCIS lesions.[37] In another study, all 33 invasive ductal carcinomas had a membranous staining for E-cadherin, and all 15 infiltrating lobular carcinomas did not.[38]

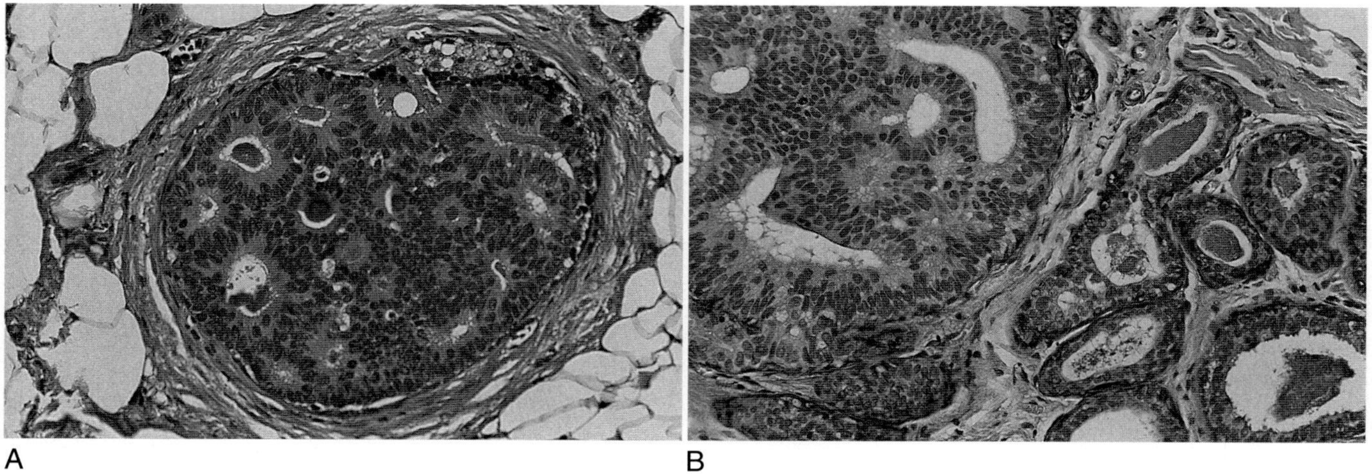

A B

Figure 19–15. **A,** Cribriform ductal carcinoma in situ. **B,** Immunohistochemical stain for smooth muscle actin reveals a complete layer of myoepithelial cells in the area of ductal hyperplasia (*right field*). In contrast, the area of ductal carcinoma in situ shows only a few myoepithelial cells remaining in the periphery of the duct.

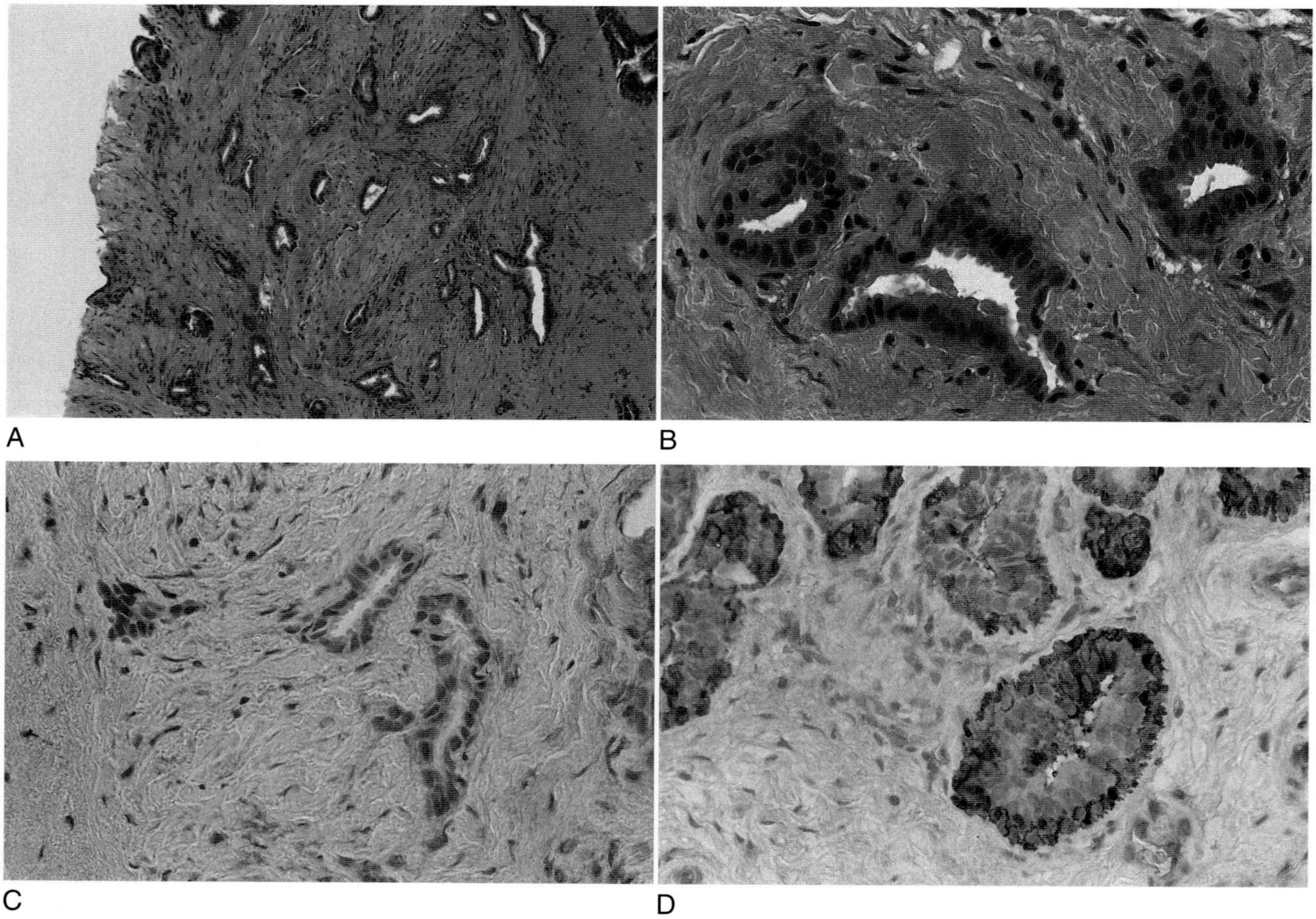

A B

C D

Figure 19–16. **A,** A well-differentiated tubular carcinoma in a core needle biopsy specimen. **B,** Higher-magnification view reveals irregular glands lined by a layer of tall columnar cells with only minimal nuclear atypia. **C,** Immunohistochemical stain for smooth muscle demonstrates no myoepithelial cells to confirm the diagnosis of tubular carcinoma. **D,** In benign ductal hyperplasia and sclerosing adenosis, abundant myoepithelial cells are present.

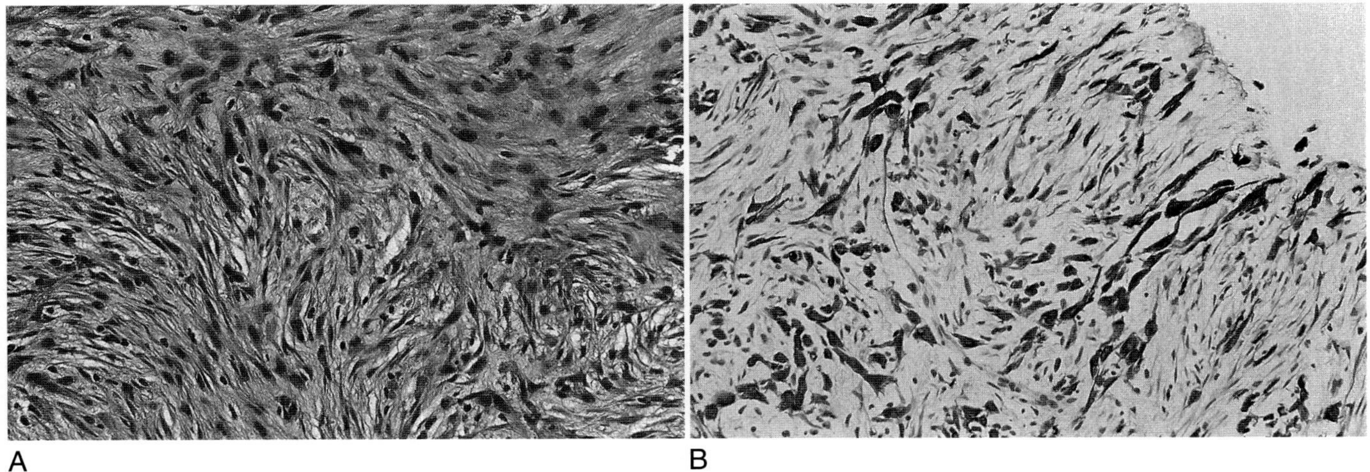

Figure 19–17. A, This breast mass consists of tumor cells with elongated nuclei suggestive of fibrosarcoma. **B,** Immunohistochemical stain of tumor cells for keratin is positive, confirming their epithelial origin and thus the diagnosis of metaplastic spindle cell carcinoma.

Immunohistochemical stain for keratin is useful to separate metaplastic spindle cell carcinoma from various sarcomas (Fig. 19–17). Endothelial cell markers and factor VIII are used to confirm angiosarcoma.

Prognostication and Prediction of Therapeutic Responses

IHC stains are used for estrogen receptor (ER), progesterone receptor (PR), and HER-2/neu oncogene to improve prognostication and to predict therapeutic responses. Currently, IHC assay for ER and PR has replaced the earlier ligand-binding biochemical assay, which requires immediate deep-freeze of fresh tissue. Most laboratories use commercially available monoclonal antibodies for IHC assay of ER and PR. There is no uniform standard for scoring and reporting the results. Most laboratories report percentage of positively responding tumor cells and arbitrarily use 10% immunoreactivity as the cutoff (Fig. 19–18). Ideally the cutoff for the IHC assay should be calibrated by clinical outcome or biochemical assay.[39] The agreement between biochemical and IHC assays is 90% or higher.

Sixty percent to 70% of invasive breast carcinomas express ER on biochemical or IHC assay. The expression of ER is a weak, favorable prognostic indicator for women not receiving adjuvant therapy, as indicated by a 10% difference in 5-year disease-free survival rates for women with ER-positive and ER-negative tumors. In contrast, ER status has a much stronger predictive value for women receiving endocrine therapy for metastatic disease. Women whose breast cancer is ER-positive have a 60% overall response rate, and a 30% higher 5-year disease-free survival rate compared with those whose breast cancer is ER-negative. Women with ER-positive tumors have an average of 20% to 30% lower recurrence or mortality rate with adjuvant endocrine therapy. Thus, the prognostic value of ER on IHC assay is widely accepted.[40]

ER and PR detections are often performed together because of the added predictive value of PR status. In the earlier studies using biochemical assays, the response rates for women with metastatic breast cancer receiving endocrine therapy were 77% if both ER and PR responses were positive, 27% if the ER response was positive and the PR response negative, 46% if the ER response was negative and the PR response positive, and 11% if both ER and PR responses were negative. Later studies using IHC assay found the 5-year disease-free survival rates to be 20% higher if the PR response is positive, confirming PR as a useful predictor for endocrine therapy response.[40]

ER evaluation by IHC detects primarily ER-α. In one study, ER-β has been detected by IHC in 17% of all breast cancers and 47% of ER-negative tumors. Although there was no correlation with overall survival rates, women with ER-β–positive tumors receiving adjuvant therapy with tamoxifen were found to have better survival, among both node-positive and node-negative women, compared with women with ER-β–negative tumors.[41]

HER-2/neu oncogene is located on chromosome 17q12-21.32, encoding a 185-kilodalton (kd) transmembrane protein (p185). It has 50% homology with epidermal growth factor in the tyrosine kinase receptor family. Since Slamon and associates[42] reported the relationship of HER-2/neu amplification and breast cancer prognosis in 1987, additional studies have addressed this issue.

Currently, IHC stains for HER-2/neu oncogene are based on commercially available antibodies, only a

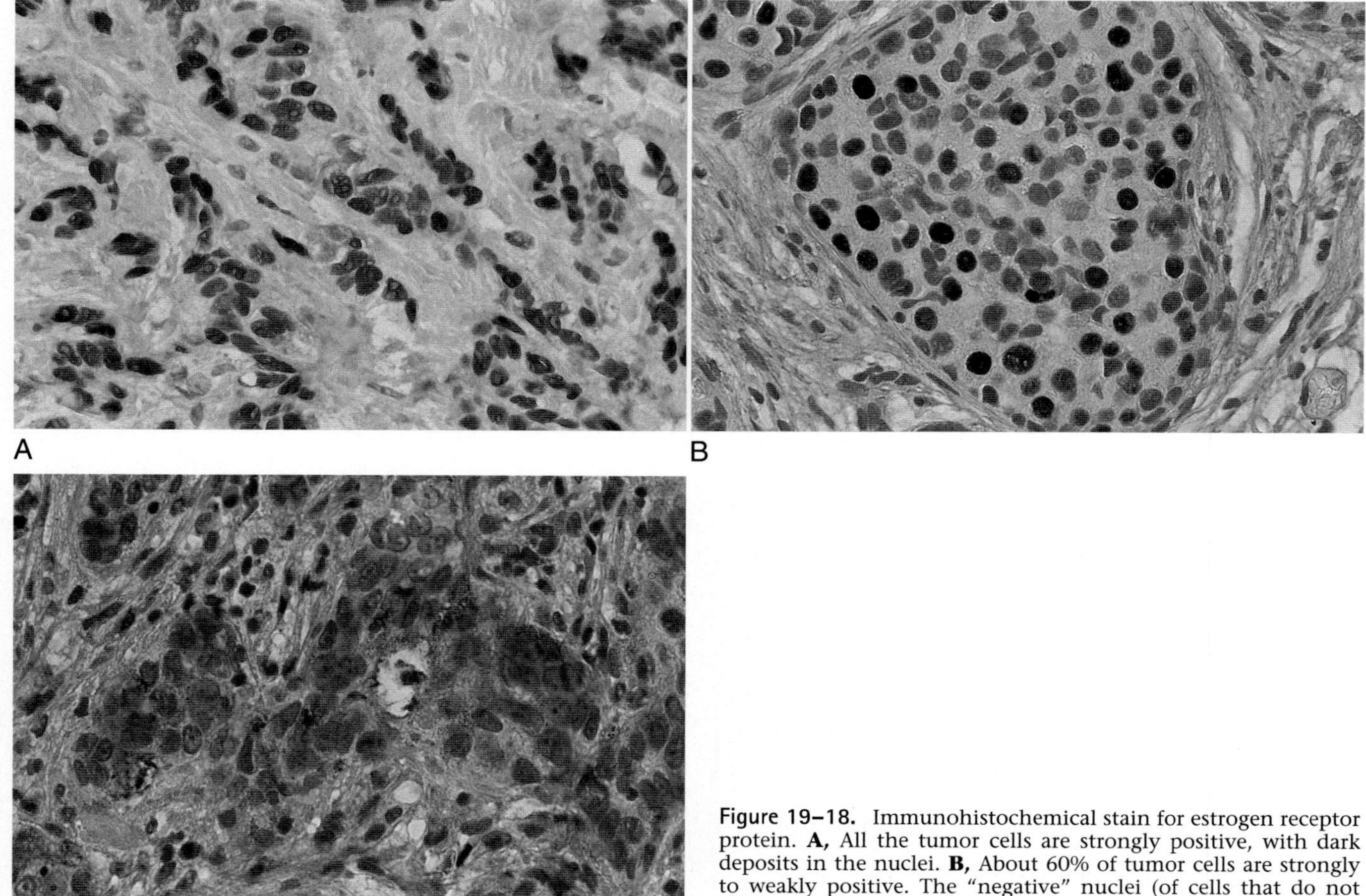

Figure 19–18. Immunohistochemical stain for estrogen receptor protein. **A,** All the tumor cells are strongly positive, with dark deposits in the nuclei. **B,** About 60% of tumor cells are strongly to weakly positive. The "negative" nuclei (of cells that do not contain the protein) do not stain. **C,** Tumor cells are entirely negative.

few of which are approved by the U.S. Food and Drug Administration (FDA). HercepTest is based on an FDA-approved polyclonal antibody manufactured by DakoCytomation. The immunoreactivity is scored by the intensity and quantity of membranous staining. Immunoreactivity of 2+ or 3+ is indicative of HER-2/neu over-expression (positive), whereas a score of 0 or 1+ is considered negative (Fig. 19–19). The alternative method is fluorescent in-situ hybridization (FISH), which is suitable for cells in frozen section, permanent tissue section, or cytologic smears. Polymerase chain reaction (PCR) is used by only a minority of investigators.[43]

Review of literature shows that the prognostic significance of HER-2/neu over-expression in node-negative breast cancers has remained controversial.[44,45] Some of the discrepant results are probably related to the different methodologies used by the investigators. Press and colleagues,[46] using the FISH method on archival paraffin-embedded "node-negative" breast cancers, found HER-2/neu amplification to be a significant predictor of early and late relapse and of disease-related death independent of tumor size, tumor grade, and ER status. The prognostic significance of HER-2/neu in node-negative breast cancers evaluated by IHC was less consistent among the studies. In addition to the two entirely different technologies, there are also issues of interpretation and laboratory consistency.

For "node-positive" breast cancers, the majority of studies have found that HER-2/neu over-expression correlates with progressive disease and is an indicator of likely response to therapy (i.e., cancers are resistant to cyclophosphamide, methotrexate, 5-fluorouracil, hormonal therapy, and radiotherapy but sensitive to doxorubicin [Adriamycin]).[44,45]

For women with HER-2/neu–amplified tumors, Slamon and colleagues[47] reported the use of Herceptin (trastuzumab) in combination with paclitaxel alone or anthracycline plus cyclophosphamide to slow tumor progression, reduce tumor size, and improve response to chemotherapy. There was no tumor progression in 28% of women treated with Herceptin and chemotherapy, compared with 14% of women treated with chemotherapy alone.

There is a strong correlation between IHC and FISH for negative (immunoreactivity 0 to 1+) and strongly immunoreactive (3+) tumors in the range of 98%.

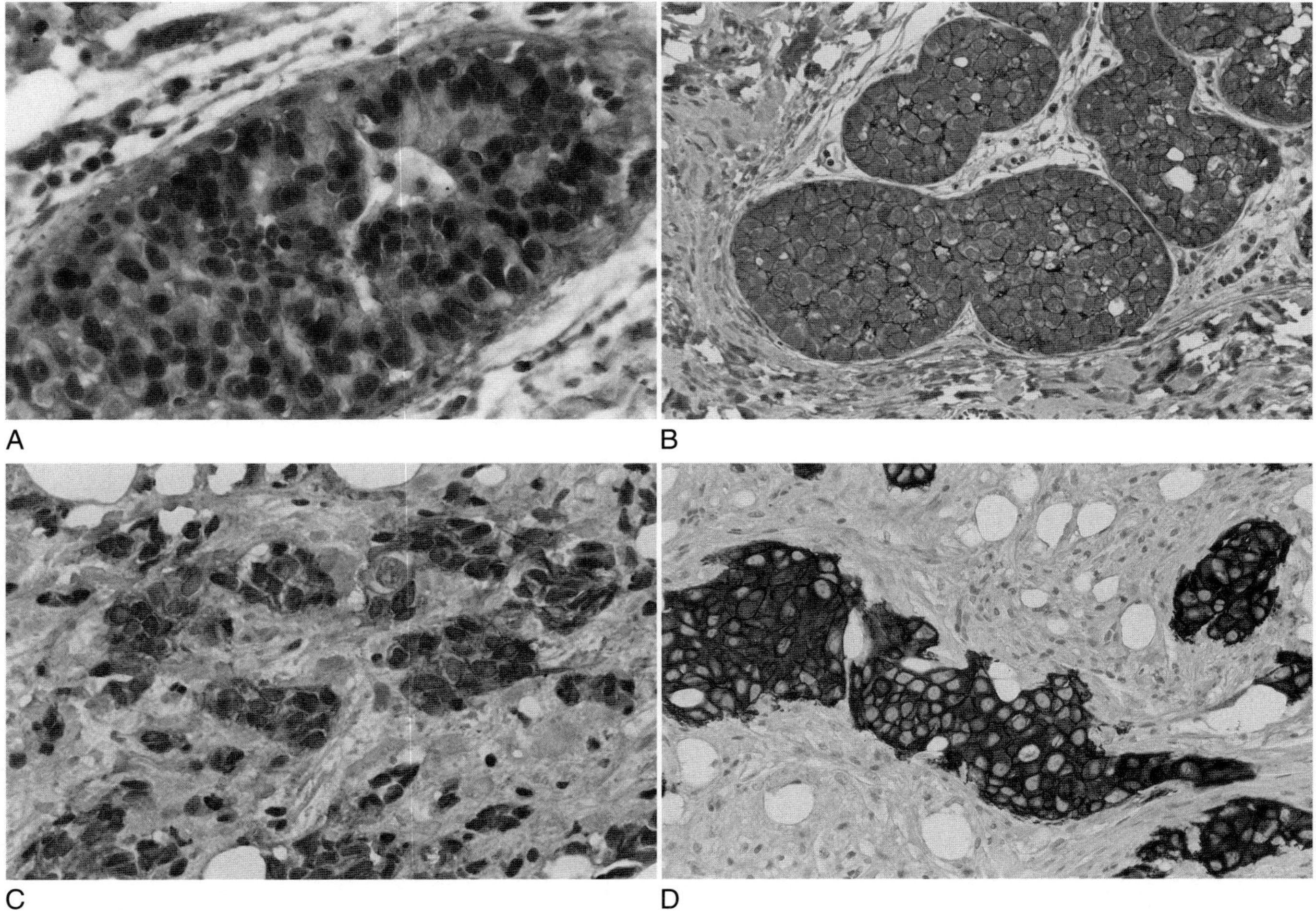

Figure 19–19. Immunohistochemical stain for HER-2/neu oncogene (HercepTest). **A,** No immunoreactivity. **B,** Immunoreactivity 1+ with a faint membranous staining in part of the membrane, not indicative of over-expression of the oncogene. **C,** Immunoreactivity 2+ with a moderate complete membranous staining in more than 10% of tumor cells, indicative of over-expression, according to the instructions given by the test manufacturer, DakoCytomation. **D,** Immunoreactivity 3+ with strong, complete membranous staining (appearing here as *dark areas*) in most tumor cells, indicative of over-expression.

However, Ridolfi and coworkers reported that only 36% of tumors with 2+ immunoreactivity were amplified by FISH.[48] With FISH amplification, 40 nuclei were analyzed from two different areas of tumor. A mean signal count of greater than four was considered to be amplified.[48] Apparently, some of the tumors with 2+ immunoreactivity have low gene copies, three to four per nucleus, resulting from chromosome 17 polysomy (polyploidy) rather than amplification of HER-2/neu.[49] When immunoreactivity is 2+ on IHC, further study with FISH is recommended to determine HER-2/neu amplification status.

HER-2/neu over-expression is correlated with the Bloom-Richardson histologic grade of ductal carcinoma. It is positive in 34% of grade 3, 11.4% of grade 2, and 3.2% of grade 1 tumors, as well as in 3.2% of lobular carcinomas.[48]

Investigation of Breast Cancer

Most studies report poor prognosis with p53 mutation for women with both "node-negative" and "node-positive" tumors.[40] IHC for p53 is particularly useful in identifying high-risk cases. Of 107 women with "node-negative" breast cancers, tumors testing positive for p53 and HER-2/neu were associated with lower overall survival and disease-free survival rates. O'Malley and associates[50] found these two parameters to be the most important prognostic variables on multivariate analysis. In their study, p53 was determined by PCR technique and HER-2/neu by IHC using monoclonal antibody CB11.[50]

In a study by Rudolph and coworkers,[51] 261 invasive breast cancers were studied by IHC for HER-2/neu, p53, and the proliferative cell nuclear antigen Ki-67. A monoclonal antibody, Ki-S2, detecting S and

G2M cells was used to determine cycling ratio (CR). Tumors with positive p53 and HER-2/neu had high CR. Univariate analysis showed tumor size, ER and PR status, Bloom-Richardson grade, HER-2/neu and Ki-67 responses, and CR to be significant predictors of outcome. A multivariate model revealed CR to be the most important independent predictor of overall and disease-free survivals.

The prognostic value of flow cytometry for DNA ploidy pattern was investigated by Bergers and colleagues[52] in 1301 freshly frozen breast cancer specimens. Although diploid versus non-diploid pattern was a significant predictor of both overall survival and disease-free survival, it failed to improve the prognostic power of lymph node status and tumor size on multivariate analysis.

Report for Breast Cancer Specimens

For mammographically detected lesions with calcifications, the pathology report should indicate whether microcalcifications are identified in the histologic sections. Table 19–1 lists pathologic findings in breast cancer that should be included in the pathology report. When in situ carcinoma and invasive carcinoma coexist, the percentage of each component should be mentioned; this finding is especially important in a small tumor. The grading method used should be specified. The Bloom-Richardson (Elston Modified) grading method, based on tubular formation (T), nuclear pleomorphism (N), and mitotic counts (M), has been widely accepted. In the evaluation of surgical margins, *positive margins* refers to the presence of tumor cells on the inked border. When the tumor cells are close to the margin, the distance is expressed as numbers of low-power or high-power microscopic fields or in millimeters. We have found it useful to use a checklist to ensure uniformity of reporting, especially in a teaching institution with multiple trainees and staff members. Data necessary for staging should be included if available.

Quality control is a critical element of laboratory operation. In a study of more than 1000 major breast specimens at a teaching hospital, the pathologic findings by the resident and faculty staff were compared. The faculty identified major errors in 5% of the specimens. The most common errors were failure to detect cancers, lymph node metastasis, and skin involvement.[53] This study emphasizes the importance of meticulous inspection of the specimens and a close collaboration of all laboratory staff.

SUMMARY

This chapter describes the proper handling of different specimens to achieve high accuracy and to optimize clinical management of breast cancer patients.

Table 19–1. Checklist for Reporting Invasive Breast Cancer Specimens

1. Tumor size
2. Tumor character: gross appearance, tumor borders, texture
3. Location: central, specific quadrant, not stated
4. Histologic type:
   - Infiltrating ductal carcinoma, specify type
   - Infiltrating lobular carcinoma
   - If in situ carcinoma present, specify type and percent of tumor area
5. Bloom/Richardson (Elston Modification) Grading Method:*

Tubular Formation	Score
>75%	1
10%-75%	2
<10%	3
Nuclear Pleomorphism	**Score**
Small and uniform	1
Moderate variation in size and shape	2
Marked variation in size and shape	3
Mitotic Counts (per 10 high power fields)	**Score**
Field diameter 0.44 mm/0.152 mm^2:	
Low (0-5 mitotic figures)	1
Moderate (6-10 mitotic figures)	2
High (>11 mitotic figures)	3
Field diameter 0.59 mm/0.274 mm^2:	
Low (0-9 mitotic figures)	1
Moderate (10-19 mitotic figures)	2
High (> 20 mitotic figures)	3
Final Grade	**Score**
Grade I, well-differentiated	3-5 points
Grade II, moderately differentiated	6-7 points
Grade III, poorly differentiated	8-9 points

6. Necrosis in infiltrative component: absent, present
7. Lymphoplasmacytic response: absent, mild, moderate, marked
8. Vascular, lymphatic invasion: absent, present
9. Nipple, skin, muscle involvement: absent, present
10. Other diseases of breast: atypical hyperplasia, papilloma, Paget's disease
11. Surgical margins:
    - Positive for tumor
    - Negative for tumor: Specify clear within one high-, low-power field or within millimeters
12. Axillary lymph node status:
    - Total number examined
    - Number and location of metastasis
    - Specify if extracapsular extension present
13. Estrogen and progesterone receptors, HER-2/neu, flow DNA ploidy
14. Ductal carcinoma in situ; if present, specify:
    - Nuclear grade: high, intermediate, low
    - Architectural type: cribriform, micropapillary, papillary, solid
    - Necrosis: present, absent
    - Calcification: present, absent
    - Surgical margins: negative, positive, close
15. TNM staging:†

    T = Tumor
    - Tis: in situ
    - T1: ≤2 cm
    - T2: 2-5 cm
    - T3: >5 cm
    - T4: chest wall/skin involvement

    N = Nodes
    - N0: no metastasis
    - N1: movable axillary metastasis
    - N2: fixed axillary metastasis
    - N3: internal mammary metastasis

    M = Metastases
    - M0: no distant metastases
    - M1: distant metastases, including to ipsilateral supraclavicular lymph nodes

*See Elston CW, Ellis IO: Pathological prognostic factors in breast cancer. I: The value of histological grade in breast cancer: Experience from a large study with long-term follow-up. Histopathology 1991;5:403-410.

†See American Joint Committee on Cancer: Breast. In Beahrs OH, Henson DE, Hutter RVP, Kennedy BJ (eds): Manual for Staging of Cancer, 4th ed. Philadelphia, JB Lippincott, 1992, pp 149, 150.

References

1. Connolly JL, Schnitt SJ: Evaluation of breast biopsy specimens in patients considered for treatment by conservative surgery and radiation therapy for early breast cancer. Pathol Annu 1988;(Pt 1):1-23.
2. Kline TS, Kline IK: Guides to Clinical Aspiration Biopsy. Breast. New York, Igaku-Shoin, 1989.
3. Koss LG: The palpable breast nodule: A cost-effective analysis of alternative diagnostic approaches. The role of the needle aspiration biopsy. Cancer 1993;72:1499-1502.
4. Layfield LJ, Chrischilles EA, Cohen MB, Bottles K: The palpable breast nodule: A cost-effective analysis of alternate diagnostic approaches. Cancer 1993;72:1642-1651.
5. Lofgren M, Anderson I, Lindholm K: Stereotactic fine-needle aspiration for cytologic diagnosis of nonpalpable breast lesions. AJR Am J Roentgenol 1990;154:1191-1195.
6. Bedard YC, Pollett AF: Breast fine-needle aspiration. A comparison of ThinPrep and conventional smears. Am J Clin Pathol 1999;111:523-527.
7. Parker SH, Loven JD, Jobe WE, et al.: Nonpalpable breast lesions: Stereotactic automated large-core biopsies. Radiology 1991;180:403-407.
8. Ioffe OB, Berg WA, Silverberg SG, Kumar D: Mammographic-histopathologic correlation of large-core needle biopsies of the breast. Mod Pathol 1998;11:721-727.
9. Sharifi S, Peterson MK, Baum JK, et al: Assessment of pathologic prognostic factors in breast core needle biopsies. Mod Pathol 1999;12:941-945.
10. Rosen PP: Breast Pathology: Diagnosis by Needle Core Biopsy. Philadelphia, Lippincott Williams & Wilkins, 1999.
11. Lee KC, Chan JKC, Ho LC: Histologic changes in the breast after fine-needle aspiration. Am J Surg Pathol 1994;18:1039-1047.
12. Youngson BJ, Cranor M, Rosen PP: Epithelial displacement in surgical breast specimens following needling procedures. Am J Surg Pathol 1994;18:896-903.
13. Carter BA, Jensen RA, Simpson JF, Page DL: Benign transport of breast epithelium into axillary lymph nodes after biopsy. Am J Clin Pathol 2000;113:259-266.
14. Casey M, Rosenblatt R, Zimmerman J, Fineberg S: Mastectomy without malignancy after carcinoma diagnosed by large-core stereotactic breast biopsy. Mod Pathol 1997;10:1209-1213.
15. Gonzalez JEG, Caldwell RG, Valaitis J: Calcium oxalate crystals in the breast: Pathology and significance. Am J Surg Pathol 1991;15:586-591.
16. Association of Directors of Anatomic and Surgical Pathology: Immediate management of mammographically detected breast lesions. Am J Pathol 1993;17:850-851.
17. Zarbo RJ, Hoffman GG, Howanitz PJ: Interinstitutional comparison of frozen section consultation: A College of American Pathologists Q-Probe Survey of 79,647 consultations in 297 North American institutions. Arch Pathol Lab Med 1991;115: 1187-1194.
18. Owings D, Hann L, Schnitt SJ: How thoroughly should needle localization breast biopsies be sampled for microscopic examination? A prospective mammographic-pathologic correlative study. Am J Surg Pathol 1990;14:578-583.
19. Schnitt SJ, Wang HH: Histologic sampling of grossly benign breast biopsies. How much is enough? Am J Surg Pathol 1989;13:505-512.
20. Abraham SC, Fox K, Fraker D, et al: Sampling of grossly benign breast reexcisions. Am J Surg Pathol 1999;23:316-322.
21. Frazier TE, Wong R, Rose D: Implications of accurate pathologic margins in the treatment of primary breast carcinoma. Arch Surg 1989;124:37-38.
22. McCormick B, Kinne D, Petrek J, et al: Limited reaction for breast cancer: A study of inked specimen margins before radiotherapy. Int J Radiat Oncol Biol Phys 1987;13:1667-1671.
23. Schmidt-Ullrich R, Wazer DE, Tercilla O, et al: Tumor margin assessment as a guide to optimal conservation surgery and irradiation in early stage breast carcinoma. Int J Radiat Oncol Biol Phys 1989;17:733-738.
24. Schnitt SJ, Connolly JL, Khettry U, et al: Pathologic findings on re-excision of the primary site in breast cancer patients considered for treatment by primary radiation therapy. Cancer 1987;59:675-681.
25. Solin LJ, Fowble B, Katz RL, et al: Results of re-excisional biopsy of the primary tumor in preparation for definitive irradiation of patients with early stage breast cancer. Int J Radiat Oncol Biol Phys 1986;12:721-725.
26. Connolly JL, Boyages J, Nixon AJ, et al: Predictors of breast recurrence after conservative surgery and radiation therapy for invasive breast cancer. Hum Pathol 1998;11:134-139.
27. Schnitt SJ: Specimen processing. In Tavassoli FA (ed): Pathology of Breast. New York, Elsevier, 1992.
28. Tavassoli FA: Pathology of the Breast. New York, Elsevier, 1992.
29. Liberman L: Pathologic analysis of sentinel lymph nodes in breast carcinoma. Cancer 2000;88:971-977.
30. Weaver DL, Krag DN, Ashikaga TA, et al: Pathologic analysis of sentinel and nonsentinel lymph nodes in breast carcinoma. Cancer 2000;88:1099-1107.
31. Turner RR, Ollila DW, Krasne DL, et al: Histopathologic validation of the sentinel lymph node hypothesis for breast carcinoma. Ann Surg 1997;226:271-278.
32. Turner RR, Hansen NM, Stern SL, Giuliano AE: Intraoperative examination of the sentinel lymph node for breast carcinoma staging. Am J Clin Pathol 1999;112:627-634.
33. Turner RR, Ollila DW, Stern S, Giuliano AE: Optimal histopathologic examination of the sentinel lymph node for breast carcinoma staging. Am J Surg Pathol 1999;23:263-267.
34. Pfeier JD: Sentinel lymph node biopsy. Am J Clin Pathol 1999;112:599-602.
35. Cohen LF, Breslin TM, Kuerer HM, et al: Identification and evaluation of axillary sentinel lymph nodes in patients with breast carcinoma treated with neoadjuvant chemotherapy. Am J Surg Pathol 2000;24:1266-1272.
36. Fitzgibbons PL, LiVolsi VA: Recommendations for handling radioactive specimens obtained by sentinel lymphadenectomy. Surgical Pathology Committee of the College of American Pathologists, and the Association of Directors of Anatomic and Surgical Pathology. Am J Surg Pathol 2000;24: 1549-1551.
37. Goldstein NS, Bassi D, Watts JC, et al: E-cadherin reactivity of 95 noninvasive ductal and lobular lesions of the breast. Am J Clin Pathol 2001;115:534-542.
38. Lehr H-A, Folpe A, Yaziji H, et al: Cytokeratin 8 immunostaining pattern and E-cadherin expression distinguish lobular from ductal breast carcinoma. Am J Clin Pathol 2000;114;190-196.
39. Cheng L, Binder SW, Fu YS, Lewin KJ: Demonstration of estrogen receptors by monoclonal antibody in formalin-fixed breast tumors. Lab Invest 1988;58:346-353.
40. Allred DC, Harvey JM, Berardo M, Clark GM: Prognostic and predictive factors in breast cancer by immunohistochemical analysis. Mod Pathol 1998;11:155-168.
41. Mann S, Laucirica R, Carlson N, et al: Estrogen receptor beta expression in invasive breast cancer. Hum Pathol 2001;32:113-118.
42. Slamon DJ, Clark GM, Wong SG, et al: Human breast cancer: Correlation of relapse and survival with amplification of HER-2/neu oncogene. Science 1987;235:177-182.
43. Hanna WM, Kahn HJ, Pienkowska M, et al: Defining a test for HER-2/neu evaluation in breast cancer in the diagnostic setting. Mod Pathol 2001;14:677-685.
44. Hanna W, Kahn HJ, Trudeau M: Evaluation of HER-2/neu (erbB-2) status in breast cancer: From bench to bedside. Mod Pathol 1999;12:827-834.
45. Ross JS, Fletcher AJ: HER-2/neu (c-erb-B2) gene and protein in breast cancer. Am J Clin Pathol 1999;112:S53-S67.
46. Press MF, Bernstein L, Thomas PA, et al: HER-2/neu gene amplification characterized by fluorescence in-situ hybridization: Poor prognosis in node-negative breast carcinomas. J Clin Oncol 1997;15:2894-2904.
47. Slamon D, Leyland-Jones B, Shak S, et al: Addition of Herceptin (humanized anti-HER-2-overexpressing metastatic breast cancer (HER-2+/MBC) markedly increases anticancer activity: A randomized, multinational controlled phase III trial [abstract]. Proc ASCO 1998;17:98a.

48. Ridolfi RL, Jamehdor MR, Arber JM: HER-2/neu testing in breast carcinoma: A combined immunohistochemical and fluorescence in situ hybridization approach. Mod Pathol 2000; 13:866-873.
49. Jimenez RE, Wallis T, Tabasczka P, Visscher DW: Determination of Her-2/neu status in breast carcinoma: Comparative analysis of immunohistochemistry and fluorescent in situ hybridization. Mod Pathol 2000;13:37-45.
50. O'Malley FP, Saad Z, Kerkvliet N, et al: The predictive power of semiquantitative immunohistochemical assessment of p53 and c-erb B-2 in lymph node-negative breast cancer. Hum Pathol 1996;27:955-963.
51. Rudolph P, Alm P, Olsson H, et al: Concurrent overexpression of p53 and c-erbB-2 correlates with accelerated cycling and concomitant poor prognosis in node-negative breast cancer Hum Pathol 2001;32:311-319.
52. Bergers E, Baak JPA, van Diest PJ, et al: Prognostic value of DNA ploidy using flow cytometry in 1301 breast cancer patients: Results of the prospective multicenter morphometric mammary carcinoma project. Mod Pathol 1997;10:762-768.
53. Wiley EL, Keh P: Diagnostic discrepancies in breast specimens subjected to gross reexamination. Am J Surg Pathol 1999;23:876-879.

Other Ultrasonographically Guided Interventional Procedures

Valerie P. Jackson and Handel E. Reynolds

Ultrasonography is an efficient, low-cost guidance modality for the performance of invasive procedures such as cyst aspiration, preoperative needle localization, fine-needle aspiration biopsy, large-core needle biopsy, directional vacuum-assisted needle biopsy, and placement of marker clips before neoadjuvant chemotherapy. The various percutaneous needle biopsy techniques are covered in Chapter 17. This chapter deals with the remaining ultrasonographically guided interventional procedures.

The use of ultrasonography for guidance during breast interventional procedures has many advantages. It is widely available and relatively low in cost. This lower cost can be passed on to patients who have interventional procedures. Ultrasonographically guided procedures involve no ionizing radiation and are often quicker and more comfortable (no breast compression is involved) than the same procedures performed with mammography or stereotactic guidance. The technique of ultrasonographic guidance for interventional procedures in the breast is similar to that employed in other anatomic sites, so that for most radiologists familiar with the technique, the learning phase involved is relatively brief. Most important, ultrasonography is the only modality that allows real-time visualization of the procedure being performed.

The one significant drawback to the use of ultrasonography in interventional procedures is that its use is limited to lesions that are visible on ultrasonography. This drawback is especially problematic with needle biopsy and preoperative needle localization. Most isolated clusters of microcalcifications are not visible on ultrasonography. Most other suspicious masses, however, can be demonstrated on ultrasonography, particularly with equipment using 12-MHz or 13-MHz transducers. Another, less important limitation is the fact that some radiologists find the bimanual coordination necessary for ultrasonographic guidance difficult to master.

TECHNICAL CONSIDERATIONS

High-resolution, real-time ultrasonography machines are appropriate for performing ultrasonographically guided procedures in the breast. As in diagnostic breast ultrasonography, it is important to use a high-frequency linear array transducer (10 to 13 MHz) to maximize resolution. For ease of operation, the ultrasonography transducer should be small and comfortable to hold. It is not necessary to use needles with specially designed echogenic surfaces in ultrasonographically guided breast procedures. Standard needles, even as small as 25 gauge, are easily seen with 10- to 13-MHz transducers.

TECHNIQUE

Two techniques are commonly used for targeting lesions using ultrasonographic guidance. The first involves the use of needle guides, small devices that attach to the transducer and allow the passage of a needle into the breast at a fixed angle. This technique does not require much bimanual coordination, because the alignment of the needle with the transducer is maintained by the needle guide. The major limitation of this technique is that the operator is restricted to a single angle of approach that may not be appropriate or convenient for all lesions and procedures.

The second method, the "freehand" technique, allows the operator a great deal of flexibility in the actual approach to the lesion. Typically, the transducer is held in the operator's nondominant hand and the needle in the dominant hand, although this arrangement may be reversed depending on the location of the lesion. The transducer hand maintains the lesion in an appropriate location on the screen, and the needle hand aligns the needle with the ultrasonography beam for maximum needle visibility as the needle is advanced toward the lesion. With this technique, it is possible to make moment-by-moment position corrections by altering the orientation of the transducer or the needle to achieve the best possible approach to the lesion. The freehand technique obviously requires good hand-eye and bimanual coordination, but, once mastered, it is the most useful technique available. Some people use a technique in which an assistant, such as a technologist, holds the transducer while the radiologist maneuvers the needle. In our experience, this approach makes needle adjustment more difficult because it reduces the radiologist's knowledge of the exact position of both the transducer and the needle.

Although the freehand technique allows limitless angles of approach, these can be reduced to three basic types: the oblique needle approach, the horizontal needle approach, and the vertical needle approach. In the *oblique approach* (Fig. 20–1), the needle pierces the skin adjacent to the short end of the transducer and is advanced toward the lesion along the plane of the ultrasonography beam. The

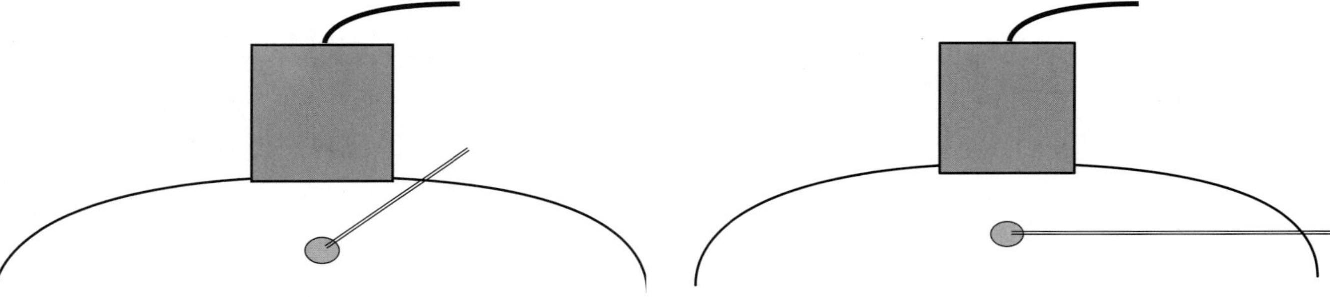

Figure 20–1. The oblique approach. See text for details.

Figure 20–2. The horizontal approach. See text for details.

path of the needle intersects the ultrasonography beam at an oblique angle, which depends on the location of the lesion. This approach allows reasonably short needle travel and relatively good needle visualization, although not as good as with the horizontal approach. Because the path of the needle causes it to intersect the chest wall if advanced too far, the oblique approach is slightly more risky for deep lesions than for lesions in the anterior aspect of the breast. Deep lesions can be more safely targeted using the horizontal approach.

In the *horizontal approach* (Fig. 20–2), the skin is pierced in a location chosen so that the needle can be advanced into it using a horizontal path. The needle travels within the plane of the ultrasonography beam and intersects it at a perpendicular angle. Because of this geometry, excellent visualization of the needle is possible once it comes into view. However, because the needle entry site is farther from the transducer than in the oblique approach, the entire needle path is not visualized—only the last several centimeters. This feature makes lining up the needle and transducer more difficult. A good alternative is to start with the oblique approach and then push the hub of the needle down after advancing it approximately 1 cm within the skin, to place the needle in a more horizontal position as it is advanced to the lesion (Fig. 20–3). The horizontal approach is well suited to deep lesions because the needle travels parallel to the chest wall.

The *vertical approach* (Fig. 20–4) involves targeting the lesion from the side, rather than the end, of the transducer.[1] Thus, if the transducer is centered on the lesion, the needle will not be seen until it is within the lesion. This technique allows the shortest needle path of the three and therefore is well suited to needle localization. Its disadvantage is that it shows the needle only in cross-section, and thus one cannot see the entire length of the needle and its tip. Therefore, it is a somewhat more difficult technique to master. With this approach, ultrasonography is used to document the presence of the needle in the lesion rather than to guide its progress toward the lesion.

SPECIAL CONSIDERATIONS

Performing breast interventional procedures using ultrasonographic guidance creates some unique problems not encountered with mammography or stereotactic guidance. The vast majority of lesions subjected to ultrasonographically guided intervention are found first on mammography. It is important to ensure that the lesion seen on ultrasonography is the same lesion identified on the mammogram. In most cases, the question can be easily answered by paying close attention to the size, shape, and location of the lesion. Occasionally, however, some confusion may exist, as when there are multiple lesions in a given region or lesions that

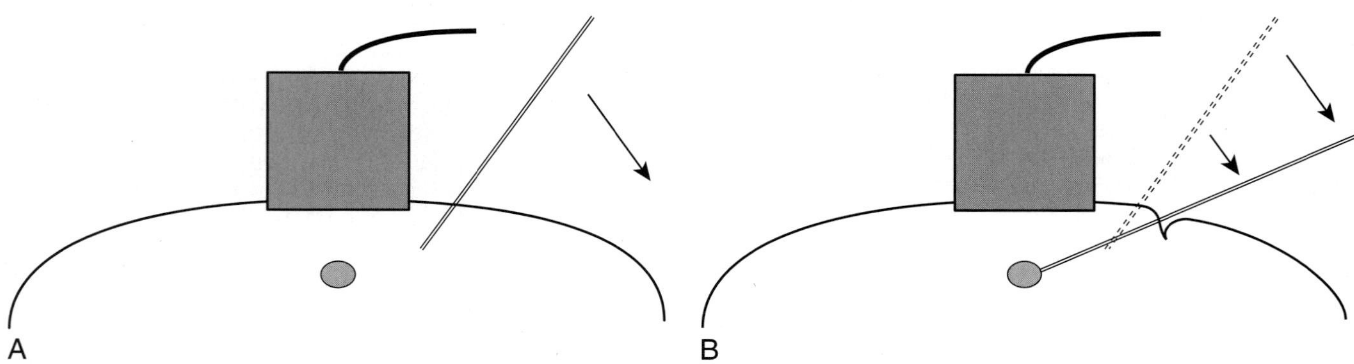

Figure 20–3. The modified oblique approach to give a more horizontal needle path. **A,** The needle is passed obliquely or even vertically to 1 to 2 cm deep to the skin. **B,** The hub is pushed down (*arrows*) as the needle is advanced though the deeper tissue in a more horizontal plane. The skin is usually stretched and indented with this maneuver, effectively displacing the skin entry site.

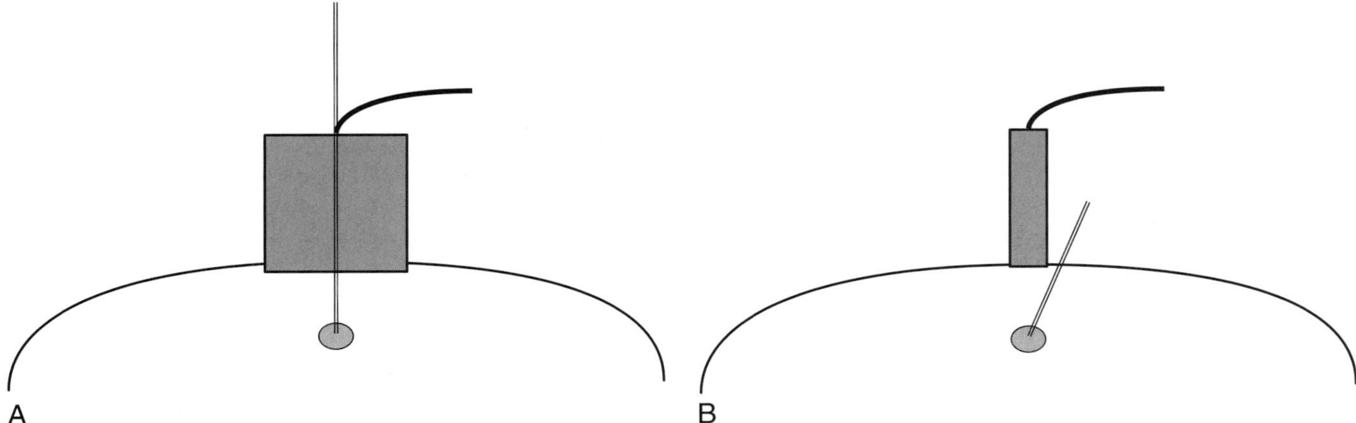

Figure 20–4. The vertical approach. **A,** View from side of transducer. **B,** View from end of transducer.

are poorly visualized on ultrasonography. This is an important issue, especially if needle localization or needle biopsy is contemplated. A simple solution is to place a fine (25-gauge) needle into the suspected lesion under ultrasonographic guidance and then perform orthogonal mammography to confirm that the two areas are the same lesion. This step adds about 10 minutes to the procedure but can mean the difference between a satisfying, successful endeavor and frustrating failure.

Because the ultrasonography transducer is a critical tool in the procedure and is invariably in the sterile field, it must be cleansed appropriately. A variety of antiseptic solutions are available for this purpose. The ultrasonographic equipment manufacturer should be consulted for suggestions. Once the transducer and a length of cord have been cleansed, they may safely be placed in the sterile field. An alternative to cleansing the transducer is placing it in a specially designed sterile plastic sheath or sterile glove containing coupling gel. During the procedure, acoustic coupling at the skin can be achieved by use of sterile gel or a small amount of alcohol or antiseptic soap.

Before the procedure, one should perform nonsterile scanning of the area of interest to plan an appropriate approach. It is our practice to mark the location of the lesion and the expected skin entry site with a permanent marker. Patient positioning for the procedure follows the same rules as for routine ultrasonography; the area of interest is flattened as much as possible, and the lesion is placed in the most anterior position possible. Thus, medial lesions can be approached with the patient supine, whereas lateral lesions require more of a decubitus or oblique positioning with a foam wedge placed under the ipsilateral shoulder and upper body. The ipsilateral arm should be abducted above the head. The position of the targeted lesion in the field of view depends on the type of procedure to be performed. For ultrasonographically guided needle biopsy with an automated "true-cut" device, it is critical to visualize as much of the needle path as possible; therefore, the lesion should be placed on the *far* side of the field of view from the skin entry site (Fig. 20–5). For procedures such as cyst aspiration and marker placement, lesion placement is less critical because needle control is better, so the lesion can be placed in the center of the field of view (Fig. 20–6). For ultrasonographically guided presurgical needle localization, it is important to minimize the distance the wire travels through the breast parenchyma, so the lesion should be placed in the field of view *near* the skin entry site (Fig. 20–7).

LEARNING THE TECHNIQUE

Many breast phantoms on the market are designed to allow practitioners to gain skill in these various techniques before applying them to their patients.[2,3]

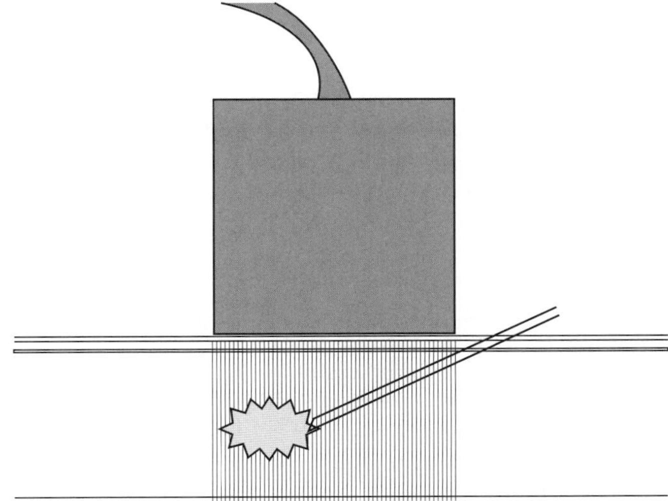

Figure 20–5. Placement of lesion in field of view for ultrasonographically guided core needle biopsy. Because of the rapid throw of the needle when the device is fired, it is important to visualize as much of the needle path as possible. Thus, the lesion should be placed at the far side of the field of view from the skin entry site.

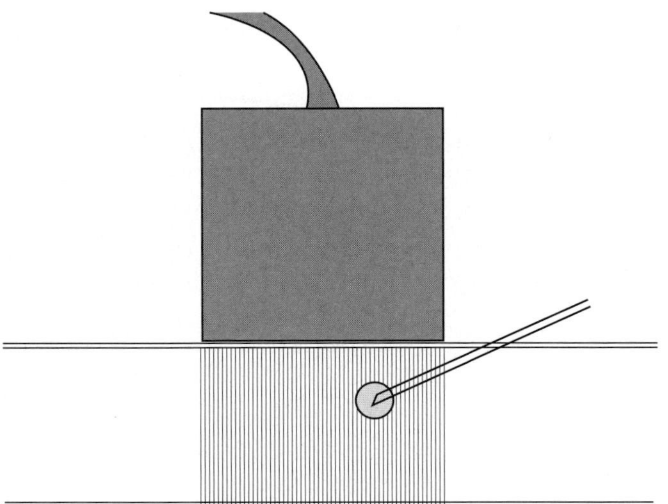

Figure 20–6. Placement of lesion in field of view for ultrasonographically guided cyst aspiration or metallic marker placement. Needle control and length of travel through the breast are not as important, so the lesion can be placed in the center of the field of view.

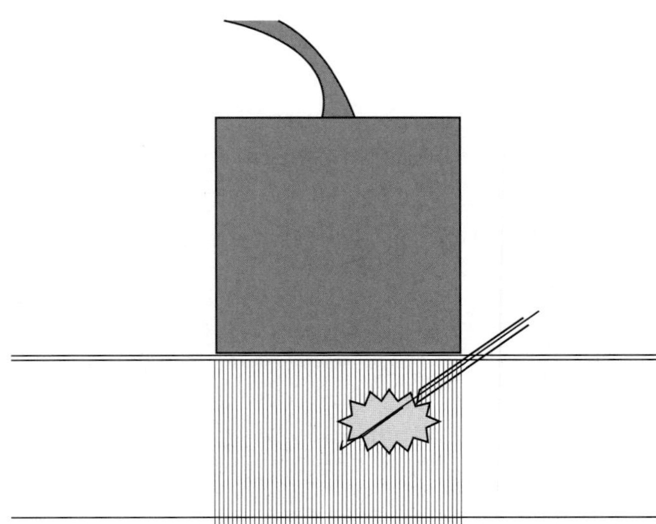

Figure 20–7. Placement of lesion in field of view for ultrasonographically guided preoperative needle localization. To minimize the distance the needle-wire passes through the breast, the mass should be placed in the field of view close to the skin entry site.

Each has its own strengths and weaknesses. A particularly useful teaching tool is the turkey breast model developed at the University of Cincinnati by Georgian-Smith and colleagues.[2] The turkey breast resembles a human breast in terms of size and ultrasonographic appearance. This model, which can easily be made at home, uses a split turkey breast (split down the center of the sternum), into which are placed simulated cystic and solid masses. The targets are placed, under water to prevent air pockets, into an easily identified muscle plane accessed from the lateral edge of the turkey breast. The solid targets are large olives with pimento, and the cystic targets are the tied-off fingers of a water-filled glove. The model can be made quickly and inexpensively and allows the operator to practice the techniques of ultrasonographically guided cyst aspiration, needle localization, and needle biopsy. Olives with pimento are used so that when the red pimento is seen in the specimen chamber after core needle biopsy, the operator is assured that a biopsy through the center of the target has been achieved.

ULTRASONOGRAPHICALLY GUIDED CYST ASPIRATION

Indications

A common indication for breast ultrasonography is to distinguish cystic from solid breast masses. Ultrasonography is a highly reliable tool in the diagnosis of simple breast cysts, which usually require no intervention. However, some clinical situations exist in which aspiration is indicated (Table 20–1). Painful cysts are often aspirated for relief of symptoms. If such cysts are nonpalpable, ultrasonographic guidance is essential. Cystic lesions that do not have the classic appearance of simple cysts on ultrasonography may be aspirated, particularly if new or palpable. Typically, these are lesions that have low-level internal echoes or slight wall irregularity. Often, these are cysts that have become complicated by infection or hemorrhage or may appear to contain internal echoes owing to improper scan parameters.

Sometimes the patient or her physician requests aspiration of a simple cyst. Some patients find it intolerable to have a mass of any kind in the breast. Large, palpable cysts are usually aspirated by clinicians under direct palpation. Ultrasonographic guidance is indicated in these cases if the clinician is unsure of the physical findings or if the patient has breast implants. Complex masses containing both cystic and solid components may be managed with needle biopsy or excision, depending on the size of the solid component. Aspiration alone of a complex mass is generally not indicated, because tissue sampling of the solid component is required, and cytologic evaluation of the fluid component has been shown to have an unacceptably high false-negative rate.[4,5]

Table 20–1. Indications for Cyst Aspiration Using Ultrasonographic Guidance

Painful cysts
Ultrasonographic appearance not classic for simple cyst
Patient or physician request
Palpable cysts in the presence of implants or questionable physical findings

Technique

Although mammography can be used to guide cyst aspiration, it is rarely used today because ultrasonographically guided cyst aspiration is a quick and relatively painless procedure. It can be performed in 5 to 10 minutes in most cases. The area of interest is cleansed with surgical soap, and a small fenestrated drape or sterile towels are used to define a sterile field. Lidocaine mixed with sodium bicarbonate (8:2 mixture) is used for local anesthesia. If one is facile and the cyst is relatively large, very little local anesthetic is needed. However, for small cysts or less experienced operators, it is helpful to use 5 to 10 mL of local anesthetic mixture, because pushing or redirection of the needle may be required, causing greater discomfort for the patient.

Some cysts can be aspirated with the 25-gauge needle used for injection of the lidocaine. Most cysts can be aspirated with a 21-gauge needle, but some contain viscous fluid or fluid laden with particulate matter that requires a larger (19- or 18-gauge) needle for successful aspiration. The needle, with an attached syringe, is advanced into the lesion under direct ultrasonographic visualization, and negative pressure is applied when the needle tip enters the cyst. It is important to inspect the fluid in the hub of the needle at the beginning of aspiration, because if blood is found, the aspiration should be stopped. If the fluid has a benign appearance, the aspiration is performed to completion (Fig. 20–8). Parker and Stavros[6] have suggested the use of a 21-gauge Vacutainer (Becton-Dickinson & Co, Franklin Lakes, NJ) needle, which is attached to a standard redtop tube after the skin is punctured, for cyst aspiration. This system automatically drains the cyst. However, if bloody fluid is encountered with this technique, it is difficult, if not impossible, to prevent complete drainage of the cyst. Complete drainage is a problem because a cyst that contains blood requires excisional biopsy, and it may be difficult to localize the lesion for surgery if has been completely drained.

It may be difficult to advance the needle through the wall of the cyst using ultrasonographic guidance, particularly if the cyst is surrounded by firm fibrous tissue. The needle may deform or displace the cyst. A quick, firm jabbing motion is often necessary to pass the needle through the cyst wall. It is important to use ultrasonography to document the amount of residual fluid, if any, within the cyst after the procedure.

If the lesion turns out to be a solid mass, the procedure can be converted to ultrasonographically guided fine-needle aspiration or core needle biopsy. If one suspects that the lesion may be solid, it is useful to obtain informed consent for both procedures initially to avoid delays once the procedure is under way.

Fluid Disposition and Patient Management

The issue of fluid disposition has been a contentious one over the years—some physicians advocating that all fluids be submitted for cytologic evaluation,[7] others believing that none should be,[4,5] and still others proposing that only bloody aspirates be evaluated.[8] Several studies, all of which have involved palpable cysts, have looked at this issue. It is not clear whether their conclusions are directly applicable to the small, nonpalpable cysts that are typically approached with ultrasonography. Cyst fluid varies in color from clear to amber to shades of green and is usually of a thin consistency. In a series of 6872 consecutive aspirations reported by Ciatto and coworkers,[8] 6747 nonbloody aspirates were present, among which there were no instances of suspicious cytologic findings, and no cancers developed in the region of the cyst through an extensive follow-up period. Thus, the yield from routine cytologic

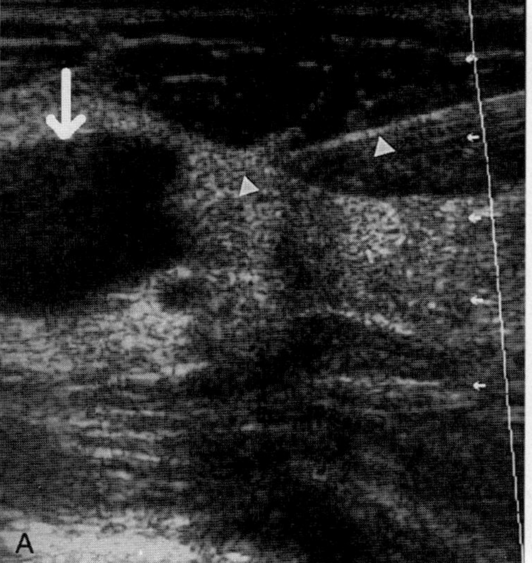

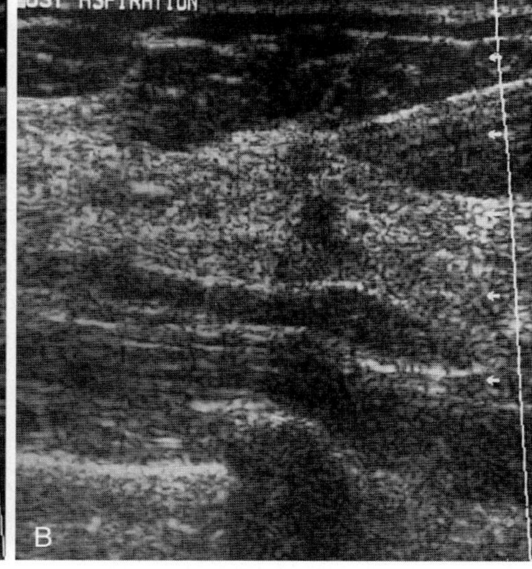

Figure 20–8. Ultrasonographically guided cyst aspiration. **A,** Before aspiration. The needle (*arrowheads*) is close to the thick fibrous wall of the cyst (*large arrow*). **B,** After successful aspiration, the cyst has been completely evacuated. The greenish fluid was discarded.

analysis of nonbloody aspirates is exceedingly low, so the practice does not appear to be justified. If no residual palpable or ultrasonographically demonstrable mass is present, the fluid can be discarded, and the patient can be reassured that she has benign disease. The presence of a residual mass is an indication for biopsy.

A bloody aspirate has several possible causes. Fresh blood is probably due to a traumatic "tap." Dark (old) blood may be due to an intracystic tumor (papilloma or carcinoma) or aspiration of the necrotic center of a solid tumor. The latter generally results in a residual mass after aspiration that should undergo biopsy, even in the absence of bloody fluid. Intracystic carcinomas are rare, seen in approximately 0.1% of cysts[5] and constituting 0.5% to 2.0% of all breast cancers.[9-12] They are typically large palpable lesions. Intracystic papillomas are much more commonly the cause of bloody aspirates.

In the study by Ciatto and colleagues,[8] 125 blood-stained aspirates were found, of which only one was cytologically suspicious. This was found at biopsy to be an intracystic papilloma. Only one "cancer" (a case of lobular carcinoma in situ) was found, being detected incidentally in a biopsy performed because of a blood-stained aspirate and an abnormal pneumocystogram. The cyst itself was benign on histologic analysis. Five intracystic papillomas were found. All of these had bloody aspirates. Four had negative or inconclusive cytologic findings, and one was suspicious. Thus, an atraumatic aspiration that yields blood-stained fluid may be due to an intracystic papilloma or carcinoma, but cytologic examination is not likely to be helpful in making this distinction. In 222 aspirates reported by Kinnard,[4] 212 were found to have normal cytologic findings. Among these were four cancers (false-negative cytologic results) diagnosed at biopsy. Biopsy was prompted by the presence of old blood and a residual mass in all cases. Nine cases of suspicious cytologic findings were found. These were all benign at surgery (false-positive cytologic results). One frankly malignant fluid was identified on cytologic examination; the aspirate was old blood, and a residual mass was seen. Cancer was confirmed at biopsy.

McSwain and coworkers[7] reported a series of 595 aspirations. Cytologic findings in 567 aspirates were negative. The one false-negative finding was an aspirate from a 150-mL cyst with dark brown fluid that promptly refilled after aspiration. Nine aspirates were suspicious, yielding five cancers at biopsy. Five were malignant, but only four cancers were found. (The fifth was a papilloma.) The researchers of this study pointed out that in most of the cancers found, there were reasons to indicate a biopsy other than cytologic findings. Two of the 10 cancers, however, had nonbloody aspirates and left no residual mass; this is a most unusual occurrence.

There are two undisputed indications for biopsy based on findings at cyst aspiration. The first is the presence of a residual mass, whether palpable or nonpalpable, that is ultrasonographically visible. The second is the presence of old blood in the aspirate. If the lesion is small and nonpalpable and no residual fluid or visible mass is left after aspiration, a marker clip should be placed immediately. Otherwise, localizing the area for biopsy becomes difficult or impossible. If a marker clip is not placed, the patient should be rescanned to check for recurrence. Cystic malignancies often recur within a few days to weeks, so follow-up imaging should be performed at 3 to 4 weeks and then 4 months after the procedure. If recurrence is documented, localization of the lesions for excisional biopsy is indicated.

Some surgeons perform biopsy on recurrent cysts, but the number of allowed recurrences varies widely. Others aspirate as often as the cyst recurs as long as no other indications for biopsy are present.[13] Cyst recurrence is not uncommon, and patients should be advised of this fact. We do not follow up routine aspirations (nonbloody fluid, no residua) of nonpalpable cysts. If a recurrence is noted the next time the patient presents for breast imaging and the cyst fulfills the criteria for a simple cyst, it is left alone.

Postaspiration Pneumocystography

Routine pneumocystography after cyst aspiration has been promoted as a means of preventing cyst recurrence and of demonstrating intracystic masses.[14-19] Intracystic masses are demonstrated very well by ultrasonography,[20-24] and as mentioned previously, true intracystic tumors are rare. The usefulness of pneumocystography in decreasing the recurrence rate of cysts remains controversial. Gizienski and associates[15] retrospectively reviewed 113 cysts aspirated in 90 women, 88 of which underwent air injection. The recurrence rate for cysts with air injection was 16%, whereas the recurrence rate was 80% for cysts not treated with pneumocystography. Thurfjell[19] reviewed the recurrence rate of 206 nonpalpable cysts and found no difference in recurrence between those cases in which pneumocystography was performed and those in which it was not. However, he did find that complete aspiration of fluid from the cyst was significantly associated with complete remission, whether or not pneumocystography was performed. Therefore, there seems to be little or no role for pneumocystography in modern breast imaging.

ULTRASONOGRAPHICALLY GUIDED PREOPERATIVE NEEDLE LOCALIZATION

Preoperative needle localization involves the placement of a hook or J-shaped wire into the area of interest. When the lesion is visible on ultrasonography, the procedure can be performed with ultrasonographic guidance.[25]

Indications

All lesions that can be seen on ultrasonography can be targeted ultrasonographically. Ultrasonographic guidance allows the procedure to be performed more quickly and comfortably than with mammographic guidance. Ultrasonographic guidance may allow a shorter approach than mammographic guidance and does not expose the patient to ionizing radiation. Ultrasonographically detected lesions that are occult or poorly seen on mammography obviously are well suited to ultrasonographic guidance. Finally, lesions that are in difficult or inaccessible locations for mammographic localization, such as the high axillary tail and deep in the breast, can be successfully targeted with ultrasonography (Table 20–2).

Technique

Any standard needle-wire localization system may be employed in the ultrasonography technique. The wire should be after-loaded once the needle is within the lesion. As mentioned previously, the vertical approach usually offers the shortest access to the lesion, but it is technically more challenging than the others and may be more risky for deep lesions. The operator should place the lesion in the field of view near the skin entry site, minimizing the distance from the entry site to the lesion and allowing use of the oblique approach (see Fig. 20–7). The horizontal approach should be considered for very deep lesions adjacent to the chest wall. Once the needle has been placed through the lesion, the wire is deployed so that the hook is just beyond the lesion (Fig. 20–9). Often the wire can be seen easily with ultrasonography. Placing an "X" on the skin directly over the lesion with a permanent marker is helpful to the surgeon. One could also mark the path of the wire in a similar fashion. After successful localization, orthogonal mammography should be performed to confirm wire placement and to provide a guide for the surgical team. After excision, it is essential that a specimen radiograph be performed. Even if the lesion was not well seen on preoperative mammography, it may be visible on specimen radiography once it has been removed from the surrounding breast tissue. If radiography fails to reveal the lesion, specimen ultrasonography should be performed.[26,27]

Table 20–2. Indications for Ultrasonographically Guided Needle Localization

Suspicious lesions that are ultrasonographically visible
Lesions that are poorly visible or occult on mammography
Lesions in difficult locations for mammography localization

Results

An early study of this technique, reported by Laing and coworkers,[28] found that seven of nine mammographically suspicious masses ranging in size from

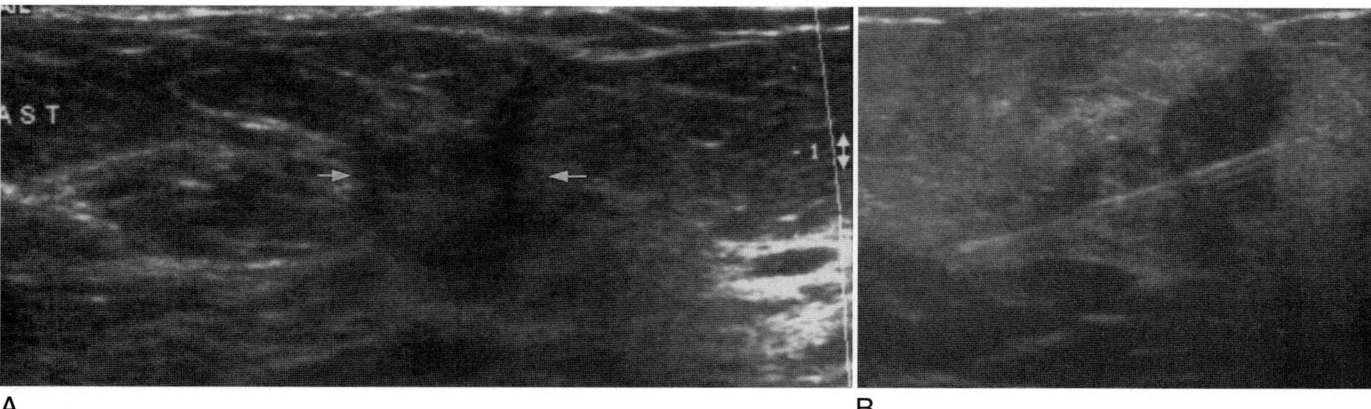

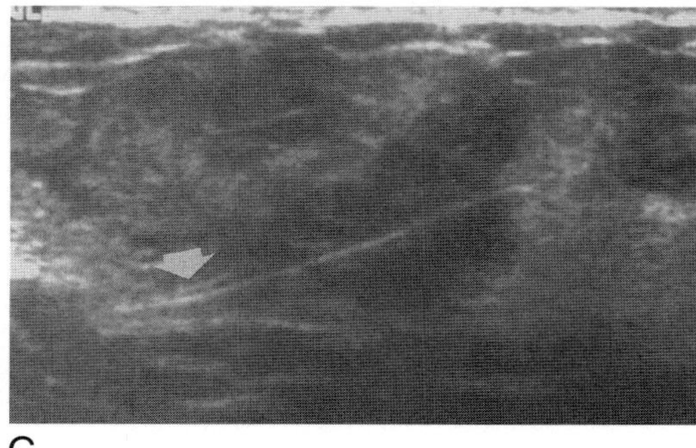

Figure 20–9. Ultrasonographically guided needle localization. **A,** Preliminary longitudinal ultrasonogram of needle biopsy–proven invasive ductal carcinoma (*arrows*). **B,** Localizing needle within the mass. **C,** Wire passing through mass. The hook of the wire (*arrow*) is just beyond the mass.

5 to 30 mm could be seen on ultrasonography well enough to be localized. The localization did not actually employ direct ultrasonographic guidance. The lesion was simply identified with ultrasonography, the skin overlying the lesion marked, and the needle placed vertically to the expected depth of the lesion. Despite the limitations of this technique, the localizing wire was within the lesion or within 1 cm of the lesion on the first attempt in all cases, and no complications occurred.

In a later study, Rissanen and colleagues[29] described the results of 102 ultrasonographically guided needle localization procedures. Ultrasonography was used primarily because of the preference of the radiologist (81 cases), although in 16 cases the lesion was mammographically occult, and in 3 cases the lesion was in a difficult location for mammographic guidance. The technique used was stated to be a "vertical or slightly oblique" approach without further elaboration or illustration. In all but eight cases, the localizing wire was placed within the lesion or within 5 mm of the lesion on the first attempt. The 8 remaining cases required a second wire placement. Successful excision was the rule, being documented by specimen radiography, ultrasonography, or both in 85 cases and by visual inspection of the specimen in 10. Two complications occurred. In one case, the localizing wire was placed within the pectoralis fascia, likely owing to the vertical approach employed in the procedure, and in the second case, the patient experienced vasovagal syncope during upright orthogonal mammography after wire placement. As radiologists have become more comfortable with and skilled at ultrasonographically guided interventional procedures, ultrasonographically guided needle localization procedures have become more widely used in practice without further scientific trials.

PLACEMENT OF MARKER CLIPS

Markers can easily be placed in breast masses using ultrasonographic guidance. This procedure is usually done for large, palpable, noncalcified, biopsy-proven carcinomas to undergo neoadjuvant chemotherapy (Table 20–3). When the lesion contains microcalcifications, the calcifications do not disappear even with good response to chemotherapy, so tumor marking is not necessary. For noncalcified carcinomas, if there is good response to the chemotherapy, the lesion may be shown by clinical breast examination, mammography, and ultrasonography to have disappeared completely. Because surgical excision of the tumor bed is still necessary for definitive therapy, it is important to have a marker in place to guide subsequent preoperative needle localization. This can be done using a variety of devices, such as embolization coils and commercially available metallic markers.[30-35] Marker placement is also indicated after percutaneous ultrasonographically guided biopsy of a small mass when there is concern that the lesion will be difficult to localize later[36,37] and when cyst aspiration reveals old blood and the cyst is completely or nearly completely evacuated.

Table 20–3. Indications for Ultrasonographically Guided Placement of Marker Clips

Known breast cancer prior to neoadjuvant chemotherapy
Cyst containing blood at aspiration from which all or most of the fluid was removed
Small solid mass that is difficult to see after ultrasonographically guided needle biopsy

Ultrasonographically guided placement of marker clips is an easy procedure, usually requiring only 10 to 20 minutes to complete. Ultrasonography is used to demonstrate the lesion and plan the approach. The lesion can be placed in the center of the field of view. The skin is prepared and draped in the usual fashion, and local anesthesia is achieved in the same manner as for ultrasonographically guided preoperative needle localization. The needle is advanced into the approximate geographic center of the mass using real-time ultrasonographic guidance (Fig. 20–10). After the tip of the needle is documented to be in the center of the mass, the metallic marker is deployed into the mass. Most of the metallic markers produce a strong echogenic artifact that is easily visible (Fig. 20–10C). The needle is then withdrawn, and orthogonal mammograms are obtained to document the position of the marker within the mass.

POTENTIAL COMPLICATIONS OF ULTRASONOGRAPHICALLY GUIDED INTERVENTIONAL PROCEDURES

The risks of ultrasonographically guided procedures such as needle localization and cyst aspiration are bleeding, infection, and vasovagal reaction. Bleeding is seldom a significant problem because relatively small needles are used and direct pressure can be applied as necessary to stop the bleeding. Infection is extremely uncommon if sterile technique is used. Vasovagal reactions are also rare for ultrasonographically guided procedures when the woman is supine. Nonetheless, the patient should never be left alone with a needle in her breast, and the staff should be prepared to handle any reaction.

CONCLUSIONS

Real-time ultrasonography is an inexpensive and efficient modality for guiding interventional procedures in the breast. Patient acceptance of the technique is generally quite good because the lack of breast compression makes these procedures relatively comfortable. The technique of ultrasonographic

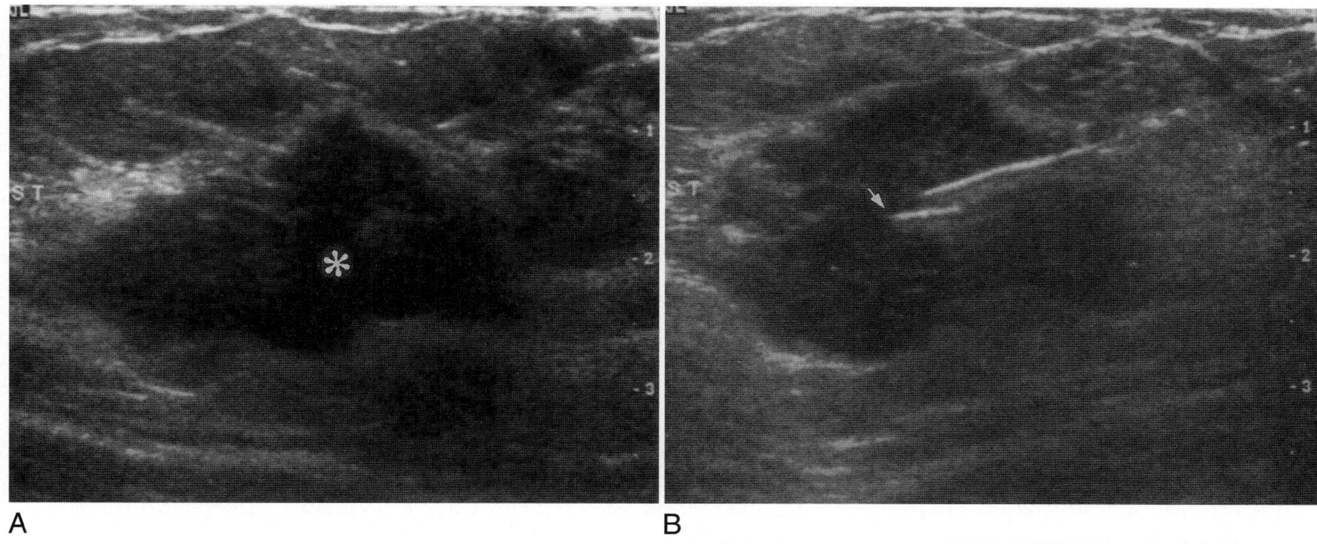

Figure 20–10. Ultrasonographically guided placement of a marker clip. **A,** Ultrasonogram of biopsy-proven invasive ductal carcinoma (*asterisk*). **B,** The needle tip is placed within the center of the mass (*arrow*), and the metallic marker is deployed. **C,** The sonogram obtained after needle removal documents the echogenic marker within the mass (*arrow*).

guidance is easy to learn regardless of the radiologist's prior level of experience with percutaneous needle procedures.

References

1. Fornage B, Coan J, David C: Ultrasound guided needle biopsy of the breast and other interventional procedures. Radiol Clin North Am 1992;30:167-185.
2. Georgian-Smith D, Shiels WE II, Lyon R, et al.: Freehand invasive sonography for breast. Radiology Suppl 1993;189:70.
3. Sisney GA, Hunt KA: A low-cost gelatin phantom for learning sonographically guided interventional breast radiology techniques. AJR Am J Roentgenol 1998;171:65-66.
4. Kinnard D: Results of cytological study of fluid aspirated from breast cysts. Am Surg 1975;41:505-506.
5. Rosemond G, Maier W, Brobyn T: Needle aspiration of breast cysts. Surg Gynecol Obstet 1969;128:351-354.
6. Parker SH, Stavros AT: Interventional breast ultrasound. In Parker SH, Jobe WE (eds): Percutaneous Breast Biopsy. New York: Raven Press, 1993, pp 129-146.
7. McSwain G, Valicenti J, O'Brien P: Cytologic evaluation of breast cysts. Surg Gynecol Obstet 1978;146:921-925.
8. Ciatto S, Cariaggi P, Bularesi P: The value of routine cytologic examination of breast cyst fluids. Acta Cytol 1987;31:301-304.
9. Czernobilsky B: Intracystic carcinoma of the female breast. Surg Gynecol Obstet 1967;124:93-98.
10. Gatchell F, Dockerty M, Clagett T: Intracystic carcinoma of the breast. Surg Gynecol Obstet 1958;106:347-352.
11. McKittrick J, Doane W, Failing R: Intracystic papillary carcinoma of the breast. Am Surg 1969;35:195-202.
12. Payne RA, Jackson DB: Cystic tumors of the breast. Ann R Coll Surg Engl 1980;62:228, 229.
13. Abramson D: A clinical evaluation of aspiration of cysts of the breast. Surg Gynecol Obstet 1974;139:531-537.
14. Dyreborg U, Blichert-Toft M, Boegh L, Kiaer H: Needle puncture followed by pneumo-cystography of palpable breast cysts. Acta Radiol Diagn 1985;26:277-281.
15. Gizienski TA, Harvey JA, Sobel AH: Breast cyst recurrence after postaspiration injection of air. Breast J 2002;8:34-37.
16. Ikeda D, Helvie M, Adler D, et al: The role of fine-needle aspiration and pneumocystography in the treatment of impalpable breast cysts. AJR Am J Roentgenol 1992;158:1239-1241.
17. Tabar L, Pentek Z: Pneumocystography of benign and malignant intracystic growths of the female breast. Acta Radiol Diagn 1976;17:829-837.
18. Tabar L, Pentek Z, Dean P: The diagnostic and therapeutic value of breast cyst puncture and pneumocystography. Radiology 1981;141:659-663.

19. Thurfjell E: Pneumocystography in nonpalpable breast cysts: Effect on remission rate. Ups J Med Sci 2001;106:111-115.
20. Estabrook A, Asch T, Gump F, et al: Mammographic features of intracystic papillary lesions. Surg Gynecol Obstet 1990;170: 113-116.
21. Fallentin E, Rothman L: Intracystic carcinoma of the male breast. J Clin Ultrasound 1994;22:118-120.
22. Knelson M, El Yousef S, Goldberg R, Ballance W: Intracystic papillary carcinoma of the breast: Mammographic, sonographic and MR appearance with pathologic correlation. J Comput Assist Tomogr 1987;11:1074-1076.
23. Reuter K, D'Orsi C, Reale F: Intracystic carcinoma of the breast: The role of ultrasonography. Radiology 1984;153:233, 234.
24. Sanders T, Morris D, Cederbom G, Gonzalez E: Pneumocystography as an aid in the diagnosis of cystic lesions of the breast. J Surg Oncol 1986;31:210-213.
25. Fornage BD, Sneige N, Edeiken BS: Interventional breast sonography. Eur J Radiol 2002;42:17-31.
26. Fornage BD, Ross MI, Singletary SE, Paulus DD: Localization of impalpable breast masses: Value of sonography in the operating room and scanning of excised specimens. AJR Am J Roentgenol 1994;163:569-573.
27. Frenna T, Meyer J, Sonnenfeld M: Ultrasound of breast biopsy specimens. Radiology 1994;190:573.
28. Laing F, Jeffrey R, Minagi H: Ultrasound localization of occult breast lesions. Radiology 1984;151:795-796.
29. Rissanen T, Makarainen H, Kiviniemi H, Suramo I: Ultrasonographically guided wire localization of nonpalpable breast lesions. J Ultrasound Med 1994;13:183-188.
30. Baron LF, Baron PL, Ackerman SJ, et al: Sonographically guided clip placement facilitates localization of breast cancer after neoadjuvant chemotherapy. AJR Am J Roentgenol 2000;174: 539-540.
31. Braeuning MP, Burke ET, Pisano ED: Embolization coils as tumor markers for mammography in patients undergoing neoadjuvant chemotherapy for carcinoma of the breast. AJR Am J Roentgenol 2000;174:251-252.
32. Dash N, Chafin SH, Johnson RR, Contractor FM: Usefulness of tissue marker clips in patients undergoing neoadjuvant chemotherapy for breast cancer. AJR Am J Roentgenol 1999; 173:911-917.
33. Edeiken BS, Fornage BD, Bedi DG, et al: US-guided implantation of metallic markers for permanent localization of the tumor bed in patients with breast cancer who undergo preoperative chemotherapy. Radiology 1999;213:895-900.
34. Kopans DB: Clip placement during sonographically guided breast biopsy. AJR Am J Roentgenol 2001;176:1076-1077.
35. Reynolds HE, Lefsnefsky MH, Jackson VP: Tumor marking before primary chemotherapy for breast cancer. AJR Am J Roentgenol 1999;173:919-920.
36. Guenin MA: Clip placement during sonographically guided large-core breast biopsy for mammographic-sonographic correlation. AJR Am J Roentgenol 2000;175:1053-1055.
37. Phillips SW, Gabriel H, Comstock CE, Venta LA: Sonographically guided metallic clip placement after core needle biopsy of the breast. AJR Am J Roentgenol 2000;175:1353-1355.

Chapter 21 Galactography

Valerie P. Jackson and Lawrence W. Bassett

Galactography (ductography) is a mammographic study involving the injection of water-soluble contrast material into a duct. It is indicated for evaluation of spontaneous bloody, serous, or clear nipple discharge that originates from one or two ducts. A hemoglobin reagent stick can be used to test the discharge for blood. Other types of discharge, such as green, yellow, and milky, are not associated with breast tumors. Most authorities stress the importance of *spontaneous* discharge rather than *expressed* discharge, because most women have some discharge when the breast and nipple are vigorously compressed.[1-3] Tabár and colleagues found a 10% incidence of carcinoma in women operated on for appropriate nipple discharge.[4] The incidence was higher for bloody discharge (13%) than for serous discharge (7%). In other series, the incidence of abnormal discharge caused by carcinoma has ranged from 3.2% to 33.3%.[2,5-9] Cytologic analysis has a high false-negative rate and is therefore unreliable for the evaluation of nipple discharge.[2,4,5,8,10] In addition, false-positive cytology results for nipple discharge have been reported.[10]

TECHNIQUE

A woman with bloody or serous nipple discharge should undergo mammography as the primary imaging modality. If no mammographic abnormalities are found to account for the discharge, ductography can be performed. Although some experts have advocated the use of ultrasonography for evaluation of nipple discharge,[11,12] there are no studies that demonstrate the efficacy of ultrasonography in this clinical situation.

Discharge must be present on the day of the ductogram, so that the discharging duct can be identified. We ask the woman to check for discharge before coming for her appointment and have her reschedule the examination if she is unable to express discharge. After the patient arrives, and before we set up the equipment for the galactogram, we attempt to express a small drop of discharge. For women known to have a scant amount of discharge, it is important to elicit only a minimal amount so that fluid will be available at the time of the actual procedure to guide cannulation of the duct.

It is unusual to find a palpable mass on physical examination to account for nipple discharge. However, physical examination is important because a "trigger point" (at which pressure will elicit the discharge) is usually found. This finding facilitates cannulation of the correct duct. The patient is often able to identify the trigger point herself, and she should be asked about this issue before the procedure.

Table 21–1 lists the equipment needed for galactography. A 27- or 30-gauge blunt, straight or curved needle-catheter system, as used for sialography, is filled with a water-soluble contrast material, such as full-strength iothalamate meglumine (e.g., Conray 60). Non-ionic contrast material can be used because of the possibility of contrast extravasation from duct perforation,[13] but this precaution is probably unnecessary because there are no reports in the literature regarding adverse effects from extravasation of ionic water-soluble contrast into the breast. The catheter is connected to a 3- or 5-mL syringe. We make this connection via a two- or three-way stopcock in order to close the system and prevent entrance of air bubbles. The system must be completely filled with contrast agent and free of air bubbles, which would appear as filling defects that may simulate intraductal tumors.

A high-intensity lamp provides additional light for better visualization in duct cannulation, and its warmth often dilates the duct orifice, making cannulation of the duct easier. Application of a warm wet cloth to the nipple also relaxes the sphincter near the duct orifice. Magnifying glasses are usually needed for optimal visualization of the duct orifice.

The patient may be supine or seated for injection of the contrast agent. The supine position may be more comfortable for the patient and allows gravity to facilitate filling of the posterior aspects of the ducts. The breast is cleaned with sterile soap or alcohol. Some soaps leave a sticky residue on the skin that may block the duct orifice. Therefore, any soap residue should be removed with alcohol. The radiologist gently expresses a very small drop of discharge onto the nipple surface. If a large drop is expressed, it will obscure the duct orifice. Because of the small size of the needle, preliminary enlargement of the duct orifice with dilators is not necessary.

The nipple should be stabilized and moved anteriorly by means of gentle pressure with the thumb and forefinger of one hand. The catheter is carefully and gently guided into the discharging duct. This often requires gradual probing of the duct orifice, with twirling and angling of the needle tip as necessary to facilitate cannulation. When entry is not readily accomplished, injection of a small amount of contrast agent when the needle tip is at the duct orifice may dilate the opening sufficiently to allow passage of the needle. Slawson and Johnson[14] recommend that if cannulation is still unsuccessful, a sterile local anesthetic gel (lidocaine) or warm compresses may be applied to the nipple-areolar complex,

Table 21–1. Equipment Needed for Galactography

Cleansing materials: gauze, sterile soap, alcohol
Dry sterile gauze
Magnifying glasses
High-intensity lamp
27-gauge to 30-gauge blunt needle-catheter system
Water-soluble contrast material
Two-way or three-way stopcock
3-mL to 5-mL syringe

and the procedure attempted again. If cannulation is still unsuccessful, they recommend that a different radiologist make another attempt. If needle placement is still not possible, the patient can be rescheduled for another attempt 1 to 2 weeks later.

If duct cannulation is not possible but a dilated duct is visible ultrasonographically, it is possible to use ultrasonography to guide placement of a needle into the duct.[15,16] Ultrasonography has also been used to guide fine-needle aspiration biopsy of intraductal masses seen on ultrasonography.[17] However, it is uncertain whether the ultrasonographically visible duct, or lesion within the duct, actually represents the source of the abnormal discharge.

When cannulation is achieved, the needle may enter only the first several millimeters of the duct, and it should not be forced because perforation may occur. The contrast injection rate will be slow because of the small needle size and the high viscosity of the contrast agent. The injection should be stopped when the patient feels fullness, discomfort, or pain or when the contrast agent refluxes onto the nipple surface. In most cases, less than 1 mL of contrast agent is used. If digital mammography is used, an early image can identify possible extravasation and document intraductal filling.

Magnification craniocaudal and 90-degree lateral (ML or LM) mammograms are obtained with mild to moderate compression. Brem and Gatewood[18] reported better filling of the ducts after the placement of a long narrow sponge or rolled cheesecloth on the posterior portion of the breast. Additional mammographic views are obtained as needed. The needle may be taped to the nipple for the mammograms or removed before filming to prevent dislodging or contamination during positioning. It is usually easy to recannulate the duct if a second injection is necessary for further duct filling or clarification of a potential abnormality. If the needle is removed, little contrast agent leaks out during the positioning for mammography.

The patient should be given sterile gauze pads to place in her bra after the procedure. She should be told that she will have increased discharge for a day or more after the procedure and that she may experience new bloody discharge during this period. She is instructed to call her referring physician or the breast imaging center immediately if she has symptoms of mastitis.

When a focal abnormality is found on galactography, the procedure can be repeated on the day of surgical biopsy, with injection of a 1:1 ratio combination of radiographic contrast agent and methylene blue or placement of a localizing device, such as a hook-wire, at the site of the suspicious lesion.[4,19-24,24a] If preoperative galactography is done with methylene blue, placement of a drop or two of collodion on the surface of the nipple will temporarily occlude the duct orifice and prevent leakage before surgery.[25] If preoperative localization of a galactographic abnormality is not performed, the radiologist, surgeon, and pathologist must cooperate and understand the imaging findings to give optimal patient management.[26]

Percutaneous imaging-guided needle biopsy is an alternative to surgery. Ultrasonography or stereotactic mammography systems can be used to guide placement of needles or directional vacuum-assisted devices for biopsy of intraductal lesions found on ultrasonography or galactography.[17,27-29]

INTERPRETATION

Normal galactography demonstrates filling of the arborizing ductal system (Fig. 21–1). Contrast agent is often seen in the lobules (Figs. 21–1 and 21–2). The normal duct caliber is variable, and normal limits

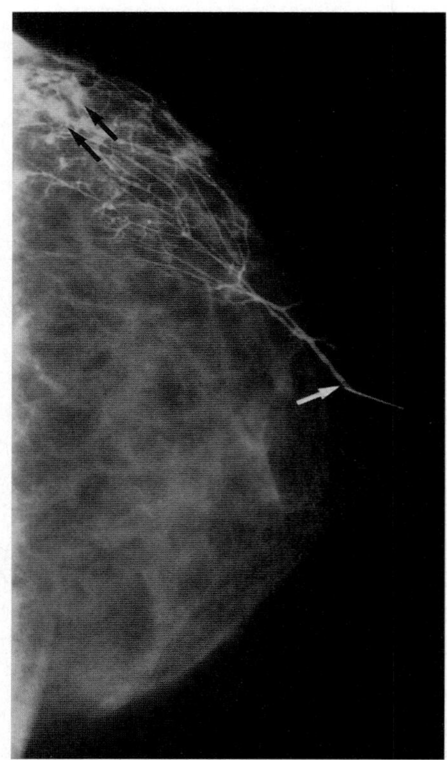

Figure 21–1. Normal galactogram (left craniocaudal projection). There is normal arborization of the ductal system, with lobular filling (*black arrows*). A small air bubble can be seen near the needle tip (*white arrow*).

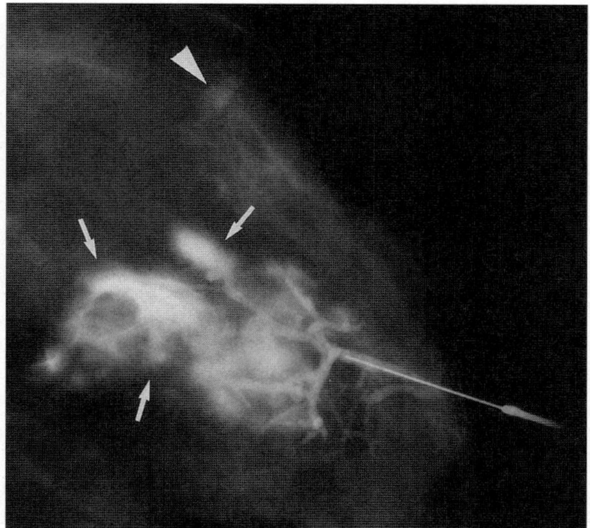

Figure 21–2. Normal left craniocaudal galactogram with intense lobular staining (*arrows*). A superficial lymphatic vessel is also filled (*arrowhead*).

have not been established.[30] Generalized duct dilatation may occur in secretory disease[3,31,32] (Fig. 21–3), and occasionally, small cysts will fill from the duct system (Figs. 21–4 and 21–5).

Papillomas are the most common cause of spontaneous bloody nipple discharge. These benign lesions are usually mammographically occult but are visible on galactography as one or more circumscribed round, oval, or lobulated filling defects within the duct (Figs. 21–6 through 21–8).[33] Papillomas may also produce duct expansion with distortion and wall irregularity. There is often dilatation of the

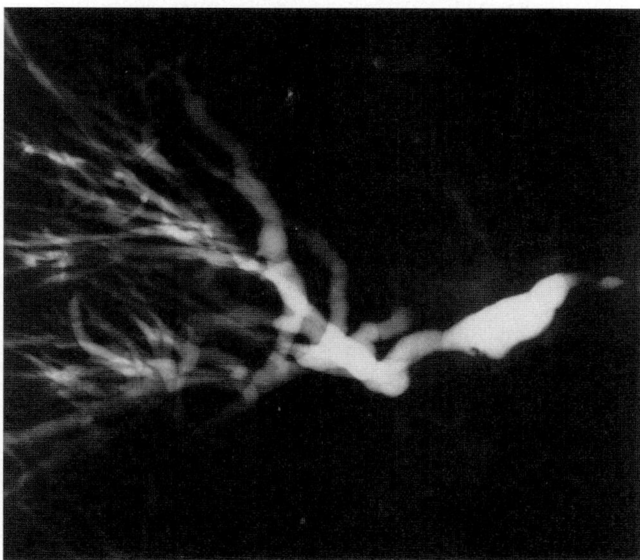

Figure 21–3. Duct ectasia. This magnification left mediolateral galactogram demonstrates diffuse mild dilatation of the ducts. There were no persistent filling defects.

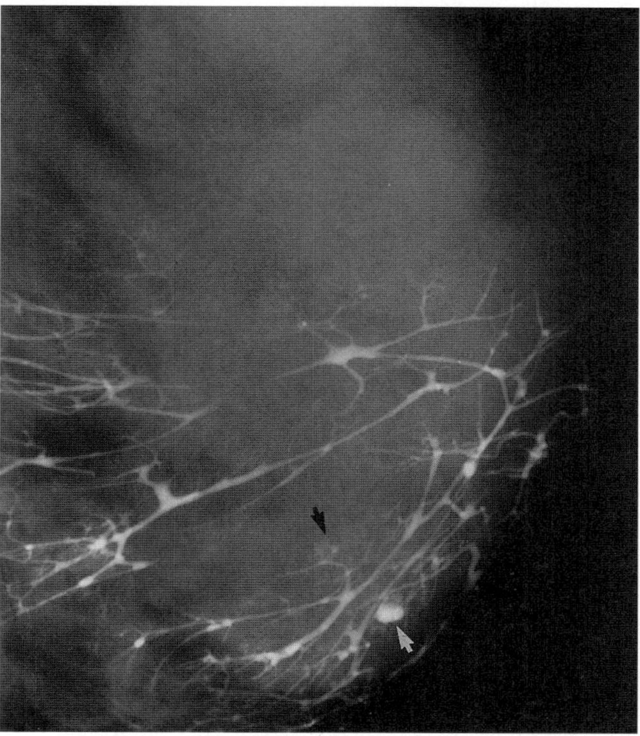

Figure 21–4. Cyst on galactography. Contrast agent fills the arborizing duct system on this left mediolateral galactogram, with filling of a few lobules (*black arrow*). A single 3-mm cyst is filled with contrast agent (*white arrow*).

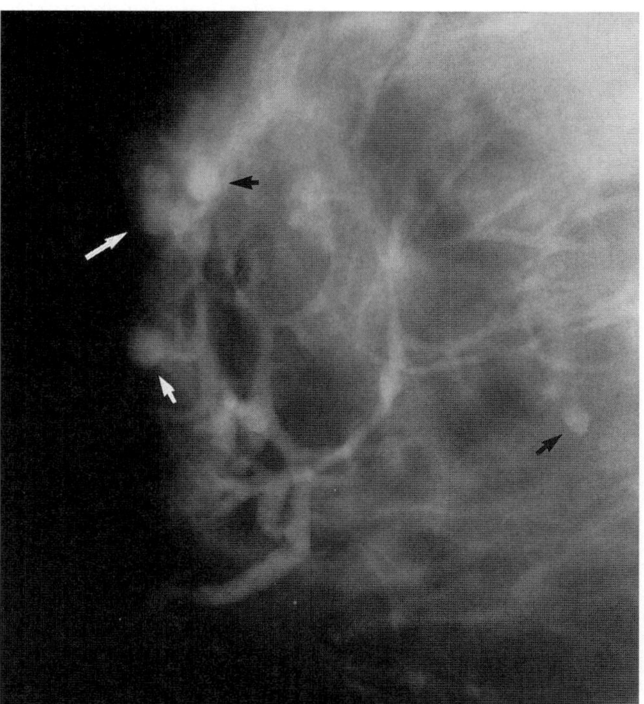

Figure 21–5. Multiple small cysts. Several 3- to 8-mm cysts (*arrows*) are filled with contrast agent on this magnification right mediolateral galactogram.

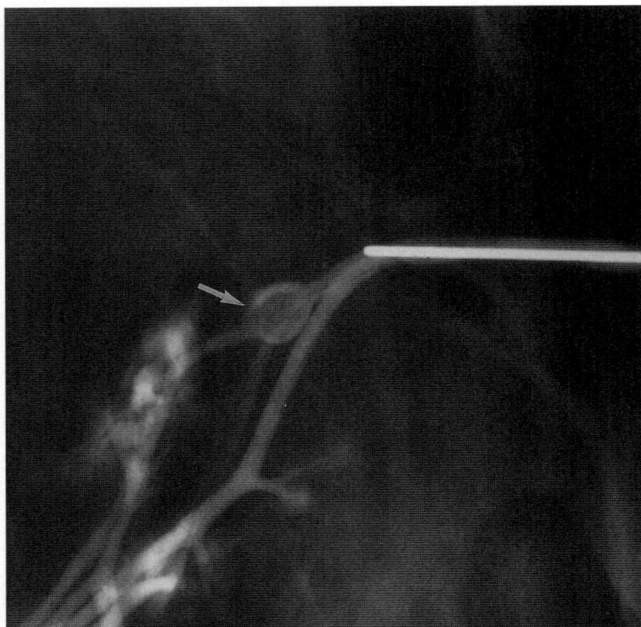

Figure 21–6. Solitary papilloma. A 49-year-old woman presented with spontaneous bloody nipple discharge. The 5-mm round circumscribed filling defect seen on galactography (*arrow*) was identified as a papilloma at excisional biopsy.

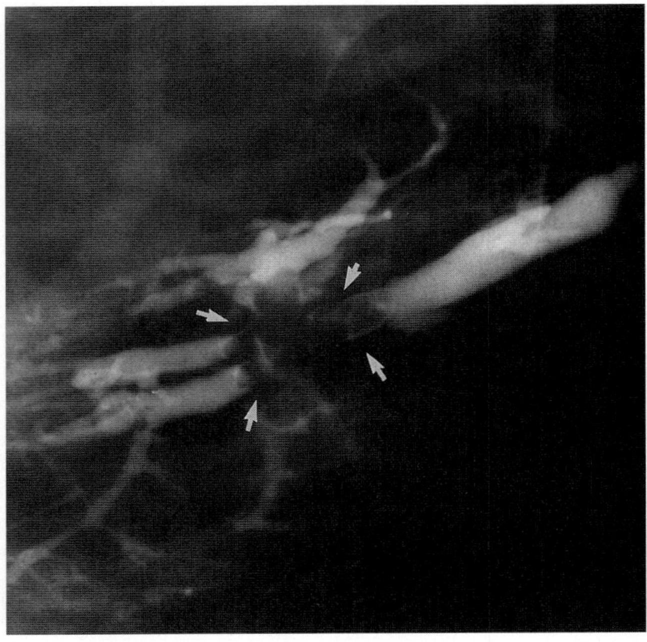

Figure 21–8. Solitary papilloma. The patient is a 65-year-old woman with bloody nipple discharge produced by a 1.5-cm circumscribed lobulated papilloma (*arrows*).

duct between the papilloma and the nipple, owing to the copious secretions produced by the tumor. Occasionally, a large papilloma may completely obstruct the duct, preventing passage of contrast agent beyond the lesion (Fig. 21–9). Other benign processes may cause filling defects on galactography that are indistinguishable from papillomas (Figs. 21–10 and 21–11). Ductal carcinoma may also produce circumscribed filling defects, wall irregularity, abrupt luminal changes, and cutoff of the

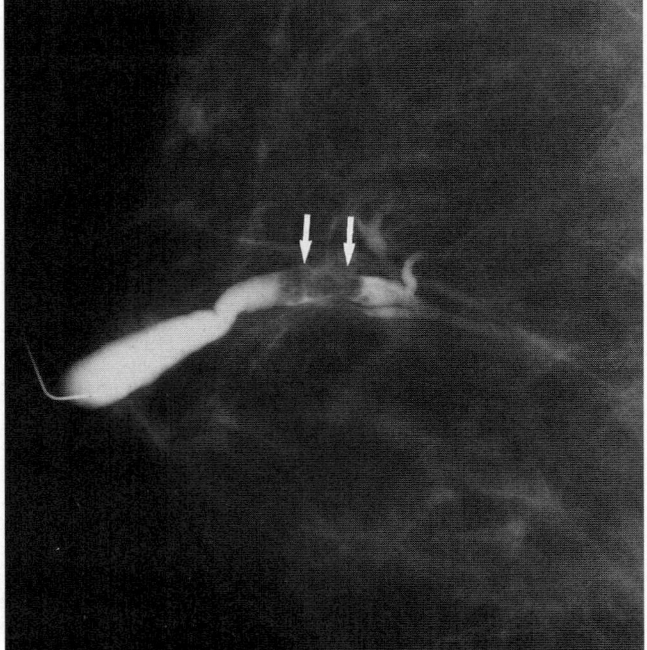

Figure 21–7. Solitary papilloma. Bloody nipple discharge in a 72-year-old woman. The 9-mm circumscribed lobulated filling defect (*arrows*) was a benign solitary papilloma at surgical biopsy.

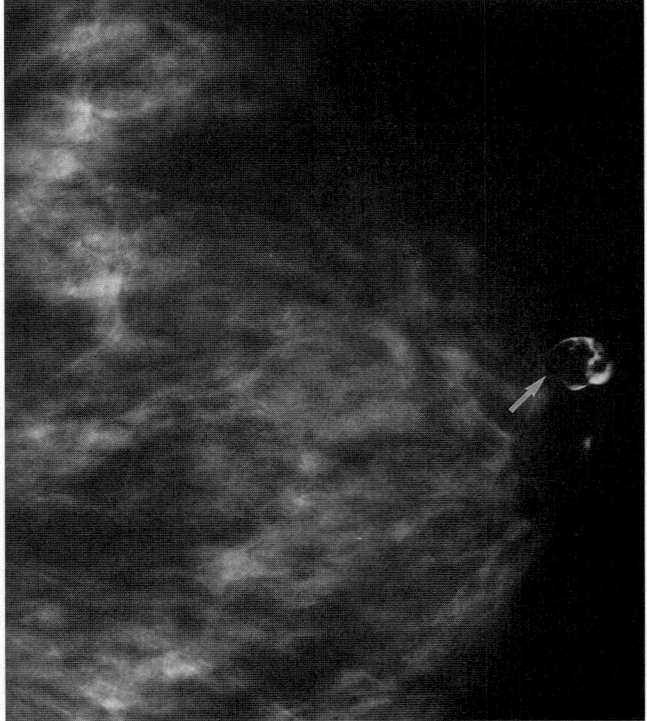

Figure 21–9. Solitary papilloma. Magnification left craniocaudal galactogram demonstrating a lobulated filling defect (*arrow*) that completely obstructs the passage of contrast agent.

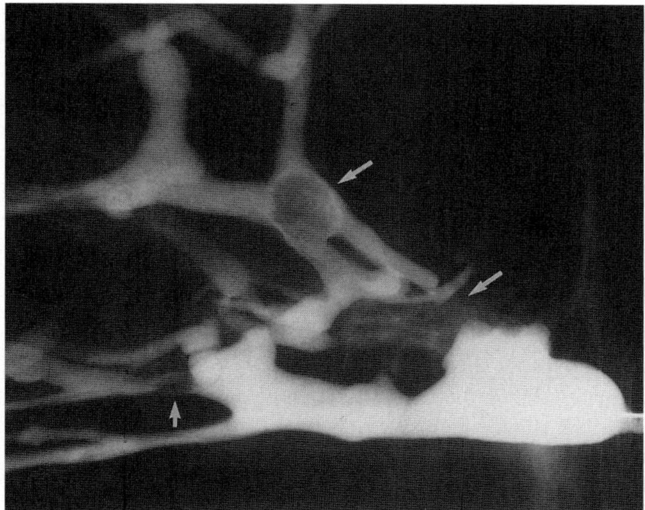

Figure 21–10. Intraductal granulation tissue in a 52-year-old woman who presented with spontaneous bloody nipple discharge. The magnification left mediolateral galactogram demonstrates multiple persistent circumscribed filling defects (*arrows*), which were found to be prominent granulation tissue at surgical biopsy.

column of contrast agent (Figs. 21–12 and 21–13).[1,3,4,22,31,32,34] It is not usually possible to differentiate between a carcinoma and a papilloma on galactography.[4,19,25,35-39]

When extravasation occurs from duct perforation, an irregular extraluminal collection of contrast agent is seen (Fig. 21–14). This occurrence prevents completion and interpretation of the galactogram on that day.

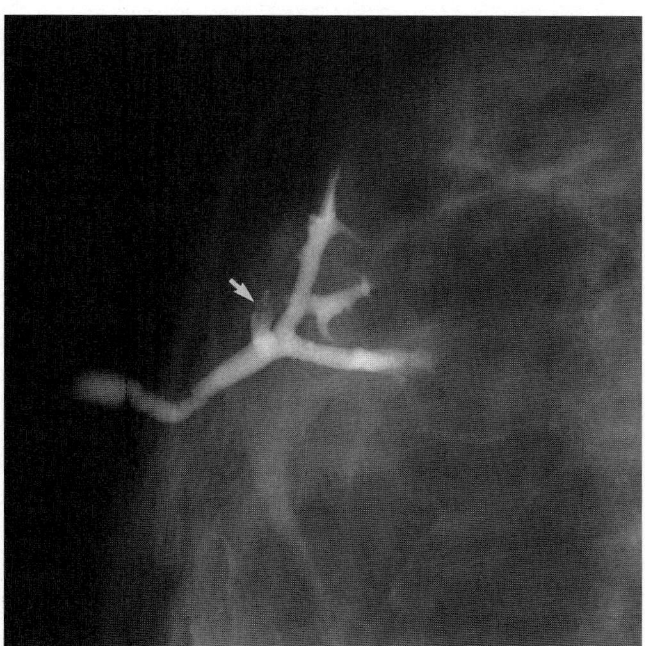

Figure 21–11. Right craniocaudal galactogram of a 50-year-old woman with bloody nipple discharge demonstrating a filling defect (*arrow*), which was found at biopsy to be apocrine metaplasia and epithelial hyperplasia.

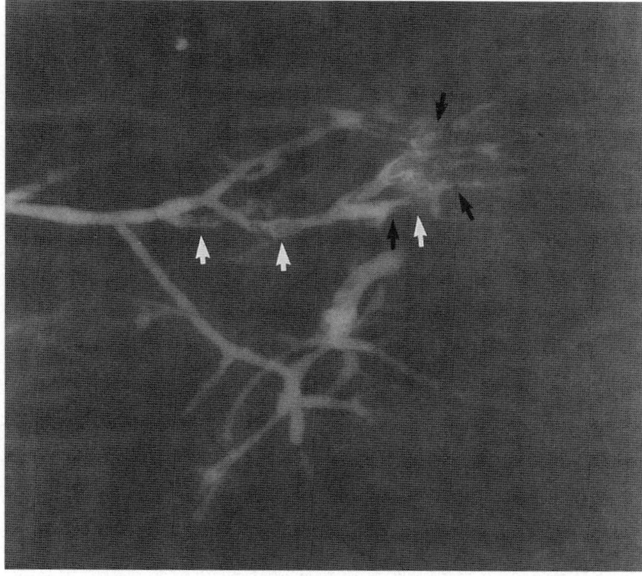

Figure 21–12. Ductal carcinoma in a 50-year-old woman with spontaneous bloody nipple discharge. The magnification right craniocaudal galactogram shows multiple small filling defects (*white arrows*), wall irregularity (*black arrows*), and abrupt cutoff of the column of contrast agent.

OTHER MODALITIES FOR THE EVALUATION OF NIPPLE DISCHARGE

As mentioned previously, ultrasonography has been used for evaluation of ducts. With the advent of 12- to 13-MHz transducers, it is possible to identify

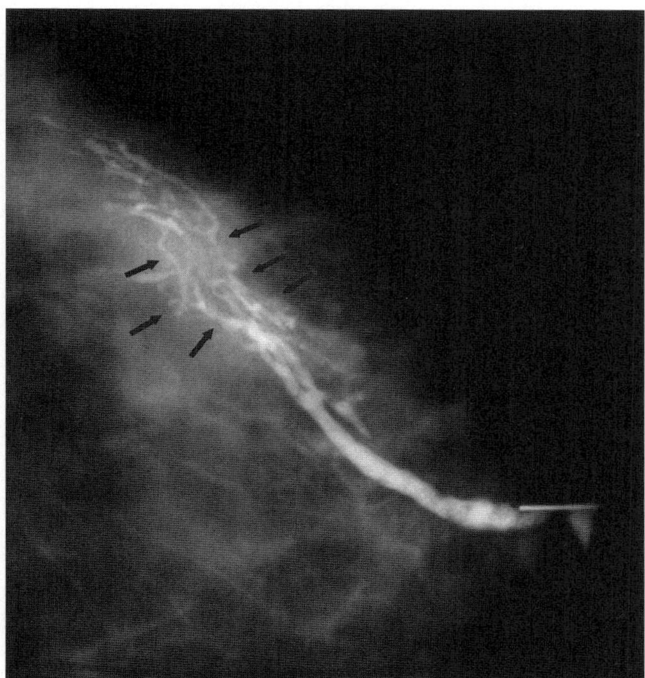

Figure 21–13. Ductal carcinoma in situ in a 60-year-old woman with bloody nipple discharge. The left craniocaudal galactogram shows wall irregularity and luminal narrowing (*arrows*).

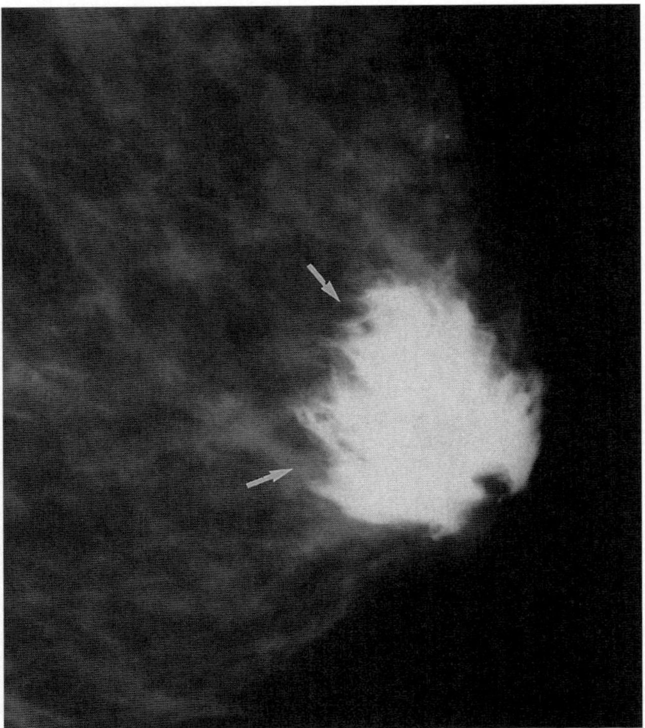

Figure 21–14. Contrast extravasation (*arrows*) from perforation of the duct in the immediate subareolar region.

intraductal abnormalities (Fig. 21–15).[11,17] However, determining whether these are the cause of the patient's discharge is often not possible.

Magnetic resonance imaging (MRI) has also been used to evaluate the ducts of the breast.[40-43] Intravenous administration of gadolinium contrast agent is used, rather than an intraductal contrast medium. There is evidence that MRI may be more sensitive than galactography for the detection of carcinoma.[40]

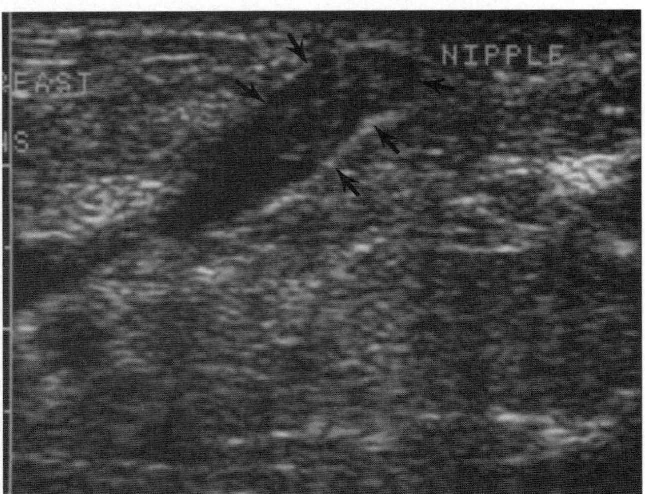

Figure 21–15. Intraductal papilloma in a 50-year-old woman with bloody nipple discharge. Ultrasonography demonstrates a 1-cm solid intraductal mass (*arrows*).

However, no specific MRI features of papillomas have been described, because contrast enhancement patterns have been variable. Therefore, specificity remains a problem. MRI could nonetheless be considered for evaluation of patients who have appropriate nipple discharge and for whom duct cannulation is not possible.[42]

CONTRAINDICATIONS, PRECAUTIONS, AND POTENTIAL COMPLICATIONS

Galactography is not indicated for evaluation of discharge that is not bloody or serous. Similarly, it is not indicated for women with any type of discharge from multiple ducts in both breasts or in pregnant or lactating women. Benign bloody discharge can occur in the second and third trimesters of pregnancy and may persist in the postpartum period.[43,44] Galactography should not be performed in a woman with active mastitis, because it may make the inflammation and infection worse.[4] In addition, this examination should not be performed in a woman with known hypersensitivity to radiographic contrast media, although there are no reports of contrast agent reactions after galactography in the literature. Additional contraindications are debilitating anxiety, an uncooperative patient, severe nipple retraction, and a history of previous nipple or areolar surgery that would disrupt the ducts.[14]

There are two major potential complications of galactography. One is perforation of the duct. This event necessitates termination of the procedure, usually before any diagnostic information has been obtained. The galactogram can be attempted again a week or more after the extravasation. There are no reports in the literature of adverse effects from contrast agent extravasation into the breast tissue, most likely because such a small amount of contrast agent is used for the procedure. The other major potential complication is inflammation or mastitis. Strict attention to sterile technique minimizes this possibility. The patient should be clearly instructed regarding the signs and symptoms of mastitis so that she can seek medical attention immediately if an infection develops.

Vasovagal reactions can occur during any interventional procedure. Although it is rare for a vasovagal reaction to occur during galactography, the patient should not be left alone during the procedure, and the staff should be prepared to treat such a reaction.

APPLICATIONS TO PATIENT CARE

The usefulness of galactography is controversial. Some surgeons prefer to dissect the discharging duct without preoperative galactography. However, many surgeons use a preoperative galactographic "road map" to guide them to the site of the tumor.

Communication between the mammographer and surgeons is necessary to determine the usefulness of galactography in an individual practice.

It is important to recognize that ductography is not a perfect test. Baker and colleagues[26] found a 20% false-positive rate and Dawes and associates[6] a 20% false-negative rate. The management of cases of abnormal discharge but normal galactographic findings remains controversial. In some published series, if a patient with spontaneous bloody nipple discharge has a normal galactogram and fluid cytology findings are normal, biopsy is not performed.[5,46] Rather, clinical follow-up is advocated. Although Ciatto and coworkers[5] found two cases of infiltrating ductal carcinoma at biopsy of patients with persistent bloody discharge but normal mammographic, ductographic, and cytologic findings, they concluded that "bloody nipple discharge alone does not justify surgical excision of the discharging duct, which should be limited to selected cases on the basis of cytology (evidence of suspect cells), or galactography (evidence consistent with breast cancer or multiple papillomas)."[5] However, most authors strongly advocate surgical duct excision for bloody discharge despite a normal ductogram.[6,47-51]

References

1. Funderburk WW, Syphax B: Evaluation of nipple discharge in benign and malignant diseases. Cancer 1969;24:1290-1296.
2. Leis HP, Cammarata A, LaRaja RD: Nipple discharge: Significance and treatment. Breast 1985;11:6-12.
3. Threatt B: Ductography. In Bassett LW, Gold RH (eds). Breast Cancer Detection: Mammography and Other Methods in Breast Imaging, 2nd ed. Orlando, Grune & Stratton, 1987, pp 119-129.
4. Tabár L, Dean PB, Pentek Z: Galactography: The diagnostic procedure of choice for nipple discharge. Radiology 1983;149:31-38.
5. Ciatto S, Bravetti P, Berni D, et al: The role of galactography in the detection of breast cancer. Tumori 1988;74:177-181.
6. Dawes LG, Bowen C, Venta LA, Morrow M: Ductography for nipple discharge: No replacement for ductal excision. Surgery 1998;124:685-691.
7. Jardines L: Management of nipple discharge. Am Surg 1996; 62:119-122.
8. Leis HP: Management of nipple discharge. World J Surg 1989; 13:736-742.
9. Paterok EM, Rosenthal H, Säbel M: Nipple discharge and abnormal galactogram: Results of a long-term study (1964-1990). Eur J Obstet Gynecol Reprod Biol 1993;50:227-234.
10. Dinkel H-P, Gassel AM, Muller T, et al: Galactography and exfoliative cytology in women with abnormal nipple discharge. Obstet Gynecol 2001;97:625-629.
11. Chung SY, Lee KW, Park KS, et al: Breast tumors associated with nipple discharge: Correlation of findings on galactography and sonography. Clin Imaging 1995;19:167-176.
12. Hild F, Duda VF, Albert U, Schulz KD: Ductal oriented sonography improves the diagnosis of pathological nipple discharge of the female breast compared with galactography. Eur J Cancer Prev 1998;7:S57-S62.
13. Fajardo LL, Jackson VP, Hunter TB: Interventional procedures in diseases of the breast: Needle biopsy, pneumocystography, and galactography. AJR Am J Roentgenol 1992;158:1231-1238.
14. Slawson SH, Johnson BA: Ductography: How to and what if? Radiographics 2001;21:133-150.
15. Hussain S, Lui DM: Ultrasound guided percutaneous galactography. Eur J Radiol 1997;24:163-165.
16. Rissanen T, Typpo T, Tikkakoski T, et al: Ultrasound-guided percutaneous galactography. J Clin Ultrasound 1993;21:497-502.
17. Sardanelli F, Imperiale A, Zandrino F, et al: Breast intraductal masses: US-guided fine-needle aspiration after galactography. Radiology 1997;204:143-148.
18. Brem RF, Gatewood OMB: Enhancement of duct filling during ductography. AJR Am J Roentgenol 1999;172:163-164.
19. Cardenosa G, Doudna C, Eklund GW: Ductography of the breast: Technique and findings. AJR Am J Roentgenol 1994; 162:1081-1087.
20. Chow JS, Smith D, Kaelin CM, Meyer JE: Galactography-guided localization of an intraductal papilloma. Clin Radiol 2001;56:72-83.
21. Saarela AO, Kiviniemi HO, Rissanen TJ: Preoperative methylene blue staining of galactographically suspicious breast lesions. Int Surg 1997;82:403-405.
22. Tabár L, Dean PB: Interventional radiologic procedures in the investigation of lesions of the breast. Radiol Clin North Am 1979;18:607-621.
23. Van Zee KJ, Perez GO, Minnard E, Cohen MA: Preoperative galactography increases the diagnostic yield of major duct excision for nipple discharge. Cancer 1998;82:1874-1880.
24. Vega Bolivar A, Landeras Alvaro RM, Ortega Garcia E: Intraductal placement of a Kopans spring-hookwire guide to localize nonpalpable breast lesions detected by galactography. Acta Radiol 1997;38:240-242.
24a. Hou M-F, Huang T-J, Huan Y-S, Hsieh J-S: A simple method of duct cannulation and localization for galactography before excision in patients with nipple discharge. Radiology 1995; 195:568-569.
25. Moskowitz M: Breast imaging. In Donegan WL, Spratt JS (eds): Cancer of the Breast. Philadelphia, WB Saunders, 1995, pp 206-239.
26. Baker KS, Davey DD, Stelling CB: Ductal abnormalities detected with galactography: Frequency of adequate excisional biopsy. AJR Am J Roentgenol 1994;162:821–824.
27. Dennis MA, Parker S, Kaske TI, et al: Incidental treatment of nipple discharge caused by benign intraductal papilloma through diagnostic Mammotome biopsy. AJR Am J Roentgenol 2000;174:1263-1268.
28. Guenin MA: Benign intraductal papilloma: Diagnosis and removal at stereotactic vacuum-assisted directional biopsy guided by galactography. Radiology 2001;218:576-579.
29. March DE, Coughlin BF, Polino JR, et al: Single dilated lactiferous duct due to papilloma: Ultrasonographically guided percutaneous biopsy with a vacuum-assisted device. J Ultrasound Med 2002;21:107-111.
30. Bjorn-Hansen R: Contrast-mammography. Br J Radiol 1965;38: 947-951.
31. Diner WC: Galactography: Mammary duct contrast examination. AJR Am J Roentgenol 1981;137:853-856.
32. Nunnerley HB, Field S: Mammary duct injection in patients with nipple discharge. Br J Radiol 1972;45:717-725.
33. Cardenosa G, Eklund GW: Benign papillary neoplasms of the breast: Mammographic findings. Radiology 1991;181:751-755.
34. Alberti GP, Troiso A: Secreting breast: The role of galactography. Eur J Gynaecol Oncol 1982;3:96-100.
35. Cardenosa G, Eklund GW: Ductography. Appl Radiol 1992;21: 24-29.
36. Dinkel H-P, Trusen A, Gassel AM, et al: Predictive value of galactographic patterns for benign and malignant neoplasms of the breast in patients with nipple discharge. Br J Radiol 2000;73:706-714.
37. Funcovics MA, Philipp MO, Lackner B, et al: Galactography: Method of choice in pathologic nipple discharge? Eur Radiol 2003;13:94-99.
38. Kindermann G, Paterok E, Weishaar J, et al: Early detection of ductal breast cancer: The diagnostic procedure for pathological discharge from the nipple. Tumori 1979;65:555-562.
39. Woods ER, Helvie MA, Ikeda DM, et al: Solitary breast papilloma: Comparison of mammographic, galactographic, and pathologic findings. AJR Am J Roentgenol 1992;159:487-491.

40. Kramer SC, Rieber A, Gorich J, et al: Diagnosis of papillomas of the breast: Value of magnetic resonance mammography in comparison with galactography. Eur Radiol 2000;10:1733-1736.
41. Orel SG, Dougherty CS, Reynolds C, et al: MR imaging in patients with nipple discharge: Initial experience. Radiology 2000;216:248-254.
42. Rovno HDS, Siegelman ES, Reynolds C, et al: Solitary intraductal papilloma: Findings at MR imaging and MR galactography. AJR Am J Roentgenol 1999;172:151-155.
43. Yoshimoto M, Kasumi F, Iwase T, et al: Magnetic resonance galactography for a patient with nipple discharge. Breast Cancer Res Treat 1997;42:87-90.
44. Kline TS, Lash SR: Bleeding nipple of pregnancy and postpartum period. Acta Cytol 1964;8:336-340.
45. LaFreniere R: Bloody nipple discharge during pregnancy: A rationale for conservative treatment. J Surg Oncol 1990;43:228-230.
46. Rubin E: Galactography in the investigation of nipple discharge. Alabama J Med Sci 1988;25:280-282.
47. DiPietro S, Coopmans de Yoldi G, Bergonzi S, et al: Nipple discharge as a sign of preneoplastic lesions and occult carcinoma of the breast: Clinical and galactographic study in 103 consecutive patients. Tumori 1979;65:317-324.
48. Osborne J: Galactography with contrast and dye: A two stage radiological/surgical approach to serous or bloody discharge. Australas Radiol 1989;33:266-269.
49. Rongione AJ, Evans BD, Kling KM, McFadden DW: Ductography is a useful technique in evaluation of abnormal nipple discharge. Am Surgeon 1996;62:785-788.
50. Sakorafas GH: Nipple discharge: Current diagnostic and therapeutic approaches. Cancer Treat Rev 2001;27:275-282.
51. Vargas HI, Romero L, Chlebowski RT: Management of bloody nipple discharge. Curr Treat Options Oncol 2002;3:157-161.

Section **V**

SCREENING MAMMOGRAPHY

The Epidemiology of Breast Cancer

Robert A. Smith, Louise A. Brinton, Joan L. Kramer, and Ahmedin Jemal

The American Cancer Society (ACS) estimated that 211,300 women would be diagnosed with invasive breast cancer and that 55,700 women would be diagnosed with ductal or lobular carcinoma in situ in 2003.[1] When cancers of the skin are excluded, invasive breast cancer is the most commonly diagnosed malignancy among women in the United States. In recent years, breast cancer has accounted for nearly 1 in 3 newly diagnosed cancers in women, exceeding the combined estimated incidence of lung cancer (80,100 new cases) and colorectal cancer (74,700 new cases) in 2003. It is the second leading cause of death from cancer among women, with an estimated 39,800 deaths in 2003, nearly 1 in 6 cancer deaths.

Death from breast cancer is the leading cause of premature death from cancer among women. On average, a woman dying of breast cancer has lost 18.6 years of life that she might have had if she had not died of this disease.[2] According to current incidence and mortality estimates, approximately 1 in every 7 women in a hypothetical cohort will be diagnosed with breast cancer in their lifetimes, and 1 in 30 will die from this disease.[2] Breast cancer is far less common among men. In 2003, it was estimated that there would be 1300 newly diagnosed cases and 400 deaths among men, less than 1% of the annual incidence and mortality for both sexes.[1] The focus of this chapter is female breast cancer, and the numbers and rates relating to incidence and mortality given here are limited to women in the United States.

The statistics just cited speak to the importance of breast cancer as a public health problem. During the past two decades, the use of mammography screening has steadily increased,[3] resulting in a progressively greater proportion of incident tumors being diagnosed while they are still localized.[2] This rapid growth in participation in screening in the United States had a pronounced effect on trends in incidence in the 1980s[4] and has been a major factor in the later observation of a decline in the mortality rate from breast cancer among women in the United States.[5] Thus, at this time, the greatest potential for reducing morbidity and mortality from breast cancer depends on early detection.

Although we know a great deal about the epidemiology of breast cancer, few of the known risk factors, alone or in combination, offer a behavioral strategy that has proven or practical potential to reduce risk measurably. Risk reductions in women at elevated risk have been demonstrated through chemoprevention with tamoxifen,[6] but the possibility of serious side effects in some women limits the potential of this strategy.[7,8] However, insofar as breast cancer is among women's greatest health concerns, it is important to look to the epidemiologic research for strategies that may reduce risk or may offer more protective surveillance strategies.

BREAST CANCER STATISTICS: NUMBERS AND RATES

Each year, the ACS estimates the number of newly diagnosed cases and deaths for the United States on the basis of incidence data from the National Cancer Institute (NCI) Surveillance Epidemiology and End-Results (SEER) program. The annual number of newly diagnosed cases for the nation is an estimate, because there is no national system to enumerate actual cases of breast cancer. Annual numbers of deaths are also estimated each year for comparison with the estimated number of newly diagnosed cases. Because deaths are enumerated by the Division of Vital Statistics of the National Center for Health Statistics (NCHS), the actual numbers of deaths in the United States from breast cancer are usually available within 2 to 3 years of the current calendar year.

Although the estimated annual numbers of new cases and deaths are important summary statistics, rates (events per population at risk) are better measures for comparisons over time and between population groups, because the size of a population and its age composition influence the number of new cases and deaths from breast cancer. To remove the effect of different age distributions in populations, or trends in the same population over time, crude rates (number of cases per midyear unit of population) are standardized to a specific population distribution. An *age-standardized rate* is a weighted average of age-specific rates in a given population, in which the weights are the proportion of persons in a standard population in the corresponding age groups.[9]

The value of age standardization for comparison of trends in breast cancer incidence and mortality rates is especially evident for U.S. trends, because the average age of the population is increasing. Those women born in the first year of the postwar birth cohort reached 40 years of age in 1985, and each year a growing number of women enter age cohorts in which screening is recommended and age-specific breast cancer incidence and mortality are higher. Because breast cancer incidence and mortality rates increase with increasing age, crude rates increase over time in an aging population on that basis alone, whereas trends in age-standardized incidence and mortality rates portray the underlying epidemiology of disease as well as trends in breast cancer detection and treatment. As a population's underlying age distribution and varying age distributions of subpopulations (i.e., different ethnic groups) grow increasingly different from the standardized distribution, the true rates and age-standardized rates may become correspondingly dissimilar. For example, in 1992, the crude incidence rate of female breast cancer in the U.S. was 128.2 per 100,000, compared with an age-adjusted rate of 110.6 per 100,000 when standardized to the 1970 U.S. population, a difference of +16%.[10] As this example shows, apart from comparisons among different populations or a population over time, the adjusted rate for any one year has no inherent meaning as a standalone measure of disease burden.

Because of the aging of the U.S. population, U.S. agencies elected to change the standard population used from 1970 to 2000, to better reflect the current distribution of the U.S. population.[11] Beginning with the 1999 U.S. incidence and mortality data, incidence and mortality rates are adjusted to the 2000 U.S. population and now more closely approximate true underlying rates. These new rates are not comparable to rates adjusted to the 1970 U.S. population, however, so comparisons between the new age-standardized rates and rates in prior publications should be made with caution. For example, the 1998 age-adjusted incidence rate standardized to the 1970 U.S. population was 118.1 per 100,000 females,[12] whereas the 1998 incidence rate standardized to the 2000 U.S. population was 140.3 per 100,000 females,[2] a rate that more closely approximates the actual number of new cases per 100,000 females in that year. Unless otherwise specified (i.e., age-specific rates), rates for U.S. women in these discussions are expressed as the annual number of cases per 100,000 women, age-adjusted to the 2000 U.S. population, and derive from the NCI's *SEER Cancer Statistics Review*.[2]

Age-specific rates, commonly calculated for 5-year age groups, are crude rates—that is, they are not age adjusted. Generally, age-specific rates are regarded as directly comparable within and between populations without age standardization because the adjustment for such a narrow age range generally adds little precision to the estimate.

INTERNATIONAL TRENDS

Breast cancer is the most common cancer in women throughout the world, accounting for more than 1 million new cases annually.[13] In developed countries, breast cancer is the most common malignancy diagnosed among women, and in developing regions, it typically ranks second to either cervical cancer or stomach cancer. Table 22–1 shows incidence data, estimated for the year 2000 and age-standardized to the world standard population, for a select group of countries. Note that the highest incidence rates are in North America, followed by western European countries. The lowest incidence rates in this series are from India and China. The magnitude of these differences is illustrated by the fact that the age-standardized incidence rate among these U.S. and European populations is three to four times higher than the rates in Japan and China.

Table 22–1. Year 2000 Estimated Average Annual Female Breast Cancer Incidence Rates per 100,000 Women in Select Locations*

Location	Rate
United States	91.39
Canada	81.78
Sweden	81.03
Finland	78.38
United Kingdom	74.93
Italy	64.87
Russian Federation	48.76
Japan	31.38
Costa Rica	28.32
India	19.10
China	16.39

*Rates are standardized to the world standard population.
From GLOBOCAN 2000: Cancer Incidence, Mortality and Prevalence Worldwide, Version 1.0. IARC CancerBase No. 5. Lyon, IARC Press, 2001.

Breast cancer is also the leading cause of cancer death among women in the majority of industrialized nations.[14] Worldwide mortality rates reported in 2000 vary considerably and follow trends similar to those observed in the comparison by incidence, although the rankings are not strictly parallel (Table 22–2). For example, although geographic areas in the U.S. rank first in incidence, mortality in the United States ranks 16th compared with mortality rates from 46 other countries. Because the mortality rate is a function of both incidence and survival rates over time, differences in a country's comparative mortality ranking are influenced not only by the magnitude of breast cancer incidence in a country but also by patterns of detection and treatment. In addition, the comparative reliability of the medical diagnosis,

Table 22–2. Year 2000 Estimated Average Annual Female Breast Cancer Mortality Rates per 100,000 Women in Select Locations*

Location	Rate
United Kingdom	26.81
Canada	22.75
United States	21.22
Italy	20.66
Finland	17.89
Sweden	17.48
Russian Federation	16.72
Costa Rica	11.65
India	9.91
Japan	7.72
China	4.51

*Rates are standardized to the world standard population.
From GLOBOCAN 2000: Cancer Incidence, Mortality and Prevalence Worldwide, Version 1.0. IARC CancerBase No. 5. Lyon, IARC Press, 2001.

reporting, and ascertainment of incident and mortality cases also influences these rates and rankings.

An analysis of cancer mortality in 15 industrialized countries conducted in 1992 found that the breast cancer mortality rate was increasing in all regions and in most age-specific groups.[15] The average annual percentage change between 1969 and 1986 ranged from 0.3% in two regions (the United States and the combined rate in New Zealand and Australia) to 1.2% in the combined average for three Eastern European countries (former German Democratic Republic, Czechoslovakia, and Hungary). In most countries, the greatest percentage increase was observed among women aged 65 to 74 years.

Comparisons of differences in international rates and of trends over time have focused not only on known risk factors for breast cancer but also on apparent lifestyle differences between cultures as a basis for hypothesis generation. However, what is most notable is that the breast cancer incidence is increasing worldwide, with the most dramatic increases occurring in countries in which Western lifestyles are becoming more prevalent. For example, although Japan stands apart from other affluent countries in having a low breast cancer incidence rate, the more widespread adoption of a Western lifestyle has resulted in a steady increase in breast cancer incidence and mortality.[13] Breast cancer incidence doubled between the 1960s and 1980s, with greater increases observed in urban versus rural areas and age-specific trends becoming more similar to those in North America and Europe.[16-18]

UNITED STATES TRENDS IN INCIDENCE, MORTALITY, AND SURVIVAL

Incidence

The analysis of long-term trends in the incidence of breast cancer in the United States has relied on data from the few geographic areas that have supported cancer registries over a long period. Incidence data before 1973 are usually drawn from the Connecticut Tumor Registry or from five geographic areas (Atlanta, Connecticut, Detroit, Iowa, and Oakland).[2,19,20] Data from Connecticut (available since 1935), data from the five geographic regions (from 1950 to 1985), and data from 1973 to 1980 from SEER show a gradual annual increase over this period in the age-adjusted incidence rate of invasive breast cancer of less than 1% per year.[20] However, between 1980 and 1987, the age-adjusted incidence rate of breast cancer rose from 102.1 to 134.4 per 100,000, a relative increase in the incidence rate over the period of 27%, or an average increase of approximately 4% per year (Fig. 22–1). Between 1987 and 2000, rates have fluctuated somewhat, but in 1996 they began to climb again, resulting in an overall annual percentage increase since 1987 of 0.4% per year.

Particularly noteworthy in the mid-1970s was the short-term increase in the incidence rate observed in 1974, which is believed to be primarily due to an increase in the numbers of women who either received breast examinations for screening or complained of symptoms after Betty Ford and Happy Rockefeller were diagnosed with breast cancer. This phenomenon was a brief preview of what was to be experienced in the mid-1980s: an increase in the annual incidence rate due to an increase in the rate of case detection. However, the trend was brief, as is clear from the subsequent decline in incidence rates after 1975 and the return to the earlier trend. This brief period of rising and declining incidence rates is consistent with a screening effect; that is, the observed short-term increase in the incidence rate is not due to a change in the underlying epidemiology of disease but to a change in the rate of case detection. Because these cases were detected before they would have become clinically apparent, an eventual decline in the incidence rate can be anticipated.[21]

Trends in Incidence

The trend in incidence (see Fig. 22–1), specifically the significant increase in rates between 1980 and 1987, has received considerable attention because of the interest in understanding the degree to which it represents a true increase in disease, a screening effect, or some combination of these two factors. There is little question that the dramatic 1980 to 1987 increase in incidence occurred during a period of rapid increase in the use of breast cancer screening with mammography.[4,22] According to Howard,[23] an evaluation of national surveys conducted between 1978 and 1983 indicated that only about 15% to 20% of American women had ever had a mammogram. In 1987, estimates from the National Health Interview Survey (NHIS) indicated that 39% of women aged 40 years and older had ever had a mammogram.[24] In 1992, according to estimates from the Mammography Attitudes and Usage Survey conducted by the Jacobs Institute of Women's Health, that number had increased to 74%.[25] During this time, a number of factors contributed to the greater utilization of mammography, including the growth of scientific support for the value of the procedure,[26-28] growing acceptance of the procedure by providers[29,30] as well as by women,[31] and improving access as measured by the growth in the number of installed dedicated mammography units.[31] Also during this period, an increasing number of women reported that they were screened on a regular basis according to recommended guidelines or whenever their doctor recommended the test.[25] Thus, the evidence supports the likelihood that increasing rates associated with screening largely represent the added detection of occult cases that otherwise would have given rise to symptoms in subsequent years.

Some analyses, however, have also concluded that the entirety of the increase in breast cancer incidence

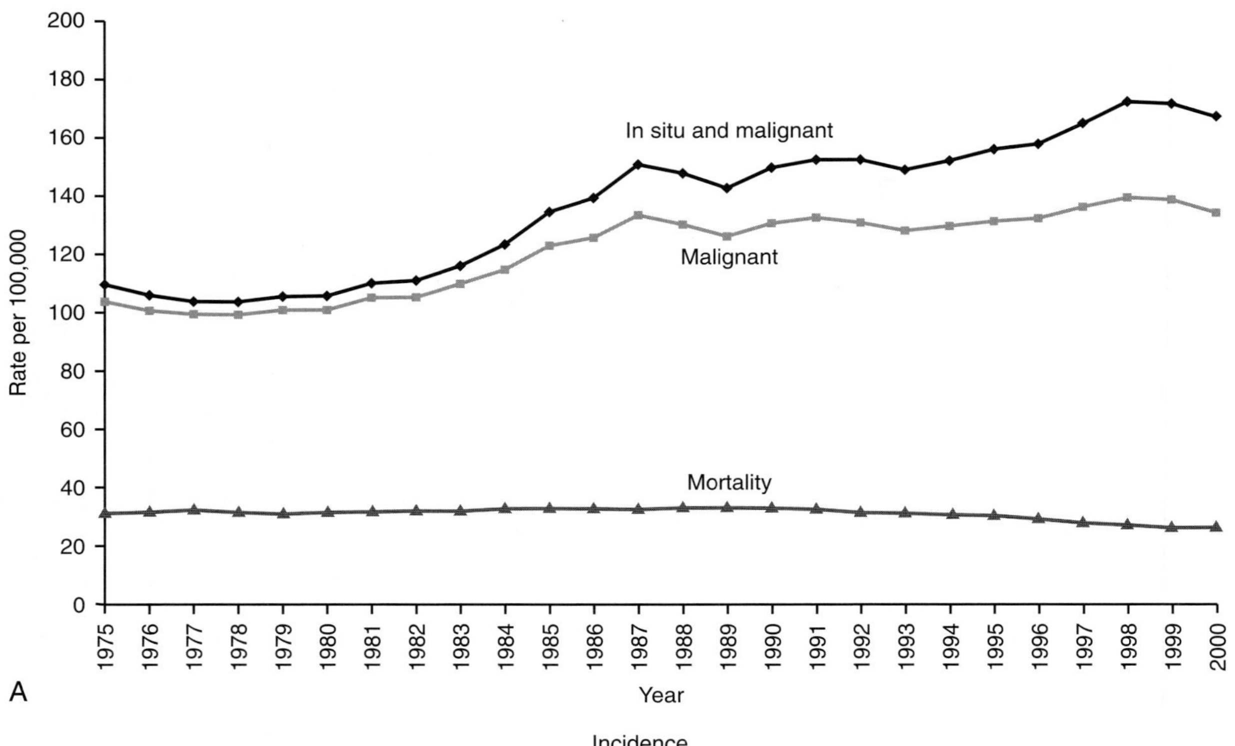

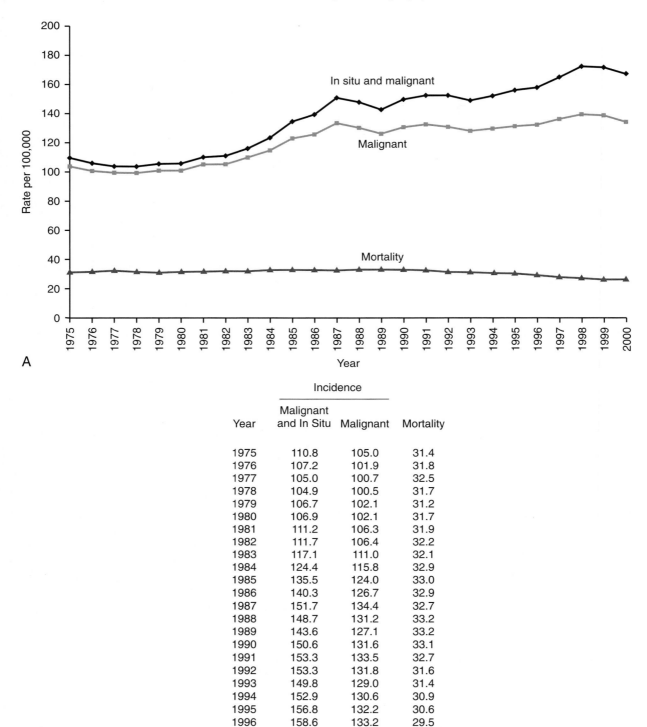

Year	Incidence: Malignant and In Situ	Incidence: Malignant	Mortality
1975	110.8	105.0	31.4
1976	107.2	101.9	31.8
1977	105.0	100.7	32.5
1978	104.9	100.5	31.7
1979	106.7	102.1	31.2
1980	106.9	102.1	31.7
1981	111.2	106.3	31.9
1982	111.7	106.4	32.2
1983	117.1	111.0	32.1
1984	124.4	115.8	32.9
1985	135.5	124.0	33.0
1986	140.3	126.7	32.9
1987	151.7	134.4	32.7
1988	148.7	131.2	33.2
1989	143.6	127.1	33.2
1990	150.6	131.6	33.1
1991	153.3	133.5	32.7
1992	153.3	131.8	31.6
1993	149.8	129.0	31.4
1994	152.9	130.6	30.9
1995	156.8	132.2	30.6
1996	158.6	133.2	29.5
1997	165.5	137.1	28.2
1998	173.0	140.3	27.5
1999	172.3	139.6	26.6
2000	167.8	135.1	26.7

B

Figure 22–1. Breast cancer incidence and mortality rates in U.S. women, 1975 to 2000. Rates are per 100,000 age-adjusted to the 2000 U.S. standard population. (From Ries L, Eisner M, Kosary C, et al: SEER Cancer Statistics Review, 1975-2000. Bethesda, MD, National Cancer Institute, 2003.)

is not due solely to an increase in case detection. White and colleagues[32] have concluded that an increase in screening accounts for the increase in incidence in women between the ages of 55 and 64 years but not entirely for women younger than 55 or older than 65 years. Likewise, Liff and coworkers[33] concluded that the growth was accounted for by both an increase in the use of mammography and a true increase in the rate of disease. There is little question that a true increase in disease is a factor in the recent increase in incidence. As noted earlier, an average annual growth of slightly less than 1% per year has been observed from Connecticut Tumor Registry data long before the widespread availability and use of mammography. In addition, using Connecticut data, Holford and colleagues[34] have shown higher age-specific incidence for successive cohorts of women born since 1870, again providing evidence that a true underlying increase in disease has contributed in part to the recent increase in the incidence trend.

Incidence and Age

The incidence of breast cancer grows with patient age (Fig. 22–2). The diagnosis of breast cancer is rare before age 25 years and begins to increase measurably after that age. Between the ages of 20 and 44 years, the incidence rate for breast cancer increases rapidly, more than doubling in each successive 5-year age group. Near the age of menopause, and observable in the age-specific incidence rates after age 45, the rate of increase in incidence rates in successive age groups is slower compared with the pattern observed in premenopausal women. This pattern has been observed in other countries, although the increase in age-specific rates after the age of menopause appears to be greater in Western countries than in Asian countries.[35]

Earlier trends—shown in Figure 22–2 as average age-specific rates during 1975 to 1979, 1985 to 1989, and 1996 to 2000—provide a clear picture of the pattern of incidence by age before the influence of screening on the incidence rate, which is evident in the age-specific rates for 1985 to 1989 and 1996 to 2000. Before 1980, the breast cancer incidence rate was higher with each successive age group. Data for the period after 1985, however, reveal a peak at the age group 75 to 79 years, followed by a decline in age-specific incidence, a pattern that was first observed in 1984 and has endured since that time.

Precise causes of this pattern are not known, but it is likely due to the interplay of several factors. First, the shift in the age-specific pattern since the mid 1980s, specifically among older women, may be explained simply by different participation rates in screening and the interaction of age and lead time gained.[4] The introduction of screening should lead to a visible increase in the incidence rate due largely to the increase in case finding in the pool of occult cases detectable on mammography. Because the average *sojourn time* for breast cancer (i.e., the average period of time that breast cancer is detectable with mammography before the onset of clinical symptoms) is longer in postmenopausal women,[36,37] a more visible increase in the incidence rate should be observed in older compared with younger women owing to the comparatively larger pool of detectable cases. This is evident in the age-specific trends in Figure 22–2. Furthermore, a higher rate of case findings in the initial years of a screening program also should lead to a more visible decline in the incidence rate in subsequent years. In contrast, a shorter sojourn time in younger women will contribute to a less visible increase in incidence and hence a smaller decline in the incidence rates in subsequent age cohorts after an increase in screening.

Second, this change in the pattern of age-specific incidence rates among older women may also be influenced by the steady decline of screening rates as women get older.[38] Age-specific incidence rates among women aged 80 years and older have not increased during the past decade at the same rate as those in women aged 60 to 79 years, so the shift in the historical trend of higher incidence with higher age may be accounted for by higher rates of screening in women younger than 75 years. It is likely that some combination of these two explanations is at work, and whether one influence is more dominant remains to be determined.

Although age-adjusted incidence rates have increased since the early 1970s, it is evident from the patterns shown in Figures 22–2 and 22–3 that age-specific changes have not been uniform. Among women younger than 40 years, the incidence of breast cancer has generally declined somewhat. Among women between the ages of 40 and 59 years, an increase in incidence between 11% and 16% is apparent, whereas among women aged 55 to 79 years, the increase in incidence has exceeded 45%. After age 85 years, a much smaller increase in incidence is seen.

Although age-specific rates in younger women have not changed much, the stability in these rates contrasts with the growth in the number of newly diagnosed cases in these age groups, as increasingly larger numbers of women born since 1945 pass their 30th birthday. Although the rate of disease may not have substantially changed, the numbers of women from whom these rates are calculated are larger. In 1970, approximately 11,550,000 women were between the ages of 30 and 39 years, whereas in 1990, it is estimated that 21,060,000 women were in that age group, roughly a doubling of the size of this age group over this 20-year period. Here, although age-specific incidence rates have been stable, the growth in the size of the population at risk resulted in a near doubling of the annual number of cases in that age group over this period. A similar pattern will be seen in subsequent age groups of women as this cohort enters and leaves successive age groups.

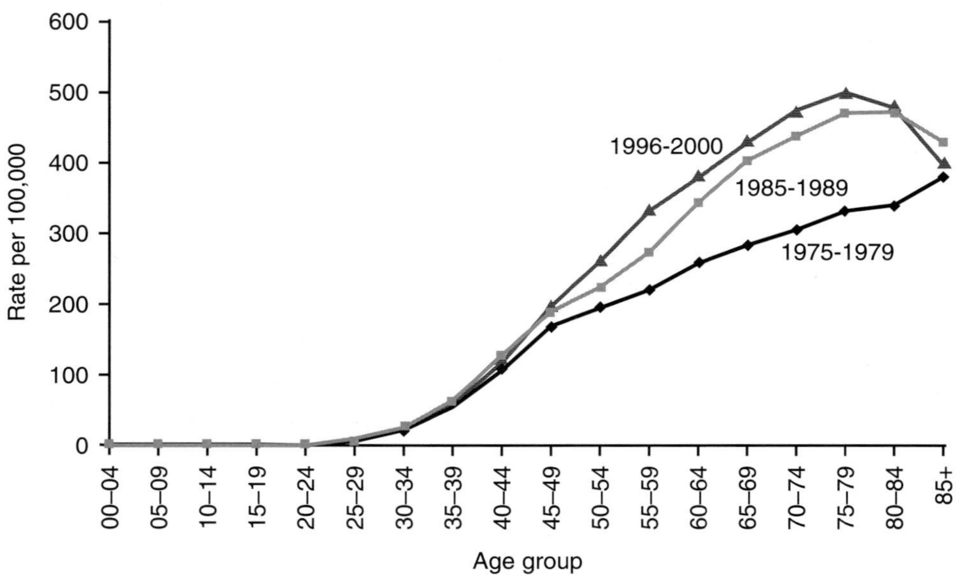

A

Age	1975–1979	1985–1989	1996–2000
00–04	0.0	0.0	0.0
05–09	0.0	0.0	0.0
10–14	0.0	0.0	0.0
15–19	0.2	0.0	0.2
20–24	1.2	0.9	1.4
25–29	8.5	7.9	7.8
30–34	25.9	26.9	25.4
35–39	57.8	65.1	61.0
40–44	108.6	127.5	121.1
45–49	171.7	191.9	198.1
50–54	197.0	225.7	263.5
55–59	221.2	275.0	333.1
60–64	260.4	346.5	380.6
65–69	284.4	408.4	430.1
70–74	306.1	439.1	476.1
75–79	332.9	472.5	499.0
80–84	342.6	471.6	477.8
85+	380.8	429.5	401.7

B

Figure 22–2. Age-specific breast cancer incidence rates, U.S. women, 1975 to 2000. Rates are per 100,000 women within the specified age group. (From Ries L, Eisner M, Kosary C, et al: SEER Cancer Statistics Review, 1975-2000. Bethesda, MD, National Cancer Institute, 2003.)

Incidence and Race

White women have higher age-adjusted incidence rates than black women (140.9 vs. 116.3 per 100,000), albeit notable differences are evident in age-specific rates and trends over time. Among women aged 40 years and younger, age-specific incidence rates are higher in black women than in white women, a difference that is especially evident among women aged 20 to 34 years (see Tables 22–3 and 22–4). In comparison, among women aged 45 years and older, age-specific incidence rates are 9% to 35% higher in white women than in black women. Likewise, the trend in incidence between 1975 and 2000 has been similar in black and white women aged 50 years and older (+37.6% vs. +33.1%, respectively), but in women younger than 50 years, the proportional increase in incidence over the same time is four times as high in black women as in white women (+25.1% vs. +6.3%).

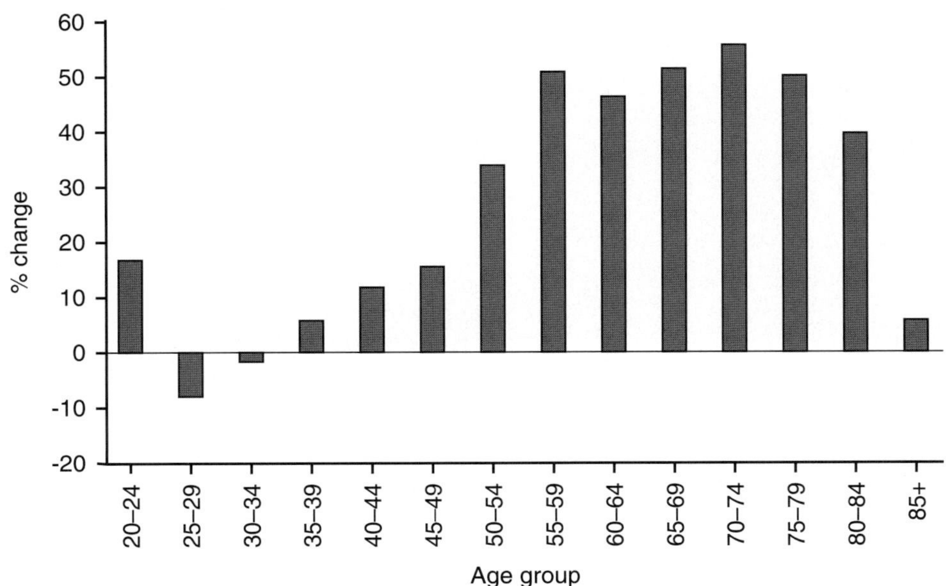

*Percent change is based on rates per 100,000 women within the specified age group.

A

Age	Initial 1975–1979	1985–1989	Final 1996–2000	% Change
00–04	0.0	0.0	0.0	0.0
05–09	0.0	0.0	0.0	0.0
10–14	0.0	0.0	0.0	0.0
15–19	0.0	0.0	0.0	0.0
20–24	1.2	0.9	1.4	16.6
25–29	8.5	7.9	7.8	–8.2
30–34	25.9	26.9	25.4	–1.9
35–39	57.8	65.1	61.0	5.5
40–44	108.6	127.5	121.1	11.5
45–49	171.7	191.9	198.1	15.3
50–54	197.0	225.7	263.5	33.7
55–59	221.2	275.0	333.1	50.5
60–64	260.4	346.5	380.6	46.1
65–69	284.4	408.4	430.1	51.2
70–74	306.1	439.1	476.1	55.5
75–79	332.9	472.5	499.0	49.8
80–84	342.6	471.6	477.8	39.4
85+	380.8	429.5	401.7	5.4

B

Figure 22–3. Percentage change in age-specific breast cancer incidence rates between 1975-1979 and 1996-2000 in U.S. women. Percentage change is based on rates per 100,000 women within the specified age group. (From Ries L, Eisner M, Kosary C, et al: SEER Cancer Statistics Review, 1975-2000. Bethesda, MD, National Cancer Institute, 2003.)

Mortality

Until 1987, breast cancer was the leading cause of cancer death among women, but now it is the second leading cause of death from cancer. The mortality rate from breast cancer was remarkably stable for several decades before the 1990s, ranging from 31.9 deaths per 100,000 women in 1950 to 33.3 per 100,000 in 1990, and from an average of 32.0 per 100,000 for 1956 to 1958 to 33.11 per 100,000 for 1986 to 1990 (see also Fig. 22–1).[2]

Racial and age-specific differences and differences in trends in mortality between 1975 and 2000 are noteworthy (see Tables 22–3 and 22–5). Overall, age-

Table 22–3. Age-Specific Female Breast Cancer Incidence and Mortality Rates by Race in the United States, 1996 to 2000

	Incidence		Mortality	
Age Group (yr)	White	Black	White	Black
0-4	*	*	*	*
5-9	*	*	*	*
10-14	*	*	*	*
15-19	*	*	*	*
20-24	1.1	*	0.1	*
25-29	7.5	12.1	0.8	1.9
30-34	24.4	32.8	3.3	7.3
35-39	60.5	66.3	8.2	16.5
40-44	122.7	120.0	16.0	29.0
45-49	203.3	184.3	26.8	46.9
50-54	272.1	236.7	41.3	64.4
55-59	346.0	282.3	54.7	79.5
60-64	398.8	318.6	67.9	88.1
65-69	453.8	357.9	82.8	97.7
70-74	499.8	393.6	102.8	119.9
75-79	521.7	415.8	120.8	135.4
80-84	496.9	385.0	146.8	158.0
85+	416.7	339.3	200.7	209.6

*Statistic not displayed due to less than 25 cases.
Underlying mortality data provided by NCHS (www.cdc.gov/nchs). Rates are per 100,000 and age-adjusted to the 2000 U.S. (18 age groups) standard.
From Ries L, Eisner M, Kosary C, et al: SEER Cancer Statistics Review, 1975-2000. Bethesda, MD, National Cancer Institute, 2003.

adjusted mortality rates for 1996 to 2000 are higher in black women (35.9 per 100,000) than in white women (27.2 per 100,000). Age-specific rates increase steadily with age for both black and white women, and unlike the incidence pattern showing a peak at age 75 to 79 years, age-specific mortality rates are considerably higher among women aged 80 to 84 years and 85 years and older than in women aged 70 to 79. Black females have higher age-specific incidence rates before age 40 and lower rates thereafter in comparison with white women. In contrast, age-specific mortality rates are higher in black women than in white women at every age (see Tables 22–3 and 22–5).

Age-adjusted breast cancer mortality has declined by 2.5% per year since 1990 among white women and by 1.0% per year since 1991 among black women. Rates began to decline earlier and declined faster in the younger (<40 years) than in the older age groups (40 years and older). Further examination of the age-specific trend among whites demonstrated that age-specific mortality rates are declining in all age groups except in that of 80 years and older (Fig. 22–4). This finding may reflect a lower rate of screening, substandard treatments, or both for women 80 years and older.

Stage at Diagnosis and Survival

The trend in the past decade of greater participation in mammography is reflected in trends in stage at diagnosis over the same period. As shown in Figure 22–5, the rate of cases diagnosed in situ and at stage I has continued to increase since the 1980s, a period when the use of mammography has been growing. As can be seen in Tables 22–6 and 22–7, a significantly greater proportion of incident cases are being detected at more favorable stages. In fact, the pro-

Table 22–4. Trends in U.S. Women: Incidence of Invasive Breast Cancer by Race and Age, 1975 to 2000

	All Races			White Women			Black Women		
Year	All ages	<40 yr	40+ yr	All ages	<40 yr	40+ yr	All ages	<40 yr	40+ yr
1975	105	12.4	227.6	107.3	11.8	233.7	93.4	18.4	192.6
1976	101.9	12.3	220.5	104.8	12.5	226.9	85.2	11.8	182.3
1977	100.7	13	216.8	103.4	12.6	223.5	86.7	16	180.2
1978	100.5	12.9	216.5	103.5	12.9	223.5	86	15.6	179.3
1979	102.1	12.1	221.1	104.7	11.8	227.7	87	15.9	181.2
1980	102.1	13.3	219.6	104.9	13.1	226.4	89.6	15.7	187.5
1981	106.3	14.1	228.3	109.8	13.9	236.7	94.2	18.7	194
1982	106.4	14.3	228.4	109.9	14.3	236.4	93.5	15.1	197.3
1983	111	13.7	239.9	114.4	13.9	247.4	103.2	14.8	220.2
1984	115.8	14.5	249.9	119.8	14.5	259.1	101.5	18.5	211.4
1985	124	14.4	269.1	127.7	14	278.2	111.6	20	232.8
1986	126.7	14.1	275.9	130.2	13.9	284.2	114.6	17.2	243.7
1987	134.4	13.8	294	140.3	13.8	307.8	109	16.3	231.8
1988	131.2	13.1	287.5	136.2	13.2	299	118.5	12.7	258.5
1989	127.1	12.6	278.7	132.2	12.5	290.7	105.1	15.7	223.4
1990	131.6	13.4	288	136.1	13.2	298.8	118.2	14.8	255.1
1991	133.5	14.1	291.5	138.5	13.8	303.7	116.7	17.5	248
1992	131.8	13	289.2	135.5	12.9	297.7	122.8	14	266.7
1993	129	12.7	282.9	133	12.6	292.4	118.7	14	257.4
1994	130.6	11.6	288.1	135.3	11.1	299.8	121.7	15.4	262.4
1995	132.2	12.6	290.5	137.1	12.4	302.1	123.1	15	266.2
1996	133.2	12.4	293	137.4	12.1	303.3	122.8	14.4	266.3
1997	137.1	12.9	301.4	141.8	12.8	312.6	123	16.1	264.7
1998	140.3	13.1	308.7	145.4	12.7	321.1	120	15.6	258.3
1999	139.6	13	307.3	144.7	13.2	318.8	122.3	13.3	266.7
2000	135.1	13	296.7	140.9	12.3	311.1	116.3	16.9	247.9

From Ries L, Eisner M, Kosary C, et al: SEER Cancer Statistics Review, 1975-2000. Bethesda, MD, National Cancer Institute, 2003.

Table 22–5. Trends in U.S. Women: Mortality of Invasive Breast Cancer by Race and Age, 1975 to 2000*

	All Races			White			Black Women		
Year	All ages	<40 yr	40+ yr	All ages	<40 yr	40+ yr	All ages	<40 yr	40+ yr
1975	31.4	2.6	69.6	31.8	2.6	70.5	29.5	3.6	63.8
1976	31.8	2.5	70.6	32.2	2.5	71.5	30.5	3.2	66.5
1977	32.5	2.6	72	32.7	2.5	72.6	32.8	3.8	71.1
1978	31.7	2.5	70.4	31.9	2.4	71	32.1	3.9	69.5
1979	31.2	2.6	69.1	31.5	2.5	69.9	30.8	3.9	66.5
1980	31.7	2.7	70.1	31.9	2.6	70.8	31.7	3.6	68.8
1981	31.9	2.6	70.7	32.1	2.5	71.3	32.6	3.8	70.7
1982	32.2	2.7	71.3	32.3	2.5	71.7	33.7	4	73.1
1983	32.1	2.5	71.2	32.2	2.4	71.6	33.5	3.7	73
1984	32.9	2.8	72.7	32.9	2.7	72.9	35.9	4.2	78
1985	33	2.6	73.2	33.1	2.5	73.7	34.9	4.1	75.6
1986	32.9	2.7	72.8	32.9	2.5	73.3	35.4	4.6	76.2
1987	32.7	2.7	72.3	32.6	2.5	72.3	36.7	4.5	79.5
1988	33.2	2.6	73.7	33.1	2.4	73.7	37.8	4.7	81.5
1989	33.2	2.5	74	33.2	2.3	74.2	36.6	4.1	79.6
1990	33.1	2.4	73.8	33	2.2	73.8	38	4	83
1991	32.7	2.4	72.8	32.4	2.2	72.5	38.3	3.9	83.7
1992	31.6	2.3	70.5	31.4	2.1	70.3	37.1	3.9	81
1993	31.4	2	70.2	31.1	1.8	69.8	38	3.8	83.4
1994	30.9	2.2	69	30.6	2	68.4	37.7	3.6	82.9
1995	30.6	2.1	68.2	30.1	2	67.3	38.2	3.6	84
1996	29.5	2	65.9	29	1.8	65.2	37.1	3.8	81.3
1997	28.2	2	63	27.6	1.8	61.8	37.4	3.7	82.1
1998	27.5	2	61.4	27	1.7	60.5	35.5	3.6	77.9
1999	26.6	1.8	59.5	26	1.5	58.3	35.2	3.4	77.3
2000	26.7	1.8	59.8	26.3	1.6	58.9	34.6	3.1	76.2

*Rates are per 100,000 and age-adjusted to the 2000 U.S. (18 age groups) standard.
From Ries L, Eisner M, Kosary C, et al: SEER Cancer Statistics Review, 1975-2000. Bethesda, MD, National Cancer Institute, 2003.

portion of cancers detected at the in situ stage has nearly doubled among white and black women, and the proportion of cancers detected at stage I has increased by more than 25% for both racial groups for cases diagnosed between 1988 and 2000. The distribution of stage at detection by race for 1996 to 2000 is shown in Table 22–8. Although the trend in detection at more favorable stages has improved during the past decade for both black and white women, a greater proportion of cancers in black women are still diagnosed at less favorable stages.

The latest 5-year survival rate (i.e., for cases diagnosed from 1992 through 1999) for all stages of invasive disease is 86.6%.[2] When calculated by stage at detection, it is evident that survival is also much improved if breast cancer is diagnosed early. The 5-year survival rate for invasive disease diagnosed at a localized stage is currently 97% for cases diagnosed during 1992 to 1999. Figure 22–6 shows 5-year survival rates by stage (extent of disease) and the comparative distribution of cases diagnosed at that stage for 1992 to 1999. As can be seen, breast cancers diagnosed at the regional or distant stage have a much poorer prognosis.

Table 22–6. Percentage Change in Incidence of Female Breast Cancer by Stage Between 1988 and 2000, by Age and Race

	Age < 40 years		Age 40+ years	
Stage	Whites	Blacks	Whites	Blacks
In situ	35.3	10.5	88.4	86
Stage I	5.3	82.4	33	28.5
Stage II	−3.3	20.3	0.1	−1.9
Stage III-IV	14.3	−6.7	−8.6	−17.7
Unknown	−55	106	−45.3	−36.2

Overall, 5-year survival rates are lower in black women (73.5%) than in white women (87.9%), and poorer survival is seen at each stage of disease detection.[2] The overall poorer survival among black women is largely due to later stage at diagnosis. An earlier analysis by Eley and associates[39] suggested that most, though not all, of the racial differences in survival could be explained by differences in prognostic factors, which may be due to a later stage at diagnosis. However, most of the difference attributable to race is a function of higher poverty rates among black women than among white women. Of particular relevance is the influence of social class on both overall survival and disease-free survival. An analysis by Gordon and colleagues[40] showed that taken alone, non-white women have shorter disease-free and overall survival, but after adjustment of data for the socioeconomic status of the patient, race ceased to be a significant factor. Later analyses by Shavers and colleagues[41] observed racial variation in clinical presentation, treatment, and survival in women aged 35 and younger, with black women tending to present with more advanced disease, being less likely to receive state-of-the-art treatment, and having poorer survival than white women. Other investigators have shown similar multifactorial explanations for

Text continued on p. 356

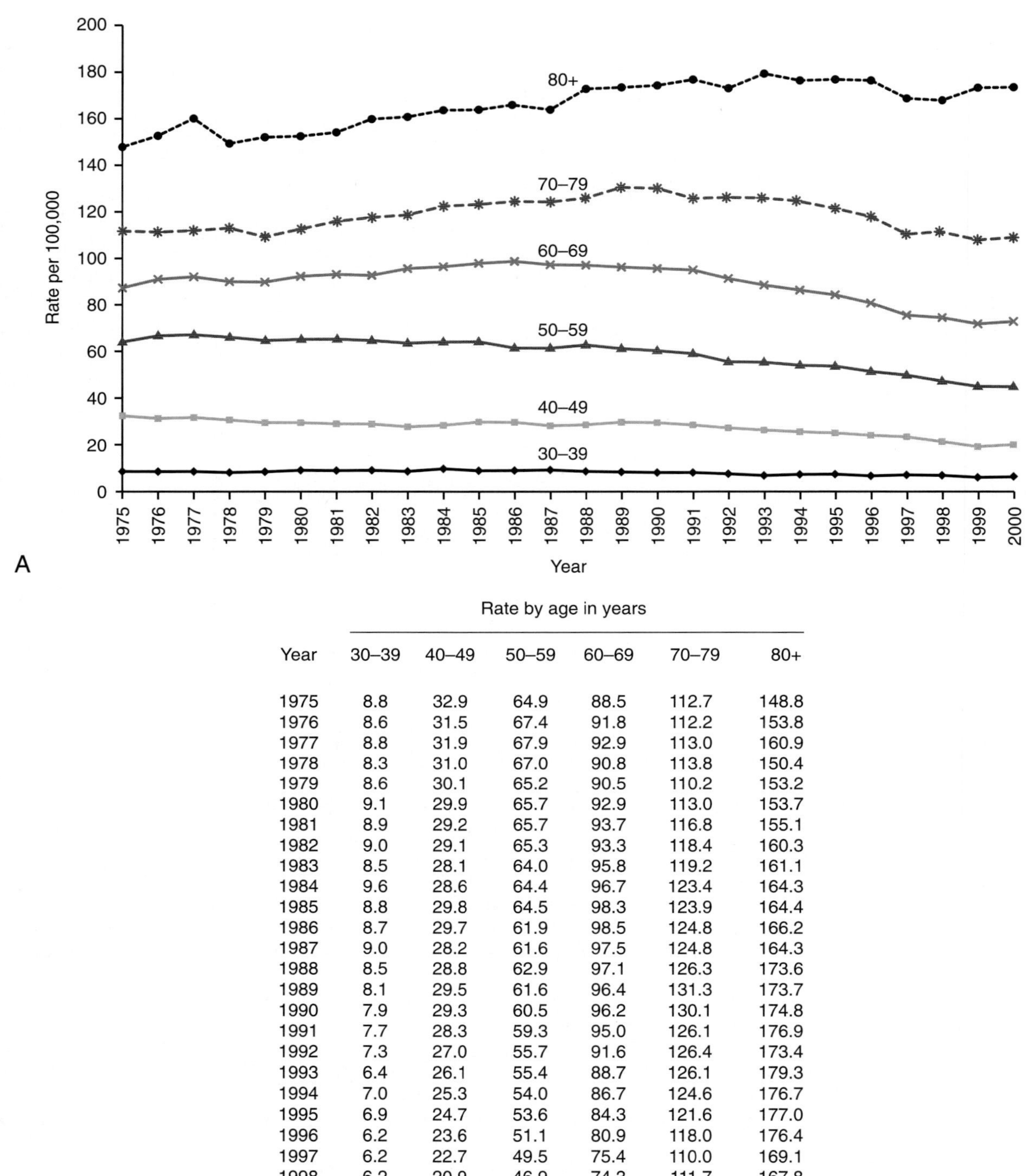

Rate by age in years

Year	30–39	40–49	50–59	60–69	70–79	80+
1975	8.8	32.9	64.9	88.5	112.7	148.8
1976	8.6	31.5	67.4	91.8	112.2	153.8
1977	8.8	31.9	67.9	92.9	113.0	160.9
1978	8.3	31.0	67.0	90.8	113.8	150.4
1979	8.6	30.1	65.2	90.5	110.2	153.2
1980	9.1	29.9	65.7	92.9	113.0	153.7
1981	8.9	29.2	65.7	93.7	116.8	155.1
1982	9.0	29.1	65.3	93.3	118.4	160.3
1983	8.5	28.1	64.0	95.8	119.2	161.1
1984	9.6	28.6	64.4	96.7	123.4	164.3
1985	8.8	29.8	64.5	98.3	123.9	164.4
1986	8.7	29.7	61.9	98.5	124.8	166.2
1987	9.0	28.2	61.6	97.5	124.8	164.3
1988	8.5	28.8	62.9	97.1	126.3	173.6
1989	8.1	29.5	61.6	96.4	131.3	173.7
1990	7.9	29.3	60.5	96.2	130.1	174.8
1991	7.7	28.3	59.3	95.0	126.1	176.9
1992	7.3	27.0	55.7	91.6	126.4	173.4
1993	6.4	26.1	55.4	88.7	126.1	179.3
1994	7.0	25.3	54.0	86.7	124.6	176.7
1995	6.9	24.7	53.6	84.3	121.6	177.0
1996	6.2	23.6	51.1	80.9	118.0	176.4
1997	6.2	22.7	49.5	75.4	110.0	169.1
1998	6.2	20.9	46.9	74.3	111.7	167.8
1999	5.4	18.7	44.5	71.3	107.3	172.6
2000	5.6	19.4	44.4	72.3	108.3	173.1

Underlying mortality data provided by NCHS (www.cdc.gov/nchs).
Rates are per 100,000 and are age adjusted to the 2000 U.S.
B (18 age groups) standard.

Figure 22–4. Age-specific breast cancer mortality rates, U.S. white women, 1975-2000. Rates given are per 100,000 women, age-adjusted to the 2000 U.S. standard population. (From Ries L, Eisner M, Kosary C, et al: SEER Cancer Statistics Review, 1975-2000. Bethesda, MD, National Cancer Institute, 2003.)

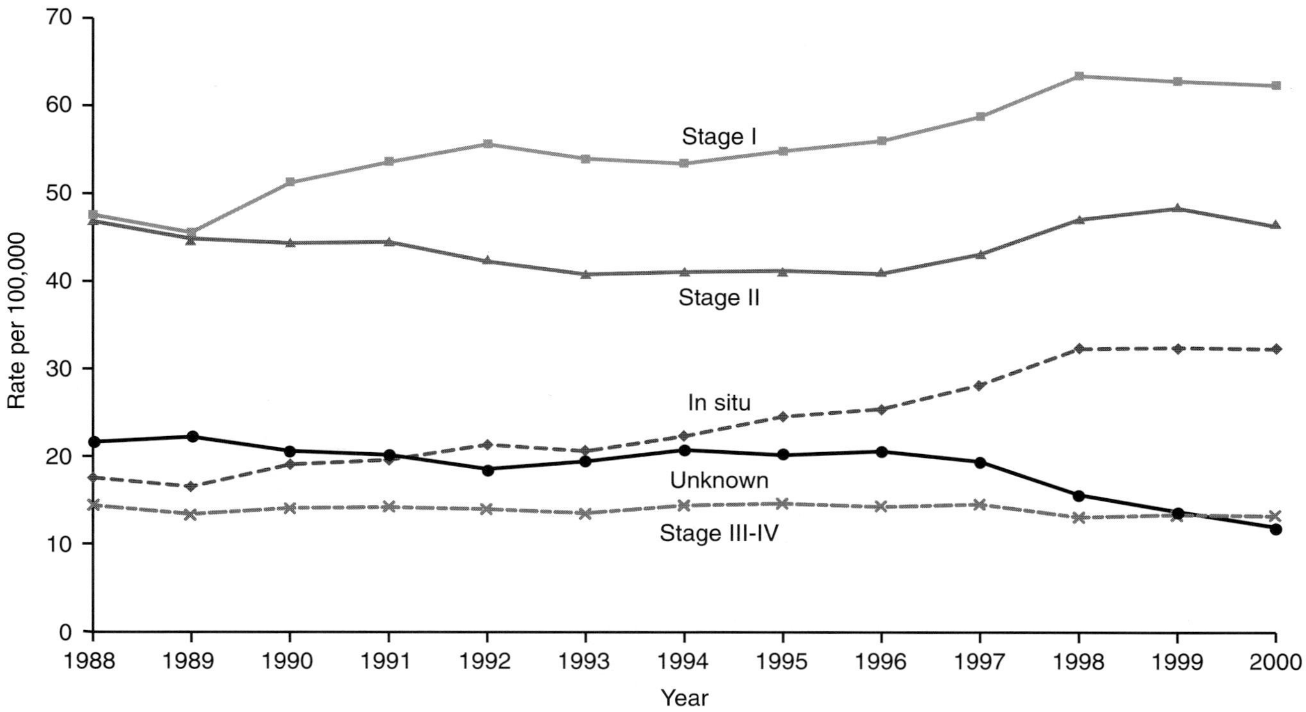

A

	Rate				
Year	In Situ	Stage I	Stage II	Stage III–IV	Unknown
1988	17.6	47.8	47.0	14.4	21.9
1989	16.6	45.8	45.0	13.5	22.6
1990	19.2	51.7	44.7	14.1	20.9
1991	19.9	53.9	44.8	14.4	20.4
1992	21.6	56.0	42.7	14.2	18.8
1993	20.9	54.3	41.2	13.7	19.6
1994	22.5	53.7	41.3	14.6	20.9
1995	24.8	55.3	41.4	14.8	20.6
1996	25.6	56.3	41.3	14.5	20.9
1997	28.4	59.1	43.4	14.7	19.8
1998	32.7	63.7	47.4	13.3	15.8
1999	32.7	63.1	48.7	13.6	14.2
2000	32.7	62.7	46.9	13.3	12.2

B

Figure 22–5. Breast cancer incidence rates by American Joint Committee on Cancer (AJCC) stage in U.S. women, 1988 to 2000. Rates given are per 100,000 women, age-adjusted to the 2000 U.S. standard population. (From Ries L, Eisner M, Kosary C, et al: SEER Cancer Statistics Review, 1975-2000. Bethesda, MD, National Cancer Institute, 2003.)

HISTORICAL STAGE DISTRIBUTION AND 5-YEAR RELATIVE SURVIVAL RATES BY STAGE, U.S. WOMEN, 1992–1999

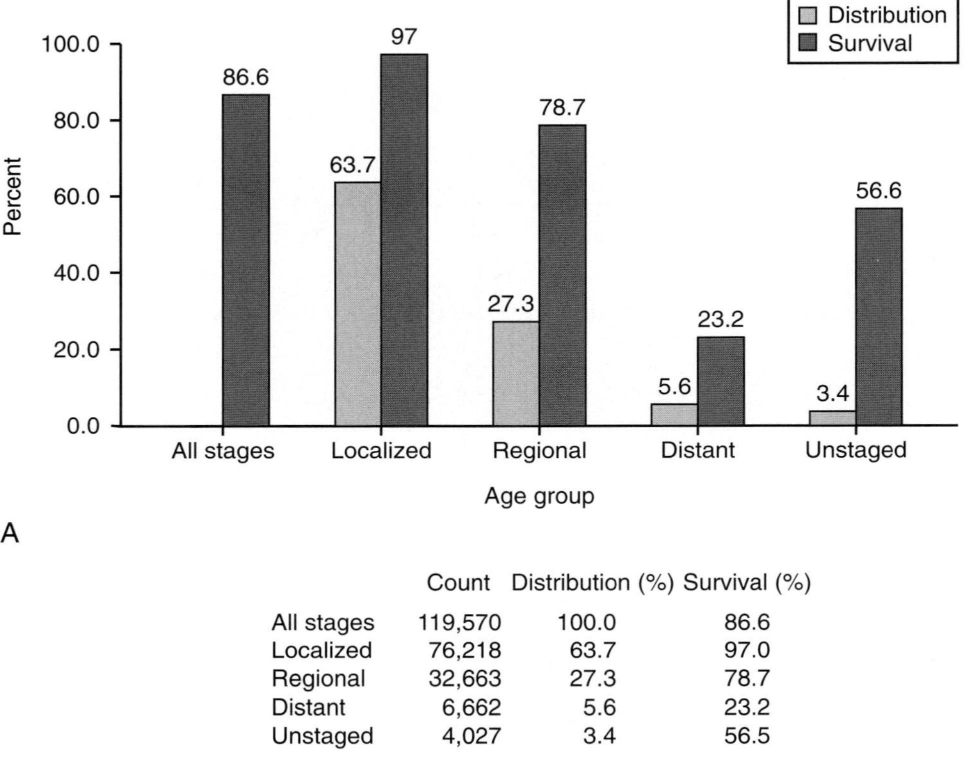

	Count	Distribution (%)	Survival (%)
All stages	119,570	100.0	86.6
Localized	76,218	63.7	97.0
Regional	32,663	27.3	78.7
Distant	6,662	5.6	23.2
Unstaged	4,027	3.4	56.5

Figure 22–6. Historical stage distribution and 5-year relative survival rates by stage in U.S. women, 1992 to 1999. (From Ries L, Eisner M, Kosary C, et al: SEER Cancer Statistics Review, 1975-2000. Bethesda, MD, National Cancer Institute, 2003.)

Table 22–7. Trend in Female Breast Cancer Incidence by AJCCS Stage, Race, and Age in the United States 1988 to 2000*

	In Situ				Stage I				Stage II				Stage III–IV				Unknown			
	<40 yr		40+ yr		<40		40+		<40		40+		<40		40+		<40		40+	
Year	*White*	*Black*	*White*	*Black*	*White*	*Black*	*White*	*Black*	*White*	*Black*	*White*	*Black*	*White*	*Black*	*White*	*Black*	*White*	*Black*	*White*	*Black*
1988	1.7	1.9	39.8	35.1	3.8	1.7	113.5	64.6	6.0	6.4	104.9	91.4	1.4	3.0	30.1	53.8	2.0	1.6	50.3	49
1989	1.5	1.3	38.0	32.2	3.9	2.5	107.8	58.8	5.3	8.1	100.7	85.6	1.6	2.2	29.2	38.4	1.7	2.9	52.7	41
1990	1.9	1.4	44.0	33.2	4.1	3.0	123.7	69.3	5.6	5.9	99.2	90.6	1.4	3.3	29.9	42.5	2.1	2.6	45.7	53
1991	1.8	2.4	45.5	32.4	4.0	3.5	128.2	66.9	6.3	8.6	98.5	90.1	1.7	2.4	30.9	46.0	1.7	2.9	45.8	45
1992	1.8	0.5	49.4	43.5	4.1	2.7	132.6	78.9	5.9	7.6	93.2	91.3	1.4	1.8	30.2	48.0	1.5	2.0	41.5	49
1993	1.6	1.4	48.0	37.0	4.2	2.7	129.1	71.2	5.3	6.3	90.4	92.5	1.6	2.7	29.4	42.9	1.4	2.3	43.3	51
1994	1.7	1.1	51.3	45.0	3.2	2.0	129.3	73.2	5.1	6.5	92.1	86.1	1.4	3.7	31.5	46.5	1.4	3.2	46.5	57
1995	1.8	1.3	55.9	50.5	3.7	3.3	131.4	83.5	5.3	5.9	92.5	86.0	1.7	2.8	31.5	43.7	1.7	2.9	46.6	53
1996	1.7	1.5	58.5	49.6	4.1	2.8	133.2	82.2	5.1	6.8	91.2	88.0	1.5	2.6	31.2	43.9	1.3	2.2	47.5	52
1997	2.0	2.1	64.6	61.3	3.8	2.3	139.9	84.4	5.5	7.6	96.5	86.0	1.7	3.5	31.5	44.4	1.7	2.7	44.6	50
1998	2.2	1.5	75.3	66.0	3.9	3.3	151.4	91.6	6.2	7.5	104.1	97.1	1.4	3.2	28.9	35.8	1.1	1.7	36.5	34
1999	2.2	2.0	73.7	65.2	4.4	2.3	150.3	90.6	6.4	7.4	106.8	101.6	1.4	2.9	29.1	41.2	1.0	0.6	32.4	33
2000	2.3	2.1	75.0	65.3	4.0	3.1	150.9	83.0	5.8	7.7	105.0	89.7	1.6	2.8	27.5	44.3	0.9	3.3	27.5	31
Percentage change†	35.3	10.5	88.4	86.0	5.3	82.4	33.0	28.5	–3.3	20.3	0.1	–1.9	14.3	–6.7	–8.6	–17.7	–55.0	106.3	–45.3	–36.2

*Rates are per 100,000 and age-adjusted to the 2000 U.S. (18 age groups) standard.
†Percent change in incidence rates between 1988 and 2000.
AJCCS, American Joint Committee on Cancer Staging.

Table 22–8. Female Breast Cancer Stage Distribution by Race in United States, 1996 to 2000

	White		Black	
	Count	Percentage	Count	Percentage
In Situ	16,562	17.6	1,716	18.4
Stage I	35,228	37.4	2,386	25.6
Stage II	25,207	26.7	2,850	30.6
Stage III	4,359	4.6	735	7.9
Stage IV	3,101	3.3	512	5.5
Unknown	9,782	10.4	1,106	11.9
Total	94,239	100.0	9,305	100.0

poorer survival among black women,[42-45] but some data suggest that black women may be more likely to be diagnosed with hormone receptor–negative tumors.[44]

The most current survival data available for women diagnosed with breast cancer show a statistically significant improvement ($P < 0.05$) in 5-year survival for women with breast cancer diagnosed in 1992 to 1999, compared with average survival for women diagnosed between 1974 and 1976 (86.6 % vs. 74.7%).[2] This improvement in the trend can be seen in the comparison of 5-year survival rates for women diagnosed with breast cancer in 1975 to 1979 with those in 1987 and in 1995, as shown in Figure 22–7. This difference is primarily due to greater improvements in average survival observed in white women between the periods 1974 to 1976 and 1992 to 1999 (from 75.3% to 87.9%) than in black women (from 63.2% to 73.5%).

The historical trend in long-term survival should not be taken as the expected rate of survival for cases diagnosed today, and caution should be used in citing 5-, 10-, and 15-year survival data because each of those estimates is based on cases diagnosed the corresponding number of years before the proportion surviving in 1999. Over this period, considerable improvements have been made in the overall stage at diagnosis and in the treatment of breast cancer.

CUMULATIVE RISK AND RELATIVE RISK

Cumulative risk and relative risk are two fundamentally different measurements of the probability that a woman will be diagnosed with breast cancer. According to current estimates, approximately 1 in every 7 women, or 13.5% of a hypothetical cohort alive today, will be diagnosed with breast cancer in their lifetimes.[2] The reference to estimate has become customary as a symbolic expression of the magnitude of the risk women face. *Lifetime risk* is a measure of absolute risk, or *cumulative risk*, over a period defined as a lifetime for a population based on current estimates of incidence. *Relative risk* is based on the occurrence of disease among women with a particular characteristic, or risk factor, in comparison with the occurrence among those without the characteristic. Measures of relative risk may also be adjusted for other known risk factors to eliminate the known or possible effects of confounding variables. The magnitude of the ratio is the relative risk, and it is expressed as a comparative likelihood of development of the disease or in terms of the protective effect associated with the risk factor. However, apart from the specific comparison, the measure and its magnitude have no inherent probabilistic meaning.

Each measurement, cumulative risk and relative risk, has the potential to be misunderstood in the context of individual behaviors and individual risk. For example, the estimate of lifetime risk is an estimate of the proportion of a cohort who will have been diagnosed with breast cancer by a certain age. The proportion consists of women whose lifetime risks are both lower and higher than 1 in 7. Further, the 1-in-7 lifetime risk is cumulative, and because the incidence of breast cancer is lower when women are younger, the majority of the cumulative risk is delayed until later years of life. Thus, absolute risk over intervals of 10 and 20 years is considerably less, especially before age 65.

With respect to relative risks, risk approximations are made on the basis of relative risks identified in the epidemiologic literature. However, the use of relative risk as a basis of estimating individual risk can be misleading for the simple reason that it is a comparative measure—that is, it is a measure of risk for individuals with a known risk factor compared with the risk for individuals without the risk factor. Furthermore, the relative risk does not directly approximate the underlying probability of a diagnosis of breast cancer. Although relative odds may be greater by a factor of two or three times for a woman with a particular risk factor, the more important estimate is her absolute risk during particular time intervals, for example, within 1 year, during one or more decades, or during a lifetime. A rather large relative risk for breast cancer at an age when the absolute risk is very low will result in very few excess new cases, whereas a more modest relative risk applied to women at an age when the absolute risk is high will lead to a significant number of excess cases. For example, Gail and Benichou[46,47] estimated the relative risk of breast cancer for a 40-year-old nulliparous woman whose mother had breast cancer and who had no other risk factors to be 2.76 compared with women without that risk profile. Her absolute risk of developing breast cancer between age 40 and age 70 years was estimated to be 11.6%. Over that 30-year period, the risk of breast cancer as estimated in the lifetime risk calculations (which are based on a hypothetical cohort of women representing all risk profiles) was 7.47%.[48] Although these two estimates are not directly comparable because they derive from different populations, they are useful to illustrate that relative risk estimates alone may inflate the perception of risk for women with a certain risk profile. On the other hand, risk between ages of 40 and 70 years

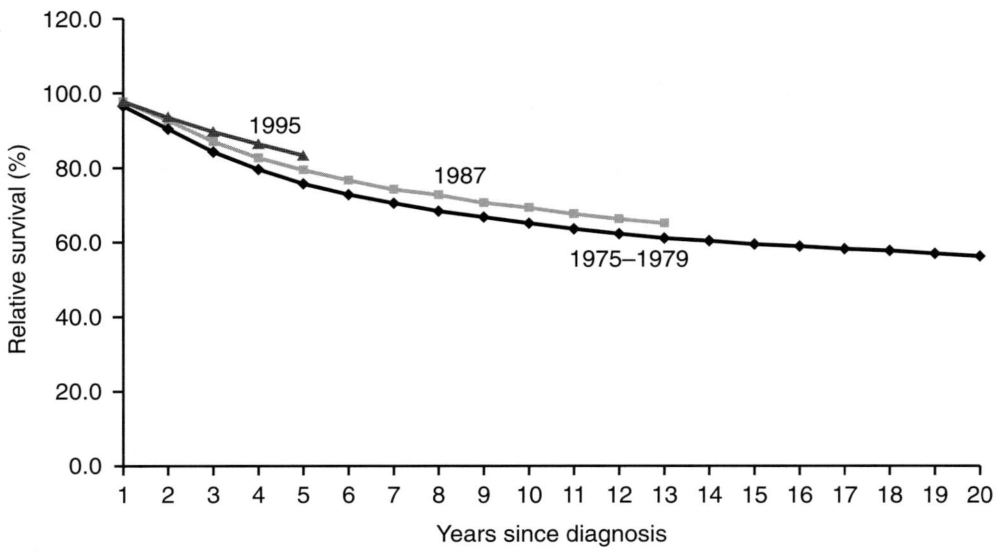

*Survival rates are relative rates expressed as percentages.

A

Years since diagnosis	1975–1979	1987	1995
1	96.8	98.1	98.0
2	90.9	92.6	93.7
3	84.6	87.1	89.8
4	80.0	83.0	86.4
5	76.1	79.5	83.6
6	73.2	77.0	
7	70.7	74.6	
8	68.7	73.0	
9	66.8	71.0	
10	65.3	69.5	
11	63.9	67.9	
12	62.4	66.4	
13	61.3	65.4	
14	60.6		
15	59.7		
16	59.0		
17	58.4		
18	57.8		
19	57.1		
20	56.3		

B

Figure 22–7. Breast cancer survival rates by years since diagnosis in U.S. women. Survival rates are relative rates expressed as percentages. (From Ries L, Eisner M, Kosary C, et al: SEER Cancer Statistics Review, 1975-2000. Bethesda, MD, National Cancer Institute, 2003.)

for a woman with a family history of breast cancer in two first-degree relatives can be estimated to be 21% and will be higher if the disease was diagnosed premenopausally in either or both relatives. In this instance, the use of this kind of counseling may serve to heighten both the woman's and her provider's attention to the importance of a program of routine screening at regular intervals.

Because women are concerned about breast cancer and their individual risks, it is important that clinicians and others understand these measurements and are equipped to appropriately counsel women.[49] It has been argued that such understanding and ability to counsel are especially important because women significantly overestimate their risk of disease and the overestimation contributes to avoidable anxiety.[50,51] This is an important issue, especially if attention to techniques of effective communication about breast cancer risk can reduce levels of anxiety. However, we should be mindful that it is unrealistic to expect that risk perceptions should correspond to actual risk or that the meaning women place on their risk should be proportional to their actual risk. The fact that women are more concerned about breast cancer than heart disease has more to do with the meaning they attach to each disease than with perceptions of actuarial likelihood.

Lifetime Risk

In 1940, a woman's risk of breast cancer up to age 85 years was 1 in 20, or 5%. By 1989, the risk to age 85 years was estimated to be 1 in 9, or 11.1%.[52] Today, risk to age 85 years is estimated to be 13.5%.[2,53] The lifetime risk of breast cancer has changed during the last five decades, largely because of the long-term trend of increasing breast cancer incidence and parallel trends in increasing longevity. Life expectancy for cohorts of women born between 1900 and 1902 was 51 years, compared with 74 years for those born between 1959 and 1961.[54] Likewise, since the decades in which the earliest cancer registries were established (1930s to 1940s), the age-specific incidence rate has increased, but most notably among women 40 years and older. The combination of increasing incidence and increasing longevity has meant a steadily growing lifetime, or absolute, risk of breast cancer. Lifetime risk is a cumulative probability, and it is the function of two factors that vary at different ages—the underlying incidence rate of disease and the rate of survival or withdrawal from the interval due to death from other causes.[48,52]

Risk of being diagnosed with breast cancer can be estimated for an interval from birth (or any age) to some end point, such as one or more decades, or some age arbitrarily defined as a lifetime (i.e., 90 years) or for the combined lifetimes of the entire cohort. Lifetime risk represents the accumulated risk over successive intervals, each with a higher probability of a diagnosis of breast cancer than the previous interval, consistent with trends in age-specific rates. As noted previously, this observation highlights the problem of internalizing the lifetime risk as near-term risk. For example, as seen in Figure 22–8, the average risk for a white woman aged 30 years for the 10-year interval between age 30 and 40 years is estimated to be 0.40%, or 1 in 250, compared with a lifetime risk from birth to "eventually" of 13.51%, or 1 in 7.4. A 60-year-old woman's risk of having breast cancer between the ages of 60 and 70 years is estimated to be 3.81%, or 1 in 26. Because lifetime risk is cumulative, the course of accumulated risk can be shown more clearly in Figure 22–9. In the first 50 years of life, a woman's cumulative probability to age 50 years is only about 1.85%, or 1 in 54 (most of which is due to the risk between ages 40 and 50 years), and risk to age 65 years is less than half of the potential lifetime risk, as measured to age 95 years and older.[2] For women who are concerned about breast cancer risk, these estimates may provide a measure of reassurance that average risk over periods of 10 and 20 years is considerably less than the frequently expressed estimate, 1 in 8 (0 to age 85 years).

Risk Factors for Breast Cancer

Despite the fact that breast cancer has been well studied epidemiologically, it is estimated that the established risk factors explain only slightly more than half of cases.[55] This estimate, which is based on a model that incorporates the accepted risk factors of advancing age, family history of breast cancer in a first-degree relative, early age at menarche, late age at menopause, nulliparity and late age at first full-term birth, and history of prior breast biopsies, does not account for some more recently recognized risk factors. These include fairly consistent increases in risk linked with lack of breastfeeding, obesity (for postmenopausal-onset disease only), and physical

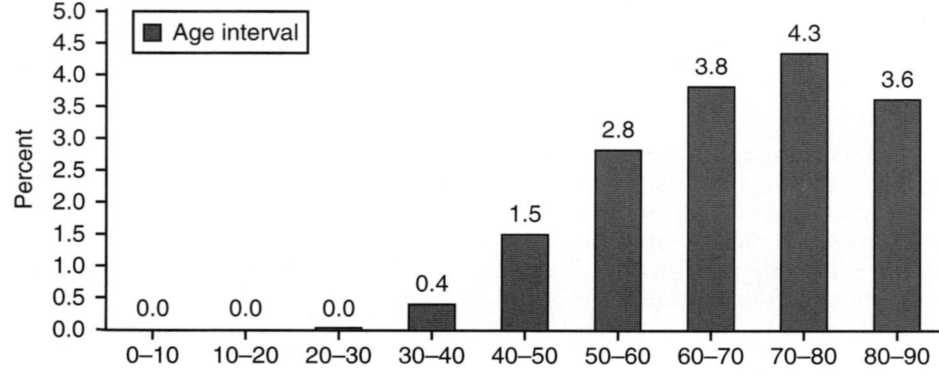

Figure 22–8. Probability of development of invasive breast cancer during specific age intervals, Surveillance Epidemiology and End-Results (SEER) areas, 1998 to 2000. (From Feuer EJ, Wun LM: DevCan: Probability of Developing or Dying of Cancer Software [computer program], version 5.0. Bethesda, MD, National Cancer Institute, 1999.)

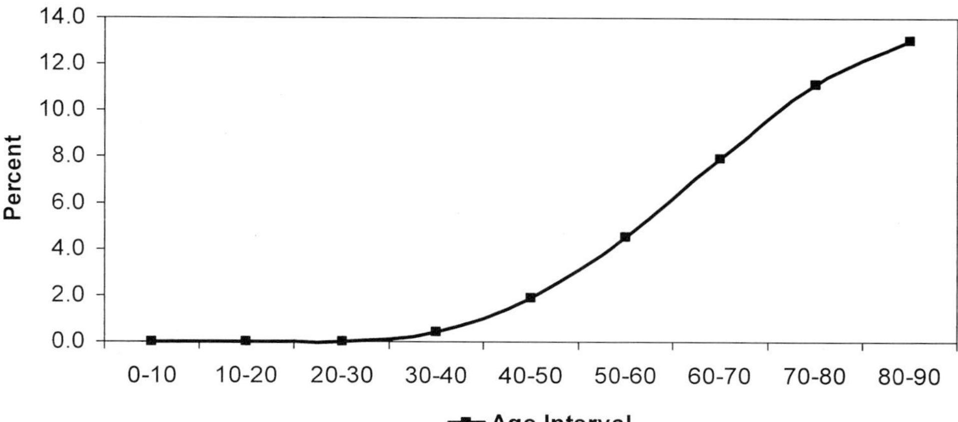

Figure 22–9. Cumulative probability of development of invasive breast cancer in white women, Surveillance Epidemiology and End-Results (SEER) areas, 1998 to 2000. (From Feuer EJ, Wun LM: DevCan: Probability of Developing or Dying of Cancer Software [computer program], version 5.0. Bethesda, MD: National Cancer Institute, 1999.)

inactivity. Although dietary factors have received extensive attention (particularly dietary fat), few components have been definitely linked to breast cancer risk. The one exception is higher alcoholic beverage consumption, which has been consistently linked with elevations in risk. Exogenous hormones have also been intensively studied, with the latest results indicating increases in risk with certain patterns of usage of both oral contraceptives and menopausal hormones, and beneficial effects of exposure to selective estrogen receptor modulators. Prediction models are currently being developed to incorporate additional risk factors, and such models are anticipated to allow a fuller understanding of the occurrence of breast cancer on a population basis.

A further complication in the understanding of the occurrence of breast cancer relates to our limited knowledge of the biologic processes underlying most of the identified risk factors. Although the important role of estrogens in the etiology of breast cancer has been recognized for some time,[56] it is clear that other biologic processes must also be taken into account. Growing attention is being focused on other hormones, such as androgens and progestogens, as well as a variety of proteins, such as insulin-like growth factors.[56-58] In addition, it is increasingly being recognized that breast cancer is a heterogeneous disease, for which there may be subsets with distinct causes. Some studies have attempted to assess etiologic variation by a variety of tumor markers, most notably hormone receptor status.[59] New technologies, including tissue microarray,[60] may be particularly useful for expanding our knowledge of the causes of this complex disease.

Most of the identified risk factors for breast cancer are associated with relatively low magnitudes of relative risk (Table 22–9). Many of the identified risk factors for breast cancer are also ones that are not readily amenable to change. It is encouraging that some of the more recently identified risk factors are ones that could be considered modifiable. It therefore appears worthwhile to review some of the results relating to these factors.

Breastfeeding

The relationship of breastfeeding to breast cancer risk has long been debated, and researchers initially assumed that any associations would merely reflect the effects of other reproductive variables. A later report of a large collaborative project involving data from 47 epidemiologic studies,[61] however, showed that in addition to a 7% reduction in risk associated with each birth, a 4.3% reduction in risk was associated with every 12 months of breastfeeding. It was further estimated that the cumulative incidence of breast cancer in developed countries could be reduced by more than half, from 6.3 to 2.7 per 100 women by age 70, if women had the average number of births and lifetime duration of breastfeeding that women in many developing countries experience.

Table 22–9. Selected Risk Factors for Breast Cancer

Factors Influencing Risk	Approximate Relative Risks
Older age (65-69 yr versus 30-34 yr)	17
Residency in North America or Europe versus Asia	4-5
Residency in urban areas	1.5
Higher education status or family income	1.5
Mother or sister with breast cancer	2-3
Nulliparity or late ages at first birth (≥30 yr versus <20 yr)	2-3
Absence of breastfeeding for long durations	1.5
Early ages at menarche (<12 yr versus ≥15 yr)	1.5
Late ages at menopause (≥55 yr versus natural menopause at <45 yr or removal of ovaries at a comparable age)	2
Biopsy-confirmed proliferative disease	2-4
Mammographically dense breasts	2-4
Obesity (postmenopausal only) (≥200 lb versus <125 lb)	2
Tallness (≥68 inches versus <62 inches)	1.5-2
Radiation to chest in moderate to high doses	2-4
History of breast cancer in one breast	2-4
History of primary cancer in endometrium, ovary	1.4-2

Body Size

The relationship of body size to breast cancer risk has been extensively investigated, with differing associations having been observed for premenopausal and postmenopausal diseases. For postmenopausal-onset disease, both weight and body mass index (BMI) (defined as weight in kilograms divided by the square of height in meters) have been fairly consistently related to increases in risk. In a large case-control study, subjects in the upper quartile of BMI were at a 40% higher risk than those in the lower quartile.[62] This relationship is believed to be due to the ability of adipose tissue to convert precursor substrates to estrogens. Although particular attention has focused on obesity during adolescence, weight gain at older ages has more consistently been shown to be associated with breast cancer risk,[63] an encouraging finding from the perspective of prevention.

In contrast to relationships with postmenopausal breast cancer, body mass appears to be inversely related to premenopausal disease, with thin women being at highest risk. In one meta-analysis, a BMI difference of 8 (i.e., the difference between a thin person and someone morbidly obese) resulted in a relative risk of 0.70 (95% confidence interval [CI], 0.5 to 0.9).[64] Although this difference in risk was initially thought to be due to difficulties in detecting breast lesions in young, heavy women, this reasoning does not appear to explain the relationship entirely. Irregular anovulation and, consequently, less exposure to endogenous hormones have been proposed as additional mechanisms underlying the inverse association of body size to premenopausal breast cancer risk.

Among postmenopausal women, body fat distribution also appears to influence risk.[65,66] In a number of studies, women whose fat was distributed abdominally (i.e., around their waists) were at higher risk than those with peripheral fat distribution (including fat accumulation on the hips). This effect appeared to be independent of total body size. In the few studies in which body fat distribution has been examined for premenopausal women, inconsistent relationships have been observed.

Physical Activity

There has been much enthusiasm regarding a potential beneficial effect of physical activity on breast cancer risk, especially given the modifiable nature of this factor. The relationship appears to be biologically plausible, given that physical activity has been associated with changes in endogenous hormones, menstrual patterns, body fat distribution patterns, and other biologic repercussions that could benefit breast cancer risk (e.g., change in immunologic parameters).[67] The strongest support for physical activity as a potential preventive mechanism derives from a study of early-onset breast cancers, in which reductions in risk associated with regular physical activity were found to be independent of body size.[68] Additional studies, however, have produced conflicting results.[69-75] The need for more precision in the approach to measuring physical activity has been stressed, including obtainment of objective measures of physical activity, collection of information on timing and intensity of activity levels, and consideration of all sources of activity (including physical activity resulting from household chores).

Alcohol Consumption

Although the relationship of breast cancer risk to most dietary factors remains unresolved, fairly consistent data have emerged regarding a potential adverse effect of consumption of alcoholic beverages. Longnecker,[76] in a meta-analysis of 38 case-control and cohort studies, showed a progressive increase in the risk of breast cancer with amount of alcohol consumed; women who consumed three or more drinks per day were at a 40% higher risk than non-drinkers. Results were consistent among case-control and cohort studies. Adjustment for known breast cancer risk factors and dietary variables had little impact on observed relationships.

An important unanswered question is whether a reduction in alcohol consumption would lead to less adverse effect on breast cancer risk. One report showed that women who drank only early in life (before age 30) experienced a risk similar to those who continued to drink.[77] However, in another study, recent adult drinking appeared to be more important than drinking patterns earlier in life.[78] This finding would be consistent with the finding that alcohol is most strongly related to late-stage tumors,[79] implying that it acts at a late stage in breast carcinogenesis.

Both intervention and cross-sectional studies have shown alterations in endogenous estrogens associated with alcohol consumption,[80,81] providing a possible biologic explanation for the association of alcohol with breast cancer risk. There is also support for several other possible biologic mechanisms, including alcohol-induced changes in folate levels, increased cell permeability, and direct effects of contaminants in the alcoholic beverages (e.g., nitrosamines). Further research is needed to clarify biologic mechanisms underlying the association of alcohol intake and breast cancer risk, particularly as related to levels of consumption and types of alcoholic beverages. Despite the enthusiasm for the possibility that cessation of alcohol consumption may be a means of reducing breast cancer risk, it appears that this measure would have only a minimal impact. Because of the modest association between alcohol consumption and breast cancer and the generally moderate level of alcohol intake among U.S. women, the proportion of breast cancer attributable to alcohol intake appears relatively small, being only 2.1% in one analysis.[82]

Use of Exogenous Hormones

Given the recognition of the importance of ovarian hormones in the etiology of breast cancer, much attention has focused on the relationship to risk of exogenous hormones, including oral contraceptives and menopausal hormones.

Oral Contraceptives

Oral contraceptives have been extensively studied in relation to breast cancer risk, with varying conclusions. Although the majority of studies have not confirmed an overall excess risk associated with use of oral contraceptives, a number of studies (including several meta-analyses) have suggested that long-term use of oral contraceptives is associated with a higher risk for early-onset cancers, usually defined as those occurring before age 45 years.[83-86] In the largest analysis, which involved the pooling of data from 54 studies of 53,297 women with breast cancer and 100,239 without breast cancer, current and recent users were at increased risk (relative risk [RR], 1.24; 95% CI, 1.15-1.33), with no evidence of an effect with the duration of use.[87] The higher risk associated with recent use of oral contraceptives subsided within 10 years of cessation of oral contraceptive use. These findings suggest that the increased risk of breast cancer observed among young, long-term users may have been due primarily to recent use, increasing the possibility that oral contraceptives might act as late-stage promoters.

Given that the influence of oral contraceptives on the breast has been hypothesized to be greatest before the cellular differentiation that occurs with a first pregnancy, a number of investigations have evaluated effects of the use of oral contraceptives prior to a first pregnancy. In the pooled analysis, a significant trend of growing risk with first use of oral contraceptives before age 20 years was observed.[87] Among women diagnosed at 30 to 34 years of age, the relative risk associated with recent oral contraceptive use was 1.54 if they began using oral contraceptives before age 20 years and 1.13 if they began at older ages. However, in several studies not included in the meta-analysis, no such increase in risk was observed.[86,88]

Studies have also attempted to determine whether the effects of oral contraceptives are influenced by the presence of other breast cancer risk factors. Of particular interest is whether effects are different in subjects with a family history of breast cancer. However, neither this factor nor various other factors (including weight and alcohol use) appear to modify relationships with oral contraceptives. Several studies have indicated that oral contraceptives may increase the risk of breast cancer more in subjects who are either *BRCA1* or *BRCA2* carriers, a suggestion requiring further confirmation with larger numbers.[88a,89]

There has also been interest in whether specific formulations of oral contraceptives have unique influences on breast cancer risk. No consistent relationships have been seen with either dose of the progestin or estrogen considered, although methodologically it has been difficult to define this information and to consider it in a systematic fashion. Only limited data on the newer formulations of pills are available.[87] Also of interest is whether injectable progestogen contraceptives are associated with alterations in breast cancer risk. In a study in South Africa, no association was found with this exposure in either older or younger women.[90]

Menopausal Hormones

The relationship of menopausal hormones to breast cancer risk was assessed in a re-analysis of data from 51 epidemiologic studies encompassing 52,705 women with breast cancer and 108,411 controls from 21 countries.[91] This study showed a 2.3% (95% CI, 1.1–3.6%) increase in the relative risk of breast cancer for each year of use of hormone replacement therapy (HRT). This increase corresponded to an RR of 1.35 for users of 5 or more years and to a cumulative excess for women who began using hormones at age 50 of approximately 2 cases per 1000 women for 5 years of HRT use, 6 cases per 1000 women for 10 years of use, and 12 cases per 1000 women for 15 years of use. This increase was comparable with the effect on breast cancer risk of later menopause. The increased risk, however, was restricted to recent users, with no material excess observed 5 or more years after discontinuation of HRT.

Although it has increasingly been accepted that recent long-term estrogen use is associated with some elevation in breast cancer risk, whether the addition of progestins to estrogens affects risk is less resolved. This regimen has become increasingly common because of its recognized advantages in terms of a reduction in endometrial cancer risk,[92] but there is evidence that added progestins may adversely affect breast cancer risk. Notably, in vitro studies have shown that breast mitotic activity is higher during the luteal phase of the menstrual cycle, when progesterone levels are at their highest. A number of studies have provided support for the notion of a more deleterious effect of combined therapy. These include results from two large cohort studies, the Nurses Health Study[93] and the follow-up study of participants in the Breast Cancer Detection Demonstration Project (BCDDP).[94] Both studies showed a relative risk of 1.4 for combined therapy, compared with RRs of 1.3 and 1.2 for estrogens alone. In the BCDDP study, the increased risk was limited to women who had used HRT within the prior 4 years and was largely confined to thin women, with the latter relationship possibly reflecting a smaller effect among heavier women because of their higher levels of endogenous hormones.

A potentially adverse effect of combined therapy has also been noted in two case-control studies, in Sweden[95] and Los Angeles County.[96] The Los Angeles study found an RR of 1.24 (95% CI, 1.1–1.4) for each 5 years of use of combined therapy, compared with an RR of 1.06 (95% CI, 0.9–1.2) for each 5 years of estrogen use. The Swedish study also supported a notion of a duration effect, with the risk increasing to 2.4 for women using HRT for 10 or more years. The latest data confirming an adverse relationship with combined therapy derive from the large Women's Health Initiative,[97] a controlled trial that was terminated because of unexpected adverse events, including a 26% increase in the risk of invasive breast cancers after 5.2 years of follow-up. Findings from an observational study also suggest that combined therapy predisposes to the risk of lobular breast cancers,[98] possibly explaining observed increases in this tumor type.[99]

Selective Estrogen Receptor Modulators

Given the recognized adverse effects of HRT, much attention has focused on assessing alternative approaches to treating menopause, including the use of tamoxifen and other selective estrogen receptor modulators (SERMs). These agents are recognized as anti-estrogens, so they presumably will offer many of the same advantages as HRT while eliminating some of the disadvantages (i.e., no increase in breast cancer risk). Data indicate that these agents offer substantial advantages in terms of reducing breast cancer risk, with the most convincing data deriving from the National Surgical Adjuvant Breast and Colorectal Project (NSABP).[6] This trial, which focused on women at an increased risk of breast cancer, found after 69 months of follow-up that those who had received tamoxifen had a 49% lower risk of invasive breast cancer than women who had received placebos. The beneficial effect pertained to women of all ages but was most apparent among women with a history of lobular carcinoma in situ or atypical hyperplasia; in addition, the risk reduction was limited to estrogen receptor–positive tumors. Two other trials, however, one in Britain[100] and the other in Italy,[101] did not find an effect of tamoxifen on breast cancer risk. These results may have reflected limited sample sizes, high dropout rates, or use of other drugs (including HRT) among trial participants.

Studies are also beginning to evaluate the relationship of other SERMs to breast cancer risk. In the Multiple Outcomes of Raloxifene Evaluation (MORE) trial of osteoporotic women, raloxifene daily decreased breast cancer risk by 76%.[102]

A trial is currently under way to evaluate the relative effectiveness of tamoxifen and raloxifene in reducing breast cancer risk.[103] Given that tamoxifen has previously been linked to a higher risk of endometrial cancer[6] and raloxifene has been associated with an increased risk of thromboembolic disease,[102] the Study of Tamoxifen and Raloxifene (STAR) trial will also assess the relative adversity of the two drugs. Trials are also beginning to evaluate the chemopreventive effects of other SERMs. In addition, there is growing enthusiasm for the potential preventive effects of phytoestrogens, which some call "natural" SERMs.[104]

Histologic and Mammographic Markers of Breast Cancer Risk

Noncancerous lesions of the breast have long been reported to be associated with an increased risk of breast cancer. Resolution of whether certain lesions are more predictive of risk than others has been complicated by the lack of uniformity of histologic classifications of benign breast disease. Dupont and Page[105] proposed diagnostic criteria that separate benign breast disease into the following three categories:

1. Nonproliferative changes, including normal breast tissue, cysts, apocrine metaplasia, and mild ductal hyperplasia.
2. Proliferative disease without atypia, including papillomas, sclerosing adenosis, fibroadenoma, and moderate to florid ductal hyperplasia of the usual type.
3. Atypical hyperplasia of either ductal or lobular type, defined as epithelial proliferations with some features of ordinary hyperplasia and some features of carcinoma in situ.

In a retrospective study of 3303 women in whom breast biopsy showed benign breast disease, these researchers found that 70% of women had nonproliferative lesions that were not associated with an increased risk of breast cancer.[105] The risk in women with proliferative disease without atypical hyperplasia was 1.9, and the risk in women with atypical hyperplasia was 5.3 compared with the risk in women without proliferative disease.

The mammographic appearance of the breast has also been found to be a predictor of subsequent breast cancer risk. A parenchymal pattern classification system, which takes into account the amount of the breast composed of ductal prominence, was initially proposed.[106] Direct measurements of dense areas of the breast have been found to be a less subjective and stronger indicator of risk. In one study, breasts with areas of density of 75% or more were associated with nearly a fivefold elevation in risk, a magnitude of risk as great as, if not greater than, most other established risk factors.[107] The finding of a heritable component to mammographic density[108] suggests that a focus on identifying genes responsible for the phenotype could assist in furthering our understanding of etiologic processes. However, it is also clear that environmental factors can influence mammographic densities; notable findings in this regard relate to higher mammographic densities associated with combined estrogen-progestin therapy.[109]

Family History and Risk Assessment

The proportion of women in the population with a family history of breast cancer in a first-degree relative (mother or sister) has been estimated to be approximately 8%[110]; in series of patients with breast cancer, the proportion approaches 14%.[110,111] Of those who cite a family history of breast cancer in first-degree relatives, only 1% have more than one affected relative, and 0.1% of individuals have three or more first-degree relatives with breast cancer.[110] In general, approximately 5% to 10% of all breast cancer can be accounted for by known hereditary breast cancer susceptibility disorders.[112-114] Thus, a true genetic predisposition to breast cancer is distinctly uncommon, and its presence generally is not signaled by the presence of only one affected family member. Because most women do not have a family history to suggest increased breast cancer risk, clinicians must be cautious not to underestimate overall breast cancer risk among women without a family history, because other risk factors account for the majority of breast cancers in the general population.

Although the majority of women in the population do not have a family history of breast cancer, family history has long been recognized as a key risk factor for the development of this disease. The magnitude of risk has been shown to vary with the degree of relatedness, because the RR associated with having a first-degree relative with breast cancer is higher than that associated with having a second-degree relative with this history (i.e., RR = 2.1 and 1.5, respectively).[115] Risk also increases as the number of affected family members increase, so that having three or more affected first-degree relatives is associated with an RR of 3.9.[110] Having a relative who was diagnosed with breast cancer at an earlier age than usual (which is typically defined as younger than 50 years) is also associated with a higher risk.[115,116]

For accurate assessment of an individual's genetic risk of breast cancer, it is essential to take a detailed history of cancer occurrence in relatives in both maternal and paternal lineages, ideally for a minimum of three generations. This history should include cancers of all types, not only breast cancer, because the hereditary breast cancer syndromes often include an increased risk for other malignancies, such as ovarian cancer. Details regarding the breast cancer diagnosis, such as age at onset, tumor characteristics, and bilaterality, should also be collected and should be confirmed when possible with pathology reports.[117] It is useful to know that the accuracy of a reported history of breast cancer is surprisingly high, often in the range of 90% or more.[118-121]

This information can allow women with a family history of breast cancer to be stratified into two groups, those at moderate risk and those at high risk.[117] Women from families with a history of breast cancer that is most often postmenopausal, is unilateral, affects one or two family members, and is not associated with a history of ovarian cancer or other genetically related malignancies are considered to be at moderate risk. These families make up a heterogeneous group, which comprises families with breast cancer related to multiple susceptibility factors or environmental exposures, including reproductive and lifestyle risk factors, families with several (coincidental) sporadic cases of cancer, and some families that carry a mutation in a dominantly transmitted susceptibility factor with low penetrance. Several models for individual risk assessment have been developed and may be useful in counseling moderate-risk families.[122,123]

High-risk women have families with a multigenerational history of breast cancer with an early age at onset, bilateral or multifocal disease, and three or more first-degree relatives with breast or ovarian cancer, or a combination of these two cancers. The presence of both breast and ovarian cancers in the same person is a particularly strong clue to the possible presence of an inherited susceptibility. Women of Ashkenazi Jewish heritage with a significant family history are also at greater risk of carrying an altered breast cancer gene. Such a history indicates a substantial probability of having a mutation in a dominantly inherited breast cancer susceptibility gene with high penetrance.[116,124] The prevalence of dominant breast cancer–related mutations in the population is estimated to be 0.33%.[125] Women with a high-risk family history account for 5% to 7% of all breast cancer cases; they also account for 33% of women diagnosed with breast cancer before age 30.[113]

Individuals from high-risk families should be referred to multidisciplinary centers that provide genetic counseling and access to genetic testing. Risk management strategies range from earlier and more intensive surveillance to risk-reducing surgical procedures (such as bilateral mastectomy and oophorectomy).

GENES AND SYNDROMES ASSOCIATED WITH AN INCREASED RISK OF BREAST CANCER

BRCA1 and *BRCA2*

Although breast cancer is associated with a number of family cancer syndromes, the majority of multiple-case families (at least four cases of breast cancer) studied to date have demonstrated mutations in the gene *BRCA1* or *BRCA2*. Linkage to these two genes has been found in approximately 95% of the families with hereditary breast and ovarian cancer (HBOC) studied by the Breast Cancer Linkage Consortium, with linkage to *BRCA1* more common than to *BRCA2*.[126] The majority of families with both male and female breast cancer could be linked to *BRCA2*.[126]

Studying family clusters of breast and ovarian cancer led to the discovery[127,128] and subsequent cloning[129] of the *BRCA1* gene, which is located on the long arm of chromosome 17. *BRCA1* is a large gene with 24 exons that encodes for a protein that is 1863 amino acids in length. Disease-associated mutations have been found scattered throughout the span of this large gene.[130] *BRCA1* acts as a tumor suppressor gene and is inherited in an autosomal dominant pattern. The initial estimates of the lifetime risk of breast cancer associated with *BRCA1* mutations approached 90%, because they were based on data from the multiple-case families that were used to map and clone the gene.[131]

Subsequent estimates of breast cancer risk, obtained from less highly selected populations, have varied from 45% to 68%,[114,132-136] depending on the populations studied. Ovarian cancer risk is also increased markedly in carriers of *BRCA1* mutations, who have a lifetime risk in the range of 40% to 60%.[126,133,134]

Studying HBOC kindreds with no evidence of linkage to the *BRCA1* gene led to the discovery of a second predisposition locus on chromosome 13, designated *BRCA2*.[137] Like *BRCA1*, *BRCA2* is a large gene with multiple disease-associated mutations documented as scattered across its span.[130] Estimates of the cumulative risk of breast cancer in carriers of *BRCA2* mutations have also varied from a low of 28% to a high of 84%.[126,138] An analysis of the data from 22 previous studies found an average cumulative risk of 45% by age 70[132] among women with a *BRCA2* mutation. *BRCA2* is also associated with an increased risk of cancers of the ovary, male breast, pancreas, and (likely) prostate.[126]

Most HBOC families with germline mutations in *BRCA1/2* have their own "private" mutations (i.e., nearly 1000 distinct mutations have been identified in each of these two genes)[130]; in some populations, however, one or a small number of mutations account for the vast majority of the mutations identified. These are termed "founder mutations"; their high frequency is due to the presence of that gene mutation in a single ancestor or small number of ancestors.

For example, in the Ashkenazi Jewish community, three specific mutations (*BRCA1* 185delAG & 5382insC, and *BRCA2* 6174delT) account for 85% to 90% of all *BRCA* mutations that occur.[139-141] Surveys in the general Ashkenazi population have suggested that 2.0% to 2.5% of all Ashkenazim carry one of these three mutations, regardless of their personal or family history of cancer.[139-141] By comparison, the prevalence of *BRCA* mutations in the general white population in the United States is estimated to be between 1 in 400 and 1 in 800.[114,142]

The term "founder mutation" is a general concept of which the Ashkenazi *BRCA* mutations are a specific example. In fact, many other populations are known to have their own founder mutations in the *BRCA* genes. For example, specific French Canadian,[143] Icelandic,[144] Dutch,[145] and Japanese[146] founder mutations have been documented. The existence of one or several founder mutations that account for the majority of mutations in a given population allows for an altered testing strategy designed to efficiently rule out those specific *BRCA* mutations before moving on to more costly and labor-intensive direct sequencing.

Li-Fraumeni Syndrome

Li-Fraumeni syndrome is a rare autosomal dominant cancer susceptibility syndrome that is characterized by sarcomas of the bone and soft tissue, brain tumors, leukemia, adrenocortical carcinoma, and breast cancer.[147-149] These malignancies manifest in childhood and early adulthood in affected individuals, and many persons are affected with multiple independent primary cancers.[149] There appears to be an increased risk of radiation-related second primary cancers within the radiation treatment field among carriers of the mutation. Germline mutations in the *p53* tumor suppressor gene have been documented in the majority of families with this syndrome.[150-154] In one large series, cancer risk among those with germline *p53* mutations was estimated at 80% by age 50, with women at greater risk than men (93% in women by age 50 versus 68% in men). The incidence of female breast cancer in this series was 100 times that in the general population.[151] In some of the families with Li-Fraumeni syndrome that do not show linkage to *p53*, a different gene, *CHEK2* (previously known as *hCHK2*), has been implicated.[155]

Cowden Syndrome

Cowden syndrome, initially described in 1963,[156] is an autosomal dominant disorder associated with mutations in the gene *PTEN*, which is located on the long arm of chromosome 10.[157,158] Because the signs of Cowden syndrome can be subtle, the published prevalence for this syndrome, 1 in 200,000, is thought by some investigators to be an underestimate. Manifestations of Cowden syndrome include multiple benign hamartomatous lesions of the skin, mucous membranes (including the gastrointestinal tract), thyroid, and breast. Macrocephaly is one of the more visible clues to the presence of the syndrome. Syndromic malignancies include cancers of the breast, gastrointestinal tract, and thyroid, with the risk of breast cancer estimated to be as high as 50%.[159]

Peutz-Jeghers Syndrome

Peutz-Jeghers syndrome is an autosomal dominant disorder linked to mutations in the *STK11* gene on chromosome 19.[160,161] Its cardinal features are pigmented oral lesions and multiple gastrointestinal polyps (both hamartomatous and adenomatous). The polyps seen in Peutz-Jeghers syndrome can occur throughout the gastrointestinal tract, including the stomach, small intestine, and large intestine, and may lead to intussusception, bleeding, or even malignant transformation. Individuals with the syndrome have a markedly increased risk of cancers of the breast, colon, stomach, and pancreas as well as of sex cord stromal tumors of the ovary.[161,162] The cumulative lifetime risk of breast cancer in these patients has been estimated at 50%.[163]

Ataxia-Telangiectasia

Ataxia-telangiectasia is a rare autosomal recessive disorder caused by the *ATM* gene, which is on the long arm of chromosome 11.[164-166] The cardinal manifestations of this disorder are progressive neurologic disease and oculocutaneous telangiectasias, with affected individuals also displaying immunodeficiency, greater sensitivity to ionizing radiation, and higher risk of cancer (particularly lymphoid malignancies).[167-170] Ataxia-telangiectasia is rare (estimated incidence 3 per 1,000,000 live births) because it requires two copies of the abnormal gene to express the syndrome, but heterozygote carriers for this disorder (i.e., those with only one altered copy of *ATM*) are relatively common. They are estimated to constitute 1% of the U.S. population.[171] Although *ATM* carriers are generally asymptomatic, investigators have found evidence of a greater in vitro sensitivity to ionizing radiation, at a level intermediate between that of normal persons and *ATM* homozygotes.[172,173]

Family studies have revealed a two- to three-fold higher risk of having[174] and dying from[175] cancer among *ATM* carriers. In particular, female carriers of *ATM* mutations have a significantly increased risk of breast cancer, with studies estimating that risk at 4 to 15 times that of the general population.[176-179] Occasional studies have found a greater frequency of germline *ATM* mutations in familial breast cancer cases, although this gene does not appear to account for a significant proportion of familial breast cancer clusters.[179-181] However, the modest elevation in breast cancer risk in ataxia-telangiectasia heterozygotes, when coupled with the relatively high frequency of *ATM* mutation carriers in the general population already mentioned, has produced estimates that 6% to 7% of U.S. breast cancer cases could be accounted for by ataxia-telangiectasia heterozygosity,[176] a proportion rivaling that seen with *BRCA* mutations.

The *CHEK2* Gene

CHEK2, located on the long arm of chromosome 22, is a gene that encodes a cell checkpoint kinase that has interactions with other gene products known to influence breast cancer risk, such as *p53*, *ATM*, and *BRCA1*.[182-184] It is estimated that 0.3% to 1.4% of the U.S. population carries a specific truncating mutation in *CHEK2* , known as 1100delC.[185-187] This mutation has been found at a higher frequency in individuals with bilateral breast cancer and in people with a positive family history of breast cancer.[186] Studies have indicated that about 5% of familial breast cancer cases that are not associated with *BRCA* mutations[186,187] are associated with the *CHEK2**1100delC mutation, and that this mutation is even more common in families with cases of male breast cancer. As indicated previously, mutations in *CHEK2* have been implicated in some cases of Li-Fraumeni syndrome.[155,188,189] Current estimates indicate that this *CHEK2* mutation is associated with a twofold increase in breast cancer risk.[187] Consequently, it is considered a low-penetrance breast cancer susceptibility allele, which is not generally found in families carrying *BRCA1/2* mutations.

CONCLUSION

With the exception of family history and age, none of the identified risk factors for breast cancer is particularly strong, either alone or in combination. Further, any discussion of risk factors with patients should not be framed strictly in terms of relative risks because such statistics provide little information about probability of the development of breast cancer over time, and also because some relative risks are transitory over time. Genetic susceptibility results in highly elevated risk but is rare.

Although a majority of women have at least one confirmed risk factor for breast cancer,[190] most women diagnosed with breast cancer do not have a risk profile that readily distinguishes them from women who do not have breast cancer. Thus, to date, efforts to design screening programs based on risk factor profiles have not proved productive because estimates of the effectiveness of targeting women on the basis of a handful of key risk factors, such as family history, age at menarche, and parity, have shown that such a program would miss the majority of incident cases. The majority of risk factors that influence a woman's risk of breast cancer, such as heredity, age, and age at onset of menarche and menopause, are beyond her control. Others, such as the timing of pregnancy, or her parity, are not easily or practically modifiable for obvious reasons. Lifestyle modifications (e.g., prudent diet, exercise, healthy BMI, and reducing alcohol intake) have not been convincingly associated with decreased breast cancer risk but can be advised on the basis of inferential evidence of possible benefit and because healthier lifestyles are consistent with good overall general health.

For women at average risk of breast cancer, *routine* screening according to recommended guidelines is the most important strategy to ensure early detection and to reduce the risk of being diagnosed with an advanced breast cancer. For women at greater than average risk of breast cancer, intensified screening and chemoprevention have been proposed as protective methods. For women at exceptionally higher risk, heightened surveillance, chemoprevention, and prophylactic surgeries may be considered. With increases in risk, clinicians face a greater responsibility to support shared decision-making with their patients. Thus, from a public health standpoint, all women in appropriate age categories should be counseled about the importance of routine breast cancer screening, and providers must recognize the important role they play in the achievement of a regular program of surveillance and in helping women make informed decisions.

References

1. Jemal A, Murray T, Samuels A, et al: Cancer statistics, 2003. CA Cancer J Clin 2003;53:5-26.
2. Ries LAG, Eisner MP, Kosary CL, et al: SEER Cancer Statistics Review, 1975-2000. Bethesda, MD, National Cancer Institute, 2003.
3. Breen N, Wagener DK, Brown ML, et al: Progress in cancer screening over a decade: Results of cancer screening from the 1987, 1992, and 1998 National Health Interview Surveys. J Natl Cancer Inst 2001;93:1704-1713.
4. Kessler LG: The relationship between age and incidence of breast cancer: Population and screening program data. Cancer 1992;69:1896-1903.
5. Weir HK, Thun MJ, Hankey BF, et al: Annual report to the nation on the status of cancer, 1975-2000, featuring the uses of surveillance data for cancer prevention and control. J Natl Cancer Inst 2003;95:1276-1299.
6. Fisher B, Costantino JP, Wickerham DL, et al: Tamoxifen for prevention of breast cancer: Report of the National Surgical Adjuvant Breast and Bowel Project P-1 Study. J Natl Cancer Inst 1998;90:1371-1388.
7. Freedman AN, Graubard BI, Rao SR, et al: Estimates of the number of US women who could benefit from tamoxifen for breast cancer chemoprevention. J Natl Cancer Inst 2003;95:526-532.
8. Gail MH, Costantino JP, Bryant J, et al: Weighing the risks and benefits of tamoxifen treatment for preventing breast cancer [see comments] [published erratum appears in J Natl Cancer Inst 2000;92:275]. J Natl Cancer Inst 1999;91:1829-1846.
9. Curtin L, Klein R: Direct Standardization (Age-Adjusted Death Rates). Healthy People 2000 Statistical Notes No. 6—Revised March 1995. Washington, DC, U.S. Department of Health and Human Services, 1995.
10. Surveillance, Epidemiology, and End Results (SEER) Program (www.seer.cancer.gov) SEER*Stat Database: Incidence—SEER 9 Regulations Public-Use, Nov 2003 Sub (1973-2001), National Cancer Institute, DCCPS, Surveillance Research Program, Cancer Statistics Branch, released April 2004, based on the November 2003 submission.
11. Edwards BK, Howe HL, Ries LAG, et al: Annual report to the nation on the status of cancer, 1973-1999, featuring implications of age and aging on U.S. cancer burden. Cancer 2002;94:2766-2792.
12. Ries LAG, Eisner MP, Kosary CL, et al: SEER Cancer Statistics Review, 1973-1998. Bethesda, MD, National Cancer Institute, 2001.
13. Ferlay J, Bray P, Pisani P, Parkin DM: Globocan 2000: Cancer Incidence, Mortality, and Prevalence Worldwide. Lyon, IARC Press, 2001.
14. Parkin DM, Pisani P, Farley J: Global cancer statistics. CA Cancer J Clin 1999;49:33-64.
15. Hoel DG, Davis DL, Miller AB, et al: Trends in cancer mortality in 15 industrialized countries, 1969-1986. J Natl Cancer Inst 1992;84:313-320.
16. Nagata C, Kawakami N, Shimizu H: Trends in the incidence rate and risk factors for breast cancer in Japan. Breast Cancer Res Treat 1997;44:75-82.
17. Tominaga S, Kuroishi T: Epidemiology of breast cancer in Japan. Cancer Lett 1995;90:75-79.
18. Wakai K, Suzuki S, Ohno Y, et al: Epidemiology of breast cancer in Japan. Int J Epidemiol 1995;24:285-291.
19. Devesa SS, Silverman DT, Young JL Jr, et al: Cancer incidence and mortality trends among whites in the United States, 1947-84. J Natl Cancer Inst 1987;79:701-770.
20. Kosary C, Hankey B, Brinton L, et al: 1995 Cancer Statistics Review. Bethesda, MD, National Cancer Institute, 1995.
21. Morrison A: Screening in Chronic Disease. Oxford, UK, Oxford University Press, 1992.
22. Smith RA, Haynes S: Barriers to screening for breast cancer. Cancer 1992;69:1968-1978.
23. Howard J: Using mammography for cancer control: An unrealized potential. CA Cancer J Clin 1987;37:33-48.
24. Dawson DA, Thompson GB: Breast cancer risk factors and screening: United States, 1987. Vital Health Stat 1990;10: 1-60.
25. Horton JA, Romans MC, Cruess DF: Mammography Attitudes and Usage Study, 1992. Womens Health Issues 1992;2:180-186; discussion 187-188.
26. American Cancer Society: Mammography: Two statements of the American Cancer Society. American Cancer Society Professional Education Publication. Atlanta, American Cancer Society, 1983.
27. Dodd GD: American Cancer Society guidelines on screening for breast cancer: An overview. Cancer 1992;69:1885-1887.
28. Shapiro S: Evidence on screening for breast cancer from a randomized trial. Cancer 1977;39:2772-2782.
29. American Cancer Society: Survey of physicians' attitudes and practices in early cancer detection. CA Cancer J Clin 1985; 35:197-213.
30. American Cancer Society: Survey of physicians' attitudes and practices in early cancer detection. CA 1990;40:77-101.
31. Brown ML, Kessler LG, Rueter FG: Is the supply of mammography machines outstripping need and demand? An economic analysis [see comments]. Ann Intern Med 1990;113:547-552.
32. White E, Lee CY, Kristal AR: Evaluation of the increase in breast cancer incidence in relation to mammography use. J Natl Cancer Inst 1990;82:1546-1552.
33. Liff JM, Sung JF, Chow WH, et al: Does increased detection account for the rising incidence of breast cancer? Am J Public Health 1991;81:462-465.
34. Holford TR, Roush GC, McKay LA: Trends in female breast cancer in Connecticut and the United States. J Clin Epidemiol 1991;44:29-39.
35. Ursin G, Bernstein L, Pike M: Breast cancer. Cancer Surv 1994;19/20:241-264.
36. Duffy SW, Chen HH, Tabar L, Day NE: Estimation of mean sojourn time in breast cancer screening using a Markov chain model of both entry to and exit from the preclinical detectable phase. Stat Med 1995;14:1531-1543.
37. Tabar L, Vitak B, Chen HH, et al: The Swedish Two-County Trial twenty years later: Updated mortality results and new insights from long-term follow-up. Radiol Clin North Am 2000;38:625-651.
38. Peek ME: Screening mammography in the elderly: A review of the issues. J Am Med Womens Assoc 2003;58: 191-198.
39. Eley JW, Hill HA, Chen VW, et al: Racial differences in survival from breast cancer: Results of the National Cancer Institute Black/White Cancer Survival Study [see comments]. JAMA 1994;272:947-954.
40. Gordon NH, Crowe JP, Brumberg DJ, Berger NA: Socioeconomic factors and race in breast cancer recurrence and survival. Am J Epidemiol 1992;135:609-618.
41. Shavers VL, Harlan LC, Stevens JL: Racial/ethnic variation in clinical presentation, treatment, and survival among breast cancer patients under age 35. Cancer 2003;97: 134-147.
42. Chu KC, Lamar CA, Freeman HP: Racial disparities in breast carcinoma survival rates: Separating factors that affect diagnosis from factors that affect treatment. Cancer 2003; 97:2853-2860.
43. Jatoi I, Becher H, Leake CR: Widening disparity in survival between white and African-American patients with breast carcinoma treated in the U. S. Department of Defense Healthcare system. Cancer 2003;98:894-899.
44. Joslyn SA: Hormone receptors in breast cancer: Racial differences in distribution and survival. Breast Cancer Res Treat 2002;73:45-59.

45. Joslyn SA: Racial differences in treatment and survival from early-stage breast carcinoma. Cancer 2002;95:1759-1766.
46. Gail M, Benichou J: Assessing the risk of breast cancer in individuals. Cancer Prev 1992;June:1-15.
47. Gail M, Benichou J: Epidemiology and biostatistics program of the National Cancer Institute. J Natl Cancer Inst 1994;86: 573-575.
48. Feuer E, Wun L, Boring C: Probability of developing cancer. In Miller B, Ries LAG, Hankey BF, et al (eds): Cancer Statistics Review 1973-90. (NIH Pub. No. 93-2789.) Bethesda, MD, National Cancer Institute, 1992.
49. Vogel VG: Management of the high-risk patient. Surg Clin North Am 2003;83:733-751.
50. Absetz P, Aro AR, Sutton SR: Experience with breast cancer: Pre-screening perceived susceptibility and the psychological impact of screening. Psychooncology 2003;12:305-18.
51. Rimer BK: Putting the "informed" in informed consent about mammography [editorial; comment]. J Natl Cancer Inst 1995;87:703-704.
52. Seidman H, Mushinski MH, Gelb SK, Silverberg E: Probabilities of eventually developing or dying of cancer—United States, 1985. CA Cancer J Clin 1985;35:36-56.
53. Feuer EJ, Wun LM: DevCan: Probability of Developing or Dying of Cancer Software [computer program], version 5.0. Bethesda, MD, National Cancer Institute, 1999.
54. National Center for Health Statistics: Lifetables. In Vital Statistics of the United States, 1990, vol 2, sec 6. Washington, U.S. Public Health Service, 1994.
55. Bruzzi P, Green SB, Byar DP, et al: Estimating the population attributable risk for multiple risk factors using case-control data. Am J Epidemiol 1985;122:904-914.
56. Endogenous sex hormones and breast cancer in postmenopausal women: Reanalysis of nine prospective studies. The Endogenous Hormones and Breast Cancer Collaborative Group. J Natl Cancer Inst 2002;94:606-616.
57. Hankinson SE, Willett WC, Colditz GA, et al: Circulating concentrations of insulin-like growth factor-I and risk of breast cancer. Lancet 1998;351:1393-1396.
58. Kaaks R, Lundin E, Rinaldi S, et al: Prospective study of IGF-I, IGF-binding proteins, and breast cancer risk, in northern and southern Sweden. Cancer Causes Control 2002;13: 307-316.
59. Britton JA, Gammon MD, Schoenberg JB, et al: Risk of breast cancer classified by joint estrogen receptor and progesterone receptor status among women 20-44 years of age. Am J Epidemiol 2002;156:507-516.
60. Hyman E, Kauraniemi P, Hautaniemi S, et al: Impact of DNA amplification on gene expression patterns in breast cancer. Cancer Res 2002;62:6240-6245.
61. Breast cancer and breastfeeding: Collaborative reanalysis of individual data from 47 epidemiological studies in 30 countries, including 50,302 women with breast cancer and 96,973 women without the disease. Collaborative Group on Hormonal Factors in Breast Cancer. Lancet 2002;360:187-195.
62. Trentham-Dietz A, Newcomb PA, Storer BE, et al: Body size and risk of breast cancer. Am J Epidemiol 1997;145:1011-1019.
63. Trentham-Dietz A, Newcomb PA, Egan KM, et al: Weight change and risk of postmenopausal breast cancer (United States). Cancer Causes Control 2000;11:533-542.
64. Ursin G, Longnecker MP, Haile RW, Greenland S: A meta-analysis of body mass index and risk of premenopausal breast cancer. Epidemiology 1995;6:137-141.
65. Ballard-Barbash R, Schatzkin A, Carter CL, et al: Body fat distribution and breast cancer in the Framingham Study. J Natl Cancer Inst 1990;82:286-290.
66. Hall IJ, Newman B, Millikan RC, Moorman PG: Body size and breast cancer risk in black women and white women: The Carolina Breast Cancer Study. Am J Epidemiol 2000;151: 754-764.
67. Hoffman-Goetz L, Apter D, Demark-Wahnefried W, et al: Possible mechanisms mediating an association between physical activity and breast cancer. Cancer 1998;83:621-628.
68. Bernstein L, Henderson BE, Hanisch R, et al: Physical exercise and reduced risk of breast cancer in young women. J Natl Cancer Inst 1994;86:1403-1408.
69. Britton JA, Gammon MD, Schoenberg JB, et al: Risk of breast cancer classified by joint estrogen receptor and progesterone receptor status among women 20-44 years of age. Am J Epidemiol 2002;156:507-516.
70. Friedenreich CM, Thune I, Brinton LA, Albanes D: Epidemiologic issues related to the association between physical activity and breast cancer. Cancer 1998;83:600-610.
71. Moradi T, Nyren O, Zack M, et al: Breast cancer risk and lifetime leisure-time and occupational physical activity (Sweden). Cancer Causes Control 2000;11:523-531.
72. Rockhill B, Willett WC, Hunter DJ, et al: A prospective study of recreational physical activity and breast cancer risk. Arch Intern Med 1999;159:2290-2296.
73. Shoff SM, Newcomb PA, Trentham-Dietz A, et al: Early-life physical activity and postmenopausal breast cancer: Effect of body size and weight change. Cancer Epidemiol Biomarkers Prev 2000;9:591-595.
74. Verloop J, Rookus MA, van der Kooy K, van Leeuwen FE: Physical activity and breast cancer risk in women aged 20-54 years. J Natl Cancer Inst 2000;92:128-135.
75. Wyshak G, Frisch RE: Breast cancer among former college athletes compared to non-athletes: A 15-year follow-up. Br J Cancer 2000;82:726-730.
76. Longnecker MP: Alcoholic beverage consumption in relation to risk of breast cancer: Meta-analysis and review. Cancer Causes Control 1994;5:73-82.
77. Harvey EB, Schairer C, Brinton LA, et al: Alcohol consumption and breast cancer. J Natl Cancer Inst 1987;78:657-661.
78. Longnecker MP, Newcomb PA, Mittendorf R, et al: Risk of breast cancer in relation to lifetime alcohol consumption. J Natl Cancer Inst 1995;87:923-929.
79. Swanson CA, Coates RJ, Malone KE, et al: Alcohol consumption and breast cancer risk among women under age 45 years. Epidemiology 1997;8:231-237.
80. Hankinson SE, Willett WC, Manson JE, et al: Alcohol, height, and adiposity in relation to estrogen and prolactin levels in postmenopausal women. J Natl Cancer Inst 1995;87:1297-1302.
81. Reichman ME, Judd JT, Longcope C, et al:. Effects of alcohol consumption on plasma and urinary hormone concentrations in premenopausal women. J Natl Cancer Inst 1993; 85:722-727.
82. Tseng M, Weinberg CR, Umbach DM, Longnecker MP: Calculation of population attributable risk for alcohol and breast cancer (United States). Cancer Causes Control 1999;10:119-123.
83. Brinton LA, Daling JR, Liff JM, et al: Oral contraceptives and breast cancer risk among younger women. J Natl Cancer Inst 1995;87:827-835.
84. Hankinson SE, Colditz GA, Manson JE, et al: A prospective study of oral contraceptive use and risk of breast cancer (Nurses' Health Study, United States). Cancer Causes Control 1997;8:65-72.
85. Romieu I, Berlin JA, Colditz G: Oral contraceptives and breast cancer: Review and meta-analysis. Cancer 1990;66:2253-2263.
86. White E, Malone KE, Weiss NS, Daling JR: Breast cancer among young U.S. women in relation to oral contraceptive use. J Natl Cancer Inst 1994;86:505-514.
87. Breast cancer and hormonal contraceptives: Collaborative reanalysis of individual data on 53 297 women with breast cancer and 100 239 women without breast cancer from 54 epidemiological studies. Collaborative Group on Hormonal Factors in Breast Cancer. Lancet 1996;347:1713-1727.
88. Wingo PA, Lee NC, Ory HW, et al: Age-specific differences in the relationship between oral contraceptive use and breast cancer. Obstet Gynecol 1991;78:161-170.
88a. Narod SA, Dube MP, Klijn J, et al: Oral contraceptives and the risk of breast cancer in BRCA1 and BRCA2 mutation carriers. J Natl Cancer Inst 2002;94:1773-1779.

89. Ursin G, Henderson BE, Haile RW, et al: Does oral contraceptive use increase the risk of breast cancer in women with BRCA1/BRCA2 mutations more than in other women? Cancer Res 1997;57:3678-3681.
90. Shapiro S, Rosenberg L, Hoffman M, et al: Risk of breast cancer in relation to the use of injectable progestogen contraceptives and combined estrogen/progestogen contraceptives. Am J Epidemiol 2000;151:396-403.
91. Breast cancer and hormone replacement therapy: Collaborative reanalysis of data from 51 epidemiological studies of 52,705 women with breast cancer and 108,411 women without breast cancer. Collaborative Group on Hormonal Factors in Breast Cancer. Lancet 1997;350:1047-1059.
92. Effects of hormone replacement therapy on endometrial histology in postmenopausal women: The Postmenopausal Estrogen/Progestin Interventions (PEPI) Trial. The Writing Group for the PEPI Trial. JAMA 1996;275:370-375.
93. Colditz GA, Hankinson SE, Hunter DJ, et al: The use of estrogens and progestins and the risk of breast cancer in postmenopausal women. N Engl J Med 1995;332:1589-1593.
94. Schairer C, Lubin J, Troisi R, et al: Menopausal estrogen and estrogen-progestin replacement therapy and breast cancer risk. JAMA 2000;283:485-491.
95. Magnusson C, Baron JA, Correia N, et al: Breast-cancer risk following long-term oestrogen- and oestrogen-progestin-replacement therapy. Int J Cancer 1999;81:339-344.
96. Ross RK, Paganini-Hill A, Wan PC, Pike MC: Effect of hormone replacement therapy on breast cancer risk: Estrogen versus estrogen plus progestin. J Natl Cancer Inst 2000; 92:328-332.
97. Rossouw JE, Anderson GL, Prentice RL, et al: Risks and benefits of estrogen plus progestin in healthy postmenopausal women: Principal results from the Women's Health Initiative randomized controlled trial. JAMA 2002;288:321-333.
98. Li CI, Weiss NS, Stanford JL, Daling JR: Hormone replacement therapy in relation to risk of lobular and ductal breast carcinoma in middle-aged women. Cancer 2000;88:2570-2577.
99. Li CI, Anderson BO, Porter P, et al: Changing incidence rate of invasive lobular breast carcinoma among older women. Cancer 2000;88:2561-2569.
100. Powles T, Eeles R, Ashley S, et al: Interim analysis of the incidence of breast cancer in the Royal Marsden Hospital tamoxifen randomised chemoprevention trial. Lancet 1998;352: 98-101.
101. Veronesi U, Maisonneuve P, Costa A, et al: Prevention of breast cancer with tamoxifen: Preliminary findings from the Italian randomised trial among hysterectomised women. Italian Tamoxifen Prevention Study. Lancet 1998;352:93-97.
102. Cummings SR, Eckert S, Krueger KA, et al: The effect of raloxifene on risk of breast cancer in postmenopausal women: Results from the MORE randomized trial. Multiple Outcomes of Raloxifene Evaluation. JAMA 1999;281:2189-2197.
103. Ford LG, Minasian LM, McCaskill-Stevens W, et al: Prevention and early detection clinical trials: Opportunities for primary care providers and their patients. CA Cancer J Clin 2003;53:82-101.
104. Brzezinski A, Debi A: Phytoestrogens: The "natural" selective estrogen receptor modulators? Eur J Obstet Gynecol Reprod Biol 1999;85:47-51.
105. Dupont WD, Page DL: Risk factors for breast cancer in women with proliferative breast disease. N Engl J Med 1985; 312:146-151.
106. Wolfe JN, Saftlas AF, Salane M: Mammographic parenchymal patterns and quantitative evaluation of mammographic densities: A case-control study. AJR Am J Roentgenol 1987;148: 1087-1092.
107. Byrne C, Schairer C, Wolfe J, et al: Mammographic features and breast cancer risk: Effects with time, age, and menopause status. J Natl Cancer Inst 1995;87:1622-1629.
108. Boyd NF, Dite GS, Stone J, et al: Heritability of mammographic density, a risk factor for breast cancer. N Engl J Med 2002;347:886-894.
109. Greendale GA, Reboussin BA, Slone S, et al: Postmenopausal hormone therapy and change in mammographic density. J Natl Cancer Inst 2003;95:30-37.
110. Familial breast cancer: Collaborative reanalysis of individual data from 52 epidemiological studies including 58,209 women with breast cancer and 101,986 women without the disease. Collaborative Group on Hormonal Factors in Breast Cancer. Lancet 2001;358:1389-1399.
111. Pharoah PD, Lipscombe JM, Redman KL, et al: Familial predisposition to breast cancer in a British population: Implications for prevention. Eur J Cancer 2000;36:773-779.
112. Anglican Breast Cancer Study Group: Prevalence and penetrance of BRCA1 and BRCA2 mutations in a population-based series of breast cancer cases. Anglican Breast Cancer Study Group. Br J Cancer 2000;83:1301-1308.
113. Claus EB, Schildkraut JM, Thompson WD, Risch NJ: The genetic attributable risk of breast and ovarian cancer. Cancer 1996;77:2318-2324.
114. Ford D, Easton DF, Peto J: Estimates of the gene frequency of BRCA1 and its contribution to breast and ovarian cancer incidence. Am J Hum Genet 1995;57:1457-1462.
115. Pharoah PD, Day NE, Duffy S, et al: Family history and the risk of breast cancer: A systematic review and meta-analysis. Int J Cancer 1997;71:800-809.
116. Claus EB, Risch N, Thompson WD: Autosomal dominant inheritance of early-onset breast cancer: Implications for risk prediction. Cancer 1994;73:643-651.
117. Hoskins KF, Stopfer JE, Calzone KA, et al: Assessment and counseling for women with a family history of breast cancer: A guide for clinicians. JAMA 1995;273:577-585.
118. Eerola H, Blomqvist C, Pukkala E, et al: Familial breast cancer in southern Finland: How prevalent are breast cancer families and can we trust the family history reported by patients? Eur J Cancer 2000;36:1143-1148.
119. Kerber RA, Slattery ML: Comparison of self-reported and database-linked family history of cancer data in a case-control study. Am J Epidemiol 1997;146:244-248.
120. Parent ME, Ghadirian P, Lacroix A, Perret C: The reliability of recollections of family history: Implications for the medical provider. J Cancer Educ 1997;12:114-120.
121. Sijmons RH, Boonstra AE, Reefhuis J, et al: Accuracy of family history of cancer: Clinical genetic implications. Eur J Hum Genet 2000;8:181-186.
122. Benichou J: A computer program for estimating individualized probabilities of breast cancer. Comput Biomed Res 1993; 26:373-382.
123. Gail MH, Brinton LA, Byar DP, et al: Projecting individualized probabilities of developing breast cancer for white females who are being examined annually. J Natl Cancer Inst 1989;81:1879-1886.
124. Lynch HT, Watson P: Early age at breast cancer onset—a genetic and oncologic perspective. Am J Epidemiol 1990;131: 984-986.
125. Claus EB, Risch N, Thompson WD: Genetic analysis of breast cancer in the cancer and steroid hormone study. Am J Hum Genet 1991;48:232-242.
126. Ford D, Easton DF, Stratton M, et al: Genetic heterogeneity and penetrance analysis of the BRCA1 and BRCA2 genes in breast cancer families. The Breast Cancer Linkage Consortium. Am J Hum Genet 1998;62:676-689.
127. Hall JM, Lee MK, Newman B, et al: Linkage of early-onset familial breast cancer to chromosome 17q21. Science 1990; 250:1684-1689.
128. Narod SA, Feunteun J, Lynch HT, et al: Familial breast-ovarian cancer locus on chromosome 17q12-q23. Lancet 1991;338:82-83.
129. Miki Y, Swensen J, Shattuck-Eidens D, et al: A strong candidate for the breast and ovarian cancer susceptibility gene BRCA1. Science 1994;266:66-71.
130. Frank TS, Deffenbaugh AM, Reid JE, et al: Clinical characteristics of individuals with germline mutations in BRCA1 and BRCA2: Analysis of 10,000 individuals. J Clin Oncol 2002;20: 1480-1490.
131. Ford D, Easton DF, Bishop DT, et al: Risks of cancer in BRCA1-mutation carriers. Breast Cancer Linkage Consortium. Lancet 1994;343:692-695.
132. Antoniou A, Pharoah PD, Narod S, et al: Average risks of breast and ovarian cancer associated with BRCA1 or BRCA2 mutations detected in case series unselected for family

history: A combined analysis of 22 studies. Am J Hum Genet 2003;72:1117-1130.
133. Brose MS, Rebbeck TR, Calzone KA, et al: Cancer risk estimates for BRCA1 mutation carriers identified in a risk evaluation program. J Natl Cancer Inst 2002;94:1365-1372.
134. Easton DF, Ford D, Bishop DT: Breast and ovarian cancer incidence in BRCA1-mutation carriers. Breast Cancer Linkage Consortium. Am J Hum Genet 1995;56:265-271.
135. Risch HA, McLaughlin JR, Cole DE, et al: Prevalence and penetrance of germline BRCA1 and BRCA2 mutations in a population series of 649 women with ovarian cancer. Am J Hum Genet 2001;68:700-710.
136. Satagopan JM, Boyd J, Kauff ND, et al: Ovarian cancer risk in Ashkenazi Jewish carriers of BRCA1 and BRCA2 mutations. Clin Cancer Res 2002;8:3776-3781.
137. Wooster R, Neuhausen SL, Mangion J, et al: Localization of a breast cancer susceptibility gene, BRCA2, to chromosome 13q12-13. Science 1994;265:2088-2090.
138. Warner E, Foulkes W, Goodwin P, et al: Prevalence and penetrance of BRCA1 and BRCA2 gene mutations in unselected Ashkenazi Jewish women with breast cancer. J Natl Cancer Inst 1999;91:1241-1247.
139. Oddoux C, Struewing JP, Clayton CM, et al: The carrier frequency of the BRCA2 6174delT mutation among Ashkenazi Jewish individuals is approximately 1%. Nat Genet 1996; 14:188-190.
140. Roa BB, Boyd AA, Volcik K, Richards CS: Ashkenazi Jewish population frequencies for common mutations in BRCA1 and BRCA2. Nat Genet 1996;14:185-187.
141. Struewing JP, Abeliovich D, Peretz T, et al: The carrier frequency of the BRCA1 185delAG mutation is approximately 1 percent in Ashkenazi Jewish individuals. Nat Genet 1995;11:198-200.
142. Whittemore AS, Gong G, Itnyre J: Prevalence and contribution of BRCA1 mutations in breast cancer and ovarian cancer: Results from three U.S. population-based case-control studies of ovarian cancer. Am J Hum Genet 1997;60:496-504.
143. Tonin PN, Mes-Masson AM, Futreal PA, et al: Founder BRCA1 and BRCA2 mutations in French Canadian breast and ovarian cancer families. Am J Hum Genet 1998;63:1341-1351.
144. Arason A, Jonasdottir A, Barkardottir RB, et al: A population study of mutations and LOH at breast cancer gene loci in tumours from sister pairs: Two recurrent mutations seem to account for all BRCA1/BRCA2 linked breast cancer in Iceland. J Med Genet 1998;35:446-449.
145. Petrij-Bosch A, Peelen T, van Vliet M, et al: BRCA1 genomic deletions are major founder mutations in Dutch breast cancer patients. Nat Genet 1997;17:341-345.
146. Sekine M, Nagata H, Tsuji S, et al: Mutational analysis of BRCA1 and BRCA2 and clinicopathologic analysis of ovarian cancer in 82 ovarian cancer families: Two common founder mutations of BRCA1 in Japanese population. Clin Cancer Res 2001;7:3144-3150.
147. Li FP, Fraumeni JF Jr, Mulvihill JJ, et al: A cancer family syndrome in twenty-four kindreds. Cancer Res 1988;48:5358-5362.
148. Li FP, Fraumeni JF Jr: Soft-tissue sarcomas, breast cancer, and other neoplasms: A familial syndrome? Ann Intern Med 1969;71:747-752.
149. Hisada M, Garber JE, Fung CY, et al: Multiple primary cancers in families with Li-Fraumeni syndrome. J Natl Cancer Inst 1998;90:606-611.
150. Frebourg T, Barbier N, Yan YX, et al: Germ-line p53 mutations in 15 families with Li-Fraumeni syndrome. Am J Hum Genet 1995;56:608-615.
151. Hwang SJ, Lozano G, Amos CI, Strong LC: Germline p53 mutations in a cohort with childhood sarcoma: Sex differences in cancer risk. Am J Hum Genet 2003;72:975-983.
152. Kleihues P, Schauble B, zur Hausen A, et al: Tumors associated with p53 germline mutations: A synopsis of 91 families. Am J Pathol 1997;150:1-13.
153. Malkin D, Li FP, Strong LC, et al: Germ line p53 mutations in a familial syndrome of breast cancer, sarcomas, and other neoplasms. Science 1990;250:1233-1238.
154. Varley JM, McGown G, Thorncroft M, et al: Germ-line mutations of TP53 in Li-Fraumeni families: An extended study of 39 families. Cancer Res 1997;57:3245-3252.
155. Bell DW, Varley JM, Szydlo TE, et al: Heterozygous germ line hCHK2 mutations in Li-Fraumeni syndrome. Science 1999;286:2528-2531.
156. Lloyd K, Dennis M: Cowden's disease, a possible new symptom complex with multiple system involvement. Ann Intern Med 1963:136-142.
157. Nelen MR, van Staveren WCG, Peeters EAJ, et al: Germline mutations in the PTEN/MMAC1 gene in patients with Cowden disease. Hum Molec Genet 1997;6:1383-1387.
158. Nelen MR, Kremer H, Konings IB, et al: Novel PTEN mutations in patients with Cowden disease: Absence of clear genotype-phenotype correlations. Eur J Hum Genet 1999;7: 267-273.
159. Eng C: Will the real Cowden syndrome please stand up: Revised diagnostic criteria. J Med Genet 2000;37:828-830.
160. Hemminki A, Markie D, Tomlinson I, et al: A serine/threonine kinase gene defective in Peutz-Jeghers syndrome. Nature 1998;391:184-187.
161. Jenne DE, Reimann H, Nezu J, et al: Peutz-Jeghers syndrome is caused by mutations in a novel serine threonine kinase. Nat Genet 1998;18:38-43.
162. Spigelman AD, Murday V, Phillips RK: Cancer and the Peutz-Jeghers syndrome. Gut 1989;30:1588-1590.
163. Giardiello FM, Brensinger JD, Tersmette AC, et al: Very high risk of cancer in familial Peutz-Jeghers syndrome. Gastroenterology 2000;119:1447-1453.
164. Savitsky K, Sfez S, Tagle DA, et al: The complete sequence of the coding region of the ATM gene reveals similarity to cell cycle regulators in different species. Hum Mol Genet 1995; 4:2025-2032.
165. Savitsky K, Bar-Shira A, Gilad S, et al: A single ataxia telangiectasia gene with a product similar to PI-3 kinase. Science 1995;268:1749-1753.
166. Byrd PJ, McConville CM, Cooper P, et al: Mutations revealed by sequencing the 5′ half of the gene for ataxia telangiectasia. Hum Mol Genet 1996;5:145-149.
167. Boder E: Ataxia-telangiectasia: Some historic, clinical and pathologic observations. Birth Defects Orig Artic Ser 1975;11: 255-270.
168. Boder E, Sedgwick RP: Ataxia-telangiectasia. (Clinical and immunological aspects). Psychiatr Neurol Med Psychol Beih 1970;13-14:8-16.
169. Reed WB, Epstein WL, Boder E, Sedgwick R: Cutaneous manifestations of ataxia-telangiectasia. JAMA 1966;195:746-753.
170. Epstein WL, Fudenberg HH, Reed WB, et al: Immunologic studies in ataxia-telangiectasia. I: Delayed hypersensitivity and serum immune globulin levels in probands and first-degree relatives. Int Arch Allergy Appl Immunol 1966;30: 15-29.
171. Swift M, Morrell D, Cromartie E, et al: The incidence and gene frequency of ataxia-telangiectasia in the United States. Am J Hum Genet 1986;39:573-583.
172. Weeks DE, Paterson MC, Lange K, et al: Assessment of chronic gamma radiosensitivity as an in vitro assay for heterozygote identification of ataxia-telangiectasia. Radiat Res 1991;128:90-99.
173. Weil MM, Kittrell FS, Yu Y, et al: Radiation induces genomic instability and mammary ductal dysplasia in Atm heterozygous mice. Oncogene 2001;20:4409-4411.
174. Swift M, Sholman L, Perry M, Chase C: Malignant neoplasms in the families of patients with ataxia-telangiectasia. Cancer Res 1976;36:209-215.
175. Su Y, Swift M: Mortality rates among carriers of ataxia-telangiectasia mutant alleles. Ann Intern Med 2000;133:770-778.
176. Athma P, Rappaport R, Swift M: Molecular genotyping shows that ataxia-telangiectasia heterozygotes are predisposed to breast cancer. Cancer Genet Cytogenet 1996;92:130-134.
177. Swift M, Reitnauer PJ, Morrell D, Chase CL: Breast and other cancers in families with ataxia-telangiectasia. N Engl J Med 1987;316:1289-1294.
178. Stankovic T, Kidd AM, Sutcliffe A, et al: ATM mutations and phenotypes in ataxia-telangiectasia families in the British

Isles: Expression of mutant ATM and the risk of leukemia, lymphoma, and breast cancer. Am J Hum Genet 1998;62: 334-345.

179. Chenevix-Trench G, Spurdle AB, Gatei M, et al: Dominant negative ATM mutations in breast cancer families. J Natl Cancer Inst 2002;94:205-215.
180. Larson GP, Zhang G, Ding S, et al: An allelic variant at the ATM locus is implicated in breast cancer susceptibility. Genet Test 1997;1:165-70.
181. Teraoka SN, Malone KE, Doody DR, et al: Increased frequency of ATM mutations in breast carcinoma patients with early onset disease and positive family history. Cancer 2001;92: 479-487.
182. Matsuoka S, Huang M, Elledge SJ: Linkage of ATM to cell cycle regulation by the Chk2 protein kinase. Science 1998; 282:1893-1897.
183. Chehab NH, Malikzay A, Appel M, Halazonetis TD: Chk2/hCds1 functions as a DNA damage checkpoint in G(1) by stabilizing p53. Genes Dev 2000;14:278-288.
184. Hirao A, Kong YY, Matsuoka S, et al: DNA damage-induced activation of p53 by the checkpoint kinase Chk2. Science 2000;287:1824-1827.
185. Offit K, Pierce H, Kirchhoff T, et al: Frequency of CHEK2*1100delC in New York breast cancer cases and controls. BMC Med Genet 2003;4:1.
186. Vahteristo P, Tamminen A, Karvinen P, et al: p53, CHK2, and CHK1 genes in Finnish families with Li-Fraumeni syndrome: further evidence of CHK2 in inherited cancer predisposition. Cancer Res 2001;61:5718-5722.
187. Meijers-Heijboer H, van den Ouweland A, Klijn J, et al: Low-penetrance susceptibility to breast cancer due to CHEK2(*)1100delC in noncarriers of BRCA1 or BRCA2 mutations. Nat Genet 2002;31:55-59.
188. Lee SB, Kim SH, Bell DW, et al: Destabilization of CHK2 by a missense mutation associated with Li-Fraumeni Syndrome. Cancer Res 2001;61:8062-8067.
189. Vahteristo P, Bartkova J, Eerola H, et al: A CHEK2 genetic variant contributing to a substantial fraction of familial breast cancer. Am J Hum Genet 2002;71:432-438.
190. Seidman H, Stellman SD, Mushinski MH: A different perspective on breast cancer risk factors: Some implications of the nonattributable risk. CA Cancer J Clin 1982;32:301-313.

Screening Results, Controversies, and Guidelines

Stephen A. Feig

Screening is the periodic examination of a population to detect previously unrecognized disease. Breast cancer screening is usually performed by means of mammography, physical examination, and breast self-examination (BSE), alone or in combination. By definition, a breast cancer screening test is performed only on women who have no clinical abnormality to suggest breast cancer, although they may be at increased risk because of factors such as age, family history, and nulliparity. When the same test, such as mammography or physical examination, is performed to evaluate a clinical sign or symptom or to evaluate an abnormality detected at screening, it is referred to as a *diagnostic (problem-solving) test*. Diagnostic testing is performed on an individual woman to answer a specific clinical question, such as the nature of her breast lump or nipple discharge, but screening is performed on large segments of the population as a public health measure.

Requirements for a screening test differ from those for a diagnostic test and include adequate sensitivity to detect early disease, acceptable specificity to minimize false-positive results, low risk, acceptable cost and cost-benefit ratio, availability of necessary equipment, and interpretive and performance expertise. Because the ultimate goal of screening is reduction in the number of deaths from breast cancer, demonstration of a statistically significant reduction in breast cancer mortality in a randomized clinical trial (RCT) may be considered another requirement. Thus far, this result has been documented for mammography but not for physical examination or BSE alone.

SCREENING MODALITIES

Mammography, physical examination, and BSE are complementary screening methods: Each should be capable of detecting cancers that are missed by one or both of the other modalities. Detection by physical examination or BSE depends on appreciation of tactile differences between a tumor and surrounding tissue. Presence of these tactile characteristics does not necessarily mean that a correspondingly visible mammographic finding will be present, especially in mammographically dense fibroglandular breasts. BSE may be advantageous in that it can be performed on a monthly basis and may detect interval cancers that surface between annual mammographic and clinical screenings. However, smaller tumors with higher survival rates are more likely to be detected by mammography than by physical examination or BSE.[1]

The Breast Cancer Detection Demonstration Project (BCDDP), sponsored by the American Cancer Society (ACS) and National Cancer Institute (NCI), was a program that screened 280,000 women throughout the United States with both mammography and physical examination from 1973 to 1981. In this program, 39% (1375) of the 3548 cancers were found by mammography alone, 7% (257) by physical examination alone, and 51% (1805) by both mammography and physical examination. Moreover, the rate of detection at physical examination was lowest for earlier-stage lesions. Of the 983 minimal cancers (invasive carcinoma measuring less than 1 cm and all ductal carcinoma in situ [DCIS]), 54% (484) were detected by mammography alone, 5% (42) by physical examination alone, and 38% (340) by both mammography and physical examination.[2]

Mammography is currently the most sensitive means of early detection. However, among women screened by both mammography and physical examination , about 5% to 10% of detected cancers are found by physical examination alone. BSE has been less efficient than mammography and physical examination.[3] Nevertheless, screening is most effective when all three modalities are used. The relative efficacy of any detection method depends on the quality of the examination being practiced. Major improvements in mammography since 1985 and especially since 1990 have enabled earlier detection of lesions than was possible in the BCDDP.[4]

Both ultrasonography and magnetic resonance imaging (MRI) have shown capability to detect some cancers missed by mammography and are currently under investigation to determine whether they might be effective as supplementary screening tests, especially in women who are at high risk or have dense breasts.[5,6] However, many questions regarding detection rates, false-positive biopsy rates, costs, and examination and interpretation time need to be answered before ultrasonography or MRI can be recommended for screening.

Digital mammography may be used for screening because its sensitivity and specificity have been shown to be comparable to those of conventional mammography. A large multicenter screening study of digital mammography is currently in progress to obtain a more precise comparison (see Chapter 13).

Other modalities, such as thermography, which measures variation in breast temperature; light scanning (transillumination), which records transmission of light through the breast; and scanning with radionuclides such as technetium Tc 99m (^{99m}Tc) sestamibi, should not be used for screening because they are much less effective than mammography in detecting very small lesions.

HIGHER SURVIVAL RATES AMONG WOMEN WITH SCREENING-DETECTED CANCERS

Two related factors—tumor size and stage at time of diagnosis—represent the major determinants of survival rates among patients with breast cancer. Smaller cancers with no histologic evidence of spread to the regional lymph nodes have the best prognosis. The 20-year relative survival rates in the BCDDP were 80.5% (overall), 85% for cancers detected by mammography alone, 82% for cancers detected by physical examination alone, and 74% for cancers detected by both mammography and physical examination. Twenty-year relative survival rates were highly dependent on lesion size. The rate was 96% for in situ carcinomas. For invasive cancers, the rates were 88% for those measuring 0.1 to 0.9 cm, 78% for cancers 1.0 to 1.9 cm, 68% for cancers 2.0 to 4.9 cm, and 58% for cancers 5.0 to 9.9 cm.[7] These rates can be compared with survival data from the Surveillance Epidemiology and End Results (SEER) Program of the NCI, a population-based network of cancer registries that monitors cancer trends throughout the United States. Women with breast cancer entered into the SEER database during the BCDDP era (1973-1978), consisting largely of women who were not being screened, had a 20-year relative survival rate of 53%.[8]

Criteria for Benefit from Screening: Longer Survival versus Decreased Mortality

There are several reasons why "improved" survival rates among women who volunteer to be screened do not necessarily establish benefit from screening. They include selection bias, lead-time bias, length bias, and interval cancers.[9] Thus, differences in survival rates may be influenced by variables other than the screening process itself.

Selection bias refers to the possibility that women who volunteer for screening differ from those who do not volunteer in ways that may alter the outcome of their diseases, such as health status and behavioral factors. Therefore, survival rates in screened and nonscreened women may be influenced by variables other than the screening process itself.

Lead-time bias implies that screening may affect the date of detection but not the date of death from breast cancer. Let us suppose that a woman who has never been screened finds her breast cancer serendipitously in 2004. She dies from her disease 5 years later, in 2009. If this same woman had been screened, her cancer might have been detected by mammography in the year 2001. Although small, the cancer detected in this woman by mammography has microscopic dissemination beyond the breast. Despite screening, the woman will die from her disease in the year 2009. Because of screening, however, she is said to have survived for 8 years instead of 5 years. Nevertheless, the seeming 3-year "improvement" in survival is not real.

Length bias sampling postulates that cancers detected at screening contain a disproportionate number of less aggressive lesions. Their growth rates are so slow that in the absence of screening they might never reach sufficient size to surface clinically. Even if undetected, such cancers might never result in death.

Finally, more favorable survival rates for screen-detected cancers may be negated by lower survival rates for faster-growing *interval cancers* that are undetected by mammography and that surface clinically between screens.

Considering these potential biases, benefit from screening cannot be proven by observation of "improved" survival rates. Rather, such proof requires prospective comparison of breast cancer death rates among study group women offered screening and control group women not offered screening in an RCT. Apart from the offer to be screened, these groups should not differ in any other substantial way. A statistically significant difference in breast cancer deaths between the groups on follow-up may be considered proof of benefit. Observation of lower mortality for the screened group in a well-designed and well-conducted RCT is not affected by selection bias, lead-time bias, length bias, or interval cancers.

RESULTS OF RANDOMIZED TRIALS

Seven population-based trials of breast cancer screening by mammography alone or in combination with physical examination have been conducted: the Health Insurance Plan of Greater New York (HIP) trial,[10] the Swedish Two-County Trial consisting of Kopparberg and Östergötland counties,[11] the Malmö (Sweden) Mammographic Screening Trial,[12] the Stockholm (Sweden) trial,[13,14] the Gothenburg (Sweden) Breast Screening Trial,[15] and the Edinburgh (Scotland) trial.[16] There has been one non–population-based RCT, the National Breast Screening Study (NBSS) of Canada.[17-19] In a population-based RCT, study and control groups are randomly selected from a predefined population. In a non–population-based RCT, study and control groups are randomly selected from women who volunteer to participate.

Protocols and results for women of all ages at entry into RCTs are shown in Table 23–1. Mortality reduction is equal to 1 minus the relative risk (RR) of dying from breast cancer in the study group women versus the control group. The HIP trial, the first RCT ever conducted, found a 23% reduction in breast cancer deaths (RR = 0.77) among women aged 40 to 64 years who were offered screening mammography and physical examination.[10]

Table 23–1. Randomized Trials of Mammography Screening: Results for All Ages Combined

Trial (Years)*	Age at Entry (Years)	No. of Views	Frequency of Mammography (Months)	Rounds (No.)	CBE	Follow-up (Years)	RR (95% CI)	Mortality Reduction
Health Insurance Plan of Greater NY trial (1963-1969)[10]	40-64	2	12	4	Annual	18	0.77 (0.61-0.97)	23%†
Malmö Mammographic Screening Trial (1976-1986)[12]	45-69	1-2	18-24	5	None	12	0.81 (0.62-1.07)	19%
Swedish Two-County Trial, Kopparberg and Östergötland counties (1979-1988)[11]	40-74	1	23-33	4	None	20	0.68 (0.59-0.80)	32%†
Edinburgh trial (1979-1988)[16]	45-64	1-2	24	4	Annual	14	0.71 (0.53-0.95)	29%†
Canadian National Breast Screening Study (1980-1987)[18]	50-59	2+ CBE versus CBE	12	5	Annual	13	1.02 (0.78-1.33)	–2%
Stockholm trial (1981-1985)[14]	40-64	1	28	2	None	8	0.80 (0.53-1.22)	20%
Gothenburg Breast Screening Trial (1982-1988)[15]	40-59	2	18	4	None	14	0.77 (0.60-1.00)	23%

CBE, Clinical breast examination; CI, confidence interval; HIP, Health Insurance Plan Project; RR, relative risk of death from breast cancer in study group/control group. Mortality reduction = 1 – RR.
*Superscript numbers indicate chapter references.
†Statistically significant.

The Two-County Swedish Trial was the first to demonstrate a statistically significant benefit from screening by mammography alone. The latest 20-year follow-up for this trial found a 32% reduction in breast cancer deaths among women aged 40 to 74 years at entry.[11] In the Edinburgh trial, screening by annual physical examination and biennial mammography resulted in a statistically significant 29% decrease in breast cancer deaths among women aged 45 to 64 years at entry.[16] The Gothenburg Breast Screening Trial had a 23% reduction in deaths from breast cancer among women aged 40 to 59 years at entry into screening, a finding that had marginal statistical significance.[15]

Two Swedish screening mammography trials reported benefits that were not statistically significant. The Malmö Mammographic Screening Trial found a 19% reduction in breast cancer deaths among women who began screening between ages 45 and 69 years.[12] The Stockholm trial described a 20% reduction in breast cancer deaths among women screened between 40 and 64 years of age.[14]

Combined results from a 15.8-year follow-up of women aged 38 to 75 years at entry into four Swedish trials (Malmö, Östergötland, Stockholm, and Gothenburg) showed a statistically significant 21% reduction in breast cancer mortality with screening.[20]

The Canadian NBSS failed to show any benefit for mammography screening in women aged 50 to 59 years. In that trial, women undergoing annual mammography and physical examination were compared with those being screening by physical examination alone.[17,18] Possible explanations for the variance between NBSS results and those of the seven other randomized trials include technical quality of mammography,[21-23] study design,[24-27] and control group contamination.[28]

In summary, of the eight randomized screening trials, seven showed evidence of benefit from screening. Breast cancer mortality reduction was statistically significant in each of three trials (HIP, Swedish Two-County, and Edinburgh) and in combined results from the Stockholm, Malmö, Östergötland, and Gothenburg trials, and marginally significant in the Gothenburg trial. Only one trial, the NBSS, found no evidence of benefit.

How the Controversy Regarding Screening Women 40 to 49 Years Old Began

Initial reports from the HIP trial found a difference in breast cancer death rates between study and control groups for women 50 years and older at entry that was apparent by year 4. Such a difference for women aged 40 to 49 years did not, however, emerge until 7 to 8 years of follow-up. By 18 years of follow-up, the reduction in breast cancer deaths among study women aged 40 to 49 years at entry was 23%, the same as that for women aged 50 to 64 years at entry. Yet even by that time, benefit for younger women was still not statistically significant according to Shapiro and colleagues,[10] who conducted and reported on the trial. This lack of statistical significance was a consequence of the relatively smaller number of younger women enrolled and the lower breast cancer incidence. Nevertheless, the apparent lack of statistically significant benefit led to controversy regarding screening of women in their 40s.[9,29,30]

The HIP trial, however, was designed to determine the efficacy not of screening separate age groups but rather of screening a single group of all women aged 40 to 65 years. Attempts to subdivide the study group reduced statistical power. The observation that results for younger women lacked statistical significance was often cited in the screening debate. The fact that the data for women aged 50 to 59 years and 60 years and older at entry, when analyzed separately, also lacked statistical significance was largely ignored.[10,31] Moreover, Chu and associates,[32] using a different method of analysis, subsequently found statistically significant mortality reductions of 24% for women aged 40 to 49 years and 21% for those aged 50 to 64 years at entry into the HIP trial.

Despite the report by Chu and associates,[32] some observers were still not convinced that screening would benefit women in their 40s, for several reasons. First, in all the trials, the reduction in the breast cancer death rates for younger women did not appear until several years after appearance of the reduction for women older than 50 years.[10] Second, results for younger women were not statistically significant for any other individual trial until 1997.

The controversy intensified in 1992 with publication of the 7-year follow-up report from the NBSS.[33] This study found no evidence of benefit among women aged 40 to 49 years who were offered five annual screenings by mammography and physical examination. There are several explanations for these disappointing results. First, the technical quality of mammography was poor. During most of the trial, more than 50% of the mammograms were poor or completely unacceptable, even as assessed by the standards of the day.[22,23,34] Second, the randomization process through which women were assigned to study and control groups was flawed.[25,34,35] All women were given a physical examination before randomization. This protocol may have allowed preferential allocation of women with breast masses and, thereby, late-stage breast cancers to the study group. As a likely consequence, an excess of late-stage breast cancers and breast cancer deaths was found in the study group compared with the control group throughout the trial.[23,27]

Proof of Benefit for Screening Women Aged 40 to 49 Years

Beginning in 1993, several successive meta-analyses of combined data for multiple RCTs were performed in order to accrue a greater number of women-years of follow-up than possible from any one RCT alone. However, the earliest meta-analyses, published in 1993 and 1995, suggested little if any benefit from screening women younger than 50 years.[36-38]

Subsequent meta-analyses published by Smart and colleagues[39] in 1995 and the Falun Meeting Committee[40] in 1996 included later follow-up data. These studies showed statistically significant mortality reduction, 24%, for women aged 40 to 49 years at entry into the seven population-based RCTs (Table 23–2). They also found a 15% to 16% mortality reduction that barely missed statistical significance when the NBSS, a non–population-based RCT, was also included. A meta-analysis of these trials, published by Hendrick and colleagues[41] in 1997, found statistically significant mortality reductions among women invited to undergo screening in their 40s: 18% for all eight RCTs and 29% for the five Swedish RCTs (see Table 23–2). Thus, with increasing length of follow-up, successive meta-analyses have shown progressively greater and statistically significant mortality reductions for women who began screening between 40 and 49 years of age. Regardless of whether NBSS results are included or excluded, meta-analyses for screening women aged 40 to 49 years now show statistically significant benefit.

Moreover, meta-analyses are no longer necessary to prove the benefit of screening younger women. Two RCTs besides the HIP trial have now shown statistically significant benefit for women aged 40 to 49 years (Table 23–3). Bjurstam and coworkers[42] reported a statistically significant 45% mortality reduction for women aged 39 to 49 years at randomization in the Gothenburg trial. Andersson and Janzon[43] reported a statistically significant 35% breast cancer mortality reduction for women in the Malmö trial who began screening mammography at age 45 to 49 years.

Should Women 75 Years and Older Be Screened?

The question of mammographic screening for elderly women is clinically relevant because there are almost 10 million women 75 years and older in the United States. The average life expectancy for a woman at age 75 is 13 years.[44] Women with good general health

Table 23–2. Meta-Analyses of Randomized Clinical Trials of Mammography Showing Statistically Significant Mortality Reduction for Women Aged 40 to 49 Years

Trials	Follow-up (yrs)	Mortality Reduction (%)
All eight trials*	10.5-18.0	18
Seven trials†	7.0-18.0	24
Five Swedish trials‡	11.4-15.2	29

*Health Insurance Plan of Greater New York (HIP), five Swedish trials, Edinburgh trial, and National Breast Screening Study of Canada (NBSS-1).
†All trials except NBSS-1.
‡Malmö Mammographic Screening Trial; Swedish Two-County Trial, Kopparberg and Östergötland; Stockholm trial; and Gothenburg Breast Screening Trial.
Data from references 39 to 41.

Table 23–3. Follow-up of Randomized Clinical Trials of Mammography Showing Statistically Significant Breast Cancer Mortality Reduction for Women Aged 40 to 49 Years

Trial (years)*	Age at Entry (yrs)	No. of Views	Frequency of Mammography (mos)	Clinical Breast Exam	Follow-up (yrs)	Mortality Reduction (%)
Health Insurance Plan of Greater NY (1963-1969)[32]	40-49	2	12	Annual	18.0	24
Malmö Mammographic Screening Program (1976-1990)[43]	45-49	1-2	18-24	None	12.7	36
Gothenburg Breast Screening Trial (1982-1988)[42]	39-49	2	18	None	12.0	45

*Superscript numbers indicate chapter references.

have a longer than average life expectancy. It is reasonable to expect that elderly women will benefit from screening. Reduction in breast cancer mortality among women aged 50 years and older becomes apparent within 4 years of entry into RCTs.[45] Therefore, for many older women with screening-detected breast cancer, death from another illness will not occur before they experience the benefit from screening.[46]

Strictly speaking, benefit from screening women 75 years and older has not been proven because this age group was not included in any RCT. Nevertheless, there is no biologic reason why early detection should not be effective for these women. Survival rates according to stage of disease are almost as high in older as in younger women.[47] The detection sensitivity of mammography is higher in the elderly because of their generally more fatty breast composition.[48,49] Therefore, screening mammography should be performed in women 75 years and older if their general health and life expectancy are good.[50,51]

Why Do Randomized Trials Underestimate the Benefit from Screening?

There are at least six reasons why results from all RCTs have underestimated the benefit to an individual woman undergoing screening with modern mammography, as follows:

- Mammographic image quality below today's standards
- Use of only one mammographic view per breast
- Noncompliance of some study group women
- Contamination of the control group
- Excessively long screening intervals
- Inadequate number of screening rounds

First, there have been many technical improvements in mammographic technique since the early 1980s, when nearly all the trials were conducted. These innovations in mammographic equipment, screen film systems, and processing allow images to have better sharpness, exposure, and contrast.[52,53] Better image quality facilitates early detection of breast cancer.[4,54]

Second, women in the RCTs were mostly screened with one view per breast. Today's standard, two views per breast examination, has been shown to detect 3% to 11% (mean 7%) more cancers than found using a mediolateral oblique (MLO) view alone.[55-60] Of the seven population-based RCTs, only the HIP and Gothenburg trials used two views on all examinations.[10,42] The Malmö trial used two views in the first two screenings and a MLO view alone on all subsequent screenings except in patients with dense breasts.[12] The Edinburgh trial used two views on the initial screening and one view on all subsequent screenings.[61] The Stockholm and Swedish Two-County trials used a single MLO view in all screenings.[11,13]

Two fundamental reasons why RCTs underestimate the benefit from screening are that (1) not all study group women accept the invitation to be screened *(noncompliance)* and (2) some control group women obtain mammography screening outside the trial *(contamination)*. Yet, in order to avoid selection bias, an RCT must compare the breast cancer death rate among all study group women, both screened and nonscreened, with that among all control group women, including those who are screened on their own initiative. Thus both noncompliance of some study women and contamination of control group women reduce the calculated benefit from RCTs.

Among the RCTs, the noncompliance rate ranged from 10% to 39%.[62] Studies performed on data from the individual trials have estimated that if all women in the study group had attended each screening round, there would have been at least an additional 10% reduction in breast cancer deaths.[63,64] Data from the Gothenburg, Malmö, and Swedish Two-County trials as well as the NBSS indicate that the rate of control group contamination ranged from 13% to 25%.[62]

Randomized trials have also underestimated the potential benefit because screening intervals have been too long. Aside from the HIP trial, screening intervals in RCTs have been longer than the annual intervals now recommended.[65] For example, women in the Swedish Two-County Trial were screened every 24 to 33 months,[11] and those in the Edinburgh trial every 24 months.[16,61] Numerous studies indicate that greater benefit should result from annual screening, especially for women aged 40 to 49 years, in whom breast cancer growth rates appear to be faster.[66-69] On the basis of a tumor growth rate model, Michaelson[70] calculated that annual screening would result in a 51% reduction in the rate of distant metastatic disease compared with a 22% reduction at a screening interval of 2 years.

It has been estimated that the use of annual screening in the Swedish Two-County Trial could have resulted in an additional 18% mortality reduction for women aged 40 to 49 years at entry, who were screened every 2 years, and an additional 12% mortality reduction for women aged 50 to 59 years at entry, who were screened every 33 months.[40] For women aged 39 to 49 at entry into the Gothenburg trial, who were screened every 18 months, it has been estimated that annual screening could have resulted in an additional 20% mortality reduction.[64]

Several investigators have used mathematical models of actual RCT data to calculate the benefit to an "average" woman who is screened every year and for whom results are not affected by noncompliance and contamination.[40,63,64,71] For example, on the basis of an observed 45% reduction in breast cancer mortality among women aged 39 to 49 years offered screening every 18 months in the Gothenburg trial, Feig[64] calculated that the mortality reduction could have been as high as 65% with annual screening at the observed 80% compliance rate and as high as 75% at a 100% compliance rate.

Finally, the fact that no randomized trial had more than four or five screening rounds represents a sixth reason why such trials may underestimate the potential benefits of screening. Such relatively short durations limit the mortality reduction estimates that can be made using standard methods of measurement. Screening must be performed not only frequently but also over much longer periods in order to reach a "steady state" at which the greatest mortality reduction will be apparent. Using a new method of moving averages, Miettinen and Henschke[72] showed that for women aged 55 to 69 years at entry into the Malmö Mammographic Screening Trial, mortality reduction was highest between 8 and 11 years of follow-up. For that period, they calculated a 55% reduction in breast cancer deaths. This value was much higher than the 26% mortality reduction reported by Andersson and Nystrom,[73] who had included data from before year 8, when benefit had not yet peaked, and from after year 11, when benefit was being diluted.

SCREENING MAMMOGRAPHY GUIDELINES

Breast cancer incidence is decidedly lower for women in their thirties than among women aged 40 to 49, being 0.4 versus 1.6 cases per 1000 women per year, respectively. Less than 5% of all breast cancers occur before age 40 and less than 0.3% before age 30, compared with 19% for ages 40 to 49. Therefore, screening mammography is not advised for most women until age 40. Screening in their thirties may be considered only for those very few women who have extremely high risk for development of breast cancer at an early age.[65]

The time between screenings can affect the benefits. Because mortality rate reduction from screening is now well established, the goal should be to optimize the benefit by using the most appropriate screening intervals. Mounting evidence indicates that cancer in younger women has a shorter sojourn time and consequently a shorter lead time than cancer in older women.[63,67,69,74,75] *Sojourn time* is the maximum time between the earliest possible detection at screening and clinical finding in the absence of screening. *Lead time* is the average time between actual detection at screening and clinical finding in the absence of screening. If the interval between screenings is too long, many rapidly growing tumors will be detected by screening only shortly before they would have become clinically apparent, thereby reducing the benefit of screening.

Accordingly, many major medical organizations, including the American Cancer Society, the American College of Radiology, the American Medical Association, and the Society for Breast Imaging, now recommend that women aged 40 to 49 years be screened annually (Table 23–4).[65,75,76] This recommendation replaces the previous recommendation that women in this age group receive screening mammography every 1 to 2 years and is justified by the more rapid growth of breast tumors among younger women. These societies continue to recommend that women 50 years and older be screened annually. Some authorities suggest that the interval between screenings can be lengthened as a women ages. Nevertheless, it is likely that even in older women, some faster-growing cancerous tumors will become clinically apparent between biennial screenings, reducing the screening benefit. Women and their physicians should be aware that the major reason for accepting a longer screening interval at any age is a presumed reduction in screening cost, but that some consequent reduction in screening benefit will occur.

Screening guidelines offered by other medical organizations are also shown in Table 23–4. Both the NCI and the U.S. Preventive Services Task Force now recommend screening every 1 to 2 years beginning at age 40.[77] The American College of Obstetricians and Gynecologists recommends screening every 1 to 2 years between ages 40 and 49 and annually thereafter. The American Academy of Family Physicians and the American College of Preventive Medicine do not advise screening before age 50 but do recommend mammography every 1 to 2 years after that age.

Breast cancer advocacy groups, such as the National Alliance of Breast Cancer Organizations (NABCO) and the Susan B. Komen Foundation, both advise women to begin annual screening at age 40.

Table 23–4. Current Guidelines for Screening Mammography

Group (Date)	Screening Frequency (Yrs) For Women 40-49 Yrs Old	Screening Frequency (Yrs) For Women 50 Yrs and Older
Government and foundations:		
American Cancer Society (2003)	1	1
National Cancer Institute (2002)	1-2	1-2
US Preventive Services Task Force (2002)	1-2	1-2
Medical specialty societies:		
American Academy of Family Physicians (2001)	No	1-2*
American College of Obstetricians and Gynecologists (2000)	1-2	1
American College of Preventive Medicine (1996)	No screening	1-2
American College of Radiology (1998)	1	1
Society of Breast Imaging (2000)	1	1
Advocacy groups:		
National Alliance of Breast Cancer Organizations (2002)	1	1
Susan B. Komen Foundation (2002)	1	1

*American Academy of Family Physicians does not recommend screening after age 70 years.

The Newest Screening Controversy

On the basis of results from RCTs conducted over the past quarter of a century and involving more than 500,000 women, consensus has been reached in the medical community in favor of screening mammography. In the face of such near-unanimous agreement, two articles made the seemingly incredible claim that none of the trials provided any convincing evidence that screening prevents breast cancer deaths.[78,79] The authors of these articles, Gotzsche and Olsen, asserted that only two of the eight screening trials—the Malmö Mammographic Screening Trial and the NBSS—were valid, and that neither of these trials found evidence of benefit. The articles received enormous publicity because of the sensational nature of their claim, which questioned the widely held belief in the efficacy of early detection through mammography screening.

The only points on which Gotzsche and Olsen and all other observers agree are that the NBSS (1) failed to find benefit for screening in women aged 50 to 70 years with mammography and clinical examination versus clinical examination alone[18] and (2) found no benefit for mammographic screening of women aged 40 to 49 years.[19,33] At that point, however, advocates of screening part ways with Gotzsche and Olsen because their explanations for the negative NBSS results are vastly different.

Because serious deficiencies at the NBSS have been well documented, it is preposterous that Gotzsche and Olsen view the NBSS as the paradigm of a well-conducted study, for several reasons. First, independent reviews found that the technical quality of mammography in the NBSS was poor even when measured by the standards of the 1980s, when the trial was conducted.[21-23] Second, performance of clinical breast examination before randomization of trial subjects may have allowed channeling of symptomatic women into the study group. The finding of an excess of advanced cancers in the study group aged 40 to 49 years suggests that randomization was not performed blindly.[23-26]

Third, NBSS was not a population-based trial. Rather, participants were self-selected volunteers. Because self-selected women are more likely to be symptomatic, adequate randomization of such subjects is more problematic, especially when clinical examination has already been performed. Self-selected asymptomatic women may have higher survival rates than randomly selected asymptomatic women. Thus, benefit may be harder to demonstrate in a trial with such subjects than in a population-based trial. Contrary to the sentiments of Gotzsche and Olsen, almost any of these fatal flaws in trial design and implementation render the NBSS incapable of providing meaningful results.

The statement by Gotzsche and Olsen that the Malmö trial showed no evidence of benefit is even more astonishing. For some inexplicable reason, Gotzsche and Olsen considered only an early report of a small, insignificant 5% mortality reduction among women aged 45 to 70 years.[12] They totally ignored later reports of breast cancer mortality reductions of 19% for women aged 45 to 70 years, 26% for women aged 55 to 70 years,[73] and 36% for women aged 45 to 50 years at entry into the Malmö trial.[43] Moreover, several months after publication of the second Olsen and Gotzsche paper,[79] Miettinen and Henschke[72] reported using 3-year moving averages of relative risk estimates to estimate that the true mortality reduction from the Malmö trial was 55% for women aged 55 to 69 years and 60% for women aged 45 to 57 years at entry into screening.

Gotzsche and Olsen also claimed to have identified age differences of 1 to 5 months between study and control groups in the HIP and Edinburgh trials and all Swedish trials aside from the Malmö trial. These writers suggested that the observed reductions in breast cancer death rates were due to these age differences rather than to the screening process itself. Gotzsche and Olsen were unaware that when screening trials use cluster randomization rather than individual randomization, such relatively small age differences are not only expected but also acceptable.[80,81]

Screening trials and therapeutic trials are different in nature and may be different in design. In therapeutic trials, all participants have disease. The main variables are treatment versus no treatment and dose regimen. Study and control groups are small. Individual randomization is required, and small age differences are significant to the study. In screening mammography trials, there is low disease prevalence, so extremely large study and control groups are necessary. For this reason, individual randomization may not be practical, and cluster randomization is usually necessary.

The age difference between the two groups that Gotzsche and Olsen purported to have discovered in the Swedish Two-County Trial had been acknowledged by Tabár and colleagues[82] in 1989. In fact, after adjustment for age, mortality rates were only minimally different: 31% versus 30% for women aged 40 to 70 years in the Swedish Two-County Trial[81] and 45% instead of 46% for women aged 39 to 49 years in the Gothenburg trial.[83] Thus, there was no way that these small differences in age could have altered the overall conclusion that screening results in a substantial reduction in deaths from breast cancer.

In another criticism, Gotzsche and Olsen suggested that assignment of the cause of death among women in the Swedish screening trials might have been inaccurate. Accurate assignment of cause of death is, of course, critical to proper assessment of trial results. Death in a woman with breast cancer may be either causally related or unrelated to her malignancy. Because screening trials compare deaths due to breast cancer in women in study groups and control groups, attribution of the cause of death must be performed in a consistent and unbiased manner. However, the criticism by Gotzsche and Olsen was baseless. The methods for cause of death assignment in the Swedish trials had been previously described in detail by Nystrom and associates.[84] The process consisted of independent blind evaluation by four physicians and resulted in unanimous agreement in a remarkable 93% of cases.[20,84-86]

Gotzsche and Olsen also observed that no statistically significant decrease in death rates from all causes combined had yet been shown in any of the Swedish trials. They interpreted this observation to mean that any benefit from reduction in breast cancer deaths would be countered by increased deaths from other causes. This incorrect conclusion disregarded the fact that breast cancer accounts for only about 5% of total mortality. Thus, even the largest individual trial would be unlikely to demonstrate any statistically significant decrease in all-cause mortality. On this issue, too, Gotzsche and Olsen were proven wrong. Subsequent to publication of the second Olsen and Gotzsche paper,[79] Nystrom and associates[20,86] were, in fact, able to find a 2% decrease in all-cause mortality among study group women in five Swedish trials combined. Additionally, Tabár and colleagues[87] observed a significant 19% reduction in deaths from all causes among breast cancer cases in the group invited to screening in the Swedish Two-County Trial. Thus, the Gotzsche and Olsen conjecture regarding all-cause mortality was incorrect.

To further their thesis that data from the Swedish Two-County trial was unreliable, Gotzsche and Olsen asserted that the reported study group size was different in the articles by Tabár and colleagues. In response to this criticism, Duffy and Tabár[88] acknowledged that the study population size did in fact differ among their published reports. In fact, Tabár and colleagues[82] had previously noted that these differences were due to progressive identification and exclusion of women diagnosed with breast cancer before the trial began. This is an acceptable and, in fact, commendable practice. This observation had escaped Gotzsche and Olsen, who obviously did not read the articles thoroughly and did not appreciate the rationale for such fastidious data collection. The irony of this unjustified criticism is that Tabár and colleagues were faulted for practicing good science.

In their papers, Gotzsche and Olsen also reiterated the conclusion of a study by Sjonell and Stahle,[89] which claimed that widespread screening in Sweden had not affected breast cancer mortality in the population. The basic mistake by Sjonell and Stahle[89] in this claim was they had measured death rates too early after screening was started. Decreased mortality should not be expected until 5 to 8 years after the start of screening. Sjonell and Stahle[89] had mistakenly begun to tally breast cancer deaths before the beginning of the service screening programs that they were attempting to assess.[86,90] Additionally, their calculations did not consider the increase in breast cancer incidence over time.

Although the report by Gotzsche and Olsen received considerable publicity in the U.S. media, no medical organization or government has changed its screening policy on the basis of their conclusions. Indeed, after review of the Gotzsche and Olsen paper, 10 leading medical organizations—American Academy of Family Physicians, American Cancer Society, American College of Obstetricians and Gynecologists, American College of Physicians–American Society of Internal Medicine, American College of Preventive Medicine, American Medical Association, Cancer Research Foundation of America, National Medical Association, Oncology Nursing Society, and the Society of Gynecologic Oncologists—reaffirmed their support of screening in a full-page public service announcement published in the *New York Times* on January 31, 2002. Also, the NCI and the U.S. Preventive Services Task Force concluded that despite Gotzsche and Olsen's contentions, the results from RCTs of screening were still valid.

In addition, the Swedish National Board of Health and Welfare,[91] the Danish National Board of Health, the Health Council of the Netherlands,[92] the European Institute of Oncology,[93] and the World Health Organization[94] dismissed Gotzsche and Olsen's arguments and concluded that the evidence for benefit of screening for breast cancer was convincing.

Service Screening Results

After the success of the Swedish randomized trials, organized service screening mammography became routine in nearly all Swedish counties by the 1990s. Unlike randomized trials, which are conducted primarily as clinical research studies, service screening is performed mainly as a public health initiative. Nevertheless, results from service screening projects have provided strong confirmation that screening mammography is effective in reducing mortality from breast cancer.[95]

Jonsson and coworkers[96] compared excess breast carcinoma mortality rates for the Swedish study group and control group counties. Study group counties were those in which screening was initiated between 1986 and 1987; control group counties were those in which screening was initiated in 1993 or later. Only women aged 50 to 69 years were evaluated because only half the counties began screening at age 40 years and some counties did not invite women to undergo screening after age 69 years. Women aged 50 to 69 years were thus invited to undergo screening in all counties. A 20% reduction in excess mortality from breast carcinoma was evident in the study group after a mean individual follow-up time of 8.4 years.[96]

A study by Tabár and colleagues[97] measured the effect of mammography in a population in which service screening is offered to all women 40 years and older. They compared breast cancer death rates in two Swedish counties over three periods: 1968 to 1977, when virtually no women were screened (prescreening era); 1978 to 1987, when half the population was offered screening in the RCT; and 1988 to 1996, after completion of the trial, when screening was offered to all women and 85% of the population was being screened. Compared with breast cancer death rates among women aged 40 to 69 years in the prescreening era, breast cancer death rates in 1988 to 1996 were 63% lower for screened women and 50% lower for the entire population (85% screened + 15% not screened) (Table 23–5). During this time, reductions in death rates from breast cancer for screened women were similar to those for women screened during the trial (63% versus 57%, respectively). However, during the RCT trial period (1978 to 1987), only half of the population was offered screening; for that era, breast cancer death rate reduction in the entire population was only 21%.

It seems probable that screening rather than advances in treatment was responsible for nearly all the benefit. The RRs of breast cancer death among nonscreened women aged 40 to 69 years were similar during the three consecutive periods (1.0, 1.7, and 1.19, respectively). Moreover, the breast cancer death rate for women aged 20 to 39 years, virtually none of whom were screened, showed no significant difference (1.0, 1.10 and 0.81, respectively) during these three consecutive periods.

Table 23–5. Reduction in Population Death Rates from Breast Cancer in Women Diagnosed Between Ages 40 and 69 Years in Two Swedish Counties*

Screening Status	1978-1987 (Randomized Trial)	1988-1996 (Service Screening)
Screened	57%	63%
Invited to screening	43%	48%
Screened plus non-screened	21%	50%

*Time of diagnosis either 1978-1987 or 1988-1996 compared with death rates from cancers diagnosed during 1969-1977 before screening began. All results were statistically significant at 95% confidence level.

Data from Tabar L, Vitak B, Chen HH, et al: Beyond randomized controlled trials: Organized mammographic screening substantially reduces breast cancer mortality. Cancer 2001;91:1724-1731.

Possibly, women who agree to be screened have selection bias factors that apart from the screening process improved their survival rates. Even assuming the maximum effect of selection bias, screening was shown to reduce breast cancer deaths by at least 50%.

A study by Duffy and Tabár[98] assessed the effect of service screening in seven Swedish counties.[98] Among women aged 40 to 69 years, breast cancer mortality was 44% lower for screened women and 39% lower for women offered screening compared with the prescreening era. On the basis of breast cancer mortality trends, it was estimated that only 12% of the mortality reduction was due to improved therapy and patient management apart from the screening process.

Garne and aassociates[99] found similar results for women in Malmö, Sweden. Between 1977 and 1992, breast cancer mortality among women 45 years and older in Malmö decreased 43%. During that same period, breast cancer deaths among women in this age group in the rest of Sweden diminished by only 12%. There was no change in mortality among women younger than 45 years. The decrease in mortality occurred in temporal relationship to the introduction of screening mammography and adjuvant therapy, consistent with a causal relationship. The Malmö trial (1976 to 1986) offered screening mammography to women aged 45 to 69 years. The screening compliance rate was estimated at 79%, and approximately 24% of control group women obtained screening outside the trial.[12]

In another service screening study, Lenner and Jonsson[100] found a 28% decrease in breast cancer mortality among women aged 40 to 74 years in two northern Swedish counties. Two adjacent counties where screening was not yet offered and that until that time had identical breast cancer mortality rates served as controls.

In Finland, nationwide population-based breast carcinoma screening for women aged 50 to 59 years was introduced gradually between 1987 and 1991. Women born in even years began screening in 1987 or 1988. Women born in odd years, who began screening between 1989 and 1991, served as controls. An effect of screening emerged after 3 to 4 years of follow-up and rapidly diluted as controls were screened. For this narrow window of time, Hakama and colleagues[101] found that mortality from breast carcinoma was 24% lower among women who were offered screening and 33% lower among women who were actually screened.[101]

Results from these many service screening studies indicate that the reductions in breast cancer mortality found in the RCTs can be obtained and exceeded in non-research, organized service screening settings. These programs effectively refute the claim by Gotzsche and Olsen that the benefits seen in the RCTs of screening were not real because of supposed flaws in randomization and ascertainment of cause of death.[102]

ADVERSE CONSEQUENCES AND COSTS OF SCREENING

A woman whose breast cancer is detected through screening is on average 50% less likely to die of the breast cancer.[95,98] However, only a tiny fraction of the population being screened each year benefits from mammographic examination, because the annual incidence of breast cancer is low and not all cases are detected by mammography. Breast cancer is a chronic disease, so the benefit from early detection may not be apparent for many years. In contradistinction, adverse consequences such as false-positive biopsy results occur sooner rather than later and affect more women. An even greater number of women may experience some anxiety that their examination may detect cancer. Moreover, the economic costs of screening are borne by nearly all members of society. All these benefits and risks must be carefully weighed in the determination of guidelines and policies for mammography screening.

That mammography produces benefit should no longer be subject to debate, because numerous randomized trials and service screening studies have produced unequivocal proof that screening can substantially lower the number of deaths due to breast cancer. Comparison of screening benefits with costs and adverse consequences, however, may reveal legitimate concerns. Such comparisons, like those discussed in the remainder of this chapter, can help determine when screening should begin and how often it should be performed. Analysis of risks from screening can lead to ways of reducing those risks without affecting cancer detection rates.

Breast Compression

The benefits of breast compression include the ability to obtain sharper images, with better exposure and more contrast, at lower radiation doses.[103] Improvements in breast compression devices and techniques over the past 30 years have allowed higher cancer detection rates and more comfortable examinations.[4]

When properly performed, mammography usually is not painful.[104] Following some simple recommendations can minimize discomfort. First, vigorous compression is not necessary; rather, the breast should be compressed only until the skin is taut.[105] The patient should first be informed why compression is necessary and told that compression will be automatically released as soon as the exposure is taken. Also, pressure should be applied gradually, with manual fine-tuning for the final degree of compression. The patient should then let the technologist know of any excessive discomfort so that no further compression will be applied. Patients who experience tenderness just before their menstrual periods may want to schedule mammography at some other time, and taking a mild analgesic before mammography may be helpful. It is important to minimize any discomfort from mammography so that women will not be reluctant to undergo periodic screening.

Recall Rates

When screening mammograms are "batch-interpreted," the patient leaves the imaging center immediately after her standard two-views-per-breast screening mammogram has been performed and checked for image quality by the technologist. The images are then placed on a rotating film viewer and interpreted in batches by a radiologist at some later time. Patients receive their results by mail. If mammographic findings indicate that supplementary views or ultrasonography is needed, the patient must return another day.

Because batch reading is much more efficient and cost-effective than on-line interpretation, it is the only practical way to perform screening mammography in the current environment of low reimbursement levels and high demand for screening.[106] In contradistinction, on-line interpretation is necessary for diagnostic mammography because of the high percentage of abnormal study findings and the need to tailor each examination to the patient's clinical problem.

Recall rate refers to the percentage of patients asked to return for additional imaging evaluation after batch interpretation of screening mammography. Batch interpretation can be performed successfully only if recall rates are kept within acceptable limits. Recall rates that are too high cause patient inconvenience and anxiety as well as raise the cost and reduce the efficiency of the screening process. Excessive recall rates represent a disincentive for women to undergo screening, for referring physicians to advise screening, and for medical care payers to support screening. If recall rates are too low, some subtle cancers may be missed, and some benign lesions may be subjected to biopsy unnecessarily because supplementary views and ultrasonography were not performed.

On the basis of published reports of recall rates for well-conducted screening programs, the American College of Radiology recommends that recall rates be maintained at 10% or less.[107] This upper limit value should probably be less for women in whom a previous mammogram has been performed recently. Hunt and colleagues found that recall rates for such women could be 30% lower than those for women having their initial mammogram.[108] These recommendations receive support from a study by Yankaskas and coworkers,[109] who found that a recall rate of 4.9% to 5.5% represents the best trade-off between detection sensitivity (the percentage of cancers that are detected by screening mammography) and biopsy positive predictive value (PPV; the percentage of biopsies that reveal malignancy).

There are several common misconceptions regarding recall rates. First, recall rates are not really false-positive rates, because most recalled patients do not undergo biopsy. Second, recall rates for 10 screenings are not 10 times the rate for the initial screening, which has a higher recall rate than subsequent screenings. Such misconceptions have appeared in the literature[110] and need to be corrected.[111]

False-Positive Biopsy Results

An excessive rate of biopsies leads to anxiety, discomfort, and pain for the patient and also increases the cost and potentially decreases the use of screening mammography. The American College of Radiology recommends that the PPV when biopsy is recommended (PPV_2) should be 25% to 40%.[107] PPV results are affected by patient age, risk factors, and presence of clinical signs and symptoms. Results from several centers have found that the PPV_1 (number of cancers detected per number of biopsies performed) is about 22% for screening women aged 40 to 49 years, 35% for those aged 50 to 59 years, 45% for those aged 60 to 69 years, and 50% for those 70 years and older.[112-115] Although the PPV is lower for women aged 40 to 49 years, it is still acceptable. A complete imaging work-up, including supplementary mammographic views and ultrasonography, follow-up rather than biopsy for lesions that appear probably benign, and the seeking of second opinions for problematic cases, can reduce false-positive biopsy rates.

Ductal Carcinoma In Situ

Coincident with the increasing use of mammography has been a marked increase in the incidence of ductal carcinoma in situ (DCIS). Before the era of mammographic screening, DCIS represented less than 5% of all malignancies of the breast.[116] DCIS now accounts for between 20% and 40% of all nonpalpable cancers detected at screening.[116] With appropriate treatment, the survival rate for patients with DCIS should be 99.5%.[116] DCIS may be considered a frequent but nonobligate precursor of fatal breast cancer. In other words, all cases of invasive ductal carcinoma are believed to develop from DCIS, but not all cases of DCIS may progress to invasive ductal carcinoma.

Justification for the use of DCIS as an index of the benefit of screening depends on how often and how rapidly DCIS evolves into invasive ductal carcinoma. As of yet, no direct method exists for determining the natural progression of DCIS. If patients with DCIS were never to undergo biopsy and the DCIS were left to develop into invasive ductal carcinoma, there would be no way to establish that the initial lesion was DCIS. If DCIS is completely excised, then its natural history has been stopped and there is no proof that it would have evolved into invasive ductal carcinoma.

Results from autopsy studies of women with no clinical evidence of breast cancer show a 6% to 14% prevalence of DCIS.[116] These rates have been used to suggest that most cases of DCIS may never become clinically apparent. However, there are reasons why this conclusion is not justified. First, most (45% to 56%) of the autopsy-detected cases of DCIS could not be identified by radiography of the surgical specimen.[116] Undoubtedly, an even higher percentage would not have been seen at mammography. Therefore, the DCIS found at autopsy is not representative of the type of DCIS detected by screening mammography, which would be larger, calcified, and therefore a faster-growing lesion. Second, detection rates for invasive ductal carcinoma at prevalence screening are 2 to 3 times higher than the expected incidence, consistent with a 2- to 3-year detection lead time. In the absence of screening, many cases of high-grade DCIS will not surface clinically as DCIS but rather as invasive carcinoma. Thus, it would not be surprising if the prevalence of mammographically visible DCIS at autopsy were even 10 to 20 times higher than the expected incidence of DCIS. Moreover, some cases classified as "DCIS" in the autopsy studies, which took place in the 1980s, would be reclassified as "atypical hyperplasia" according to current diagnostic criteria.

Several follow-up studies of DCIS treated with biopsy alone also shed light on the invasive potential of DCIS. The lesions in these studies were categorized as benign at initial histologic review, and so wide excision was not performed. In one study, researchers found development of invasive ductal carcinoma at the biopsy site in 53% of cases within 9.7 years.[116] Another study showed development of invasive ductal carcinoma in 28% of cases by 10 years and 36% of cases within 24 years.[116] Recurrence rates for DCIS in series such as these have suggested to some observers that DCIS is unlikely to progress to invasive disease.

There are two reasons, however, why these studies should lead to just the opposite conclusion. First, these studies underestimate the invasive potential of DCIS because they involved only cases of low-grade DCIS, that is, all histologic subtypes of DCIS except for comedocarcinoma, the most aggressive subtype. Comedocarcinoma typically accounts for 32% to 50% of all cases of DCIS detected at mammographic screening.[116] Second, these studies included some cases in which the DCIS lesion was completely removed and other cases in which some DCIS remained in the breast because biopsy margins were not sufficiently wide. Invasive ductal carcinoma would be expected only in this latter subgroup.

Screening Benefits versus Risks for Woman Aged 40 to 49 Years

Because the benefit of screening for women aged 40 to 49 years has now been established, the remaining screening issues for this age group are the smaller absolute reduction in breast cancer deaths and the higher relative rate of risks and procedures per cancer detected. However, differences in benefits between women aged 40 to 49 years and women aged 50 to 59 years are small. So are the differences in risks. Such changes occur gradually with age rather than abruptly at age 50.[112,113,117]

Women aged 40 to 49 years have a lower incidence of breast cancer, a faster rate of breast cancer growth, and a tendency to have denser, more fibroglandular breast tissue, for which mammography is less sensitive. As a consequence, screening detection rates for women in their 40s are somewhat lower than those for women in succeeding decades. Biopsy PPV is also lower for women in their 40s. However, both detection rates and PPVs for women aged 40 to 49 years are well within acceptable limits (Table 23–6).

Some investigators have used inappropriate methods of comparison to suggest that detection rates are too low and false-positive rates are too high to support screening of women aged 40 to 49 years. Methods such as pooling data for women aged 40 to 49 years with data from younger women, pooling data for women aged 50 to 59 yeas with data from older women, and the exclusive use of data from the initial (prevalence) screening result in an inaccurate portrayal of screening outcomes for women in their 40s. Such improper assessment led Kerlikowske and associates[118] to make the misleading statement that screening of women younger than 50 years will detect only 20% as many cancers per 1000 women screened, will require 4 times as many diagnostic procedures per cancer detected, and will cause 2.5 times as many false-positive biopsy results for each cancer detected as screening of older women.[118]

Proper assessment of the accuracy of screening mammography for women aged 40 to 49 years requires comparison of data for that age group only with data for women aged 50 to 59 years. The use of data from initial (prevalence) screening alone may be misleading. The use of data from subsequent (incidence) screening alone is preferred, but combined data from prevalence and incidence screenings may also be used. Such an assessment indicates that screening of women aged 40 to 49 years detects at least 63% to 80% as many cancers, requires 1.7 times as many diagnostic imaging procedures, and results in 1.3 to 1.4 times as many false-positive biopsy results for cancers detected (Table 23–7).[117]

The increase in sensitivity and specificity from screening in women aged 50 to 59 years compared with screening in women aged 40 to 49 years is similar to that of screening in women aged 60 to 69 years compared with women aged 50 to 59 years and also to that of screening in women 70 years or older compared with women aged 60 to 69 years. Although

Table 23–6. Detection Rates and Accuracy of Mammography at Three Service Screening Programs According to Age

	Age Range (yrs)				
Parameter	30–39	40–49	50–59	60–69	70–79
Cancer detection rates*:					
MGH	NA	2.4	3.0	3.9	5.0
UCSF	2.9	3.4	5.4	7.5	9.5
NM	NA	3.5	4.8	7.0	9.5
Biopsy PPV†:					
MGH	NA	0.17	0.24	0.32	0.40
UCSF	0.16	0.26	0.35	0.43	0.55
NM	NA	0.25	0.32	0.41	0.60
Screening recall rates‡:					
MGH	NA	7.0	6.9	6.0	5.6
UCSF	2.3	2.0	1.9	2.0	1.4

*Cancers per 1000 women screened at first and subsequent screens combined.
†Cancers detected/biopsies performed at first and subsequent screens at MGH, subsequent screens only at UCSF.
‡Percentage of screening patients requiring supplemental imaging at first and subsequent screens at MGH, subsequent screens only at UCSF.
MGH, Massachusetts General Hospital; NA, not applicable; NM, X-ray Associates of New Mexico (private practice group); PPV, positive predictive value; UCSF, University of California at San Francisco.
Data from references 112-115, 117, 118.

Table 23–7. Relative Benefits and Risks of Screening According to Age Groups Being Compared

	Age Groups Being Compared (yrs)	
	30–49 vs 50–69*	40–49 vs 50–59†
Detection rates	20%	63% to 80%
Diagnostic procedures per cancer detected	4 ×	1.7×
False-positive biopsy results per cancer detected	2.5×	1.3×-1.4×

*Prevalent screen data.
†Prevalent and incident screen data.
Data from Feig SA: Age-related accuracy of screening mammography: How should it be measured? Radiology 2000;214:633-640.

mammography becomes more accurate as the age of the subject increases, there is no abrupt change in accuracy at the age of 50 years.[112,113,117]

Radiation Exposure

Misperceptions regarding radiation risk from mammography persist even though no woman has ever been shown to have experienced breast cancer as a result of mammography, not even from multiple examinations over many years' time at doses much higher than the current dose of 0.40 rad (0.004 Gy) for a two-view-per-breast examination. Such concern is based on the observation that some groups of women, such as Japanese atomic bomb survivors and North American women who were given radiation therapy for benign breast conditions such as postpartum mastitis or were monitored with multiple chest fluoroscopies during treatment for tuberculosis before 1940, were found to be at increased risk of breast cancer.[119-121] Among these women, excess risk was observed for doses from 100 to more than 1000 rad (1 to 10 Gy).

The hypothetical risk for mammography is based on a linear extrapolation from these high-dose studies. If there is any risk from mammography, it is extremely low and is lowest for those who are exposed when older than 35 years. The current mean breast dose of 0.4 rad (0.004 Gy) from mammography is markedly less than the mean glandular dose of 3.2 rad (0.032 Gy) from the mammography film systems that were used at most facilities until 1973.[121]

Screening benefits can be compared with radiation risks. On the basis of results from screening trials, we know that annual screening can reduce deaths from breast cancer detected among women aged 40 to 49 years by at least 35% and deaths from breast cancer detected among women 50 years and older by at least 46%.[120] Possible deaths from radiation exposure due to mammography can be estimated through the use of a linear RR extrapolation of risk found among populations that received extremely high doses. Calculations based on these assumptions indicate that 18,900 deaths from breast cancer can be averted when 1,000,000 women are screened annually from age 40 years until age 74 years, and that at most, 21.6 excess deaths might be caused by radiation (Table 23–8). Thus, even if there is a risk from multiple mammographic examinations at a dose of 0.4 rad (0.004 Gy) each, the benefit from annual screening for women 40 years and older exceeds that theoretical risk by at least 875 to 1.[120]

Using similar assumptions, one can conclude that five biennial screenings between the ages of 40 to 50 years will result in 323.3 years of life expectancy gained per year of life lost; the corresponding benefit-to-risk ratio for 10 annual screenings is 243.3 years of life expectancy gained per year of life lost.[121] Including benefits from earlier detection of cancers potentially caused by radiation, screening after age 50 would increase these respective benefit-to-risk ratios to 539.0 (for biennial screening) and 405.5 for annual screening.[121] Benefit-to-risk ratios for biennial screening are approximately 1.3 times higher than those for annual screening.[119] However, the net benefits minus the risks are 1.5 times higher for annual screening than for biennial screening.[119] These calculations favor annual over biennial screening.

Table 23–8. Detection Benefits and Radiation Risks from Annual Screening Mammography of 1,000,000 Women from Age 40 to Age 74 years

Parameter	No. of women
Lives saved	18,900
Possible deaths caused	21.6
Benefit-risk ratio	875:1
Net benefit in lives	18,878

Data from Feig SA: Risk, benefit and controversies in mammographic screening. In Haus AG, Yaffe MJ (eds): Physical Aspects of Breast Imaging—Current and Future Considerations: 1999 Syllabus, Categorical Courses in Radiology Physics. Oak Brook, IL, Radiological Society of North America, 1999, pp 99-108.

Economic Costs of Screening

Many investigators have calculated the cost-effectiveness of screening mammography. Their estimates have varied because they have used different assumptions for benefits and costs and different methods of calculation. Many of these studies, such as one published by Salzmann and associates[122] in 1997, are no longer valid because the benefits, particularly those for women aged 40 to 49 years, are now known to be much higher than previously believed.

A later study by Rosenquist and Lindfors[123] estimated that annual screening mammography beginning at age 40 years and continuing until age 79 years would cost $18,800 per year of life expectancy saved.[123] The assumption in that study was that annual screening would reduce breast cancer deaths by 36% for cancers detected in women aged 40 to 49 years and by 45% for cancers detected in women 50 to 79 years. The assumed costs included mammography at $64, core biopsy at $850, excisional biopsy of a nonpalpable lesion at $2400, and definitive treatment for breast cancer at $6100. Their final estimate for the cost-effectiveness of screening mammography is in the same general range as that for other commonly accepted interventions, such as screening for cervical cancer and osteoporosis (Table 23–9). The cost per year of life gained from annual screening mammography is higher than that for screening for colorectal cancer but is much lower than that for the use of seat belts and airbags in automobiles.

Although the cost per year of life gained for screening mammography is less than that for renal dialysis or heart transplants, these latter interventions are needed for only a tiny fraction of the population. Because screening mammography is advised for all

Table 23–9. Median Cost Per Life-Year Saved for Annual Mammographic Screening of Women Aged 40 to 79 Years and Other Selected Types of Lifesaving Interventions

Intervention	Median Cost per Year of Life Saved ($)
Colorectal screening	3000
Cholesterol screening	6000
Cervical cancer screening	12,000
Antihypertensive drugs	15,000
Osteoporosis screening	18,000
Mammography screening	18,800
Coronary artery bypass surgery	26,000
Automobile seat belts and air bags	32,000
Hormone replacement therapy	42,000
Renal dialysis	46,000
Heart transplant	54,000
Cholesterol treatment	154,000

Data on non-mammographic interventions from Tengs TO, Adams M, Pliskin J, et al: Five hundred life-saving interventions and their cost-effectiveness. Risk Anal 1995;15:369-390. Cost-effectiveness estimate for screening mammography from Rosenquist CJ, Lindfors KK: Screening mammography beginning at age 40 years: A reappraisal of cost-effectiveness. Cancer 1998;82:2235-2240.

women 40 years and older, its total program cost must also be considered. In the United States, 62.6 million women are 40 to 89 years old. If every one of these women obtained an annual screening mammogram at a cost of $90, the total cost would come to $5.6 billion per year. The total annual cost for all U.S. health care expenditures, however, is even more staggering: $1.3 trillion for the year 2000. Thus, even if every woman 40 to 89 years old obtained an annual mammogram, the total cost would be only 0.43% of the national expenditure on health care. At present, 59% of all U.S. women 40 to 89 years old report having had a screening mammogram in the past year. At this compliance rate, screening mammography at a cost of $90 would account for 0.25% of all U.S. health care expenditure.[124]

In a related comparison, 19,136,000 women aged 65 to 89 years are currently living in the United States. If all of these women were screened every year at $90 per mammogram, the annual cost would be $1.7 billion. This cost, however, represents only 0.68% of all Medicare expenditures, which were $244 billion in the year 2000.[124] Assuming the current 59% compliance rate for obtaining an annual mammogram, the cost would be $1.013 billion, or 0.41% of all Medicare expenditures.[124]

This year, breast cancer will develop in 192,200 women in the United States, and 40,200 women will die from previously diagnosed breast cancer. It is often stated that when women living to age 85 are included, 1 of every 8 U.S. women will have breast cancer during her lifetime. Because of screening mammography and early treatment, most women who have breast cancer today will not die from their disease. Breast cancer, though the most common cancer among women and the second most common cause of cancer death among women, accounts for only 3.9% of all causes of death among women in the United States.[124] Nevertheless, allocation of 0.4% of all national health expenditures (or approximately 0.8% of all national health expenditures for women) to substantially reduce the death rate from a disease that accounts for 3.9% of all deaths among women would seem to be a reasonable policy. Moreover, early detection can also reduce other health care expenditures, such as treatment of advanced primary cancers, diagnosis and treatment of distant metastases or recurrent disease, loss of work productivity, short-term disability, long-term disability, and terminal-care costs.

Summary

The main risks and other adverse consequences from screening include discomfort or pain from breast compression, the need to recall patients for additional imaging, and false-positive biopsy results. Although these risks affect a larger number of women than the number who benefit from screening, the risks are far less consequential than the life-sparing benefits from early detection. Detection of DCIS is a benefit rather than a risk from screening. Radiation risk, even for multiple screenings, is negligible at current mammography doses.

References

1. Senie RT, Lesser M, Kinne DW, et al: Method of tumor detection influences disease-free survival of women with breast carcinoma. Cancer 1994;73:1666-1672.
2. Seidman H, Gelb SK, Stilverberg E, et al: Survival experience in the breast cancer detection demonstration project. CA Cancer J Clin 1987;37:258-290.
3. Feig SA: Should breast self-examination be included in a mammographic screening program? Recent Results Cancer Res 1990;119:151-164.
4. Feig SA: Screening mammography: Effect of image quality on clinical outcome. AJR Am J Roentgenol 2002;178:805-807.
5. Leconte I, Feger C, Galant C, et al: Mammography and subsequent whole-breast sonography of nonpalpable breast cancer: The importance of radiologic breast density. AJR Am J Roentgenol 2003;180:1675-1679.
6. Warner E, Plewes DB, Shumak RJ, et al: Comparison of breast magnetic resonance imaging, mammography, and ultrasound for surveillance of women at high risk for hereditary breast cancer. J Clin Oncol 2001;19:3524-3531.
7. Smart CR, Byrne C, Smith RA, et al: Twenty-year follow-up of the breast cancers diagnosed during the Breast Cancer Detection Demonstration Project. CA Cancer J Clin 1997; 47:134-149.
8. Ries L, Kosary C, Hankey B, et al: SEER Cancer Statistics Review, 1973-1998. Bethesda, MD, National Cancer Institute, 2001.
9. Feig SA: Methods to identify benefit from mammographic screening. Radiology 1996;201:309-316.
10. Shapiro S, Venet W, Strax P, et al: Periodic Screening for Breast Cancer: The Health Insurance Plan Project and its Sequelae, 1963-1986. Baltimore, Johns Hopkins University Press, 1988.
11. Tabár L, Vitak B, Chen H-H, et al: The Swedish Two-County Trial twenty years later. Radiol Clin North Am 2000;38:625-652.
12. Andersson I, Aspegren K, Janzon L, et al: Mammographic screening and mortality from breast cancer: The Malmö

Mammographic Screening Trial. BMJ Brit Med J 1988;297: 943-948.
13. Frisell J, Eklund G, Hellstrom L, et al: Randomized study of mammography screening: Preliminary report on mortality in the Stockholm trial. Breast Cancer Res Treat 1991;18:49-56.
14. Frisell J, Lidbrink E, Hellstrom L, Rutqvist LE: Follow-up after 11 years: Update of mortality results in the Stockholm mammographic screening trial. Breast Cancer Res Treat 1997;45:263-270.
15. Bjurstam N, Bjorneld L, Warwick J, et al: The Gothenburg Breast Screening Trial. Cancer 2001;97:2387-2396.
16. Alexander FE, Anderson TJ, Brown HK, et al: 14 years of follow-up from Edinburgh randomized trial of breast cancer screening. Lancet 1999;353:1903-1908.
17. Miller AB, Baines CJ, To T, et al: Canadian National Breast Screening Study. II: Breast cancer detection and death rates among women aged 50-59 years. Can Med Assoc J 1992; 147:1477-1488.
18. Miller AB, To T, Baines CJ, Wall C: Canadian National Breast Screening Study—2: 13-year results of a randomized trial in women aged 50-59 years. J Natl Cancer Inst 2000;92:1490-1499.
19. Miller AB, To T, Baines CJ, Wall C: The Canadian National Breast Screening Study—1: Breast cancer mortality after 11-16 years of follow-up: A randomized trial of mammography in women age 40 to 49 years. Ann Intern Med 2002;137:305-312.
20. Nystrom L, Andersson I, Bjurstam N, et al: Long-term effects of mammography screening: Updated overview of the Swedish randomized trials. Lancet 2002;359:909-919.
21. Baines CJ, Miller AB, Kopans DB, et al: Canadian National Breast Screening Study: Assessment of technical quality by external review. AJR Am J Roentgenol 1990;155:743-747.
22. Kopans DB: The Canadian Screening Program: A different perspective. AJR Am J Roentgenol 1990;155:748-749.
23. Kopans DB, Feig SA: The Canadian National Breast Screening Study: A critical review. AJR Am J Roentgenol 1993;161: 755-760.
24. Bailar JC III, MacMahon B: Randomization in the Canadian National Breast Screening Study: A review of evidence for subversion. Can Med Assoc J 1997;156:193-199.
25. Boyd NF: The review of randomization in the Canadian National Breast Screening Study: Is the debate over? Can Med Assoc J 1997;156:207-209.
26. Boyd NF, Jong RA, Yaffe MJ, et al: A critical appraisal of the Canadian National Breast Screening Study. Radiology 1993; 189:661-663.
27. Tarone RE: The excess of patients with advanced breast cancer in young women screened with mammography in the Canadian National Breast Screening Study. Cancer 1995;75:997-1003.
28. Sun J, Chapman J, Gordon R: Survival from primary breast cancer after routine clinical use of mammography. Breast J 2002;8:199-208.
29. Fletcher SW, Black W, Harris R, et al: Report of the International Workshop on Screening for Breast Cancer. J Natl Cancer Inst 1993;85:1644-1656.
30. Smith RA: Breast cancer screening among women younger than age 50: A current assessment of the issues. CA Cancer J Clin 2000;50:312-336.
31. Hurley SF, Kaldor JM: The benefits and risks of mammographic screening for breast cancer. Epidemiol Rev 1992;14: 101-130.
32. Chu KC, Smart CR, Tarone RE: Analysis of breast cancer mortality and stage distribution by age for the Health Insurance Plan clinical trial. J Natl Cancer Inst 1998; 80:1125-1132.
33. Miller AB, Baines CJ, To T, et al: Canadian National Breast Screening Study. I: Breast cancer detection and death rates among women aged 40-49 years. Can Med Assoc J 1992;147:1477-1488.
34. Warren-Burhenne LJ, Burhenne HJ: The Canadian National Breast Screening Study: A Canadian Critique. AJR Am J Roentgenol 1993;161:761-763.
35. Mettlin CJ, Smart CR: The Canadian National Breast Screening Study: An appraisal and implications for early detection policy. Cancer 1993;72:1461-1465.
36. Elwood JM, Cox B, Richardson AK: The effectiveness of breast cancer screening in younger women. Online J Curr Clin Trials 1993;Feb 25:Doc 32.
37. Glasziou PP, Woodward AJ, Mahon CM: Mammographic screening trials for women aged under 50: A quality assessment and meta-analysis. Med J Australia 1995;162:625-629.
38. Kerlikowske K, Grady D, Rubin SM, et al: Efficacy of screening mammography: A meta-analysis. JAMA 1995;273:149-154.
39. Smart CR, Hendrick RE, Rutledge JH III, et al: Benefit of mammography screening in women ages 40-49 years: Current evidence from randomized controlled trials [erratum appears in Cancer 75:2788]. Cancer 1995;75:1619-1626.
40. Falun Meeting Committee and Collaborators: Falun meeting on breast cancer screening with mammography in women aged 40-49 years: Report of the organizing committee and collaborators. Int J Cancer 1996;68:693-699.
41. Hendrick RE, Smith RA, Rutledge JH III, et al: Benefit of screening mammography in women aged 40-49: A new meta-analysis of randomized controlled trials. Monogr Natl Cancer Inst 1997;33:87-92.
42. Bjurstam N, Bjorneld L, Duffy SW: The Gothenburg Breast Screening Trial: First results on mortality, incidence, and mode of detection for women ages 39-49 years at randomization. Cancer 1997;20:2091-2099.
43. Andersson I, Janzon L: Reduced breast cancer mortality in women under 50: Updated results from the Malmö Mammographic Screening Program. Monogr Natl Cancer Inst 1997;22:63-68.
44. U.S. Bureau of the Census: Statistical Abstract of the United States, 203rd ed. Washington, DC, U.S. Government Printing Office, 2003.
45. Feig SA: Mammographic screening of elderly women. JAMA 1996;276:446.
46. Mandelblatt JS, Wheat ME, Monane M, et al: Breast cancer screening for elderly women with and without comorbid conditions. Ann Intern Med 1992;116:722-730.
47. Yancik R, Reis LG, Yates JW: Breast cancer in women: A population based study of contrasts in stage, survival, and surgery. Cancer 1989;163:976-981.
48. Faulk RM, Sickles EA, Sollito RA, et al: Clinical efficacy of mammographic screening in the elderly. Radiology 1995;194:193-197.
49. Wilson TE, Helvie MA, August DA: Breast cancer in the elderly patient: early detection with mammography. Radiology 1994;190:203-207.
50. Costanza ME: Issues in breast cancer screening in older women. Cancer 1994;74:2009-2015.
51. Walter LC, Covinsky KE: Cancer screening in elderly patients: A framework for individual decision making. JAMA 2001;285:2750-2756.
52. Conway BJ, Suleiman OH, Reuter FG, et al: National survey of mammographic facilities in 1985, 1988, and 1992. Radiology 1994;191:323-330.
53. Haus AG: Dedicated mammography x-ray equipment, screen-film processing-systems, and viewing conditions for mammography. Semin Breast Dis 1999;2:30-54.
54. Young K, Wallis MG, Ramsdale ML: Mammographic film density and detection of small breast cancers. Clin Radiol 1994;49:461-465.
55. Andersson I, Hildell J, Muhlow A, Pettersson H: Number of projections in mammography: Influence on detection of breast disease. AJR Am J Roentgenol 1978;130:349-51.
56. Anttinen I, Pamilo M, Roiha M, et al: Baseline screening mammography with one versus two views. Eur J Radiol 1989;9:241-243.
57. Bassett LW, Bunnell DH, Jahanshahi R, et al: Breast cancer detection: One versus two views. Radiology 1987;165: 95-97.
58. Muir BB, Kirkpatrick AE, Roberts MM, Duffy SW: Oblique-view mammography: Adequacy for screening. Radiology 1984;151:39-41.

59. Sickles EA, Weber WN, Galvin HB, et al: Baseline screening mammography: One vs. two views per breast. AJR Am J Roentgenol 1986;147:1149-53.
60. Thurfjell G, Taube A, Tabár L: One-versus two-view mammography screening: A prospective population based study. Acta Radiol 1994;35:340-344.
61. Roberts MM, Alexander FE, Anderson TJ, et al: Edinburgh trial of screening for breast cancer: Mortality at seven years. Lancet 1990;335:241-246.
62. Humphrey LL, Helfant M, Chan BKS, Woolf SH: Breast cancer screening: A summary of the evidence for the U S Preventive Services Task Force. Ann Intern Med 2002;137: 347-360.
63. Feig SA: Estimation of currently attainable benefit from mammographic screening of women aged 40-49 years. Cancer 1995;75:2412-2419.
64. Feig SA: Increased benefit from shorter screening mammography intervals for women ages 40-49 years. Cancer 1997; 80:2035-2039.
65. Smith RA, Saslow D, Sawyer KA, et al: American Cancer Society Guidelines for Breast Cancer Screening: Update 2003. CA Cancer J Clin 2003;53:141-169.
66. Feig SA: Determination of mammographic screening intervals with surrogate measures for women aged 40-49 years. Radiology 1994;193:311-314.
67. Moskowitz M: Breast cancer: Age specific growth rates and screening strategies. Radiology 1986;161:37-41.
68. Pelikan S, Moskowitz M: Effects of lead-time, length bias, and false-negative reassurance on screening for breast cancer. Cancer 1993;71:1998-2005.
69. Tabár L, Fagerberg G, Day NE, et al: What is the optimum interval between screening examinations? An analysis based on the latest results of the Swedish two-county breast cancer screening trial. Br J Cancer 1987;55:547-551.
70. Michaelson JS, Halpern E, Kopans DB: Breast cancer computer simulation method for estimation of optimal intervals for screening. Radiology 1999;212:551-560.
71. Tabár L, Fagerberg G, Chen H-H: Efficacy of breast cancer screening by age: New results from the Swedish Two-County Trial. Cancer 1995;75:2507-2517.
72. Miettinen OS, Henschke CI, Pasmantier MW, et al: Mammographic screening: No reliable supporting evidence? Lancet 2002;359:404-406.
73. Andersson I, Nystrom L: Mammography screening. J Natl Cancer Inst 1995;87:1263-1264.
74. Duffy SW, Day NE, Tabár L, et al: Markov models of breast tumor progression: Some age-specific results. Monogr Natl Cancer Inst 1997;22:93-98.
75. Feig SA, D'Orsi CJ, Hendrick RE, et al: American College of Radiology Guidelines for Breast Cancer Screening. AJR Am J Roentgenol 1998;171:29-33.
76. Council on Scientific Affairs: Mammography screening for asymptomatic women. Report No. 16. Chicago, American Medical Association, 1999.
77. U.S. Preventive Services Task Force: Screening for breast cancer: Recommendations and rationale. Ann Intern Med 2002;137:344-346.
78. Gotzsche PC, Olsen O: Is screening for breast cancer with mammography justifiable? Lancet 2000;355:129-1134.
79. Olsen O, Gotzsche PC: Cochrane review on screening for breast cancer with mammography. Lancet 2001;358:1340-1342.
80. de Koning HJ: Assessment of nationwide cancer-screening programmes. Lancet 2000;355:80-81.
81. Duffy SW: Interpretation of the breast screening trials: A commentary on the recent paper by Gotzsche and Olsen. Breast 2001;10:209-212.
82. Tabár L, Fagerberg G, Duffy SW, Day NE: The Swedish two county trial of mammographic screening for breast cancer: Recent results and calculation of benefit. J Epidemiol Comm Health 1989;43:107-114.
83. Bjurstam N, Bjorneld L, Duffy SW, Prevost TC: The Gothenburg Breast Screening Trial [authors' reply]. Cancer 1998; 83:188-190.
84. Nystrom L, Larsson L-G, Rutqvist L-E, et al: Determination of cause of death among breast cancer cases in the Swedish randomized mammography screening trials: A comparison between official statistics and validation by an end point committee. Acta Oncol 1995;34:145-152.
85. Nystrom L, Rutqvist L-E, Wall S, et al: Breast cancer screening with mammography: Overview of Swedish randomized trials [published erratum appears in Lancet 1993;342:1372]. Lancet 1993;341:973-978.
86. Nystrom L: Screening mammography re-evaluated [letter to the editor]. Lancet 2002;355:748-749.
87. Tabár L, Duffy SW, Warwick J, et al: All cause mortality among breast cancer patients in a screening trial: Support for breast cancer mortality as an endpoint. J Med Screening 2002;9:159-162.
88. Duffy SW, Tabár L: Screening mammography re-evaluated [letter to the editor]. Lancet 2000;355:747-748.
89. Sjonell G, Stahle L: Mammography screening does not reduce breast cancer mortality [Swedish]. Lakartidningen 1999;96: 904-913.
90. Rosen M, Rehnqvist N: No need to reconsider breast screening programme on basis of results from defective study [letter to the editor]. Br Med J 1999;318:809-810.
91. Swedish Board of Health and Welfare: Vilka Effekter Har Mammografic screening? Referat av ett expertmote anordnat av Socialstyrelsen och ancerfonden i; Stockholm den 15 Februari 2002.
92. The Benefit of Population Screening for Breast Cancer with Mammography. The Hague, Health Council of the Netherlands, 2002.
93. Veronisi U, Forrest P, Wood W: Statement from the chair: Global Summit on Mammographic Screening, European Institute of Oncology, June 3-5, 2002, Milan.
94. International Agency for Research on Cancer: Mammography Screening Can Reduce Deaths from Breast Cancer. Lyon, France, IARC Press, 2002.
95. Feig SA: Effect of service screening mammography on population mortality from breast carcinoma. Cancer 2002;95:451-457.
96. Jonsson H, Nystrom L, Tornberg S, Lenner P: Service screening with mammography of women aged 50-69 years in Sweden: Effects on mortality from breast cancer. J Med Screen 2001;8:152-160.
97. Tabár L, Vitak B, Chen H-H, et al: Beyond randomized controlled trials: Organized mammographic screening substantially reduces breast carcinoma mortality. Cancer 2001;91:1724-1731.
98. Duffy SW, Tabár L, Chen H-H, et al: The impact of organized mammography service screening on breast cancer mortality in seven Swedish counties: A collaborative evaluation. Cancer 2002;95:458-469.
99. Garne JP, Aspegren K, Balldin G, Ranstam J: Increasing incidence of and declining mortality from breast carcinoma: Trends in Malmö, Sweden, 1961-1992. Cancer 1997;79:69-74.
100. Lenner P, Jonsson H: Excess mortality from breast cancer in relation to mammography screening in northern Sweden. J Med Screen 1997;4:6-9.
101. Hakama M, Pukkala E, Heikkila M, Kallio M: Effectiveness of the public health policy for breast cancer screening in Finland: A population based cohort study. Brit Med J 1997; 314:864-867.
102. Feig SA: How reliable is the evidence for screening mammography? Recent Results Cancer Res 2003; 163:129-139.
103. Feig SA: Mammography equipment: Principles, features, selection. Radiol Clin North Am 1987;15: 897-911.
104. Stomper PC, Kopans DB, Sadowsky NL, et al: Is mammography painful? A multicenter patient study. Arch Intern Med 1988;148:521-524.
105. American College of Radiology: Mammography Quality Control Manual. Reston, VA, American College of Radiology, 1999.
106. Feig SA: Economic challenges in breast imaging: A survivor's guide to success. Radiol Clin North Am 2000;38:843-852.
107. ACR BI-RADS Committee: Breast Imaging Reporting and Data System—Mammography, 4th ed. Reston, VA, American College of Radiology, 2003, p 234.
108. Hunt KA, Rosen EL, Sickles EA: Outcome analysis for women undergoing annual versus biennial screening mammogra-

phy: A review of 24,211 examinations. AJR Am J Roentgenol 1999;173:285-289.
109. Yankaskas BC, Cleveland RJ, Schell MJ, et al: Association of recall rates with sensitivity and positive predictive values of screening mammography. AJR Am J Roentgenol 2001; 177:543-549.
110. Elmore JG, Barton MB, Moceri VM, et al: Ten-year risk of false positive screening mammograms and clinical breast examinations. New Engl J Med 1998;338:1089-1096.
111. Feig SA: A perspective on false positive screening mammograms. ACR Bulletin 1998;54:8-13.
112. Kopans DB, Moore RH, McCarthy KA, et al: Positive predictive value of breast biopsy performed as a result of mammography: There is no abrupt change at age 50 years. Radiology 1996;200:357-360.
113. Kopans DB, Moore RH, McCathy KA, et al: Biasing the interpretation of mammography screening data by age grouping: Nothing changes abruptly at age 50. Breast J 1998;4:139-145.
114. Linver MN, Paster SB: Mammography outcomes in a practice setting by age: Prognostic factors, sensitivity, and positive biopsy rate. Monogr Natl Cancer Inst 1997;33:113-117.
115. Sickles EA: Auditing your practice. In Kopans DB, Mendelson EB (eds): Syllabus: A Categorical Course in Breast Imaging. Oak Brook, IL, Radiological Society of North America, 1995, pp 81-91.
116. Feig SA: Ductal carcinoma in situ: Implications for screening mammography. Radiol Clin North Am 2000;38:653-668.
117. Feig SA: Age-related accuracy of screening mammography: How should it be measured? Radiology 2000;214:633-640.
118. Kerlikowske K, Grady D, Barclay J, et al: Positive predictive value of screening mammography by age and family history of breast cancer. JAMA 1993;270:2444-2450.
119. Feig SA: Mammographic screening of women age 40-49, 1994: Benefit, risk, and cost considerations. Cancer 1995;76: 2097-2016.
120. Feig SA: Risk, benefit and controversies in mammographic screening. In Haus AG, Yaffe MJ (eds): Physical Aspects of Breast Imaging—Current and Future Considerations: 1999 Syllabus, Categorical Courses in Radiology Physics. Oak Brook, IL, Radiological Society of North America, 1999, pp 99-108.
121. Feig SA, Hendrick RE: Radiation risk from screening mammography of women aged 40-49 years. Monogr Natl Cancer Inst 1997;22:119-124.
122. Salzmann P, Kerlikowske K, Phillips K: Cost-effectiveness of screening mammography of women aged 40-49 years of age. Ann Intern Med 1997;127:955-965.
123. Rosenquist CJ, Lindfors KK: Screening mammography beginning at age 40 years: A reappraisal of cost-effectiveness. Cancer 1998;82:2235-2240.
124. Feig SA: Projected benefits and national health care costs from screening mammography. Semin Breast Dis 2001;4:62-67.

Section VI

Normal Breast and Benign and Malignant Conditions

Chapter 24 The Normal Breast

Karin L. Fu, Yao S. Fu, January K. Lopez, Seth Y. Cardall, and Lawrence W. Bassett

EMBRYOLOGY AND DEVELOPMENT

In the fifth week of fetal life, a pair of primitive milk streaks (milk lines) develop, extending from the axilla to the groin.[1] All of this primitive tissue undergoes regression, except in the thoracic region, where it develops into two mammary glands. In each gland, the ectoderm forms 15 to 20 branching epithelial cords extending into the mesoderm. The mesoderm develops into fibrous and adipose tissue. In the last 8 weeks of fetal life, the solid epithelial columns become canalized and open to a depressed area on the epidermis. At birth, this depression becomes a recognizable nipple with eversion of the underlying lactiferous ducts. These early ducts develop very slowly until puberty.

In the female, the onset of menstrual cycles and the secretion of sex hormones at puberty stimulate the ducts to proliferate and the lobules to form. The stroma accumulates fatty tissue. In the male, the breast tissue usually remains rudimentary, except in cases of gynecomastia.

ANATOMY AND HISTOLOGY

The base of the adult female breast extends from the second to the sixth rib in the midclavicular line and lies almost completely on the pectoralis major muscle (Fig. 24–1). The breast tissue spreads from the lateral edge of the sternum to the anterior axillary line and often extends into the axilla as the tail of Spence. The presence of axillary breast tissue is important because it signifies the possibility of benign and malignant lesions in the axilla. Fibrous strands that extend from the deep dermis into the underlying breast tissue, called the suspensory ligaments of Cooper, provide support to the breast and attach the breast to the underlying fascia and pectoral muscles.

On gross examination, the breast consists of 15 to 20 segments or lobes (Fig. 24–2). A lobe comprises all of the lobules and excretory ducts that drain via one lactiferous duct at the nipple. The branching system ends at the terminal duct lobular unit (TDLU), which consists of an interlobular duct and an associated lobule (Fig. 24–3). The lobule itself is composed of terminal ducts and acini (sometimes called ductules and terminal ductules, respectively). The number of acini is highly variable within the breast and among individual women. The secretory product drains sequentially from the acini to the terminal ducts, interlobular ducts, excretory ducts, lactiferous sinus, lactiferous duct, and nipple.

We should point out that the terminology used to describe the various components of the glandular system is not standardized and varies among different writers. For example, some writers reserve the term *acinus* for the terminal secretory units only during active lactation and refer to the terminal units as *terminal ductules* in the resting phase. In this textbook, the term *acinus* is used for both the active lactating and resting stages.

The histology of breast tissue in reproductive women is highly variable and depends on whether the breast is lactating or in the resting phase. Nonetheless, important basic histologic features are present. All normal glandular tissue, including the ducts, terminal ducts, and acini, have a two-cell epithelial layer—an inner layer of secretory cells and an outer layer of myoepithelial cells (Fig. 24–4). The myofilaments in the myoepithelial layer provide contractility to squeeze the secretory product toward the nipple. The fibrous supporting tissue of the lobule appears more "loose," more cellular, and hormonally more responsive compared with that of the duct.

The lobule is the functional unit of the breast. Histologically it is composed of terminal ducts and acini (Fig. 24–5A). During the resting phase, acini may become inconspicuous, and the lobules may be composed largely of terminal ductules.[2] During the secretory phase of the menstrual cycle, the lobule undergoes hyperplasia. After childbirth, the hyperplastic lobules begin to produce milk. Myoepithelial cells in the outer layer of ducts and acini can be identified by immunohistochemical stains for smooth muscle actin and S-100 protein (Fig. 24–5B). After menopause, atrophy results in a decrease in the size and number of lobules and a relative increase in stromal hyalinization and fibrosis (Fig. 24–6A) in comparison with the perimenopausal lobule (Fig. 24–6B).

COMPOSITION OF BREAST TISSUE

The sensitivity of mammography is inversely related to the tissue composition, or ratio of dense tissue to fatty tissue. The fatty breast tissue serves as a lucent background against which radiodense abnormalities can be identified, whereas normal tissue can obscure a mass. Therefore, the tissue composition is important for the referring physician to know because it correlates with the ability of mammography to detect

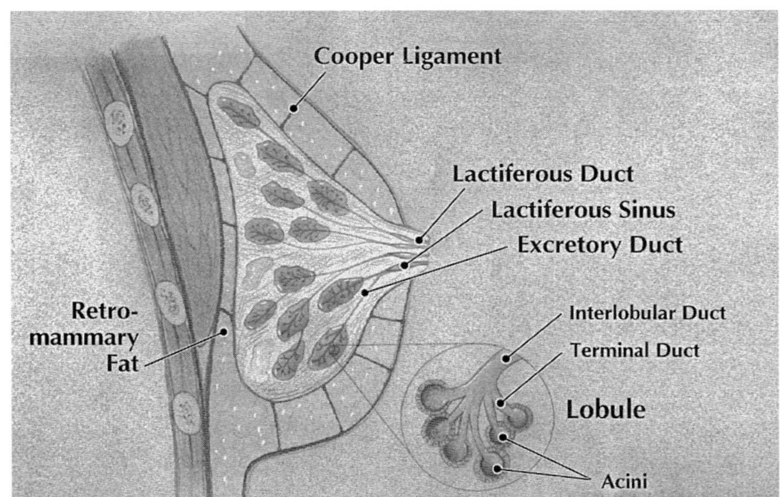

Figure 24–1. Sagittal section of the breast. The breast lies primarily on the pectoralis muscle and extends from approximately the second to the sixth rib. Retroglandular fat lies behind the fibroglandular tissue. The pyramid of fibroglandular tissue contains the ducts, which extend from the nipple posteriorly as lactiferous ducts, lactiferous sinuses, and excretory ducts, dividing and subdividing to end in the lobule. The functional unit of the breast, the lobule is composed of terminal ducts and acini. Cooper ligaments are supporting ligaments that extend from the deep fascia to the skin of the breast.

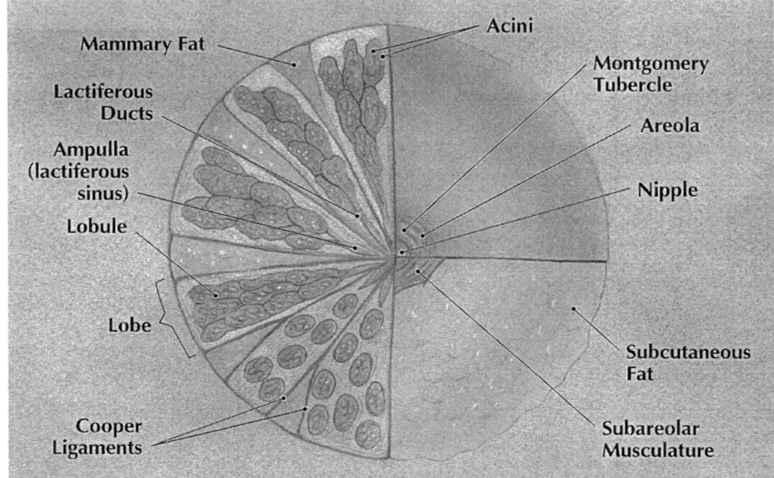

Figure 24–2. Frontal section of the breast. A lobe includes all of the ducts that terminate at a single orifice at the nipple. In reality, the lobes are poorly defined subdivisions that may overlap and have no real anatomic delineation. The tubercles of Montgomery are small, rounded elevations on the surface of the areola.

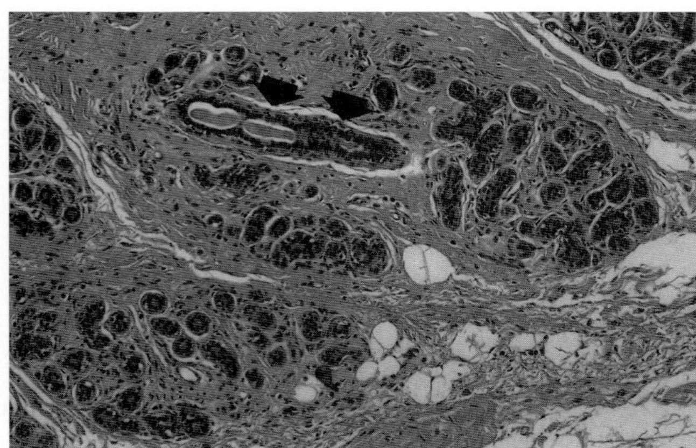

Figure 24–3. A low-power view of an interlobular duct (*arrowheads*). Note the two cell layers in the terminal duct lobular units (TDLUs).

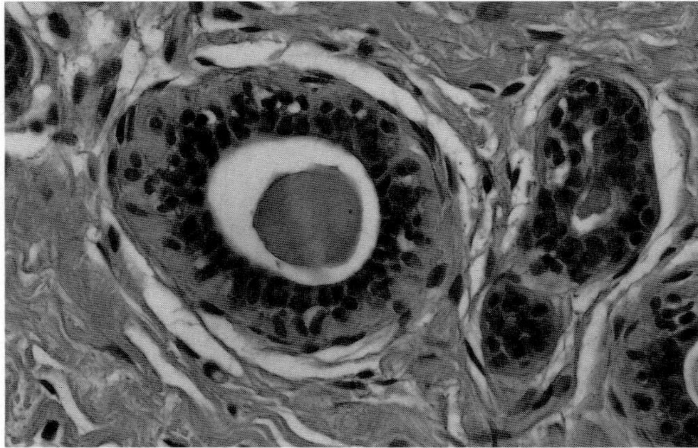

Figure 24–4. High-power view of a duct showing two cell layers of epithelial lining. All normal glandular tissues, including ducts and acini, are characterized by an inner layer of either cuboidal or columnar cells and an outer layer of myoepithelial cells.

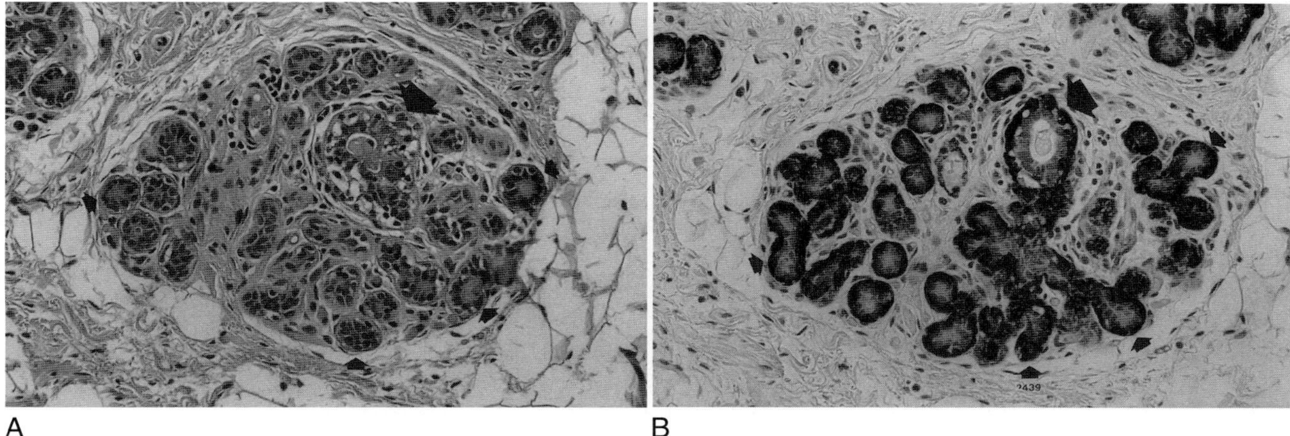

Figure 24–5. **A,** The terminal duct lobular unit consists of a terminal duct (*large arrowhead*) and acini (*small arrowheads*). **B,** Immunohistochemical stain for smooth muscle actin identifies myoepithelial cells in the black outer layer of the duct and acini.

lesions in the breast. The four categories of tissue composition are (1) almost entirely fat, (2) scattered fibroglandular densities, (3) heterogeneously dense tissue (in which the sensitivity of mammography may be lower), and (4) extremely dense tissue (which could obscure a lesion on a mammogram). As tissue density increases, sensitivity of mammography decreases (Fig. 24–7).

NORMAL VARIANTS

Normal anatomic variations in the breast can be seen on mammography and are important to recognize. Accessory breast tissue can be seen anywhere along the milk line but is most often observed in the axilla (Fig. 24–8). It can be either in continuity with or separate from the breast.[3]

A triangular or flame-shaped density sometimes seen along the medial aspect of the breast on the craniocaudal view represents the sternalis muscle (Fig. 24–9). This muscle runs parallel to the sternum and is not seen on the mediolateral oblique projection because it is rarely pulled into view. This variant is present in less than 10% of people.[3]

NORMAL ULTRASONOGRAPHIC ANATOMY

We described the normal anatomy of the breast here to provide a foundation for the understanding of breast ultrasonography (Fig. 24–10). The normal skin measures 3 mm or less and consists of parallel white lines beneath the lines produced by the transducer. Below the skin is a layer of subcutaneous fat, followed by intervening layers of fibroglandular tissue

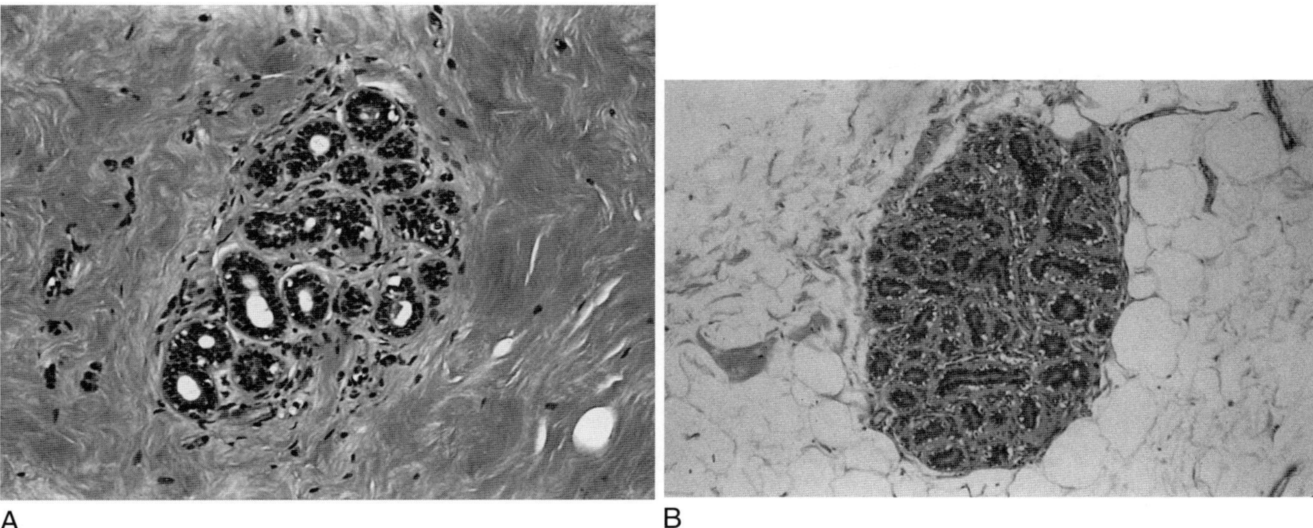

Figure 24–6. **A,** Lobule in postmenopausal woman. The lobule is involuted with a smaller number of acini and less sclerosis of surrounding stroma compared with the perimenopausal lobule. **B,** Lobule in a perimenopausal woman.

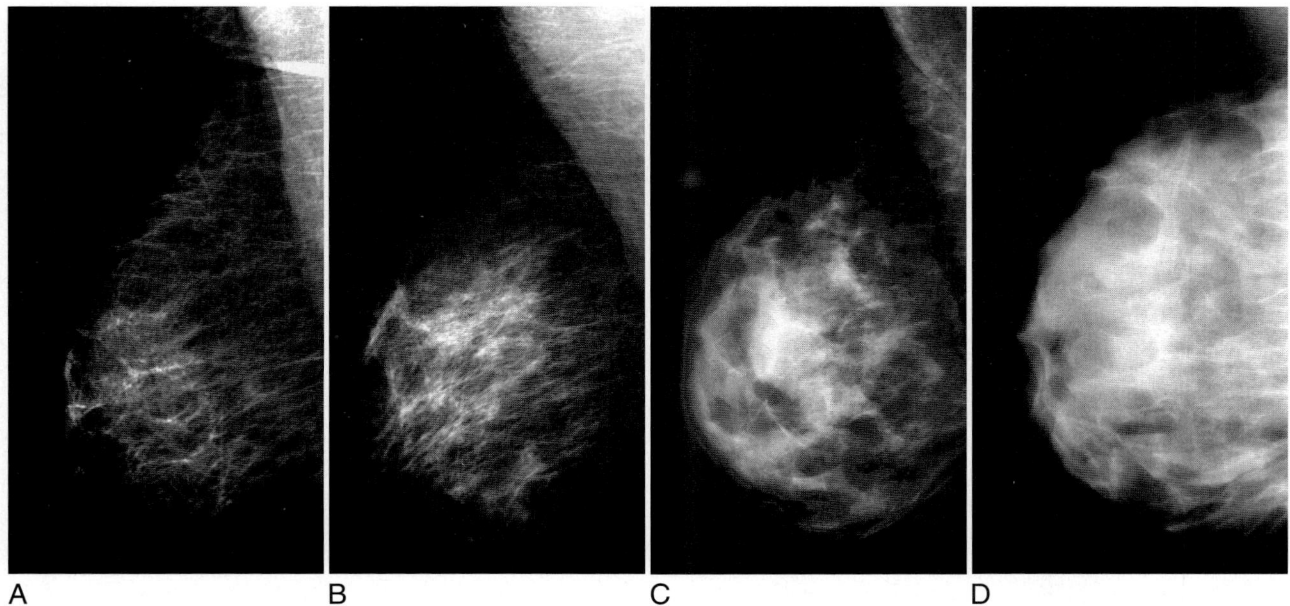

Figure 24–7. Mediolateral oblique mammograms demonstrating four types of tissue composition (percentage of breast composed of fibroglandular density). **A,** Almost entirely fat (0-25%). **B,** Scattered fibroglandular densities (25%-50%). **C,** Heterogeneously dense (50%-75%). **D,** Extremely dense (75%-100%). As tissue density increases, mammogram sensitivity decreases.

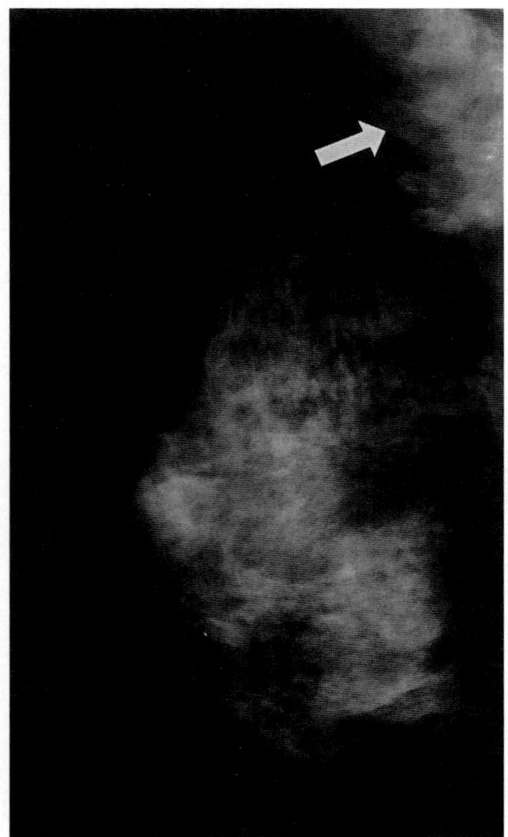

Figure 24–8. Mediolateral oblique mammogram depicting accessory breast tissue in the axilla (*arrow*), where it is most often seen; it can, however, be found anywhere along the milk line.

and fat. The fibroglandular tissue is hyperechoic (white) compared with the fatty tissue (gray to black). Beneath the fibroglandular tissue is the retromammary fat, which is superficial to the chest wall. The chest wall contains the pectoralis muscle, the ribs, and the parietal pleura that encases the thoracic cavity. These structures can be readily identified with ultrasonography.

PATHOLOGY OF THE BREAST

We discuss only basic pathology of the breast here; more detailed pathologic descriptions of common entities appear in following chapters. Benign and malignant epithelial proliferations can be divided into ductal and lobular. It should be emphasized that this classification system does not necessarily correspond to the histogenetic origin of the lesions. For example, cells of infiltrating lobular carcinoma do not necessarily originate in the lobules. The ductal proliferations are epitheliosis, papillomatosis, ductal hyperplasia, intraductal carcinoma, and various types of invasive ductal carcinomas. Proliferations of the lobules include lactational change, sclerosing adenosis, lobular hyperplasia, and in-situ and invasive lobular carcinomas.

Because the breast is the end target organ of many hormones, especially estrogen, progesterone, and prolactin, the epithelium and the stroma of the breast undergo proliferation or involution throughout life, depending on the levels of hormones and the local responses. Some women complain of breast tenderness, pain, and palpable lesions during their

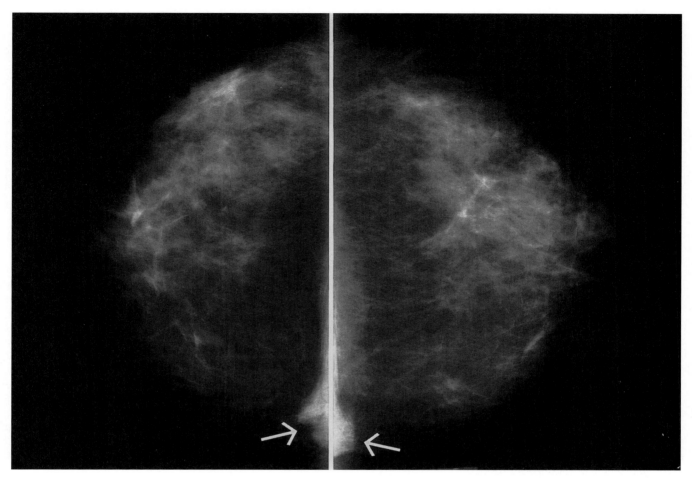

Figure 24–9. Bilateral craniocaudal mammograms demonstrating triangular densities (*arrows*) along the medial aspects of the breasts, which represent the sternalis muscle, a variant present in less than 10% of the population.

menstrual cycles. When these lesions undergo biopsy, a wide range of morphologic changes is encountered. These changes have been referred to as fibrocystic disease, chronic cystic mastitis, indurative mastopathy, and various other entities. Most experts regard these findings as physiologic responses to hormonal fluctuations rather than actual disease and prefer the terms *fibrocystic changes, lumpy breasts,* or *physiologic nodularity* to describe them.[4]

The failure to define uniform criteria for fibrocystic changes has contributed to controversy regarding the risk of cancer in women with these findings.[5] Dupont and Page[6] reviewed more than 10,500 consecutive breast biopsy specimens for benign diseases. More than 3300 cases were followed for a median period of 17 years. Seventy percent of the original specimens demonstrated no epithelial proliferation. In the remaining 30% of women whose specimens had epithelial proliferation, 26% had no evidence of nuclear atypia on later biopsies, and 4% had atypia. Follow-up data led to the conclusion that women with nonproliferative change have no increased risk

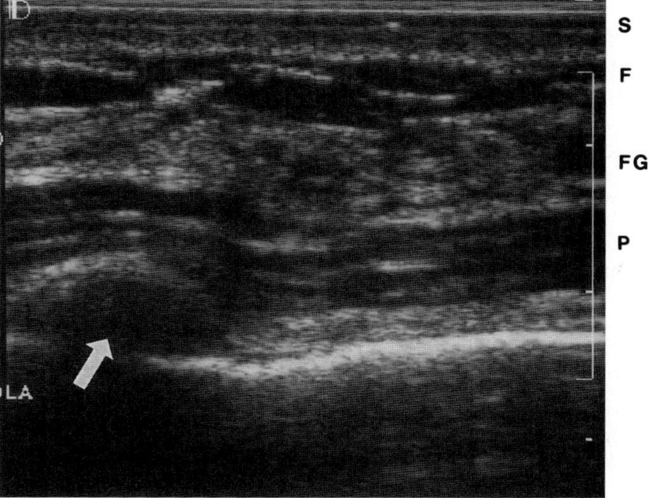

Figure 24–10. An ultrasonogram of a normal breast. F, subcutaneous fat; FG, fibroglandular tissue with intervening fatty tissue; P, pectoralis muscle; S, skin. The hypoechoic region beneath the pectoralis muscle represents a rib (*arrow*).

Table 24–1. Relative Risks of Breast Cancer for Proliferative Lesions

No proliferative disease: 1.0×	Adenosis Apocrine change Ductal ectasia Mild epithelial hyperplasia of usual type
Proliferative disease without atypia: 1.5×-2.0×	Hyperplasia of usual type, moderate or florid Multiple papillomas Sclerosing adenosis
Proliferative disease with atypia: 4×-5×	Atypical ductal hyperplasia Atypical lobular hyperplasia
Carcinoma in situ: 8×-10×	Ductal carcinoma in situ Lobular carcinoma in situ

Modified from Page DL, Dupont WD: Premalignant conditions and markers of elevated risk in the breast and their management. Surg Clin North Am 1990;70:831-851.

Table 24–2. Histologic Classification of Breast Carcinoma

Ductal carcinoma
- Intraductal carcinoma or ductal carcinoma in situ
  - Low, intermediate, and high grades
- Invasive ductal carcinoma
- Not otherwise specified
- Special variants
  - Colloid, papillary, medullary, tubular, cribriform, inflammatory, secretory carcinoma, adenoid cystic carcinoma, squamous cell carcinoma, and metaplastic carcinoma

Lobular carcinoma
- Lobular carcinoma in situ
- Invasive lobular carcinoma

Stromal tumors

for breast cancer. Those with proliferative change without atypia have a slightly higher relative risk, of 1.5 to 2 times that of women with no proliferative changes. The relative risk for women with atypical hyperplasia is approximately 4 to 5 times that of women with no proliferative disease (Table 24–1). When this finding is combined with other known risk factors, about 20% of women who have atypical hyperplasia and a family history of breast cancer will experience breast cancer over a 15-year follow-up period, compared with 8% of women with atypical hyperplasia but no family history. The comparable rates are 4% for women with proliferative changes without atypia and 2% for women without any evidence of proliferative changes. In subsequent studies, Dupont and Page[7] and Page[8] reported that the highest risk for the development of invasive breast carcinoma in these women occurs during the first 10 years after biopsy, and the risk decreases thereafter.

We agree that when the term *fibrocystic changes* is used, the presence or absence of epithelial proliferation and atypia should be indicated. The morphologic criteria for various hyperplasias and atypical hyperplasias have been illustrated.[9] The importance of atypical hyperplasia as a biologic marker for increased risk of invasive breast cancer has been confirmed in a multicenter study involving more than 280,000 women.[10] In this book, we have followed the morphologic criteria and definitions proposed by Dupont and Page.[6,11]

Histologically, breast carcinomas are classified into ductal and lobular types. Each type is further divided into in-situ and invasive (or infiltrating) categories on the basis of stromal invasion. Ductal carcinoma in situ (DCIS) may be of low, intermediate, or high grade (Table 24–2). Breast carcinomas are generally believed to progress from carcinomas in situ to early invasive carcinomas and then to frankly invasive carcinomas. In invasive ductal carcinoma, malignant cells break through the duct wall and invade the surrounding stroma, adjacent breast tissue, and lymphatic and vascular spaces. In the earliest stages, intraductal carcinoma often coexists with microinvasive carcinoma ($T1_{mic}$). With time, the invasive component predominates and may leave few or no in-situ foci.

The majority of invasive ductal carcinomas are of the not otherwise specified type, manifested by heterogeneous microscopic patterns. Mucinous (or colloid), papillary, tubular, and medullary are specialized variants of ductal carcinoma that have distinct morphologies and more favorable prognoses than the not otherwise specified, usual ductal carcinoma (see Table 24–2).[12,13] Inflammatory carcinoma is also recognized as a distinct entity because of its characteristic clinical presentation, dermal lymphatic invasion, and dismal outcome.

Lobular carcinoma in situ is characterized by solid filling of the lobules with relatively small, uniform cells. Invasive lobular carcinoma has a tendency to spread diffusely or between the collagen fibers. The latter results in tumor cells arranged in a single layer, the so-called Indian file pattern. The individual cells of invasive lobular carcinoma have small, round nuclei and scanty cytoplasm. Variants of lobular carcinomas include signet-ring, alveolar, solid, and pleomorphic types.

Unfortunately, in relatively few American women who present with palpable breast cancers are the lesions detected at the in-situ or early invasive stage, suggesting that most cancers are invasive. In a survey of 24,000 new breast cancers in 1978, only 0.84% were intraductal carcinomas.[14] Of the 2072 stage I and stage II breast cancer specimens studied by the National Surgical Adjuvant Breast Project, only 78 (3.8%) were intraductal carcinomas.[15] However, with mammographic screening, the cancers detected can be "shifted" toward those in the in-situ or early invasive stages. Approximately 50% of mammographically detected cancers are at a potentially curable in-situ or early invasive stage. In one study of 62 nonpalpable breast cancers detected at screening mammography, 20 (32%) were intraductal carcinomas, 5 (8%) lobular carcinomas in situ, 7 (11%) minimal invasive ductal carcinomas, and 30 (48%) invasive ductal carcinomas.[16]

Do mammographically detected asymptomatic breast carcinomas differ from symptomatic clinical lesions? In a study by Walker and associates,[17] 79 cases of pure DCIS detected by mammography, which included 5 cases with microinvasion and 8 cases with 1 to 2 mm of invasion, were compared with 59 cases of pure DCIS detected clinically, which included 8 cases with microinvasion and 7 cases with 1 to 2 mm of invasion. The only statistically significant difference in DCIS between the two groups was smaller tumor size in the screening group (50% less than 20 mm versus 30% in the clinical group). There were also fewer cases of overexpression of the oncogene HER-2/neu in the screening group (42% versus 59%, respectively).

In a second study, 39 screening-detected, 3- to 5-mm cancers were compared with 78 consecutive clinical cancers that were all 10 mm or larger. The types of coexisting in-situ components were similar in the groups, but the mammographically detected group had a higher incidence of tubular carcinoma (12.8% versus 3.8%, but not statistically significant). Significant differences included lower nuclear and architectural grades, fewer mitotic cells, fewer tumors positive for p53, lower microvessel density, and more diploid tumors in the screening group than in the clinical group.[18] Distribution of estrogen and progesterone receptors (ER/PR) was similar. These findings suggest that breast cancers detected by screening and nonscreening modalities are the same disease that progresses with increasing tumor size.[16,18]

Nonepithelial tumors of the breast are rare; they include granular cell tumor, stromal cell sarcoma, lymphoma, hemangioma, and angiosarcoma. Metastatic tumors to the breast from extramammary carcinomas occur but are not common; they must be differentiated from spread of carcinoma from the other breast.

SUMMARY

This chapter describes the anatomic, histologic, and pathologic terminology used in this textbook.

References

1. Sadler TW: Langman's Medical Embryology, 5th ed. Baltimore, Williams & Wilkins, 1985.
2. Wellings SR: A hypothesis of the origin of human breast cancer from the terminal ductal lobular unit. Pathol Res Pract 1980;166:515-535.
3. Kopans D: Breast Imaging, 2nd ed. Philadelphia, Lippincott-Raven, 1998.
4. Love SM, Gelman RS, Silen W: Fibrocystic "disease" of the breast: A nondisease? N Engl J Med 1982;307:1010-1014.
5. Page DL, Dupont WD: Premalignant conditions and markers of elevated risk in the breast and their management. Surg Clin North Am 1990;70:831-851.
6. Dupont WD, Page DL: Risk factors for breast cancer in women with proliferative breast disease. N Engl J Med 1985;312:146-151.
7. Dupont WD, Page DL: Relative risk of breast cancer varies with time since diagnosis of atypical hyperplasia. Hum Pathol 1989;20:723-725.
8. Page DL: Cancer risk assessment in benign breast biopsies. Hum Pathol 1986;17:871-874.
9. Page DL, Anderson TJ: Diagnostic Histopathology of the Breast. New York, Churchill Livingstone, 1987.
10. Dupont WD, Parl FF, Hartmann WH, et al: Breast cancer risk associated with proliferative breast disease and atypical hyperplasia. Cancer 1993;71:1258-1265.
11. Page DL, Jensen RA, Simpson JF: Premalignant and malignant disease of the breast: The role of the pathologist. Mod Pathol 1998;11:120-128.
12. Fisher ER, Gregorio RM, Fisher B, et al: The pathology of invasive breast cancer: A syllabus derived from findings of the national surgical adjuvant breast project (protocol 4). Cancer 1975;36:1-85.
13. Fu YS, Maksem JA, Huban CA, Reagan JW: The relationship of breast cancer morphology and estrogen receptor protein status. In Fenoglio CM, Wolff M (eds): Progress in Surgical Pathology, Vol. III. New York, Masson, 1981, pp 65-76.
14. Rosner D, Bedwani RN, Vana J, et al: Noninvasive breast carcinoma: Results of a national survey by the American College of Surgeons. Ann Surg 1980;192:139-147.
15. Fisher ER, Sass R, Fisher B, et al: Pathologic findings from the National Surgical Adjuvant Breast Project (protocol 6). 1: Intraductal carcinoma (DCIS). Cancer 1986;57:197-208.
16. Schwartz GF, Patchefsky AS, Feig SA, et al: Clinically occult breast cancer. Ann Surg 1980;191:8-12.
17. Walker RA, Dearing SJ, Brown LA: Comparison of pathological and biological features of symptomatic and mammographically detected ductal carcinoma in situ of the breast. Hum Pathol 1999;30:943-948.
18. Moezzi M, Melamed J, Vamvakas E, et al: Morphological and biological characteristics of mammogram-detected invasive breast cancer. Hum Pathol 1996;27:944-948.

Chapter 25

Benign Breast Lesions

Valerie P. Jackson, Yao S. Fu, and Karin L. Fu

The vast majority of lesions that occur within the breast are benign. Benign processes may be asymptomatic or have clinical manifestations, which include nodularity, thickening, a palpable mass, pain, inflammation, or nipple discharge. The location of the lesion may be a clue to its cause. Many of the signs and symptoms of breast disease are nonspecific and must be evaluated further with imaging and sometimes biopsy to determine whether the lesion is benign or malignant. High-quality mammography is required to begin the imaging workup of all breast symptoms, except in very young women, for whom ultrasound (US) is usually the initial imaging modality.

SKIN LESIONS

Skin lesions may be superimposed on the breast tissue on mammographic views, often mimicking parenchymal lesions. It is important to recognize the location of these lesions because they do not represent primary breast carcinoma, and biopsy or close-interval follow-up mammography is not indicated. Several types of skin conditions may appear on mammography, including skin pores, moles, skin tags, keloids, scars, epidermal inclusion cysts, sebaceous cysts, sebaceous gland calcifications, and foreign material on the skin. Many of these, such as skin moles, scars, and sebaceous cysts, are clinically obvious. The radiologic technologist should mark visible skin lesions with a small radiographically visible marker, such as a metallic BB, before mammography and should indicate their location on a worksheet. Other skin lesions, such as dermal calcifications and foreign material on the skin, are often not clinically apparent, and the interpreting physician should suspect their cause based on appearance or location. If a lesion seems to be in the skin but nothing is clinically apparent, a tangential view should be performed.

Skin Pores

Many women have prominent skin pores that can appear as numerous small round or oval lucencies on the mammogram (Fig. 25–1). The appearance is so typical that they should not cause confusion during mammographic interpretation.

Skin Moles and Other Raised Skin Lesions

Flat pigmented skin moles are not visible on mammography, whereas raised smooth or verrucous skin moles, warts, skin tags, and thick areas of seborrheic keratosis are frequently visible as circumscribed round, oval, or lobulated masses, which may have air in crevices (Figs. 25–2 to 25–5). A large halo of lucency is often seen around the lesion. This represents air trapped between the lesion, the skin of the breast, and the image receptor. If a wide band of lucency is present around all or a portion of the mass, or if the lesion appears to be relatively superficial on one or more mammographic views, one should suspect a skin lesion. If the cause is uncertain, a metallic BB should be placed over the mass and the mammogram repeated to prove that the lesion seen on the mammogram is truly the skin lesion.

Epidermal Inclusion Cysts and Sebaceous Cysts

Clinical Aspects

Epidermal inclusion cysts and sebaceous cysts arise from the skin and may occur in the cutaneous or subcutaneous tissues of the breast. Sebaceous cysts are retention cysts that arise from the sebaceous glands. Epidermal inclusion cysts usually arise from obstructed hair follicles, but they also may occur along embryonic lines of closure with adnexa opening into them (dermoid cysts). They may also arise from traumatic implantation or squamous metaplasia of a sweat duct.[1] These lesions are usually apparent on physical examination or during positioning of the breast for mammography and should be marked with a metallic BB before mammography.

Imaging Features

On mammography, epidermal inclusion cysts and sebaceous cysts are circumscribed, round soft-tissue density lesions that may be projected over the breast parenchyma on any view. Often, a portion of the border is ill defined (Fig. 25–6). On ultrasonography, these lesions appear to arise from the skin or immediate subcutaneous tissue of the breast, and the skin is seen surrounding the anterior part of the mass

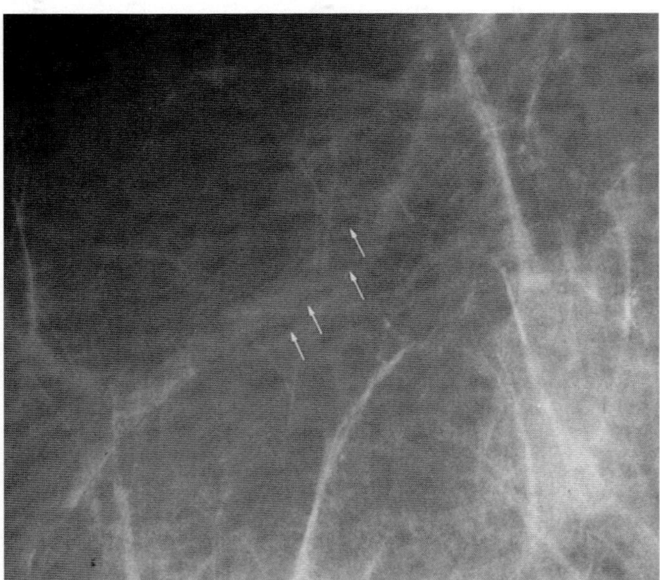

Figure 25–1. Skin pores *(arrows)*. The radiolucencies are caused by air trapped between the pores and the image receptor.

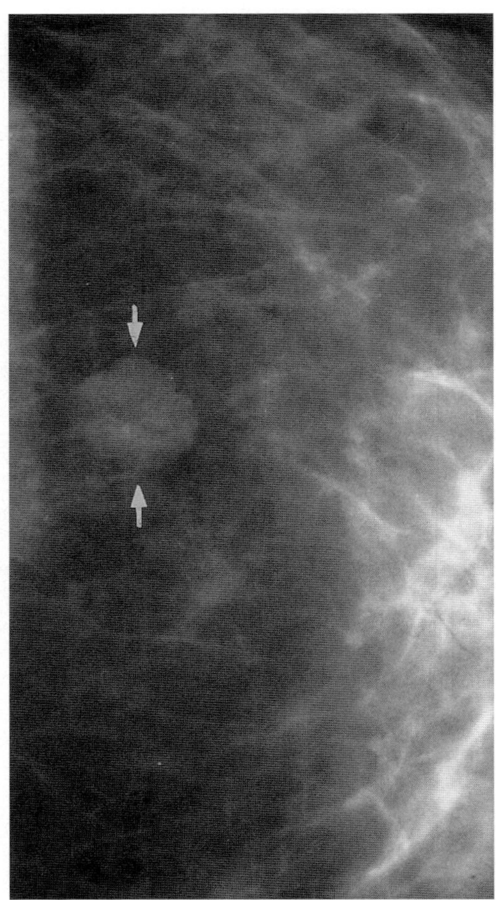

Figure 25–2. A 1-cm verrucous skin mole *(arrows)* with air outlining the periphery of the mass.

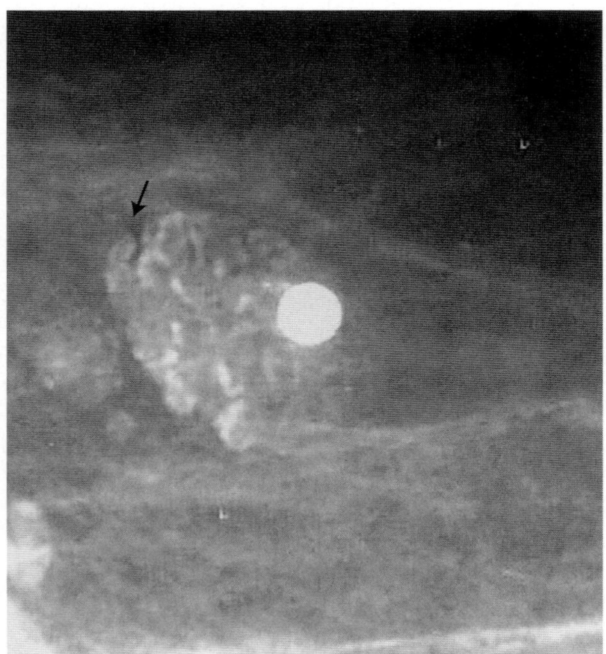

Figure 25–3. Verrucous skin mole *(arrow)* marked with metallic BB. The patient put a radiopaque ointment on the mole, and the ointment and air are trapped within the crevices of the mole.

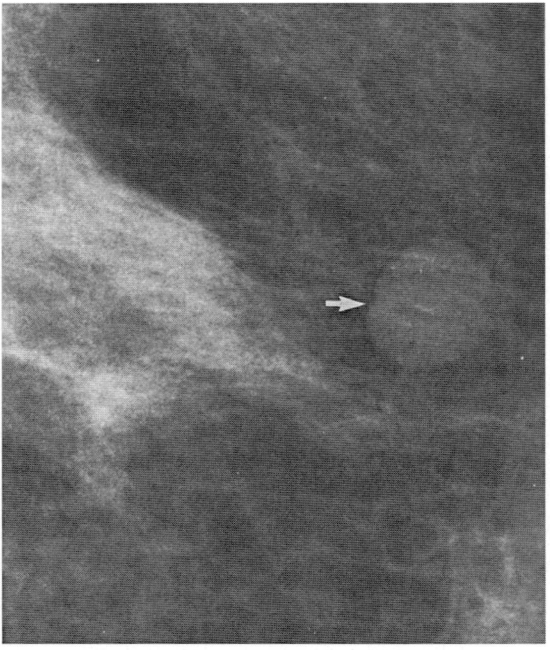

Figure 25–4. An 8-mm round raised skin mole *(arrow)* with thin surrounding halo of lucent air.

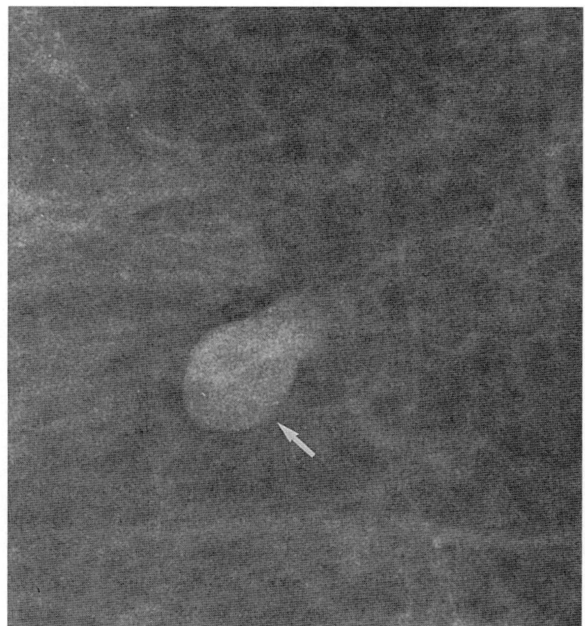

Figure 25–5. Pedunculated skin tag *(arrow).*

instead of being flattened or displaced, as would happen with a breast parenchymal lesion. Most are circumscribed and contain low-level internal echoes, produced by the thick material within these lesions (Fig. 25–7).

Neurofibromas and Neurilemmomas

Clinical Aspects

Neurofibromas and neurilemmomas are nerve sheath tumors that may involve the breast. Neurilemmomas

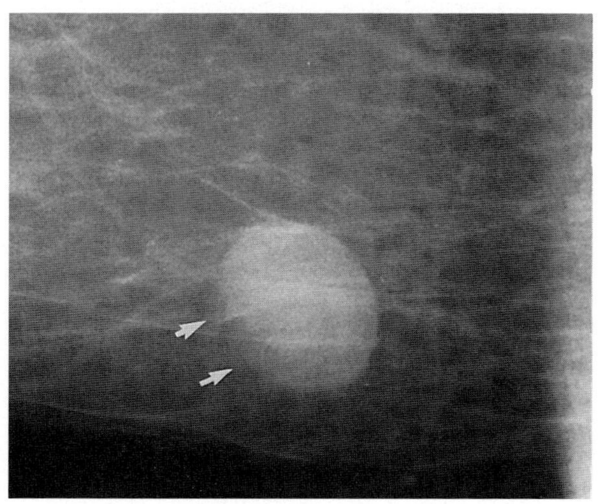

Figure 25–6. Epidermal inclusion cyst. On the mammogram, the lesion is predominantly circumscribed, but a portion of the border is ill defined *(arrows).*

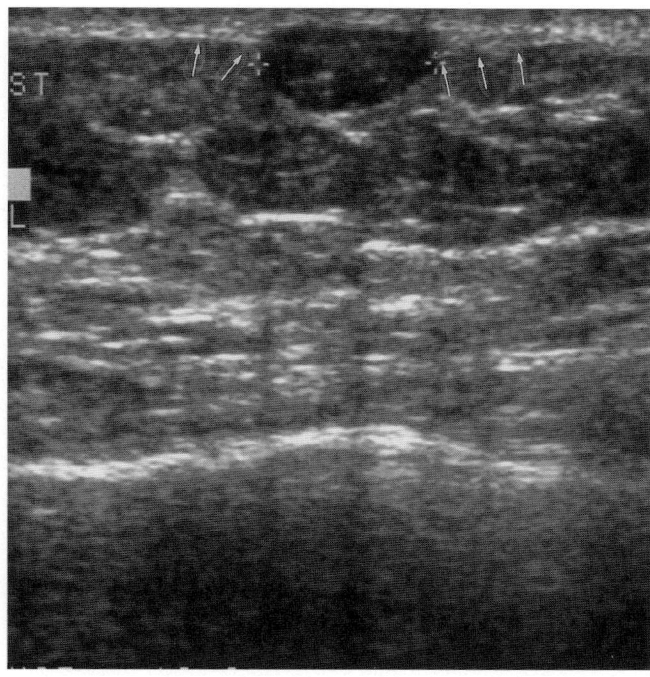

Figure 25–7. Epidermal inclusion cyst. On ultrasound, the intracutaneous lesion (*calipers*) contains low-level internal echoes. The skin forms a "claw sign" around the mass *(arrows),* indicating that the mass originates from the skin and is benign.

are usually single lesions not associated with neurofibromatosis. Women with neurofibromatosis often have multiple neurofibromas involving the breasts, especially in the periareolar region.

Imaging Features

On mammography, these raised skin lesions are sharply circumscribed peripheral lesions with a surrounding halo of lucency (air) that suggests their location in the skin. Unless very numerous, clinically apparent lesions should be marked with radiopaque markers before mammography so that they are not misinterpreted as parenchymal masses.

Steatocystoma Multiplex

Clinical Aspects

Steatocystoma multiplex is an uncommon inherited disorder of multiple cystic lesions involving the skin, particularly on the upper anterior aspect of the trunk. Affected individuals have multiple soft, freely movable cutaneous lesions that appear in adolescence or early adulthood and often later increase in size and number. The lesions are within the dermis, are composed of keratinizing epithelium, and contain either a clear oily liquid or a cheesy white material.[2]

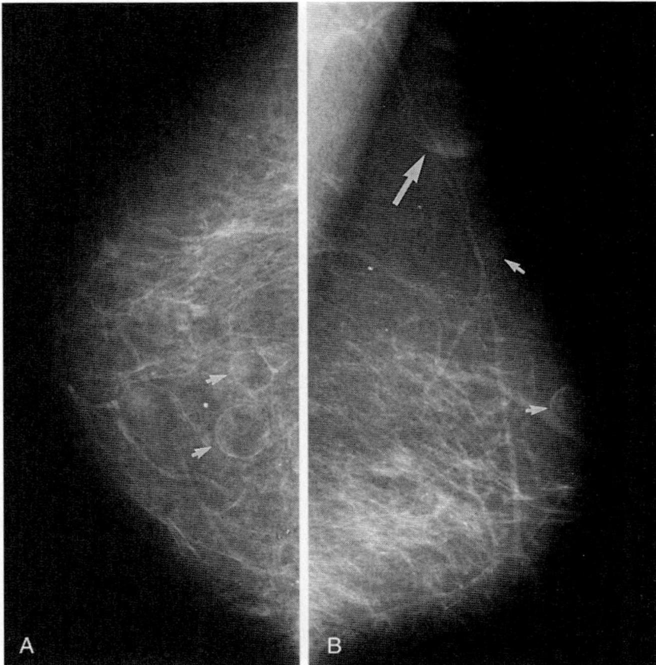

Figure 25–8. Steatocystoma multiplex. Right craniocaudal **(A)** and left mediolateral oblique (MLO) **(B)** views demonstrate multiple circumscribed fat-containing masses (*small arrows*). The left axillary tail lesion (*large arrow*) contains a fat/fluid level on the MLO view.

Imaging Features

The characteristic mammographic appearance is multiple circumscribed fat-density masses with thin capsules.[3-5] Most lesions range in size from 0.2 to 2.0 cm. The lesions are superficial, but many are projected over the parenchyma on all mammographic views. On horizontal beam films, it is not unusual to see a fat-fluid meniscus within the larger lesions (Fig. 25–8). A similar mammographic appearance has been reported in severe nodulocystic acne.[6] Although ultrasound features have been described,[5] the mammographic features are so typical that ultrasonography is not indicated. These lesions are always benign, and there is no increased risk for breast carcinoma in affected women.

Dermal Calcifications

Calcifications often occur within the sebaceous glands of the skin. They are not visible on inspection of the skin during physical examination and are of no clinical consequence. They may, however, cause confusion on mammography. Depending on their location, dermal calcifications may be projected peripherally on one or more mammographic views, or they may appear to be within the parenchyma. The most common appearance on mammography is faint spherical or polygonal lucent-centered calcifications, which are frequently clustered (Figs. 25–9 and 25–10).[7] They occur most often in the inferior and medial aspect of the breasts.

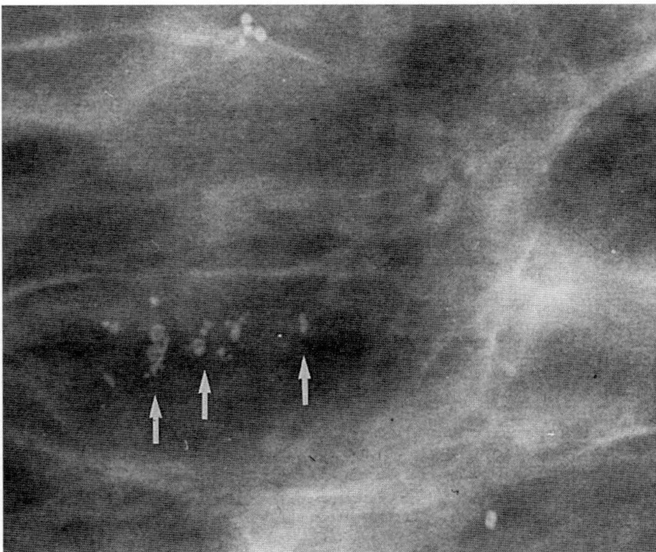

Figure 25–9. Dermal calcifications with typical polygonal shapes and lucent centers *(arrows)*.

Some dermal calcifications do not have a characteristic appearance and appear only as nonspecific clustered microcalcifications.[7] Skin calcifications should be suspected when the calcifications appear to be quite superficial on at least one view. In these cases, further workup is necessary to determine whether they are dermal or parenchymal in location. This is most easily done by the use of a fenestrated mammographic compression paddle.[8] The standard mediolateral oblique (MLO) and craniocaudal (CC)

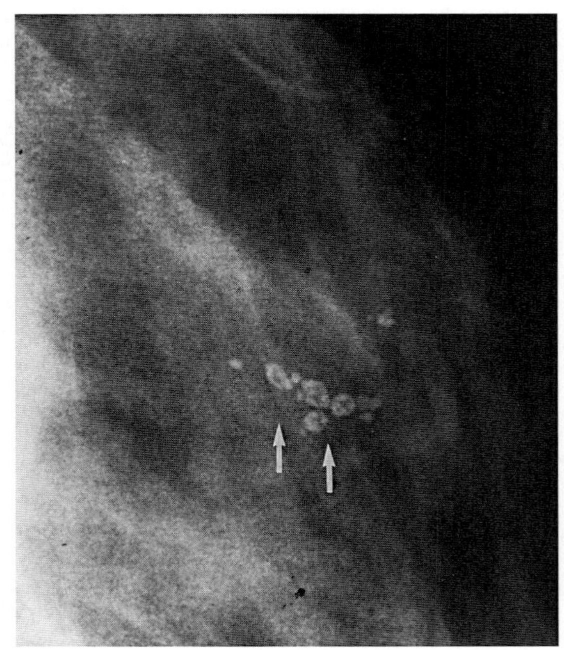

Figure 25–10. Dermal calcifications *(arrows)*.

views are reviewed to determine the skin surface closest to the calcifications (Fig. 25–11A and B), and the woman is placed in the mammography unit with the fenestrated compression paddle against that skin. A film in this projection is processed and reviewed while the woman remains in compression (Fig. 25–11C). The coordinates of the calcifications are used to guide placement of a metallic BB on the skin before a tangential view is obtained (Fig. 25–11D).

It is important to distinguish between dermal and parenchymal calcifications if recommendation for biopsy is contemplated, because dermal calcifications are always benign and breast biopsies do not usually include skin. Thus, specimen radiographs do not include the calcifications. Unnecessary biopsies can be avoided at the time of stereotactic needle biopsy by noting that the targeted calcifications are at the same depth as the skin, or at the time of presurgical

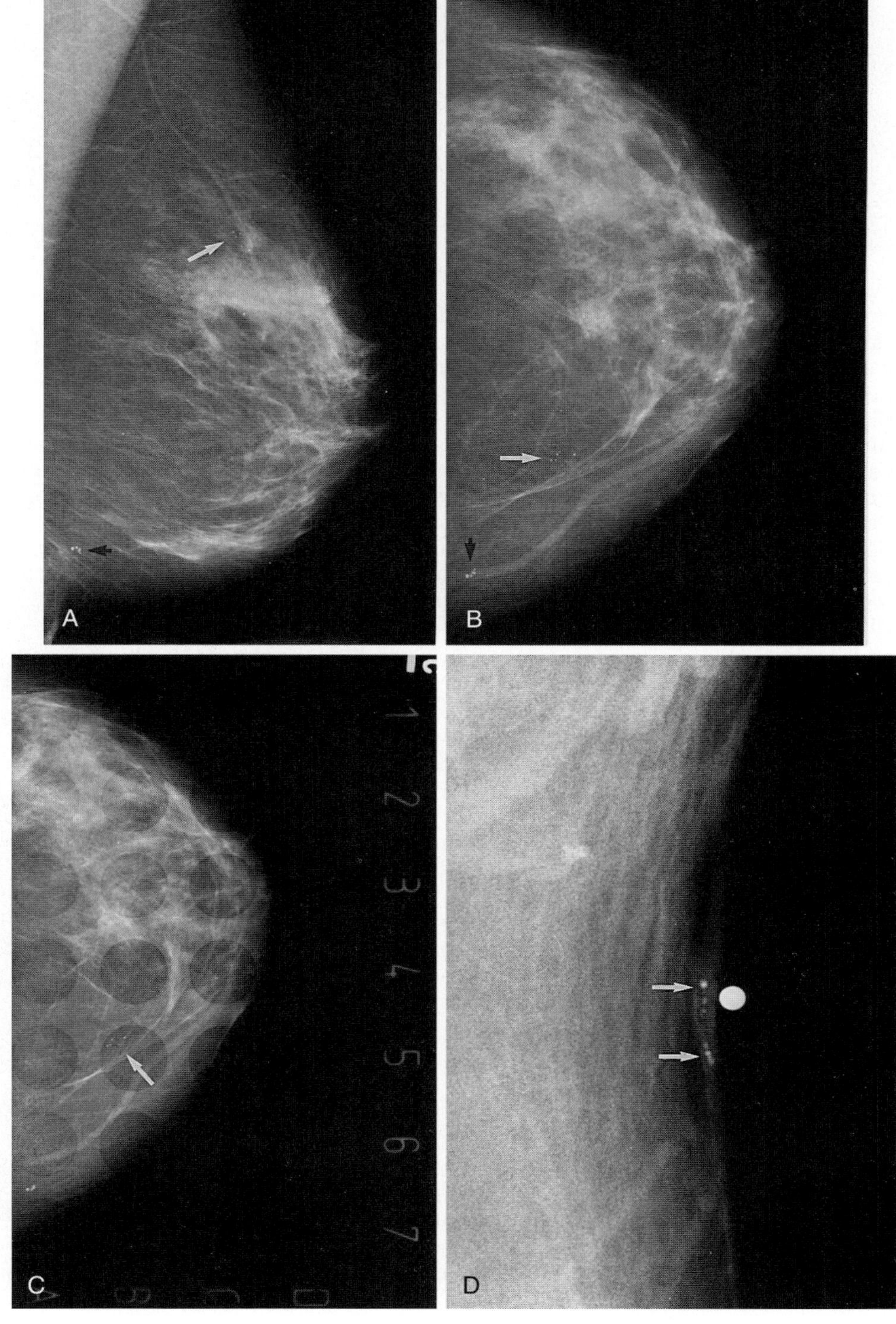

Figure 25–11. Atypical dermal calcifications. On the left mediolateral oblique **(A)** and craniocaudal **(B)** mammograms, there is a cluster of microcalcifications of indeterminate cause in the upper-inner quadrant *(white arrows)*. Obvious dermal calcifications are present in the left lower-inner quadrant *(black arrows)*, which raised the suspicion that the indeterminate calcifications might be dermal in location. The patient was placed in the mammography unit with the fenestrated compression paddle against the superior aspect of the breast, which was the skin surface closest to the calcifications **(C,** *arrow*). A metallic BB was placed at the appropriate coordinates of the calcifications and a tangential view **(D)** was obtained, which confirmed that the calcifications *(arrows)* were in the skin and did not require biopsy.

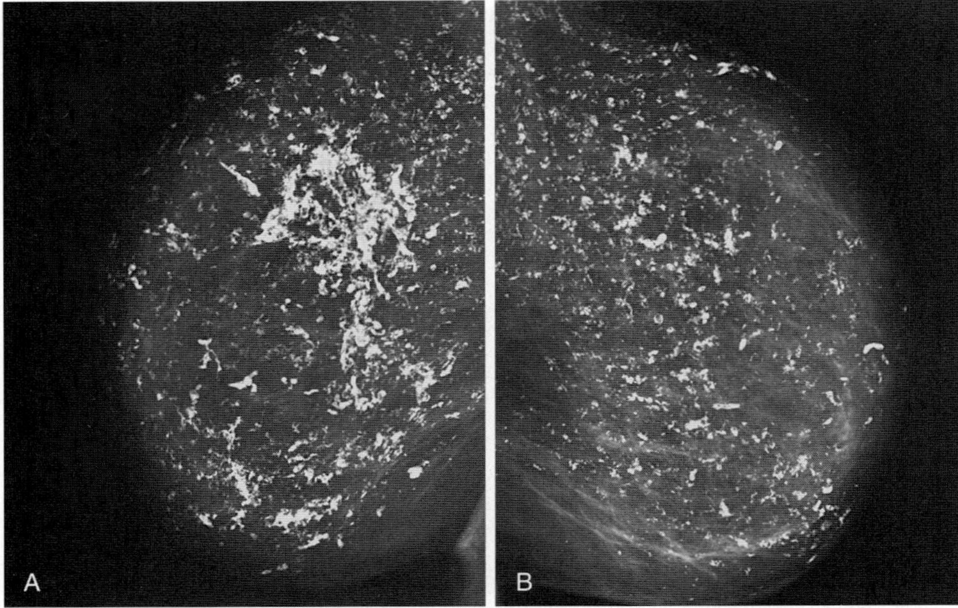

Figure 25–12. Dermatomyositis. Right **(A)** and left **(B)** mediolateral oblique views demonstrate diffuse bizarre superficial calcifications.

needle localization by placing a metallic BB at the skin entry site of the localizing needle. If the calcifications are located within the skin, their location will be obvious when the orthogonal view for needle placement is obtained with the BB in tangent. The needle then can be withdrawn and the biopsy canceled.[9] Unfortunately, some women have multiple unsuccessful surgical biopsies to remove clusters of dermal calcifications when the true location has not been recognized. Even today, some women are subjected to unnecessary anxiety if stereotactic biopsy is recommended for calcifications that are not recognized as dermal in location.

Dermatomyositis

Dermatomyositis is a condition of diffuse inflammation and degeneration involving the skeletal muscles and skin. It most frequently affects middle-aged women and may be manifested on mammography as subcutaneous calcifications. The calcifications are large, dense, clearly benign, and often bizarre (Figs. 25–12 and 25–13).[10] Approximately 15% to 25% of patients with dermatomyositis also have a malignancy. This situation most commonly occurs in men. In women, breast cancer has been reported to be one of the associated malignancies.[11,12]

Substances on the Skin

A number of materials that are applied to the skin are radiopaque. The best known is underarm antiperspirant, which contains a metallic compound with aluminum (Fig. 25–14). Plain deodorant does not contain metallic material and therefore is not visible on mammography. Although most facilities recommend that women not use antiperspirant before mammography, not all women follow this recommendation, or the material may remain within skin crevices after washing. It is not difficult to determine the cause of the densities when the material is in the axilla, but some women apply it in a wide area, including the area over the axillary tail of the breast, where it may simulate parenchymal calcifications.

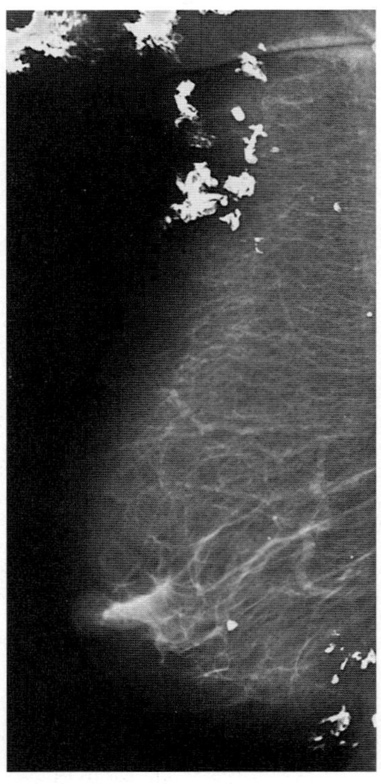

Figure 25–13. Dermatomyositis. Right mediolateral oblique view demonstrates coarse, bizarre, superficial calcifications in the axillary tail, upper arm, and inferior aspect of the breast.

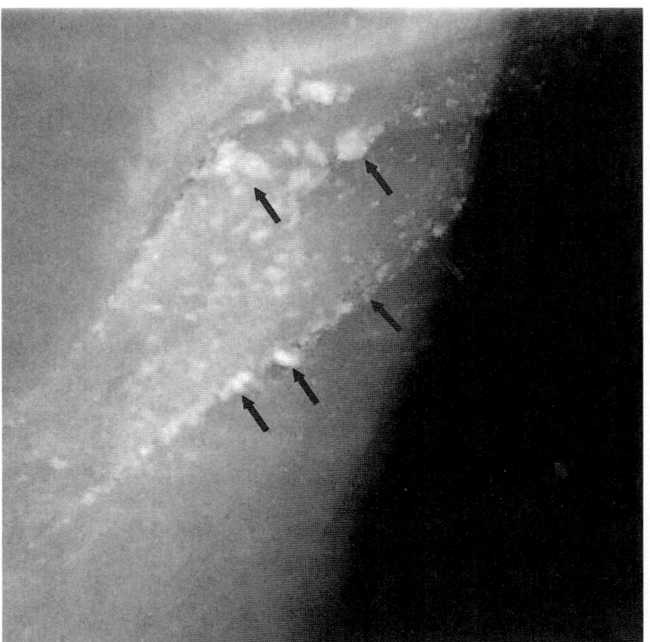

Figure 25–14. Antiperspirant *(arrows)* in axilla.

Some powders, creams, and ointments also contain radiopaque material, which can mimic suspicious microcalcifications on mammography (Fig. 25–15). Some pigments used in tattoos are radiopaque and can be mammographically visible (Fig. 25–16).[13] Substances in or on the skin should be suspected when the "calcification" is faint, has a bizarre configuration, is extremely peripheral in location, or extends into the axilla, or if the woman has skin lesions for which she might apply medication.

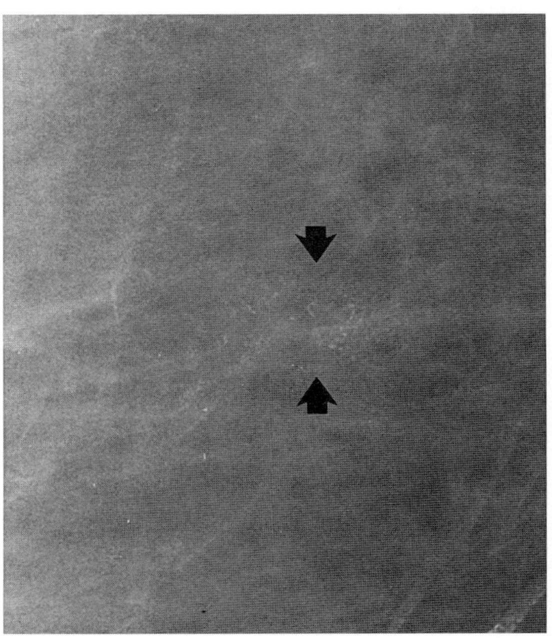

Figure 25–15. Zinc oxide–containing ointment on the skin, producing faint pleomorphic radiopaque densities *(arrows)*.

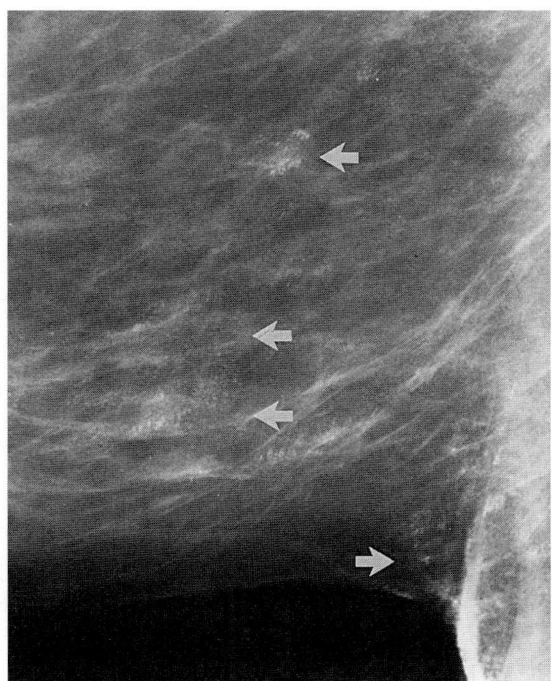

Figure 25–16. Radiopaque pigments in skin tattoos *(arrows)*.

VASCULAR LESIONS

The most common vascular lesion identified with mammography is atherosclerotic arterial calcification (Fig. 25–17). The classic "train track" appearance on mammography usually makes the diagnosis obvious. In early atherosclerosis, however, the calcification may be seen on only one wall, and it may mimic malignant ductal calcifications (Fig. 25–18).

Arterial calcification is usually a finding of advancing age. Although it occurs more commonly in diabetic than nondiabetic women, the presence of arterial calcification is not an accurate predictor for this disease.[14] Mammographic demonstration of arterial calcification has been associated with systemic cardiovascular disease and increased risk for events such as myocardial infarction and stroke.[15] Extensive diffuse bilateral arterial calcifications are often seen in women with secondary hyperparathyroidism from chronic renal failure, particularly those on dialysis (Fig. 25–19).[16,17]

The superficial veins of the breast may enlarge to provide collateral blood flow in cases of central venous obstruction. If the veins are markedly dilated, they may present clinically as soft superficial nodules. On mammography, the dilated serpiginous veins are obviously benign (Fig. 25–20).

Mondor disease is an uncommon thrombophlebitis of the subcutaneous veins of the breast, reportedly associated with trauma, surgery, excessive physical activity,[18] injections,[19] and, rarely, breast carcinoma.[20,21] The most frequently affected veins are the thoracoepigastric and the lateral thoracic.[18] The

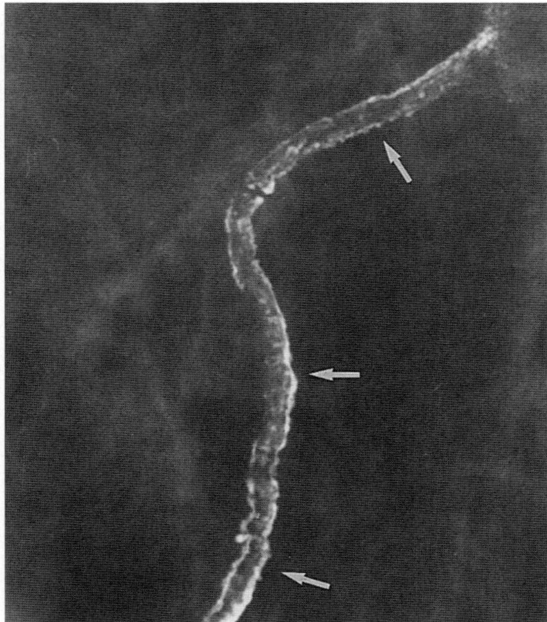

Figure 25–17. Arterial calcifications (*arrows*). Note the train track–like configuration of most portions of this heavily calcified artery.

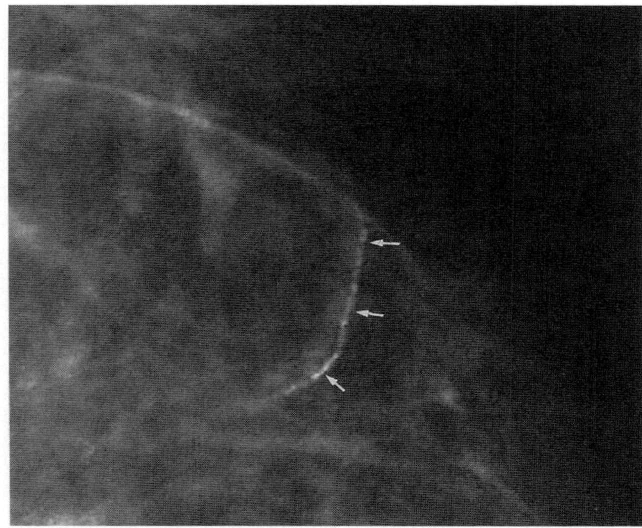

Figure 25–18. Early arterial calcifications. The calcifications *(arrows)* are seen along only one wall of the artery. Early arterial calcifications occasionally mimic malignant ductal microcalcifications of ductal carcinoma in situ. The visualization of the calcifications associated with the serpiginous vessel are the key to the diagnosis.

condition presents with pain, tenderness, and a palpable cord, usually on the lateral aspect of the breast. Associated skin dimpling or retraction often occurs. The process usually resolves completely within 6 weeks without treatment. On mammography, the thrombosed vein is a thickened, somewhat nodular, ropelike structure (Fig. 25–21A).[18] On ultrasonography, the vein appears as a superficial tubular structure filled with low-level internal echoes (Fig. 25–21B).[18] Occasionally, the thrombosed vein undergoes dense calcification (Fig. 25–22). The combination of the imaging and clinical features should be sufficient to make the diagnosis of this benign process and prevent an unnecessary biopsy. The mammogram should be carefully evaluated for any evidence of a rare associated malignancy, however.

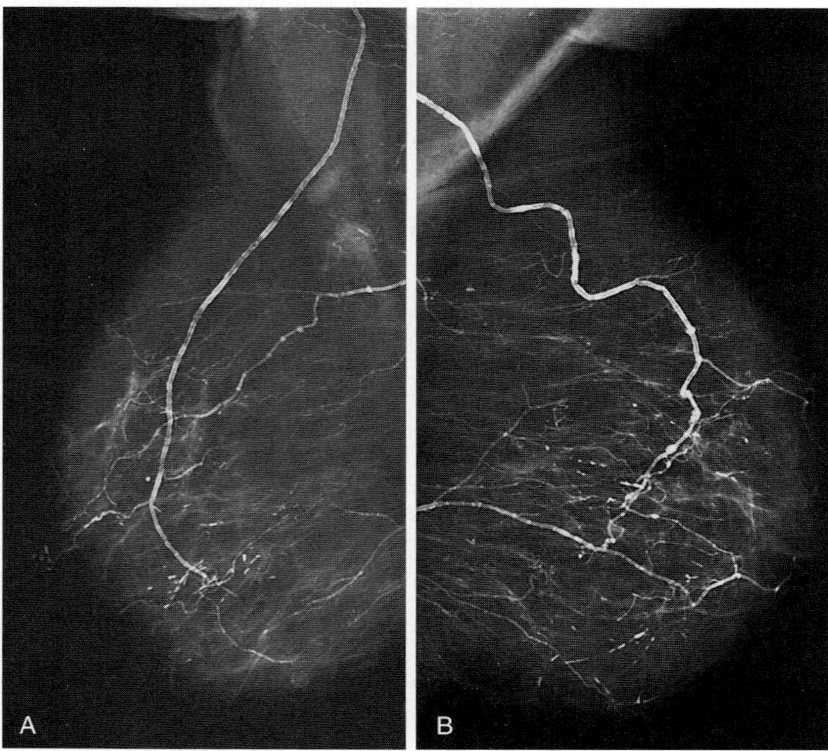

Figure 25–19. Hyperparathyroidism. Right **(A)** and left **(B)** mediolateral oblique mammograms demonstrate extensive bilateral arterial calcifications. Positioning for these mammograms was suboptimal because of the woman's debilitated condition.

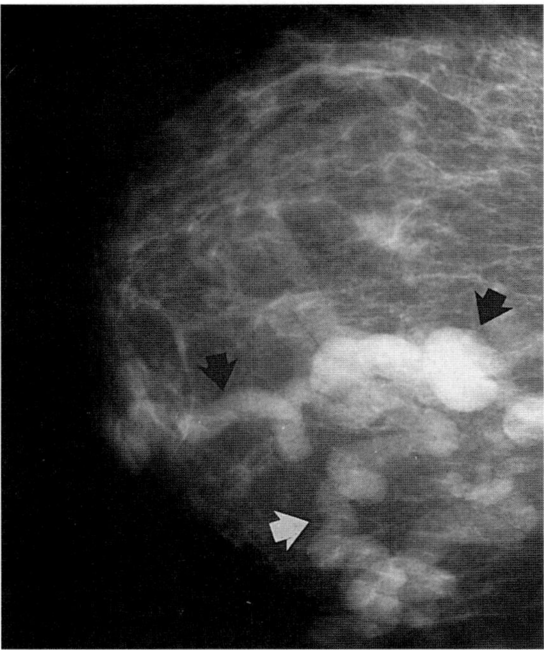

Figure 25–20. Dilated veins *(arrows)* on right craniocaudal mammogram in a young woman with superior vena caval obstruction from histoplasmosis.

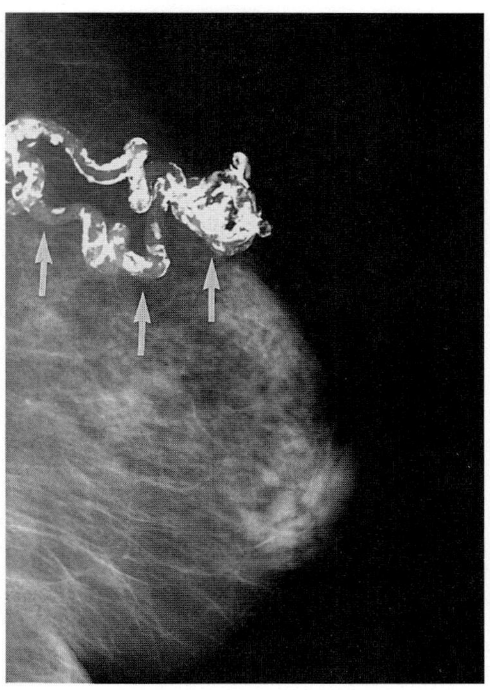

Figure 25–22. Mondor disease with calcification of chronically thrombosed vein *(arrows)*.

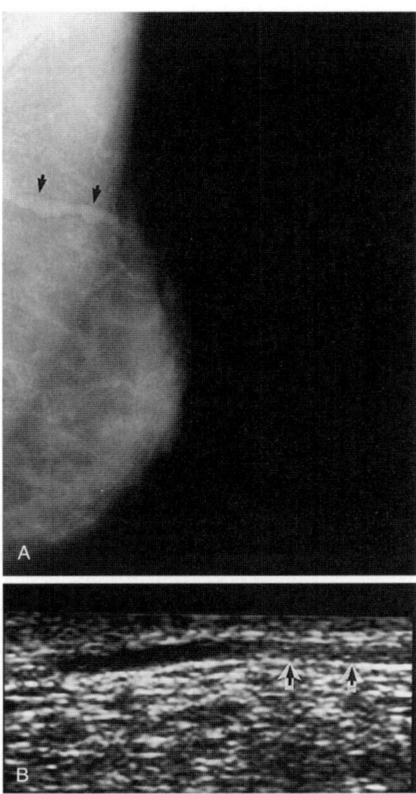

Figure 25–21. Mondor disease. **A,** The mediolateral oblique mammogram shows a somewhat nodular tubular density *(arrows)*, which is the thrombosed vein. **B,** Ultrasonography demonstrates a partly thrombosed vein. The low-level internal echoes *(arrows)* represent thrombus.

LYMPH NODES

Clinical Aspects

Lymph nodes are commonly encountered on mammograms. The vast majority seen on mammography are in the upper outer quadrant of the breast, the axillary tail, and the axilla. On histologic examination, they occur within any quadrant of the breast,[22] and they may also be detected by mammography in "atypical" locations.[23]

Imaging and Pathology Features

Lymph nodes usually appear on mammography as circumscribed oval or reniform noncalcified masses. Most intramammary lymph nodes are less than 1 cm in greatest dimension, whereas normal axillary lymph nodes may be 2 cm or more in size. The fat within the hilum of the lymph node is often seen as a lucency at the periphery when viewed in tangent (Fig. 25–23) or in the central portion of the mass when viewed en face (Fig. 25–24). This reflects the histologic finding of fat surrounded by lymphoid tissue (Fig. 25–25). Regardless of its size, when the typical mammographic appearance is seen, the lesion can be discounted as being benign, and no further workup is needed. In some cases, the diagnosis is not obvious on the standard views, and additional mammographic workup is necessary to demonstrate the fat within the mass.

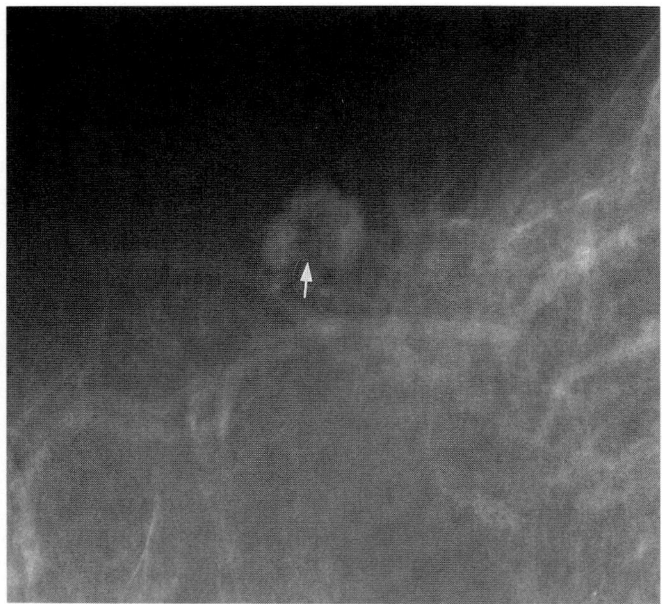

Figure 25–23. Intramammary lymph node. The peripheral fat hilum *(arrow)* is clearly visible.

When a fat hilum is not demonstrated by mammography, the lesion falls into the category of an indeterminate circumscribed noncalcified mass, and ultrasonography is indicated. In many cases, ultrasonography can demonstrate the symmetrical hypoechoic cortex and the highly echogenic fat hilum of a normal lymph node, establishing the benign diagnosis (Figs. 25–26 and 25–27).[24,25] In some normal lymph nodes, however, the fat hilum is not demonstrated by mammography or ultrasonography. In these cases, in the absence of demonstrable stability on previous mammograms, a close-interval follow-up mammogram or biopsy may be indicated (Fig. 25–28).

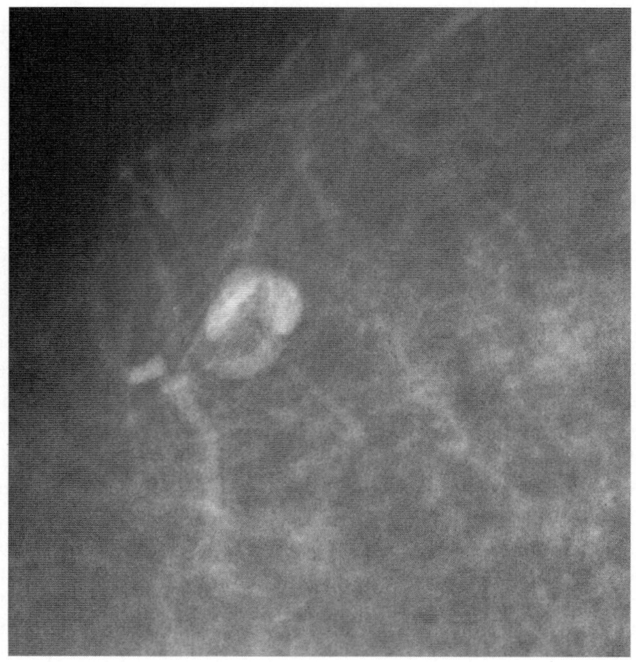

Figure 25–24. Intramammary lymph node. In this case, the fat hilum is seen en face.

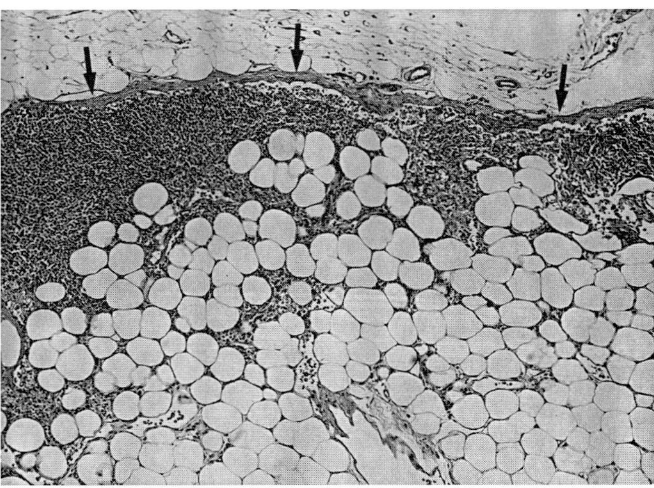

Figure 25–25. Fatty replacement of lymph node. Most of the lymph node is replaced by mature adipose tissue, with only a narrow rim of lymphoid tissue remaining under the capsule *(arrows)*.

Lymph nodes may become involved with inflammation, granulomatous processes, and metastatic carcinoma.[26-30] On mammography, most involved lymph nodes are rounded, enlarged, and abnormally dense and lack a visible fat hilum (Figs. 25–29 to 25–31). Reactive inflammatory lymph nodes usually maintain circumscribed borders. Coarse calcifications are sometimes seen in granulomatous disease involving the nodes (Fig. 25–32), such as histoplasmosis, tuberculosis, or sarcoidosis. Faint metallic deposits simulating microcalcifications have been seen in patients with rheumatoid arthritis after gold therapy injections (Figs. 25–33 and 25–34).[31] Metastatic lymph nodes may develop indistinct or spiculated margins, and microcalcifications are rarely seen. In malignancy, ultrasonography may demonstrate focal

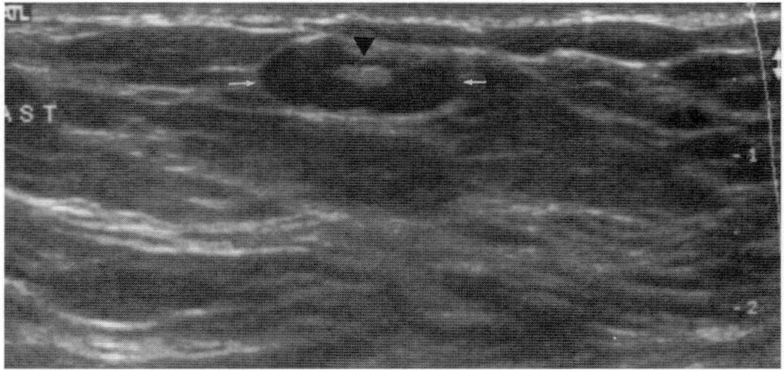

Figure 25–26. Intramammary lymph node. Ultrasonogram of normal 1-cm lymph node. The peripheral lymphoid tissue *(arrows)* is hypoechoic relative to fat and fibroglandular tissue. The fat hilum *(arrowhead)* is highly echogenic.

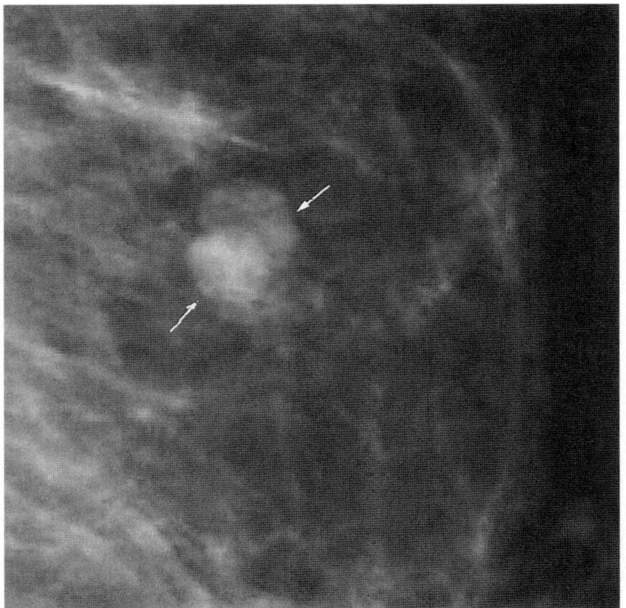

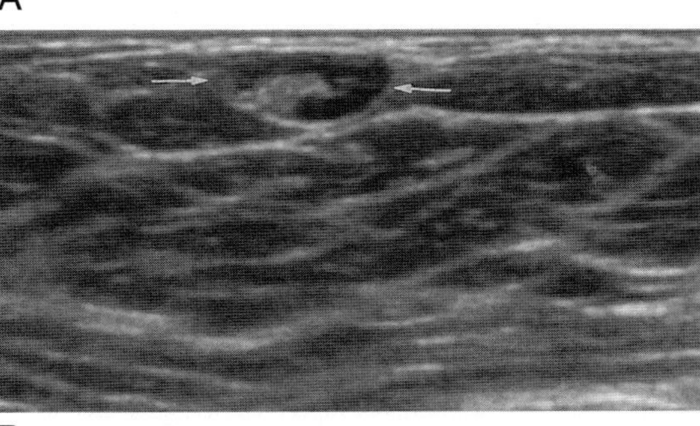

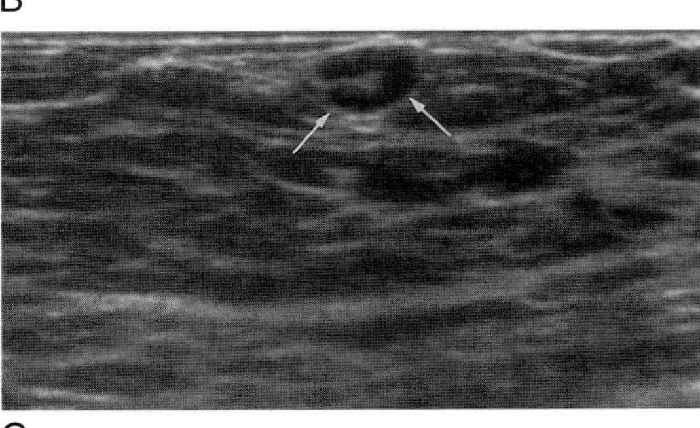

Figure 25–27. Lymph node. **A,** A 1.3-cm lobulated, circumscribed, noncalcified mass *(arrows)* is seen in the upper-outer quadrant of the left breast on mammography. Longitudinal **(B)** and transverse **(C)** ultrasonograms demonstrate the typical features of a normal intramammary lymph node *(arrows)*.

or diffuse cortical widening, and thinning, displacement, or loss of the normal echogenic hilum, whereas in reactive processes, the normal architecture tends to be preserved within the enlarged node (Fig. 25–35).[32,33]

Diffusely enlarged axillary lymph nodes may be unilateral or bilateral. Unilateral axillary adenopathy may be caused by ipsilateral breast cancer, mastitis, or inflammation involving the upper extremity. Bilateral axillary adenopathy is usually caused by a systemic process such as lymphoma, leukemia, or rheumatoid arthritis (Fig. 25–36).

POST-TRAUMATIC HEMATOMAS AND SCARS

Dermal Scars from Surgery or Trauma

Most postsurgical and post-traumatic skin scars are mammographically invisible or manifest as localized skin thickening with or without retraction. Some women form very thick skin scars (keloids), which are often mammographically visible. When these focal areas of skin thickening are viewed in tangent, their cause is obvious. When they are projected over the parenchyma on both the MLO and CC views, however, they may simulate parenchymal masses, often with bizarre shapes (Fig. 25–37). The technologist should mark scars and keloids on a worksheet and on the skin with a radiopaque marker before mammography. Within the scar, acute and chronic inflammation, granulation tissue, fat necrosis, foreign body reaction, and fibrosis occur.

Parenchymal Changes

A variety of parenchymal findings may be seen after blunt, penetrating, or surgical trauma.[34] Acutely, hematomas are frequently visible as ill-defined masses at the site of surgery or trauma (Figs. 25–38 and 25–39). Hematomas decrease in size over time and usually resolve completely. Scars are areas of fibrosis that are visible as ill-defined or spiculated masses or areas of architectural distortion (Fig. 25–40). A scar is usually at its maximal size by approximately 6 months after trauma. Thereafter, scars usually decrease in size and prominence to a variable degree (Fig. 25–41). Many women have no residual mammographic or ultrasonographic changes 1 year or more after trauma or surgery; however, many have visible sequelae for life. To make the diagnosis of a scar, it is important to compare with previous studies and, if the patient has had a surgical biopsy, to review prebiopsy mammograms to determine that the spiculated mass or architectural distortion is truly in the area of the lesion that had been removed. If there is any doubt, histologic confirmation may be required (Fig. 25–42).

FAT NECROSIS

Clinical Aspects

Fat necrosis is a common benign condition that may be asymptomatic or may present with a palpable mass, pain, or associated findings such as skin

Text continued on p. 415

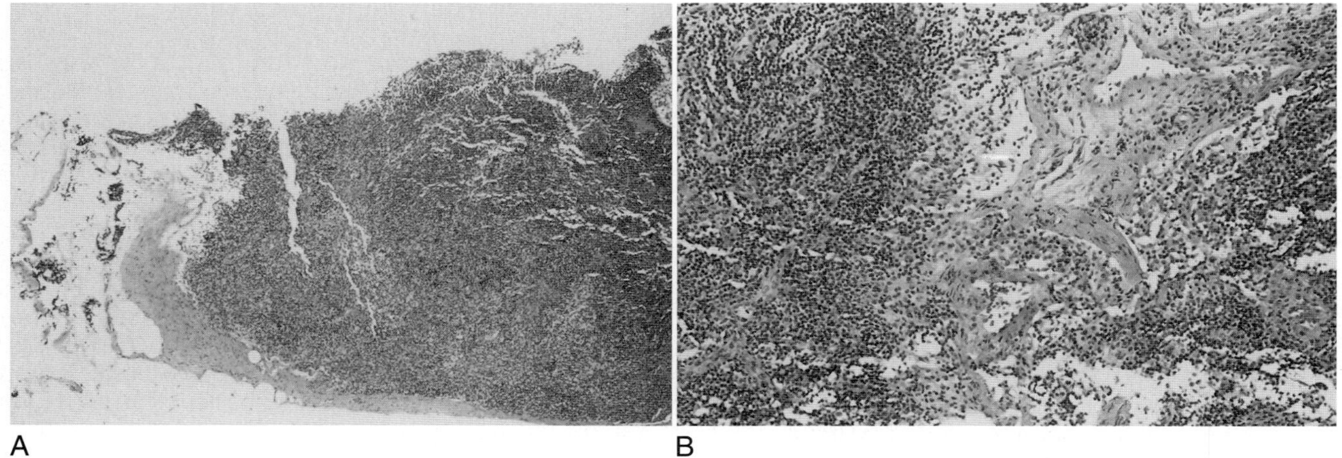

Figure 25–28. Intramammary reactive lymph node. **A,** In this core needle biopsy, the lymph node includes the capsule and benign lymphoid tissue. **B,** A higher magnification reveals subcapsular sinus histiocytosis and adjacent mature lymphocytes. No malignancy is seen.

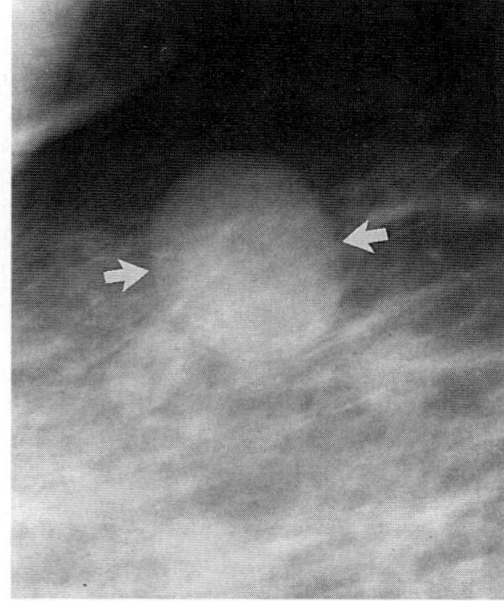

Figure 25–29. Reactive intramammary lymph node in mastitis. Mammographically, the node *(arrows)* is enlarged (3 cm in diameter) and has a round shape and no visible fat hilum.

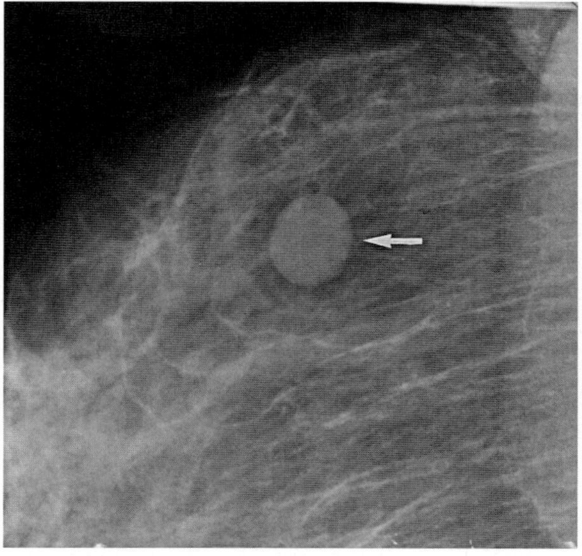

Figure 25–30. Reactive lymph node. A 1.2-cm circumscribed, enlarged, intramammary lymph node *(arrow)* in a woman with acquired immunodeficiency syndrome (AIDS).

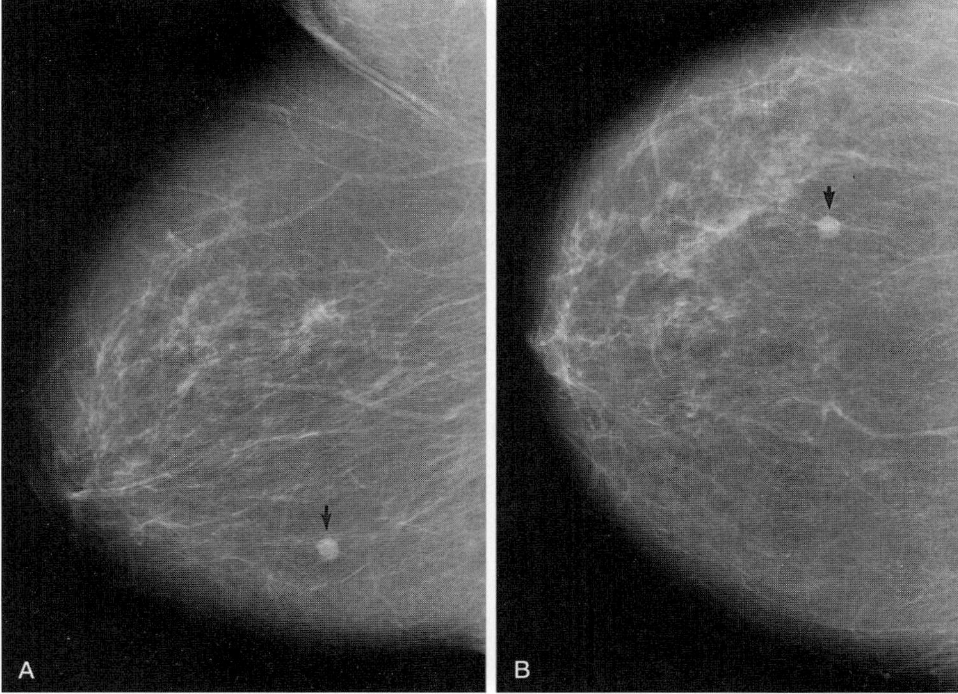

Figure 25–31. Reactive intramammary lymph node in atypical location. Mediolateral **(A)** and craniocaudal **(B)** mammograms demonstrate a new 8-mm round circumscribed nodule *(arrows)* in the lower-outer quadrant of the right breast. At biopsy, this was a reactive lymph node.

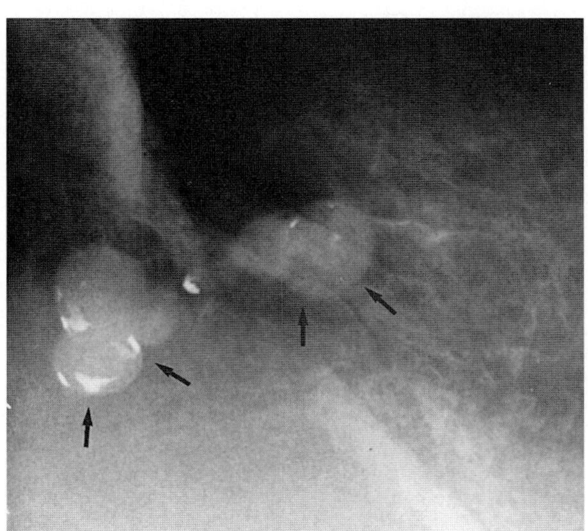

Figure 25–32. Histoplasmosis. Enlarged axillary lymph nodes with coarse peripheral calcifications *(arrows)* in a woman with a history of disseminated histoplasmosis. Other granulomatous diseases may produce identical calcifications.

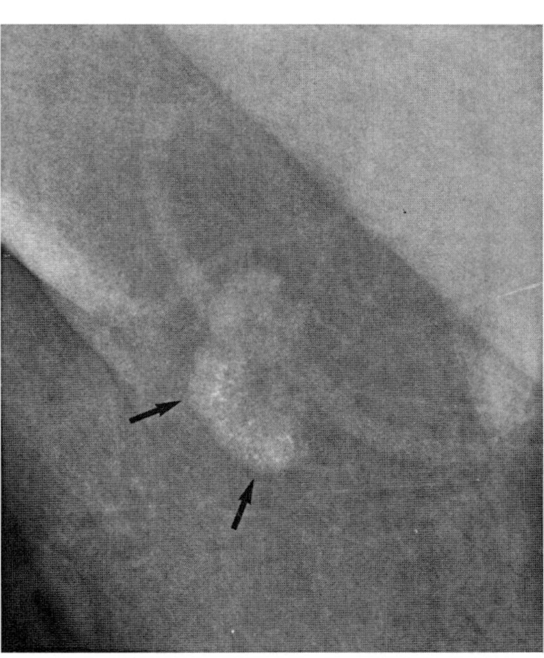

Figure 25–33. Gold deposits. This woman had gold injections for rheumatoid arthritis. The metallic particles simulate microcalcifications in a lymph node *(arrows)*.

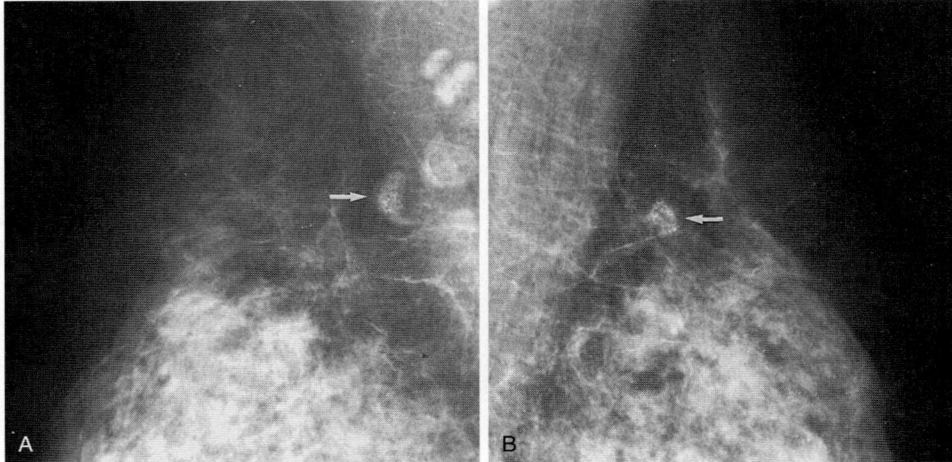

Figure 25–34. Gold deposits. Right **(A)** and left **(B)** mediolateral oblique views demonstrate gold deposits in bilateral axillary-tail lymph nodes *(arrows)* in a woman with a history of gold therapy for rheumatoid arthritis.

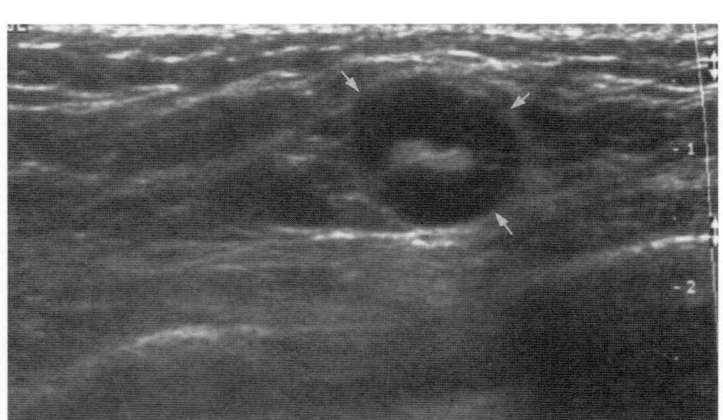

Figure 25–35. Reactive intramammary lymph node in a patient with psoriasis. On ultrasonography, the echogenic fat hilum is visible and the peripheral lymphoid tissue is diffusely thickened *(arrows)*, but the normal architecture is preserved.

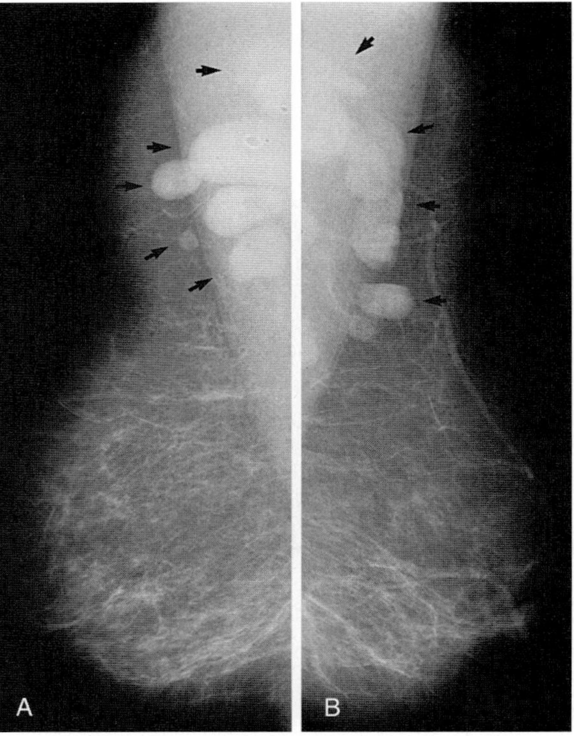

Figure 25–36. Axillary adenopathy. Bilateral axillary lymphadenopathy *(arrows)* in a woman with rheumatoid arthritis.

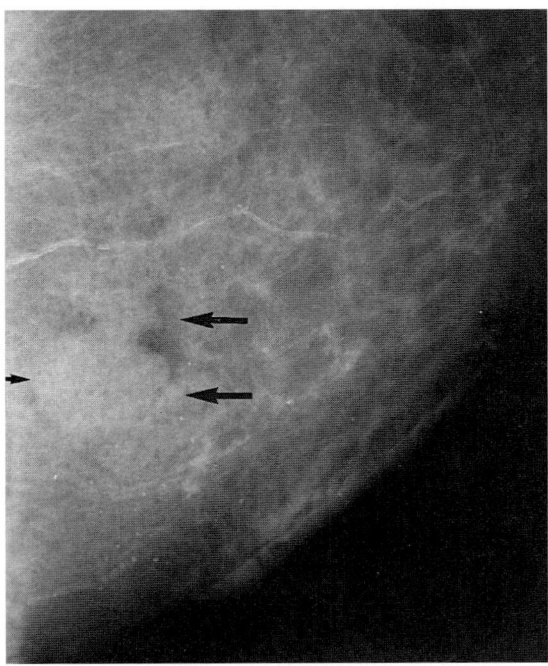

Figure 25–37. Skin keloid. The irregular thickening of the skin produces a lobular circumscribed density *(arrows)*. Note the wide margin of air surrounding a portion of the lesion.

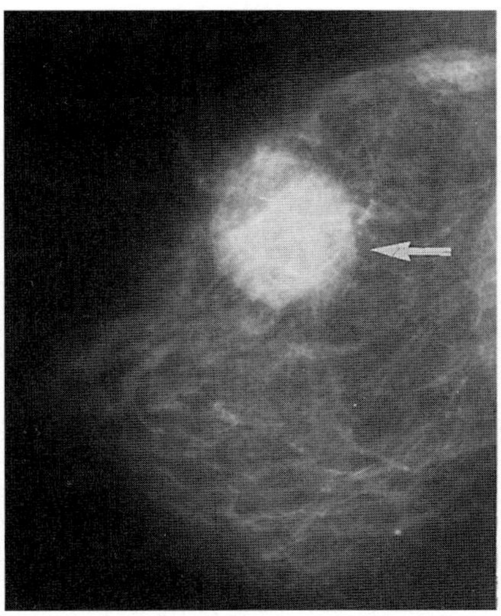

Figure 25–38. A 3-cm hematoma 2 weeks after a benign breast biopsy. The right exaggerated craniocaudal lateral mammogram demonstrates an ill-defined round mass *(arrow)* at the biopsy site.

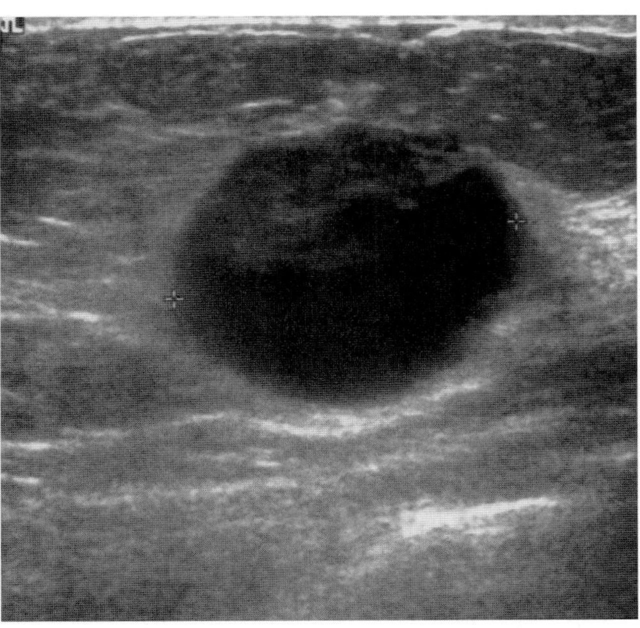

Figure 25–39. A 2.5-cm hematoma 1 week after blunt trauma to the breast. Typical ultrasonographic findings of a hematoma *(calipers)* include a round, oval, or lobular shape, indistinct margins, posterior acoustic enhancements, and both cystic and solid-appearing internal components.

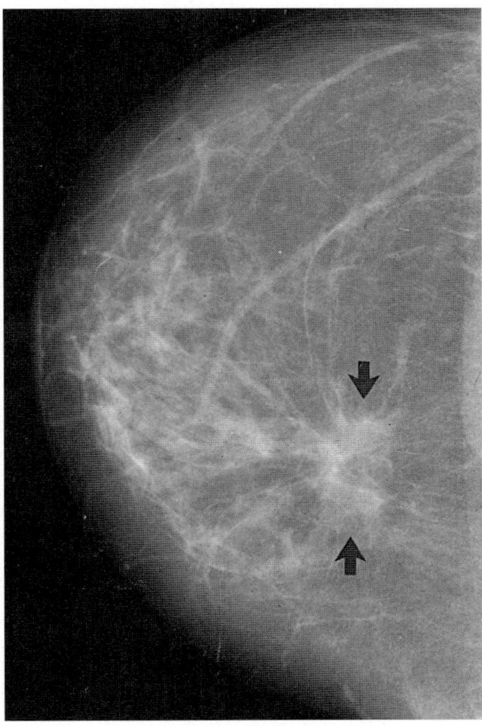

Figure 25–40. Postoperative scar *(arrows)* 3 years after benign breast biopsy. The findings mimic breast carcinoma, and an accurate history and comparison with old films are necessary to make the diagnosis.

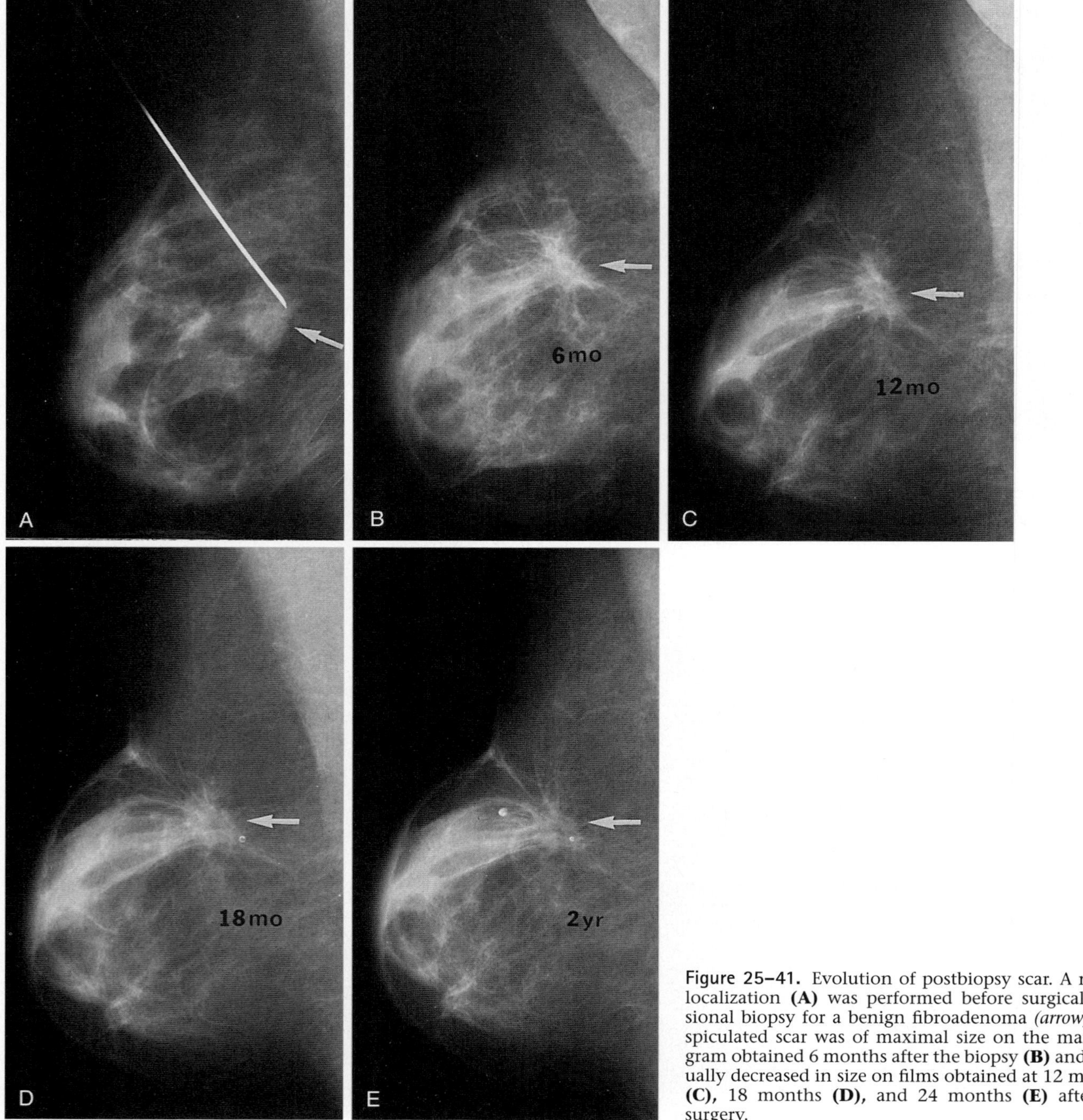

Figure 25–41. Evolution of postbiopsy scar. A needle localization **(A)** was performed before surgical excisional biopsy for a benign fibroadenoma *(arrow)*. The spiculated scar was of maximal size on the mammogram obtained 6 months after the biopsy **(B)** and gradually decreased in size on films obtained at 12 months **(C)**, 18 months **(D)**, and 24 months **(E)** after the surgery.

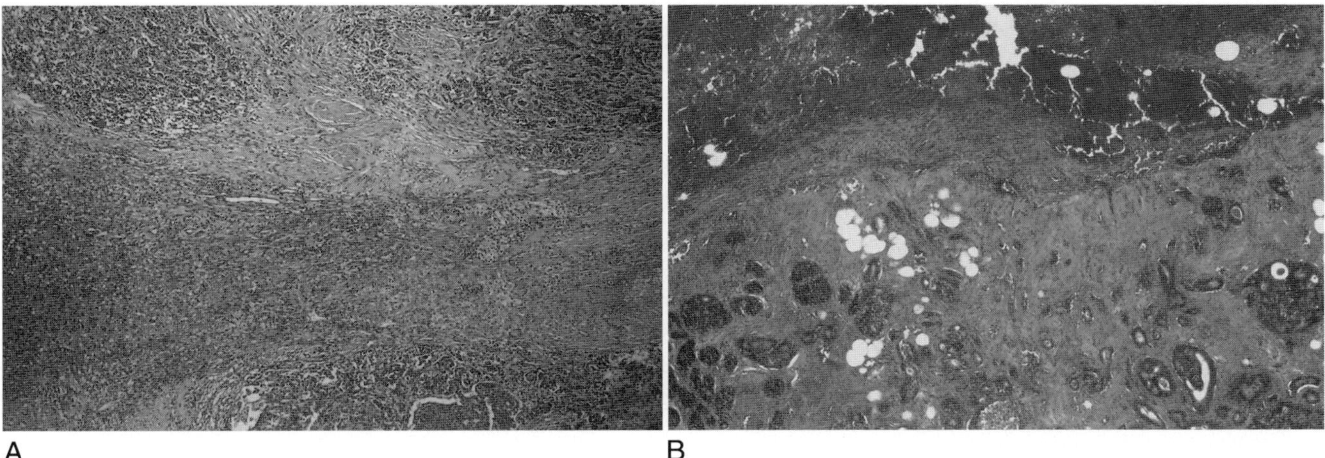

Figure 25–42. Effects of core needle biopsy. **A,** An area of fibrosis corresponding to the needle track of a previous core biopsy. **B,** An area of hemorrhage (upper field) and ductal carcinoma in situ (lower field) excised 2 weeks after core needle biopsy.

thickening or nipple retraction. The clinical findings may mimic carcinoma.

Imaging Features

Fat necrosis may have a variety of mammographic appearances. Many of the findings mimic carcinoma, including spiculated masses, microcalcifications, and architectural distortion (Figs. 25–43 and 25–44).[35] One common and characteristic finding is a radiolucent or mixed fat- and soft tissue–density circumscribed mass with a calcified or noncalcified rim, known as a lipid or oil cyst (Figs. 25–45 through 25–53).[35-37] These can be seen after any trauma to the breast, including surgery. Fat necrosis is commonly seen after lumpectomy and radiation therapy for breast carcinoma and after extensive surgery such as reduction mammoplasty. In most cases, the mammographic findings are diagnostic of a benign lesion. Early peripheral calcification may mimic microcalcification of malignancy, however. Nonetheless, in most cases, the location of the calcifications at the periphery of a fat-density circumscribed mass is sufficient to establish the benign diagnosis.

Ultrasonography is not performed when the mammographic features are typical for fat necrosis, but it is often performed for cases for which the mammogram shows a soft tissue–density mass. In our experience, early fat necrosis is usually manifest as an

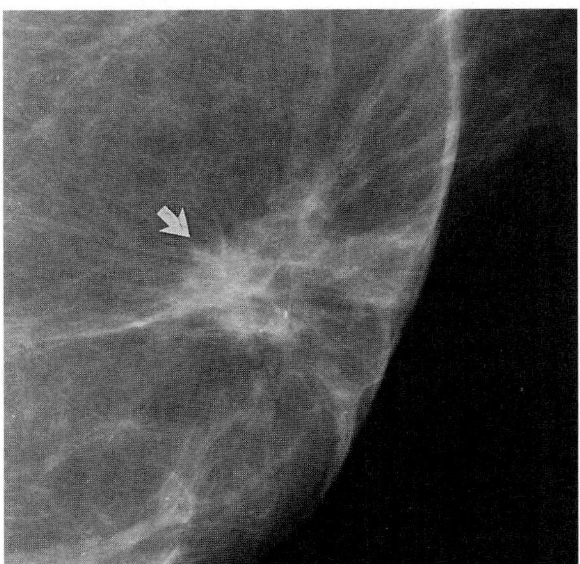

Figure 25–43. Fat necrosis *(arrow)* manifesting as a spiculated mass.

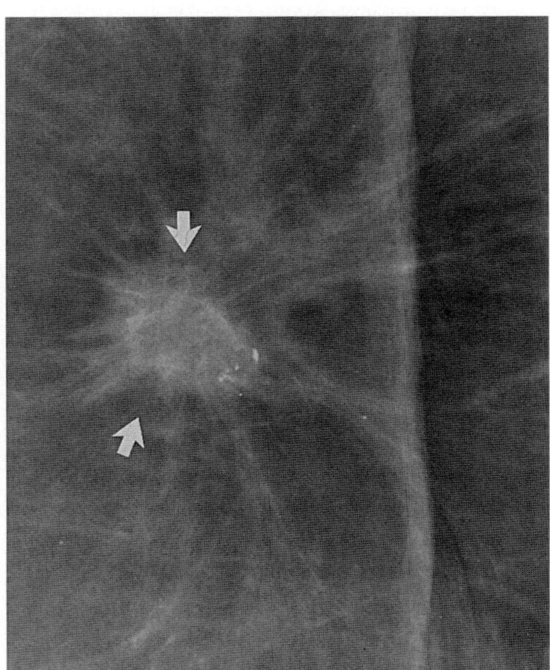

Figure 25–44. Fat necrosis. The spiculated mass *(arrows)* has a few peripheral microcalcifications.

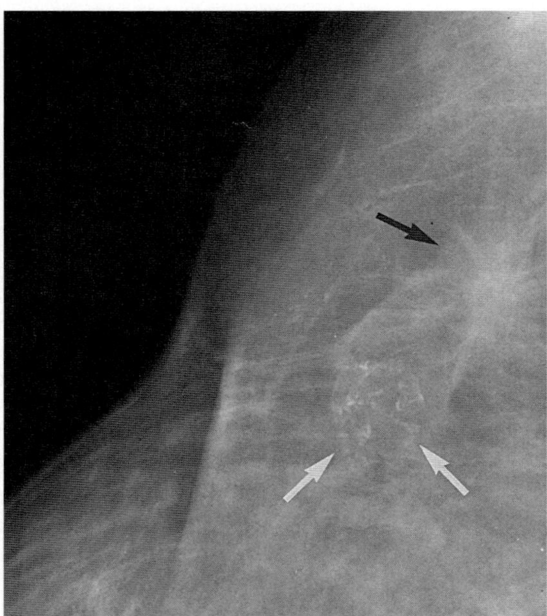

Figure 25–45. Varied appearance of fat necrosis, with a spiculated mass *(black arrow)* and an adjacent group of pleomorphic microcalcifications *(white arrows)* at the periphery of a circumscribed fat-density mass.

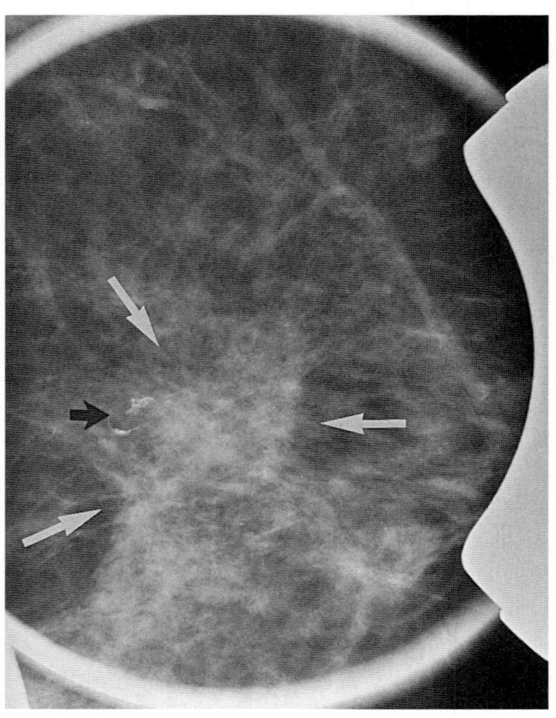

Figure 25–46. Fat necrosis with architectural distortion *(white arrows)* and a few rim calcifications *(black arrow)*.

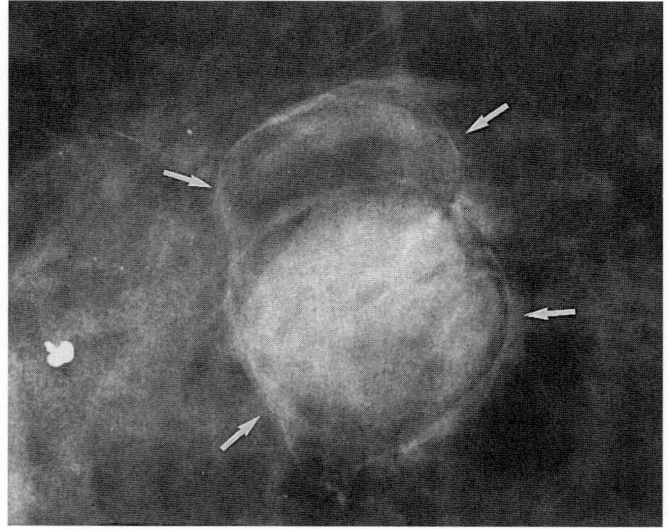

Figure 25–47. Early fat necrosis in hematoma. This woman had suffered blunt trauma to the chest wall in an automobile accident 3 weeks before the mammogram. This 2-cm lobular circumscribed mass *(arrows)* contains both fat and soft-tissue density (blood). This completely resolved within 6 months of the trauma.

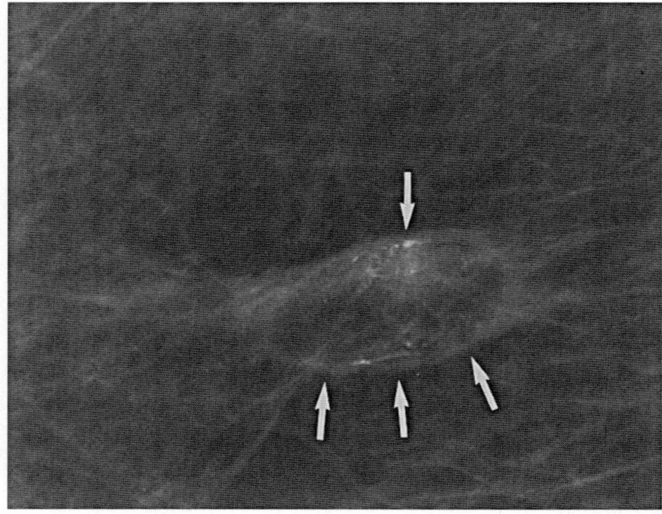

Figure 25–48. Fat necrosis. Faint peripheral calcification around fat-density mass *(arrows)*.

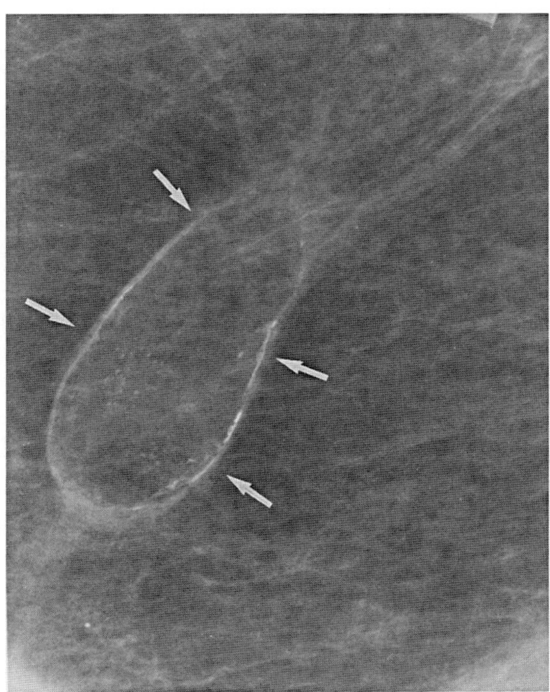

Figure 25–49. Fat necrosis *(arrows)* with rim calcification around fat-density mass.

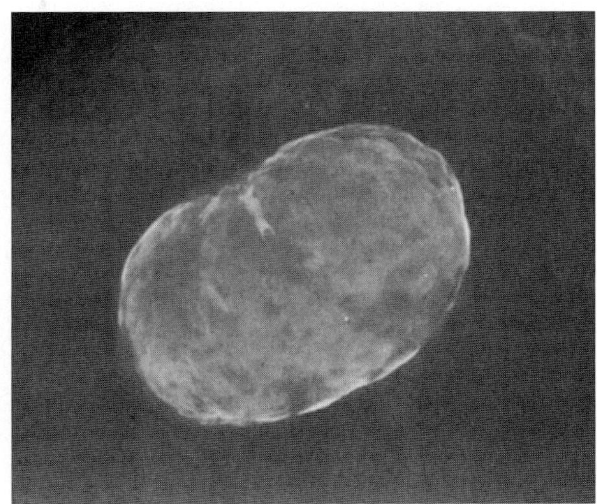

Figure 25–50. Densely calcified 3-cm area of fat necrosis 2 years after blunt trauma to the breast.

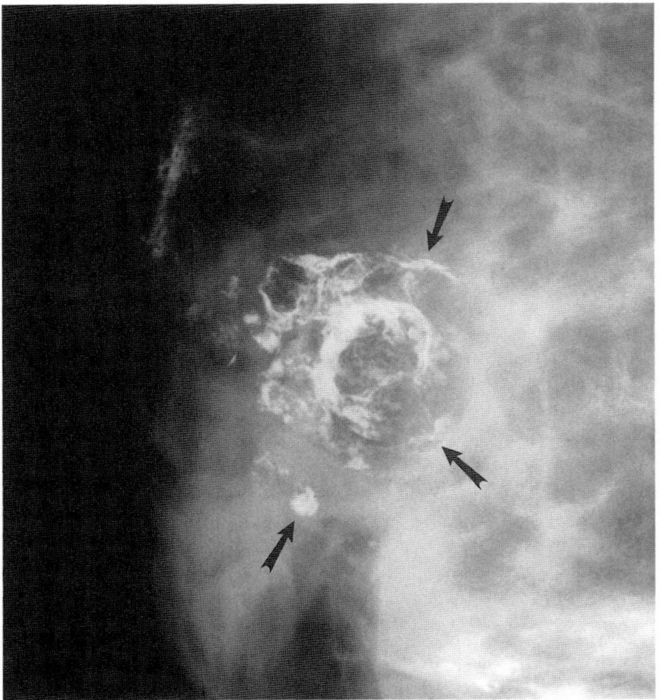

Figure 25–51. Fat necrosis with calcifications *(arrows)* after reduction mammoplasty.

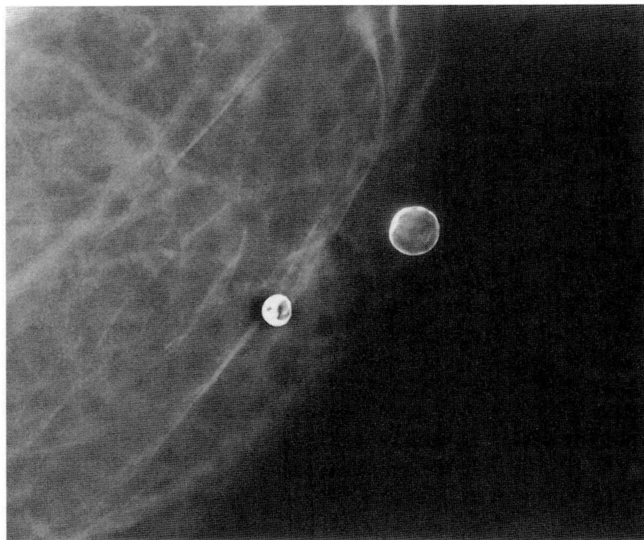

Figure 25–52. Small oil cysts from fat necrosis. This patient had no known trauma.

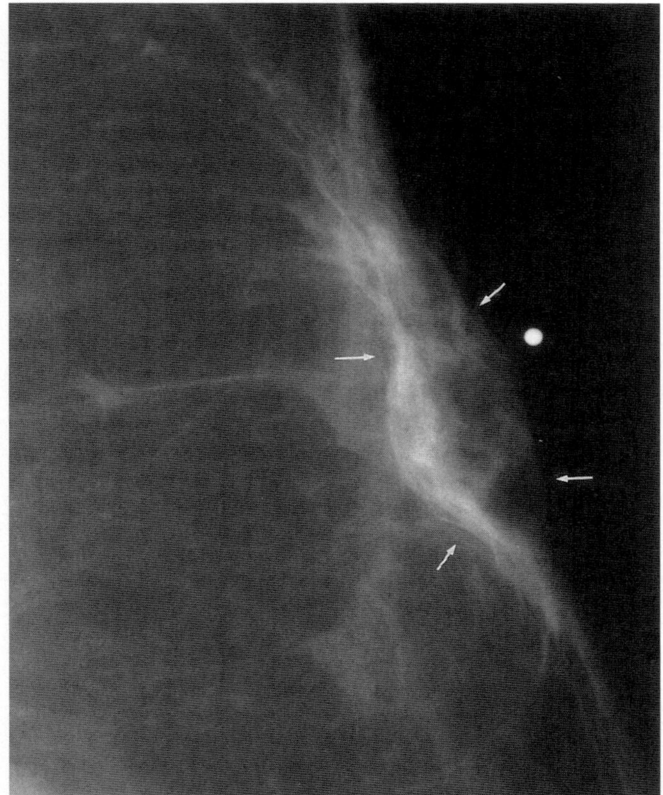

Figure 25–53. Fat necrosis after dog bite to the breast. This fat-density superficial mass *(arrows)* has peripheral fibrosis but does not contain calcification.

ill-defined uniformly hyperechoic area, usually in the superficial tissue of the breast (Fig. 25–54)

Pathology

On histologic examination, fat necrosis is recognized by the loss of nuclei, fusion of adipocytes resulting in fatty spaces of varying sizes, and accumulation of foamy histiocytes, cholesterol crystals, and calcifications (Fig. 25–55A and B). Some of the histiocytes fuse into multinucleated giant cells (Fig. 25–55C). A mixed inflammatory reaction consisting of lymphocytes, polymorphs, and plasma cells may also be seen. The fibroblasts surrounding the area of fat necrosis form a fibrous band in the periphery of the lesion, creating a zone of denser tissue in the

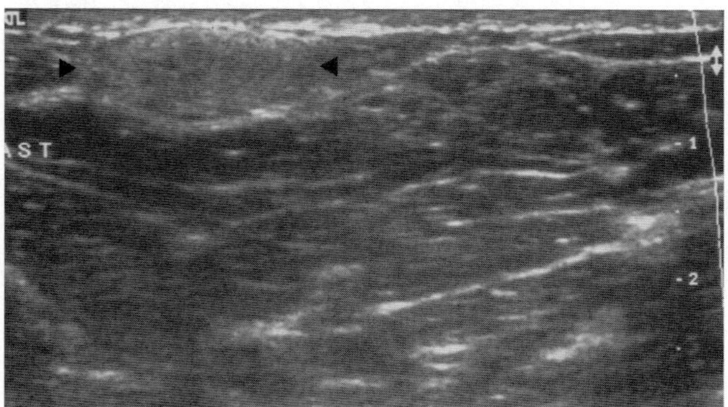

Figure 25–54. Ultrasound of fat necrosis. The superficial hyperechoic mass *(arrowheads)* developed after blunt trauma to the breast and resolved on follow-up examination.

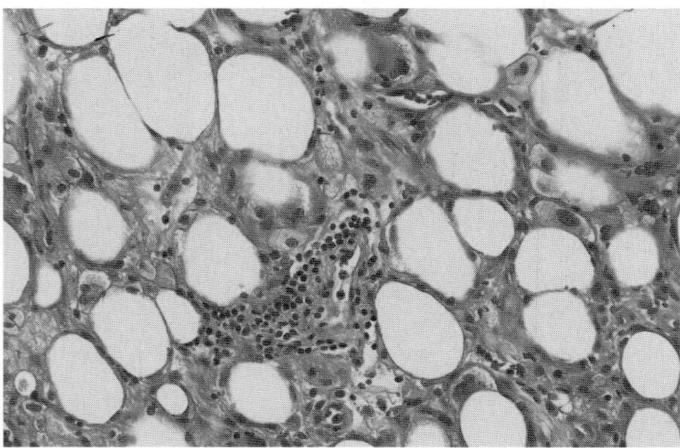

A

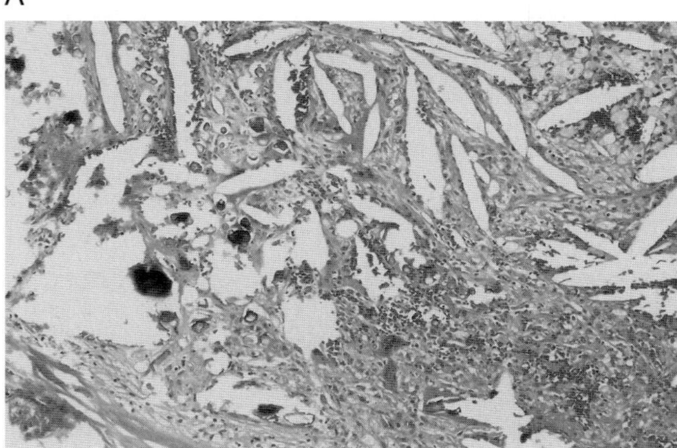

B

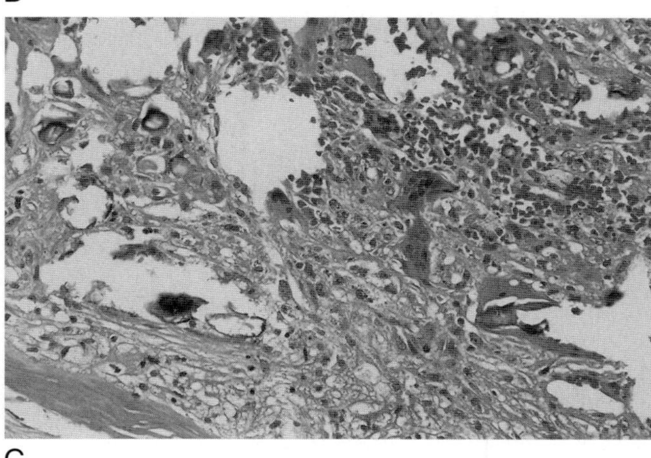

C

Figure 25–55. Fat necrosis. **A,** Disruption of the adipocytes has occurred, with the released fat forming vacuolated spaces surrounded by foamy macrophages and lymphocytes. **B,** Collections of needle-like cholesterol clefts, macrophages, and purple microcalcifications. **C,** A higher magnification reveals multinucleated giant cells, hemosiderin-laden macrophages, red blood cells, and microcalcifications.

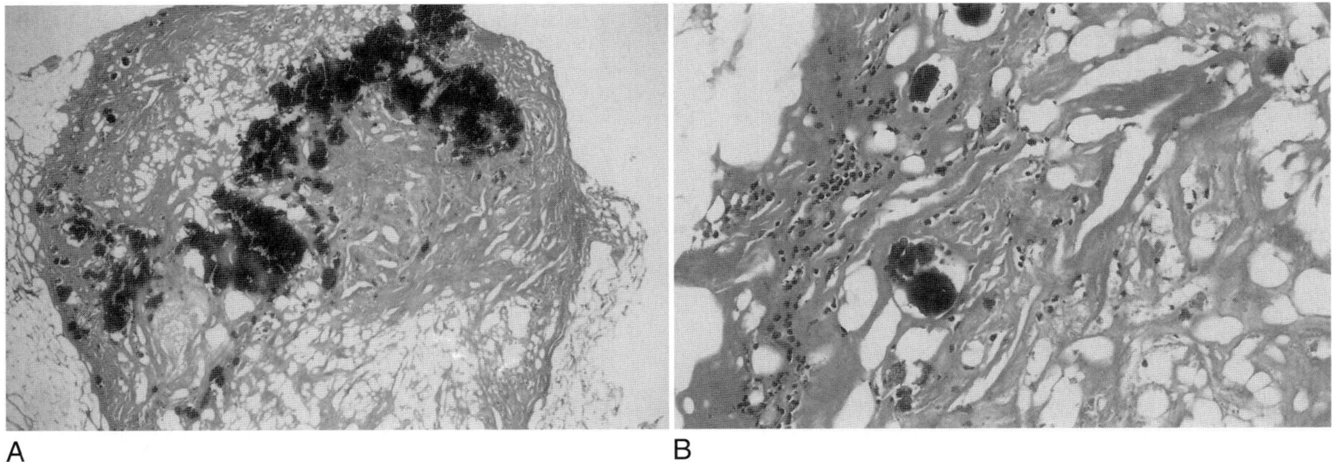

Figure 25–56. Fat necrosis in a late stage. **A,** Necrotic adipose tissue is replaced by acellular fibrous stroma and a large amount of irregular pleomorphic microcalcification. **B,** A higher magnification reveals necrotic fat (right field) and microcalcifications (left field).

periphery, with the more radiolucent necrotic area in the center. Eventually, the area of necrosis is replaced by dense fibrous tissue, with a few oil-filled vacuoles remaining. Calcification sometimes occurs within the necrotic fat (Fig. 25–56).

FOREIGN BODIES

The most common foreign bodies seen within the breast mammographically are metallic bullet fragments (Fig. 25–57). Occasionally, the particles are small enough to mimic microcalcifications, but careful attention to the very high radiographic density of the fragments should prevent confusion (see Figs. 25–57 to 25–59). Other metal objects, such as sewing needles or fragments of localizing wires, are occasionally found (Fig. 25–60). One of the few nonmetallic foreign bodies that are mammographically visible is the retained Dacron cuff of a Hickman central venous catheter, which has a characteristic appearance (Fig. 25–61).[38] Foreign body reaction or

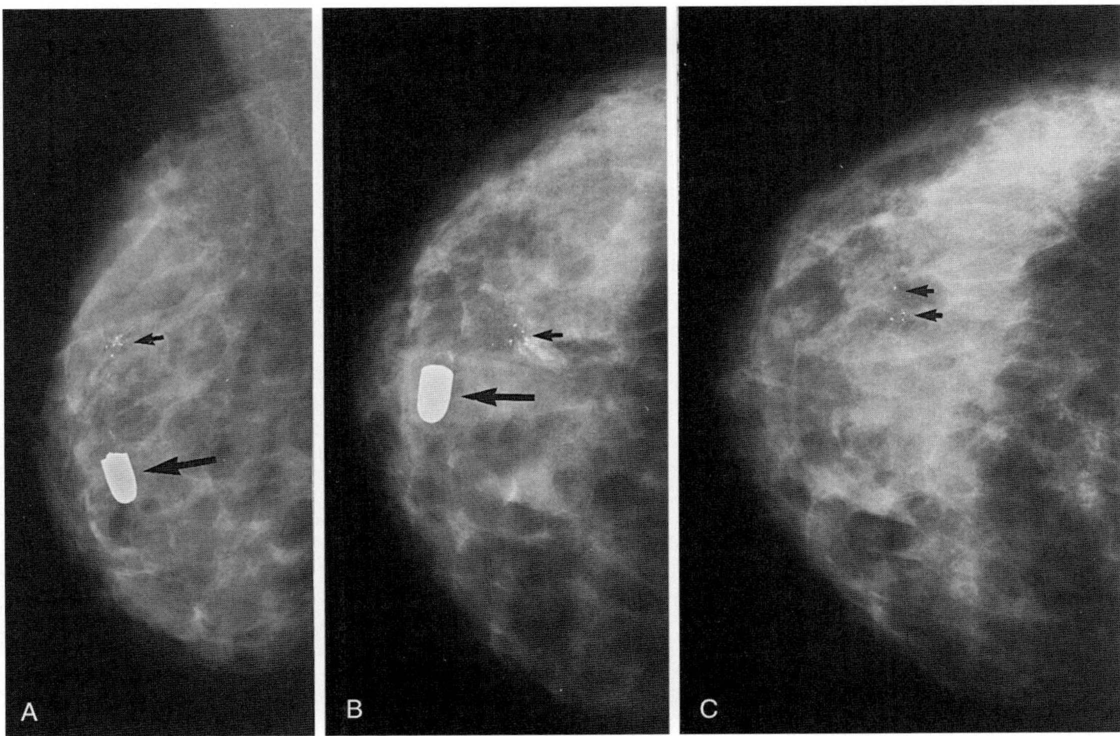

Figure 25–57. Bullet in the breast after a gunshot wound. The right mediolateral oblique **(A)** and craniocaudal (CC) **(B)** mammograms demonstrate a bullet (*large arrow*) in the subareolar region of the breast, with a cluster of small metallic bullet fragments at the 11-o'clock position of the breast (*small arrow*). On a routine screening mammogram 2 years after removal of the large bullet **(C),** the cluster of small metallic fragments *(arrows)* is more dispersed on this CC view because the woman has gained weight in the interval. The metallic fragments are too radiographically dense for their size to be calcifications.

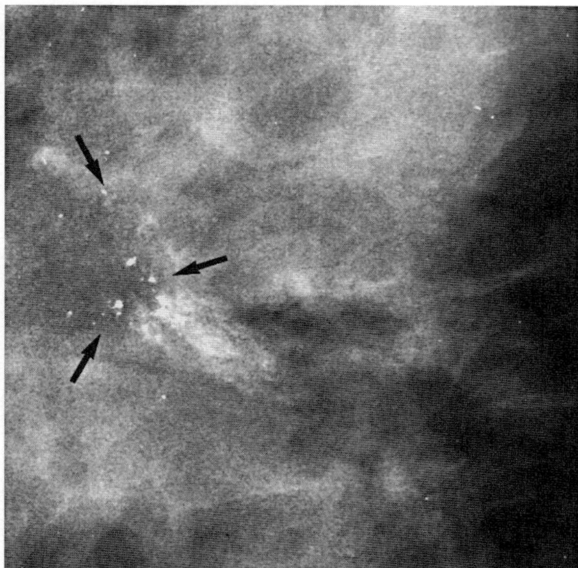

Figure 25–58. Bullet fragments. Small metallic bullet fragments in the breast after a gunshot wound *(arrows)*. In this case, the fragments range in size from approximately 0.5 to 2 mm. The fragments are too radiographically dense for their size to be calcifications.

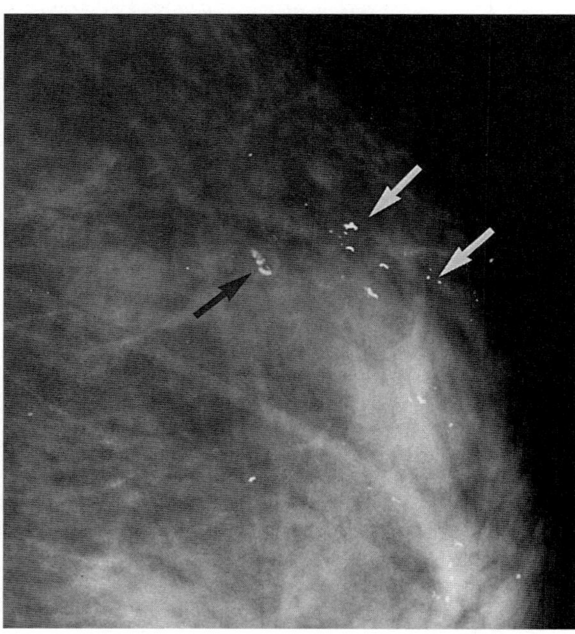

Figure 25–59. Bullet fragments. Metallic bullet fragments *(white arrows)* and benign calcifications *(black arrow)* in the same region of the breast. Note the difference in radiographic density of the two materials.

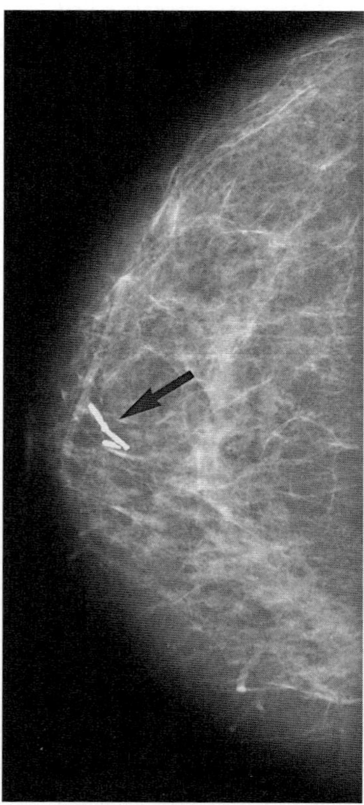

Figure 25–60. Foreign body. Fragmented sewing needle *(arrow)* in the subareolar region of the right breast.

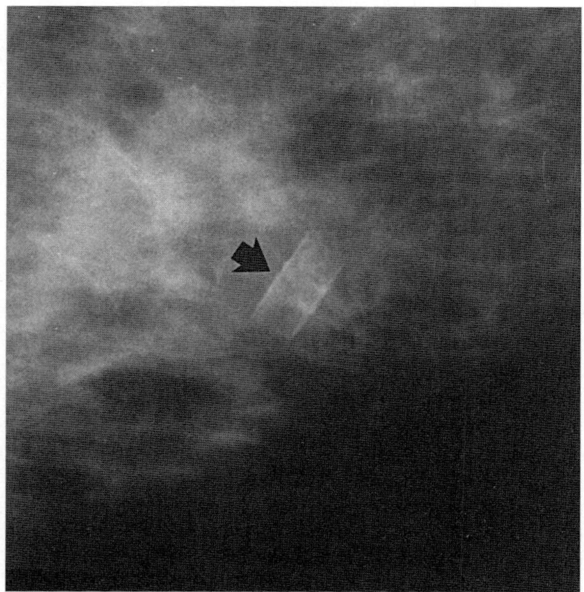

Figure 25–61. Retained Hickman catheter Dacron cuff *(arrow)*.

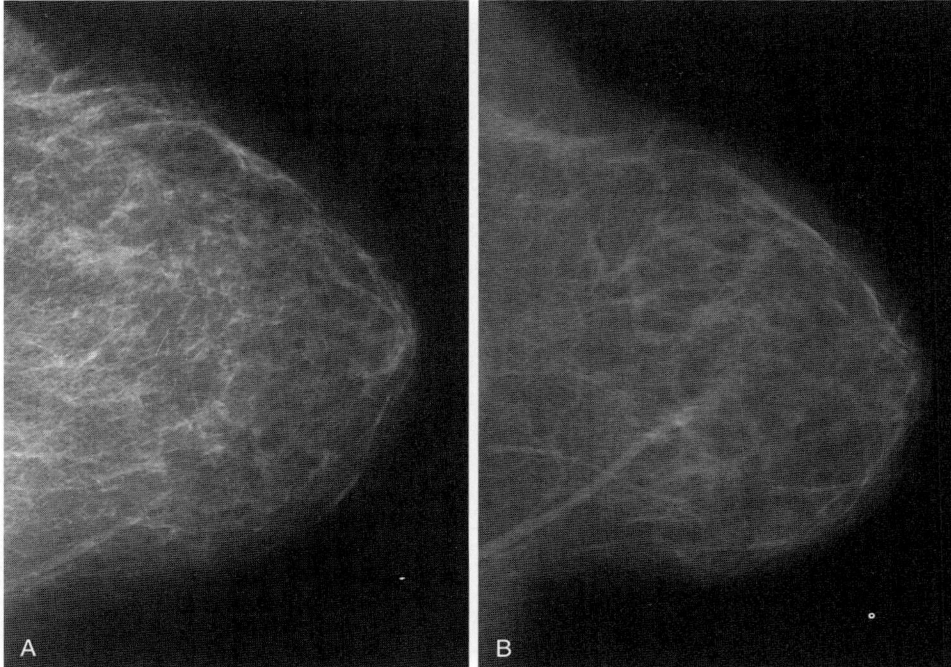

Figure 25–62. Mastitis. The right craniocaudal mammogram **(A)** obtained during the episode of mastitis demonstrates diffuse trabecular thickening, which resolved when the mammogram was repeated after treatment **(B)**.

abscess formation around foreign bodies may produce an ill-defined or spiculated mass and mimic carcinoma.[39] The visualization of the foreign object within the mass should establish the benign diagnosis.

INFECTIONS OF THE BREAST

Clinical Aspects

Most cases of mastitis and breast abscess occur during lactation and are due to *Staphylococcus aureus* and streptococcal bacteria.[40] Many infections are due to mixed flora, however.[40] The infection is due to disruption of the epithelial interface of the nipple-areolar complex with retrograde dissemination of the organisms. In streptococcal infections, a diffuse cellulitis or mastitis usually is present, with focal abscess formation in advanced stages. *S. aureus* abscesses tend to be more localized and invasive from the onset, with acute and chronic abscess formation. Women who are not lactating, particularly heavy smokers, may also develop retrograde infections with these bacteria, often with the development of relatively superficial periareolar abscesses.[40] Rarely, the breast may become infected with echinococcosis,[41,42] blastomycosis,[43] schistosomiasis,[44] loiasis,[45] tuberculosis,[46] or other granulomatous and parasitic diseases. A complete history and organism culture are necessary to make the diagnosis.

Imaging Features

When mammography is performed, the most common findings in mastitis are skin and trabecular thickening from breast edema (Figs. 25–62 to 25–64). These findings may be diffuse or focal. Pain and edema usually limit the compressibility of the breast; therefore, image quality is often compromised in these patients. When mammographically visible within the edema, abscesses are usually ill-defined

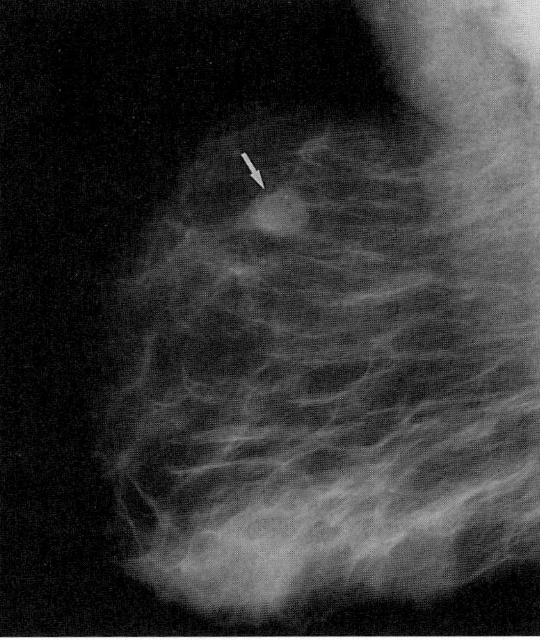

Figure 25–63. Mastitis with reactive lymph node. The right mediolateral oblique mammogram demonstrates trabecular thickening and ill-defined density inferiorly. The circumscribed mass *(arrow)* in the upper-outer quadrant was ultrasonographically shown to be a lymph node. The node returned to normal size after antibiotic therapy.

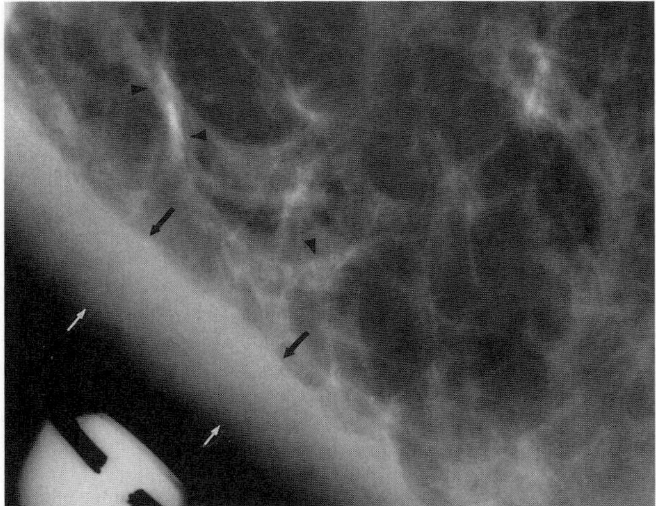

Figure 25–64. Mastitis with massive skin *(arrows)* and trabecular *(arrowheads)* thickening.

noncalcified masses (Figs. 25–65 and 25–66). Air is very rarely seen within an abscess. The differential diagnosis from the mammogram includes inflammatory carcinoma and other invasive breast carcinomas. Many physicians advocate prompt biopsy to differentiate between infection and malignancy, particularly for nonlactating women, whereas others give a trial of antibiotics. If an abscess is present, biopsy should be performed at the time of surgical or percutaneous drainage.

Ultrasonography is an ideal imaging method for the detection of focal breast abscesses.[47] Most women easily tolerate the gentle compression of the US transducer. As a cross-sectional imaging method, ultrasonography depicts abscess cavities within the area of infection and inflammation. The skin thickening and breast edema are easily seen on ultrasonographic examination (Fig. 25–67). Abscesses are usually irregular hypoechoic or anechoic masses with ill-defined margins, sometimes with fluid/debris levels and usually with posterior acoustic enhancement (see Figs. 25–67 to 25–69). Rarely, air within an abscess may produce bright specular reflections (Fig. 25–70). The size and exact location of the abscess are visible, allowing for accurate localization

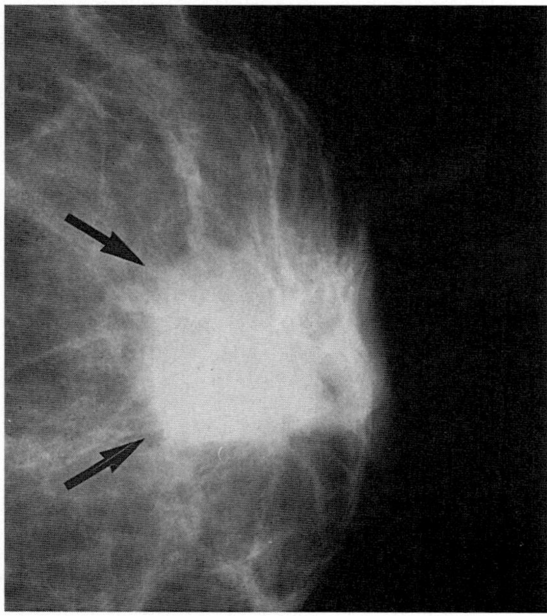

Figure 25–65. Subareolar abscess *(arrows)*. The margins are spiculated.

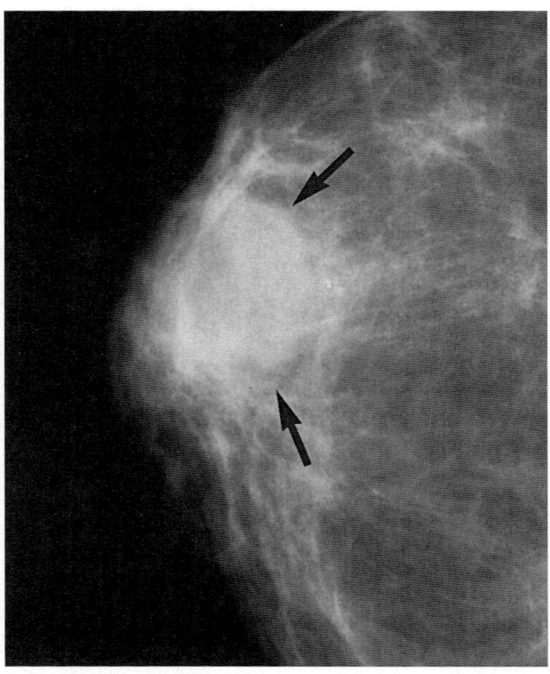

Figure 25–66. Subareolar abscess *(arrows)* with ill-defined margins.

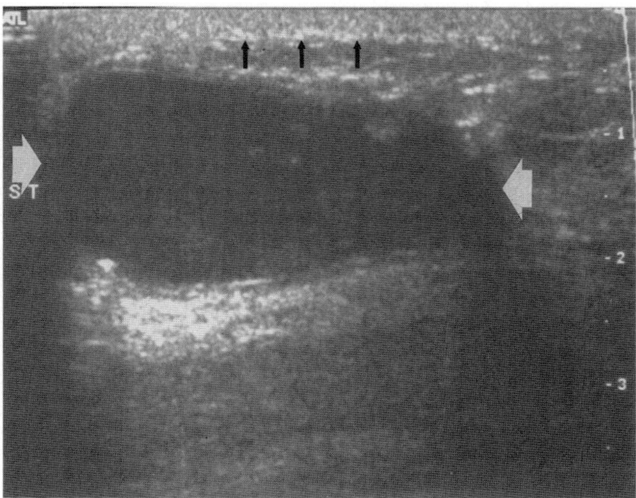

Figure 25–67. Abscess. Ultrasonogram of a 3.5-cm breast abscess *(white arrows)*. The margins are indistinct, and there are low-level internal echoes. The overlying skin is thickened *(black arrows)*.

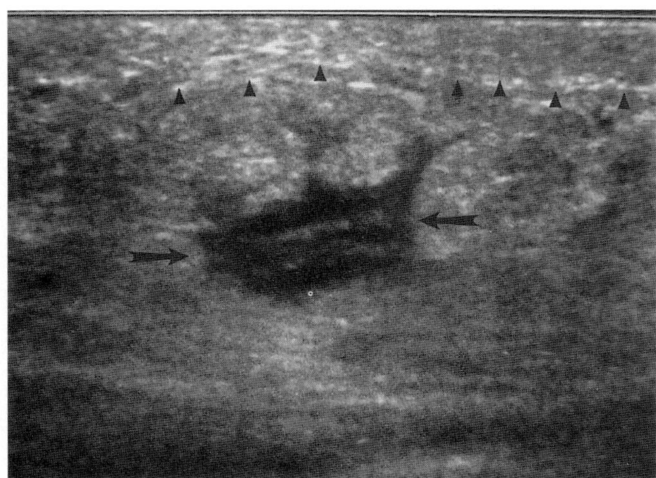

Figure 25–68. Abscess. There is a 1.5-cm irregular hypoechoic mass with angular and indistinct margins *(arrows)*. There is surrounding increased echogenicity and skin thickening *(arrowheads)*.

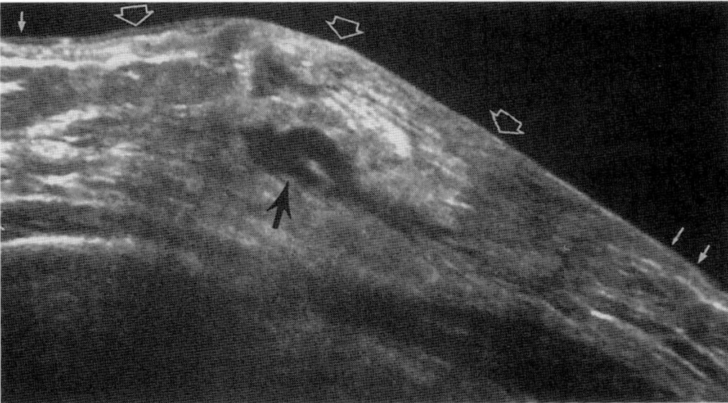

Figure 25–69. Mastitis with small abscess. Panoramic ultrasound demonstrates the transition between normal (*small white arrows*) and inflamed breast tissue (*open arrows*). The fat is abnormally echogenic, and there is loss of the normal architecture within the area of inflammation. A small irregular abscess cavity is visible within the area of mastitis *(black arrow)*.

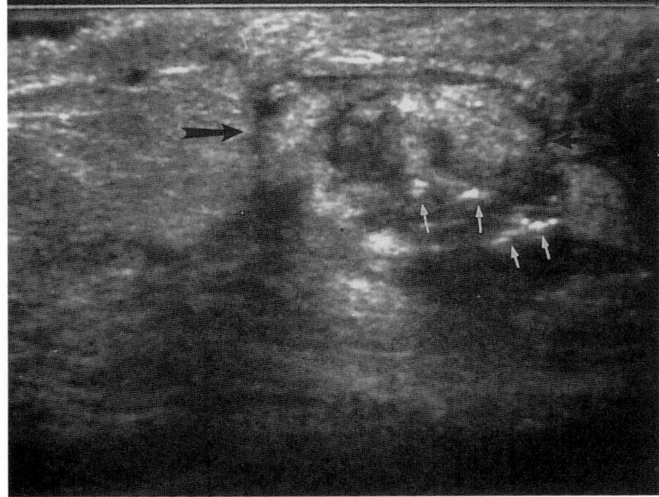

Figure 25–70. Abscess *(black arrows)* containing air. Bright specular reflections *(white arrows)* within the 2.5-cm ill-defined heterogeneous mass are from the air within the lesion.

for treatment and therapy monitoring. Although most breast abscesses are treated with surgical incision and drainage,[40] US-guided percutaneous drainage may be an acceptable alternative.[48,49]

The mammographic findings in unusual granulomatous and parasitic infections are usually nonspecific and may include diffuse breast edema, masses, and calcifications (Figs. 25–71 and 25–72). Trichinosis infection may be seen mammographically as diffuse punctate microcalcifications limited to the pectoralis muscles bilaterally (Fig. 25–73).[50]

In addition to the infectious mastitis discussed earlier, local inflammatory reaction may occur in

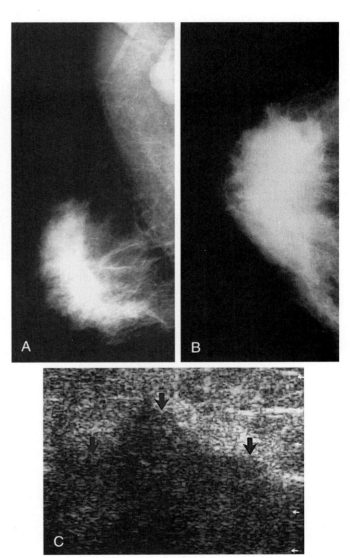

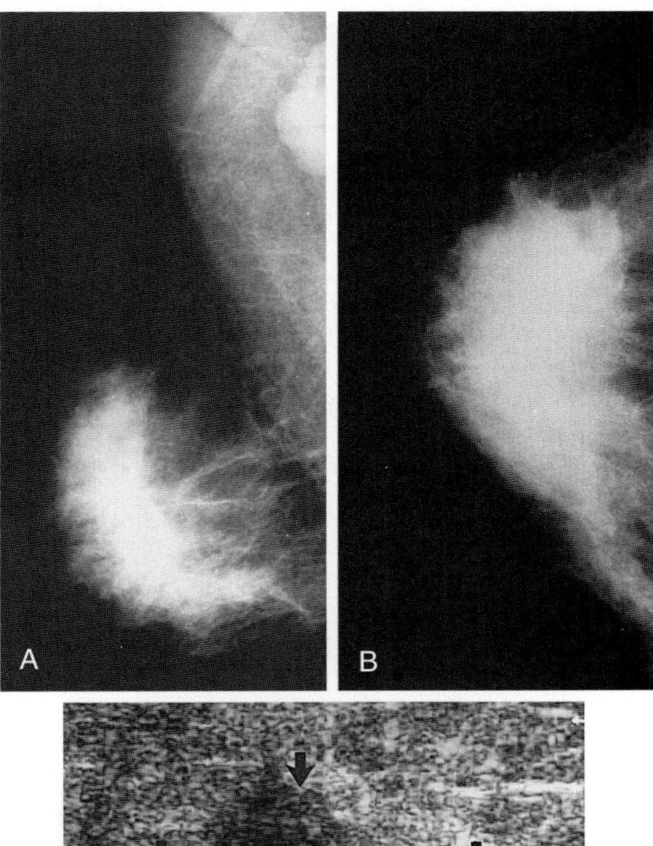

Figure 25–71. Granulomatous mastitis. A 45-year-old woman with a 1-month history of right breast swelling and increased firmness. The mediolateral oblique **(A)** and craniocaudal **(B)** mammograms demonstrate asymmetrical increased density throughout most of the right breast and right axillary adenopathy. The 7.5-MHz real-time ultrasonogram **(C)** shows mild diffuse architectural distortion with marked attenuation of the US beam *(arrows)*, without a discrete mass or fluid collection.

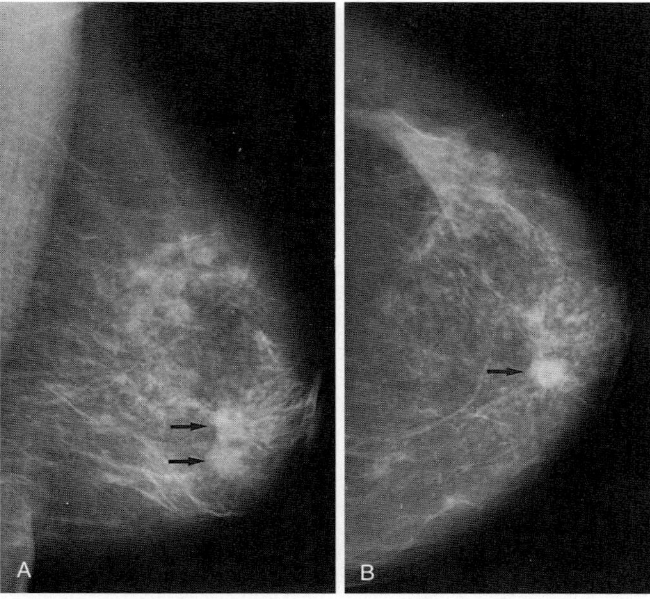

Figure 25–72. Granulomatous mastitis. A 1.5-cm spiculated mass at 9 o'clock in the medial left breast *(arrows)*.

response to inspissated secretion or an immune response with accumulation of plasma cells (plasma cell mastitis), granulomatous formation (granulomatous mastitis),[51] or lymphocytic infiltration (lymphocytic mastitis).

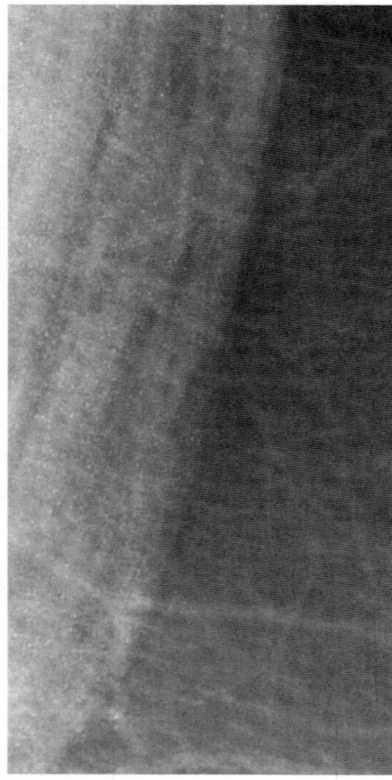

Figure 25–73. Trichinosis. Diffuse punctate microcalcifications are seen throughout the pectoralis muscle. These were bilateral, and no calcifications were present within the breast parenchyma. (Courtesy Jan Patterson, MD, San Francisco, CA.)

FIBROADENOMAS

Clinical Aspects

Fibroadenomas are the most common breast masses encountered in women younger than 35 years and the most common solid masses found in women of all ages. They usually do not develop de novo after menopause. When clinically apparent, these round, oval, or lobular circumscribed masses are usually firm and freely mobile and may change with the menstrual cycle or pregnancy. The peak age of incidence is between the ages of 20 and 30 years.[52] Most cease growth when they reach 2 to 3 cm in diameter,[53] but giant fibroadenomas may exceed 6 cm in diameter.[54] Fibroadenomas are multiple in approximately 15% to 20% of cases.[52,55] Many fibroadenomas begin to involute in the postpartum period and after menopause, with hyaline degeneration and subsequent calcification. Rarely, fibroadenomas enlarge in postmenopausal women, with or without hormone replacement therapy.[56,57] A solid mass that enlarges in a postmenopausal woman should not be assumed to be a fibroadenoma. This is suspicious for malignancy, and biopsy should be performed.

Imaging Features

On mammography, fibroadenomas are usually circumscribed round, oval, or lobular low- or equal-density radiopaque masses (Figs. 25–74 to 25–76). They are usually mammographically indistinguishable from cysts; therefore, ultrasonography is useful to demonstrate the solid nature of these lesions (Fig. 25–77). Involuting fibroadenomas have typical coarse calcification, which usually begins at the periphery of the mass and moves centrally, often completely replacing the soft-tissue mass itself (Figs. 25–78 to 25–81). When calcifications are present within the mass, obviously US is not necessary. Some fibroadenomas have "atypical" mammographic appearances, mimicking carcinoma with irregular shapes, indistinct or spiculated margins, or pleomorphic microcalcifications (Figs. 25–82 to 25–84).

Fibroadenomas have many appearances on ultrasonography. The typical US finding is an oval, circumscribed, homogeneous solid mass with internal echoes, often isoechoic or slightly hypoechoic to fat (Fig. 25–85).[58,59] Many "atypical" findings are seen, including irregular, microlobulated, or ill-defined masses (Fig. 25–86), attenuating masses, and ultrasonographically "invisible" masses.[58,60-62] In addition, other benign and malignant processes have ultrasonographic features that mimic "classic" fibroadenomas.[62,63]

Fibroadenomas account for many benign breast biopsies. Therefore, a number of researchers have tried to distinguish benign from malignant lesions, primarily using US features such as the configuration

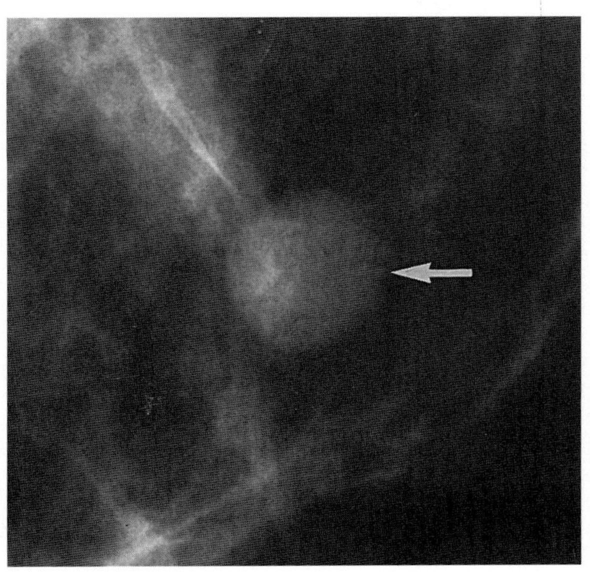

Figure 25–74. Fibroadenoma. The 1-cm mass *(arrow)* is round and has circumscribed margins.

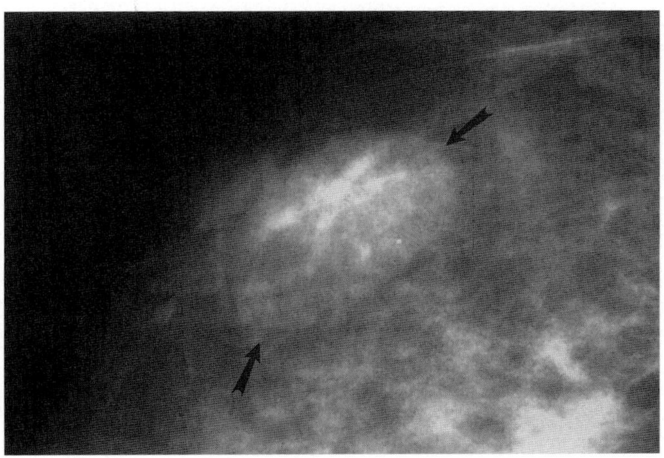

Figure 25–75. Fibroadenoma. This 2-cm oval mass *(arrows)* has circumscribed margins.

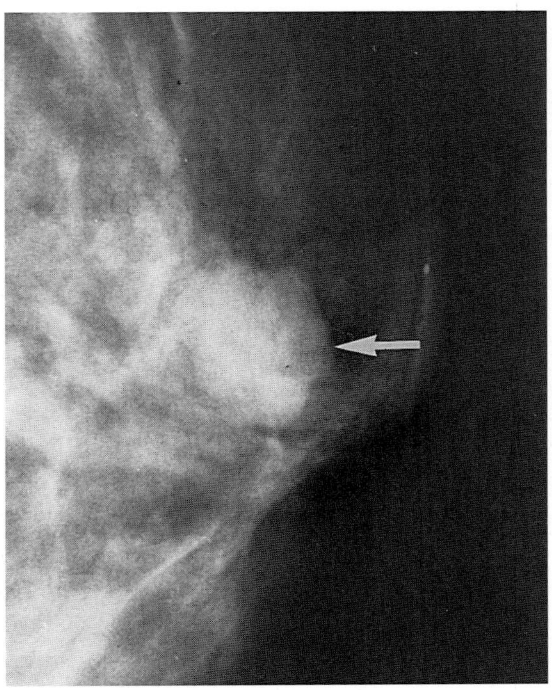

Figure 25–76. Fibroadenoma. A 1.2-cm lobular subareolar mass *(arrow)*.

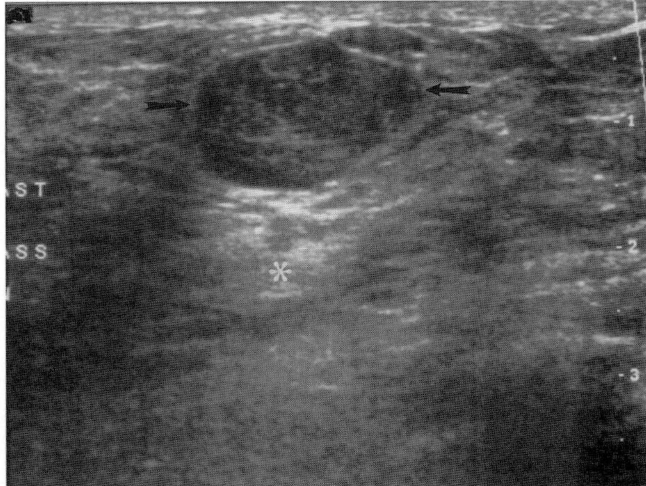

Figure 25–77. Fibroadenoma. Ultrasonogram of a 1.3-cm oval circumscribed mass *(arrows)*, which contains relatively homogeneous internal echoes. Mild posterior acoustic enhancement is seen (*asterisk*).

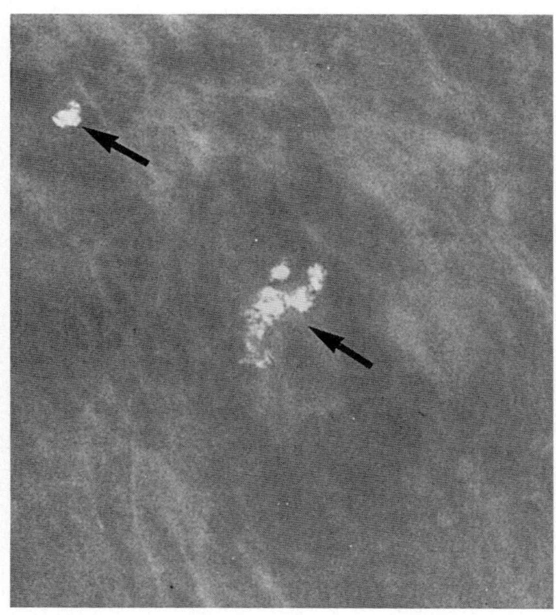

Figure 25–78. Involuting fibroadenomas. Coarse calcifications *(arrows)* are present in two involuting fibroadenomas. The soft tissue masses are no longer visible.

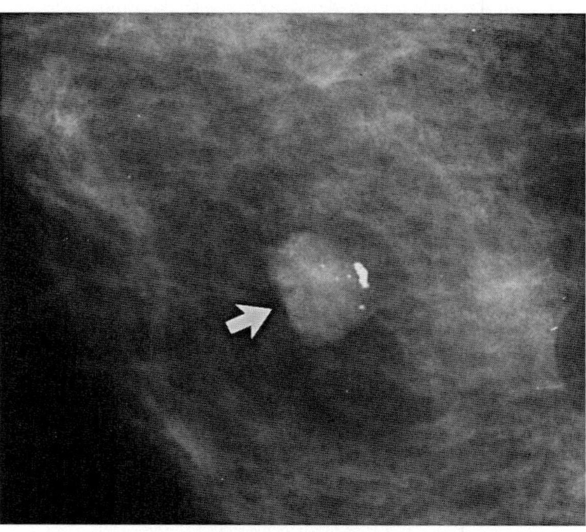

Figure 25–79. Involuting fibroadenoma. Early peripheral calcification is present in this 1-cm mass *(arrow)*.

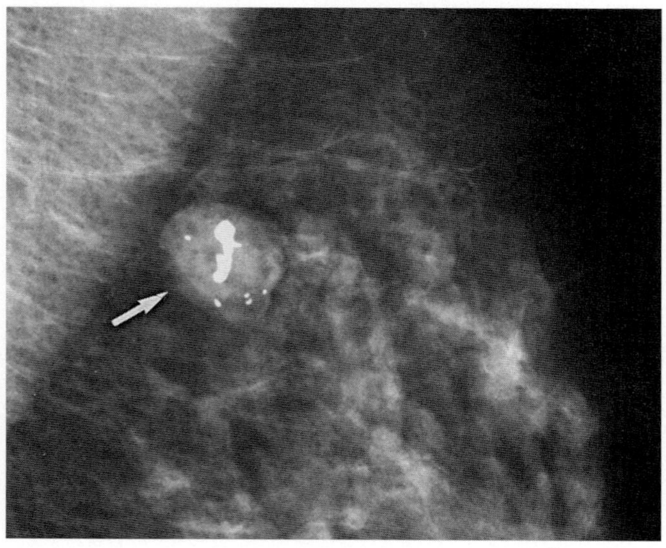

Figure 25–80. Involuting fibroadenoma. Coarse calcifications in a 2-cm involuting fibroadenoma *(arrow)*. The circumscribed soft tissue mass is clearly visible in this case.

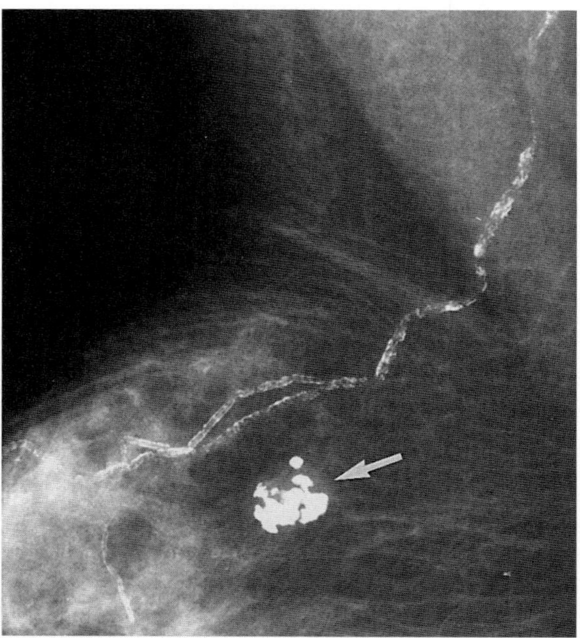

Figure 25–81. Involuting fibroadenoma. The majority of this 1.5-cm involuting fibroadenoma *(arrow)* contains coarse calcifications.

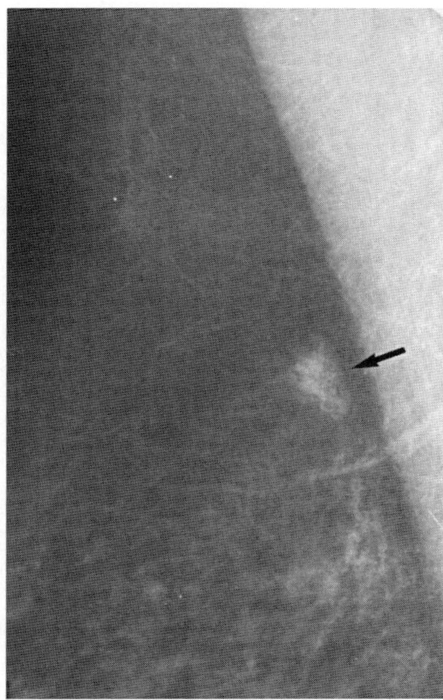

Figure 25–82. Fibroadenoma with atypical mammographic appearance. A 1-cm irregular mass with indistinct margins *(arrow)*.

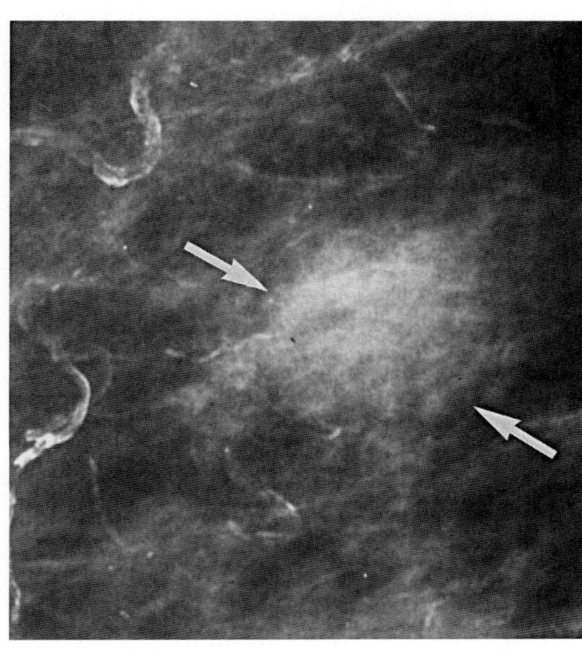

Figure 25–83. Fibroadenoma with atypical mammographic appearance. A 1.5-cm ill-defined mass *(arrows)*.

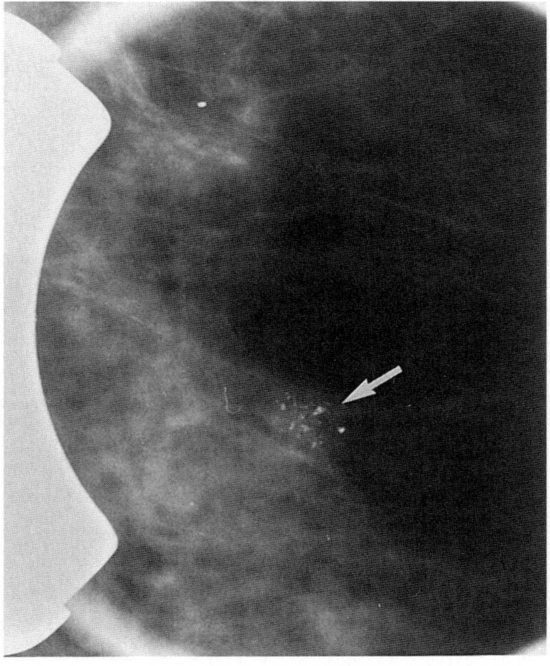

Figure 25–84. Fibroadenoma with atypical mammographic appearance. This 8-mm indistinct mass contains multiple central pleomorphic microcalcifications *(arrow)*, suspicious for malignancy.

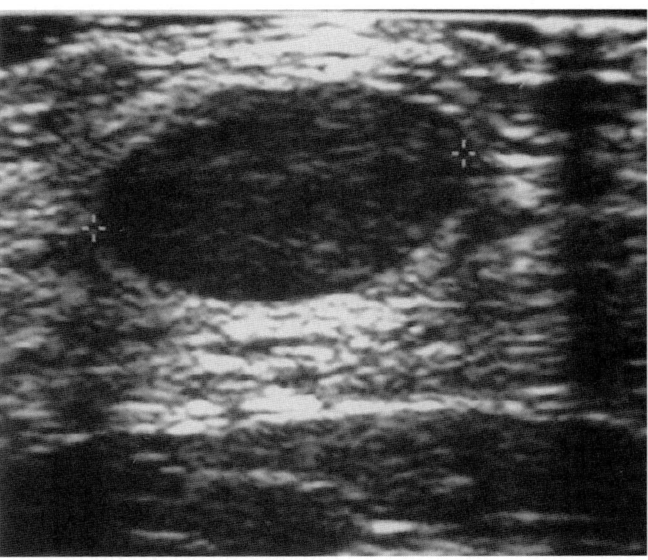

Figure 25–85. Fibroadenoma with "typical" ultrasonographic appearance. The mass (*calipers*) is circumscribed and oval and contains relatively homogeneous low-level internal echoes. In this case, posterior acoustic enhancement is seen.

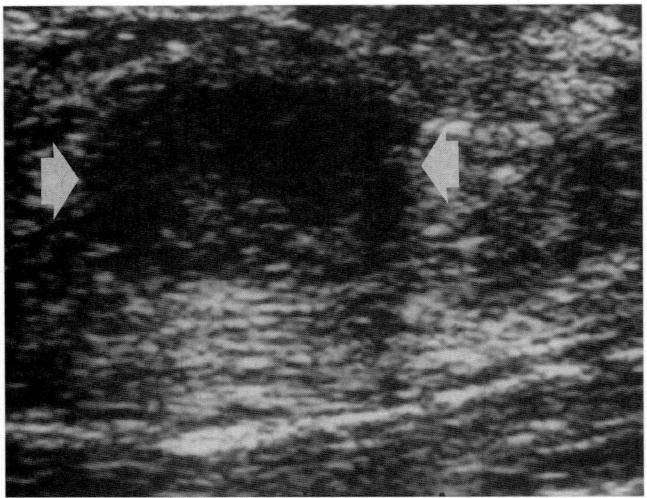

Figure 25–86. Ill-defined fibroadenoma. On ultrasonography, the 1.2-cm fibroadenoma *(arrows)* has indistinct margins and heterogeneous internal echoes.

of the lesion (parallel or not parallel to the skin), the internal echogenicity, margin and surrounding tissue characteristics, location within the breast, and Doppler flow characteristics.[59,64-72] With improved US equipment and refinement of interpretation criteria, US has potential to be clinically useful in the diagnosis of fibroadenomas.[71]

For a woman younger than 25 or 30 years with a "typical" ultrasonographic or mammographic appearance, close clinical follow-up is often an appropriate method of management. For women older than 30 years without previous mammograms for comparison, one should assess the margins of the lesion with spot-compression magnification views. If a solid lesion is completely circumscribed, the management often depends on the size of the mass and the clinical findings. Controversy exists regarding the size threshold for follow-up mammography versus immediate biopsy. In a large series, Sickles[73] showed that size need not be a basis for management decisions for completely circumscribed *nonpalpable* solid masses. Nonetheless, in many practices, close-interval follow-up is usually recommended for such lesions less than approximately 2 cm in diameter, and biopsy is often recommended for larger lesions.

Several benign lesions are related to fibroadenomas. Tubular adenomas are uncommon lesions with dominant tubular elements and minimal supporting stroma.[74] Lactating adenomas occur during pregnancy and lactation and have prominent lobular and tubular anatomy, with secretory activity.[75] Juvenile fibroadenomas occur in adolescents and are characterized by increased cellularity of the stroma or epithelium, often with rapid growth and large size.[76] All of these lesions are indistinguishable from fibroadenomas on mammography and ultrasonography.

The risk of development of carcinoma within fibroadenomas is no higher than the risk of breast carcinoma for the general population. Many of the reported cases of fibroadenomas associated with cancer have had ductal or lobular carcinoma in situ adjacent to the fibroadenoma, but several cases of carcinoma truly within fibroadenomas have been reported (Fig. 25–87).[77-79]

Pathology

Fibroadenomas are benign tumors composed of varying amounts of fibrous and epithelial elements. Gross examination shows a circumscribed rubbery nodule. Its edge is clearly demarcated from the surrounding tissue without a true capsule (Fig. 25–88). Microscopically, proliferation of both the stromal and epithelial components of the breast exists, although the fibrous component comprises most of the tumor (Fig. 25–89). Two different growth patterns have been described, intracanalicular and pericanalicular. The fibroblastic stroma can enclose the glandular elements, compressing them into slitlike spaces (intracanalicular fibroadenoma) (Fig. 25–90), or the glands may maintain their round or oval shape within the proliferating fibrous tissue (pericanalicular fibroadenoma). These different growth patterns, however, have no practical or prognostic significance.

The epithelial elements in fibroadenoma can be hyperplastic in young women but are atrophic in the postmenopausal female. The stromal component of the tumor may show considerable variation in cellularity. It may be moderately cellular with rare mitotic figures, simulating a phyllodes tumor. Its lack of nuclear atypia separates it from the phyllodes tumor. Fibroadenomas may also be myxoid and hypocellular. The less-cellular stroma with hyalinization and

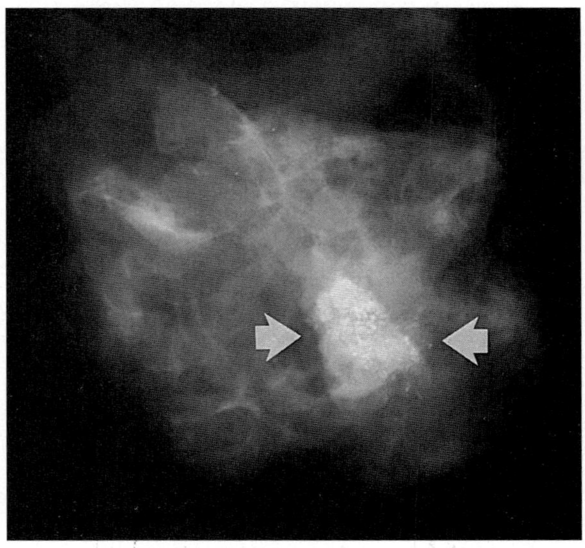

Figure 25–87. Fibroadenoma containing ductal carcinoma in situ. Specimen radiograph of an irregular mass with pleomorphic microcalcifications *(arrows)*.

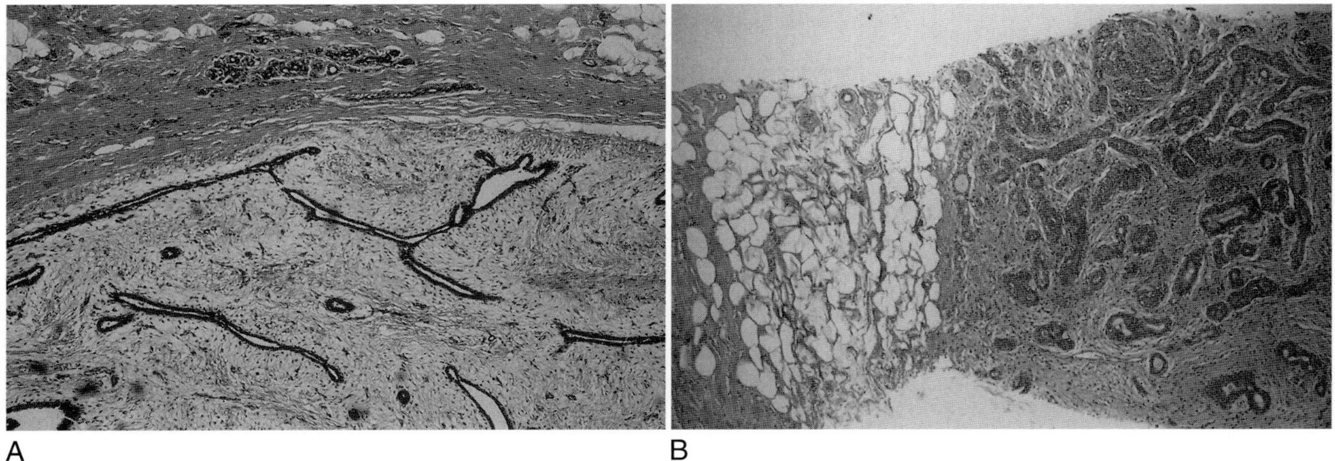

Figure 25–88. Fibroadenoma. **A,** It has a smooth border with a compressed fibrous capsule. The fibroadenoma consists of branching hyperplastic ducts and edematous, slightly cellular fibrous stroma. **B,** In a core needle biopsy, there is a smooth interface between the normal fatty breast tissue and the fibroadenoma. In the latter, branching hyperplastic ducts are surrounded by basophilic myxoid stroma in a pericanalicular growth pattern.

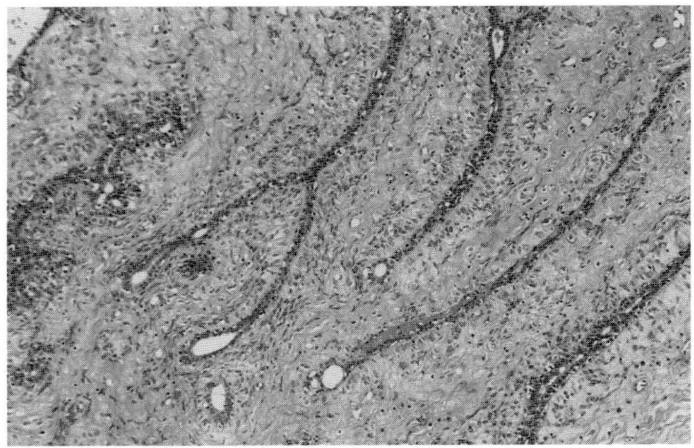

Figure 25–89. Fibroadenoma. The tumor shows predominantly an intracanalicular growth pattern, with the ducts compressed into slitlike spaces by a benign, mildly cellular fibrous stroma.

fibrosis tends to occur in older patients. Further involution can lead to calcification (see Fig. 25–90).

Several variants of fibroadenomas have been described. The giant fibroadenoma is simply a fibroadenoma that has reached a large size. No official size criteria have been set for a giant fibroadenoma, although the term is typically reserved for those larger than 6 to 8 cm. On microscopic examination, these can exhibit any of the features described previously. Juvenile fibroadenomas are also described as a separate variant. The term is reserved for fibroadenomas that occur in an adolescent. On histologic examination, they can have features of a typical fibroadenoma. They do tend to be more cellular and are often very large, which qualifies them as giant fibroadenoma.

Fibroadenomas may rarely give rise to in-situ and invasive carcinoma, most frequently lobular

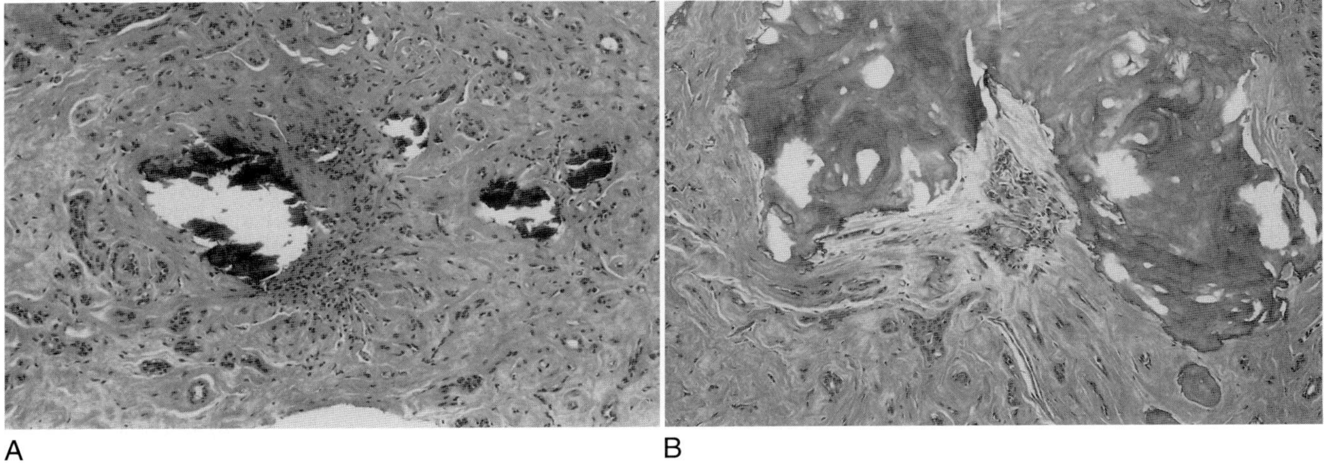

Figure 25–90. Involuting fibroadenoma with microcalcification **(A)** and ossification **(B)**. The fibrous stroma is hypocellular to acellular, and the ducts are atrophic.

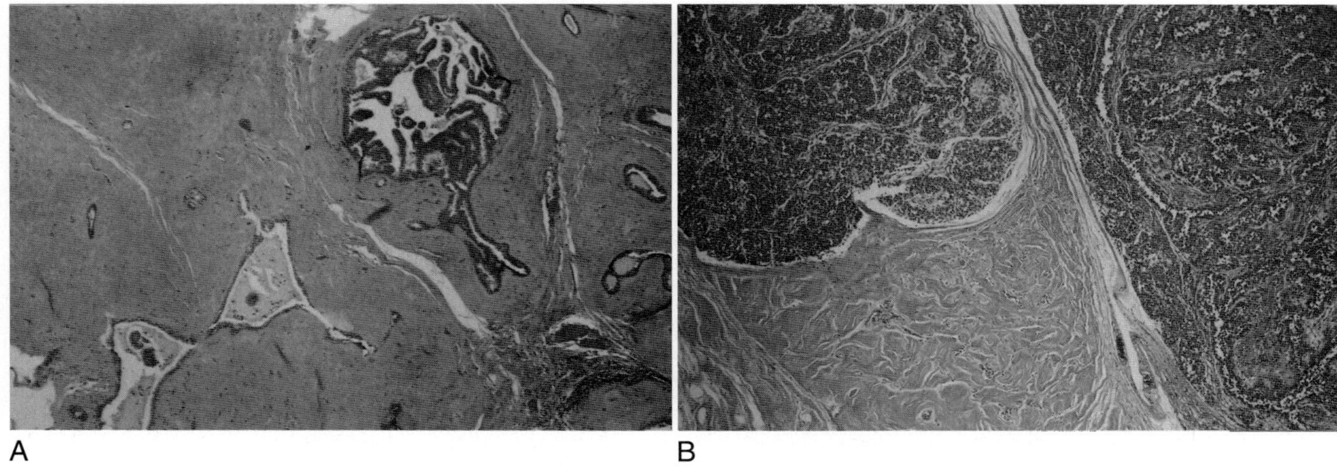

Figure 25–91. Fibroadenoma with micropapillary ductal carcinoma in situ **(A)** and lobular carcinoma in situ **(B)**.

carcinoma in situ, followed by ductal carcinoma in situ (Fig. 25–91). Invasive carcinomas within fibroadenomas are exceedingly rare.

HAMARTOMAS

Clinical Aspects

Hamartomas are unusual circumscribed benign breast lesions composed of variable amounts of fat, glandular tissue, and fibrous connective tissue.[80,81] Other names, such as *fibroadenolipoma* and *lipofibroadenoma*, have been used to reflect the dominant type of tissue within the mass. Many hamartomas are asymptomatic, but some are palpable as soft or firm masses, depending on the ratio of fat to fibroepithelial elements within the tumor. Large, predominantly fatty hamartomas are often impalpable, whereas lesions with a large fibrous component often mimic fibroadenomas or carcinomas on physical examination. The majority are detected in women older than 35 years.[82]

Imaging Features

The classic mammographic appearance of a breast hamartoma is virtually diagnostic. The lesion is circumscribed and contains both fat and soft-tissue density surrounded by a thin radiopaque capsule, which is visible when fat is identified on both sides.[80,83-85] The appearance is similar to a "cut sausage" on radiography (Figs. 25–92 and 25–93). Although many of these lesions do not have a true fibrous capsule,[82] a thin radiopaque pseudocapsule is usually seen around at least a portion of the mass (Fig. 25–94). Hamartomas containing predominantly soft-tissue density are more difficult to diagnose mammographically. Some have only a small amount of fat beneath the capsule (Fig. 25–95), and others have so little fat that they mimic a fibroadenoma or carcinoma on mammography.[84] Such atypical cases would require close-interval follow-up mammography or biopsy, depending on the lesion's size, imaging features, and clinical findings.

When the typical mammographic appearance is present, there is no indication for ultrasonography. For those lesions that present atypically as a circumscribed, completely radiopaque mass, however, ultrasonography is usually performed to distinguish between a cyst and a solid mass. The

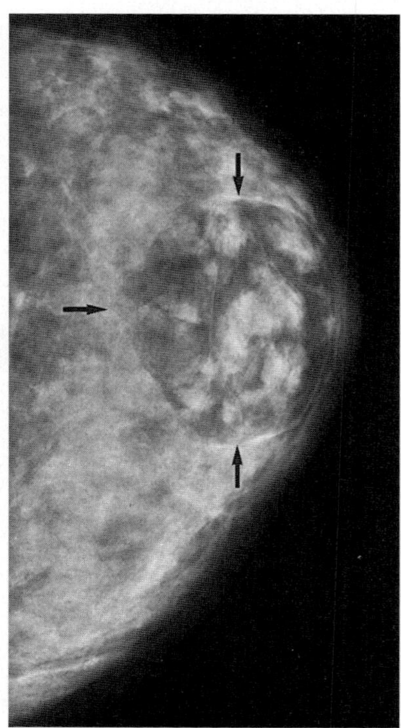

Figure 25–92. Hamartoma. A 4-cm oval circumscribed mass *(arrows)* containing both fat and soft-tissue density in the subareolar region of the left breast.

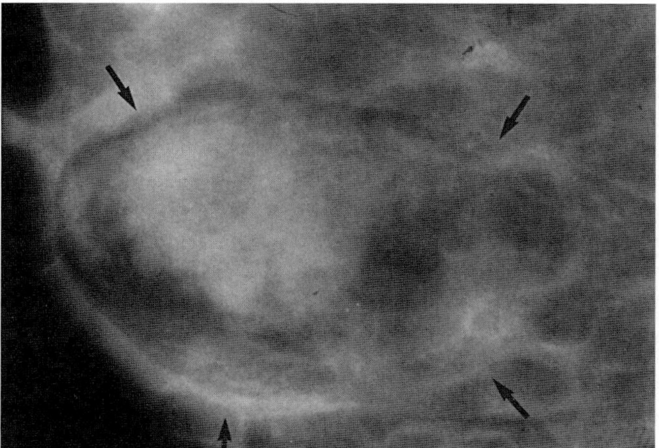

Figure 25–93. Hamartoma. A 3-cm oval circumscribed mass *(arrows)* containing both fat and soft-tissue density.

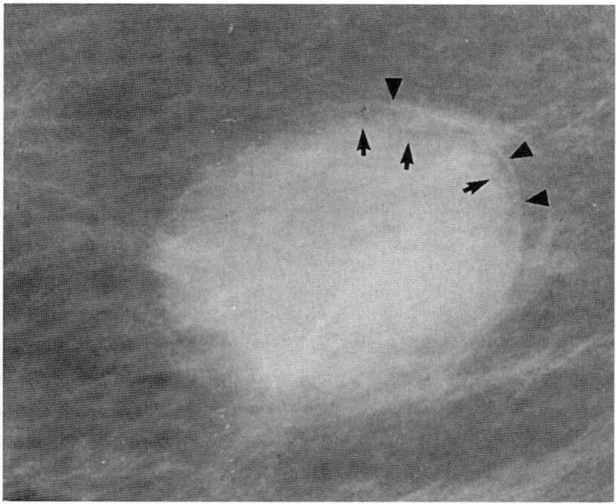

Figure 25–95. Hamartoma. This 2.5-cm oval circumscribed mass contains very little visible fat *(arrows)* beneath the pseudocapsule *(arrowheads)*.

ultrasonographic appearance is variable. The lesion may contain areas of low-level internal echogenicity interspersed with irregular areas of hyperechogenicity[86,87] or may mimic a fibroadenoma,[88,89] or, in some instances, the fatty tissue within the lesion may be highly echogenic (Fig. 25–96).[90]

When typical mammographic features are present, one can confidently make the diagnosis of a hamartoma, and no further follow-up or intervention is required. In the unusual situation in which the lesion is palpable and the patient is bothered by the mass, excision can be considered. In such cases, local excision is sufficient because there is no risk of recurrence or malignant change.[91] Malignancy within a hamartoma is so rare that an aggressive approach to the management of these lesions is not indicated.[92,93]

Pathology

On histologic examination, hamartomas contain varying amounts of adipose tissue, fibrous stroma,

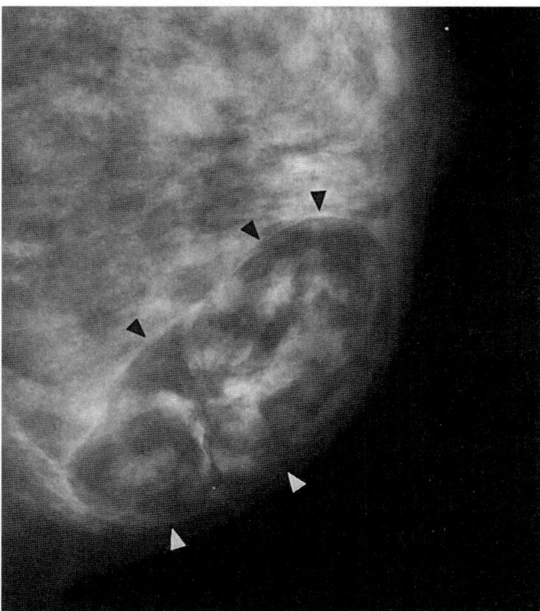

Figure 25–94. Hamartoma. The thin radiopaque pseudocapsule *(arrowheads)* is visible around most of this 4-cm oval circumscribed mass.

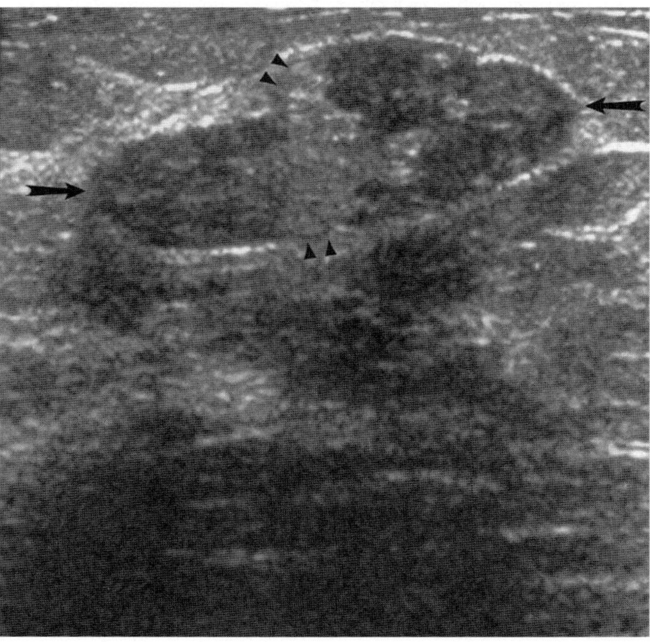

Figure 25–96. Hamartoma. Ultrasonogram demonstrates a 3-cm lobulated circumscribed mass that is predominantly hypoechoic *(arrows)*. Some of the fatty tissue within the lesion is hyperechoic *(arrowheads)*, although this is not seen in all hamartomas. (Courtesy of James Youker, MD, Milwaukee, WI.)

smooth muscle tissue, and glandular tissue, some of which may be cystic (Fig. 25–97).[94] An unusual finding in the fibrous stroma is the presence of slitlike spaces, which prove to be not of endothelial origin on immunohistochemical examination. Thus, the stroma is referred to as *pseudoangiomatous hyperplasia* (Fig. 25–97C). An important feature is the well-circumscribed margin with a partial or complete capsule. Knowledge of the radiologic findings facilitates the correct histologic diagnosis.

A

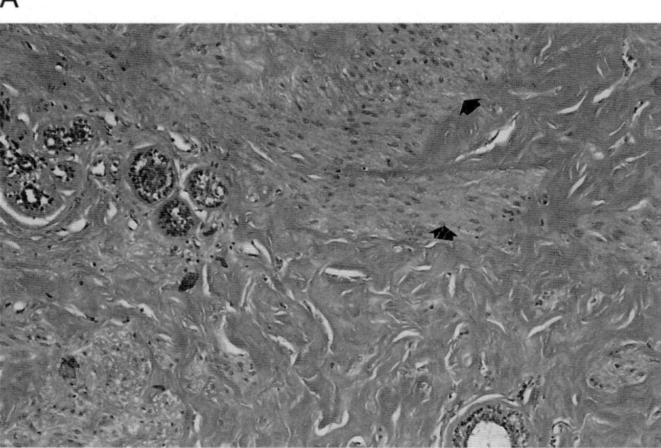

B

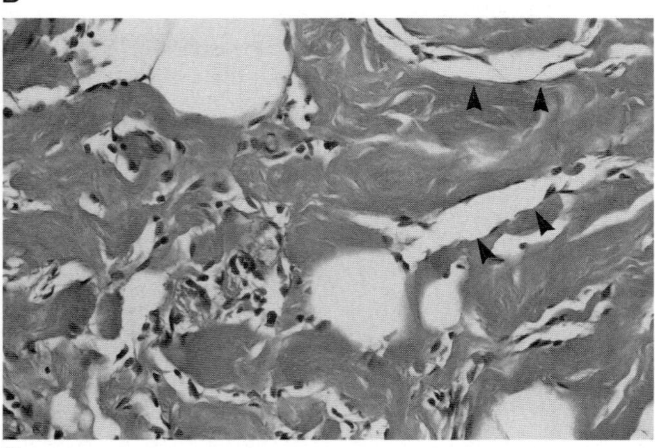

C

Figure 25–97. Hamartoma of the breast. **A,** This hamartoma has a smooth border but no capsule. Clusters of proliferating ducts are surrounded by hypocellular fibrous stroma. **B,** In the hypocellular fibrous stroma, there are bundles of smooth muscle cells *(arrows)*. **C,** Pseudoangiomatous slitlike spaces *(arrowheads)* in the stroma are distinct features of hamartoma.

FIBROCYSTIC CHANGE

Clinical Aspects

Fibrocystic change, condition, or "disease" is a common clinical and histologic diagnosis that encompasses a wide variety of normal and benign findings, including cysts, adenosis, fibrosis, and ductal hyperplasia. Despite the attempts to rename the condition, previously termed *fibrocystic disease,* this name appears to be ingrained in clinical usage. At least 50% of normal women have palpably irregular breasts, cyclic pain, and tenderness. These symptoms are commonly attributed to fibrocystic disease[95] yet are within the spectrum of normal hormone-related findings in the breast. Therefore, the term *fibrocystic disease* should not be used;[96] *fibrocystic changes* is a more appropriate term.

Pathology

The pathologic changes in the breast that fall under the designation of fibrocystic changes range from those that are entirely innocuous to those that are associated with increased risk of breast cancer. Furthermore, although these pathologic changes often coexist in the same breast, they may be found individually in a biopsy. For these reasons, the term *fibrocystic changes* should not be used as a catch-all phrase; the lesions in this category should be considered separately.

Most of the benign histologic findings within the spectrum of fibrocystic change have no associated increased risk for breast carcinoma. As shown in Table 25–1, a moderately increased risk is associated with atypical ductal or atypical lobular hyperplasia.[97,98] The individual lesions that fall under the category of fibrocystic changes are discussed separately in this chapter.

CYSTS

Clinical Aspects

Cysts are common fluid-filled masses that originate from the terminal ductal lobular unit or from an obstructed ectatic duct. They are frequently multiple and bilateral and may vary in size from microscopic to a few centimeters. Cysts are the most common breast masses in women aged 40 to 50 years.[99] Although they are often asymptomatic, many present as painful, freely mobile, palpable masses.

Table 25–1. Relative Risk for Invasive Breast Carcinoma Based on Pathologic Examination of Benign Breast Tissue

No Increased Risk
Adenosis
Apocrine metaplasia
Cysts (macrocysts and/or microcysts)
Duct ectasia
Hyperplasia, mild
Mastitis
Periductal mastitis
Squamous metaplasia
Slightly Increased Risk (1.5–2×)
Hyperplasia, moderate or florid, solid or papillary
Papilloma with fibrovascular core
Moderately Increased Risk (5×)
Atypical ductal hyperplasia
Atypical lobular hyperplasia

Modified from Hutter RVP: Cancer Committee of the College of American Pathologists: Consensus meeting: Is "fibrocystic disease" of the breast precancerous? Arch Pathol Lab Med 1986;110:171-173. Copyright 1986, American Medical Association.

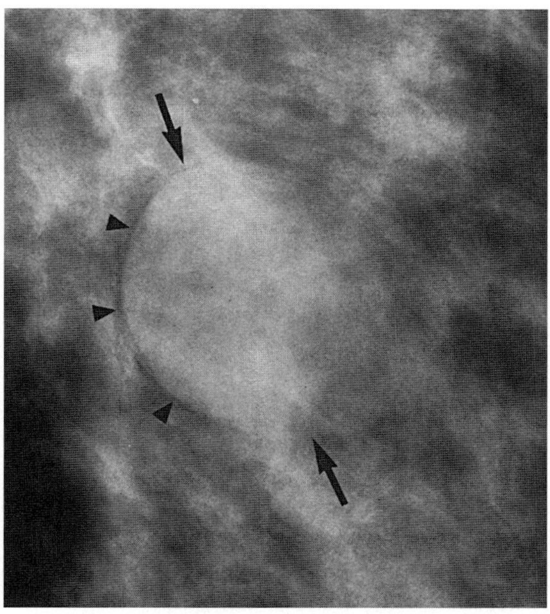

Figure 25–99. Cyst. The posterior margin of this round mass *(arrows)* is obscured, whereas the anterior margin is circumscribed with a halo sign *(arrowheads)*.

Imaging Features

On mammography, cysts are usually low- or equal-density, radiopaque, circumscribed masses that are round, oval, or lobular (Fig. 25–98). A partial or complete "halo sign" may be seen (Fig. 25–99), but this is not diagnostic for a cyst or other benign lesion.[100] Cysts may be partially or completely obscured by adjacent fibroglandular tissue or by other cysts or masses (Fig. 25–100). Most cysts are not calcified, but occasionally a thin peripheral rim of calcification occurs (Fig. 25–101), or milk of calcium collects within the dependent portion of micro- or macrocysts (Figs. 25–102 and 25–103). On horizontal beam films (mediolateral [ML] or lateromedial [LM]), layering calcifications have a linear or crescent shape, whereas on vertical beam films (CC), the calcification is rounded or not visible (Fig. 25–104).[101-104] It is critically important to obtain magnification views in the 90-degree lateral (ML or LM) and CC projections to best assess the configuration of the calcification (Fig. 25–105). When typical findings of milk of calcium are present, the benign cystic nature of the lesion is confirmed, and further evaluation (including ultrasonography) or intervention is not necessary.

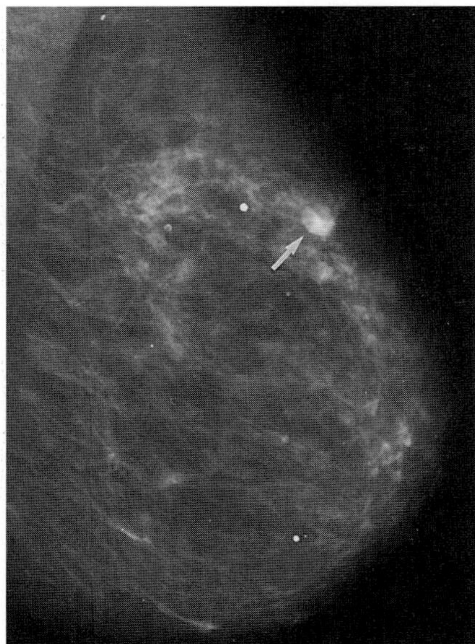

Figure 25–98. Cyst. A 1-cm round circumscribed mass on left mediolateral oblique mammogram *(arrow)*.

On mammography, noncalcified cysts are usually indistinguishable from fibroadenomas or other circumscribed solid masses. Needle aspiration or ultrasonography is required to distinguish between cysts and solid masses. The decision whether to perform US or aspiration after mammography of a palpable mass should be made by the mammographer and referring physician, and policy varies from center to center. US is the preferred method for diagnosis of nonpalpable cysts[105] and for palpable masses at most centers in the United States.

Ultrasonography is 96% to 100% accurate in the diagnosis of cysts[106-108] if one uses strict criteria. The operator should evaluate the cyst for wall irregularity or solid internal projections, which may indicate an intracystic tumor.[109-111] Most simple cysts have smooth walls, sharp anterior and posterior borders, no internal echoes, and posterior enhancement (Fig. 25–106). Angulated margins may be seen when cysts are multiple, clustered, or surrounded by fibrous tissue. A cluster of small (2- to 5-mm) cysts with thin intervening septa suggests the diagnosis of benign

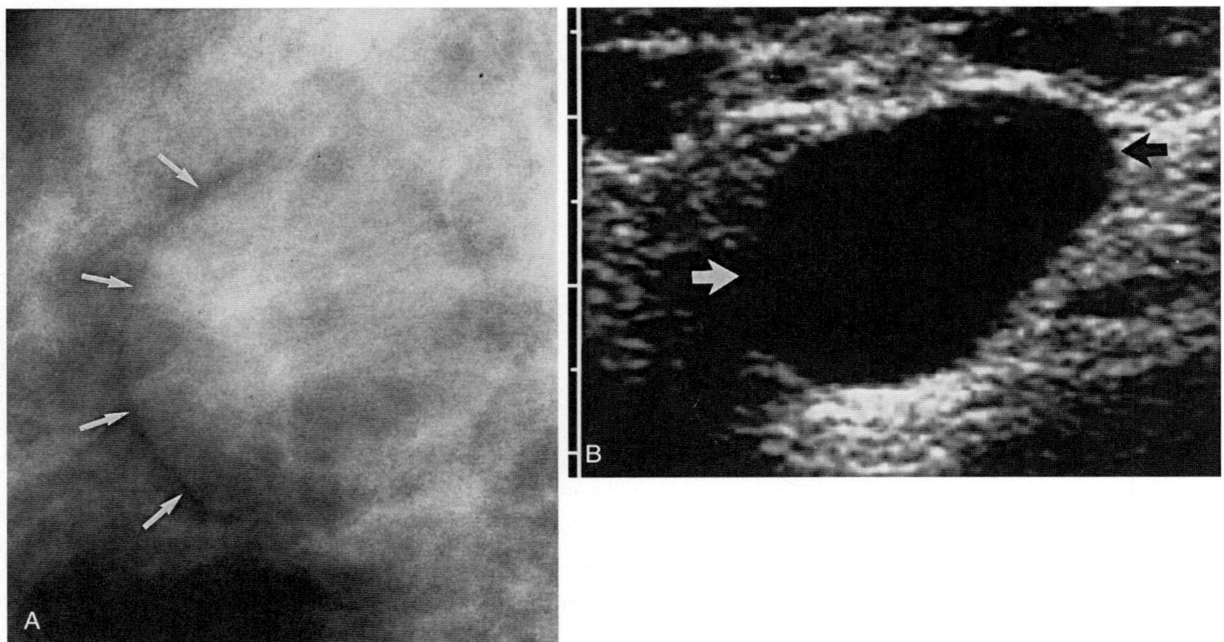

Figure 25–100. Obscured cyst. A 40-year-old woman with a 3-cm palpable mass. **A,** The anterior margin of the mass is visible on mammography *(arrows)*, whereas the remainder of the lesion is obscured by fibroglandular density. **B,** The diagnosis of a cyst *(arrows)* was made by ultrasonography.

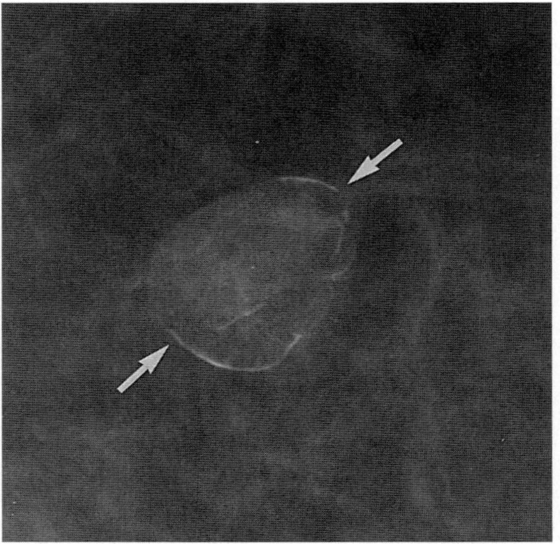

Figure 25–101. Cyst with rim calcification *(arrows)*.

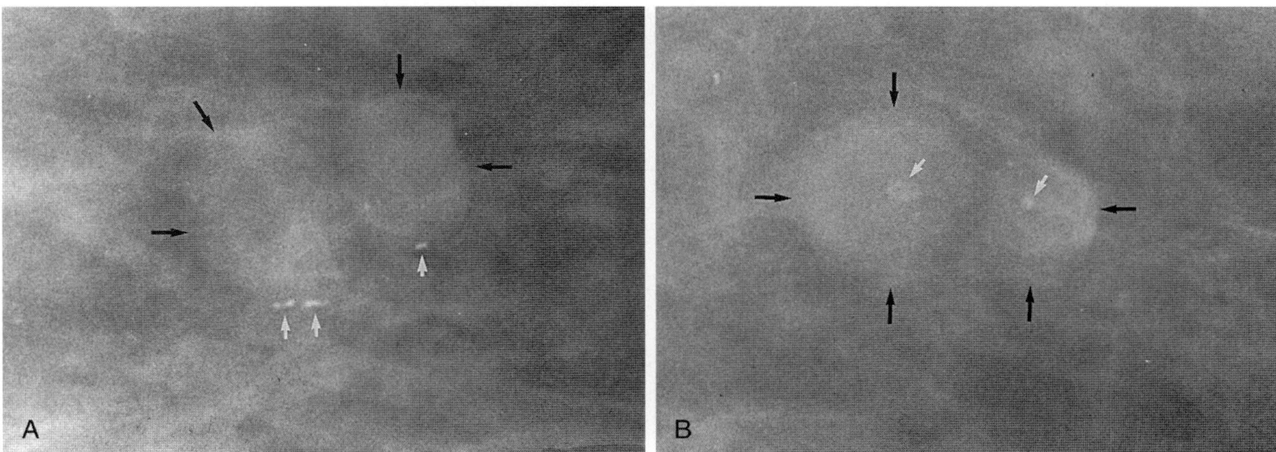

Figure 25–102. Milk of calcium in adjacent cysts. **A,** On the magnification mediolateral view, the calcifications *(white arrows)* appear linear and are in the dependent portion of the 6- and 8-mm cysts *(black arrows)*. **B,** Magnification craniocaudal view. The calcifications *(white arrows)* have round shapes and are projected near the center of the cysts *(black arrows)*.

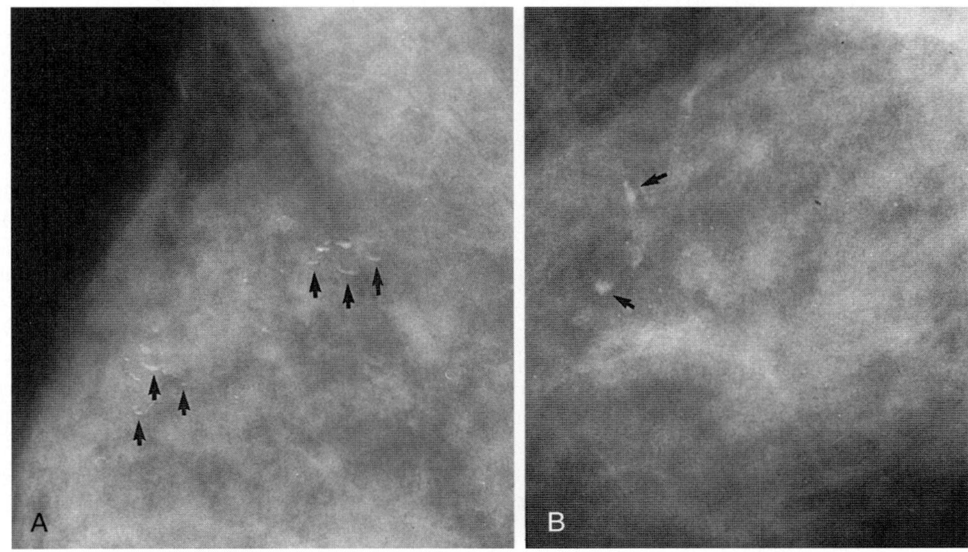

Figure 25–103. Milk of calcium in microcysts. **A,** On the lateromedial view, the calcifications are curvilinear *(arrows)*. **B,** On the craniocaudal view, many of the calcifications are not visible. The visible calcifications *(arrows)* have round shapes.

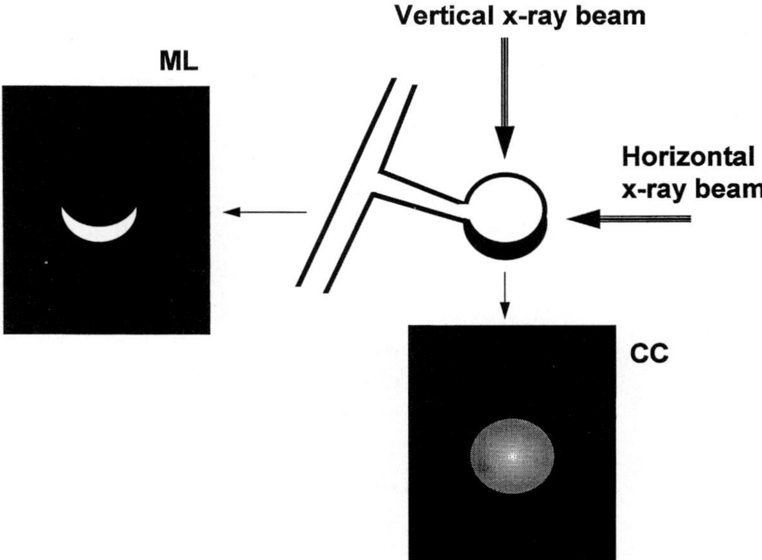

Figure 25–104. Milk of calcium. There is precipitation of calcium in the fluid within dilated lobules or cysts. On a horizontal beam film (mediolateral or lateromedial), the layered calcium appears linear or curvilinear, often likened to "teacups." On a vertical beam film (craniocaudal), if the thin layer of calcium is visible, it appears rounded.

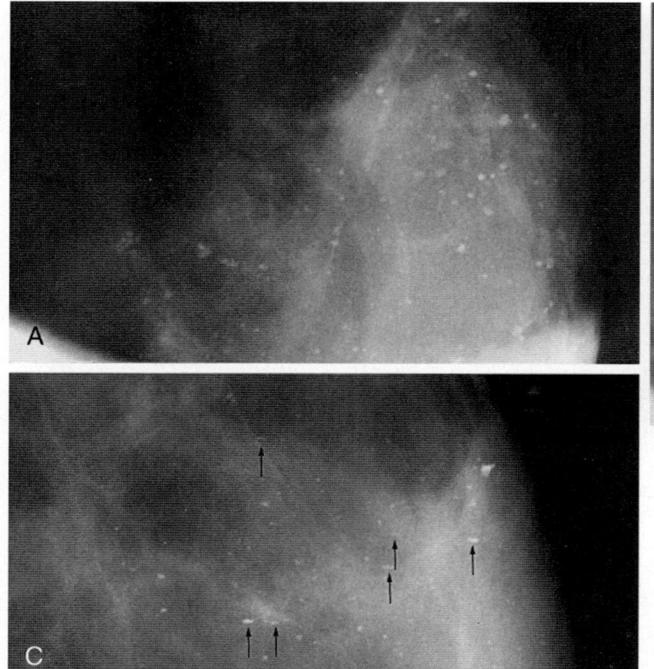

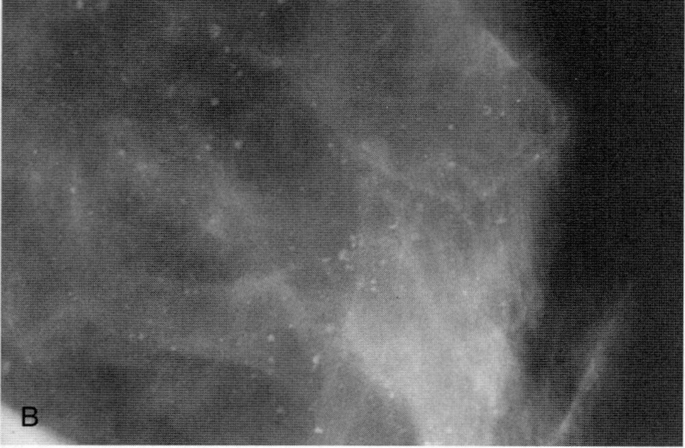

Figure 25–105. Milk of calcium in microcysts. The magnification mediolateral oblique **(A)** and craniocaudal **(B)** mammograms show a region of round calcifications. On the lateromedial view **(C)**, many of the calcifications are linear or curvilinear *(arrows)*, establishing the diagnosis of benign milk of calcium.

apocrine metaplasia (Fig. 25–107).[112] Not all simple benign cysts display the classic features described previously.[113] When internal echoes are seen within a cyst, most are the result of improper gain or power settings, reverberation, or other artifacts. When "real" echoes are found within a cyst, they are usually attributed to proteinaceous material, cellular debris, hemorrhage, infection, or cholesterol crystals (Figs. 25–108 and 25–109).[70,113] Movement of this material is often visible on real-time ultrasonography. From Berg's study,[114] it appears that aspiration is unnecessary in these cases. If there is no apparent movement of the internal echoes on real-time US examination and if color Doppler examination shows no flow within the mass, one should attempt aspiration before needle biopsy. If the fluid is completely removed and is not bloody, no residual palpable abnormality is seen, and the cyst does not recur, the lesion can be assumed to be benign.

Asymptomatic impalpable cysts with typical mammographic and ultrasonographic features require no further intervention, and the patient can return to routine mammography. If the ultrasonographic features are not diagnostic, the cyst is painful, or the woman is bothered by the palpable mass, needle aspiration is useful for both diagnosis and treatment. Cytologic examination of cyst fluid is unreliable for the diagnosis of benign and malignant intracystic tumors,[115] so most cyst fluid is discarded rather than sent to the laboratory.

Pathology

A cyst is defined as a fluid-filled space lined by epithelium. Grossly, cysts in the breast have a rounded contour and are bluish in color (blue-dome cysts) owing to contained semitranslucent, turbid fluid.

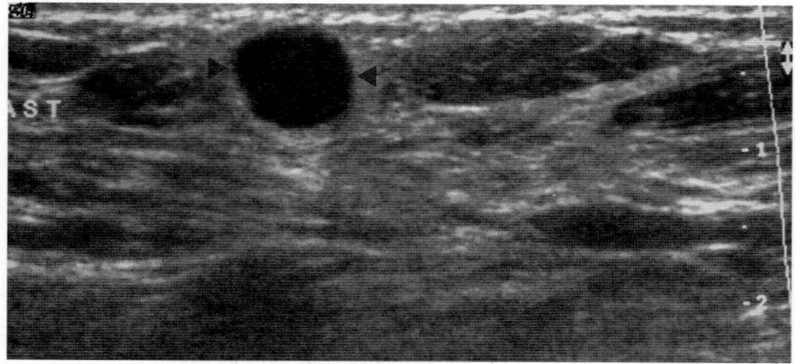

Figure 25–106. Simple cyst. The mass *(arrowheads)* is anechoic and has circumscribed margins and posterior acoustic enhancement.

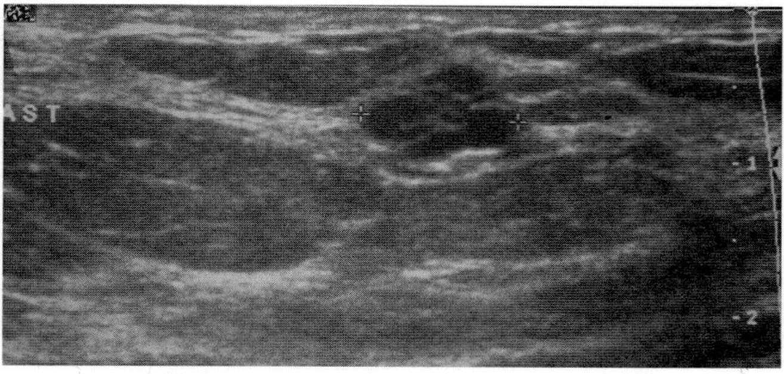

Figure 25–107. Microcysts. This cluster of small cysts with thin septations suggests the diagnosis of benign apocrine metaplasia.

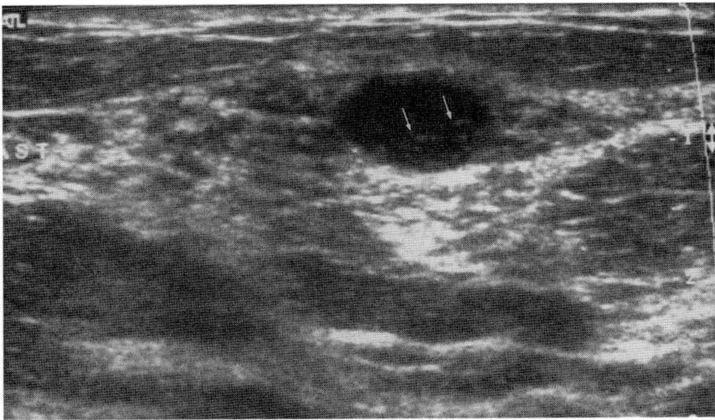

Figure 25–108. Cyst with fluid/debris level *(arrows)*. At biopsy, this was a benign cyst with internal hemorrhage.

Microscopically, the cyst lining shows a varied appearance. The epithelium may be flattened or totally atrophic. These are termed *attenuated cysts*, and biochemical correlation with histologic findings has shown a low potassium content in these cysts. Most commonly, the cyst lining shows large columnar or cuboidal cells with granular, eosinophilic cytoplasm resembling the epithelium of apocrine sweat glands. These are termed *apocrine cysts* (apocrine change or apocrine metaplasia) (Fig. 25–110A and B). The apocrine cells show rounded protrusions into the apical border, termed *apocrine snouts* (Fig. 25–110C). Within the cyst, cells with foamy cytoplasm and calcium oxalate crystals are often seen (see Fig. 25–110B and 25–111). These cysts typically have a high potassium content in the cyst fluid, with Na/K ratios less than 3. The apocrine type of cyst lining has been correlated with multiplicity and high rate of recurrence after aspiration.[116] Although the

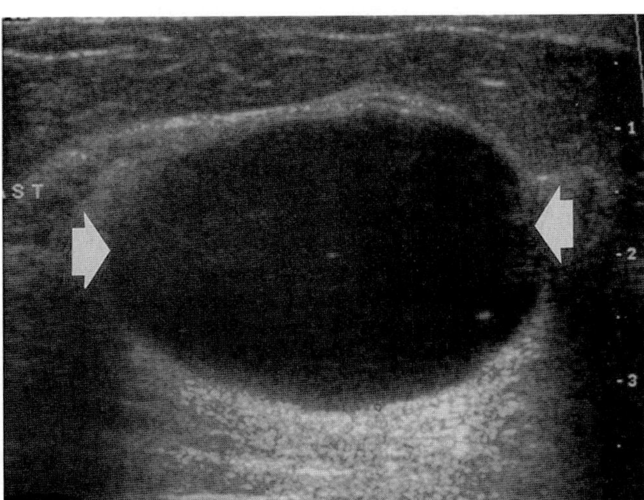

Figure 25–109. Benign cyst containing low-level internal echoes. This mass *(arrows)* was initially interpreted as being solid because of its ultrasonographic appearance. During instillation of local anesthesia for the ultrasound-guided needle biopsy procedure, clear green fluid was aspirated and the mass completely resolved, so the biopsy was canceled. The cyst has not recurred in 2 years of imaging follow-up.

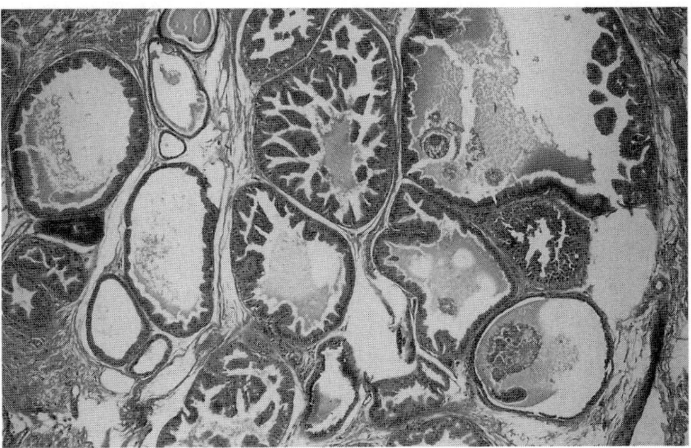

A

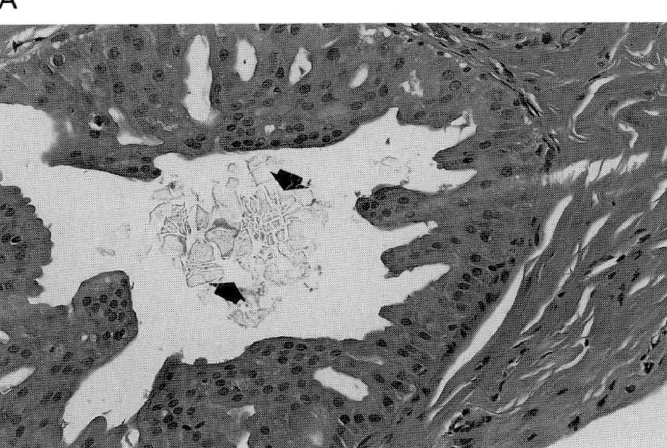

B

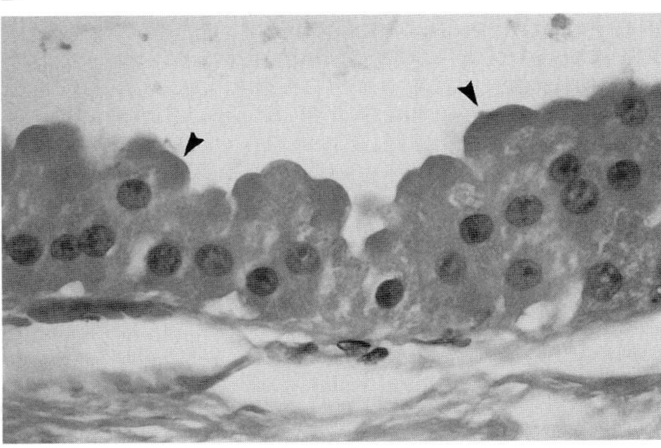

C

Figure 25–110. Fibrocystic change. **A,** Multiple cystic spaces are lined by apocrine metaplastic cells. Some of the spaces contain proteinaceous secretions. **B,** Apocrine metaplastic cells form papillary projections and cribriform spaces. In the glandular lumen, there are calcium oxalate crystals *(arrows)*. **C,** There is abundant eosinophilic granular cytoplasm and apical cytoplasmic projections, so-called apocrine snouts *(arrowheads)*. Uniformly round to oval nuclei contain small nucleoli.

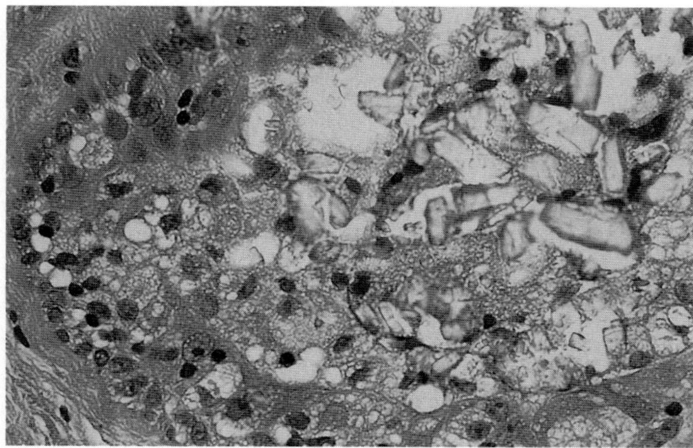

Figure 25–111. The glandular space contains foamy histiocytes and calcium oxalate with rectangular and rhomboid-shaped crystals.

apocrine epithelial lining of cysts is usually a single layer of cells, occasionally the epithelium is heaped up into papillary projections with complex interconnecting arches (see Fig. 25–110A).

GALACTOCELES

Clinical Aspects

A galactocele is a benign cyst filled with milk. This uncommon lesion almost always occurs in women during or a few months after lactation.[117,118] Rarely, galactoceles have been described in males.[119] Galactoceles are presumed to be caused by some form of ductal obstruction. The milk within the galactocele may be of normal consistency if it is fresh or may be thickened if it is older. Galactoceles usually present as nontender, firm, freely mobile palpable masses, usually without evidence of acute inflammation.[118] Needle aspiration of milk from the mass confirms the diagnosis and generally serves to treat the lesion.[120]

Imaging Features

The need for breast imaging in a pregnant or lactating woman depends on her age and clinical findings. Haagensen[120] indicated that whenever "a tumor develops in a woman who has lactated within 6 to 10 months it should be assumed that it may be a galactocele, and aspiration should be attempted." This can be a dangerous assumption, however, because breast carcinoma can occur in pregnant or lactating women, particularly as more women delay childbearing into their 30s and beyond. Because galactoceles mimic fibroadenomas or carcinomas on physical examination, imaging is often performed, particularly for women older than 30 years.

The mammographic appearance depends on the amount of fat and proteinaceous material within the milk. If the fat content is very high, the mass may be completely radiolucent, mimicking a lipoma.[121,122] The mammographic finding of a circumscribed mass with a fat-fluid level on upright horizontal beam films is diagnostic (Figs. 25–112 and 25–113). This finding will not be as apparent on an MLO view because it is not a horizontal beam film. Therefore, if this condition is suspected, an upright ML or LM view should be obtained. In Gomez and colleagues' series of 11 cases,[123] five mammograms demonstrated fat-fluid levels within the mass on horizontal beam (ML) films. In one of their cases, the fat and water densities were mixed, simulating a hamartoma. In the additional five cases, the entire lesion was water density. Thus, in 55% of cases, mammography established a benign diagnosis.

Little in the literature addresses the US features of galactoceles. Kopans[122] reported that they are circumscribed, contain low-level internal echoes, and demonstrate posterior acoustic enhancement, similar to circumscribed solid breast tumors. Salvador and coworkers[124] found a fluid-debris level on ultrasonography, with anechoic fatty liquid and highly echogenic proteinaceous material.

Pathology

A galactocele is simply cystic dilation of a duct occurring during lactation. A single duct may be affected, producing a single cyst, but more often multiple

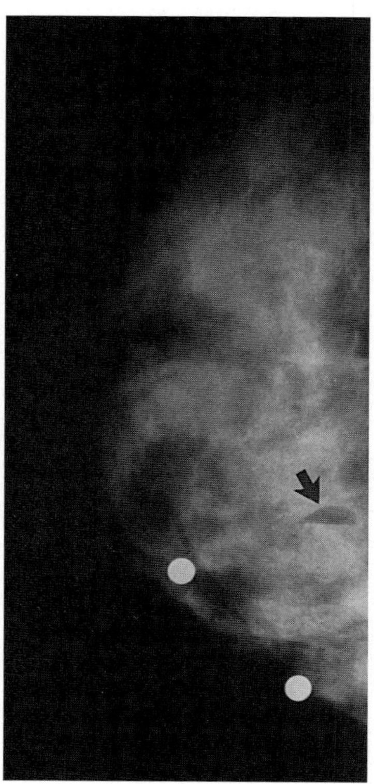

Figure 25–112. Galactocele. Mediolateral mammogram of a palpable mass in a lactating woman. The fat/fluid level in the 1-cm mass *(arrow)* is diagnostic of a galactocele.

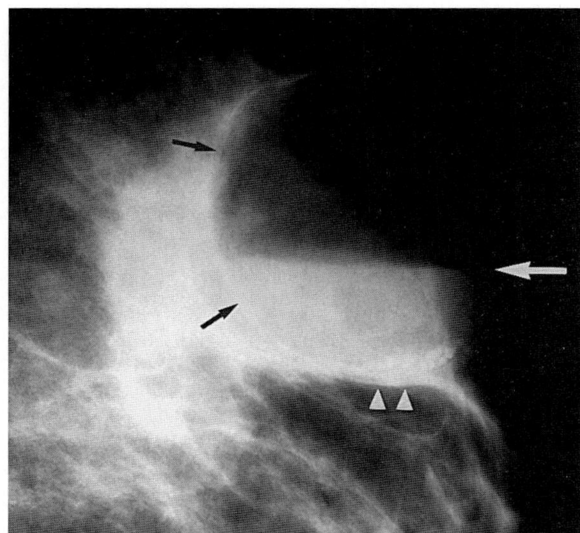

Figure 25–113. Galactocele. Mediolateral mammogram of a 4-cm palpable mass (*black arrows*) in the left breast of a lactating woman. A fat/fluid level *(white arrow)* and layering calcifications *(arrowheads)* are present. (Courtesy of Shalom Buchbinder, MD, Staten Island, NY.)

ducts are involved. Biopsy shows dilated ductal spaces that are lined by a double layer of epithelial and myoepithelial cells.

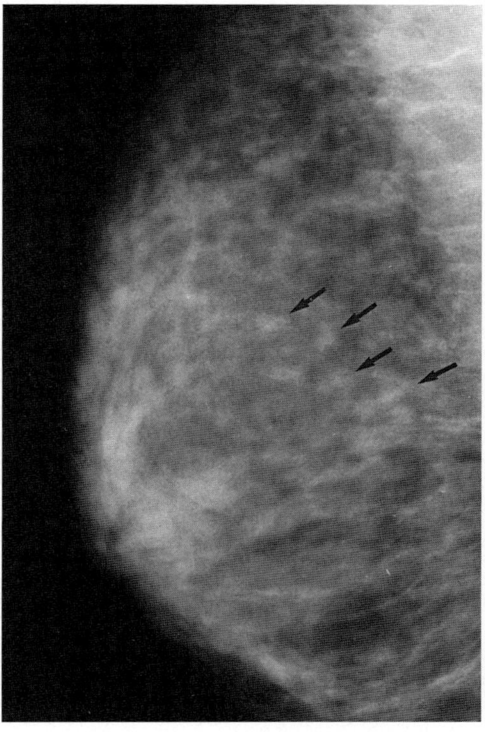

Figure 25–114. Adenosis. Diffuse, scattered, indistinct 3- to 5-mm nodules *(arrows)* were present bilaterally, caused by hyperplasia of the lobules.

ADENOSIS

Clinical Aspects

Adenosis is a spectrum of histologic lesions ranging from hyperplasia of the lobule to sclerosing adenosis with fibrosis and calcifications.

Imaging Features

The mammographic findings are usually nonspecific and include diffuse ill-defined 3- to 5-mm nodular densities (adenosis) (Fig. 25–114), multiple round or punctate calcifications (often associated with radiographically dense breast tissue in sclerosing adenosis) (Figs. 25–115 and 25–116), and focal spiculated masses with or without microcalcifications, mimicking breast carcinoma (Figs. 25–117 and 25–118). There are no typical ultrasonographic findings in adenosis. Because of the lack of definitive imaging findings, this should be considered a histologic diagnosis, rather than an imaging diagnosis. When the imaging findings mimic carcinoma, biopsy is required.

Pathology

Adenosis is an abnormality of the lobules that as stated previously includes the spectrum from lobular hyperplasia to sclerosing adenosis. The changes occur over the woman's lifetime. In the early stage of adenosis, under estrogenic stimulation, the lobules become hyperplastic and enlarged beyond the average range of 10 to 100 acini (Fig. 25–119A and B). This is essentially the change that occurs during pregnancy. The lobules contain overcrowded acini (Fig. 119C). Later, with the cessation of hormonal stimulation, the lobules regress. In addition, myoepithelial proliferation and stromal fibrosis occur, which can cause elongation and distortion of acini (Fig. 25–120). These compressed acini may simulate invasive carcinoma. It is then important to appreciate the lobular architecture under low-power magnification. On high power, the preservation of the basement membrane and normal two cell layers of the acini is indication of benignancy. Calcifications occur within the acini that may simulate malignant calcifications on mammograms (see Fig. 25–120). In the final stage, the acini become few in number, and the lobules become involuted with fibrosis, so-called sclerosing adenosis (Fig. 25–121). The stromal fibrosis can cause increased density on the mammogram, which in combination with the calcifications may simulate malignancy.

A rare form of adenosis, microglandular adenosis, deserves mention because it can be confused with tubular carcinoma on histologic examination. This lesion most often presents as a mass in women between 45 and 55 years of age. Clusters of small regular glands occur in fibrous stroma or adipose

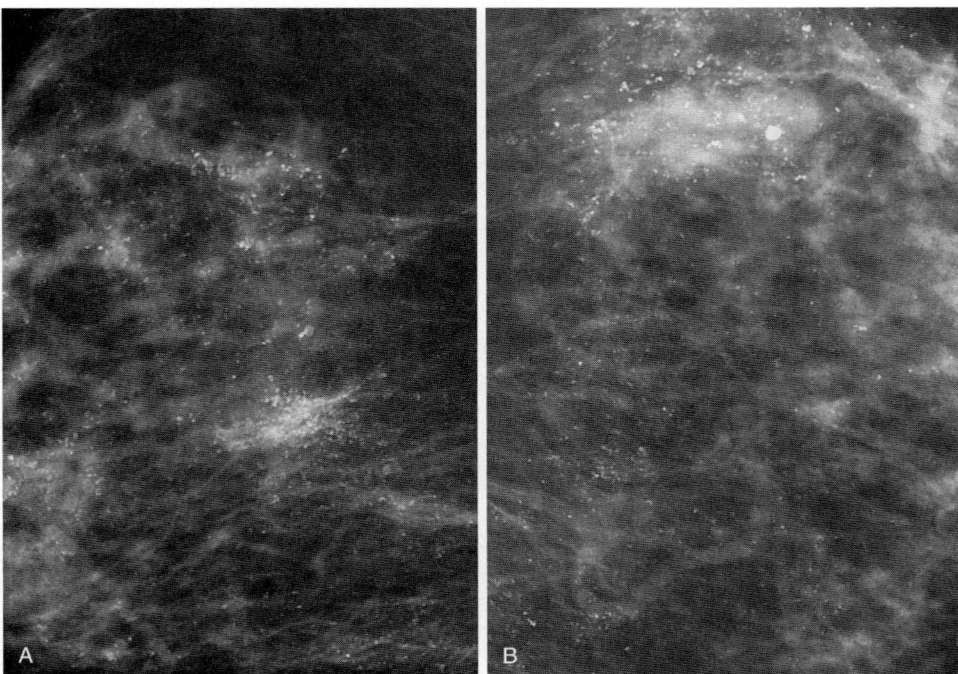

Figure 25–115. Adenosis calcifications. Diffuse round and punctate calcifications scattered throughout both right **(A)** and left **(B)** breasts. The random distribution produces apparent clustering in some areas, but the distribution of the calcifications is that of a benign process.

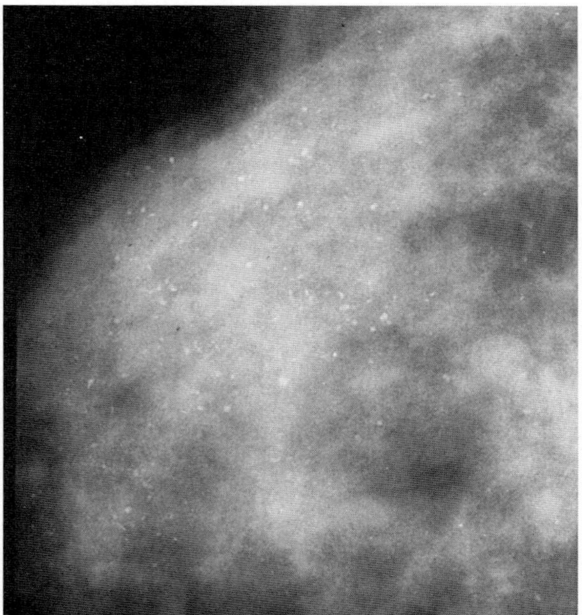

Figure 25–116. Sclerosing adenosis. Right mediolateral oblique mammogram demonstrating multiple round and punctate calcifications associated with radiographically dense breast tissue. The calcifications were present only in this region. Biopsy was performed, which established the diagnosis of sclerosing adenosis.

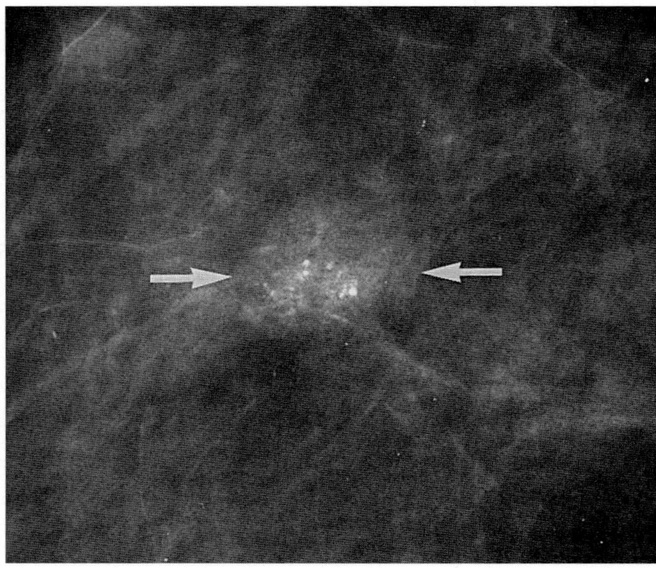

Figure 25–117. Sclerosing adenosis. A 1-cm ill-defined mass with pleomorphic microcalcifications *(arrows)*, suspicious for carcinoma. Biopsy is necessary to establish the diagnosis.

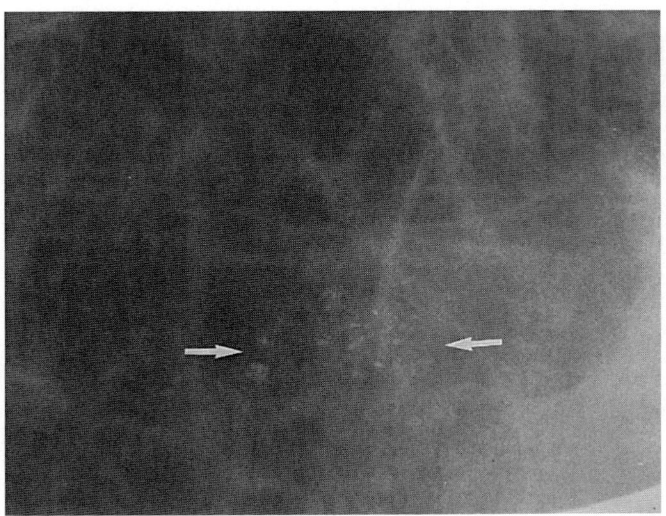

Figure 25–118. Sclerosing adenosis. A 1-cm cluster of pleomorphic microcalcifications *(arrows)*—benign sclerosing adenosis at biopsy.

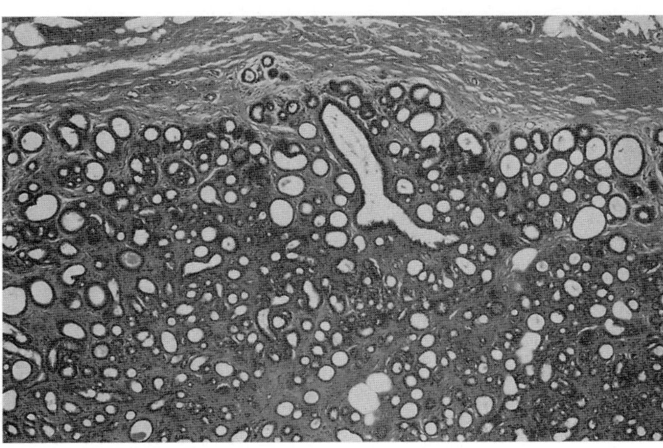

A

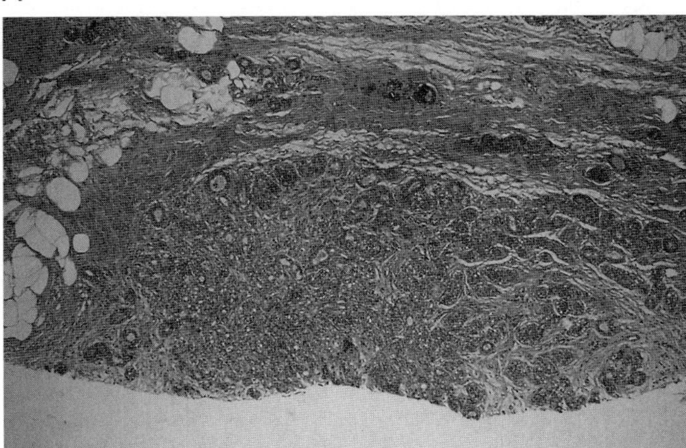

B

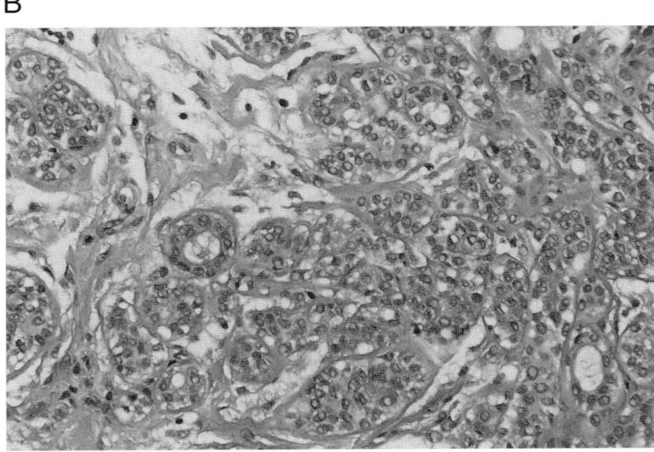

C

Figure 25–119. Early stage of florid adenosis. **A,** An expanded hyperplastic lobule consists of overcrowded acini. The smooth border helps separate it from an infiltrative carcinoma. **B,** In a core needle biopsy, the preservation of lobular architecture with a smooth border is critical for a correct histologic diagnosis. **C,** A higher magnification illustrates closely apposed crowded acini.

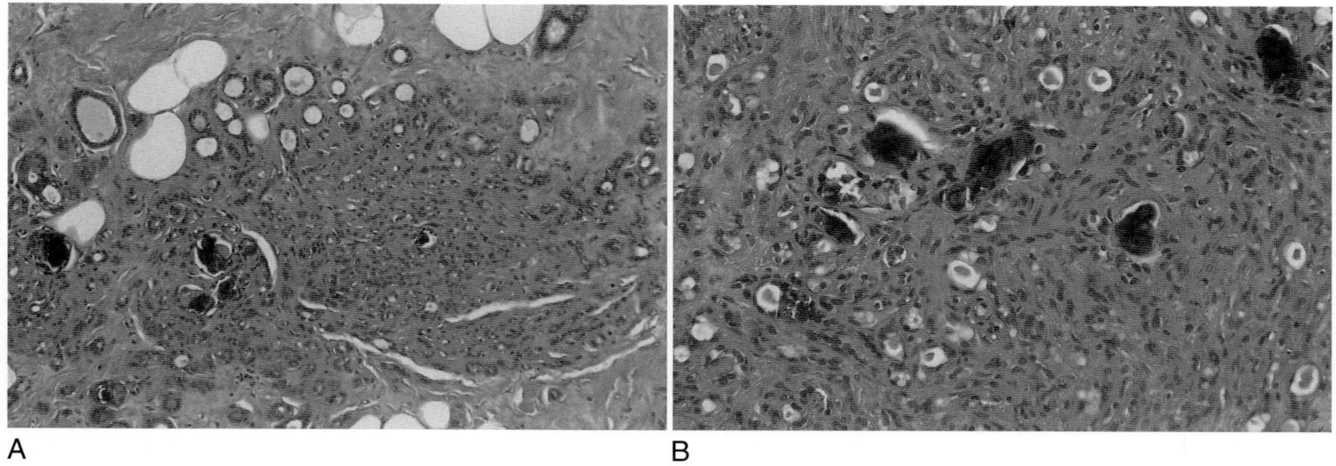

Figure 25–120. Sclerosing adenosis. **A,** The shape of the lobule is slightly irregular and distorted, owing to stromal fibrosis. The borders are circumscribed. Microcalcifications are present. **B,** Distorted acini are associated with stromal fibrosis and microcalcifications, which have a basophilic, laminated appearance characteristic of calcium phosphate.

tissue without a lobular architecture (Fig. 25–122A). These glands appear to be lined by a single layer of cuboidal to columnar cells (Fig. 25–122B). Myoepithelial cells are not readily seen on regular hematoxylin and eosin stained sections but can be demonstrated by immunohistochemical staining for S-100 protein and smooth muscle actin. A rare form of tubular adenosis has also been reported.[125]

FIBROSIS

Clinical Aspects

Fibrosis is a benign proliferation of fibrous connective tissue of the breast, which may be associated with a variety of other benign processes. Focal fibrosis may present as a palpable mass or as an impalpable mammographic abnormality.

Imaging Features

The mammographic findings are nonspecific and include ill-defined or spiculated masses or architectural distortion (Fig. 25–123) and occasionally a circumscribed mass (Fig. 25–124).[122,126-128] On ultrasonography, fibrosis is often highly echogenic and identical in appearance to normal fibroglandular tissue. It is not unusual for ultrasonography to demonstrate an oval hypoechoic mass, however.[127,128] Because of the significant false-negative rate of ultrasonography, one should not assume that a lesion is fibrosis when only echogenic tissue is seen. Because the imaging findings often mimic malignancy, biopsy should be considered unless one has a reliable history of previous biopsy or trauma to that area.

A variant of fibrosis occurs in some women with a long history of insulin-dependent diabetes mellitus. This condition is termed diabetic fibrous breast

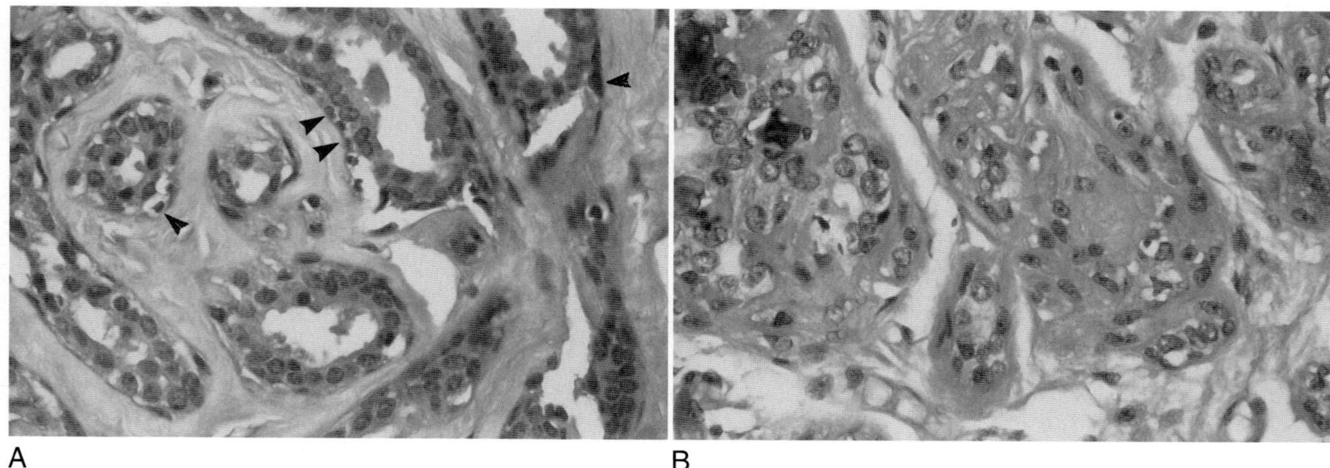

Figure 25–121. Sclerosing adenosis. **A,** In better preserved acini, two types of cells are evident: inner epithelial cells and outer small, darker myoepithelial cells *(arrowheads)*. **B,** Atrophic acini are associated with stromal fibrosis and microcalcifications (left upper corner).

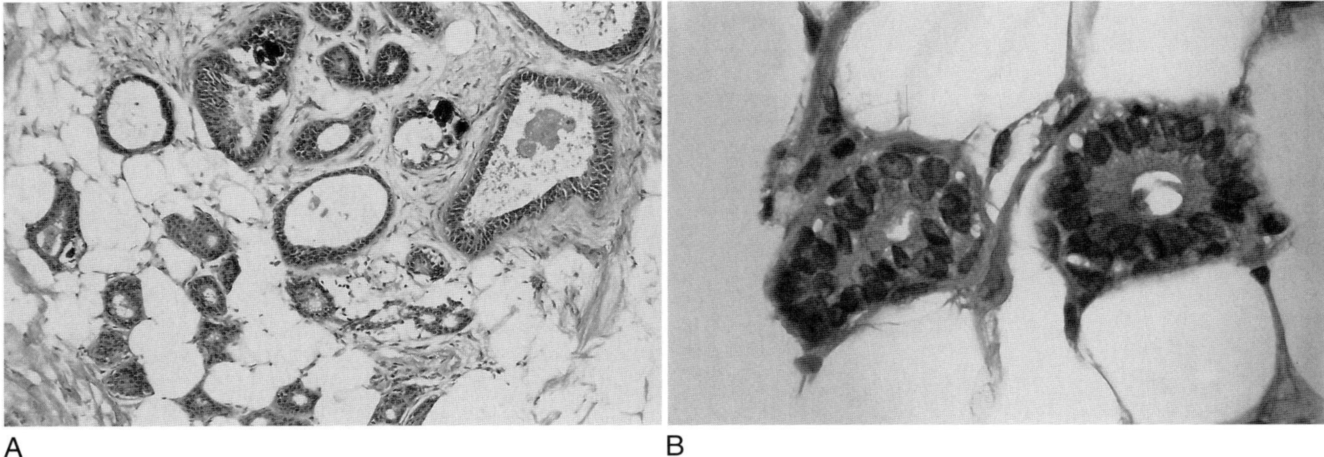

Figure 25–122. Microglandular adenosis. **A,** Isolated round ductules in a fatty stroma can simulate tubular carcinoma. Microcalcifications are also present. **B,** Isolated acini are usually lined by a single layer of benign columnar to cuboidal cells. Myoepithelial cells are indistinct. In tubular carcinoma, a greater degree of nuclear atypia and a desmoplastic stromal reaction are expected.

disease (DFBD),[122,129] and affected women have radiographically dense breast tissue and one or more hard, irregular, painful, freely mobile masses, which are obscured by fibroglandular density on mammography. The lesions are visible as areas of marked acoustical shadowing on breast ultrasonography. The imaging features of DFBD are nonspecific, and although the diagnosis can be suggested when the proper constellation of clinical and imaging findings is present, needle or excisional biopsy is required to make the diagnosis.

Pathology

On histologic examination, fibrous tissue surrounding atrophic ducts and acini is seen (Fig. 25–125). The specialized loose connective tissue surrounding the lobules is gradually replaced by the dense collagenous fibrous tissue. An inflammatory cell infiltrate may be seen. It has been suggested that the fibrous tumor is the end result of an inflammatory process that leads to atrophy and obliteration of the glandular tissue, with fibrosis accompanying and following the inflammation.[130]

DUCT ECTASIA

Clinical Aspects

Duct ectasia is a nonspecific dilation of the major subareolar ducts, with occasional involvement of the

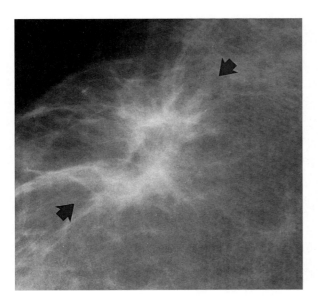

Figure 25–123. Fibrosis. A 2-cm spiculated mass *(arrows)*, simulating carcinoma.

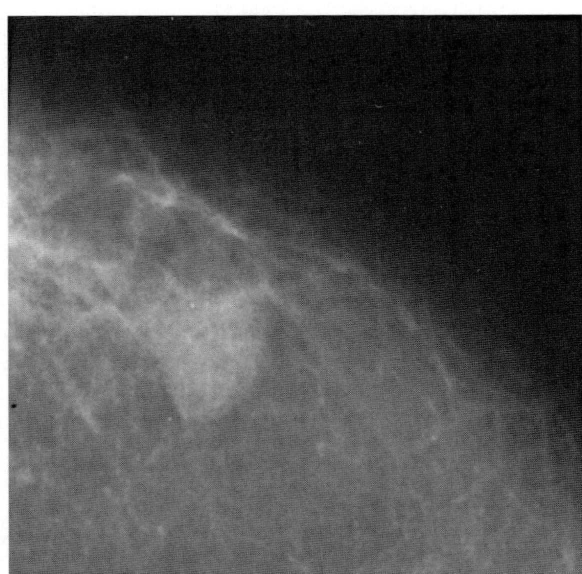

Figure 25–124. Focal fibrosis. A 1.3-cm circumscribed mass, which was a focal area of fibrosis at biopsy.

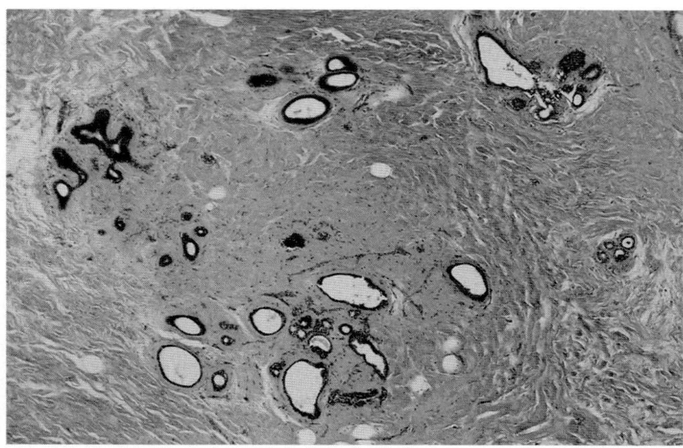

Figure 25–125. Fibrosis of the breast. Broad bands of dense fibrous stroma in which atrophic ducts and rare lobules remain.

smaller ducts. The various anatomic features of this disease have led to many different descriptive diagnostic terms, including *plasma cell mastitis, obliterative mastitis,* and *comedomastitis*. The cause of duct ectasia is unknown. It has been suggested that the initiating event is the inflammatory process, which leads to destruction of the elastic network of the duct and, hence, duct ectasia and periductal fibrosis. Others have suggested that the dilation is primary, perhaps caused by obstruction of the duct, and that the inflammation is a secondary phenomenon related to leakage of duct contents.

Imaging Features

The distended ducts may be palpable or visible on mammography (Fig. 25–126) or ultrasonography (Fig. 25–127). The ducts may be filled with fluid or with thick secretions and cellular debris.[122] The material within the ducts often calcifies, producing the typical secretory calcifications seen on mammography as dense, solid, rodlike calcifications, which are usually bilateral and diffuse (Fig. 25–128) but occasionally focal (Fig. 25–129). The calcifications may also contain internal lucencies when the calcified material is outside, rather than within, the duct (Fig 25–130). Such calcifications are asymptomatic, are of no clinical consequence to the patient, and do not elevate the woman's risk of breast cancer. Occasionally, early focal secretory calcifications may mimic malignant microcalcifications, leading to biopsy. In addition, if asymmetrically dilated ducts represent an interval change or contain pleomorphic microcalcifications, biopsy should be performed.[131]

Pathology

On histologic examination, dilated ducts with periductal inflammation exist (Fig. 25–131). The dilated ducts are filled with necrotic, acidophilic debris, foamy macrophages (Fig. 25–132), and, occasionally, cholesterol clefts. Calcification of the luminal contents leads to the characteristic rodlike calcifications described previously. The periductal inflammation can consist of lymphocytes, plasma

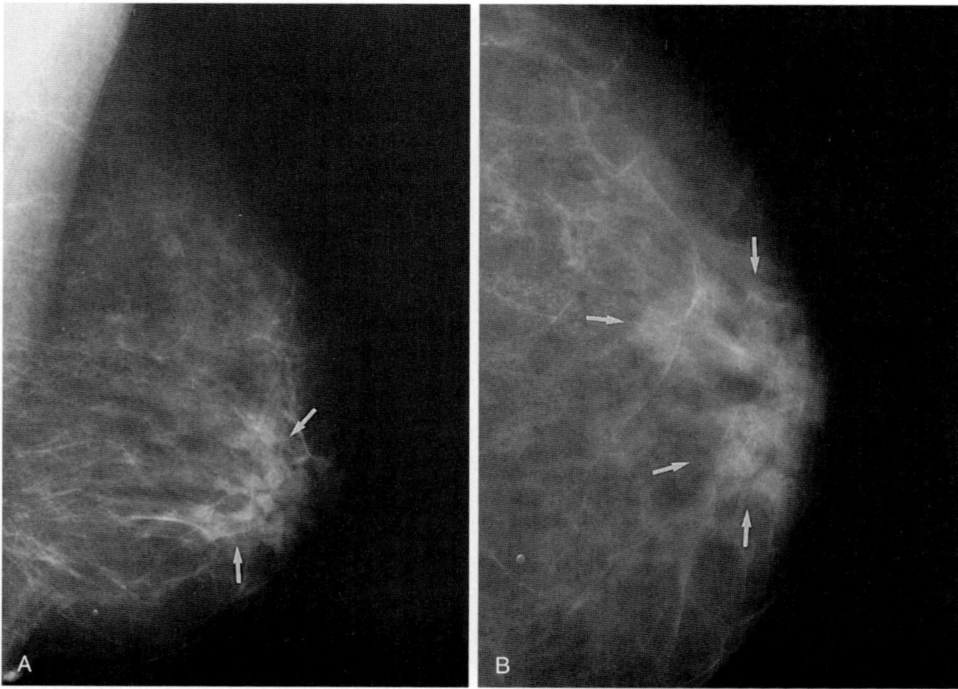

Figure 25–126. Prominent subareolar ducts. Dilated tubular structures *(arrows)* radiate from the nipple on the mediolateral **(A)** and craniocaudal **(B)** views.

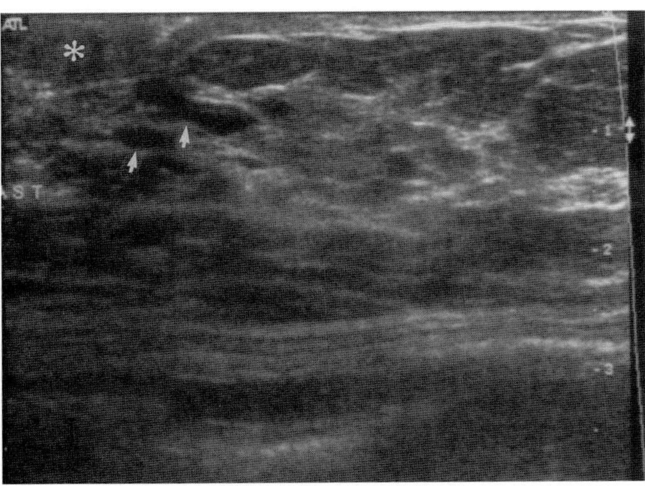

Figure 25–127. Prominent subareolar ducts on ultrasound. Fluid-filled tubular structures *(arrows)* behind the nipple *(asterisk)*.

cells, and, rarely, eosinophils. With time, the ductal epithelium can become denuded, with development of fibrosis around the ducts (see Fig. 25–132).

PAPILLOMA

Clinical Aspects and Imaging Features

Three types of benign papillary lesions involve the breast: solitary central papillomas, multiple papillomas (papillomatosis), and juvenile papillomatosis. Benign solitary papillomas can also present as intracystic lesions.

Solitary papillomas are usually located within a major duct in the subareolar or central regions of the breast. Rarely, they involve the nipple.[132] They usually present with bloody or serous discharge, are frequently nonpalpable, and are often mammographically occult because of their small size.[133,134] Although a papilloma is occasionally visible as a circumscribed nodule (Figs. 25–133 and 25–134) or a cluster of calcifications (Fig. 25–135) on mammography, galactography is usually necessary for visualization (Fig. 25–136).

Multiple papillomas develop within a group of ducts and are usually located peripherally in the breast.[132,135] Affected women tend to be younger, and the process is more often bilateral and less often associated with nipple discharge than in solitary papillomas.[136] Multiple peripheral papillomas may present on mammographic examination as multiple nodules, occasionally with microcalcifications (Fig. 25–137).[133] Multiple peripheral papillomas are associated with an increased risk for subsequent development of breast carcinoma,[133,135,137] and a high tendency for recurrence after local excision exists.[138]

Juvenile papillomatosis was described by Rosen and associates[139] in 1980 in a group of "adolescents and young women with a striking constellation of changes usually described as components of fibrocystic disease." Severe ductal papillomatosis is associated with changes usually seen in fibrocystic change in older women. Clinically, the process usually presents as a focal palpable mass in a young woman, which mimics fibroadenoma. Also called "Swiss cheese disease," this condition has been reported in women aged 10 to 48 years.[139,140] The lesion may be a marker for families at risk for breast cancer, because 28% to 33% of affected women have a family history of breast carcinoma,[140,141] and it has been suggested that the woman herself may have an increased risk of developing breast cancer later in life.[140] Bazzocchi and colleagues[141] reported coexisting carcinoma in 15% of women and atypical ductal hyperplasia in another 15% of cases.

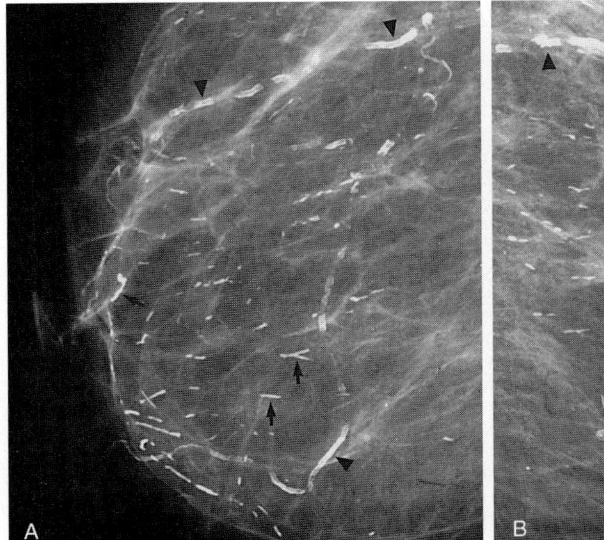

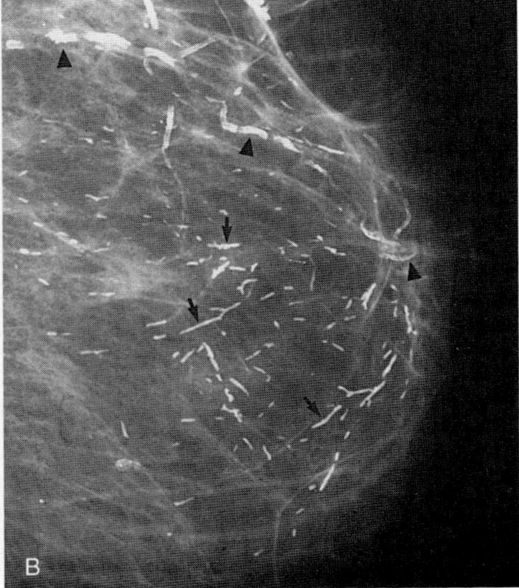

Figure 25–128. Secretory calcifications. Right **(A)** and left **(B)** mediolateral mammograms show diffuse dense linear calcifications *(arrows)*, generally oriented toward the nipple. Vascular calcifications are also present *(arrowheads)*.

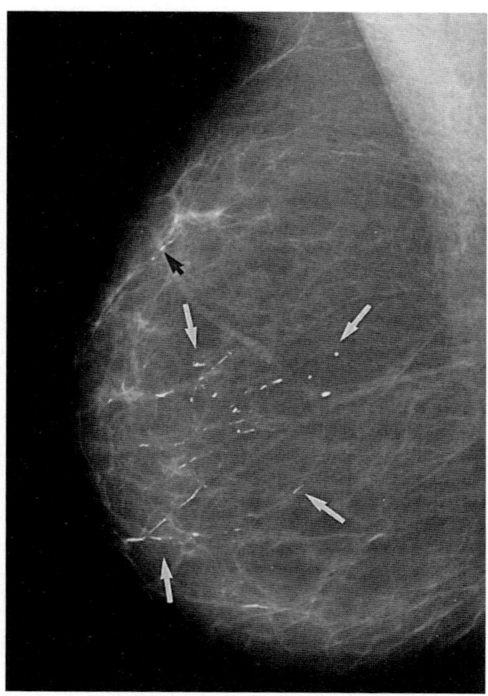

Figure 25–129. Focal secretory calcifications present in only one region of the right breast *(white arrows)*. The calcifications in the superior aspect of the right breast are vascular *(black arrow)*. No calcifications were present on the left.

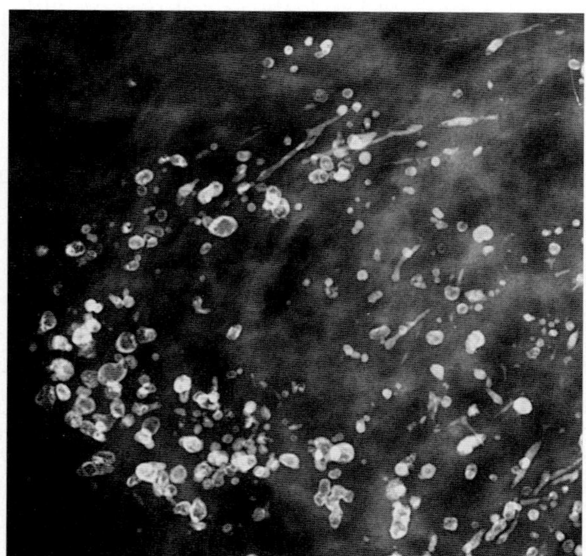

Figure 25–130. Extensive secretory calcifications with internal lucencies.

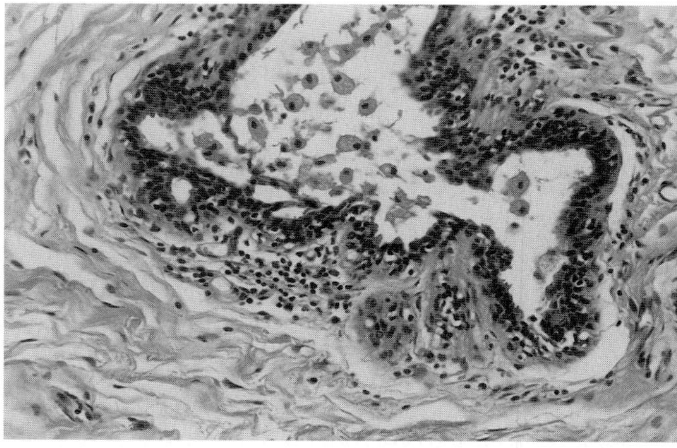

Figure 25–131. Ductal ectasia. The dilated duct contains foamy macrophages and is surrounded by lymphocytes and plasma cells.

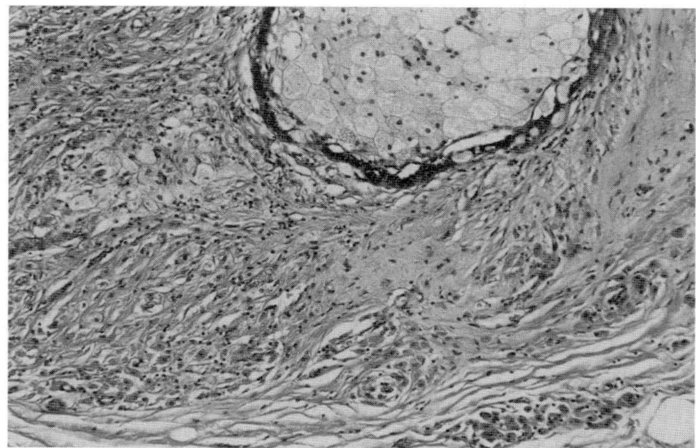

Figure 25–132. Ductal ectasia. A dilated duct contains foamy macrophages. In the periductal region, there are abundant foamy macrophages and fibrosis.

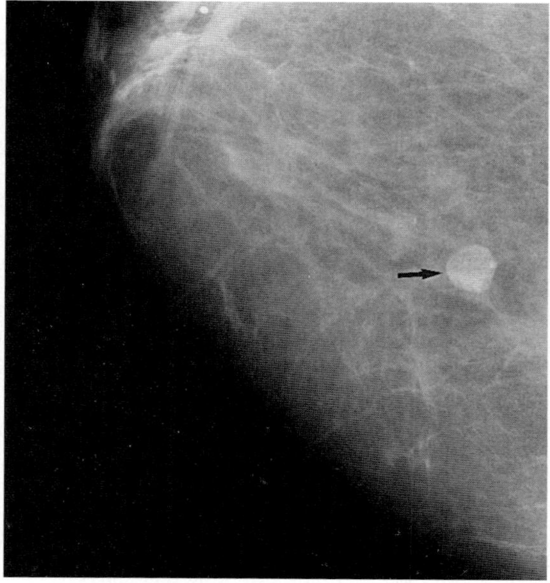

Figure 25–133. Solitary papilloma. A 7-mm circumscribed mass *(arrow)* found to be an intraductal papilloma at biopsy.

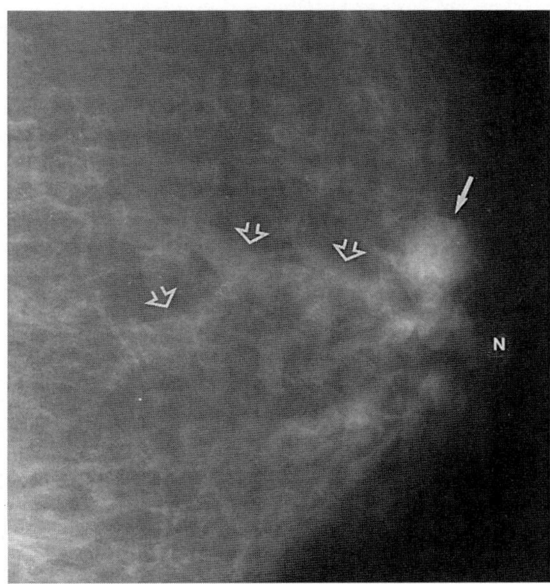

Figure 25–134. Solitary subareolar papilloma. A 1.5-cm round circumscribed mass *(solid arrow)* with associated dilated duct *(open arrows)*. N, nipple.

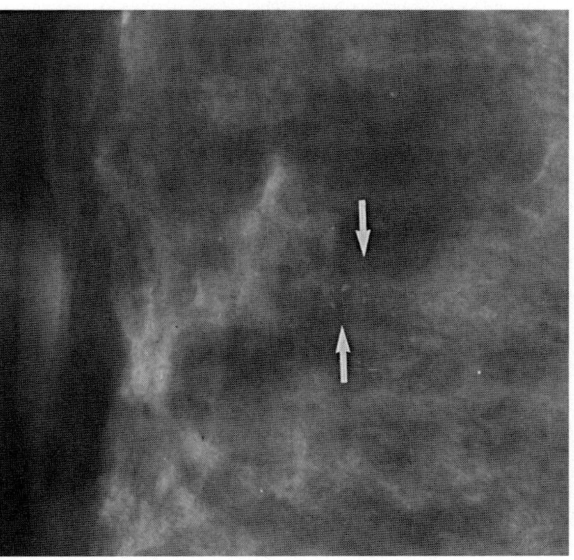

Figure 25–135. Solitary intraductal papilloma. A 7-mm cluster of faint pleomorphic microcalcifications *(arrows)*, found at biopsy to be a benign papilloma.

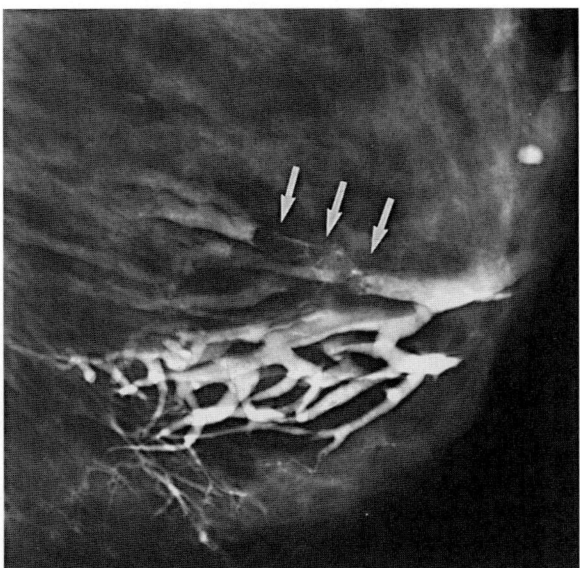

Figure 25–136. Solitary papilloma on galactography. Left craniocaudal view demonstrating a 1-cm lobular filling defect *(arrows)* in the contrast column.

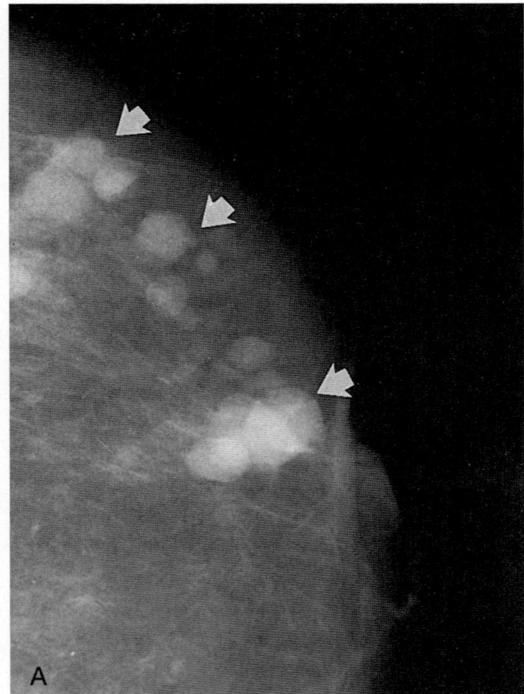

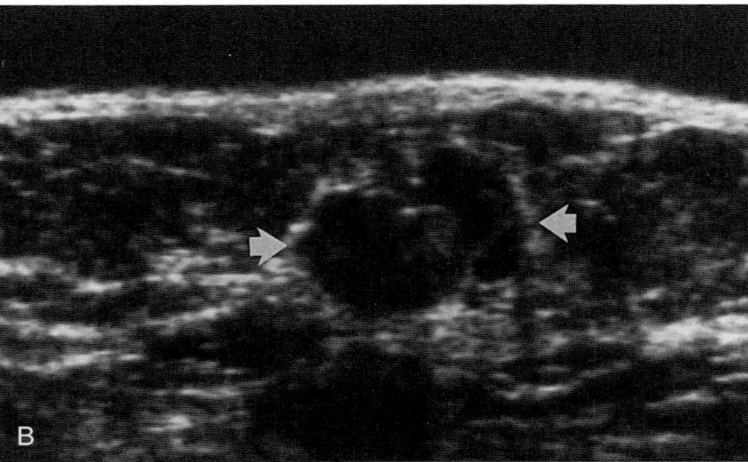

Figure 25–137. Multiple peripheral papillomas. **A,** Craniocaudal mammogram demonstrating multiple circumscribed masses *(arrows)*. **B,** Ultrasonogram of one of the larger masses *(arrows)*, demonstrating both cystic and solid components.

Because of the relatively young age of affected women, little in the literature addresses the mammographic findings of juvenile papillomatosis.[140,142] The ultrasonographic appearance has been described as an ill-defined inhomogeneous mass with one or more small ($\leq$ 0.4 cm) rounded anechoic areas, often seen in the periphery of the lesion (Fig. 25–138).[142,143] The treatment of choice is wide local excision of the lesion, with careful surveillance of the affected woman and her family members.[140,144]

Pathology

On histologic examination, papillomas have stalks covered with epithelium and a fibrovascular core attached to the wall (Figs. 25–139 and 25–140). The proliferative epithelium has the usual two cell layers with inner secretory cells and outer myoepithelial cells (Fig. 25–141). The fibrovascular stalks often undergo secondary changes in the form of hemorrhage, infarction, fibrosis, and hyalinization

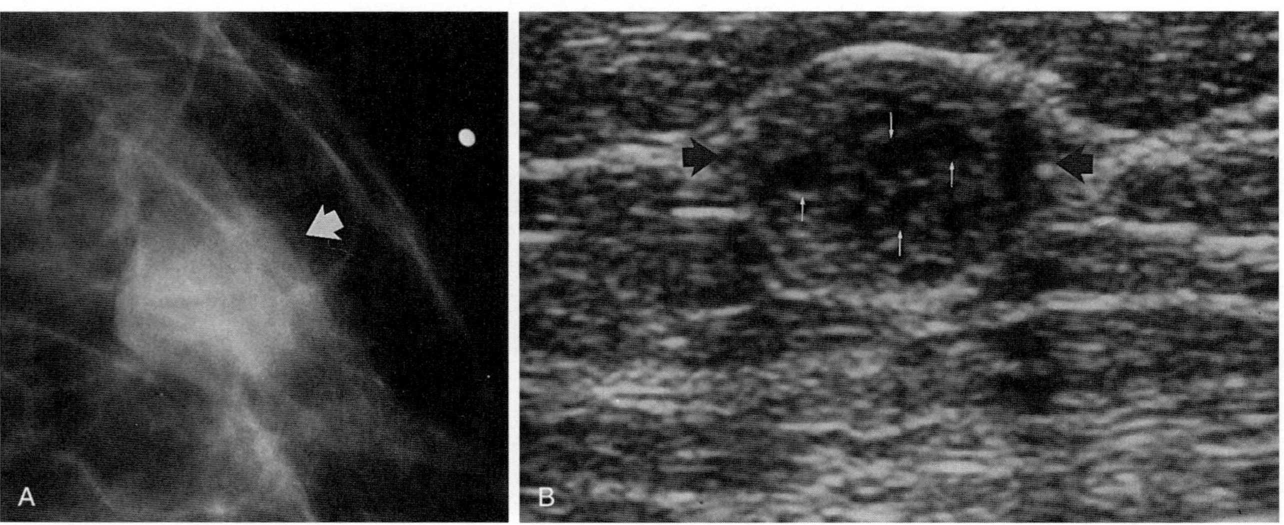

Figure 25–138. Juvenile papillomatosis. **A,** Mediolateral oblique mammogram of a 24-year-old woman with a palpable left breast mass. A 2-cm circumscribed round mass *(arrow)* is present. **B,** Ultrasonogram demonstrating a round circumscribed mass *(black arrows)* with several small internal anechoic spaces (*small white arrows*).

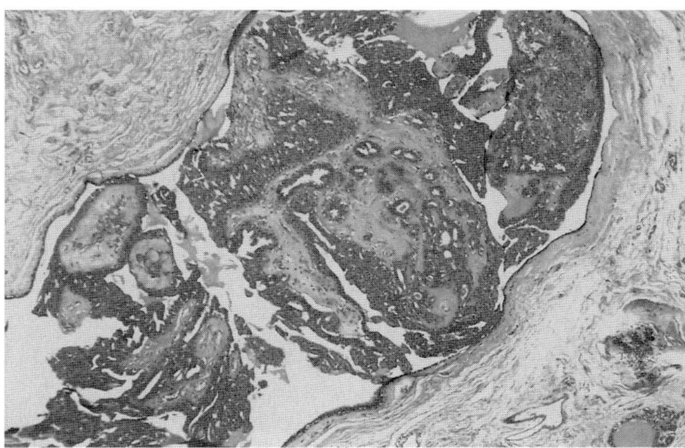

Figure 25–139. Papilloma. This papilloma occurs in a dilated duct and consists of plump papillary projections with fibrovascular cores. The proliferating ductal cells form irregular glandular spaces and solid sheets.

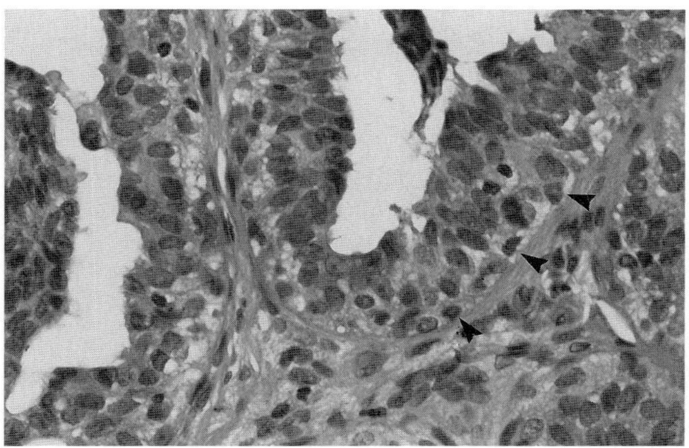

Figure 25–141. Papilloma. Proliferating cells include inner ductal epithelial cells and outer myoepithelial cells *(arrowheads)*.

(Fig. 25–142), most likely resulting from torsion of the fibrous stalks and ischemic injury. The damaged epithelium and hyalinized stroma may also deposit calcium. In core needle biopsies, potential diagnostic problems include entrapped ducts in the hyaline stroma mimicking invasive carcinoma. Nuclear atypia in papillary lesions needs careful evaluation to rule out atypical hyperplasia and ductal carcinoma in situ.

RADIAL SCAR

Clinical Aspects

Radial scar is a benign lesion known by a variety of names in the literature, including infiltrating epitheliosis, nonencapsulated sclerosing lesion, indurative mastopathy, scleroelastic lesion, sclerosing papillary proliferation, benign sclerosing ductal hyperplasia, and radial sclerosing lesion. It is almost always an asymptomatic lesion found on mammography. The cause is unknown, but it is not related to previous surgery or trauma.

Imaging Features

Most radial scars are spiculated masses or areas of architectural distortion, often with multiple long spicules and central areas of lucency (Fig. 25–143).[145-147] These findings are nonspecific, however, and may be found in invasive ductal carcinoma (Fig. 25–144), invasive lobular carcinoma, and many benign processes.[146,148-150] In addition, radial scars may have dense central regions (Figs. 25–145 and 25–146),[149,150] and microcalcifications may be mammographically visible in up to 37% of cases (Fig. 25–147).[146,148,151] In the first report in the literature of ultrasonography of radial scars, 57% showed only nonspecific posterior acoustic shadowing (Fig. 25–148).[150] Kopans showed a single case of ultrasonography of radial scar, which was an ill-defined hypoechoic mass with posterior acoustic

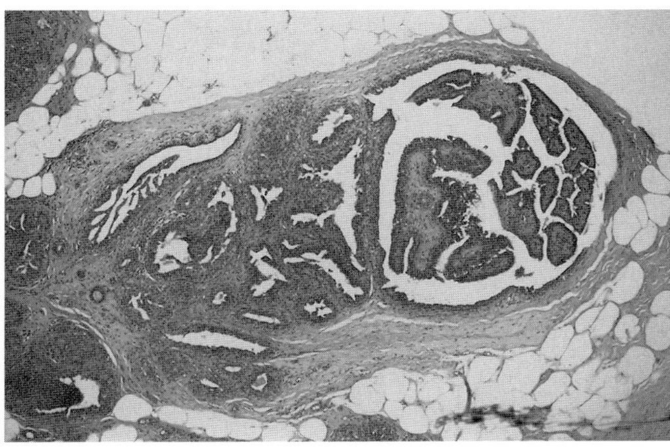

Figure 25–140. Papilloma. Proliferating ductal cells form complex papillary structures supported by fibrovascular cores.

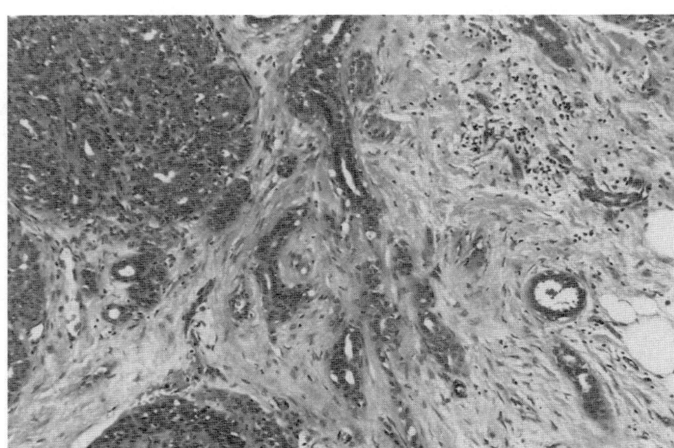

Figure 25–142. Papilloma. Stomal fibrosis in the fibrovascular cores results in entrapped ducts resembling an invasive ductal carcinoma (center field).

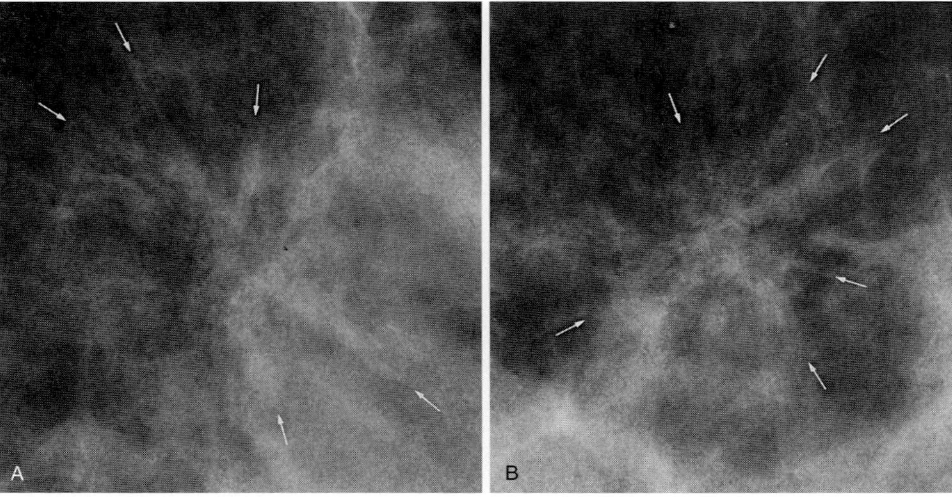

Figure 25–143. Radial scar. Magnification mediolateral oblique **(A)** and craniocaudal **(B)** views demonstrate a 2-cm area of architectural distortion with long radiating spicules *(arrows)* and areas of central lucency.

shadowing.[122] Thus, there is no known specific ultrasonographic appearance of radial scar.

It is not possible to differentiate between radial scar and breast carcinoma by imaging, and biopsy should be performed. There has been controversy over the years regarding the appropriate biopsy method for lesions for which radial scar is high in the differential diagnosis. In the past, excisional biopsy, rather than needle biopsy, was usually recommended because of the sampling error associated with the use of 14-gauge automated Tru-Cut biopsy devices; problems with differentiating between radial scar and other lesions, such as tubular carcinoma, in the small histologic specimens; and the fact that radial scar has been shown to be associated with invasive ductal carcinoma (not otherwise specified), tubular carcinoma, ductal carcinoma in situ (DCIS), lobular carcinoma in situ (LCIS), and atypical hyperplasia.[150,152-159] Today, in many practices, needle biopsy with a stereotactic 11-gauge directional vacuum-assisted device is the preferred method. Many of these lesions are carcinoma, rather than radial scar, and subsequent definitive therapy can proceed in the usual manner. For those lesions for which the histologic diagnosis is radial scar on the needle biopsy, most mammographers and pathologists recommend excision of the lesion to exclude sampling error (missing of an associated malignancy). It is possible that in the future, radial scar may be definitively diagnosed by needle biopsy, particularly when large amounts of tissue are removed with the large-gauge vacuum-assisted devices.

Pathology

Radial scar occurs in the background of benign ductal hyperplasia, intraductal papilloma, or sclerosing

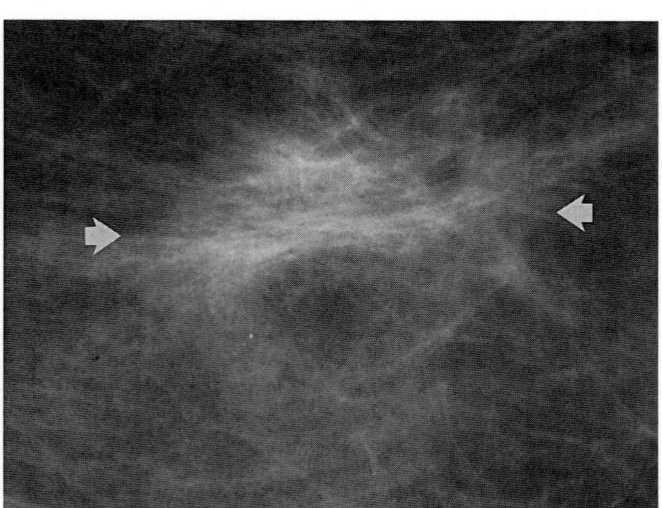

Figure 25–144. Invasive ductal carcinoma with radiating spicules and central lucencies *(arrows)*, mimicking radial scar.

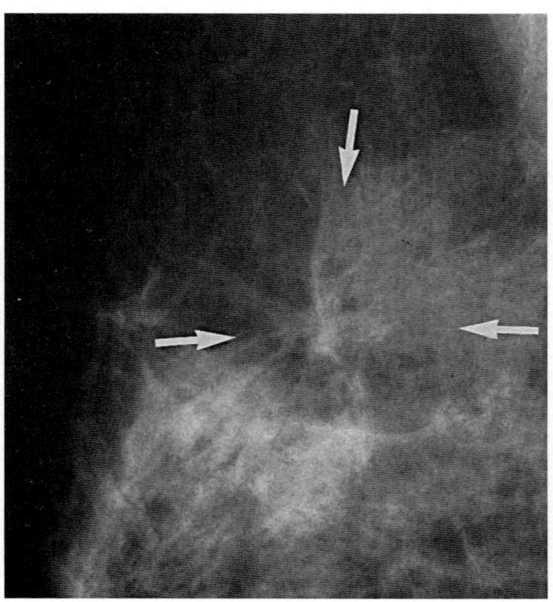

Figure 25–145. Radial scar *(arrows)* with central density.

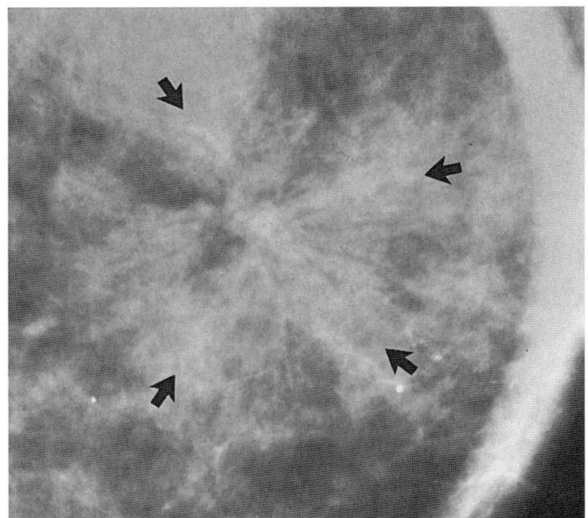

Figure 25–146. Radial scar *(arrows)* with central density.

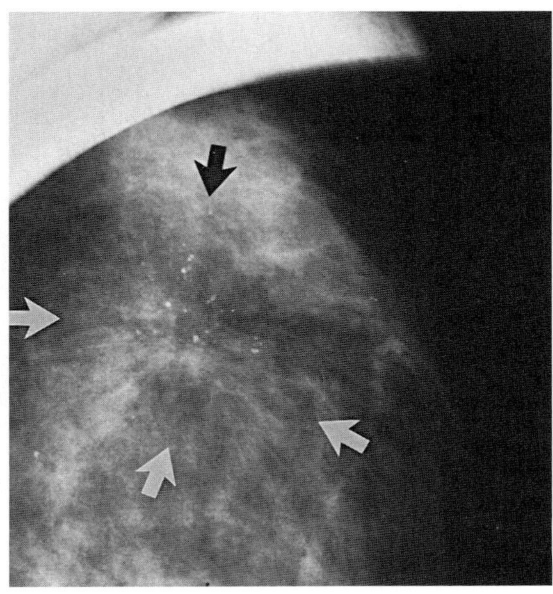

Figure 25–147. Radial scar with pleomorphic microcalcifications *(arrows)*.

adenosis. The center of the lesion undergoes fibrosis and elastosis, with resultant retraction of the periphery of the lesion (Fig. 25–149). As a result, fibrous strands with distorted entrapped ducts and ductules arranged in a radiating pattern are seen in the periphery (Fig. 25–150). Fat may be entrapped in the center of the lesion, giving rise to the central lucency seen on mammograms. The ducts entrapped in the scar may superficially resemble invasive carcinoma, particularly tubular carcinoma (Fig. 25–151). An important differentiating feature is the presence in tubular carcinoma of rounded glandular structures lined with a single layer of cells infiltrating adjacent fat. The benign ducts in radial scar retain the usual two cell layers of epithelial and myoepithelial cells without significant nuclear atypia or evidence of invasion.

EPITHELIAL HYPERPLASIAS WITH AND WITHOUT ATYPIA

The fundamental feature of epithelial hyperplasia is proliferation of the cells, with an increase in the layers of epithelium lining the glands beyond the usual double cell layer. Epithelial hyperplasia has been categorized as either ductal or lobular. This can

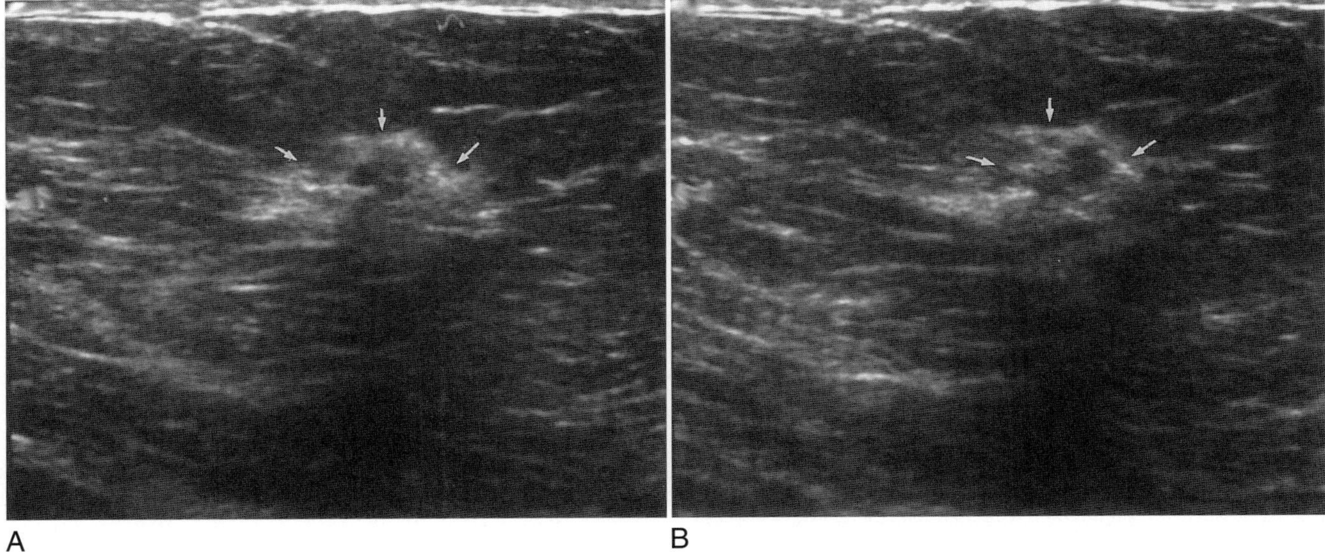

Figure 25–148. Radial scar. Radial **(A)** and antiradial **(B)** ultrasonograms demonstrate an irregular indistinct heterogeneous mass *(arrows)* with surrounding increased echogenicity and posterior acoustic shadowing.

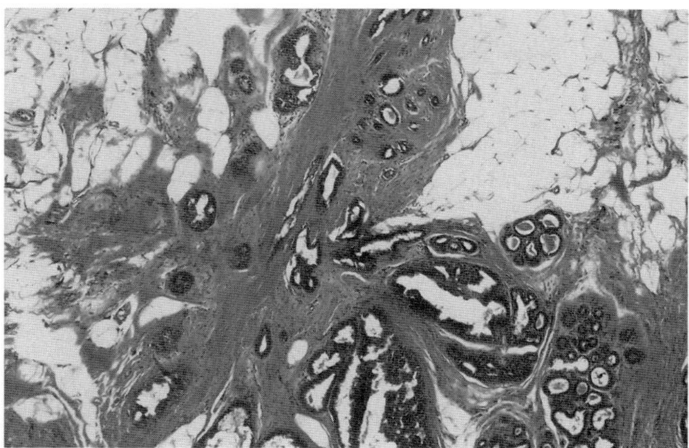

Figure 25–149. Radial scar. An area of ductal hyperplasia undergoes central fibrosis and elastosis, resulting in a spiculated lesion on mammography mimicking a malignancy.

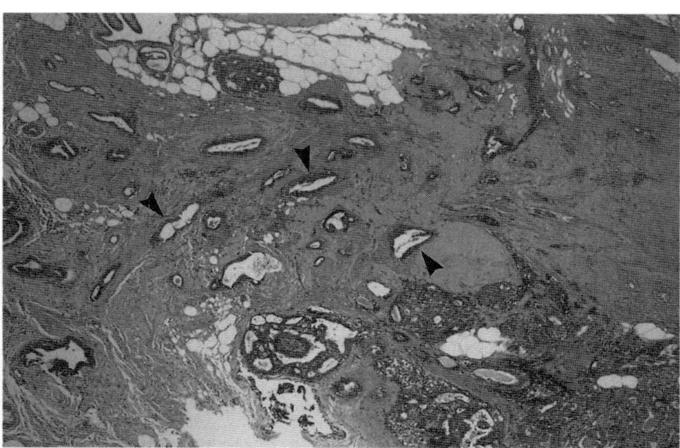

Figure 25–151. Radial scar. A broad area of fibrosis and elastosis with entrapped ducts *(arrowheads)* simulating an invasive ductal carcinoma. The fibrosis has strong eosinophilic staining, whereas the elastosis has lighter staining.

be misleading, because it tends to infer a site of origin for these lesions. Although atypical lobular hyperplasia is thought to arise from the lobular units, ductal hyperplasias do not arise solely from the ducts. In fact, these ductal-pattern lesions usually occur within the terminal duct lobular unit. For this reason, some authors prefer the term *epithelial hyperplasia of usual type* or *of no special type* rather than ductal type.[160] Each type of epithelial hyperplasia has a spectrum of morphologic changes ranging from mild, with almost no increased risk of malignancy, to severe, with patterns approaching that of carcinoma in situ. Epithelial hyperplasia without atypia has been demonstrated to carry an increased risk of subsequent invasive carcinoma of one and a half to two times that of the general population.[161] The presence of atypical ductal hyperplasia increases a woman's risk for subsequent development of breast cancer by approximately five times.[98] In addition, it can be difficult to distinguish from ductal carcinoma in situ on histologic examination and is often found in the vicinity of malignancy. Although the

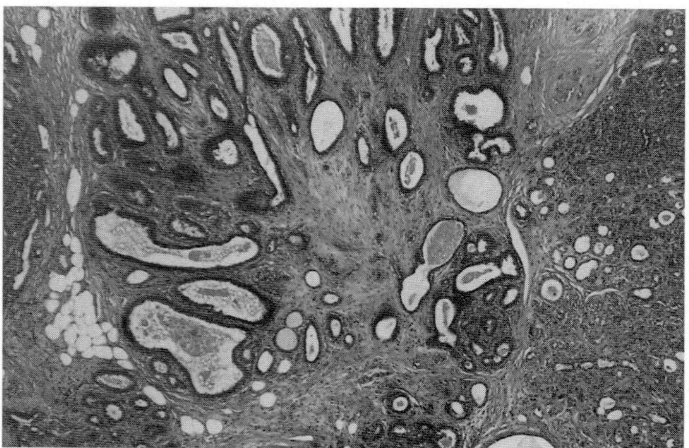

Figure 25–150. Radial scar. Central fibrosis results in a radiating pattern of the dilated ducts.

"upgrade" rate to carcinoma at surgical excision for atypical ductal hyperplasia diagnosed by 11-gauge directional vacuum-assisted devices is significantly less than for the 14-gauge automated Tru-Cut–type biopsies (which ranged from 40% to 50%), it remains high enough that an excisional biopsy should be performed when the result of atypical ductal hyperplasia is obtained on any type of needle biopsy.[162-169] Women with an *excisional* biopsy diagnosis of atypical ductal hyperplasia should have regular mammography and clinical breast examination to evaluate for the development of breast carcinoma.

Atypical lobular hyperplasia is also associated with an increased risk of developing an invasive carcinoma. The risk is less than with lobular carcinoma in situ and has been estimated to be four to five times greater than for the general population.[98,170-172] The developing carcinoma may appear in the ipsilateral or contralateral breast and is more likely to be of tubular or invasive lobular type.[170,173] The management of atypical lobular hyperplasia found on percutaneous needle biopsy remains controversial, but many researchers believe that excisional biopsy is required because some cases will be found to have malignancy present at surgery. In a recent study, the "upgrade" rate for core needle biopsy diagnosis of atypical lobular hyperplasia to malignancy was 17%.[174]

The following sections begin with a discussion of the histopathology of epithelial hyperplasias and then discuss their mammographic features.

Epithelial Hyperplasias, Ductal Type

In response to hormonal stimulation and imbalances, the ductal epithelium can undergo hyperplasia or involution. In hyperplasia, the number of cells above the basement membrane in the glandular structures increases. The proliferating cells may form a variety of histologic patterns, including papillary

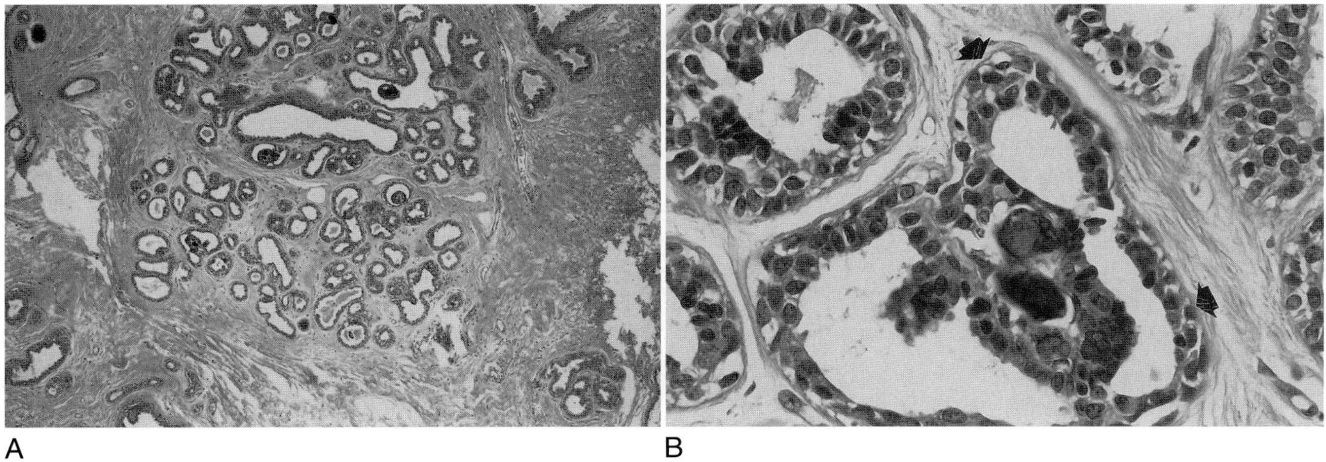

Figure 25–152. Epithelial ductal hyperplasia without atypia. **A,** A localized area of ductal hyperplasia with multiple microcalcifications. **B,** A higher magnification demonstrates laminated microcalcifications and proliferation of inner ductal epithelial cells and outer myoepithelial cells *(arrows)*. The nuclei of ductal cells contain finely granular chromatin with uniform distribution. The nucleoli are indistinct or small.

projections, cribriform spaces, or solid sheets of cells with occlusion of the ductal lumen (Fig. 25–152). Distinction from carcinoma in situ is based on many factors. One of the essential features is lack of cytologic atypia. The epithelial cells in ductal hyperplasia tend to be uniform in appearance with normochromic nuclei and inconspicuous nucleoli. Mitotic activity is low, and mitotic figures are morphologically normal. The cribriform pattern, when present, shows irregular glandular spaces. Punched-out, neatly rounded geometric spaces favor the diagnosis of carcinoma in situ. In addition, intermixed with the epithelial cells is a smaller population of myoepithelial cells. Epithelial hyperplasia is thus a polymorphic proliferation with a mixture of cell types, epithelial and myoepithelial, important in distinguishing it from carcinoma in situ.

Atypical Ductal Hyperplasia

Atypical ductal hyperplasia is defined as having some but not all the features of ductal carcinoma in situ. Atypical cells have enlargement, irregularity, and hyperchromasia of their nucleus with prominent nucleoli, all features suggestive of malignancy. These atypical cells coexist and are intermixed with benign ductal cells in the hyperplastic ductal epithelium (Fig. 25–153). Thus, atypical ductal hyperplasia lacks the homogeneous population of atypical cells seen in

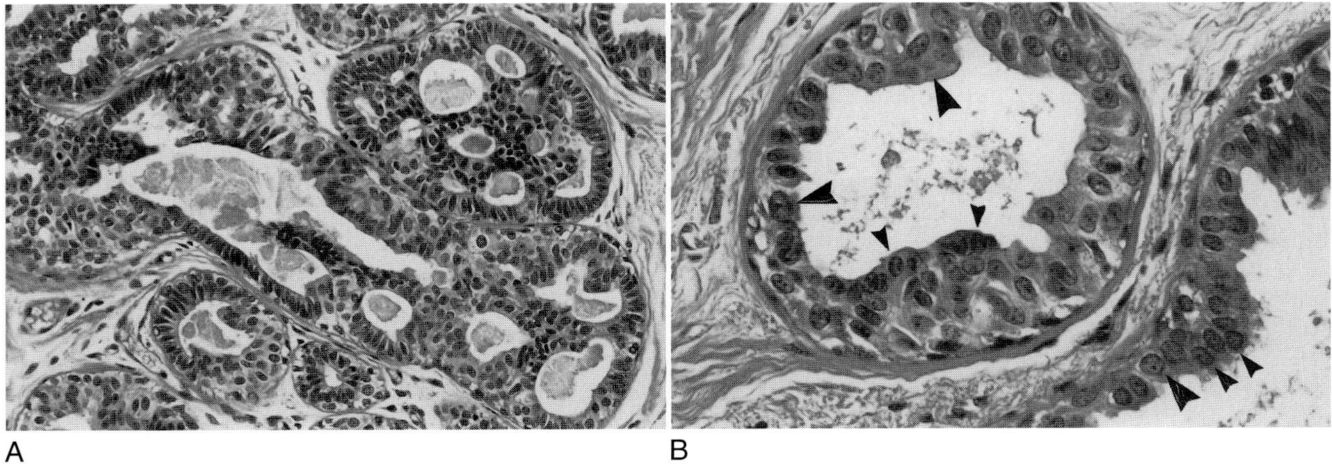

Figure 25–153. Epithelial ductal hyperplasia with atypia (atypical ductal hyperplasia). **A,** Complex cribriform glands with eosinophilic secretions in the glandular lumens. There is a mixture of ductal cells with and without nuclear atypia. In those ductal cells without atypia, the nuclei are arranged in parallel rows and are uniformly elongated. The atypical ductal cells are arranged in a disorderly fashion and have larger, more irregular nuclei. **B,** Comparison of atypical ductal cells, which have larger, more irregular nuclei, unevenly distributed chromatin, and more prominent nucleoli *(large arrowheads)* when compared with those ductal cells without nuclear atypia *(small arrowheads)*.

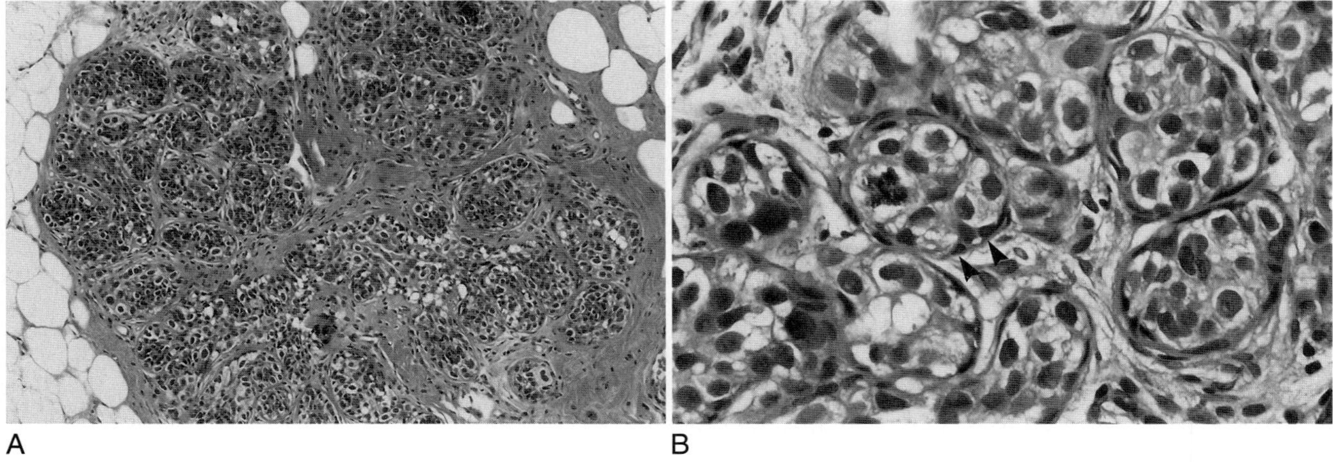

Figure 25–154. Epithelial lobular hyperplasia with atypia (atypical lobular hyperplasia). **A,** Expanded terminal ductular-lobular units. **B,** The acini are filled with atypical cells with enlarged round to oval, hyperchromatic nuclei, indistinct nucleoli, and a moderate amount of eosinophilic cytoplasm. A closer examination reveals rare myoepithelial cells with small hyperchromatic nuclei beneath the atypical lobular cells *(arrowheads)*. Their presence results in the appearance of a heterogeneous cellular population in the lobules.

ductal carcinoma in situ. The degree of atypia can vary from one part of the lesion to another, and the lesion may merge with foci of carcinoma in situ. Therefore, specimens exhibiting atypical hyperplasia should be sampled extensively.

Atypical Lobular Hyperplasia

Atypical lobular hyperplasia is used to describe hyperplasias of the terminal duct lobular unit that have some but not all of the features of lobular carcinoma in situ (Fig. 25–154). Its distinction from ductal hyperplasias described in the previous section is based on cytologic and architectural features rather than the site of origin. Differentiation between the two types of hyperplasia is important because of their different behavior, particularly with respect to multicentricity. On cytologic examination, the atypical cells in atypical lobular hyperplasia tend to be rounded or ovoid and exhibit marked uniformity with little variation in size or shape. Mitotic activity is rare. The proliferation tends to be polymorphic, as with ductal hyperplasias, with mixtures of myoepithelial and epithelial cells. Atypical lobular hyperplasia in its most severe form merges with lobular carcinoma in situ. If, on histologic examination of a specimen, any lobular unit meets the criteria for lobular carcinoma in situ, this diagnosis overrides that of atypical lobular hyperplasia.

Imaging Features

Few studies have documented the mammographic findings of epithelial hyperplasia, and these have dealt with atypical hyperplasias.[175-177] The lesion is often found within or adjacent to another benign or malignant mammographic abnormality.[177] The reported mammographic findings for these proliferative lesions include normal results, masses, architectural distortion, asymmetrical density, and, most commonly, microcalcifications (Figs. 25–155 to 25–157).[175,177] There are no reported characteristic ultrasonographic features. Therefore, the imaging findings are nonspecific, often mimic carcinoma, and require biopsy for diagnosis.

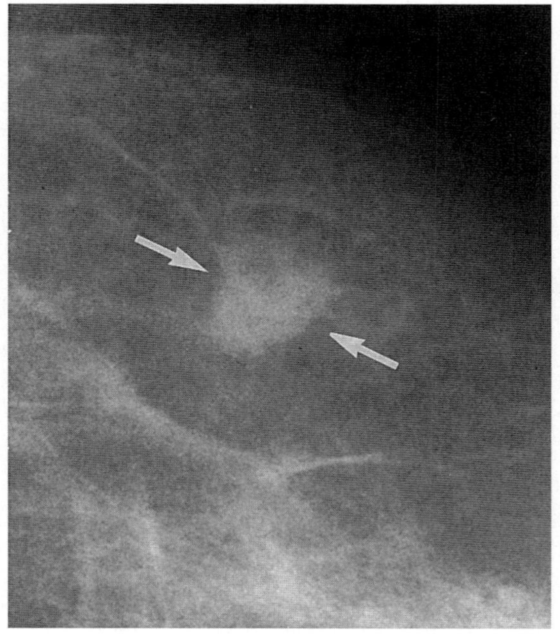

Figure 25–155. Atypical ductal hyperplasia. A 1-cm oval mass with indistinct margins *(arrows)*, simulating carcinoma.

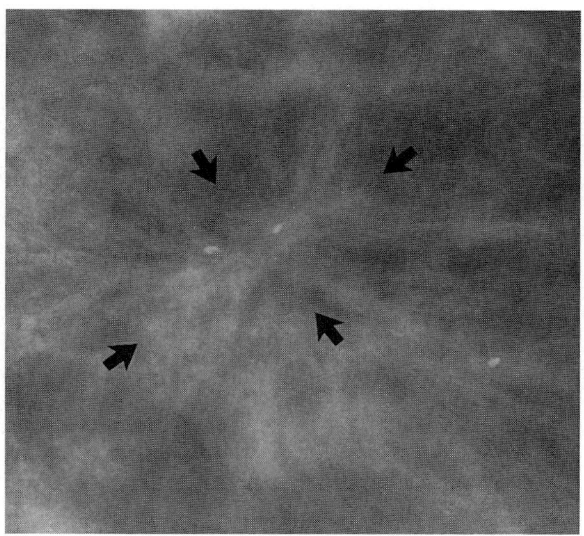

Figure 25–156. Atypical ductal hyperplasia. A 1.5-cm spiculated mass *(arrows)* containing two 1-mm calcifications.

LOBULAR CARCINOMA IN SITU, LOBULAR NEOPLASIA

Clinical Aspects and Pathology

LCIS was originally described in 1941 by Foote and Stewart.[178] No specific clinical signs or symptoms can be attributed to LCIS. Because LCIS is no longer considered a malignant lesion, the preferred term today is *lobular neoplasia*.

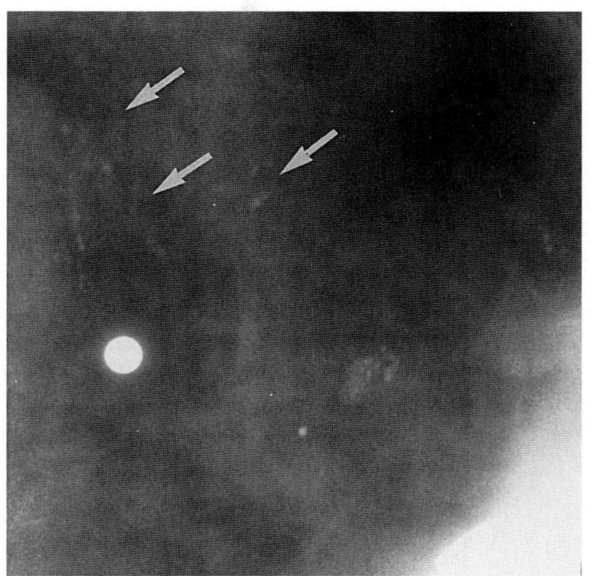

Figure 25–157. Atypical ductal hyperplasia. A 2-cm cluster of faint pleomorphic microcalcifications *(arrows)*.

Imaging Features

There are no mammographic or ultrasonographic features of lobular neoplasia.[179,180] It is an incidental finding at biopsy for another mammographic or clinical abnormality. The process is often multifocal or multicentric and may be bilateral. It is now considered to be a high-risk marker, rather than a true malignancy. A woman with lobular neoplasia has a relative risk of developing invasive carcinoma that is 8 to 11 times that of the general population and an absolute risk of 20% to 25% at 15 to 20 years after biopsy.[173,181] The subsequent invasive carcinoma may be ductal or lobular in origin and may occur at any location in either breast. The most common method of treatment of women with a biopsy result of lobular neoplasia is close clinical and mammographic surveillance, although some physicians advocate bilateral mastectomy.

The management of patients with lobular neoplasia diagnosed by imaging-guided needle biopsy remains controversial. It is important to be sure that the lesion for which biopsy was originally recommended is explained by histologic examination, because of the lack of imaging findings for lobular neoplasia. When the lesion is explained to be benign, and lobular neoplasia is found as an incidental finding, a small percentage of cases will be found to have a coexisting malignancy at surgical excision of that area. Thus, although many currently advocate surgical excision whenever lobular neoplasia is found on a needle biopsy, this varies by practice, and further studies will be required to determine the optimal management for these cases.[174,182-190]

Pathology

In LCIS, the breast lobules are expanded by atypical epithelial cells, which are small and rounded with dark nuclei, inconspicuous nucleoli, and a high nucleocytoplasmic ratio (Fig. 25–158). The cytoplasm may be clear. The epithelial cells tend to be uniform (see Fig. 25–158B), although some degree of cytologic heterogeneity may exist. Unlike atypical lobular hyperplasia, the proliferation is monomorphic with no myoepithelial cells. The cytoplasm may contain clear vacuoles (Fig. 25–159), a helpful marker, because it is frequently present in LCIS and absent in atypical lobular hyperplasia. The following criteria are recommended to achieve consistency in the diagnosis of LCIS: (1) The characteristic neoplastic cells must comprise the entire cell population in a lobular unit; (2) complete filling of the acini must be present, with no remaining spaces between the cells; and (3) at least one half of the acini in the lobular unit must be involved.[191]

In difficult cases, immunohistochemical staining for E-cadherin can be used to distinguish LCIS from lobular extension by DCIS. E-cadherin is expressed in

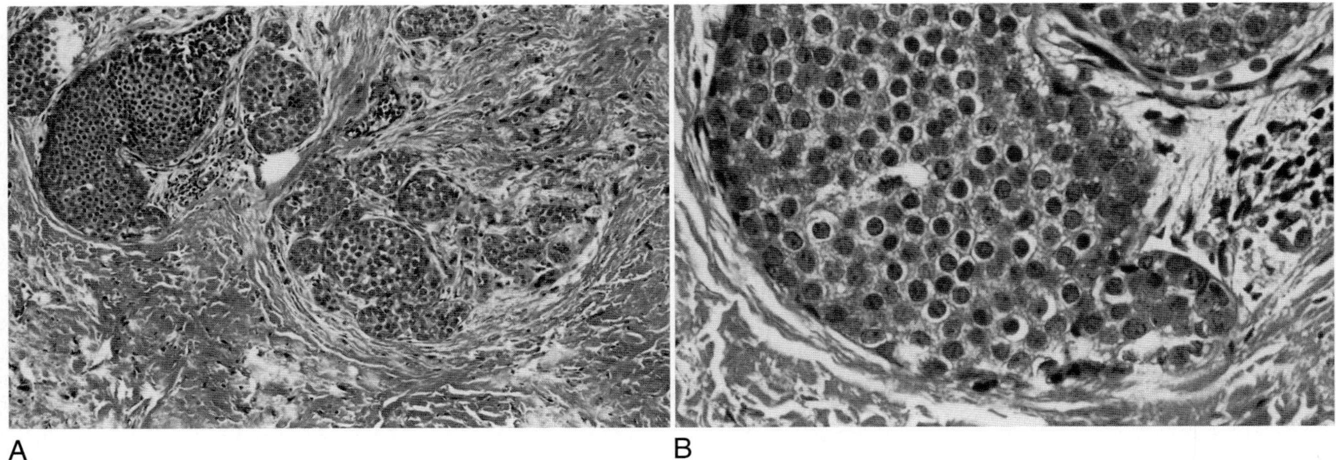

Figure 25–158. Lobular carcinoma in situ. **A,** Expanded terminal ductular-lobular unit with solid filling of atypical cells. **B,** These atypical cells have uniformly round to oval cells with mild nuclear enlargement and hyperchromasia, with a moderate amount of eosinophilic cytoplasm. Myoepithelial cells have largely disappeared, resulting in a homogeneous cell population.

only 9% of LCIS lesions, whereas all cases of DCIS are positive.[192]

PHYLLODES TUMOR

Clinical Aspects

Phyllodes tumor is an uncommon neoplasm originally described and named *cystosarcoma phyllodes* by Johannes Muller in 1838.[193] The currently preferred name is *phyllodes tumor*. This tumor occasionally has been equated with a giant fibroadenoma because both contain epithelial and mesenchymal elements, but the stroma of the phyllodes tumor is much more cellular. The average age at presentation is between 40 and 52 years, older than the average age at presentation for fibroadenomas.[194] Although small lesions are occasionally encountered, the most common clinical presentation is a large rapidly growing mass.

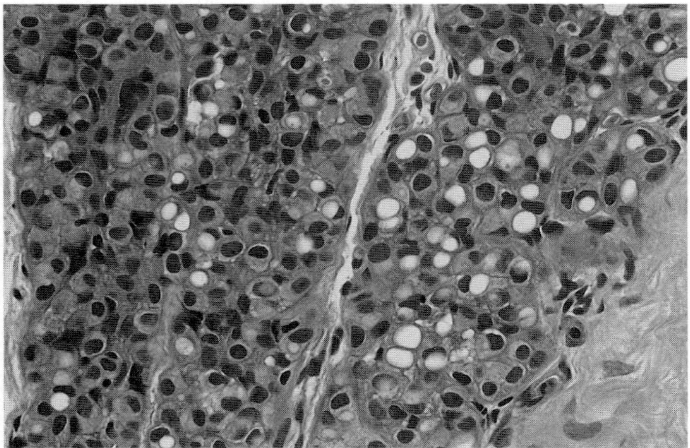

Figure 25–159. Lobular carcinoma in situ. Some of the atypical cells have a clear or vacuolated cytoplasm resembling signet-ring cells.

The clinical behavior of phyllodes tumor is unpredictable. Both benign and malignant phyllodes tumors may recur if incompletely excised. Therefore, wide local excision is required. The majority of phyllodes tumors are benign, but approximately 5% to 25% contain areas of malignancy.[195,196] Less than 20% of malignant lesions metastasize[197] via hematogenous spread, most commonly to the lung, pleura, and bone.[198,199]

Imaging Features

On mammography, most phyllodes tumors are large, circumscribed, noncalcified masses that are round, oval, or lobulated.[200-203] When small, the appearance is identical to a fibroadenoma (Fig. 25–160). When large, the size may suggest the diagnosis (Fig. 25–161). Calcifications are rare. Ultrasonography demonstrates a solid mass, often with inhomogeneous internal echoes and posterior acoustic enhancement, and sometimes containing small peripheral cystic spaces (see Figs. 25–161B and 25–162).[200,202-205] It is not possible to reliably differentiate between phyllodes tumor, fibroadenoma, and carcinoma based on the imaging features.

Pathology

Grossly, phyllodes tumor can measure up to 15 cm and have a lobular, circumscribed margin (Fig. 25–163). On microscopic examination, it is similar

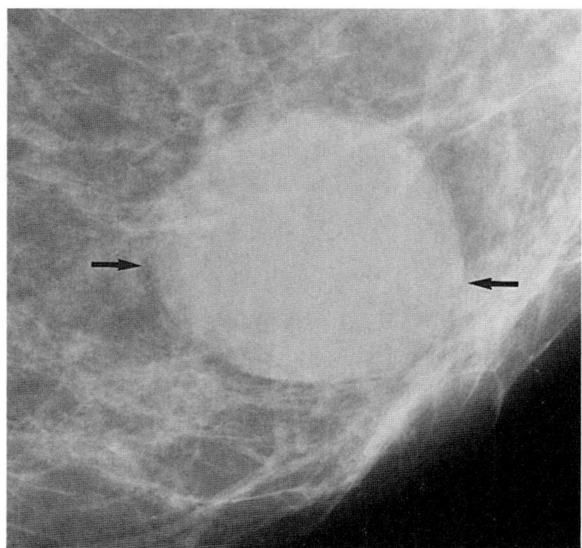

Figure 25–160. Benign phyllodes tumor. Left mediolateral oblique mammogram of a 4-cm round circumscribed mass *(arrows)*.

to a fibroadenoma, consisting of epithelial and stromal elements (see Fig. 25–163). Phyllodes tumor consists of branching, hyperplastic ducts. The stroma is mostly fibrous but is more cellular than in fibroadenoma.

Phyllodes tumor may be benign or malignant. For this reason, the designation *cystosarcoma phyllodes* has been replaced by phyllodes tumor, with the designation of benign, malignant, or borderline malignant based on histologic evaluation of the tumor. The benign phyllodes tumor characteristically has smooth, pushing borders with benign-appearing mesenchymal elements showing minimal nuclear atypia and low mitotic activity (Fig. 25–164). In contrast, malignant phyllodes tumors have infiltrative borders, moderate or severe nuclear atypia, and increased mitotic activity, usually three or more mitotic figures per 10 high-power fields (Fig. 25–165). In the presence of malignant-appearing stromal elements, it is important to adequately sample the neoplasm to determine whether ductal elements are present. In the absence of epithelial cells, the neoplasm is classified as primary stromal sarcoma of the breast.

OTHER BENIGN LESIONS

Lipoma

Lipomas are circumscribed fat-containing lesions that may occur anywhere within the breast. When palpable, they are usually soft and freely movable. On mammographic examination, a lipoma is a

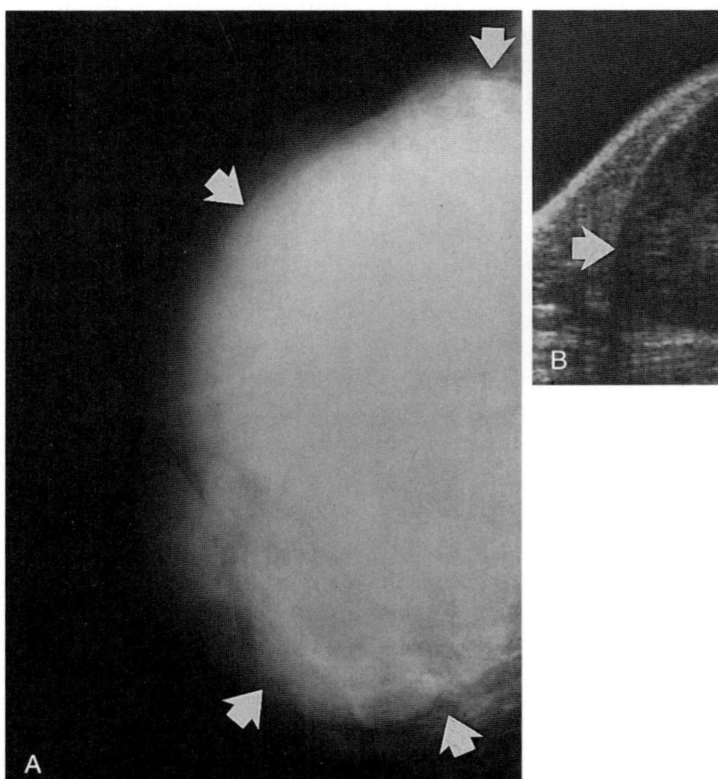

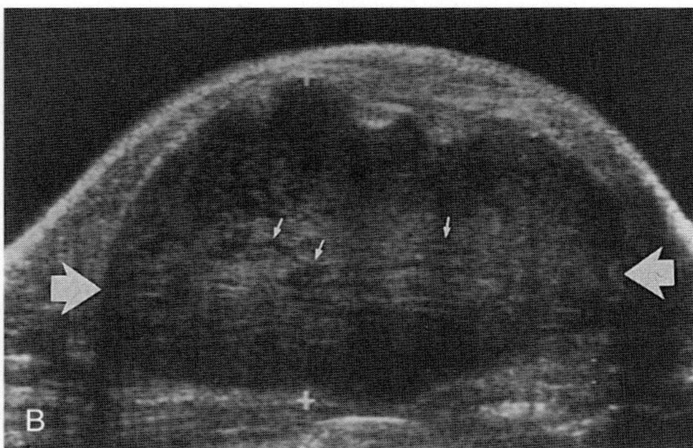

Figure 25–161. Large benign phyllodes tumor. **A,** Right mediolateral oblique mammogram shows a 9.5-cm circumscribed lobular mass filling most of the breast *(arrows)*. **B,** On ultrasonography, the mass (*large arrows*) has inhomogeneous internal echo texture. Although several anechoic slits are seen (*small arrows*), peripheral cystic spaces are not seen in this tumor.

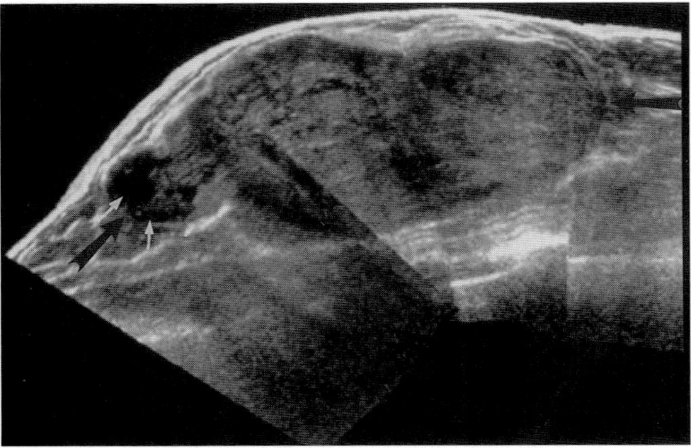

Figure 25–162. Large benign phyllodes tumor. Panoramic ultrasonogram demonstrates a 5.5-cm circumscribed lobular mass *(black arrows)* with peripheral cystic spaces *(white arrows)* as well as several internal cystic clefts.

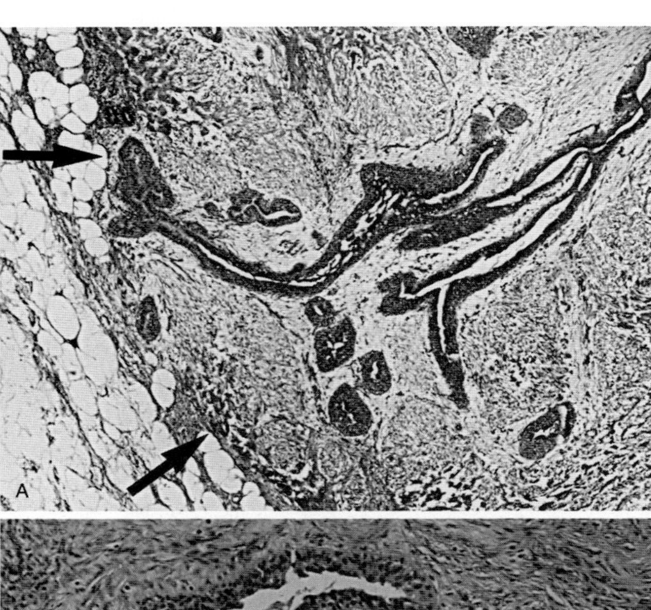

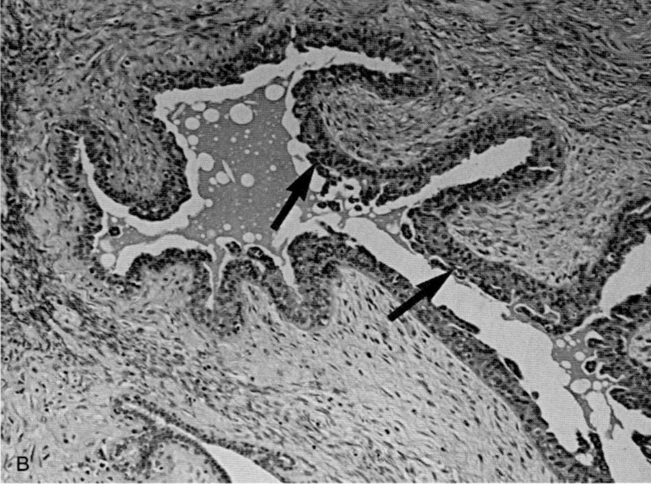

Figure 25–163. Benign phyllodes tumor. **A,** Note circumscribed margin of this tumor *(arrows)*. **B,** Classic histologic features of a phyllodes tumor are seen with abundant cellular fibrous stroma and epithelial lined clefts. Large leaflike papillary projections *(arrows)*, which push into the cystic spaces, are characteristic of this tumor.

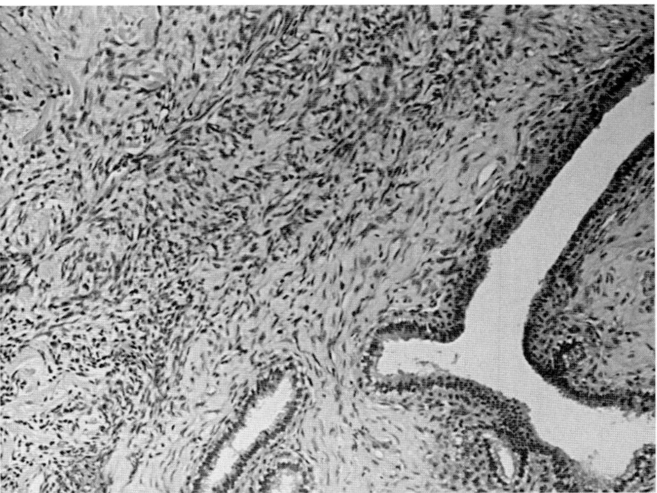

Figure 25–164. Benign phyllodes tumor. The stroma is densely cellular and consists mainly of spindle-celled fibroblasts. At higher power, no features of malignancy were seen in the stroma.

fat-containing, completely radiolucent lesion surrounded by a thin radiopaque capsule (Figs. 25–166 to 25–168). The appearance is diagnostic for a benign lesion, and further workup (including ultrasonography) or intervention is not necessary. On histologic examination, they are composed of mature adipose tissue (Fig. 25–169). The fat is normal on cytologic evaluation, and delicate encapsulation of the tumor may be present. Lipomas are not precursors to liposarcomas in the breast.

Liposarcomas are extremely rare lesions that can arise de novo or as malignant components within phyllodes tumor.[206] In a case report of liposarcoma of the pectoralis muscle, the internal density of the tumor was predominantly fat, but there were internal soft-tissue density nodules and an indistinct margin.[207] Most liposarcomas, however, are described as being radiographically dense, unless very well differentiated, because they often contain areas of hemorrhage, fat necrosis, and cystic change. The mass often becomes less circumscribed as it enlarges, so mammographic distinction between benign and malignant forms should not be a problem.[122,208]

Granular Cell Tumor

Granular cell tumor is an unusual benign lesion, first described as "granular cell myoblastoma" by Abrikossoff[209] in 1926 because he believed that it had a myogenic origin. More recently, it has become apparent that these tumors originate from Schwann cells.[122,210] Granular cell tumors occur in the tongue and many soft tissues of the body. Only approximately 6% occur in the breast.[211,212] Women are affected much more commonly than men, and the average age at the time of diagnosis is 40 years, approximately 10

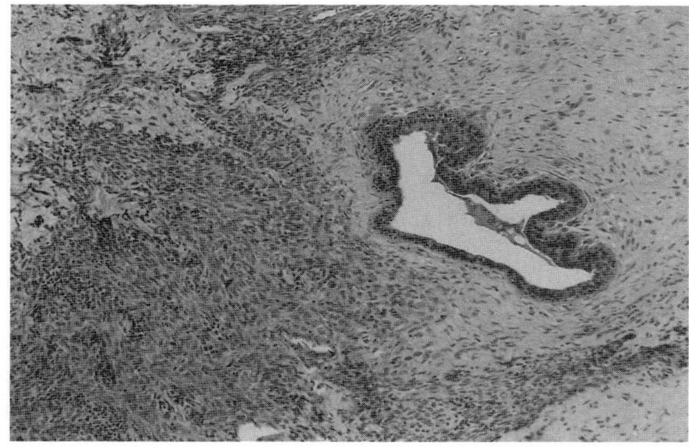

A

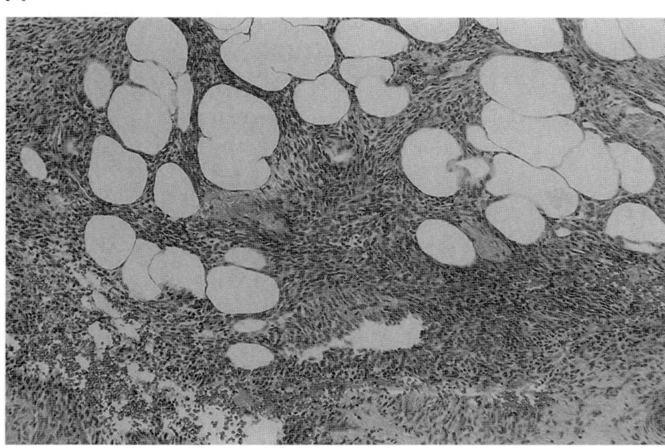

B

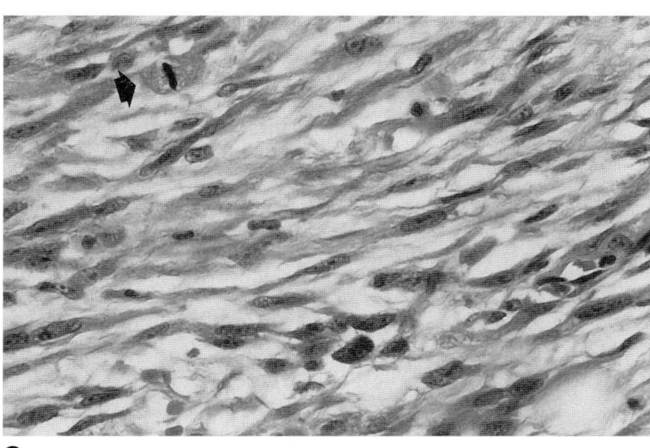

C

Figure 25–165. Malignant phyllodes tumor. **A,** A dilated hyperplastic duct and highly cellular fibrosarcomatous stroma. **B,** Fibrosarcomatous cells infiltrate the adjacent adipose tissue. **C,** A higher magnification of stromal cells demonstrates moderate nuclear atypia and mitotic figures *(arrow)*.

years younger than the mean age for breast carcinoma.[213] The majority of granular cell tumors occur in the upper-inner quadrant of the breast.[214]

Granular cell tumors usually mimic carcinoma on clinical breast examination, mammography, and ultrasonography. On physical examination, the

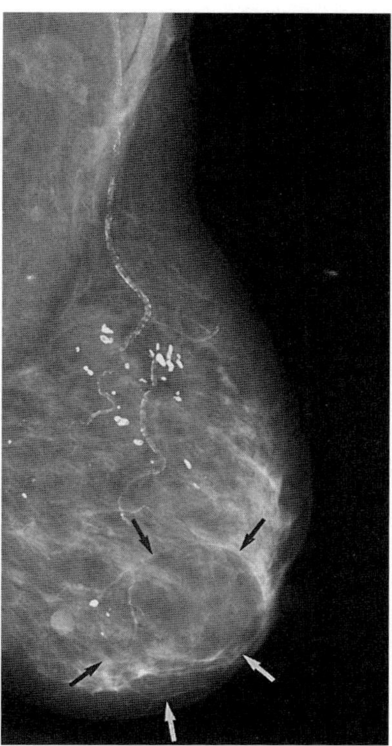

Figure 25–166. Lipoma. A 4-cm fat-density mass *(arrows)* on left mediolateral view. The soft-tissue density in the region of the mass is superimposed fibroglandular tissue located elsewhere in the breast.

lesion usually presents as a hard palpable mass, sometimes with fixation and skin ulceration. On mammography, the mass is usually round, oval, or irregular with spiculated or indistinct margins (Figs. 25–170 and 25–171).[148,211,215-217] Microcalcifications have not been reported in these lesions. For the few

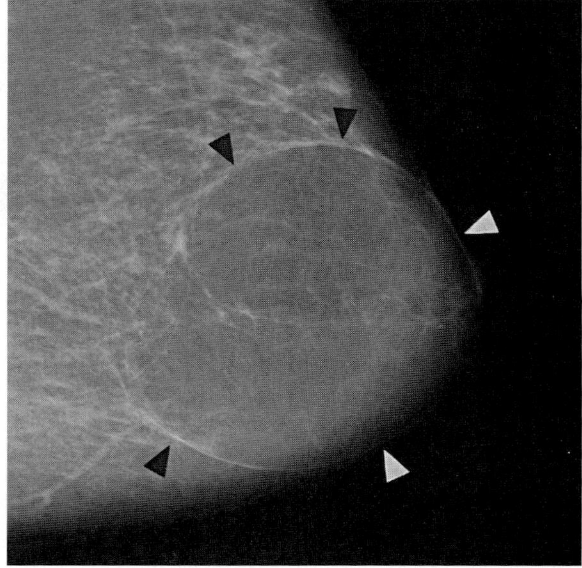

Figure 25–167. Lipoma. The radiopaque capsule *(arrowheads)* is visible around all except the most posterior aspect of the mass.

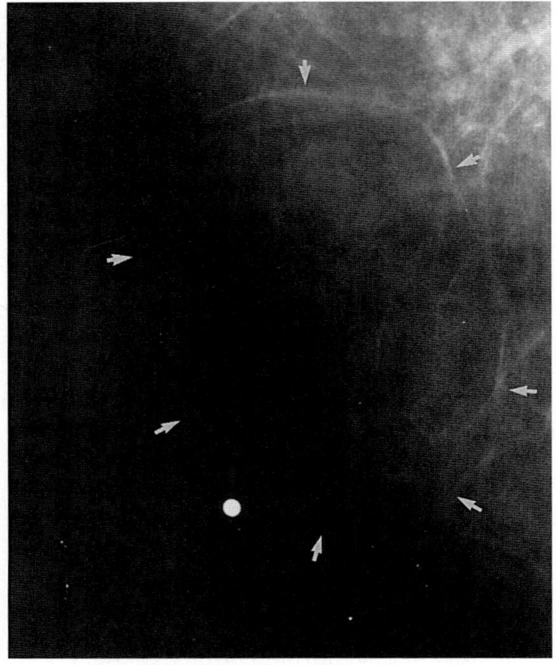

Figure 25–168. Lipoma. This woman presented with a firm palpable mass inferiorly in the right breast *(arrows)*. The mammographic appearance is diagnostic of a benign lipoma.

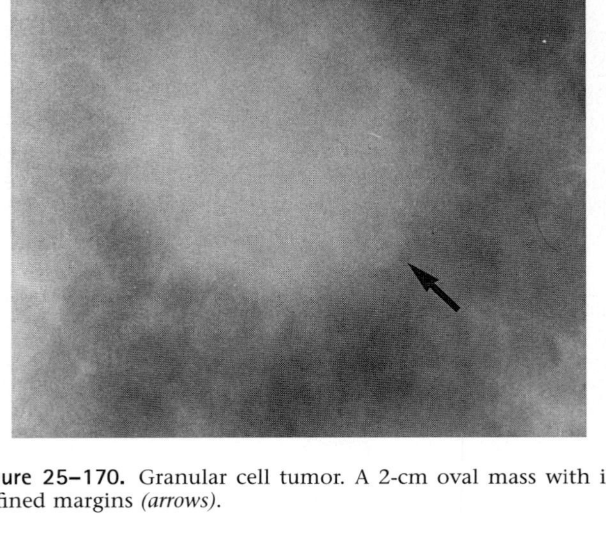

Figure 25–170. Granular cell tumor. A 2-cm oval mass with ill-defined margins *(arrows)*.

reported cases of ultrasound examination of granular cell tumors, ultrasonography has demonstrated irregular, highly attenuating masses.[216,218,219] Biopsy is therefore necessary to differentiate granular cell tumors from breast carcinoma. The distinction may be difficult on gross examination because the tumor is often firm and gritty. Histologic evaluation is necessary to make the diagnosis.

On histologic examination, the tumor cells have abundant granular eosinophilic cytoplasm and are arranged in bundles, cords, and nests in a dense fibrous stroma simulating an infiltrative carcinoma (Fig. 25–172). The granular, eosinophilic cytoplasm can mimic apocrine carcinoma. Fewer than 1% of granular cell tumors are malignant,[220] and standard treatment for histologically benign lesions is local excision.

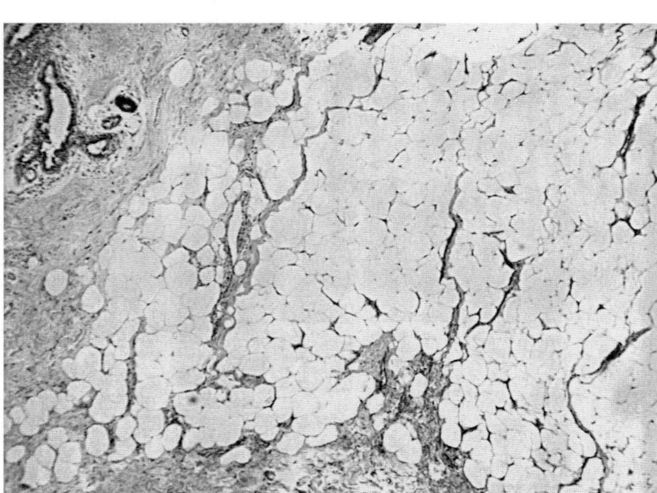

Figure 25–169. Lipoma. The tumor consists of a well-delineated mass of mature lobulated adipose tissue.

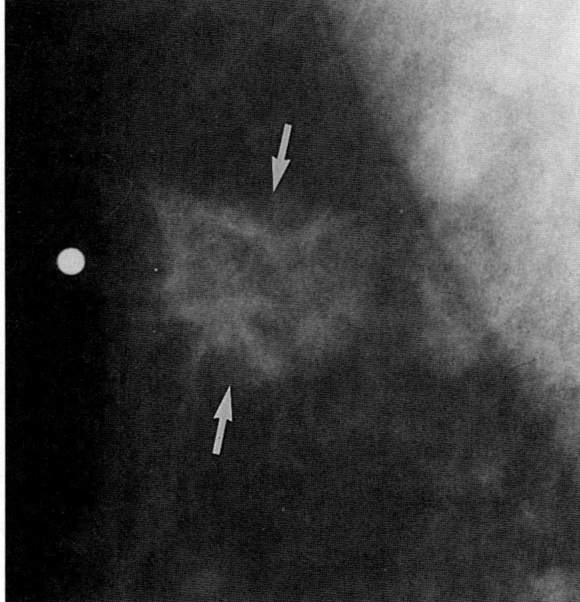

Figure 25–171. Granular cell tumor. A 1-cm ill-defined mass palpable in the right axillary tail *(arrows)*.

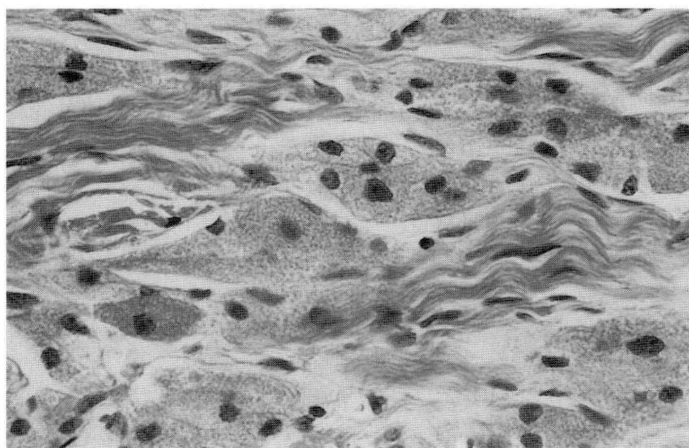

Figure 25–172. Granular cell tumor. Cords of tumor cells in a dense fibrous stroma simulate infiltrating carcinoma. The abundant eosinophilic granular cytoplasm and benign-appearing nuclei are characteristic of this tumor.

Extra-abdominal Desmoid

Extra-abdominal desmoid (fibromatosis of the breast) is an extremely rare, benign, localized proliferation of fibroblasts that usually presents as a firm, freely movable, nontender, palpable mass, with occasional skin retraction or fixation to the pectoralis muscle. On mammography, the few reported cases have been irregular, spiculated, noncalcified masses that were indistinguishable from carcinoma.[122,221-224] One report of ultrasonography of an extra-abdominal desmoid describes an irregular hypoechoic mass with posterior acoustic shadowing,[223] whereas the other reports an ill-defined hypoechoic mass,[224] both mimicking carcinoma. Therefore, biopsy is necessary to make the diagnosis.

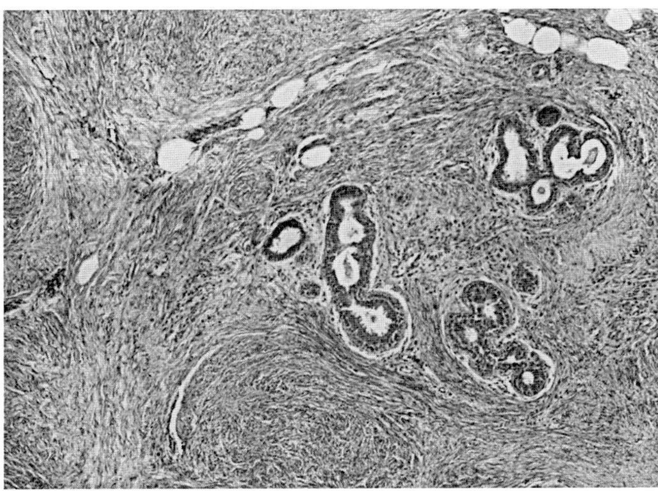

Figure 25–173. Extra-abdominal desmoid tumor. The normal lobule is infiltrated and separated by bundles of mature fibroblasts. The cellularity is much higher than in the normal fibrous stroma of the breast.

On histologic evaluation, this is an ill-defined, locally infiltrative, fibrous neoplasm consisting of mature fibroblasts arranged in interlacing bundles (Fig. 25–173). The cellularity is higher than the normal fibrous stroma. No nuclear atypia or increased mitotic activity is seen. The treatment for these lesions is wide local excision, because inadequately excised tumors have a tendency to recur. Mastectomy is sometimes necessary for recurrent tumor deep in the breast, soft tissue, or chest wall.

Acknowledgment

We wish to thank Brian D. White, MD, for his manuscript review and editorial suggestions.

References

1. Chantra PK, Tang JTC, Stanley TM, Bassett LW: Circumscribed fibrocystic mastopathy with formation of an epidermal cyst. AJR Am J Roentgenol 1994;163:831-832.
2. Magid ML, Wentzell JM, Roenigk HH: Multiple cystic lesions: Steatocystoma multiplex. Arch Dermatol 1990;126:101-102.
3. Aboody LR, Asch T, Estabrook A: Breast masses in two women with steatocystoma multiplex. Invest Radiol 1992;27:329-330.
4. Pollack AH, Kuerer HM: Steatocystoma multiplex: Appearance at mammography. Radiology 1991;180:836-838.
5. Park KY, Oh KK, Noh TW: Steatocystoma multiplex: Mammographic and ultrasonographic manifestations. AJR Am J Roentgenol 2003;180:271-274.
6. Westeren AC, Santiago ML, Cigtay OS: Severe nodulocystic acne causing "ring lesions" on mammography. AJR Am J Roentgenol 1003;160:1148.
7. Kopans DB, Meyer JE, Homer MJ, Grabbe J: Dermal deposits mistaken for breast calcifications. Radiology 1983;149:592-594.
8. Berkowitz JE, Gatewood OMB, Donovan GB, Gayler BW: Dermal breast calcifications: Localization with template-guided placement of skin marker. Radiology 1987;163:282.
9. Frenna TH, Meyer JE: Identification of atypical skin calcifications. Radiology 1993;187:584.
10. Gyves-Ray KM, Adler DD: Dermatomyositis: An unusual cause of breast calcifications. Breast Dis 1989;2:195-201.
11. Black KA, Zilko PJ, Dawkins RL, et al: Cancer in connective tissue disease. Arthritis Rheum 1982;25:1130-1133.
12. Callen JP: Dermatomyositis. Dermatol Clin 1983;1:461-473.
13. Gold RH, Bassett LW, Coulson WF: Mammographic features of malignant and benign disease. In Bassett LW, Gold RH (eds): Breast Cancer Detection: Mammography and Other Methods in Breast Imaging, 2nd ed. Orlando, FL, Grune & Stratton, 1987, pp 15-65.
14. Sickles EA, Galvin HB: Breast arterial calcification in association with diabetes mellitus: Too weak a correlation to have clinical utility. Radiology 1985;155:577-579.
15. Van Noord PA, Beijerinck D, Kemmeren JM, van der Graaf Y: Mammograms may convey more than breast cancer risk: Breast arterial calcification and arteriosclerotic related diseases in women of the DOM cohort. Eur J Cancer Prev 1996; 5:483-487.
16. Evans AJ, Cohen MEL, Cohen GF: Patterns of breast calcification in patients on renal dialysis. Clin Radiol 1992;45:343-344.
17. Sommer G, Kopsa H, Zazgornik J, Salomonowitz E: Breast calcifications in renal hyperparathyroidism. AJR Am J Roentgenol 1987;148:855-857.
18. Conant EF, Wilkes AN, Mendelson EB, Feig SA: Superficial thrombophlebitis of the breast (Mondor's disease): Mammographic findings. AJR Am J Roentgenol 1993;160:1201-1203.

19. Cooper RA: Mondor's disease secondary to intravenous drug abuse. Arch Surg 1990;125:807-808.
20. Gutman H, Kott I, Reiss R: Inflammatory carcinoma of the breast with Mondor's disease. Practitioner 1987;231:1086-1088.
21. Levi I, Baum M: Mondor's disease as a presenting symptom of breast cancer. Br J Surg 1987;74:700.
22. Egan RL, McSweeney MB: Intramammary lymph nodes. Cancer 1983;51:1838-1842.
23. Meyer JE, Ferraro FA, Frenna TH, et al: Mammographic appearance of normal intramammary lymph nodes in an atypical location. AJR Am J Roentgenol 1993;161:779-780.
24. Gordon PB, Gilks B: Ultrasonographic appearance of normal intramammary lymph nodes. J Ultrasound Med 1988;7:545-548.
25. Marchal G, Verschakelen J, Gelin J, et al: Ultrasonographic appearance of normal lymph nodes. J Ultrasound Med 1985; 4:417-419.
26. Helvie MA, Rebner M, Sickles EA, Oberman HA: Calcifications in metastatic breast carcinoma in axillary lymph nodes. AJR Am J Roentgenol 1988;151:921-922.
27. Kopans DB, Meyer JE, Murphy GF: Benign lymph nodes associated with dermatitis presenting as breast masses. Radiology 1980;137:15-19.
28. Lindfors KK, Kopans DB, McCarthy KA, et al: Breast cancer metastasis to intramammary lymph nodes. AJR Am J Roentgenol 1986;146:133-136.
29. Meyer JE, Kopans DB, Long JC: Mammographic appearance of malignant lymphoma of the breast. Radiology 1980;135: 623-626.
30. Schmidt WA, Boudousquie AC, Vetto JT, et al: Lymph nodes in the human female breast: A review of their detection and significance. Hum Pathol 2001;32:178-187.
31. Bruwer A, Nelson GW, Spark RP: Punctate intranodal gold deposits simulating microcalcifications on mammograms. Radiology 1987;163:87-88.
32. Vassallo P, Wernecke K, Roos N, Peters PE: Differentiation of benign from malignant superficial lymphadenopathy: The role of high-resolution US. Radiology 1992;183:215-220.
33. Vassallo P, Edel G, Roos N, et al: In-vitro high-resolution ultrasonography of benign and malignant lymph nodes: A ultrasonographic-pathologic correlation. Invest Radiol 1993; 28:698-705.
34. Stigers KB, King JG, Davey DD, Stelling CB: Abnormalities of the breast caused by biopsy: Spectrum of mammographic findings. AJR Am J Roentgenol 1991;156:287-291.
35. Bassett LW, Gold RH, Cove HC: Mammographic spectrum of traumatic fat necrosis: The fallibility of "pathognomonic" signs of carcinoma. AJR Am J Roentgenol 1978;130:119-122.
36. Bassett LW, Gold RH, Mirra JM: Nonneoplastic breast calcifications in lipid cysts: Development after excision and primary irradiation. AJR Am J Roentgenol 1982;138:335-338.
37. Evers K, Troupin RH: Lipid cyst: Classic and atypical appearances. AJR Am J Roentgenol 1991;157:271-273.
38. Beyer GA, Thorsen MK, Shaffer KA, Walker AP: Mammographic appearance of the retained Dacron cuff of a Hickman catheter. AJR Am J Roentgenol 1990;155:1203-1204.
39. Wakabayashi M, Reid JD, Bhattacharjee M: Foreign body granuloma caused by prior gunshot wound mimicking malignant breast mass. AJR Am J Roentgenol 1999;173:321-322.
40. Meguid MM, Kort KC, Numann PJ, Oler A: Subareolar breast abscess: The penultimate stage of the Mammary Duct Associated Disease Sequence. In Bland KI, Copeland EM: The Breast: Comprehensive Management of Benign and Malignant Disorders. Philadelphia, Saunders, 2004, pp 93-131.
41. Radhi JM, Thavanathan MJ: Hydatid cyst presenting as a breast lump. Can J Surg 1990;33:29-30.
42. Vega A, Ortega E, Cavada A, Garijo F: Hydatid cyst of the breast: Mammographic findings. AJR Am J Roentgenol 1994; 162:825-826.
43. Seymour EQ: Blastomycosis of the breast. AJR Am J Roentgenol 1982;139:822-823.
44. Gorman JD, Champaign JL, Sumida FK, Canavan L: Schistosomiasis involving the breast. Radiology 1992;185:423-424.
45. Britton CA, Sumkin J, Math M, Williams S: Mammographic appearance of loiasis. AJR Am J Roentgenol 1992;159:51-52.
46. Aguirrezabalaga J, Sogo C, Parajo A, et al: Mammary tuberculosis. Three case reports. Breast Dis 1994;7:377-382.
47. Hayes R, Michell M, Nunnerley HB: Acute inflammation of the breast—The role of breast ultrasound in diagnosis and management. Clin Radiol 1991;44:253-256.
48. Karstrup S, Solvig J, Nolsoe CP, et al: Acute puerperal breast abscesses: US-guided drainage. Radiology 1993;188:807-809.
49. Garg P, Rathee SK, Lal A: Ultrasonically guided percutaneous drainage of breast abscess. J Indian Med Assoc 1997;95:584-585.
50. Ikeda DM, Sickles EA: Mammographic demonstration of pectoral muscle microcalcifications. AJR Am J Roentgenol 1988; 151:475-476.
51. Han B-K, Choe YH, Park JM, et al: Granulomatous mastitis: Mammographic and ultrasonographic appearances. AJR Am J Roentgenol 1999;173:317-320.
52. Rosen PP: Fibroepithelial neoplasms. In Rosen PP: Rosen's Breast Pathology, 2nd ed. Philadelphia, Lippincott Williams & Wilkins, 2001, pp 163-200.
53. Haagensen CD: Adenofibroma. In Haagensen CD (ed): Diseases of the Breast, 3rd ed. Philadelphia, WB Saunders, 1986, pp 267-283.
54. Ackerman LV, Rosai J: Surgical Pathology. St. Louis, Mosby, 1974, pp 906-908.
55. Azzopardi JG: Fibroadenoma. In Azzopardi JG (ed): Problems in Breast Pathology. Philadelphia, WB Saunders, 1979, pp 39-56.
56. Meyer JE, Frenna TH, Polger M, et al: Enlarging occult fibroadenomas. Radiology 1992;183:639-641.
57. Swisher RC, Gade NR, Suk JJ, et al: Enlarging fibroadenoma in a postmenopausal woman: Case report. Radiology 1992; 184:425-426.
58. Cole-Beuglet C, Soriano RZ, Kurtz AB, Goldberg BB: Fibroadenoma of the breast: Ultrasonomammography correlated with pathology in 122 patients. AJR Am J Roentgenol 1983;140: 369-375.
59. Leucht NJ, Dagmar RR, Klaus-Dieter H: Diagnostic value of different interpretive criteria in real-time ultrasonography of the breast. Ultrasound Med Biol 1988;14:59-73.
60. Fornage BD, Lorigan JG, Andry E: Fibroadenoma of the breast: Ultrasonographic appearance. Radiology 1989;172: 671-675.
61. Heywang SH, Lipsit ER, Glassman LM, Thomas MA: Specificity of ultrasonography in the diagnosis of benign breast masses. J Ultrasound Med 1984;3:453-461.
62. Jackson VP, Rothschild PA, Kreipke DL, et al: The spectrum of ultrasonographic findings of fibroadenoma of the breast. Invest Radiol 1986;21:34-40.
63. Cosmacini P, Veronesi P, Galimberti V, et al: Ultrasonographic evaluation of palpable breast masses: Analysis of 134 cases. Tumori 1990;76:495-498.
64. Adler DD, Hyde DL, Ikeda DM: Quantitative ultrasonographic parameters as a means of distinguishing breast cancers from benign solid breast masses. J Ultrasound Med 1991;10:505-508.
65. Cosgrove DO, Kedar RP, Bamber JC, et al: Breast diseases: Color Doppler US in differential diagnosis. Radiology 1993; 189:99-104.
66. Dock W: Duplex ultrasonography of mammary tumors: A prospective study of 75 patients. J Ultrasound Med 1993;12: 79-82.
67. Fornage BD, Sneige N, Faroux MJ, Andry E: Sonographic appearance and ultrasound-guided fine-needle aspiration biopsy of breast carcinomas smaller than 1 cm^3. J Ultrasound Med 1990;9:559-568.
68. McNicholas MMJ, Mercer PM, Miller JC, et al: Color Doppler ultrasonography in the evaluation of palpable breast masses. AJR Am J Roentgenol 1993;161:765-771.
69. Pamilo M, Soiva M, Anttinen I, et al: Ultrasonography of breast lesions detected in mammography screening. Acta Radiol 1991;32:220-225.

70. Stavros AT, Dennis MA: The ultrasound of breast pathology. In Parker SH, Jobe WE (eds): Percutaneous Breast Biopsy. New York, Raven Press, 1993, pp 111-127.
71. Stavros AT, Thickman D, Rapp CL, et al: Solid breast nodules: Use of ultrasonography to distinguish between benign and malignant lesions. Radiology 1995;196:123-134.
72. Ueno EI, Tohna E, Itoh K: Classification and diagnostic criteria in breast echography. Japan J Med Ultrasonics 1986;13: 19-31.
73. Sickles EA: Nonpalpable, circumscribed, noncalcified solid breast masses: Likelihood of malignancy based on lesion size and age of patient. Radiology 1994;192:439-442.
74. Hertel BG, Zaloudek C, Kempson RL: Breast adenomas. Cancer 1976;37:2891-2905.
75. O'Hara MF, Page DL: Adenomas of the breast and ectopic breast under lactational influences. Hum Pathol 1985;16: 707-712.
76. Pike AM, Oberman HA: Juvenile (cellular) fibroadenoma. A clinicopathologic study. Am J Surg Pathol 1985;9:730-736.
77. Baker KS, Monsees BS, Diaz NM, et al: Carcinoma within fibroadenomas: Mammographic features. Radiology 1990; 176:371-374.
78. Pick PW, Iossifides IA: Occurrence of breast carcinoma within a fibroadenoma: A review. Arch Pathol Lab Med 1984;108: 590-594.
79. Yoshida Y, Takaoka M, Fukumoto M: Carcinoma arising in fibroadenoma: Case report and review of the world literature. J Surg Oncol 1985;29:132-140.
80. Andersson I, Hildell J, Linell F, Ljungqvist U: Mammary hamartomas. Acta Radiol [Diagn] 1979;20:712-720.
81. Arrigoni M, Dockerty M, Judd E: The identification and treatment of mammary hamartoma. Surg Gynecol Obstet 1971; 133:577-582.
82. Fechner RE: Fibroadenoma and related lesions. In Page DL, Anderson TJ (eds): Diagnostic Histopathology of the Breast. Edinburgh, Churchill Livingstone, 1987, pp 72-85.
83. Crothers JG, Butler NF, Fortt RW, Gravelle IH: Fibroadenolipoma of the breast. Br J Radiol 1985;58:191-202.
84. Helvie MA, Adler DD, Rebner M, Oberman HA: Breast hamartomas: Variable mammographic appearance. Radiology 1989; 170:417-421.
85. Hessler C, Schnyder P, Ozzello L: Hamartoma of the breast: Diagnostic observation of 16 cases. Radiology 1978;126:95-98.
86. Adler DD, Jeffries DO, Helvie MA: Ultrasonographic features of breast hamartomas. J Ultrasound Med 1990;9:85-90.
87. Kopans DB, Meyer JE, Proppe KH: Ultrasonographic, xeromammographic and histologic correlation of a fibroadenolipoma of the breast. J Clin Ultrasound 1982;10:409-411.
88. Tse GMK, Law BKB, Ma TKF, et al: Hamartoma of the breast: A clinicopathological review. J Clin Pathol 2002;55:951-954.
89. Wahner-Roedler DL, Sebo TJ, Gisvold JJ: Hamartomas of the breast: Clinical, radiologic, and pathologic manifestations. Breast J 2001;7:101-105.
90. Berna JD, Nieves FJ, Romero T, Arcas I: A multimodality approach to the diagnosis of breast hamartomas with atypical mammographic appearance. Breast J 2001;7:2-7.
91. Rosen PP, Oberman HA: Miscellaneous neoplasms. In Rosen PP, Oberman HA (eds): Tumors of the Mammary Gland. Washington, DC, Armed Forces Institute of Pathology, 1993, pp 343-354.
92. Baron M, Ladonne J-M, Gravier A, et al: Invasive lobular carcinoma in a breast hamartoma. Breast J 2003;9:246-248.
93. Lee EH, Wylie EJ, Bourke AG, Bastiaan De Boer W: Invasive ductal carcinoma arising in a breast hamartoma: Two case reports and a review of the literature. Clin Radiol 2003;58:80-83.
94. Daya D, Trus T, D'Souza TJ, et al: Hamartoma of the breast, an underrecognized breast lesion. Am J Clin Pathol 1995; 103:685-689.
95. Devitt JE: Clinical benign disorders of the breast and carcinoma of the breast. Surg Gynecol Obstet 1981;152:437-440.
96. Love SM, Gelman RS, Silen W: Fibrocystic "disease" of the breast: A nondisease? N Engl J Med 1982;307:1010-1014.
97. Page DL, Jensen RA, Simpson JF: Premalignant and malignant disease of the breast: The role of the pathologist. Mod Pathol 1998;11:120-128.
98. Cancer Committee of the College of American Pathologists: Consensus meeting: Is "fibrocystic disease" of the breast precancerous? Arch Pathol Lab Med 1986;110:171-173.
99. Haagensen CD: Gross cystic disease. In Haagensen CD (ed): Diseases of the Breast, 3rd ed. Philadelphia, WB Saunders, 1986, pp 250-266.
100. Swann CA, Kopans DB, Koerner FC, et al: The halo sign and malignant breast lesions. AJR Am J Roentgenol 1987;149: 1145-1147.
101. Homer MJ, Cooper AG, Pile-Spellman ER: Milk of calcium in breast microcysts: Manifestation as a solitary focal disease. AJR Am J Roentgenol 1988;150:789-790.
102. Linden SS, Sickles EA: Sedimented calcium in benign breast cysts: The full spectrum of mammographic presentations. AJR Am J Roentgenol 1989;152:967-971.
103. Pennes DR, Rebner M: Layering granular calcifications in macroscopic breast cysts. Breast Dis 1988;1:109-112.
104. Sickles EA, Abele JS: Milk of calcium within tiny benign breast cysts. Radiology 1981;141:655-658.
105. Jackson VP: The role of US in breast imaging. Radiology 1990;177:305-311.
106. Hilton SVW, Leopold GR, Olson LK, Willson SA: Real-time breast ultrasonography: Application in 300 consecutive patients. AJR Am J Roentgenol 1986;147:479-486.
107. Jellins J, Kossoff G, Reeve TS: Detection and classification of liquid-filled masses in the breast by gray scale echography. Radiology 1977;125:205-212.
108. Sickles EA, Filly RA, Callen PW: Benign breast lesions: Ultrasound detection and diagnosis. Radiology 1984;151: 467-470.
109. Kasumi F, Tanaka H: Diagnosis of intracystic tumors by ultrasound. In Jellins J, Kobayashi T (eds): Ultrasonic Examination of the Breast. Chichester, England, John Wiley & Sons, 1983, pp 283-291.
110. Omori LM, Hisa N, Ohkuma K, et al: Breast masses with mixed cystic-solid ultrasonographic appearance. J Clin Ultrasound 1993;21:489-495.
111. Reuter K, D'Orsi CJ, Reale F: Intracystic carcinoma of the breast: The role of ultrasonography. Radiology 1984;153:233-234.
112. Warner JK, Kumar K, Berg WA: Apocrine metaplasia: Mammographic and ultrasonographic appearances. AJR Am J Roentgenol 1998;170:1375-1379.
113. Khaleghian R: Breast cysts: Pitfalls in ultrasonographic diagnosis. Australas Radiol 1993;37:192-194.
114. Berg WA, Campassi CI, Ioffe CB: Cystic lesions of the breast: Ultrasonographic-pathologic correlation. Radiology 2003; 227:183-191.
115. Tabar L, Pentek Z, Dean PB: The diagnostic and therapeutic value of breast cyst puncture and pneumocystography. Radiology 1981;41:659-663.
116. Dixon JM, Scott WM, Miller WR: Natural history of cystic disease: The importance of cyst type. Br J Surg 1985;72:190-192.
117. Golden GT, Wangensteen SL: Galactocele of the breast. Am J Surg 1972;123:271-273.
118. Winkler JM: Galactocele of the breast. Am J Surg 1964;108: 357-360.
119. Bessman SP, Lucas JC: Galactocele in a male infant. Pediatrics 1953;11:109-112.
120. Haagensen CD: Abnormalities of breast growth, secretion, and lactation. In Haagensen CD (ed): Diseases of the Breast, 3rd ed. Philadelphia, WB Saunders, 1986, pp 56-74.
121. Feig SA: Breast masses: Mammographic and ultrasonographic evaluation. Radiol Clin North Am 1992;30:67-92.
122. Kopans DB: Pathologic, mammographic, and ultrasonographic correlation. In Kopans DB: Breast Imaging, 2nd ed. Philadelphia, Lippincott-Raven, 1997, pp 511-615.
123. Gomez A, Mata JM, Donoso L, Rams A: Galactocele: Three distinctive radiographic appearances. Radiology 1986;158: 43-44.

124. Salvador R, Salvador M, Jimenez JA, et al: Galactocele of the breast: Radiologic and ultrasonographic findings. Br J Radiol 1990;63:140-142.
125. Lee KC, Chan JKC, Gwi E: Tubular adenosis of the breast. Am J Surg Pathol 1996;20:46-54.
126. Hermann G, Schwartz IS: Focal fibrous disease of the breast: Mammographic detection of an unappreciated condition. AJR Am J Roentgenol 1983;140:1245-1246.
127. Venta LA, Wiley EL, Gabriel H, Adler YT: Imaging features of focal breast fibrosis: Mammographic-pathologic correlation of noncalcified breast lesions. AJR Am J Roentgenol 1999; 173:309-316.
128. Rosen EL, Soo MS, Bentley RC: Focal fibrosis: A common breast lesion diagnosed at imaging-guided core biopsy. AJR Am J Roentgenol 1999;173:1657-1662.
129. Logan WW, Hoffman NY: Diabetic fibrous breast disease. Radiology 1989;172:667-670.
130. Haagensen CD: Fibrous disease. In Haagensen CD (ed): Diseases of the Breast, 3rd ed. Philadelphia, WB Saunders, 1986, pp 125-135.
131. Huynh PT, Parellada JA, Shaw de Paredes E: Dilated duct pattern at mammography. Radiology 1997;204:137-141.
132. Haagensen CD: Solitary intraductal papilloma. In Haagensen CD (ed): Diseases of the Breast, 3rd ed. Philadelphia, WB Saunders, 1986, pp 136-175.
133. Cardenosa G, Eklund GW: Benign papillary neoplasms of the breast: Mammographic findings. Radiology 1991;181:751-755.
134. Woods ER, Helvie MA, Ikeda DM, et al: Solitary breast papilloma: Comparison of mammographic, galactographic, and pathologic findings. AJR Am J Roentgenol 1992;159:487-491.
135. Haagensen CD: Multiple intraductal papilloma. In Haagensen CD (ed): Diseases of the Breast, 3rd ed. Philadelphia, WB Saunders, 1986, pp 176-191.
136. Rosen PP: Papilloma and related benign tumors. In Rosen PP: Rosen's Breast Pathology, 2nd ed. Philadelphia, Lippincott Williams & Wilkins, 2001, pp 77-119.
137. Ohuchi N, Abe R, Kasai M: Possible cancerous change of intraductal papillomas of the breast: A 3-D reconstruction study of 25 cases. Cancer 1984;54:605-611.
138. Murad TM, Contesso G, Mouriesse H: Papillary tumors of large lactiferous ducts. Cancer 1981;48:122-133.
139. Rosen PP, Cantrell B, Mullen DL, DePalo A: Juvenile papillomatosis (Swiss cheese disease) of the breast. Am J Surg Pathol 1980;4:3-12.
140. Rosen PP, Holmes G, Lesser ML, et al: Juvenile papillomatosis and breast carcinoma. Cancer 1985;55:1345-1352.
141. Bazzocchi F, Santini D, Martinelli G, et al: Juvenile papillomatosis (epitheliosis) of the breast. Am J Clin Pathol 1986;86: 745-748.
142. Kersschott EAJ, Hermans M-E, Pauwels C, et al: Juvenile papillomatosis of the breast: Ultrasonographic appearance. Radiology 1988;169:631-633.
143. Hidalgo F, Llano JM, Marhuenda A: Juvenile papillomatosis of the breast (Swiss cheese disease). AJR Am J Roentgenol 1997;169:912.
144. Rosen PP: Breast tumors in children. In Rosen PP: Rosen's Breast Pathology, 2nd ed. Philadelphia, Lippincott Williams & Wilkins, 2001, pp 729-748.
145. Adler DD, Helvie MA, Oberman HA, et al: Radial sclerosing lesion of the breast: Mammographic features. Radiology 1990;176:737-740.
146. Ciatto S, Morrone D, Catarzi S, et al: Radial scars of the breast: Review of 38 consecutive mammographic diagnoses. Radiology 1993;187:757-760.
147. Tabar L, Dean PB: Stellate/spiculated lesions. In Tabar L, Dean PB: Teaching Atlas of Mammography, 3rd ed. Stuttgart, Thieme, 2001, pp 93-147.
148. D'Orsi CJ, Feldhaus L, Sonnenfeld M: Unusual lesions of the breast. Radiol Clin North Am 1983;21:67-80.
149. Mitnick JS, Vazquez MF, Harris MN, Roses DF: Differentiation of radial scar from scirrhous carcinoma of the breast: Mammographic-pathologic correlation. Radiology 1989;173:697-700.
150. Vega A, Garijo F: Radial scar and tubular carcinoma: Mammographic and ultrasonographic findings. Acta Radiol 1993; 34:43-47.
151. Orel SG, Evers K, Yeh I-T, Troupin RH: Radial scar with microcalcifications: Radiologic-pathologic correlation. Radiology 1992;183:479-482.
152. Frouge C, Miquel A, Adrien C, et al: Mammographic lesions suggestive of radial scars: Microscopic findings in 40 cases. In Proceedings of the 80th Scientific Assembly and Annual Meeting of the Radiological Society of North America, November 27-December 2, 1994, p 186.
153. Hassell PR, Klein-Parker HA, Worth AJ, et al: Radiologic features of radial scar. In Proceedings of the 80th Scientific Assembly and Annual Meeting of the Radiological Society of North America, November 27-December 2, 1994, p 186.
154. Vazquez MF, Mitnick JS, Pressman P, et al: Radial scar: Cytologic evaluation by stereotactic aspiration. Breast Dis 1994;7: 299-306.
155. King TA, Scharfenberg JC, Smetherman DH, et al: A better understanding of the term radial scar. Am J Surg 2000;180: 428-433.
156. Brenner RJ, Jackman RJ, Parker SH, et al: Percutaneous core needle biopsy of radial scars of the breast: When is excision necessary? AJR Am J Roentgenol 2002;179:1179-1184.
157. Cawson JN, Malara F, Kavanagh A, et al: Fourteen-gauge needle core biopsy of mammographically evident radial scars: Is excision necessary? Cancer 2003;97:345-351.
158. Bonzanini M, Gilioli E, Brancato B, et al: Cytologic features of 22 radial scar/complex sclerosing lesions of the breast, three of which are associated with carcinoma: Clinical, mammographic, and histologic correlation. Diagn Cytopathol 1997;17:353-362.
159. Sloane JP, Mayers MM: Carcinoma and atypical hyperplasia in radial scars and complex sclerosing lesions: Importance of lesion size and patient age. Histopathology 1993;23:225-231.
160. Page DL, Anderson TJ, Rogers LW: Epithelial hyperplasia. In Page DL, Anderson TJ (eds): Diagnostic Histopathology of the Breast. Edinburgh, Churchill Livingstone, 1987, pp 120-156.
161. Dupont WD, Page DL: Risk factors for breast cancer in women with proliferative breast disease. N Engl J Med 1985;312:146-151.
162. Jackman RJ, Nowels KW, Shepard MJ, et al: Stereotaxic large-core needle biopsy of 450 nonpalpable breast lesions with surgical correlation in lesions with cancer or atypical hyperplasia. Radiology 1994;193:91-95.
163. Yeh IT, Dimitrov D, Otto P, et al: Pathologic review of atypical hyperplasia identified by image-guided breast needle core biopsy. Correlation with excision specimen. Arch Pathol Lab Med 2003;127:49-54.
164. Andrales G, Turk P, Wallace T, et al: Is surgical excision necessary for atypical ductal hyperplasia of the breast diagnosed by Mammotome? Am J Surg 2000;180:313-315.
165. Cangiarella J, Waisman J, Symmans WF, et al: Mammotome core biopsy for mammary calcification: Analysis of 160 biopsies from 142 women with surgical and radiologic followup. Cancer 2001;91:173-177.
166. Mendez I, Andreu FJ, Saez E, et al: Ductal carcinoma in situ and atypical ductal hyperplasia of the breast diagnosed at stereotactic core biopsy. Breast J 2001;7:14-18.
167. Rao A, Parker S, Ratzer E, et al: Atypical ductal hyperplasia of the breast diagnosed by 11-gauge directional vacuum-assisted biopsy. Am J Surg 2002;184:534-537.
168. Harvey JM, Sterrett GF, Frost FA: Atypical ductal hyperplasia and atypia of uncertain significance in core biopsies from mammographically detected lesions: Correlation with excision diagnosis. Pathology 2002;34:410-416.
169. Dmytrasz K, Tartter PI, Mizrachy H, et al: The significance of atypical lobular hyperplasia at percutaneous biopsy. Breast J 2003;9:10-12.
170. Page DL, Dupont WD, Rogers LW, Rados MS: Atypical hyperplastic lesions of the female breast. A long term follow-up study. Cancer 1985;55:2698-2708.
171. Page DL, Vander Zwaag R, Rogers LW, et al: Relation between component parts of fibrocystic disease complex and breast cancer. J Natl Cancer Inst 1978;61:1055-1063.

172. Singletary SE: Rating the risk factors for breast cancer. Ann Surg 2003;237:474-482.
173. Haagensen CD, Lane N, Lattes R, Bodian C: Lobular neoplasia (so-called lobular carcinoma in situ) of the breast. Cancer 1978;42:737-769.
174. Foster MC, Helvie MA, Gregory NE, et al: Lobular carcinoma in situ or atypical lobular hyperplasia at core-needle biopsy: Is excisional biopsy necessary? Radiology 2004;231:813-819.
175. Helvie MA, Hessler C, Frank TS, Ikeda DM: Atypical hyperplasia of the breast: Mammographic appearance and histologic correlation. Radiology 1991;179:759-764.
176. Rubin E, Visscher DW, Alexander RW, et al: Proliferative disease and atypia in biopsies performed for nonpalpable lesions detected mammographically. Cancer 1988;61:2077-2082.
177. Stomper PC, Cholewinski SP, Penetrante RB, et al: Atypical hyperplasia: Frequency and mammographic and pathologic relationships in excisional biopsies guided with mammography and clinical examination. Radiology 1993;189:667-671.
178. Foote FW, Stewart FW: Lobular carcinoma in situ. Am J Pathol 1941;17:491-495.
179. Mackarem G, Yacoub LK, Lee AKC, et al: Effects of screening on detection of lobular carcinoma in situ of the breast: Nonspecificity of mammography and physical examination. Breast Dis 1994;7:339-345.
180. Pope TL, Fechner RE, Wilhelm MC, et al: Lobular carcinoma in situ of the breast: Mammographic features. Radiology 1988;168:63-66.
181. Rosen PP, Lieberman PH, Braun DW, et al: Lobular carcinoma in situ of the breast: Detailed analysis of 99 patients with average follow-up of 24 years. Am J Surg Pathol 1978;2:225-251.
182. Berg WA, Mrose HE, Ioffe OB: Atypical lobular hyperplasia or lobular carcinoma in situ at core-needle biopsy. Radiology 2001;218:503-509.
183. Liberman L, Sama M, Susnik B, et al: Lobular carcinoma in situ at percutaneous breast biopsy: Surgical biopsy findings. AJR Am J Roentgenol 1999;173:291-299.
184. Philpotts LE, Shaheen NA, Jain KD, et al: Uncommon high-risk lesions of the breast diagnosed at stereotactic core needle biopsy: Clinical importance. Radiology 2000;216:831-837.
185. Shin SJ, Rosen PP: Excisional biopsy should be performed if lobular carcinoma in situ is seen on needle core biopsy. Arch Pathol Lab Med 2002;126:697-701.
186. Dershaw DD: Does LCIS or ALH without other high-risk lesions diagnosed on core biopsy require surgical excision? Breast J 2003;9:1-3.
187. Baure VP, Ditkoff BA, Schnabel F, et al: The management of lobular neoplasia identified on percutaneous core breast biopsy. Breast J 2003;9:4-9.
188. Renshaw AA, Cartagena N, Derhagopian RP, Gould EW: Lobular neoplasia in breast core needle biopsy specimens is not associated with an increased risk of ductal carcinoma in situ or invasive cancer. Am J Clin Pathol 2002;117:797-799.
189. Gabriel H: The dilemma of lobular carcinoma in situ at percutaneous biopsy: To excise or to monitor. AJR Am J Roentgenol 1999;173:300-302.
190. Cohen MA: Cancer upgrades at excisional biopsy after diagnosis of atypical lobular hyperplasia or lobular carcinoma in situ at core-needle biopsy: Some reasons why. Radiology 2004;231:617-621.
191. Page DL, Anderson TJ, Rogers LW: Carcinoma in situ. In Page DL, Anderson TJ (eds): Diagnostic Histopathology of the Breast. Edinburgh, Churchill Livingstone, 1987, pp 157-192.
192. Goldstein NS, Bassi D, Watts JC, et al: E-cadherin reactivity of 95 invasive ductal and lobular lesions of the breast. Am J Clin Pathol 2001;115:534-542.
193. Muller J: Uber den feineran Bau and die Forman der Krankhaften Geschwulste. Berlin, Reimer, 1838, p 54.
194. Haagensen CD: Cystosarcoma phyllodes. In Haagensen CD (ed): Diseases of the Breast, 3rd ed. Philadelphia, WB Saunders, 1986, pp 284-312.
195. Hawkins RE, Schofield JB, Fisher C, et al: The clinical and histologic criteria that predict metastases from cystosarcoma phyllodes. Cancer 1992;69:141-147.
196. Page DL, Anderson TJ, Johnson RL: Sarcomas of the breast. In Page DL, Anderson TJ (eds): Diagnostic Histopathology of the Breast. Edinburgh, Churchill Livingstone, 1987, pp 335-353.
197. Kessinger A, Foley JF, Lemon HM, Miller DM: Metastatic cystosarcoma phyllodes: A case report and review of the literature. J Surg Oncol 1972;4:131-147.
198. Hart WR, Bauer RC, Oberman HA: Cystosarcoma phyllodes. A clinicopathologic study of 26 hypercellular periductal stroma tumors of the breast. Am J Clin Pathol 1978;70:211-216.
199. Pietrusz M, Barnes L: Cystosarcoma phyllodes. A clinicopathologic analysis of 42 cases. Cancer 1978;41:1974-1983.
200. Buchberger W, Strasser K, Heim K, et al: Phylloides tumor: Findings on mammography, ultrasonography, and aspiration cytology in 10 cases. AJR Am J Roentgenol 1991;157:715-719.
201. Page JE, Williams JE: The radiological features of phylloides tumour of the breast with clinico-pathological correlation. Clin Radiol 1991;44:8-12.
202. Liberman L, Bonaccio E, Hamele-Bene D, et al: Benign and malignant phyllodes tumors: Mammographic and ultrasonographic findings. Radiology 1996;198:121-124.
203. Lifshitz OH, Whitman GJ, Sahin AA, Yang WT: Phyllodes tumor of the breast. AJR Am J Roentgenol 2003;180:332.
204. Cole-Beuglet C, Soriano RZ, Kurtz AB, et al: Ultrasound, x-ray mammography, and histopathology of cystosarcoma phylloides. Radiology 1983;146:481-486.
205. Chao T-C, Lo Y-F, Chen S-C, Chen M-F: Phyllodes tumors of the breast. Eur Radiol 2003;13:88-93.
206. Pierson KK, Wilkinson EJ: Malignant neoplasia of the breast: Infiltrating carcinomas. In Bland KI, Copeland EM (eds): The Breast: Comprehensive Management of Benign and Malignant Diseases. Philadelphia, WB Saunders, 1991, pp 193-221.
207. So NMC, Yang WT, Metreweli C: Imaging features of liposarcoma of the pectoral muscle. AJR Am J Roentgenol 1999;172:1148-1149.
208. Odom JW, Mikhailova B, Pryce E, et al: Liposarcoma of the breast: Report of a case and review of the literature. Breast Dis 1991;4:293-298.
209. Abrikossoff A: Ueber Myome, Augesehend von der quergestreiften willkurlichen Muskulatur. Virchows Arch Pathol Anat 1926;260:215-233.
210. Ingram DL, Mossler JA, Snowhite J, et al: Granular cell tumours of the breast. Steroid receptor analysis and localization of carcinoembryonic antigen, myoglobin, and S100 protein. Arch Pathol Lab Med 1984;108:897-901.
211. Bassett LW, Cove HC: Myoblastoma of the breast. AJR Am J Roentgenol 1979;132:122-123.
212. DeMay R, Kay S: Granular cell tumor of the breast. Pathol Ann 1984;19:121-148.
213. Haagensen CD: Nonepithelial neoplasms. In Haagensen CD (ed): Diseases of the Breast, 3rd ed. Philadelphia, WB Saunders, 1986, pp 313-349.
214. Mulcare R: Granular cell myoblastoma of the breast. Ann Surg 1968;168:262-268.
215. Gold DA, Hermann G, Schwartz IS, et al: Granular cell tumor of the breast: Case report of an occult lesion simulating carcinoma. Breast Dis 1989;2:211-215.
216. Ilkhanipour ZS, Harris KM, Kanbour AI: Granular cell tumor of the breast: Two case reports mimicking carcinoma. Breast Dis 1993;6:221-225.
217. Rickard MT, Sendel A, Burchett I: Case report: Granular cell tumor of the breast. Clin Radiol 1992;45:347-348.
218. Baum JK, Robins JR, Schnitt S, Houlihan MJ: The ultrasound appearance of granular cell tumor of the breast: A case report. Breast Dis 1994;7:281-285.
219. Scatarige JC, Hsiu JG, de la Torre R, et al: Acoustic shadowing in benign granular cell tumor (myoblastoma) of the breast. J Ultrasound Med 1987;6:545-547.
220. Rosen PP: Benign mesenchymal neoplasms. In Rosen PP: Rosen's Breast Pathology, 2nd ed. Philadelphia, Lippincott Williams & Wilkins, 2001, pp 749-811.

221. Cederlund CG, Gustavsson S, Linell F, et al: Fibromatosis of the breast mimicking carcinoma at mammography. Br J Radiol 1984;57:98-101.
222. Kalisher L, Long J, Peyster RG: Extra-abdominal desmoid of the axillary tail mimicking breast carcinoma. AJR Am J Roentgenol 1976;126:903-909.
223. Leal SM, Poppiti RJ, Surujon I, Matallana R: Fibromatosis of the breast mimicking infiltrating carcinoma on mammography. Breast Dis 1989;1:277-282.
224. Greenberg D, McIntyre H, Ramsaroop R, et al: Aggressive fibromatosis of the breast: A case report and literature review. Breast J 2002;8:55-57.

Chapter 26

Noninvasive Carcinoma

Karin L. Fu, Yao S. Fu, January K. Lopez, Seth Y. Cardall, and Lawrence W. Bassett

DUCTAL CARCINOMA IN SITU

Carcinoma in situ (CIS, or noninvasive carcinoma) is a distinct lesion of the breast that has potential to become invasive cancer. CIS lesions cannot metastasize because they are by definition restricted to the glandular lumen and have no access to lymphatics or blood vessels. CIS can be divided into two major types, ductal carcinoma in situ (DCIS, or intraductal carcinoma) and lobular carcinoma in situ (LCIS). These are quite different lesions and are discussed separately (Table 26–1). The most important difference is that DCIS is considered a true preinvasive lesion, whereas LCIS is considered a risk factor for breast carcinoma. This differentiation is based on the fact that in a significant number of women, approximately 30%, whose biopsies showed DCIS without complete excision of the lesion, invasive breast cancer had subsequently developed at the surgical site at 10-year follow-up.[1,2]

Women with LCIS have invasive carcinoma of the breast in numbers approximately equal to those who have DCIS; however, the carcinomas that develop in women with LCIS can occur in any location in the ipsilateral or contralateral breast, rather than at the site of the biopsy. The estimated risk for the development of invasive cancer in women with LCIS is 1% per year.[3] These two lesions create a dilemma during calculation of the medical audit data because they lie in a gray zone between benign and malignant. Currently, we recommend that DCIS be regarded as a malignancy during calculation of the medical audit data but that LCIS be considered a high-risk lesion and that it not be included as malignancy during medical audits.[4] For this reason, the in-depth discussion of LCIS is part of the treatment of benign lesions in this textbook.

Mammography plays a key role in the detection of DCIS, because it is usually nonpalpable and is most often identified from mammographically detected microcalcifications. However, LCIS has no characteristic radiographic or clinical features, being found incidentally at the time of a biopsy for a palpable or mammographic abnormality.

Before the widespread use of screening mammography, DCIS was thought to be a relatively uncommon lesion, accounting for less than 5% of all breast carcinomas.[5] Today, DCIS makes up approximately 30% of breast malignancies detected in screening programs, and the majority of cases of DCIS are detected on mammography.[6] A major breakthrough in knowledge about DCIS occurred when Holland and Hendriks[7] described their findings in mastectomy specimens containing DCIS. They concluded that DCIS typically (1) is distributed within a single segment of the duct system and (2) is unicentric and segmental rather than multifocal or multicentric. This finding is consistent with the observation that breast cancer recurrences are usually in the region of the original tumor.[8]

Because all cases of DCIS do not confer the same likelihood for eventual invasion and metastasis, it is important to understand that DCIS comprises a spectrum of lesions. Several classification systems have been developed on the basis of the extent of the lesion, clinical findings, and histologic features. The most commonly used classification divides DCIS into two major types, the more aggressive comedo carcinoma and the more indolent noncomedo carcinoma. During examination of excised specimens containing comedocarcinoma, the involved ducts may extrude a thick material resembling that of a comedo—thus the name *comedocarcinoma*.[9] Comedocarcinoma is characterized by more aggressive malignant cytologic features and behavior. The noncomedo carcinoma subtypes are less aggressive clinically. In reality, the histologic subtypes of DCIS are often intermediate and intermixed, and the prognosis probably depends on the nuclear grade as well as other factors summarized in the pathology section of this chapter. In general, morphologically extensive, casting-type calcifications (like those seen in comedocarcinoma; see later) are associated with more aggressive DCIS and greater extent of disease.[10]

DCIS may also be associated with invasive carcinoma. Of particular interest to radiologists are those cases of invasive cancer with an extensive intraductal component (EIC–positive, or EIC+). In EIC+ cases, successful treatment often depends on knowledge of the complete extent of the nonpalpable noninvasive portion. Also of interest are those cases in which extensive DCIS is associated with microinvasion. Extensive intraductal component is discussed in more detail later.

Paget's disease of the nipple and noninvasive papillary carcinoma are subtypes of intraductal carcinoma that are also discussed in this chapter.

Table 26–1. Ductal Carcinoma In Situ versus Lobular Carcinoma In Situ

Feature	Ductal Carcinoma in Situ	Lobular Carcinoma in Situ
Method of detection	Mammography	Incidental (at biopsy)
Mammographic features	Microcalcifications	None
Relationship to invasive breast cancer	Precursor	Risk factor
Site of subsequent invasive cancer	Local	Anywhere, either breast
Medical audit	Malignant	Benign

Clinical Aspects

The majority of intraductal carcinomas do not have clinical signs or symptoms. When present, the most common clinical manifestations are palpable masses, nipple discharge, and Paget's disease.[11] Comedocarcinoma is more likely than noncomedo carcinoma to manifest as a palpable mass. Several studies have suggested that comedocarcinoma is also more commonly associated with microinvasion and lymph node involvement, reflections of its more aggressive behavior. A periductal, inflammatory reaction also can occur, leading to a mammographically dense lesion and sometimes palpability.[12]

Imaging Features

Ductal Carcinoma In Situ

DCIS is usually detected on mammography, and calcifications are the mammographic hallmark (Table 26–2).[13-15] The typical appearance is fine, linear, discontinuous, and branching calcifications with a diameter of usually less than 0.5 mm. Their appearance suggests filling of the duct lumen involved irregularly by breast cancer, or *casting* of the duct system (Fig. 26–1).

Mammographically, microcalcifications of noncomedo DCIS are granular, hazy, amorphous, or indistinct particles characterized by variable size and shape. In contrast, the individual calcifications of comedocarcinoma are likely to be larger and more coarse as well as discontinuous, linear, and branching (Fig. 26–2). However, these radiographic features are not always reliable in differentiating between the histologic subtypes of lesions.[7,15,16]

Another important feature of DCIS is the distribution of the calcifications. They are usually found in a linear, branching, or segmental distribution (Fig. 26–3). The distribution of calcifications in an individual case depends on the lesion's anatomic location. Those in major ducts are likely to be distributed in a line toward the nipple (Fig. 26–4), whereas those in smaller subdivisions of the ductal system may be distributed like the branches of the interlobular and intralobular ducts (Fig. 26–5). Interestingly, it has been observed that the visible calcifications of comedocarcinoma closely match the actual extent of the lesion, but noncomedo carcinoma may be more extensive than suggested by its calcifications. In general the discrepancy is less than 2 cm in 80% to 85% of cases.[7]

In a little more than 10% of cases, only a soft tissue mass can be appreciated in mammograms.[11,12] These changes are the manifestation of a solid mass of tumor cells or associated inflammation, edema, and fibrosis at the periphery of the involved ducts.[12,17] Other unusual manifestations of DCIS are

Table 26–2. Mammographic Manifestations of Ductal Carcinoma In Situ

Mammographic Finding	Percentage of Cases
Calcifications alone	72
Calcifications with soft tissue abnormality	12
Soft tissue abnormality alone	10
No mammography findings	6

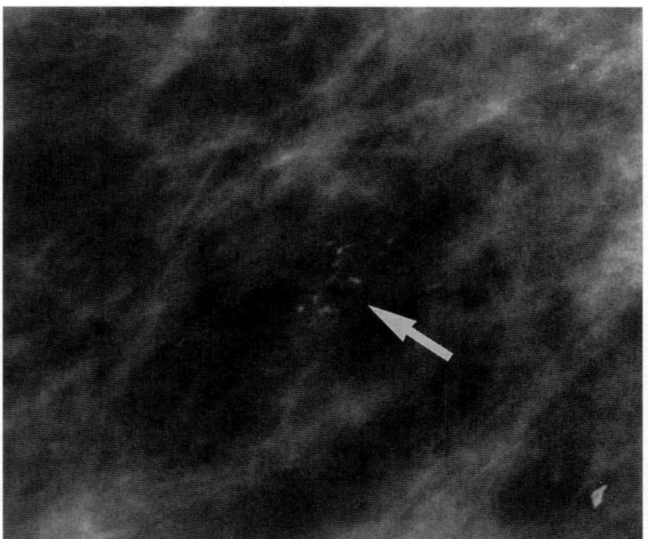

Figure 26–1. Magnification mammogram of a cluster of fine, linear branching (casting) calcifications (*arrow*). These are thin, irregular calcifications that appear linear but are discontinuous and less than 0.5 mm in width. Their appearance suggests irregular filling of the lumen of a small branching duct containing breast cancer. The white speck in the lower right corner is an artifact.

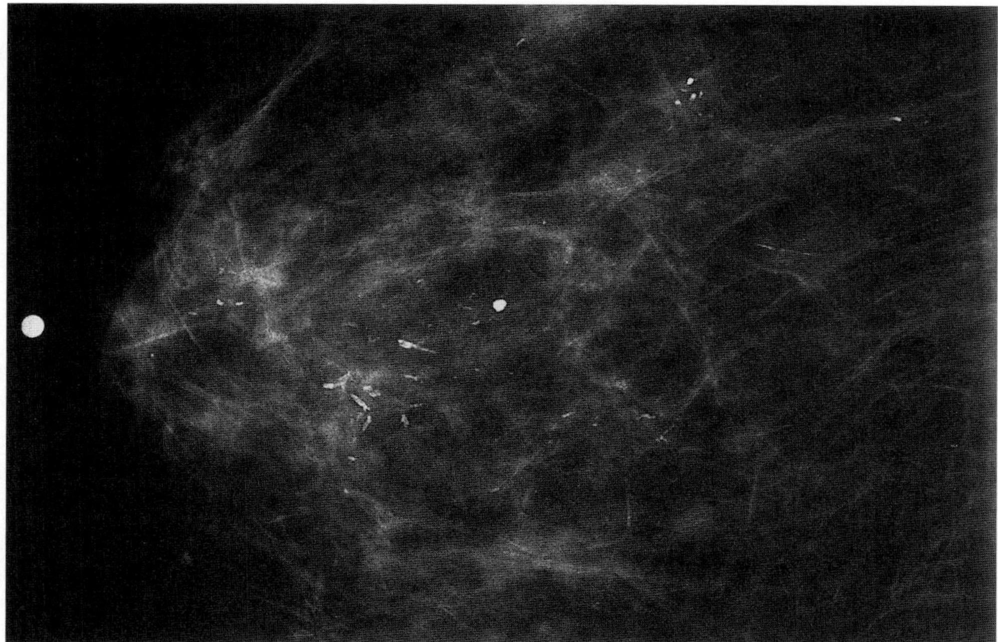

Figure 26–2. Fine, linear, and branching calcifications of comedocarcinoma make casts of the ducts.

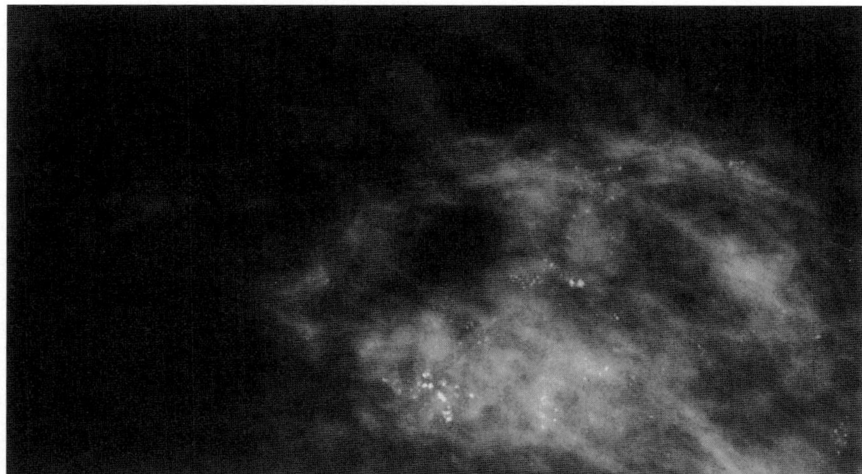

Figure 26–3. Magnification view demonstrating irregular, heterogeneous calcifications in a linear distribution. Histologic evaluation revealed comedo-type ductal carcinoma in situ.

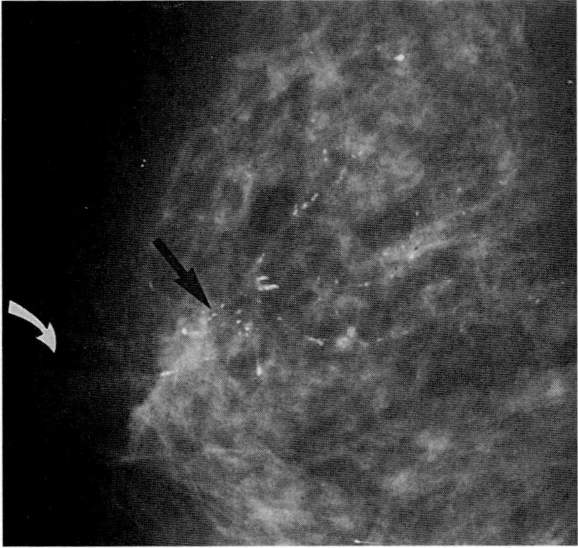

Figure 26–4. Segmental distribution of calcifications in ductal carcinoma in situ. The calcifications (*straight arrow*) are in the larger ducts, and linear patterns extend toward the nipple (*curved arrow*).

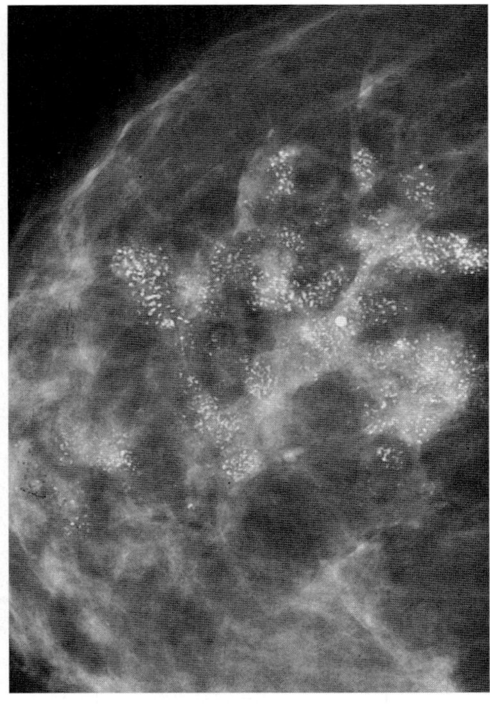

Figure 26–5. Extensive ductal carcinoma in situ (comedocarcinoma). The tumor is in the terminal branches of the ductal system and extends into the lobules. Associated soft tissue density is present.

asymmetrical density (Fig. 26–6), dilated retroareolar ducts, an ill-defined rounded tumor, architectural distortion, and a developing density.[13]

Invasive Cancer with Extensive Intraductal Component

Tumors are classified as being EIC+ if they are predominantly intraductal with small areas of invasion or if they are primarily invasive with (1) DCIS filling nonobliterated ducts within the invasive cancer or (2) DCIS in the tissue adjacent to the invasive tumor (Fig. 26–7).[18] The significance of the EIC+ designation is the greater incidence of local recurrence of breast cancer after surgical excision and radiotherapy: The incidence of recurrence for EIC+ cases is approximately 25% at 5 years, compared with 6% for cases without an EIC (EIC–).[19] These findings verify observations of others that the presence of EIC+ in DCIS is a marker for widespread residual tumor after excision.[20] However, if all of the DCIS is successfully removed, the local recurrence rate is similar to that for EIC– tumors.

Mammography plays an important role in the management of EIC+ cases. First, mammographic wire localization is essential prior to surgical excision. If the purpose of the localization procedure is to excise all of the lesion for segmental resection before radiotherapy, not just take a sample for diagnostic purposes, multiple wires are often used to identify the full extent of the lesion.[21] We refer to this procedure as "bracketing of the lesion" (Fig. 26–8). At the time of surgical excision of DCIS, a specimen radiograph should always be performed. However, it should be borne in mind that the specimen radiograph is not an adequate tool by which to ensure that all malignant calcifications have been removed (Fig. 26–9).[22]

It is usually the responsibility of the pathologist to determine whether the margins of the resected tissue are free of tumor. However, the complex branching of the breast ductal system may lead to errors as to whether intraductal tumor has been completely removed. In other words, although the margins of the surgical specimen may appear to be clear of tumor in the histologic sections, DCIS can still be present in the breast. Therefore, it is important that after surgery and before radiotherapy in women with DCIS manifested as calcifications, mammography be performed to enable a search for residual malignant calcifications. The preradiotherapy mammograms are usually obtained 3 to 4 weeks after surgery to allow as much time as possible to reduce the discomfort associated with mammographic compression. We perform the postoperative preradiotherapy examination with a wire placed over the surgical site. In addition to standard views, magnification views are obtained over the region of the wire (Fig. 26–10). If soft tissue edema obscures the surgical site, a magnification view tangential to the wire is performed to move overlying edematous skin and subcutaneous tissues away from the area of interest.

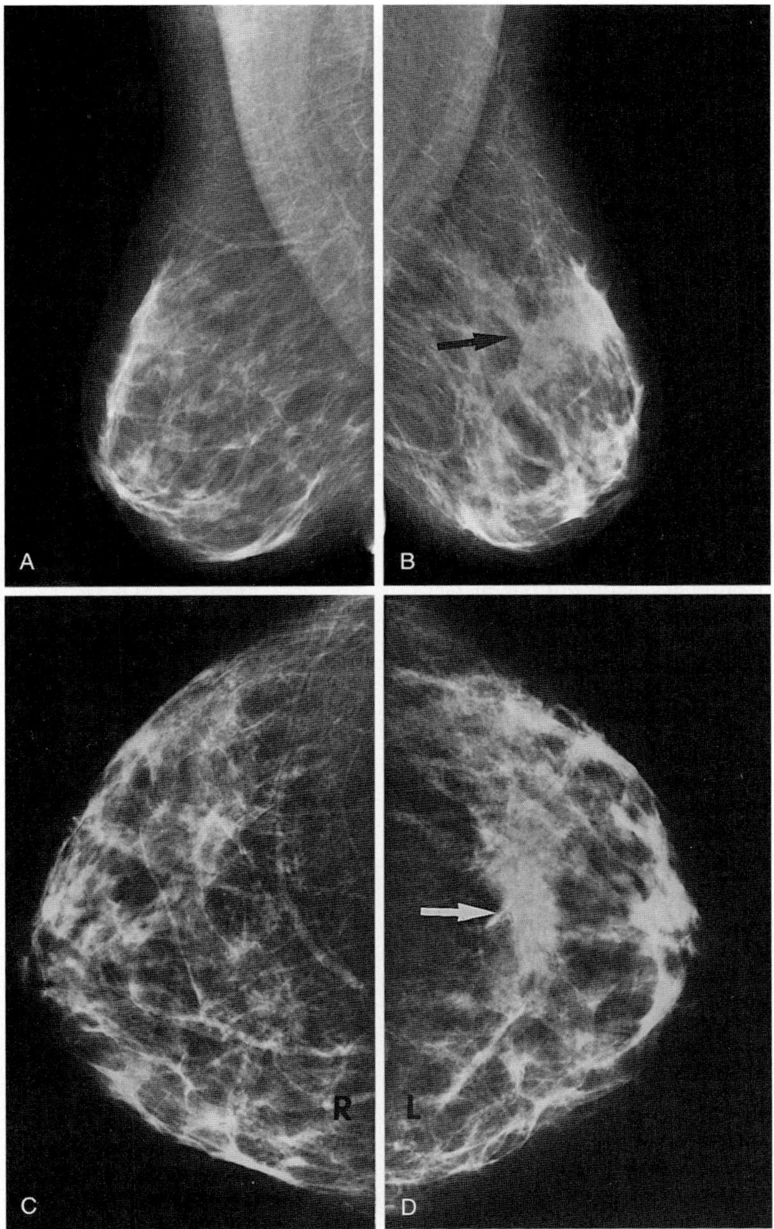

Figure 26–6. Ductal carcinoma in situ manifesting as an asymmetrical density with architectural distortion. **A** and **B,** Mediolateral oblique (MLO) views show an area of asymmetrical density (*arrow*) with distortion in the upper hemisphere of the left breast. **C** and **D,** Craniocaudal (CC) views confirm the asymmetrical density (*arrow*) in the left breast.

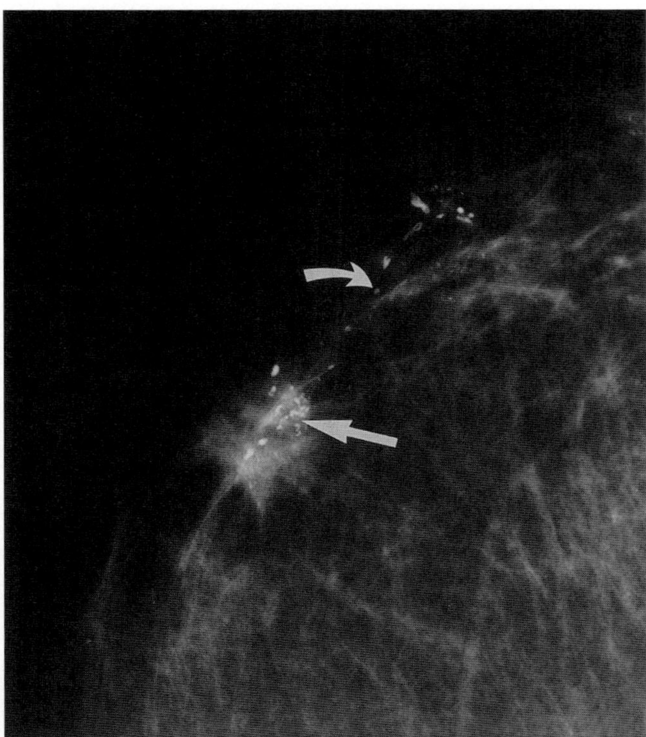

Figure 26–7. Invasive cancer with extensive intraductal component (EIC+). Close-up of a mammogram shows a spiculated invasive carcinoma accompanied by pleomorphic and fine, linear branching microcalcifications, which are present both within the tumor mass (*straight arrow*) and outside it (*curved arrow*). The calcifications outside the tumor mass are in a segmental distribution, suggesting deposits in a duct and its branches.

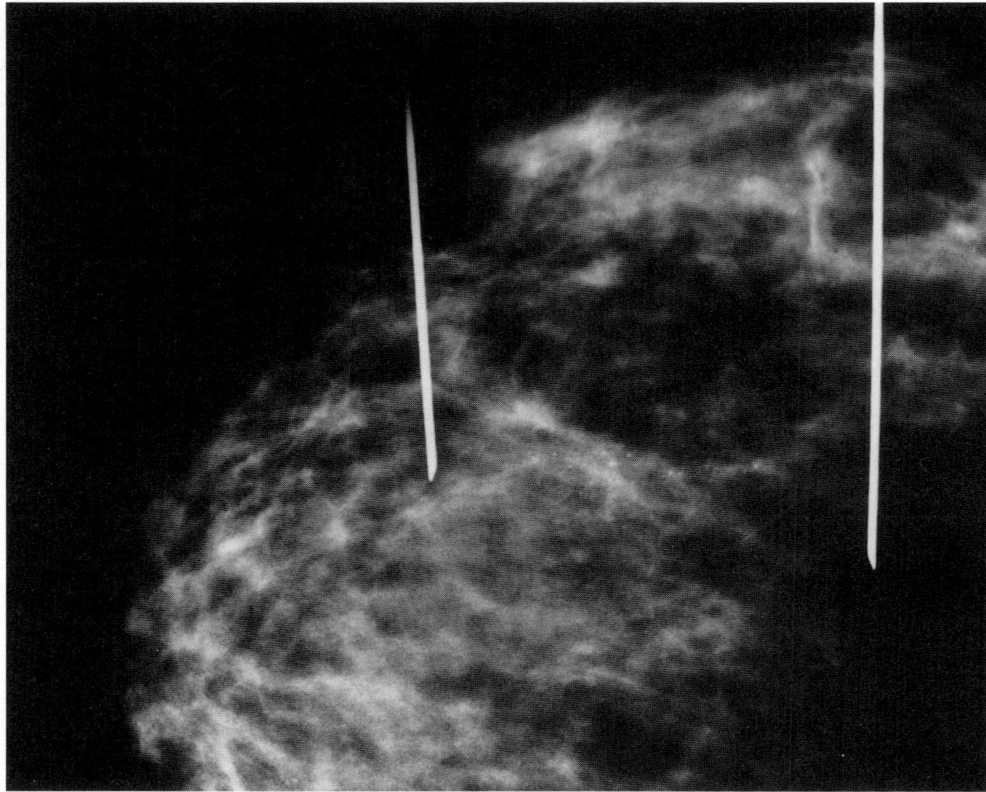

Figure 26–8. After a craniocaudal view has been obtained, the bracketing needles are adjusted so that the tip of the anterior needle is at the most medial extent of the calcifications.

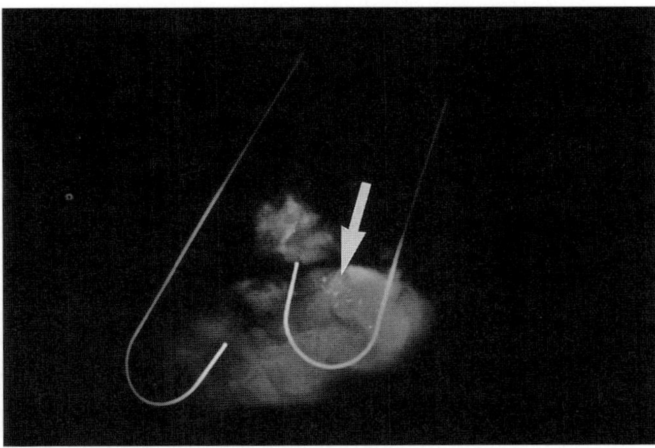

Figure 26–9. This 33-year-old patient had a palpable mass in the right breast. Excisional biopsy of the palpable mass and the nonpalpable calcifications was performed after wire localization. This specimen radiograph verifies the presence of calcifications (*arrow*). Histologic evaluation showed an invasive ductal carcinoma with extensive intraductal component (EIC+) and clear surgical margins.

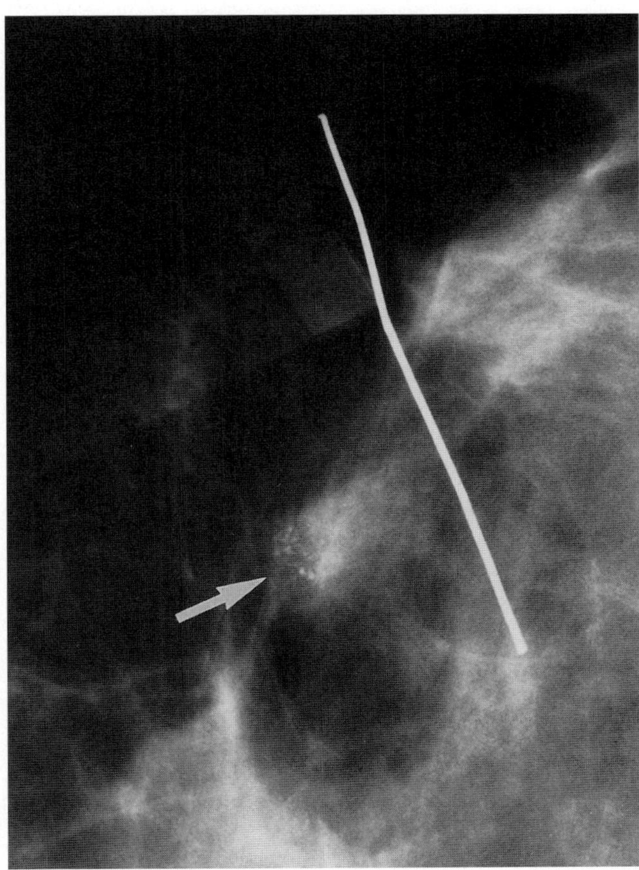

Figure 26–10. Post-lumpectomy, preradiotherapy magnification mammogram shows a small cluster of residual calcifications (*arrow*) near the surgical bed. The wire marks the location of the skin incision.

Summary

For DCIS manifested as calcifications, histologic inspection of the tumor resection margins and mammography are complementary tools in determining whether the tumor has been completely excised. The role of mammography in the evaluation of malignant calcifications is summarized in Figure 26–11.

Pathology

Ductal carcinoma in situ is defined as malignant ductal cells that proliferate within the ductal structures and basement membranes and eventually replace the benign cells within the ducts proximally and the lobules distally. Management and outcome of women with DCIS are closely related to the pathologic findings in the excised specimen.

Gross Pathology

On gross examination, most mammographically detected DCIS does not have a distinct appearance. The background breast tissue may be fatty or fibrous, and slightly firm on palpation. Occasionally, DCIS may manifest as a clinical mass. Such masses are usually extensive and associated with stromal

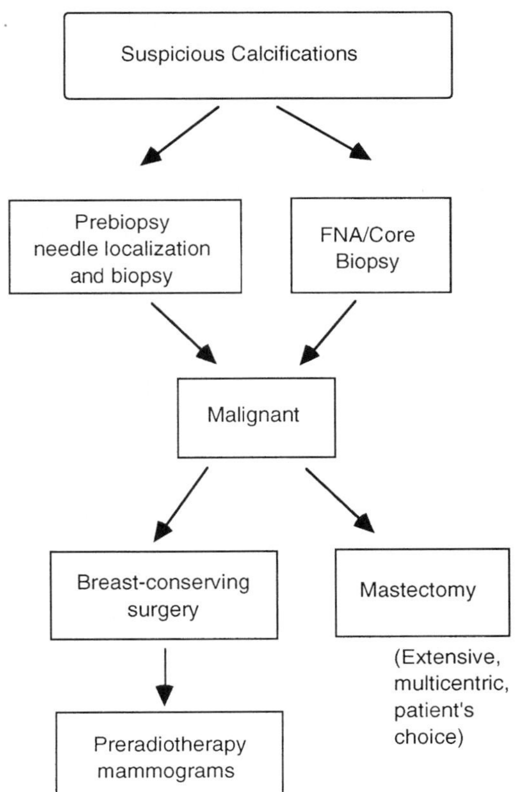

Figure 26–11. An algorithm showing the role of mammography for malignant calcifications. FNA, fine-needle aspiration.

fibrosis. Comedo-type DCIS is an example. The involved area has a firm, granular character, and when it is squeezed, necrotic material exudes from the ducts. Because the majority of DCIS lesions do not have a distinct gross appearance, all excisional specimens in which DCIS is suspected should be handled properly right from the outset.

Microscopic Pathology

DCIS comprises a heterogeneous group of lesions with different malignant potential and outcome. Although histologic diagnosis of classic comedo DCIS with high nuclear grade and typical central necrosis is straightforward, considerable variations in architecture and nuclear grade exist in the non-comedo type of DCIS. With the current mammographic screening and management of DCIS by conservation surgery and radiotherapy, it is important to adopt a classification system that defines and correlates with the behavior of DCIS. Most systems divide DCIS into three grades by architecture, nuclear grade, and tumor necrosis.[23-28]

Classification by Predominant Architecture

Architecture in most systems refers to the microscopic arrangement of tumor cells, which can be papillary-micropapillary, cribriform, or solid. There is some degree of correlation between the architecture and the nuclear grade, but there are exceptions.

The papillary-micropapillary type of DCIS is characterized by multiple isolated papillary projections, most of which lack fibrovascular stalks. Papillae become fused to form roman bridges and arches, giving the impression of rigidity. The majority of tumors have low nuclear grade. Necrosis is absent or focal. Some micropapillary tumors can be quite extensive (Fig. 26–12).

In the cribriform type of DCIS, tumor cells are arranged in a sievelike pattern with multiple small round glands growing in a larger gland or duct. These glands are confluent without fibrous walls. Sometimes the glands grow in a back-to-back fashion,

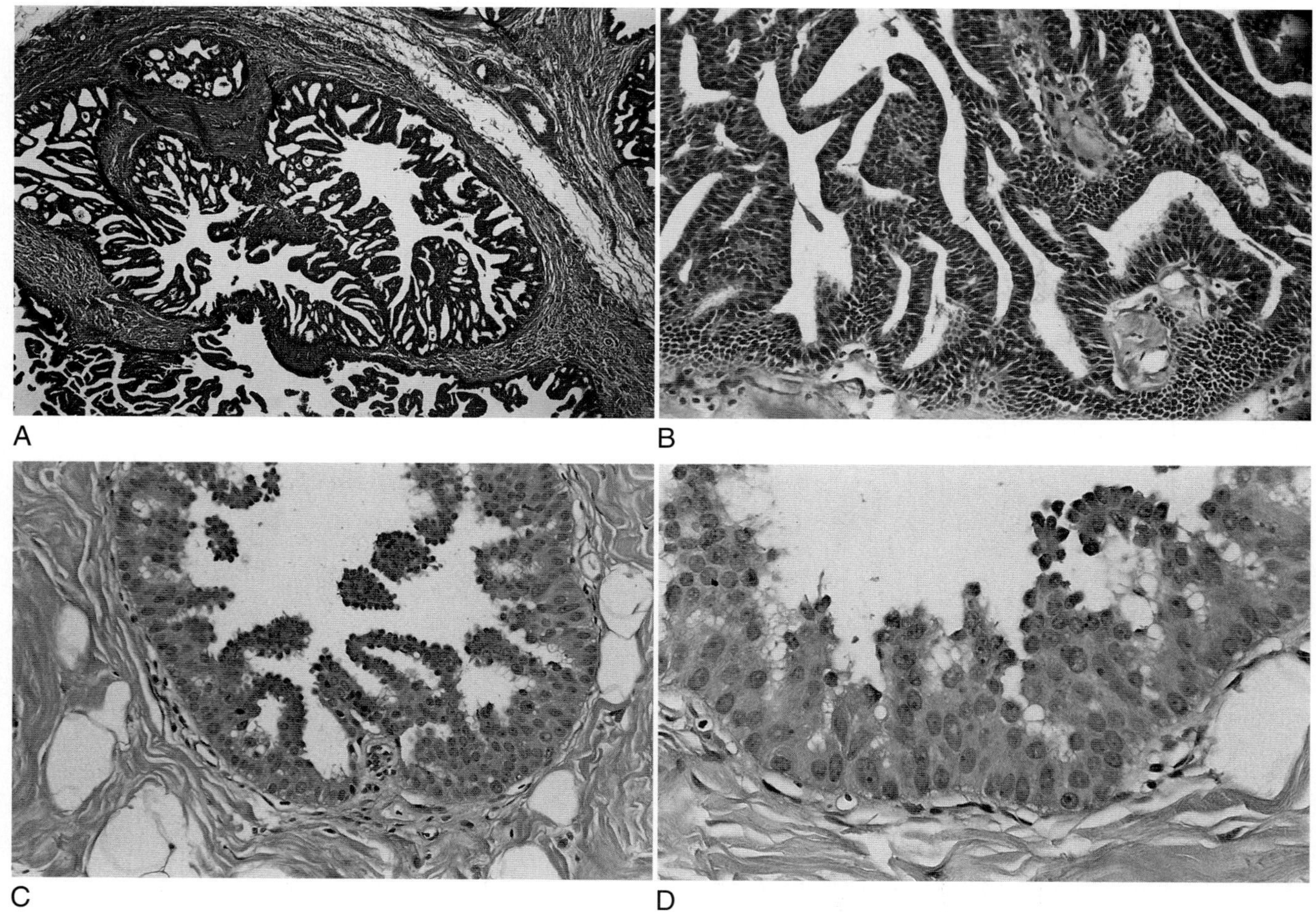

Figure 26–12. Ductal carcinoma in situ. **A,** Papillary type consisting of multiple finger-like projections, most of which are without fibrovascular cores. **B,** Higher-magnification view of **A** shows uniform tumor cells with low nuclear grade. **C,** Micropapillary type characterized by isolated projections, some of which become fused to form glandular spaces resembling roman arches. **D,** Higher-magnification view of **C** demonstrates cells with low nuclear grade.

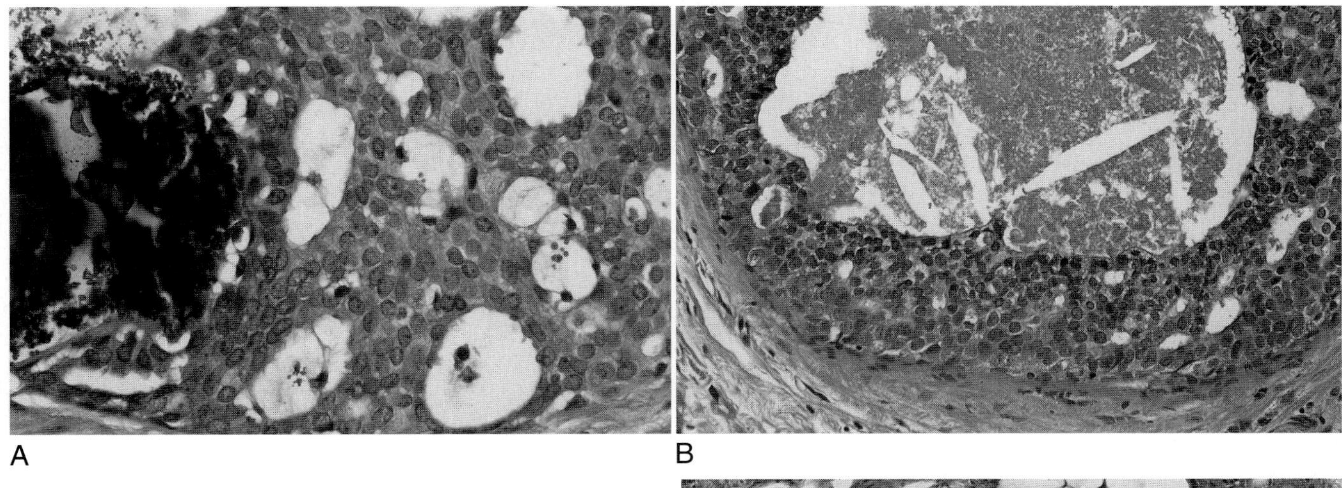

Figure 26–13. Ductal carcinoma in situ, cribriform type. **A,** Tumor cells form a sievelike space. Coarse calcifications are present in the glandular space. **B,** Eosinophilic secretions and cholesterol clefts in the glandular space. Because of the lack of necrotic cells, these changes do not represent tumor necrosis. **C,** Tumor necrosis with calcified psammoma bodies in the glandular lumens.

separated by only one layer of fibroblasts. The majority of tumor cells are of low or intermediate nuclear grade. Necrosis is usually focal (Fig. 26–13). Rare tumors have high nuclear grade and necrosis.

The solid type of DCIS manifests as solid filling of the ducts by tumor cells having high or intermediate nuclear grade. Necrosis is usually present. The typical comedo type of DCIS is a tumor with a solid growth pattern, prominent central necrosis and calcification, and high nuclear grade (Fig. 26–14). Several different growth patterns may occur within the same lesion, and the classification is based on the most prevalent pattern.

In the European Working Group classification, *architecture* refers to the radial arrangement of cellular apex toward the glandular lumen, and the tumors are graded as prominent, present or not prominent, and minimal or absent.[23]

Classification by Nuclear Features

The nuclear grade by Lagios's method divides the tumor into low, intermediate, and high grades according to the nuclear features, nucleoli, and mitotic activity (Table 26–3).[24] Other systems apply similar criteria.[27,28]

The nuclei of low-grade tumor cells are about 1 to 1.5 times the size of a red blood cell. The nuclei are uniform in size and shape and contain finely granular chromatin that is evenly distributed. Nucleoli are rare or absent; when present, they are small, indistinct, and few in number. The mitotic activity is low (Fig. 26–15).

Table 26–3. Summary of Nuclear Grade According to Lagios

Criteria	Low Grade	Intermediate Grade	High Grade
Nuclear diameter*	1.0-1.5	1.5-2.0	>2.0
Nuclear diameter (μm)	10-12	13-16	>16
Nuclear variation in size and shape	Mild	Moderate	Marked
Chromatin	Fine, even	Coarse, even	Coarse, uneven
Nucleoli	Rare to absent, small, indistinct	Some, small	Large, many
Mitotic activity	Low	Intermediate	High

*Compared with diameter of a red blood cell.

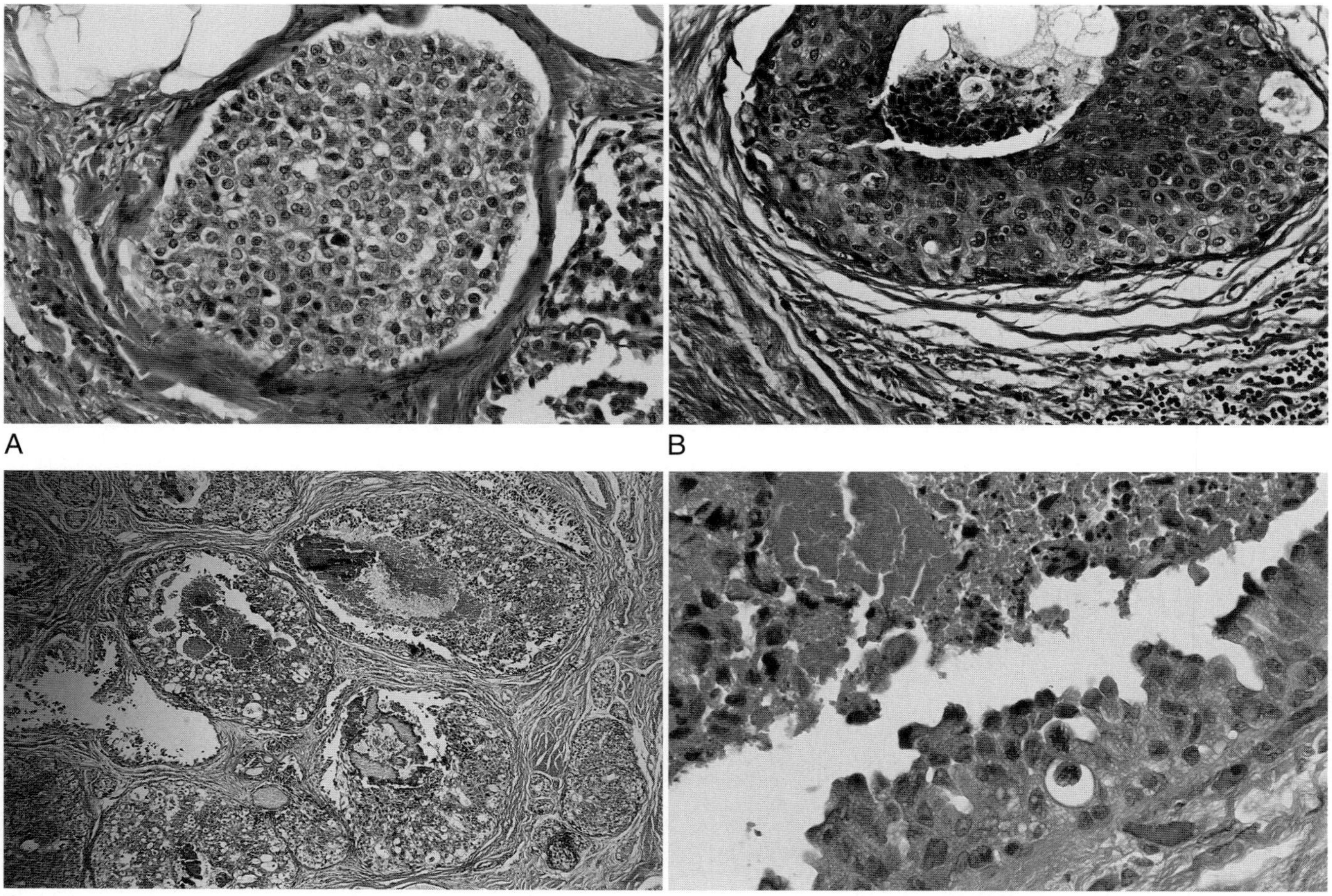

Figure 26–14. Ductal carcinoma in situ (DCIS), solid type. **A,** Tumor cells fill the dilated duct without tumor necrosis. **B** and **C,** Solid nests of DCIS with central necrosis and calcifications characteristic of comedocarcinoma. Calcifications in **C** are variable in size and shape. **D,** Higher-magnification view of **C** shows high nuclear grade and tumor necrosis consisting of necrotic cells, nuclear debris, and pyknotic nuclei.

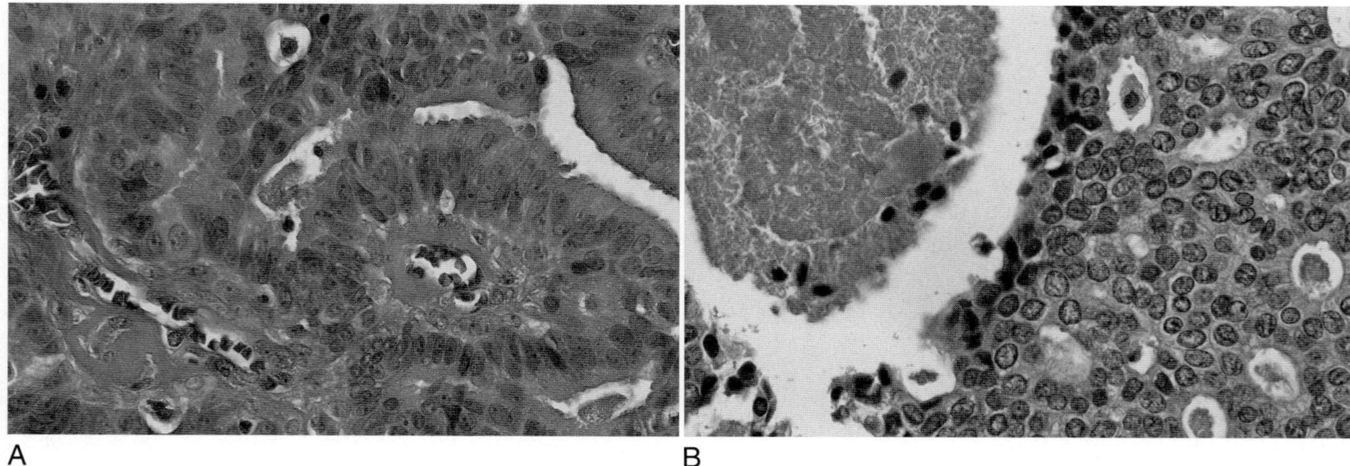

Figure 26–15. Low nuclear grade. **A,** Papillary ductal carcinoma in situ (DCIS) with elongated nuclei that are uniform in size and shape. **B,** Cribriform DCIS with round to oval, uniform nuclei and indistinct nucleoli. There are rare apoptotic cells with pyknotic nuclei mixed with eosinophilic secretions, but no necrotic cells or nuclear debris to justify the designation tumor necrosis.

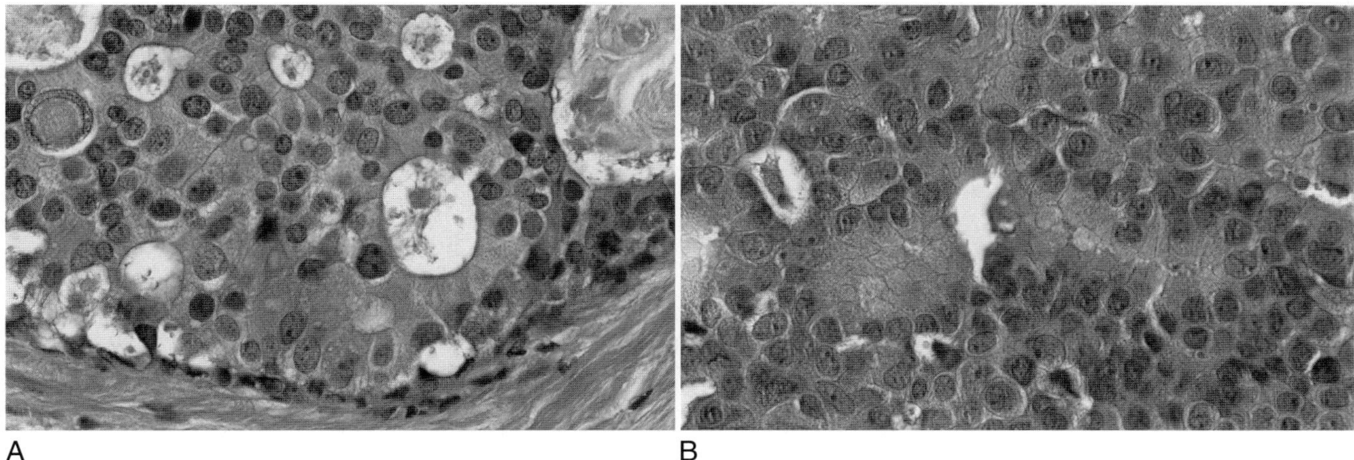

Figure 26–16. Intermediate nuclear grade. **A** and **B,** The nuclei are larger than in tumors of low nuclear grade. There is a moderate variation in nuclear size and shape. Nucleoli are small.

In the intermediate-grade tumor, the nucleus is up to 2 times the size of a red blood cell. Although the tumor cells appear relatively uniform, the nuclei reveal mild to moderate variation in nuclear size and shape. The chromatin is coarsely granular and evenly distributed. The nucleoli are infrequent and small. The mitotic activity is between that of the low- and high-grade tumors (Fig. 26–16).

The nuclei of high-grade tumors are more than 2 times the size of a red blood cell. There is a marked variation in nuclear size and shape. The coarsely granular chromatin is unevenly distributed. The nucleoli are large and multiple. The mitotic activity is high (Fig. 26–17).

Tumor Necrosis

Tumor necrosis refers to the presence of degenerated and necrotic tumor cells with nuclear pyknosis, necrotic ghost cells, and nuclear debris. Tumor necrosis may be limited, focal, or extensive. *Comedo necrosis* refers to the necrosis in the center of solid sheets, whereas punctate necrosis is nonzonal. Luminal secretion, apoptotic cells, and foamy histiocytes are insufficient to be regarded as tumor necrosis.

Final Histologic Grade

Almost all classification systems have adopted three final histologic grades—low, intermediate, and high. In the Lagios method, the final histologic grade takes into consideration the nuclear grade and presence and type of necrosis. Low-grade DCIS has low nuclear grade without necrosis. Intermediate-grade DCIS consists of tumors with intermediate nuclear grade and punctate necrosis. High-grade DCIS has high nuclear grade with comedo necrosis (Table 26–4).[24,29]

The Van Nuys system also uses a three-grade method (Table 26–5). Any DCIS with high nuclear grade is high grade. Non–high-grade DCIS is either low or intermediate grade, according to the absence or presence of tumor necrosis, respectively.[27,28]

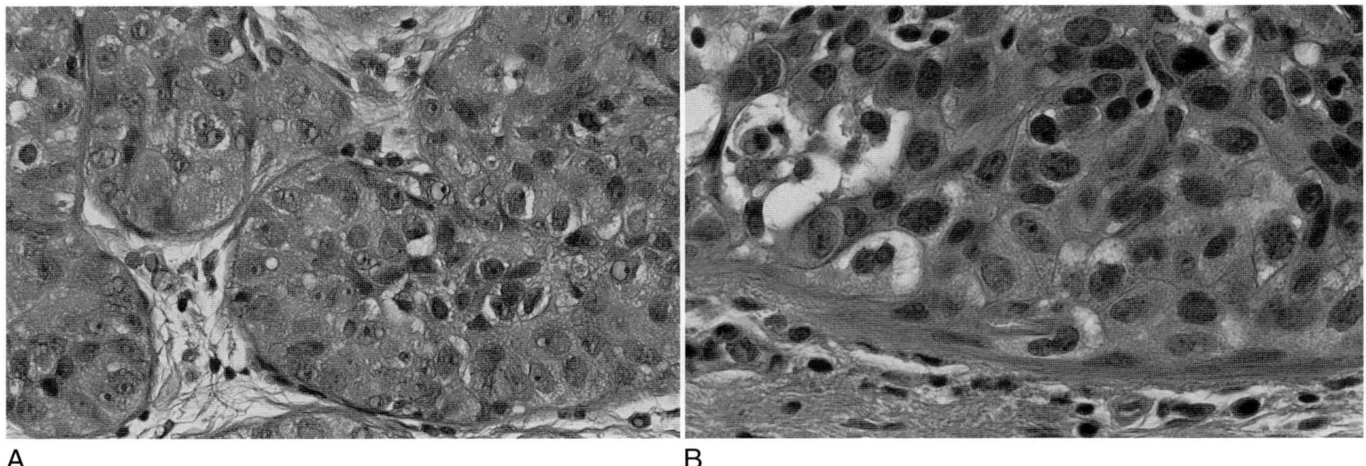

Figure 26–17. High nuclear grade. **A** and **B,** Large nuclei with marked variation in nuclear size and shape. The coarsely granular chromatin is unevenly distributed. Nucleoli are prominent.

Table 26–4. Modified Lagios Classification System

Architecture	Nuclear Grade	Necrosis	Final Grade
Comedo	High	Extensive	High
Noncomedo*	Intermediate	Focal/absent	Intermediate
Noncomedo†	Low	Absent	Low

*Often a mixture of noncomedo patterns.
†Solid, cribriform, papillary, or focal micropapillary DCIS.
From Mack L, Kerkvliet N, Doig G, O'Malley FP: Relationship of a new histological categorization of ductal carcinoma in situ of the breast with size and the immunohistochemical expression of p53, c-erb B2, bcl-2, and ki-67. Hum Pathol 1997;28:974-979.

Table 26–5. Van Nuys Prognostic Index

		Prognosis	
Group	Final Score (points)	Recurrence Rate (%)	8-Year Disease-Free Rate (%)
1	3-4	3.8	93
2	5-7	11.1	84
3	8-9	26.5	61

Adapted from Silverstein MJ, Poller DN, Waisman JR, et al: Prognostic classification of breast ductal carcinoma in situ. Lancet 1995;345: 1154-1157.

The modified Lagios grading method has received endorsement from the expert panels because of its reproducibility and its correlation with tumor size, behavior, and immunohistochemical expression of the HER-2/neu oncogene.[29-32]

Lobular Extension or Lobular Cancerization

Extension of DCIS cells from the ducts into the lobules and sclerosing adenosis are common findings, especially in extensive DCIS. The acini and ductules are solidly filled with tumor cells, sometimes associated with periglandular fibrosis. As long as the lobular pattern is maintained on low-power view, the lesion is considered DCIS (Fig. 26–18). Compared with LCIS, the tumor cells have larger, more irregular nuclei and prominent nucleoli. In LCIS, the nuclei are uniformly small and up to intermediate in size, and nucleoli are absent or indistinct. Sometimes DCIS and LCIS occur in the same lesion. In one study, the quantity of DCIS in the ducts or terminal duct and lobular units was found to correlate with residual disease in the re-excision specimens.[33]

The distinctions between atypical ductal hyperplasia and DCIS and between atypical lobular hyperplasia and LCIS are based on a homogeneous proliferation of neoplastic cells with loss of most myoepithelial cells in DCIS and LCIS. Atypical hyperplasias are discussed further in other sections.

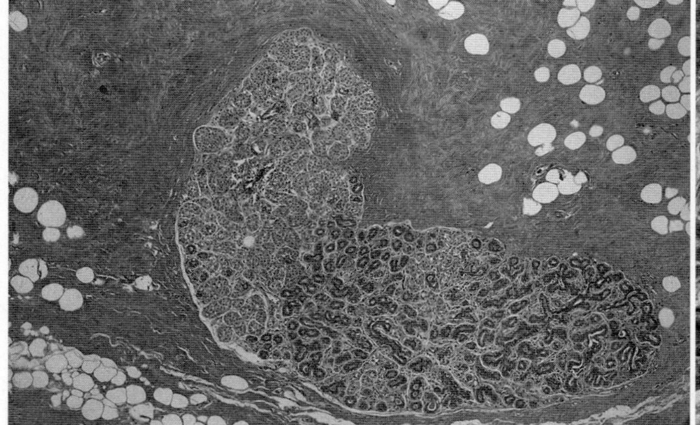

A

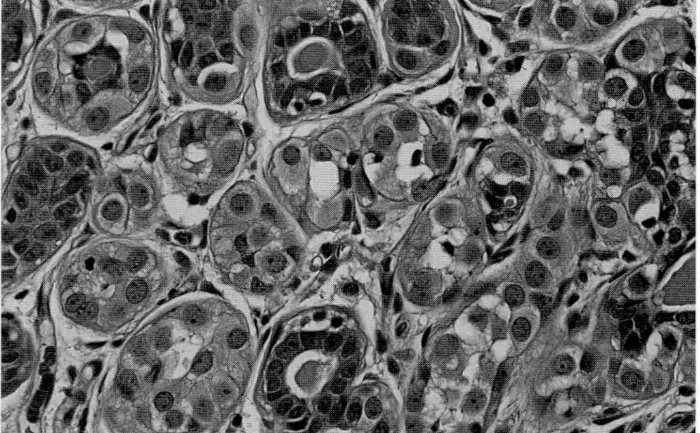

B

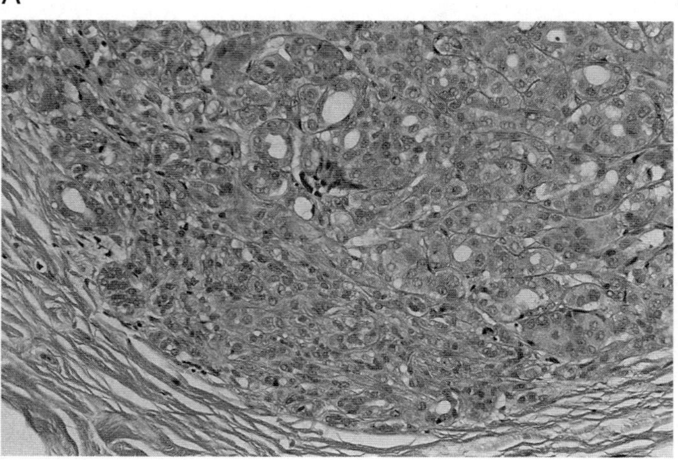

C

Figure 26–18. **A** and **B,** Ductal carcinoma in situ (DCIS) extension into lobules. The lobule involved by DCIS reveals expanded acini compared with the normal lobule. Note the smooth lobular borders. Higher-magnification view in **B** shows tumor cells with intermediate nuclear grade replacing the normal ductular cells. **C,** DCIS extension into sclerosing adenosis. Residual sclerosing adenosis consists of small glands (*left lower field*). Malignant cells distend the acini. Note the smooth borders of glandular profiles.

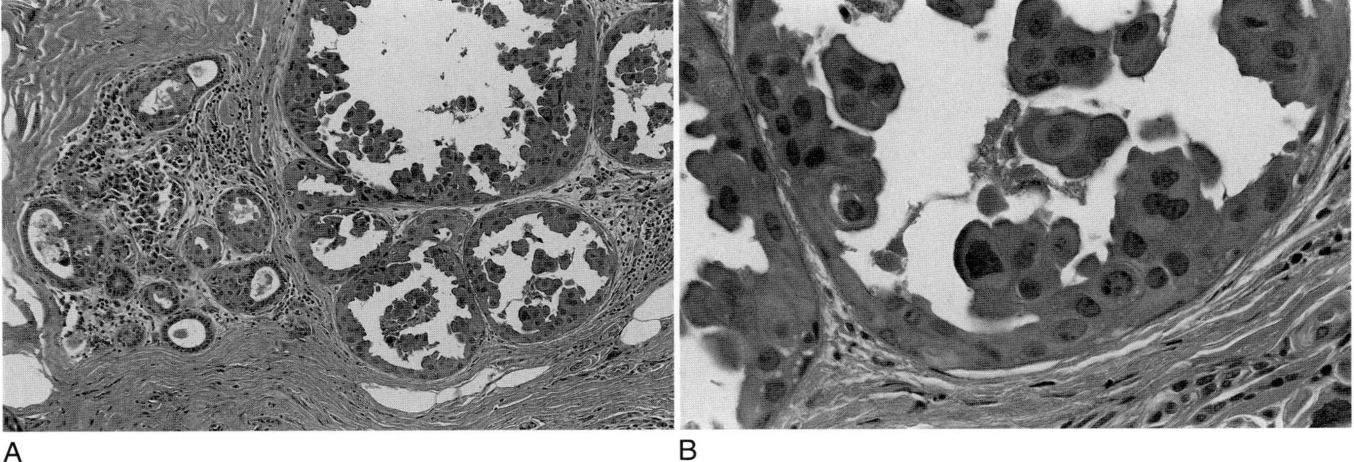

Figure 26–19. Apocrine ductal carcinoma in situ. **A,** Tumor cells form micropapillary projections involving ducts and ductules. **B,** Higher-magnification view shows tumor cells of intermediate nuclear grade without necrosis.

Prognosis Based on Combined Parameters

The prognosis of DCIS is closely related to histologic grade, status of surgical margins, and lesion size.[27,28,34] In the Van Nuys Prognostic Index, a score of 1 to 3 points is assigned to each of three features—histologic grade, surgical margin clearance, and lesion size. The final score correlates strongly with treatment outcome.[27,28] The 8-year disease-free survival rate is 97% for group 1 tumors (3-4 points), 77% for group 2 (5-7 points), and 20% for group 3 (8-9 points). The rates of recurrence of invasive carcinoma are 0 for group 1 tumors, 53% for group 2, and 38% for group 3.[28]

Special Types

Special variants of DCIS include those made up of tumor cells with special differentiation, such as apocrine (Fig. 26–19), neuroendocrine (Fig. 26–20),[35] and hypersecretory change. Intracystic papillary carcinoma (IPC) is a rare variant of DCIS. In a study of 29 cases of the variant, 31% were pure IPC, 31% IPC and DCIS, and 38% IPC and invasive carcinoma. Most of these tumors were of low or intermediate nuclear grade, all were positive for estrogen receptor expression, and all but one were HER-2/neu negative. One patient with IPC alone had a local recurrence 5 years later. Lymph node metastasis developed in a case with invasive carcinoma. IPC is a low-grade carcinoma with excellent prognosis.[36]

Noninvasive Papillary Carcinoma

Papillary carcinoma should be categorized as noninvasive or invasive. Noninvasive papillary carcinoma can occur either as a malignancy in which the epithelium proliferates into villous projections into the duct lumen or as an intracystic lesion. Bloody nipple discharge is seen in approximately 20% of cases. Correlation between histologic type and mammographic appearance has been reported.[37] Papillary carcinoma growing within a large duct usually manifests on

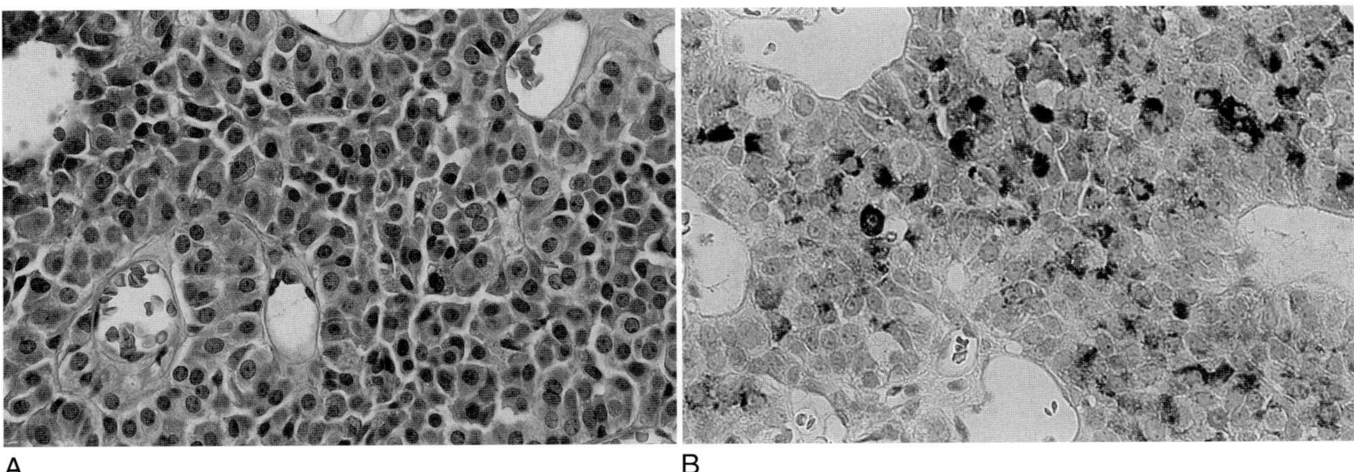

Figure 26–20. Ductal carcinoma in situ with neuroendocrine differentiation. **A,** Solid tumor cells with uniform hyperchromatic nuclei and indistinct nucleoli. **B,** Immunohistochemical stain for chromogranin shows brown immunoreactivity in the cytoplasm (appearing here as the very dark-staining structures) to indicate neuroendocrine differentiation.

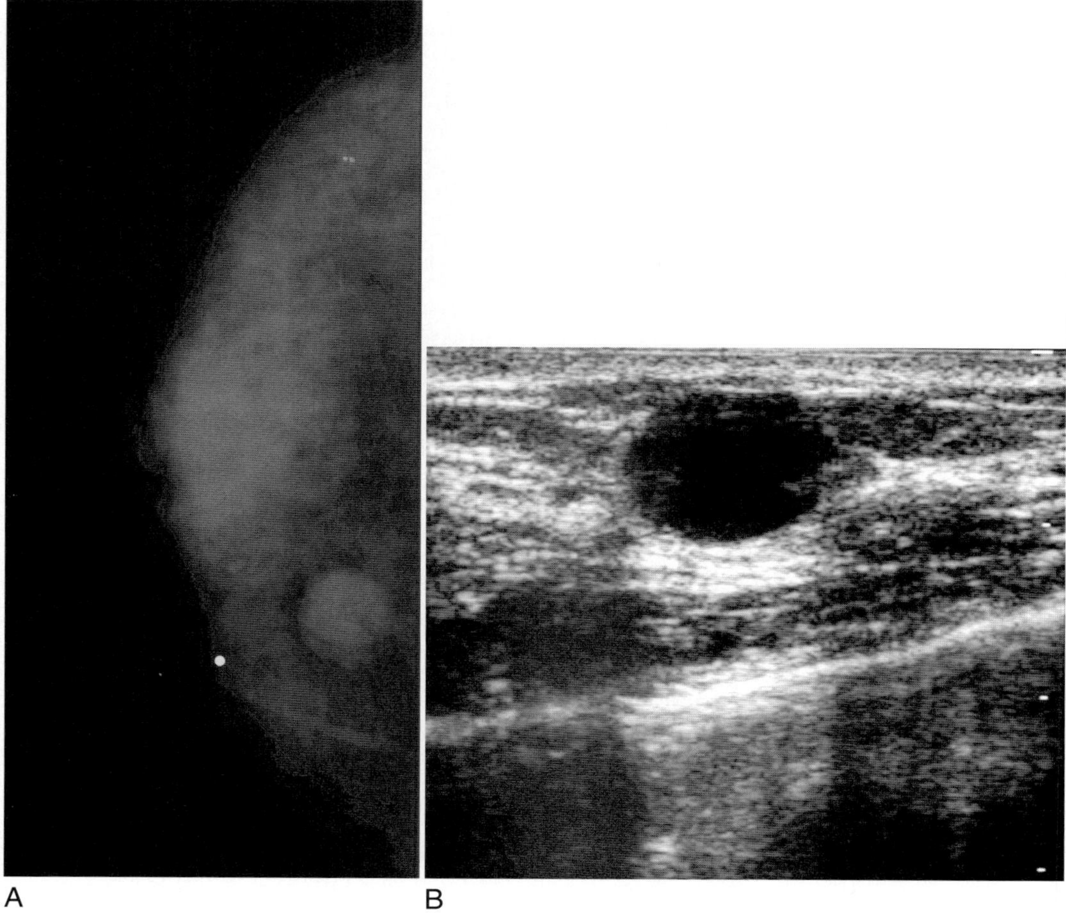

Figure 26–21. Intracystic papillary carcinoma. A large palpable mass was present. **A,** Mammography shows a round mass with circumscribed margins. **B,** Ultrasonography demonstrates a complex cyst with masses protruding from the wall of the cyst into the lumen.

mammograms as clustered calcifications. Noninvasive intracystic papillary carcinomas appear on mammograms as circumscribed masses that on ultrasonography are complex lesions with echogenic tissue projecting from the wall of the cyst into the lumen (Fig. 26–21).

Paget's Disease

Paget's disease of the nipple and areola complex is an uncommon condition in which malignant cells from intraductal or invasive ductal carcinoma migrate to the nipple skin (Fig. 26–22), resulting in the clinical

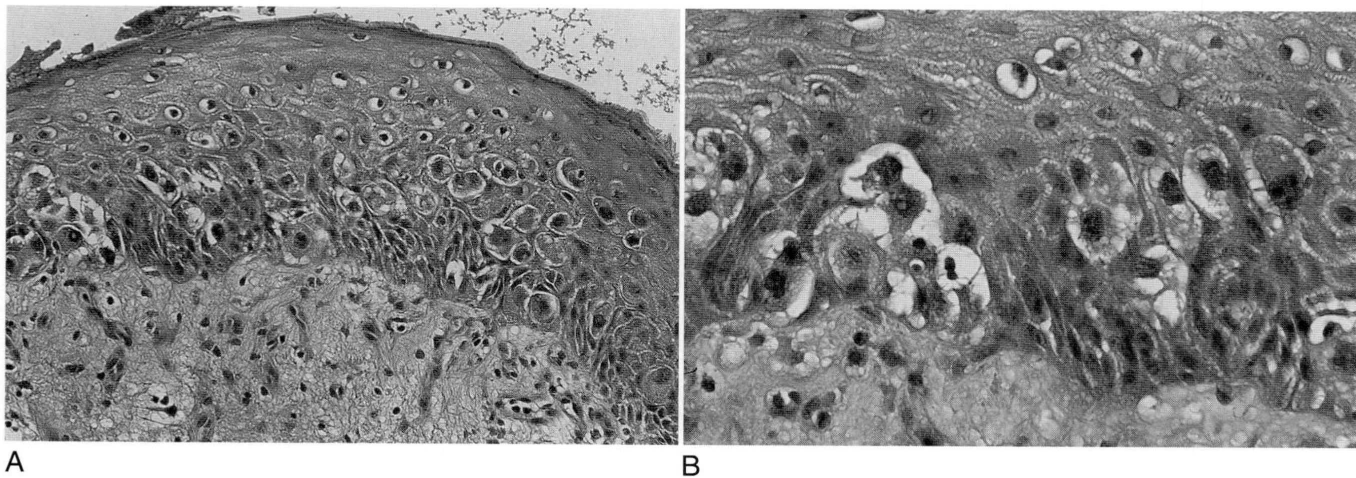

Figure 26–22. Paget's disease of the nipple. **A,** Malignant cells migrate through the epidermis in an ameboid fashion. **B,** Higher-magnification view shows large irregular hyperchromatic nuclei, prominent nucleoli, and vacuolated cytoplasm.

presentation of a chronic, moist, scaly, or erythematous eruption with symptoms such as itching, burning, oozing, and bleeding. This is a special clinical presentation of breast carcinoma that manifests earlier as a result of the changes in the nipple. A palpable or mammographically visible mass implies more aggressive treatment such as mastectomy. Patients who do not have a mammographic density or palpable abnormality do extremely well with breast-conserving surgery and radiotherapy.[38] The prognosis of a woman with Paget's disease of the nipple is also excellent if the underlying tumor is intraductal. Occasionally an invasive component of the tumor is present.

References

1. Page DL, Dupont WD, Rogers LW, Landenberger M: Intraductal carcinoma of the breast: Follow-up after biopsy only. Cancer 1982;49:751-758.
2. Rosen PP, Braun DW Jr, Kinne DW: The clinical significance of pre-invasive breast carcinoma. Cancer 1980;46:919-925.
3. Rosen PP, Lieberman PH, Braun DW Jr, et al: Lobular carcinoma in situ of the breast: Detailed analysis of 99 patients with average follow-up of 24 years. Am J Surg Pathol 1978; 2:225-251.
4. Bassett LW, Hendrick RE, Bassford TL, et al: Quality Determinants of Mammography. (Clinical Practice Guideline, No. 13; AHCPR Publication No. 95-0632.) Rockville, MD, Agency for Health Care Policy and Research, Public Health Service, U.S. Department of Health and Human Services, 1994.
5. Rosner D, Bedwani RN, Vana J, et al: Noninvasive breast carcinoma: Results of a national survey by the American College of Surgeons. Ann Surg 1980;192:139-147.
6. Bassett LW, Liu H-S, Giuliano A, Gold RH: Prevalence of carcinoma in palpable vs impalpable mammographically-detected lesions. AJR Am J Roentgenol 1991;157:21-24.
7. Holland R, Hendriks JH: Microcalcifications associated with ductal carcinoma in situ: Mammographic-pathologic correlation. Semin Diagn Pathol 1994;11:181-192.
8. Paulus DD: Malignant masses in the therapeutically irradiated breast. AJR Am J Roentgenol 1980;135:789-795.
9. World Health Organization: Histological Typing of Breast Tumors, 2nd ed. (International Histological Classification of Tumors. No 2, p 19.) Geneva, World Health Organization, 1981.
10. Zunzunegui RG, Chung MA, Oruwari J, et al: Casting-type calcifications with invasion and high-grade ductal carcinoma in situ: A more aggressive disease? Arch Surg 2003;138:537-540.
11. Stomper PC, Connolly JL, Meyer JE, Harris JR: Clinically occult ductal carcinoma in situ detected with mammography: Analysis of 100 cases with radiologic-pathologic correlation. Radiology 1989;172:235-241.
12. Kinkel K, Gilles R, Féger C, et al: Focal areas of increased opacity in ductal carcinoma in situ of the comedo type: Mammographic-pathologic correlation. Radiology 1994;192: 443-446.
13. Ikeda DM, Andersson I: Ductal carcinoma in situ: Atypical mammographic appearances. Radiology 1989;172:661-666.
14. American College of Radiology: Mammography: Breast Imaging Reporting & Data System (BI-RADS®), ed 3. Available online at www.acr.org/dyna/?doc=mammography/index.html
15. Stomper PC, Connolly JL: Ductal carcinoma in situ of the breast: Correlation between mammographic calcifications and tumor subtype. AJR Am J Roentgenol 1992;159:483-485.
16. Slanetz PJ, Giardino AA, Oyama T, et al: Mammographic appearance of ductal carcinoma in situ does not reliably predict histologic subtype. Breast J 2001;7:417-421.
17. Azzopardi JG, Laurini RN: Elastosis in breast cancer. Cancer 1974;33:174-183.
18. Schnitt SJ, Connolly JL, Khettry U, et al: Pathologic findings on re-excision of the primary site in breast cancer patients considered for treatment by primary radiation therapy. Cancer 1987;59:675-681.
19. Boyages J, Recht A, Connolly J, et al: Factors associated with local recurrence as a first site of failure following the conservation treatment of early breast cancer. Recent Results Cancer Res 1989;115:92-102.
20. Holland R, Connolly JL, Gelman R, et al: The presence of an extensive intraductal component following a limited resection correlates with prominent residual disease in the remainder of the breast. J Clin Oncol 1990;8:113-118.
21. Stomper PC, Margolin FR: Ductal carcinoma in situ: The mammographer's perspective. AJR Am J Roentgenol 1994;162:585-591.
22. Graham RA, Homer MJ, Sigler CJ, et al.: The efficacy of specimen radiography in evaluating the surgical margins of impalpable breast carcinoma. AJR Am J Roentgenol 1994;162: 33-36.
23. Holland R, Petersen JL, Millis RR, et al: Ductal carcinoma in situ: A proposal for a new classification. Semin Diagn Pathol 1994;11:167-180.
24. Lagios MD, Margolin F, Westdahl PR, Rose MR: Mammographically-detected duct carcinoma in situ: Frequency of local recurrence following tylectomy and prognostic effect of nuclear grade on local recurrence. Cancer 1989;63:618-624.
25. Lagios MD: Ductal carcinoma in situ: Pathology and treatment. Surg Clin North Am 1990;70:853-871.
26. Poller D, Silverstein M, Galea M: Ductal carcinoma in situ of the breast: A proposal for a new simplified histological classification, association between cellular proliferation and c-erb-2 protein expression. Mod Pathol 1994;7:257-262.
27. Silverstein MJ, Poller DN, Waisman JR, et al: Prognostic classification of breast ductal carcinoma in situ. Lancet 1995; 345:1154-1157.
28. Silverstein MJ, Lagios MD, Craig P, et al: A prognostic index for ductal carcinoma in situ of the breast. Cancer 1996;77: 2267-2274.
29. Mack L, Kerkvliet N, Doig G, O'Malley FP: Relationship of a new histological categorization of ductal carcinoma in situ of the breast with size and the immunohistochemical expression of p53, c-erb B2, and ki-67. Hum Pathol 1997;28:974-979.
30. Association of Directors of Anatomic and Surgical Pathology: Recommendations for the reporting of breast carcinoma. Hum Pathol 1996;27:220-224.
31. Schwartz GF, Lagios MD, Carter D, et al: Consensus conference on the classification of ductal carcinoma in situ. Hum Pathol 1997;28:1221-1225.
32. Scott MA, Lagios MD, Axelsson K, et al: Ductal carcinoma in situ of the breast: Reproducibility of histological subtype analysis. Hum Pathol 1997;28:967-973.
33. Goldstein N, Kestin L, Vicini F: Pathologic features of initial biopsy specimens associated with residual intraductal carcinoma on reexcision in patients with ductal carcinoma in situ of the breast referred for breast-conserving therapy. Am J Surg Pathol 1999;23:1340-1348.
34. Connolly JL, Boyages J, Nixon AJ, et al: Predictors of breast recurrence after conservative surgery and radiation therapy for invasive breast cancer. Hum Pathol 1998;11:134-139.
35. Tsang WY, Chan JK: Endocrine ductal carcinoma in situ (E-DCIS) of the breast. Am J Surg Pathol 1996;20:921-943.
36. Leal C, Costa I, Fonseca D, et al: Intracystic (encysted) papillary carcinoma of the breast: A clinical, pathological, and immunohistochemical study. Hum Pathol 1998;29:1097-1104.
37. Soo MS, Williford ME, Walsh R, et al: Papillary carcinoma of the breast: Imaging findings. AJR Am J Roentgenol 1995; 164:321-326.
38. Marshall JK, Griffith KA, Haffty BG, et al: Conservative management with Paget disease of the breast with radiotherapy: 10- and 15- year results. Cancer 2003;97:2142-2149.

Invasive Malignancies

Karin L. Fu, Yao S. Fu, Lawrence W. Bassett, Seth Y. Cardall, and January K. Lopez

INVASIVE BREAST CANCER

Invasive cancer is believed to evolve from an intraductal noninvasive precursor. The majority of invasive breast cancers are believed to arise in the terminal duct lobular unit. Approximately three fourths of invasive breast cancers are classified as the *not otherwise specified* (NOS) type. The NOS group has heterogeneous histologic patterns and carries the worst overall prognosis of the invasive breast cancers.[1] Special types of invasive breast carcinomas show distinctive pathologic features, which in some instances have prognostic significance. Although some clinical and mammographic findings may suggest a specific type of invasive cancer, considerable overlap occurs, and a specific diagnosis requires histologic evaluation.

This chapter discusses the general clinical and mammographic features of invasive breast cancers, specific histologic types of invasive breast cancer, malignancies arising from nonductal tissue, and metastases to the breast.

Clinical Features of Invasive Carcinomas

Clinical Breast Examination

In-depth discussion of the clinical breast examination (CBE) is provided in Chapter 11. However, it should be emphasized that a proper CBE requires both experience and time. The most common failure in CBE is not devoting enough time to the examination. Similar to the situation that occurs when mammography is performed with poor quality, an inadequate CBE can lead to a false sense of security.[2]

CBE and mammography are complementary for breast cancer detection. Although mammography is more sensitive, CBE detects some cancers not evident on mammograms. In the Breast Cancer Detection Demonstration Projects of the 1970s, the proportion of cancers detected by mammography alone was 42%, whereas the proportion detected by physical examination alone was 9%.[3] CBE has many of the same limitations attributed to mammography. For example, CBE leads to a significant number of biopsies of benign conditions and has a positive predictive value for cancer similar to that of mammography but a lower sensitivity.[4] CBE can also lead to delay in diagnosis and has been reported to incorrectly identify palpable cancers as benign in 15% of cases.[5]

Clinical signs of breast carcinoma are a palpable mass, palpable asymmetry, skin changes, nipple discharge, and pain. Several factors influence when these clinical signs become apparent.[2] For example, palpation of a mass is more likely to be delayed in a woman with large breasts than in a woman with small breasts. The location of the mass is another factor. A superficial mass is usually more readily palpated than one deep within the breast. Skin changes, such as retraction, also are evident sooner in women with a superficial tumor. Tumors located directly under the nipple can lead to nipple retraction or spontaneous nipple discharge, but the same findings would take much longer to manifest if the tumor were deeper in the breast.

Mass

A palpable mass is the most common physical sign of breast cancer.[6] The mass of invasive breast cancer is typically, but not necessarily, hard and fixed rather than soft and freely movable. However, carcinomas are occasionally freely movable and may in this way mimic benign masses. The invasive breast cancer mass may be tender, but it is usually painless. If a cyst is suspected, it can be verified by needle aspiration or ultrasonography. Cancers are usually first noticed by the woman herself. Sometimes, the discovery occurs after trauma to the breast and is therefore incorrectly attributed to the traumatic event. Malignant breast masses often seem to be larger on palpation than measured on the mammogram or ultrasonogram. This size disparity is due to the associated edema and cicatrization incited by malignant tumors and manifested on palpation.

The most likely etiology of a palpable breast mass depends to some extent on the age of the patient. In women younger than 30 years, fibroadenomas are the most common source of a palpable breast mass. In women between 30 and 50 years, cysts are more common. In women older than 50 years, the etiology of a palpable breast mass is more likely to be breast cancer. Considerable overlap is seen in the kind of lesions that occur in different age groups, and breast cancer cannot be excluded on the basis of the patient's age alone.

Asymmetry

A localized nodularity or thickening may represent breast cancer. Breast cancer can be found in up to 5% of people with palpable breast thickening.[7] However, when these findings are bilateral and symmetrical, cancer is unlikely. Therefore, clinical examination of the breast should always include a comparison of findings in the same location in the other breast.

Physiologic nodularity, which can be defined as multiple tiny localized benign nodules confined to an area of the breast, is one of the most common findings at palpation and also one of the most difficult clinical diagnoses.[8] The correct diagnosis of physiologic nodularity depends on the experience of the examiner. When an area of suspected physiologic nodularity is identified, it must be compared with the same area of the other breast. Bilaterally symmetrical nodularity is strong evidence for benignity. Physiologic nodularity is particularly likely to occur in the upper-outer quadrants.

Skin Changes

Invasive breast cancer can also cause changes in the overlying skin. Breast cancer may become attached to a suspensory ligament, and the cicatrization process associated with many breast cancers can lead to thickening and shortening of the ligament, leading to skin retraction. The skin retraction, also referred to as skin dimpling or flattening, may be difficult to see in the early stages of development. Therefore, visual inspection of the breast should be made under good light. Observing the breast in various dependent positions and having the woman raise her arms over her head are also helpful in bringing out the phenomenon of skin retraction. The breasts should be inspected with the woman upright, leaning forward, and supine. Like palpation, visual inspection should include a comparison of the two breasts, observing for asymmetry in the skin contour. Symmetric skin changes can represent "false dimpling," reflecting attachment of the normal suspensory ligaments to the skin.[2] The latter phenomenon is more likely to occur in the axillary area, where the skin is closely attached to the extensions of the tail of the breast.

Paget's disease of the nipple and areola is an uncommon condition associated with underlying carcinoma, in which the nipple has a chronic, moist, scaly, or erythematous eruption. Symptoms include itching, burning, oozing, and bleeding. The associated carcinoma is intraductal or invasive carcinoma that has spread through the subareolar ducts to the nipple skin.

Inflammatory carcinoma makes up less than 4% of total cases of invasive breast carcinoma.[9] The diagnosis is based on clinical detection of redness, heat, and edema of the skin.[10] This type of breast carcinoma has a grave prognosis.

Nipple Retraction

The nipple is often involved in invasive cancer, and a gradual flattening or retraction of the nipple is an important sign.[2] Nipple retraction should be differentiated from benign nipple inversion, which can usually be reversed by application of manual pressure around the margins of the nipple. Clinical history is also important. Therefore, if nipple retraction is observed, it is important to determine whether it is congenital, long-standing, progressive, or of recent onset. If the nipple changes are progressive or of recent onset, the chance that they are related to underlying breast cancer is greater. Nipple retraction can also be associated with fat necrosis, plasma cell mastitis, and Mondor's disease.

Nipple Discharge

Discharge from the nipple is usually of benign origin. However, if the nipple discharge is bloody or serous, coming from only one or two ducts, and spontaneous and persistent, carcinoma should be considered. Breast cancer is present in only about 2% of women with nipple discharge.[11] Discharge associated with breast cancer should test positive for hemoglobin.[12] Bloody nipple discharge can also be caused by trauma and a solitary papilloma. The likelihood that a nipple discharge is due to cancer increases with age.[13] When invasive cancer is associated with a nipple discharge, a careful clinical examination frequently uncovers an associated palpable mass.[11]

Axillary Adenopathy

Rarely, enlarged axillary lymph nodes are the first clinical evidence of invasive breast carcinoma.[14] The involved nodes are often hard or tender. Fixed nodes are particularly likely to harbor malignancy. Mammography reveals an ipsilateral carcinoma in up to 50% of women with metastatic adenocarcinoma in axillary lymph nodes.[15] Other causes of metastatic adenocarcinoma in axillary nodes are contralateral breast carcinoma, lung carcinoma, and gastrointestinal carcinoma.

Breast Pain

Pain is the only subjective symptom of breast cancer. Although breast pain is a relatively uncommon presentation, its presence does not exclude the diagnosis of cancer. Women so frequently have breast pain that the presence of this symptom is usually interpreted to mean that malignancy does not exist. In a like manner, the frequency of breast pain may be the reason that a woman does not mention it when she presents with a palpable cancer. However, the very fact that breast pain is so common is another reason that its presence does not rule out the possibility of cancer. Although generalized breast pain is usually not an indication of malignancy, a complaint of localized breast pain should be taken seriously. It has been estimated that about 15% of palpable malignant breast lumps are painful.[6]

Imaging Features of Invasive Carcinomas

The mammographic signs of invasive breast cancer are often divided into primary, secondary, and indirect signs.

Primary Signs

Mass

The most common mammographic sign of an invasive breast cancer is a mass. A *mass* has been defined as a space-occupying lesion that is seen in at least two mammographic projections.[16] In about 40% of cases, the mass is associated with malignant calcifications. Typically, the mass of an invasive breast cancer has an irregular shape, ill-defined or spiculated margins, and high radiographic density (Figs. 27–1 and 27–2).

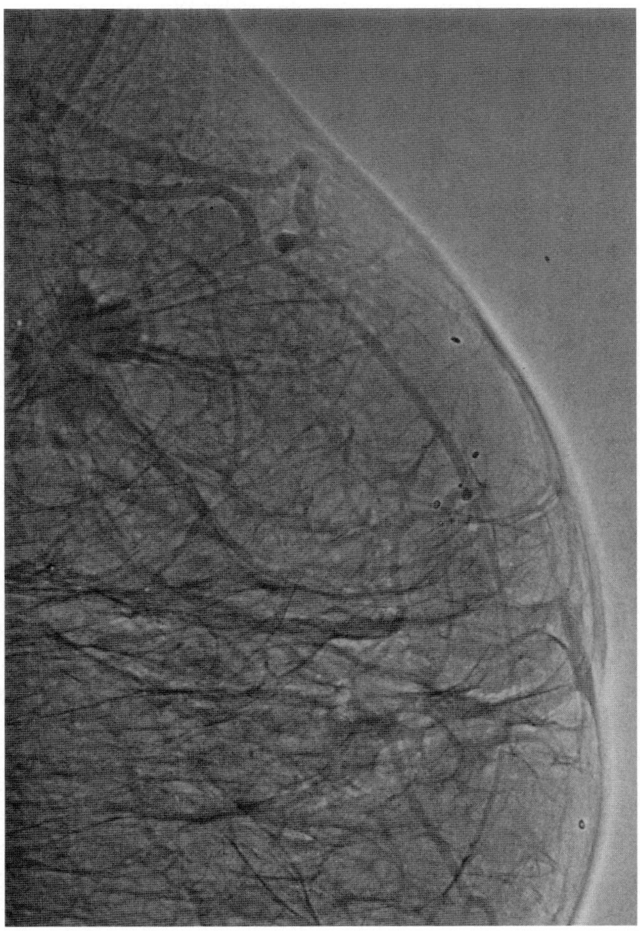

Figure 27–1. Invasive ductal carcinoma, not otherwise specified. The mass has an irregular shape, spiculated margins, and high radiographic density.

A spiculated or ill-defined margin is probably the most significant mammographic feature differentiating malignancies from benign masses. Occasionally an invasive breast cancer has a circumscribed margin (Fig. 27–3), but this feature occurs in less than 10% of cases. Furthermore, when spot compression and magnification mammography techniques are employed, a malignant lesion usually manifests partially ill-defined margins (Fig. 27–4).[17]

Radiographic density is another feature distinguishing malignant from benign masses. The term *density* is used to define the radiographic attenuation of the lesion relative to the expected attenuation of an equal volume of normal fibroglandular tissue.[16] Although this feature is not always reliable, malignant masses usually show higher radiographic density than do normal tissue or benign masses.[18]

Microcalcifications

Invasive breast cancers are commonly associated with microcalcifications, either within the tumor or adjacent to it (Fig. 27–5). The calcifications outside a malignant mass usually represent an intraductal component of the tumor. It is important that all of the calcifications are identified before excisional biopsy so that they can be completely excised (Fig. 27–6). If an extensive intraductal component (EIC) is present, the tumor is regarded as EIC+, and the prognosis for successful breast-conserving surgery diminishes. Rarely, benign-appearing solitary or coarse calcifications may be found within an invasive breast tumor, and the latter finding should not defer

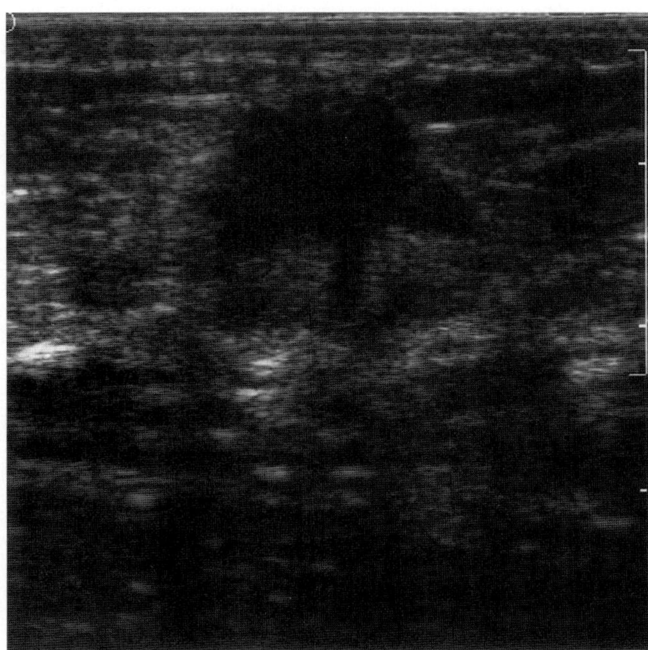

Figure 27–2. Invasive ductal carcinoma, not otherwise specified. Ultrasonography demonstrates a hypoechoic, irregular mass with angular, spiculated margins and an echogenic halo.

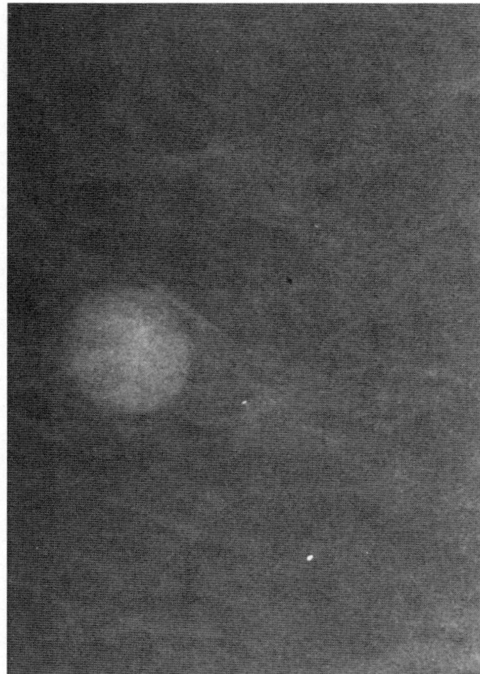

Figure 27–3. Invasive ductal carcinoma, not otherwise specified. The mass is round and has primarily circumscribed margins, suggesting benignity.

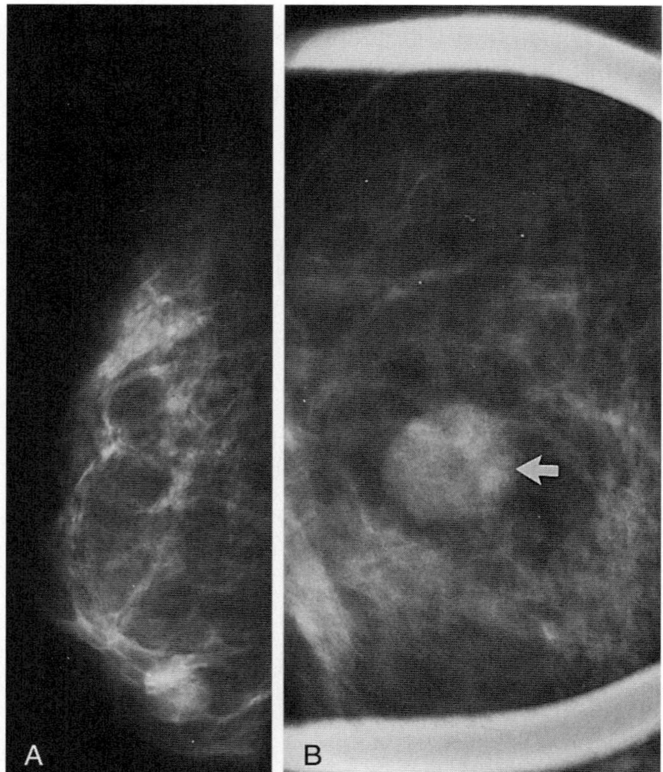

Figure 27–4. Invasive ductal carcinoma, not otherwise specified. **A,** Right mediolateral (ML) view shows a round mass in the inferior aspect of the breast. **B,** Spot compression view with magnification reveals that the posterior margin (*arrow*) of the mass is ill defined. Biopsy revealed ductal carcinoma, not otherwise specified.

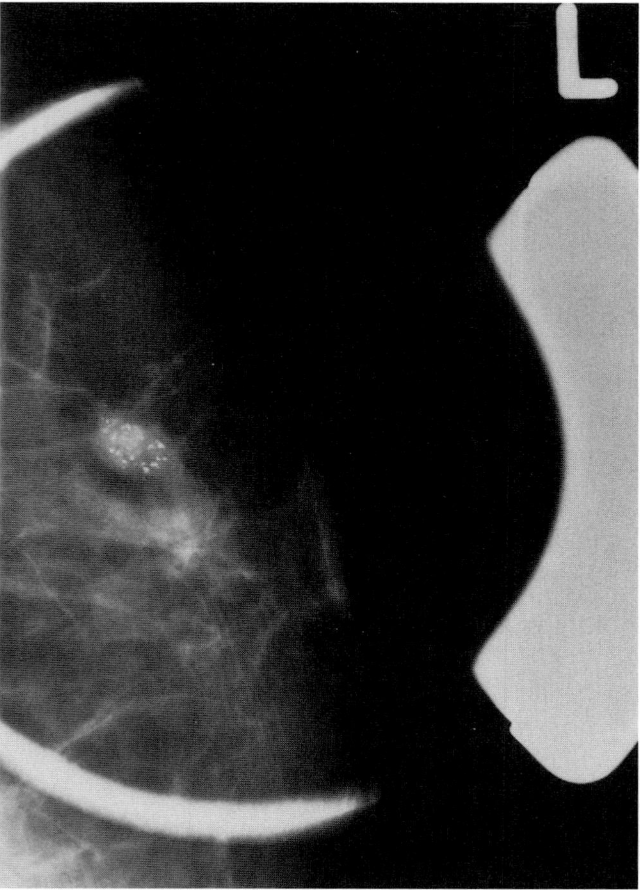

Figure 27–5. Invasive ductal carcinoma, not otherwise specified. Spot compression view with magnification shows an irregular mass containing clustered, heterogeneous microcalcifications highly suggestive of malignancy.

the decision for a biopsy if the mass is suspicious for cancer (Fig. 27–7).

Secondary Signs

Secondary signs of malignancy are usually associated with advanced cancers that are readily detected on CBE or mammography. These secondary signs are skin thickening or retraction, nipple retraction, and axillary node enlargement. When evident mammographically, these manifestations suggest a poor prognosis.

Skin Thickening

The skin is usually 0.5 to 2 mm in thickness, except at the inframammary crease, near the cleavage, and in the periareolar region, where it is normally thicker. Invasive carcinomas may be associated with localized adjacent skin thickening, which suggests infiltration of the skin by the tumor. Diffuse skin thickening may be associated with lymphatic obstruction secondary to underlying carcinoma, or metastases to axillary nodes.

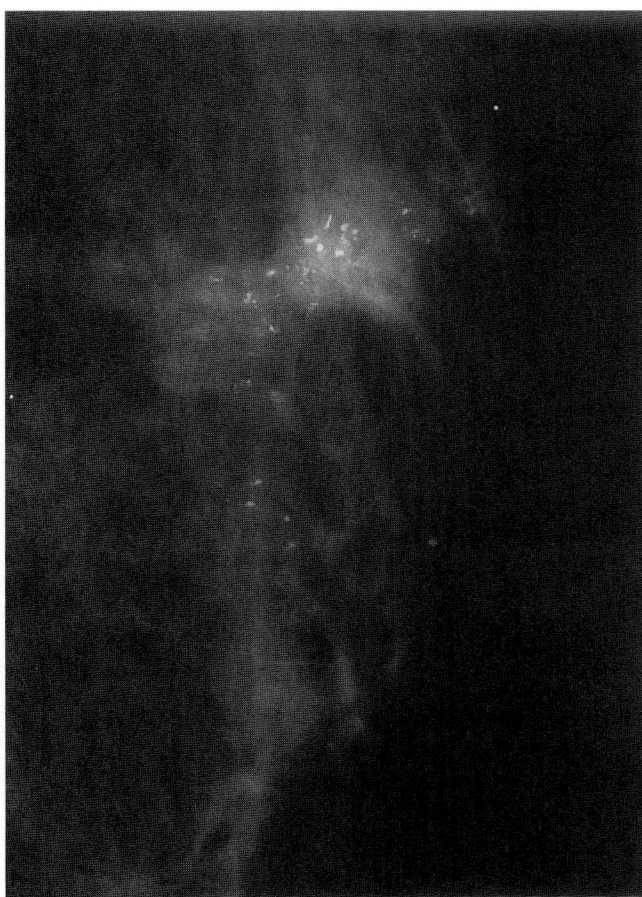

Figure 27–6. Ductal carcinoma, not otherwise specified. There is an irregular spiculated mass of high density containing suspicious calcifications. Additional microcalcifications are located adjacent to the mass. Biopsy showed invasive ductal carcinoma with an extensive intraductal component (EIC+).

Inflammatory carcinoma is a clinical diagnosis that is based on the features of an inflamed breast, which may feel hot and heavy to the patient. Skin biopsy may reveal extensive permeation of the dermal lymphatics by tumor cells. Inflammatory carcinoma is associated with diffuse skin thickening and increased radiographic density of the breast (Fig. 27–8). The differentiation between mastitis and carcinoma with lymphangitic spread (inflammatory carcinoma) may be difficult. In both conditions, the primary lesion may be completely obscured by edema. In this situation, abscess may be excluded mammographically only if typical branching malignant calcifications are present. In general, the diagnosis of inflammatory carcinoma is made clinically and through biopsy unless the mammogram reveals an obvious malignancy.

Generalized skin thickening may also be associated with an abscess, progressive systemic sclerosis, obstruction of the superior vena cava, pemphigus, nephrotic syndrome, congestive heart failure, lymphoma, lymphatic extension from a contralateral breast carcinoma, and changes secondary to radiotherapy.

Skin Retraction

Skin retraction associated with carcinoma comprises a spectrum of changes from a small local dimpling of the skin overlying a small tumor to shrinkage of the entire breast associated with a large, deeply located tumor. Skin retraction and nipple retraction are usually first observed on visual inspection of the breast. Skin retraction may be exaggerated or noticed for the first time as a result of the application of

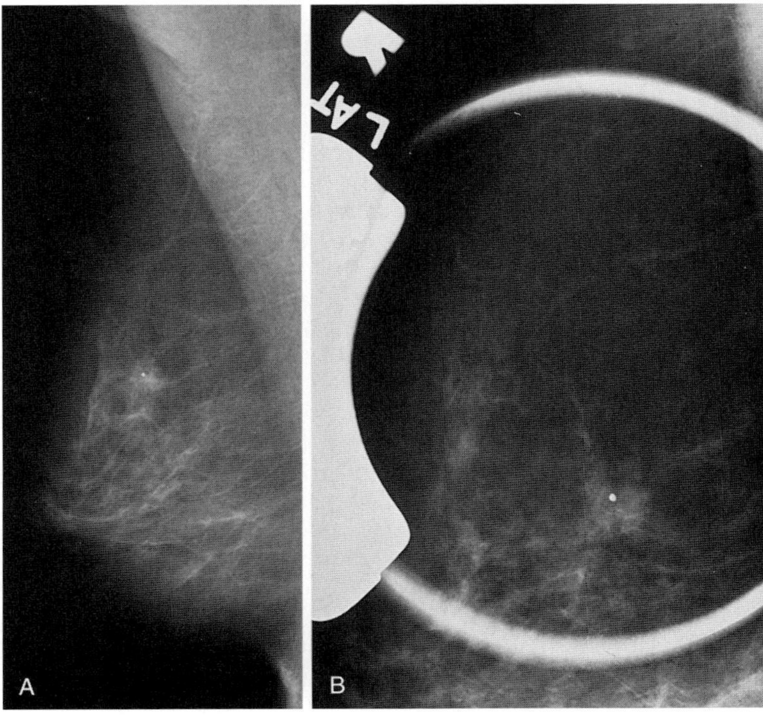

Figure 27–7. Invasive ductal carcinoma, not otherwise specified, containing a benign calcification. **A,** Right mediolateral oblique (MLO) view shows a solitary, round, dense calcification within an irregular mass. **B,** Spot compression–magnification view shows that the mass has an irregular shape and ill-defined margins. No additional calcifications were found. Biopsy demonstrated invasive ductal carcinoma.

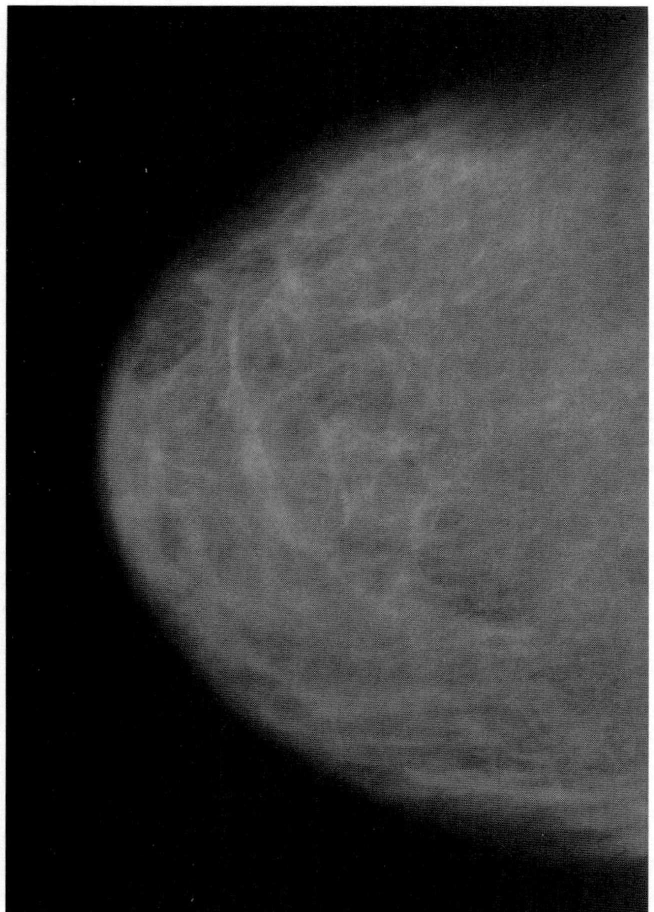

Figure 27–8. Inflammatory carcinoma. Mammogram shows diffuse skin thickening and diffusely increased radiographic density.

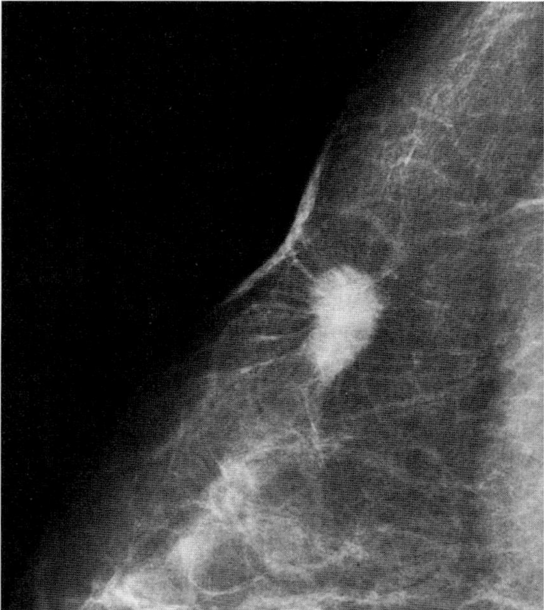

Figure 27–9. Invasive ductal carcinoma, not otherwise specified. Close-up of mammogram with x-ray beam tangential to the area of skin retraction shows the underlying carcinoma with attachment to Cooper ligaments. Skin thickening can be seen.

mammographic compression. When the x-ray beam is tangential to the involved breast surface, flattening of the breast contour or retraction can be seen on the mammogram (Fig. 27–9).

Skin retraction associated with breast cancer is attributed to the proliferation of fibrous tissue, or *cicatrization,* not only within the tumor itself but also in the surrounding breast tissue. In time, the cicatrization process results in contraction of the ligaments of Cooper, the suspensory ligaments of the breast, pulling the skin toward the lesion. Occasionally, skin retraction may occur with inflammation from bacterial infection or fat necrosis.

Nipple Retraction

Cicatrization associated with an adjacent breast cancer can lead to changes in subareolar ducts, causing them to thicken and shorten. Eventually, flattening and retraction of the nipple area occur, which can be observed on mammograms (Fig. 27–10). As mentioned previously, nipple retraction should be differentiated from nipple inversion. The latter condition is usually a long-standing process, often bilateral, that may occur in healthy women.

Retraction of the skin or nipple may also occur secondary to scarring from a previous surgical procedure or secondary to an abscess (Fig. 27–11). Thus, it is important to be aware of the exact site of any previous biopsies when viewing the mammograms. This information is usually reported by the woman on a

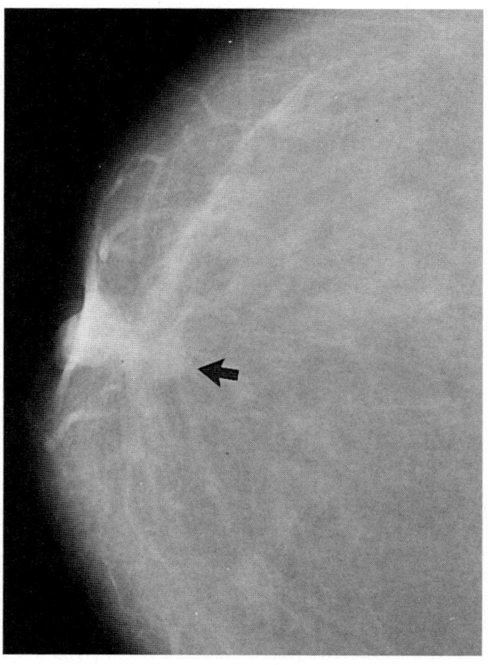

Figure 27–10. Invasive ductal carcinoma, not otherwise specified. The nipple is retracted due to underlying spiculated carcinoma (*arrow*).

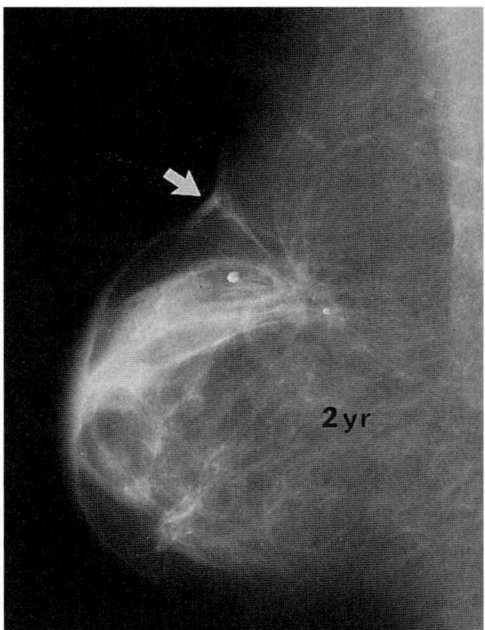

Figure 27–11. Scar, 2 years after biopsy. An architectural distortion is seen, associated with retraction and thickening of the overlying skin (*arrow*). Benign calcifications are also present. The findings are typical of a postoperative scar: The abnormality changed shape from one view to another, was not palpable, and was smaller than on the examination performed 1 year before.

history questionnaire and recorded on a diagram by the radiologic technologist. Often, a thin radiopaque wire is placed directly over the site of a biopsy scar to expedite the correlation of mammographic findings.

Axillary Lymph Node Metastases

Involvement of the axillary lymph nodes is one of the most important factors in the prognosis of an individual case of breast cancer. Routine use of the mediolateral oblique (MLO) projection assures that at least the lower axillary nodes can be visualized on a screening examination. The axillary tail view shows a greater amount of axillary tissue than does the MLO. However, radiographic evaluation of the axillary nodes has proved to be of limited clinical value.[19] Absence of radiolucent fat within a node larger than 2 cm suggests axillary node metastases (Figs. 27–12 and 27–13).

The lymph node involved by metastasis may be small, and the metastasis detectable only with microscopic examination. Malignant cells first enter the lymph node through afferent lymphatics and become entrapped in the subcapsular sinusoidal spaces (see Fig. 27–12C), where the tumor emboli proliferate and eventually destroy the sinusoidal spaces and the adjacent lymphoid tissue. This process is often associated with a desmoplastic response (see Fig. 27–12D), resulting in the increased density of the lymph node seen on mammograms. Sometimes the entire lymph node is replaced by tumor, leaving no identifiable nodal structure. The number and the size of lymph nodes with metastasis are directly related to the prognosis. The presence of extranodal spread in the form of lymphatic and vascular space involvement or tumor nodule in the perinodal fibroadipose tissue also adversely affects the prognosis (see Fig. 27–12E and F).

Enlarged axillary nodes may be seen in several benign diseases, such as sarcoid, tuberculosis, and rheumatoid arthritis.[20] Malignant conditions other than breast carcinoma that may result in enlarged

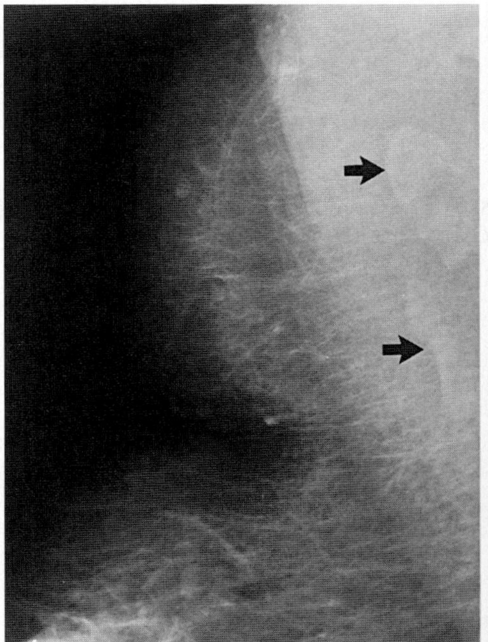

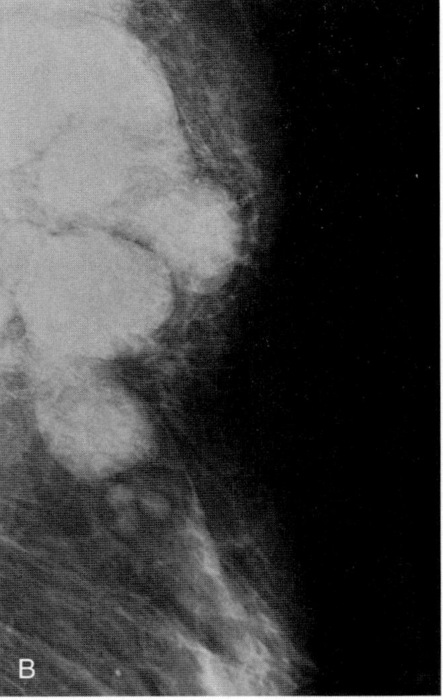

Figure 27–12. Axillary lymph node metastases from breast carcinoma. **A,** Right mediolateral oblique (MLO) view shows normal nodes (*arrows*) with radiolucent fat in hilum of nodes. **B,** Left MLO view shows enlarged, round to oval, dense axillary nodes. Biopsy showed adenocarcinoma, consistent with a primary breast tumor.

Continued

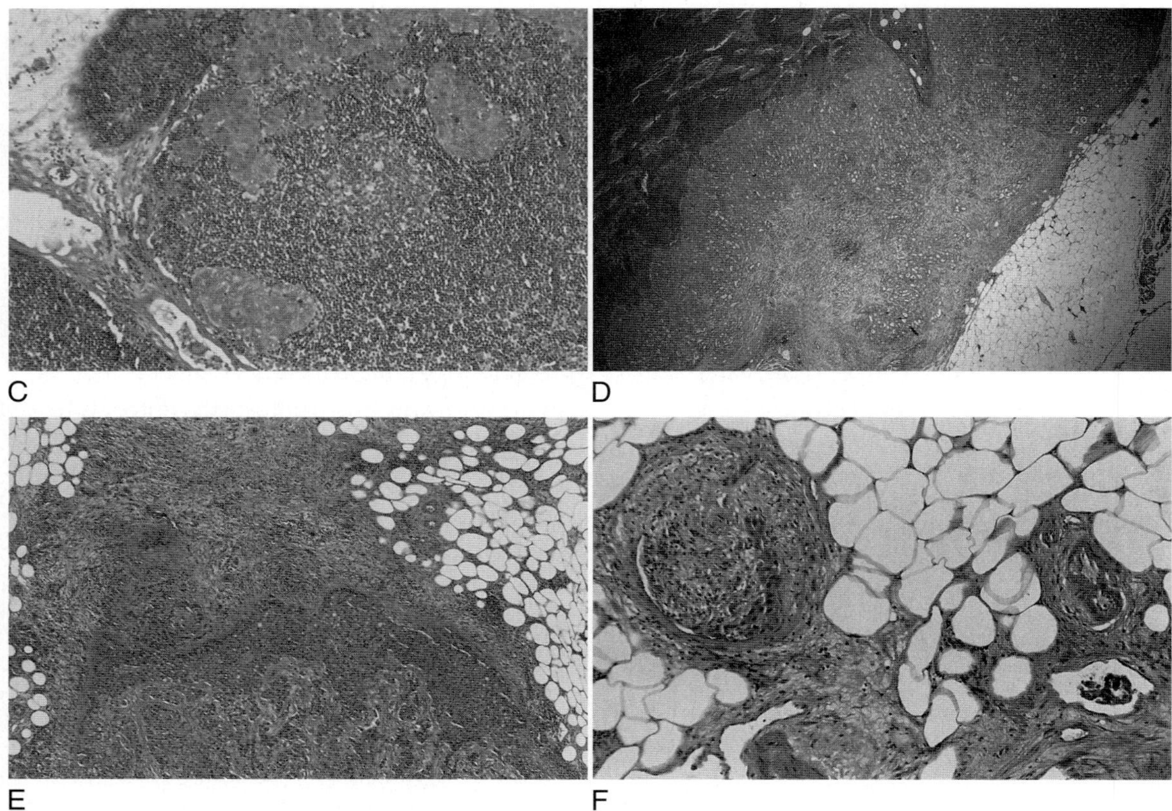

Figure 27–12, cont'd. **C** to **F**, Progression of lymph node metastasis: **C**, early metastasis in the subcapsular region of the lymph node; **D**, massive replacement of lymph node with desmoplastic stromal reaction; **E**, extracapsular soft tissue extension; **F**, extracapsular vascular invasion.

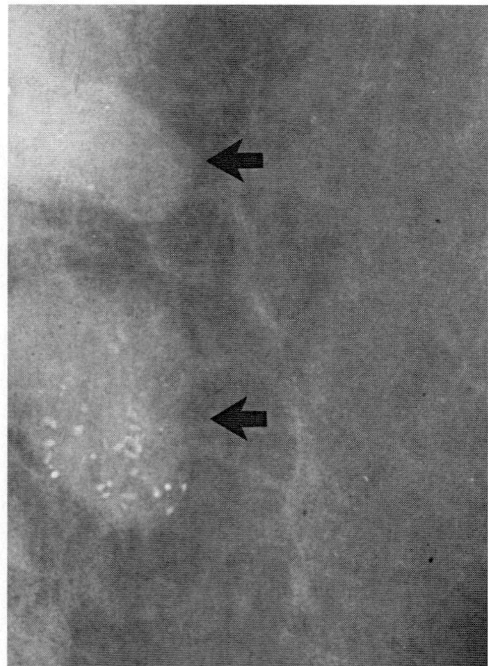

Figure 27–13. Calcified axillary node metastases from breast carcinoma. Close-up of nodes shows characteristic malignant calcifications (*arrows*) that were present in the primary breast carcinoma. The presence of calcification in metastatic nodes is uncommon.

nodes include lymphoma, leukemia, and metastases from extramammary malignancies. Furthermore, no reliable radiographic criteria exist to exclude early nodal involvement with metastases. Surgical exploration with histologic evaluation is currently the only reliable way to exclude lymph node metastases due to invasive breast carcinoma.

Indirect Signs

Although the majority of invasive breast cancers are identified as irregular masses with ill-defined or spiculated margins, some carcinomas are identifiable only from indirect mammographic signs. The indirect signs of malignancy include a developing density, architectural distortion, asymmetrical density, and a unilateral single dilated duct.[21]

Developing Density

Because the breasts of postmenopausal women are expected to undergo involution, the appearance of a new or growing density in mammograms should be considered a possible sign of early breast cancer. To identify a developing density, the radiologist must have access to previous mammograms.[22] The developing density may be classified as a *neodensity* if it cannot be recognized in previous studies (Figs. 27–14 and 27–15), or it may be an *evolving density*, which

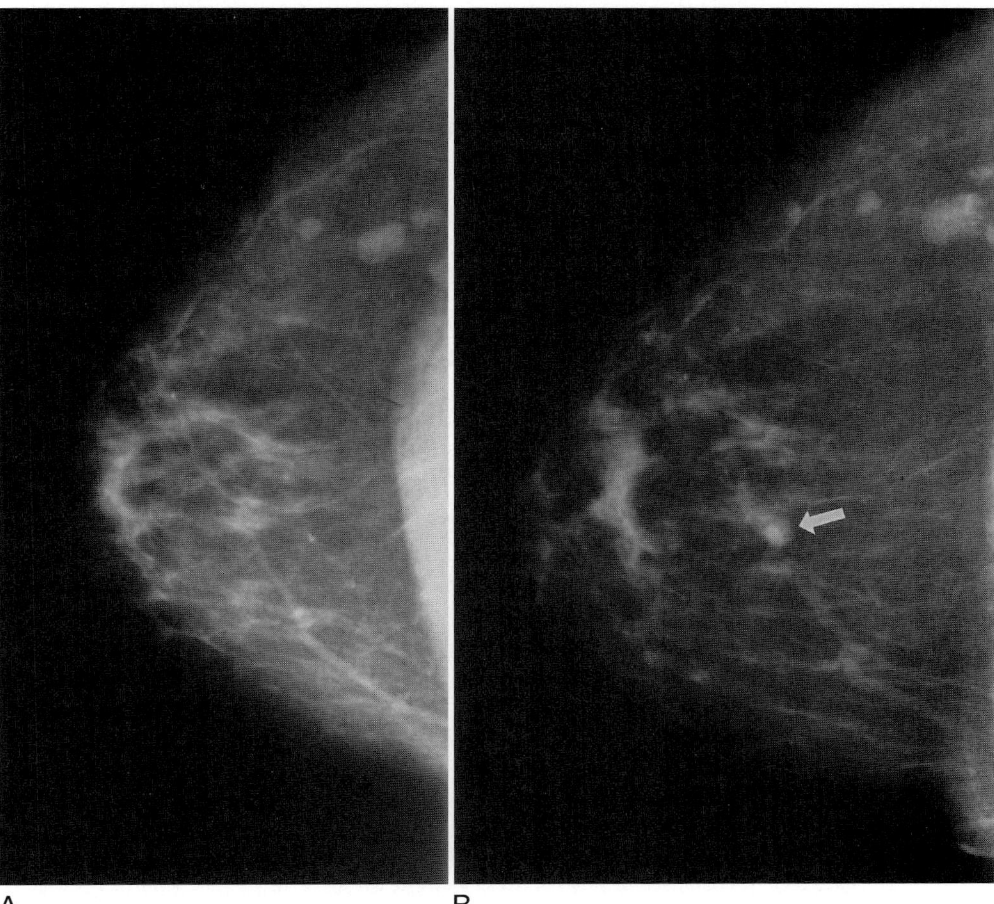

Figure 27–14. Invasive ductal carcinoma, not otherwise specified, manifested as a neodensity. **A,** Baseline mammogram showed only several benign nodules representing intramammary lymph nodes. **B,** Mammogram obtained 1 year later shows a small neodensity (*arrow*). Biopsy demonstrated invasive ductal carcinoma.

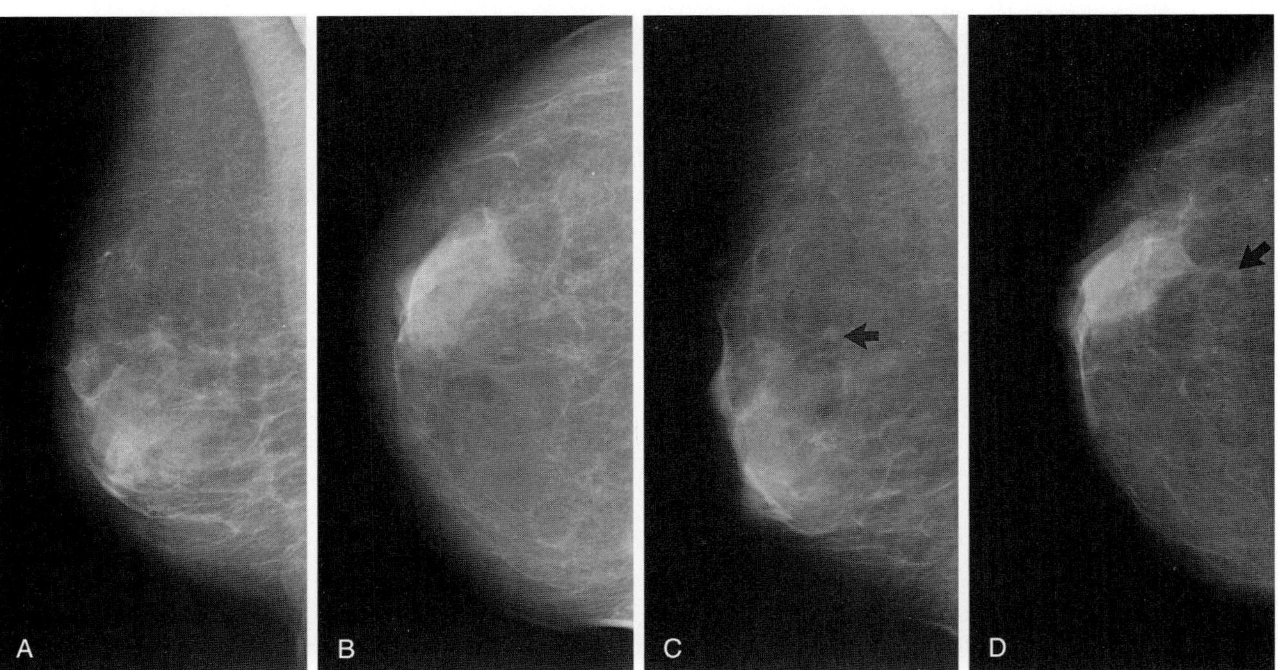

Figure 27–15. Invasive ductal carcinoma, not otherwise specified, manifested as a neodensity. Baseline mediolateral oblique (MLO) (**A**) and craniocaudal (CC) (**B**) mammograms showed no abnormalities. Screening MLO (**C**) and CC (**D**) mammograms obtained 1 year later show a 5-mm neodensity (*arrows*).

was present at the previous examination but was smaller and was not recognized as significant (Fig. 27–16). If the density has mammographic features that might indicate a cyst, ultrasonography or aspiration should be done. If a simple cyst is disclosed and it matches the site of the mammographic abnormality, no further evaluation is necessary. The presence of a cyst in a postmenopausal woman who is not receiving hormone replacement therapy (HRT) is unusual, however, and the surrounding tissue should be carefully scrutinized.

Neodensities are not uncommon in women undergoing HRT. The mammographic tissue densities due to HRT can usually be differentiated from a neodensity associated with breast cancer. The densities associated with exogenous hormone therapy usually are present in several areas of the same breast and are bilateral. If a solitary neodensity is present in a woman receiving HRT, it may be difficult to rule out breast cancer. In the latter situation, it may be useful for the HRT to be stopped for 2 months; if the neodensity persists after suspension of HRT, biopsy should be considered.

Localized Architectural Distortion

An architectural distortion may be the earliest sign of breast carcinoma (Fig. 27–17). *Architectural distortion* is a focal abnormal arrangement of the parenchymal tissues, including the ducts and ligaments. The normal architecture is distorted with no definite

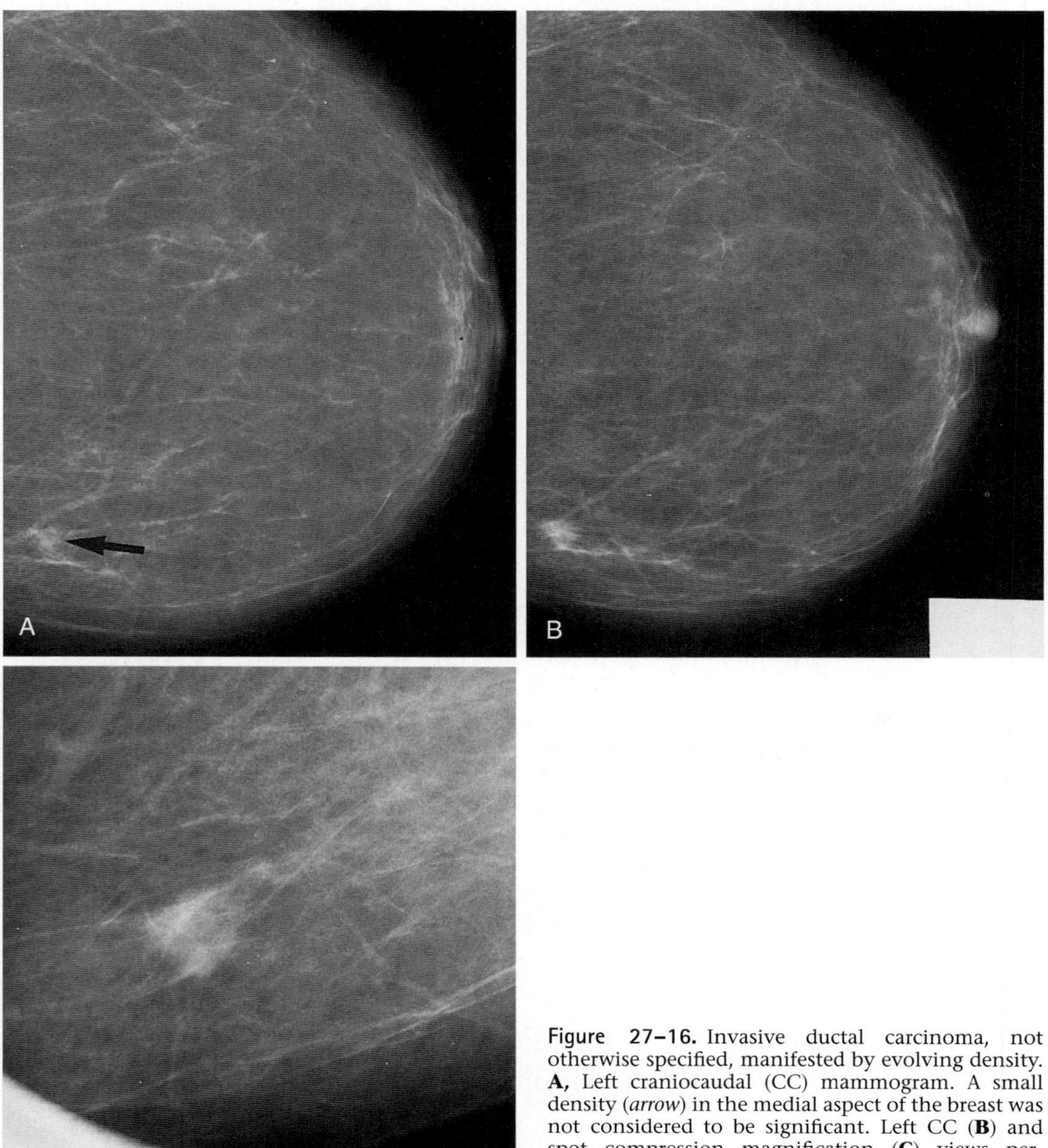

Figure 27–16. Invasive ductal carcinoma, not otherwise specified, manifested by evolving density. **A,** Left craniocaudal (CC) mammogram. A small density (*arrow*) in the medial aspect of the breast was not considered to be significant. Left CC (**B**) and spot compression magnification (**C**) views performed 1 year later reveal increased size and radiographic density of the lesion.

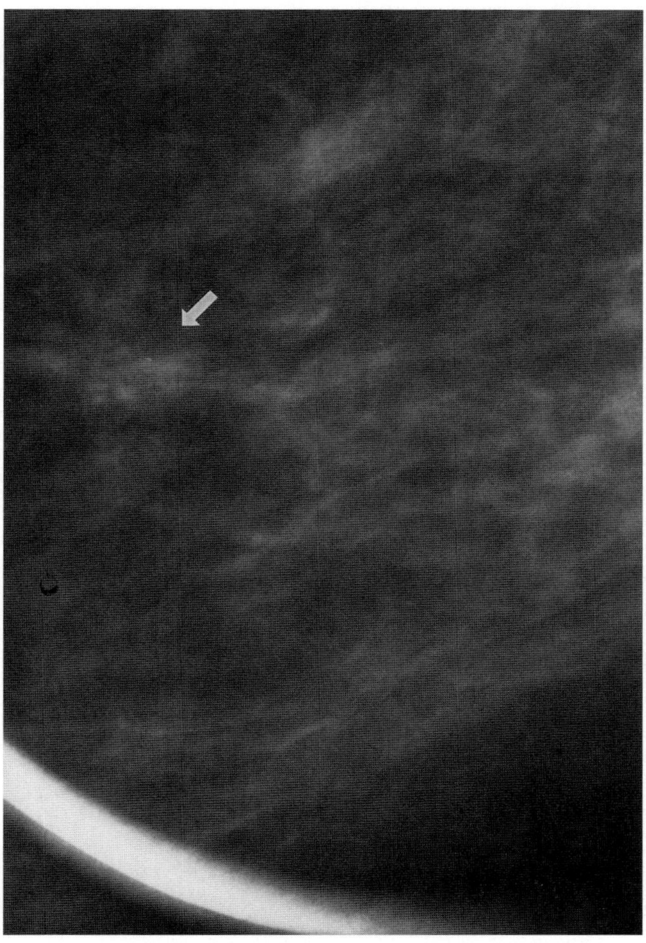

Figure 27–17. Invasive ductal carcinoma, not otherwise specified, identified by architectural distortion. Spot compression–magnification view demonstrates the architectural distortion (*arrow*) with no central mass.

mass visible.[16] The term architectural distortion includes spiculations radiating from a point and focal retraction or distortion of the edge of the parenchyma. When associated with invasive carcinoma, this finding is usually due to fibrosis. An architectural distortion may be the only indicator of a large cancer located within dense breast tissue (Fig. 27–18). Spot compression or rolled views can be helpful in verification of a suspected architectural distortion (Fig. 27–19). In addition, ultrasonography is a useful imaging modality to confirm mammographic findings.

Architectural distortions can also be associated with surgical and radial scars. Because postoperative scarring results in distortions of the parenchyma, it is important to be aware of the location of any previous operations.[23] The radiologic technologist should enter the location of visible scars on a diagram of the breast. Some radiologists find it useful for the radiologic technologist to place a wire directly over surgical scars before performing mammograms so that the exact site of the scar is indicated in the images.[24]

A radial scar, or radial sclerosing lesion (RSL), can also manifest mammographically as an architectural distortion or masslike density. Typically, a radial scar can have a radiolucent center with radiating long, thin spicules. However, exceptions to these general rules are common, and it is not possible to differentiate radial scars from breast cancers mammographically.[25]

Asymmetrical Density

Asymmetrical density refers to a relative increase in the volume of fibroglandular tissue compared with the corresponding area in the other breast. This asymmetry usually represents a normal variation in distribution of fibroglandular tissue. Rarely, however, an asymmetrical density is an indirect sign of breast cancer. To appreciate a parenchymal asymmetry, one must view the mammograms of the two breasts side by side and back to back. Because variations in the distribution of the parenchymal tissue occur normally, an unacceptably high rate of unnecessary false-negative biopsy findings would result if biopsy were performed for all asymmetrical densities.

A biopsy is not indicated unless suspicious clinical or mammographic features are associated with the asymmetrical density. Association of an asymmetrical density with a palpable abnormality is of greater concern, and a biopsy should be considered in such cases (Fig. 27–20).

When a question exists as to the nature of a localized region of asymmetrical breast tissue, additional evaluation is warranted. Spot compression views usually show whether the area of increased density is normal compressible tissue. Accessory breast tissue in the axilla is a common normal variant that should not be mistaken for a significant asymmetrical density (Fig. 27–21). In addition, ultrasonography is a useful imaging modality to confirm benignity or detect an underlying lesion such as an ultrasonographic mass or architectural distortion.

Single Dilated Duct

Dilatation of a unilateral single subareolar duct has also been reported to be an indirect sign of an early carcinoma (Fig. 27–22).[21] However, this finding is rarely the presenting sign of malignancy. More often, a single dilated duct is due to duct ectasia or an intraductal papilloma. If mammography discloses suspicious calcifications or a spiculated mass at the site of the dilated duct, a biopsy should be considered. If a persistent, spontaneous, hemoglobin-positive nipple discharge is present, ductography, aspiration cytology, or biopsy is performed.

Specific Histologic Types of Breast Cancer

Table 27–1 lists the histologic types of breast cancer and their incidence. In this section, the usual clinical, imaging, and histologic features of different types of breast carcinoma are presented.

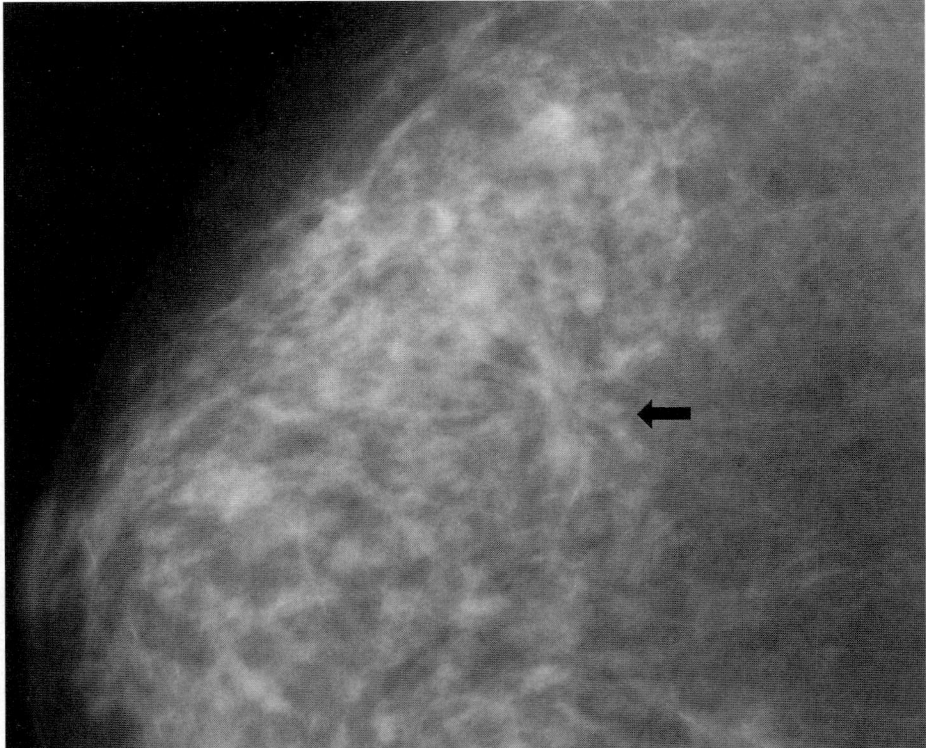

Figure 27–18. Invasive ductal carcinoma, not otherwise specified, signified by architectural distortion (*arrow*) within a dense breast.

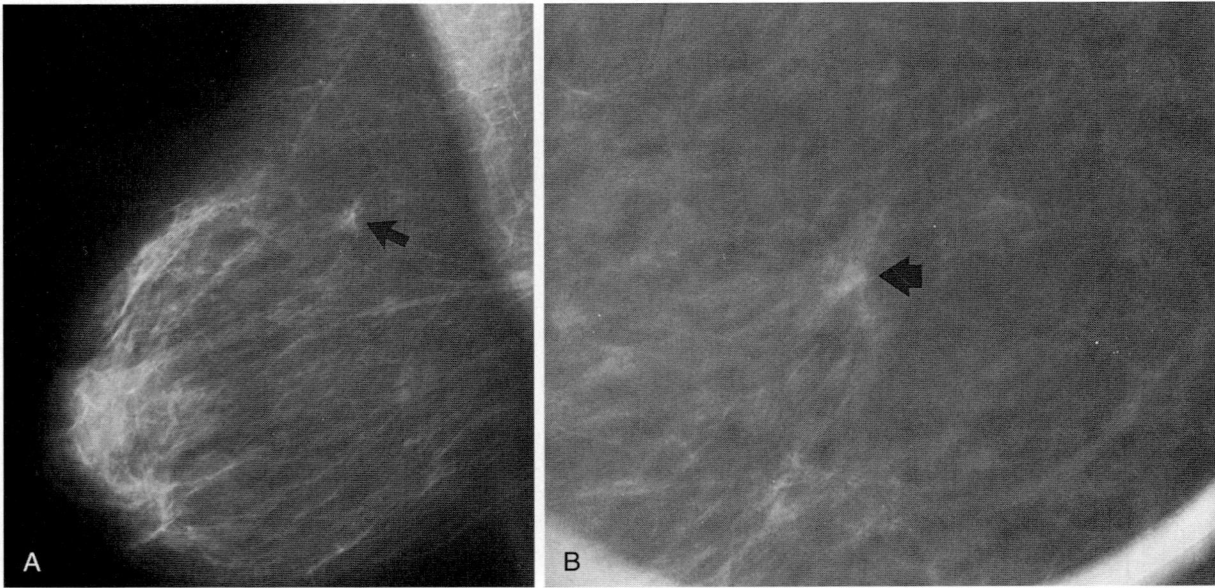

Figure 27–19. Small invasive ductal carcinoma, not otherwise specified, signified by architectural distortion. **A,** Mediolateral oblique mammogram shows an architectural distortion 8 mm in diameter (*arrow*). **B,** Close-up of spot compression view over the area of concern confirms the architectural distortion (*arrow*).

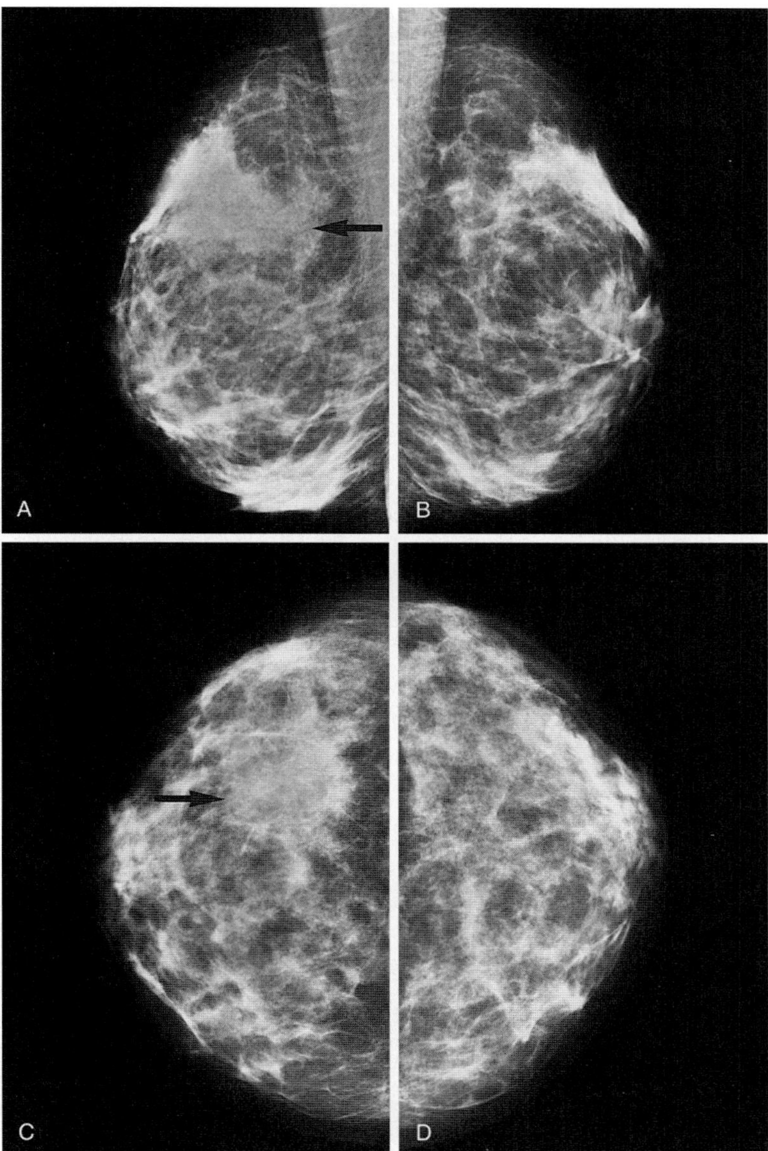

Figure 27–20. Invasive ductal carcinoma, not otherwise specified, signified by asymmetrical breast tissue. Right (**A**) and left (**B**) mediolateral oblique views show asymmetry with increased breast tissue (*arrow*) in the upper hemisphere. **C** and **D,** The asymmetrical tissue (*arrow*) is confirmed on the craniocaudal views. A clinical breast examination was performed after the mammogram demonstrated discrete "thickening" in the right upper outer quadrant. A biopsy showed invasive carcinoma.

Table 27–1. Types of Breast Carcinoma and Their Incidence*

Histologic Type	Incidence (%)
Infiltrating ductal carcinoma (NOS)	52.6
Mixed types that include NOS	28.0
Medullary	6.2
Lobular invasive	4.9
Mucinous	2.4
Paget's disease	2.3
Mixed types that do not include NOS tumors	1.6
Tubular	1.2
Adenocystic carcinoma	0.4
Papillary	0.3
Carcinosarcoma	0.1

NOS, not otherwise specified
*From 1000 reported cases.
Adapted from Fisher ER, Gregorio RM, Fisher B, et al: The pathology of invasive breast cancer: A syllabus derived from findings of the National Surgical Adjuvant Breast Project (Protocol No. 4). Cancer 1975;36:1-85.

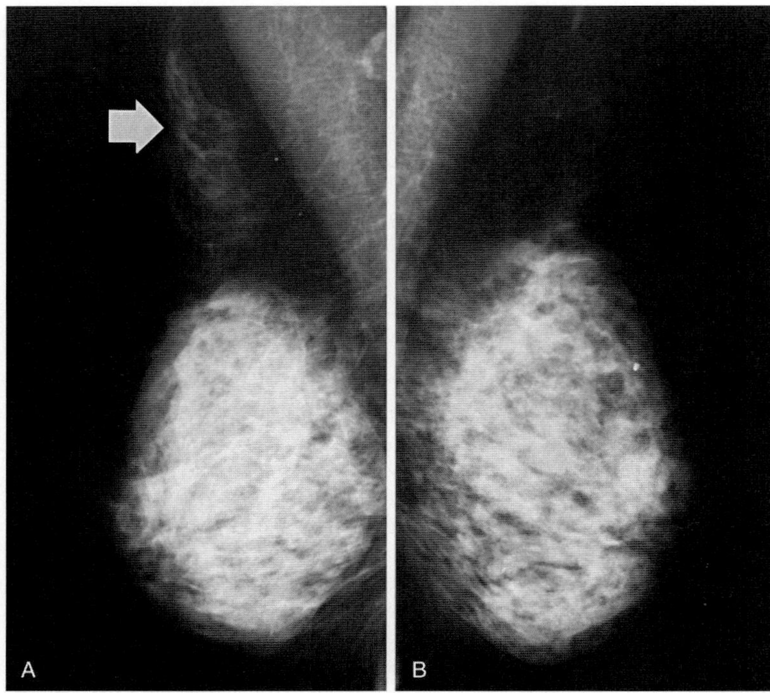

Figure 27–21. Asymmetrical breast tissue in axilla. Right (**A**) and left (**B**) mediolateral oblique views show an area of asymmetrical density (*arrow*) in the right axilla. This asymmetrical tissue is a normal variant.

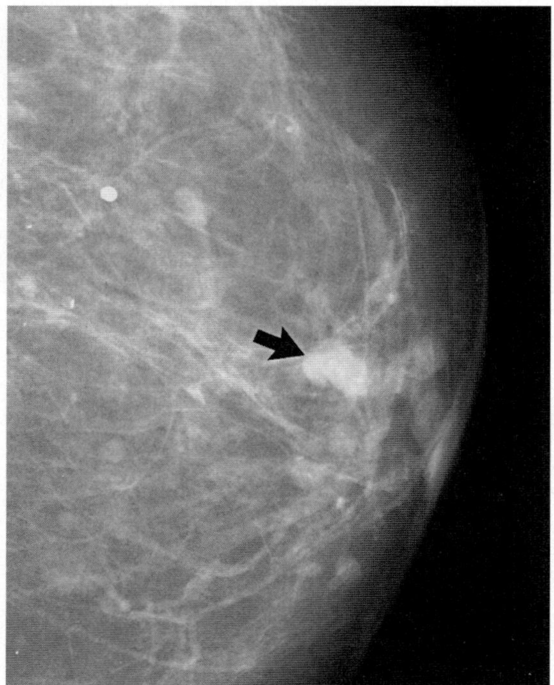

Figure 27–22. Invasive ductal carcinoma manifesting as a unilateral, solitary, dilated duct. The dilated subareolar duct (*arrow*) was tortuous and not related to nipple discharge. (Courtesy of R.J. Brenner, Los Angeles, CA.)

Invasive Ductal Carcinoma, Not Otherwise Specified

Synonyms for NOS invasive ductal carcinoma are NOS adenocarcinoma; ductal carcinoma of no special type (NST), usual or common ductal carcinoma, and scirrhous carcinoma. The NOS classification comprises a heterogeneous group of tumors. The gross feature is a poorly marginated mass that is typically hard on palpation, leading to the designation *scirrhous* (of a hard, fibrous consistency). Although less ominous histologic types may coexist with it, the prognosis is predicated on the presence of the NOS type.[26] Axillary nodal status, tumor size, and histologic differentiation as well as a variety of new tests are used to determine the prognosis in an individual case.[27,28]

Clinical Aspects

If palpable, the tumor often is solitary, stony hard, and fixed to surrounding tissues. When involvement of the skin occurs with redness and heat, inflammatory carcinoma is clinically diagnosed and may be confirmed by a biopsy showing tumor cells in the dermal lymphatics.

Imaging Features

As stated earlier, the NOS type of invasive breast cancer is characteristically irregular in shape with spiculated or ill-defined margins (see Figs. 27–1 and 27–2). It can be associated with calcifications, either within or adjacent to the tumor (see Figs. 27–5 and 27–6). The NOS type of ductal carcinoma may be associated with secondary signs, such as skin thickening and retraction (see Figs 27–9 and 27–10). However, it may also manifest as a relatively circumscribed mass (see Fig. 27–3). In fact, because of its frequency, the usual ductal type of carcinoma (NOS) makes up the majority of carcinomas that have "circumscribed" margins.

Pathology

After exclusion of special types of invasive breast carcinoma, the remaining lesions fall into the category of NOS type, which constitutes 50% to 75% of all invasive carcinomas. Within this group, about one third have pushing, smooth borders on low-power examination (Fig. 27–23). The remaining two thirds have infiltrative, irregular margins with malignant cells invading into the adjacent breast and fibroadipose tissue in a radiating pattern (see Fig. 27–23B), corresponding to the spiculated lesion seen on gross examination and mammographic images.

Under microscopic examination, the tumor cells form various structures, such as tubules, cribriform glands, papillae, irregular glands, cords, nests, and solid sheets (Fig. 27–24). These structures are often intermixed within a given tumor, although a particular pattern may predominate. The *nuclear grade* refers to the uniformity or variation of nuclear size, shape, and chromatinic aggregates; nucleoli; and mitotic activity. In general, a good correlation exists between the architecture and the nuclear features. Well-differentiated tumors with predominantly tubules, papillae, and glands tend to have uniformly small nuclei, fine chromatin, inconspicuous nucleoli, and low mitotic activity, whereas poorly differentiated tumors have mostly nests and sheets present with large, irregular nuclei, coarse chromatin, prominent nucleoli, and high mitotic activity (see Fig. 27–24A and D). The grading system using the modified Bloom-Richardson method—which is based on the percentage of tubular formation, the extent of nuclear variation, and mitotic activity—provides a reproducible approach that has prognostic significance (see Table 23–1).[29]

In response to tumor cell invasion, the fibrous stroma undergoes desmoplastic reaction with proliferation of newly formed fibroblasts in an edematous, myxomatous, or highly collagenized matrix (Fig. 27–25A). In the background, elastosis also occurs. The number of lymphocytes, plasma cells, and histiocytes is usually limited, although they can be abundant in about 20% of tumors (see Fig. 27–25B). The majority of lymphocytes are T lymphocytes, mainly T4 helper cells and T8 cytotoxic suppressor cells.[30]

The tumor cells may also gain access to the lymphatic capillary spaces (Fig. 27–26A). This finding is associated with adverse prognosis. However, tissue shrinkage due to fixation and processing can lead to a false impression of vascular lymphatic spaces filled with tumor cells. Therefore, one must clearly identify lining endothelial cells before concluding that the spaces are really of lymphatic vascular origin. Less commonly, tumor cells invade the blood vessels (see Fig. 27–26B) and perineural spaces. Studies have demonstrated a higher death rate in patients who have tumor invasion of the lymphatics, capillaries, and blood vessels with or without lymph node metastases than in patients with a similar stage of tumor without vascular space invasion.[31-33] Perineural space invasion does not have prognostic significance by itself. Dermal lymphatic space invasion is the hallmark of inflammatory breast carcinoma (see Fig. 27–26C).

About 20% to 30% of the NOS carcinomas have minor components of other histologic types, such as mucinous, tubular, and infiltrating lobular carcinomas. The prognosis of such "mixed" carcinomas depends on the predominant histologic elements. The term *infiltrating ductal carcinoma with extensive intraductal component* applies when histologic examination shows that intraductal carcinoma accounts for more than 25% of the tumor. The latter

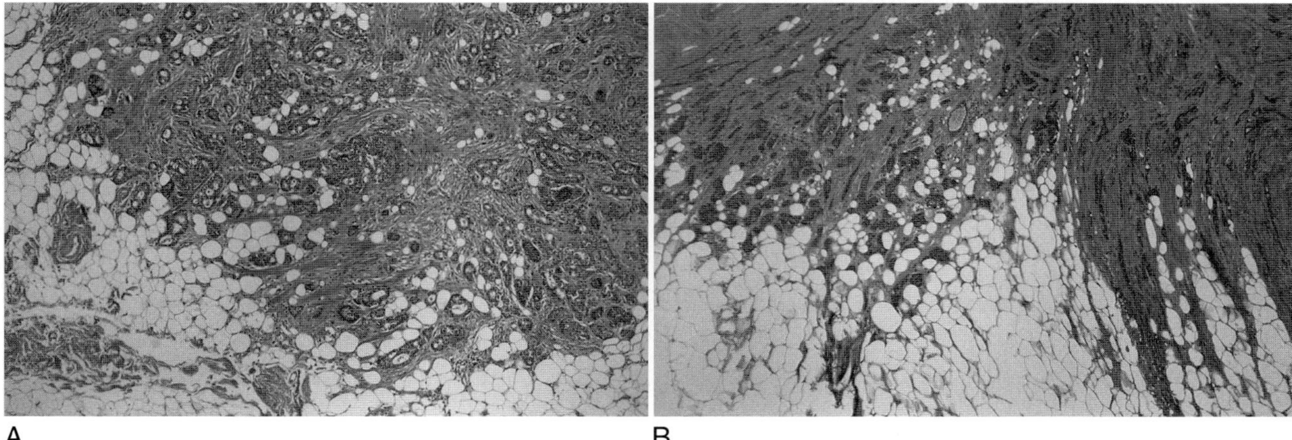

Figure 27–23. Borders of an infiltrating ductal carcinoma, not otherwise specified. **A,** Relatively smooth borders. **B,** Multiple irregular infiltrations into the adjacent adipose tissue.

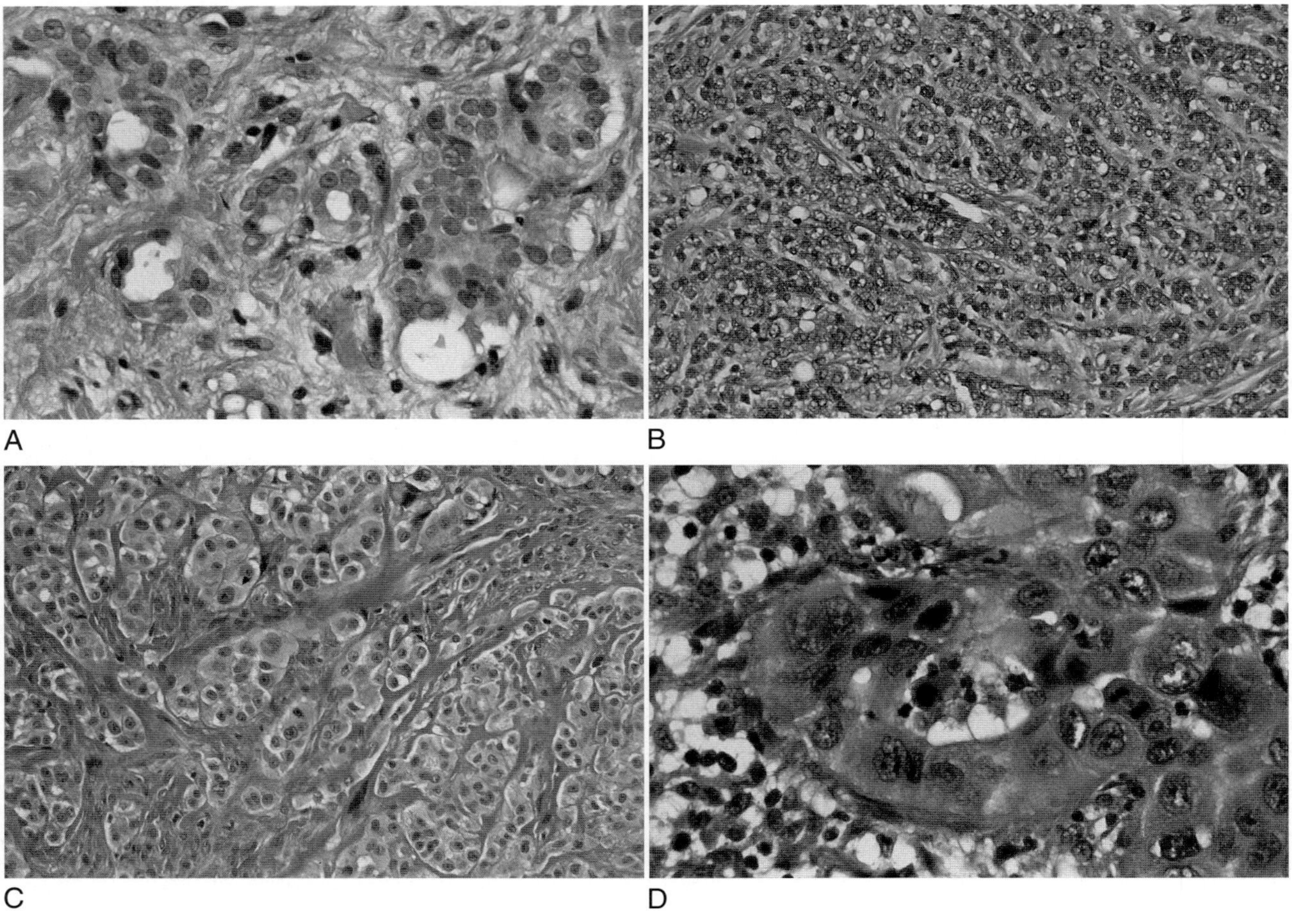

Figure 27–24. Growth patterns of infiltrating ductal carcinoma, not otherwise specified. **A,** Tubular glands. Tumor cells have uniformly round to oval nuclei and indistinct nucleoli. **B,** Cords. **C,** Solid nests. **D,** Large sheets. Tumor cells have pleomorphic nuclei and prominent nucleoli.

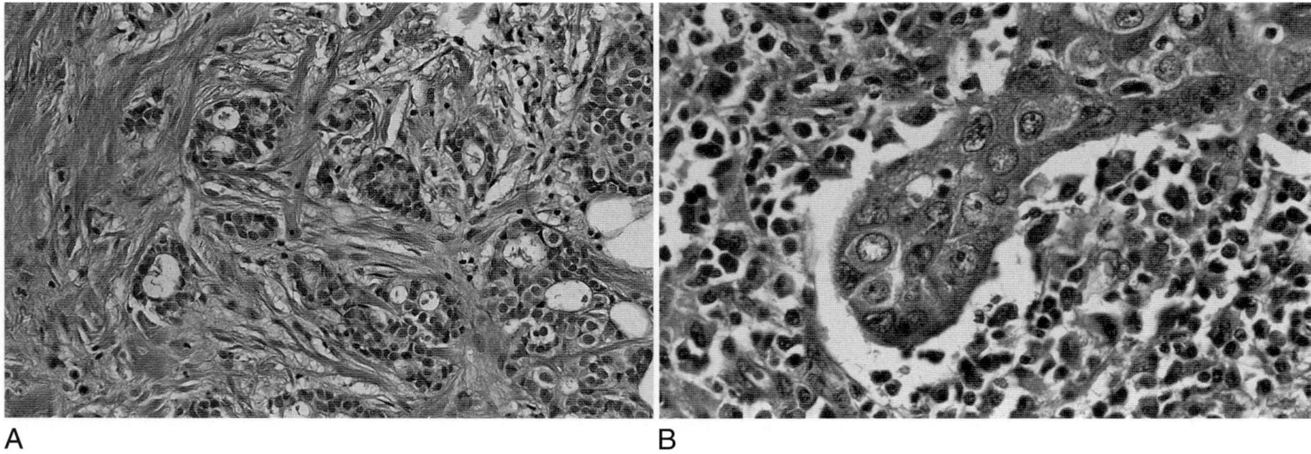

Figure 27–25. Ductal carcinoma, not otherwise specified. **A,** Desmoplastic stromal reaction with collagenous stroma. **B,** Abundant lymphocytes, plasma cells, and eosinophils in the stroma.

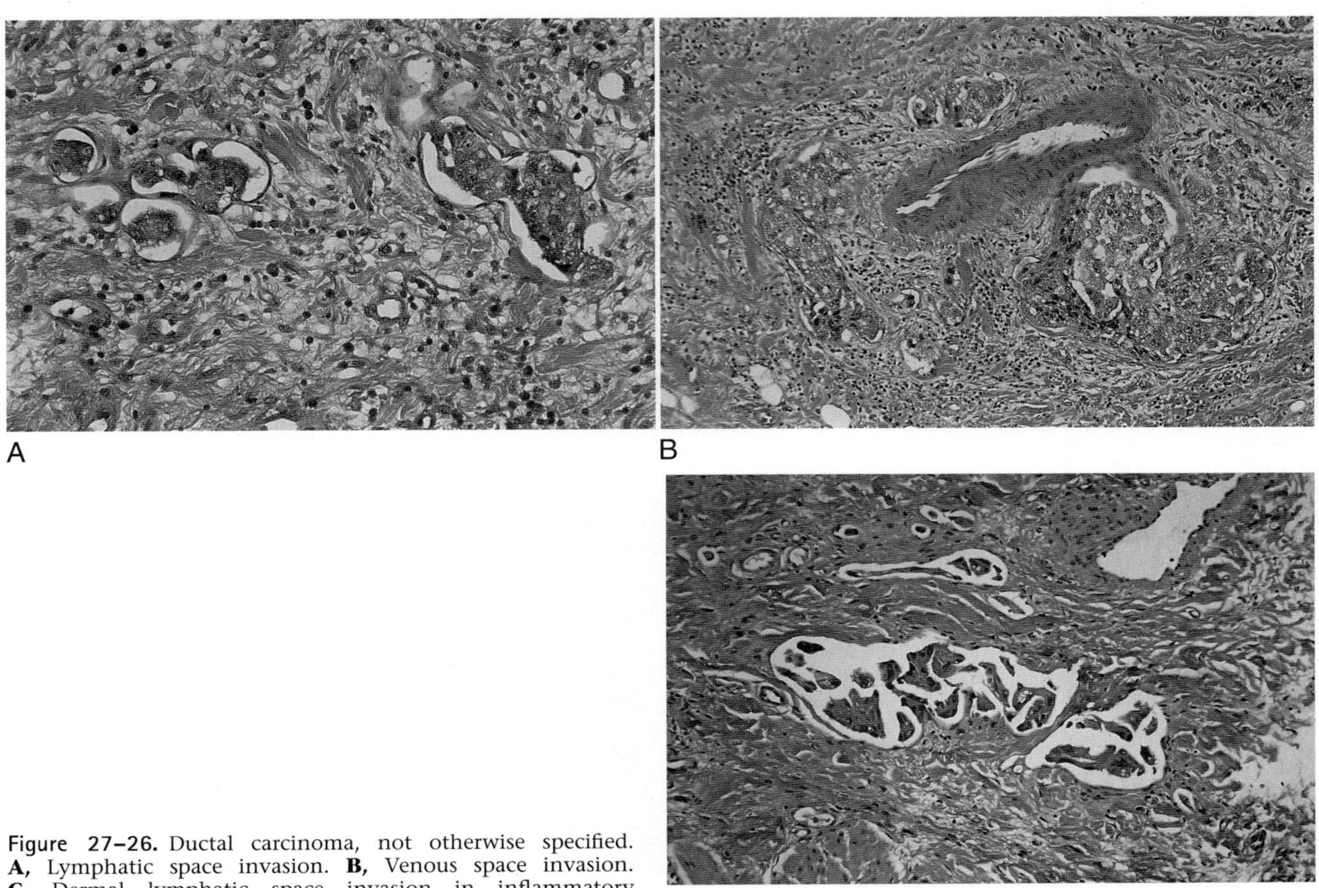

Figure 27–26. Ductal carcinoma, not otherwise specified. **A,** Lymphatic space invasion. **B,** Venous space invasion. **C,** Dermal lymphatic space invasion in inflammatory carcinoma.

designation is important because of its greater risk for local recurrence.[34]

Microinvasive Carcinoma ($T1_{mic}$)

With the use of mammographic screening, the detection of early invasive carcinoma is expected to increase. Previous reports on the definition of "microinvasive carcinoma" of the breast vary from less than 1 mm[35] to 2 mm.[36] Based on Union Internationale Contre le Cancer (UICC) TNM staging method, microinvasive carcinoma ($T1_{mic}$) is defined as 0.1 cm or less in greatest dimension.[37] Using this definition, Prasad and colleagues[38] reported a series of 21 cases, consisting of 18 ductal carcinomas and 3 lobular carcinomas; the mean age of patients was 60.9 years, and 61% of the lesions were detected on mammographic screening. In this series, microinvasive carcinoma occurred in 5.1% of ductal carcinomas in situ (DCISs) and accounted for 1% of all invasive carcinomas.

At the point of invasion, the tumor cells initially form a tonguelike protrusion and subsequently break through the basement membrane to form isolated single cells and aggregates, which are surrounded by desmoplastic stroma (Fig. 27–27). The number of microinvasive foci per case in the series reported by Prasad and colleagues[38] ranged from 1 to 7 (mean, 2). The invasion most commonly originates from the comedo type of DCIS (72%), and less commonly from solid (1 case) and papillary and micropapillary (2 each) DCIS. The nuclear grade was grade 1 in 1, grade 2 in 1, and grade 3 in 16 (89%). Two (13%) of 15 patients had lymph node metastasis. Two women experienced local recurrences, one a tumor in the chest wall and the other a DCIS.[38]

Invasive Lobular Carcinoma

Invasive lobular carcinoma is often difficult to diagnose on clinical and mammographic grounds. The most common clinical presentation is a focal hard mass fixed to surrounding tissues, but frequently, lobular carcinoma is diffusely infiltrating and does not manifest as a discrete palpable mass. It has been suggested that the elusive nature of the tumor may be due to its failure to elicit a desmoplastic reaction.[39] Lobular carcinomas have also been reported as difficult to diagnose with fine-needle aspiration cytology. Invasive lobular carcinoma also has a higher rate of multicentricity and bilaterality than the NOS type of ductal carcinoma. Despite these characteristics, the

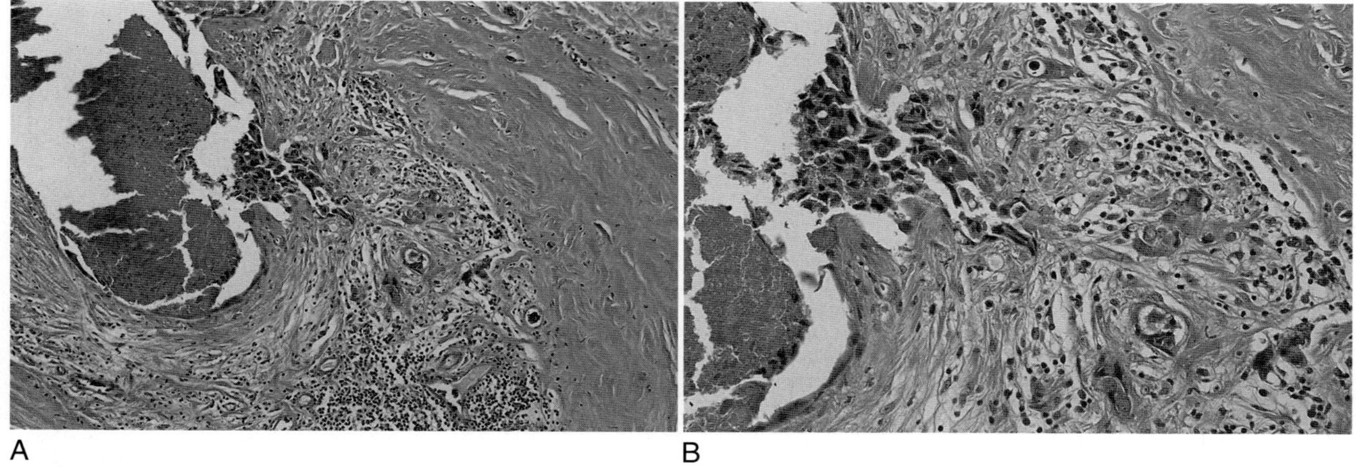

Figure 27–27. Microinvasive ductal carcinoma. **A,** Early stromal invasion arising from the periphery of comedo ductal carcinoma in situ presents as tonguelike protrusion measuring less than 1 mm in size. **B,** Higher magnification to reveal breakthrough of basement membrane and nests of tumor cells with nuclear pleomorphism.

overall survival with invasive lobular carcinoma, when detected at the same size and stage, is believed to be slightly better than that with the NOS invasive ductal type.[39,40]

Imaging Features

In the majority of cases, invasive lobular carcinoma can be seen on mammograms.[41,42] The most common presentations of invasive lobular carcinoma are a spiculated mass, an ill-defined or obscured mass, and architectural distortion (Fig. 27–28).[41,42] However, many invasive lobular carcinomas are diffusely infiltrating and may show only subtle findings or changes on mammography. In the dense breast, these tumors may be completely unrecognizable, even when they are large. As a result, invasive lobular carcinomas are considered among the most difficult cancers to detect with mammography.[43,44] Owing to the failure of mammography to depict some invasive lobular carcinomas, combining mammography with CBE as well as ultrasonography, magnetic resonance imaging (MRI), and core needle biopsy will improve the detection of these cancer.

Several explanations exist for the difficulty in diagnosis of many invasive lobular carcinomas. In addition to their diffuse infiltration, it has been observed that invasive lobular carcinomas frequently have a radiographic density equal to or lower than that of normal parenchyma.[45] In addition, associated calcifications are seen in only 20% of invasive lobular carcinomas.[43,45] However, combining mammography with ultrasonography is extremely useful in suspected cases of underlying lobular carcinomas. Ultrasonography often reveals a hypoechoic or heterogenic, irregular, solid mass.[46]

Up to a third of invasive lobular carcinomas are bilateral (Fig. 27–29).[40,43] Therefore, special attention should be paid to the contralateral breast when invasive lobular carcinoma is diagnosed. Magnetic resonance imaging also has a role in guiding treatment for infiltrating lobular carcinoma as well as in delineating the true extent of disease. Those that manifest as architectural distortion, asymmetrical density, or a normal mammographic appearance are more likely to be associated with residual disease at excision than are those that manifest as a discrete spiculated mass.[48]

Pathology

In the classic type of infiltrating lobular carcinoma, the tumor cells infiltrate between the collagen bundles in a linear fashion, the single-file pattern (Fig. 27–30A). When the tumor cells invade the wall of duct, a tagetoid pattern results (see Fig. 27–30B). Individual cells have small to medium-sized, uniformly round to oval nuclei, scant cytoplasm, inconspicuous nucleoli, and low mitotic activity (see Fig. 27–30C). Sometimes the tumor cells appear so benign as to simulate mature lymphocytes. Irregularly shaped nests and sheets of cells may also occur intermixed with the single-file pattern. Another distinct feature is the presence of signet-ring cells and cells with intracytoplasmic lumens (see Fig. 27–30D).

Several variants of infiltrating lobular carcinoma have been recognized. In the solid type, the tumor cells appear in diffuse sheets with little intervening stroma, simulating malignant lymphoma or leukemic infiltration. In the alveolar variant, loosely cohesive tumor cells form discrete aggregates and are surrounded by fibrous stroma. A tubulolobular variant consists of small tubules and rosettes. Finally, a pleomorphic variant is made up of cells with medium to large, irregular, hyperchromatic nuclei and eosinophilic cytoplasm simulating myoblasts.[49-51] Whether tubulolobular and pleomorphic types should be included with the invasive lobular group is a matter of controversy.[52]

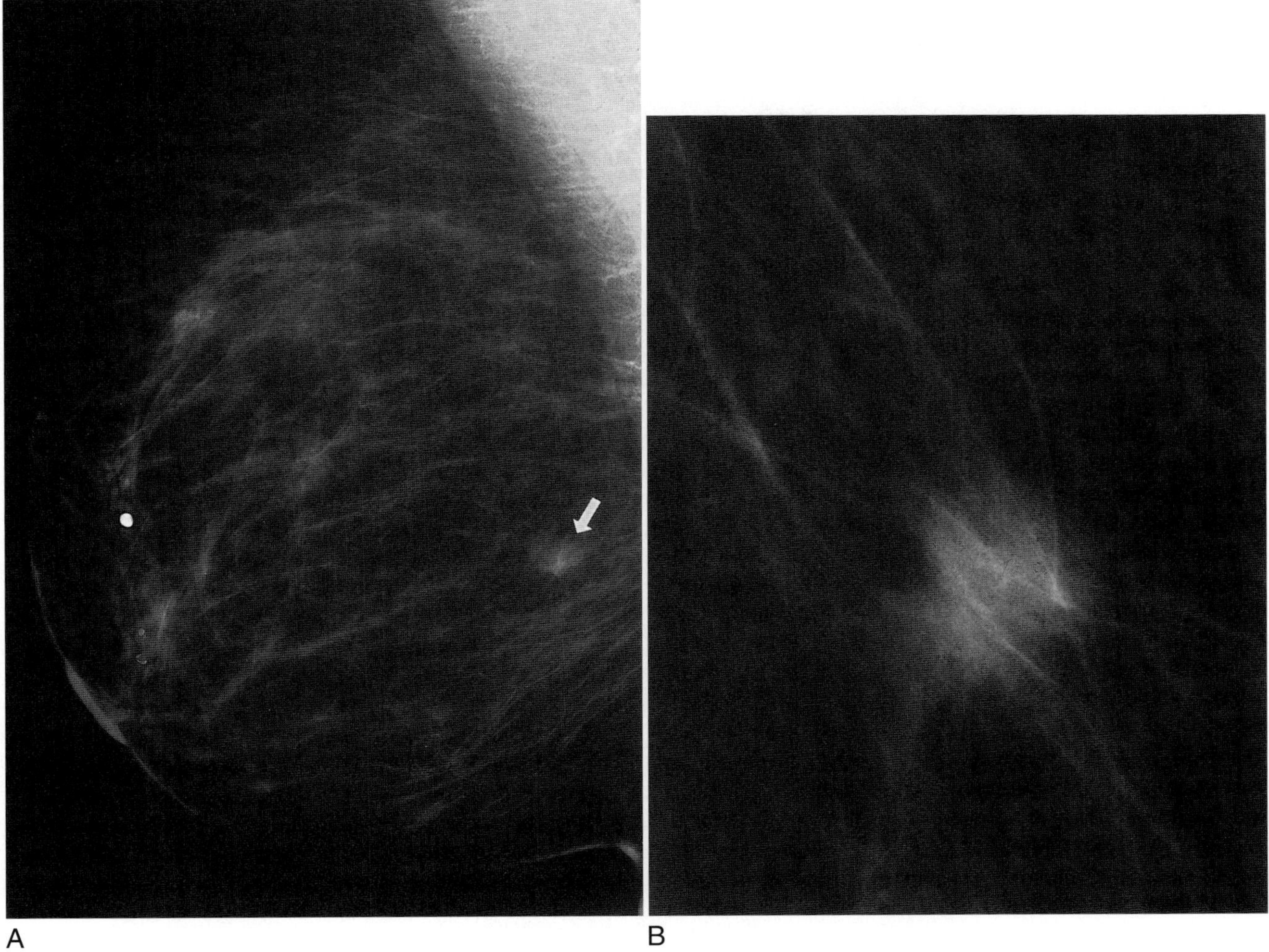

Figure 27–28. Invasive lobular carcinoma. **A,** Right mediolateral view shows a small density (*arrow*). **B,** Magnification view demonstrates persistence of the density with ill-defined margins in the posterior lower-outer quadrant of the right breast.

Medullary Carcinoma

Medullary carcinomas, also called circumscribed carcinomas, make up less than 10% of breast cancers. They can be classified into typical and atypical types.[53,54] Typical medullary carcinomas can present a clinical dilemma. For one thing, the majority of women who have them are younger than 50 years, an age group in whom breast cancer is less likely to be suspected.[55] In addition, the tumor often manifests as a rounded mass unfixed to the adjacent tissues, clinically suggesting a benign mass.

Imaging Features

To radiologists, the typical medullary carcinoma conjures up the mammographic and ultrasonographic image of a carcinoma with round, oval, or lobular shape and circumscribed margins (Figs. 27–31 and 27–32).[56] The typical margins of medullary carcinomas have led to the term *circumscribed carcinoma*.[8] Because of its clinical and radiographic features, medullary carcinoma can be mistaken for a fibroadenoma. Furthermore, the clinical and mammographic features suggesting benignity may explain why medullary carcinomas are relatively large at the time of diagnosis. In the larger medullary carcinomas, ultrasonography may show anechoic areas representing central necrosis. Despite its relatively large size, fast rate of growth, and negative hormone receptor status, the typical medullary carcinoma does have a better prognosis overall than the NOS type.[57] However, atypical medullary carcinoma, which appears radiographically and clinically to be more infiltrative, has a similar prognosis to that of the NOS type. Mammographically visible calcifications are unusual in medullary carcinoma. As with the other types, axillary nodal status is the most important prognostic indicator in an individual case.

Pathology

To be identified as a medullary carcinoma, a tumor should have (1) circumscribed, noninfiltrative

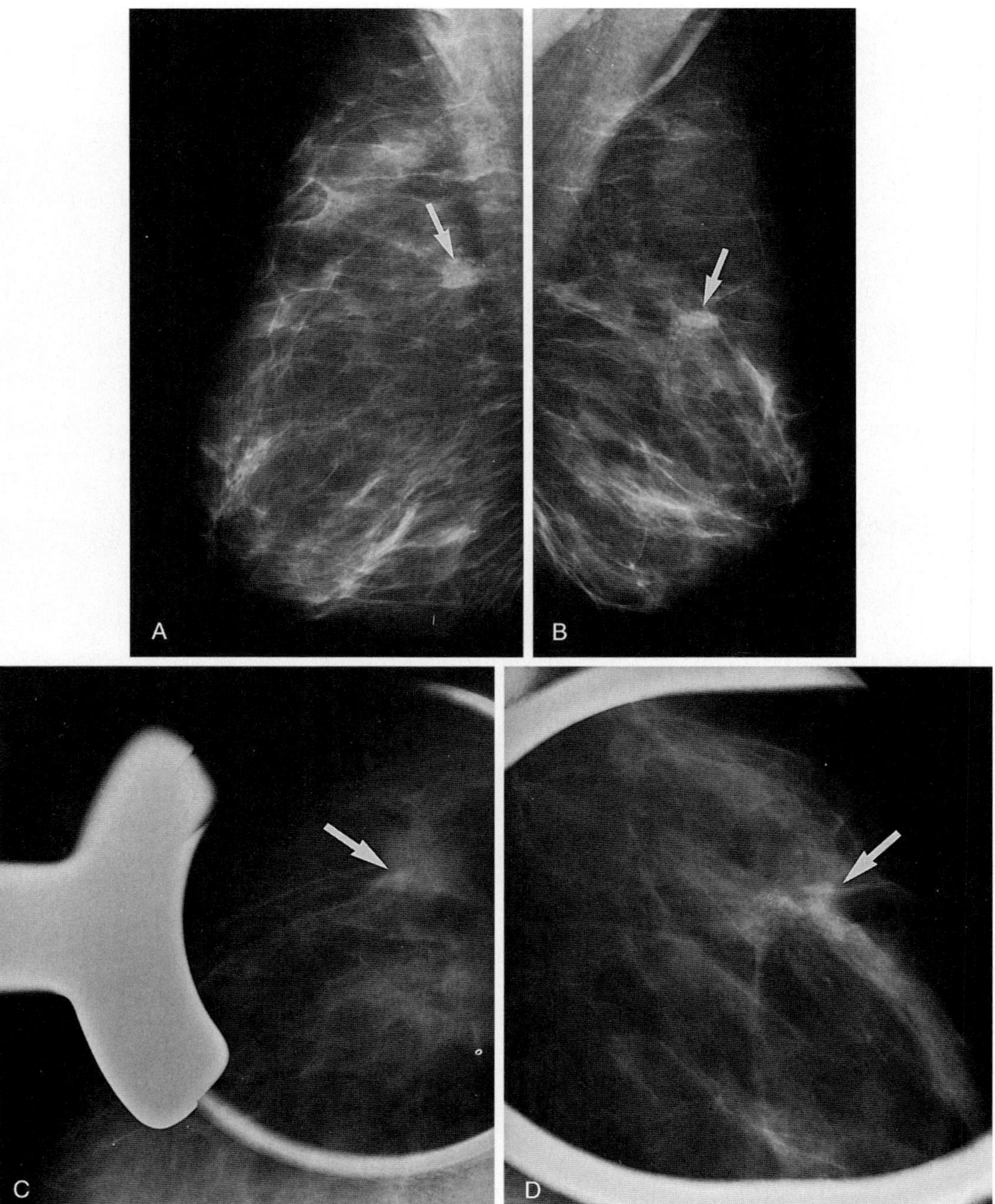

Figure 27–29. Invasive lobular carcinoma. The patient felt a vague "thickening" in the upper-outer quadrant of her right breast. **A,** Right mediolateral oblique (MLO) view shows a spiculated density (*arrow*) at the site of the palpable finding. **B,** Left MLO view also shows a possible abnormality (*arrow*). Right (**C**) and left (**D**) spot compression views in the craniocaudal projection confirm that both lesions (*arrows*) are suspicious. Excisional biopsies demonstrated bilateral invasive lobular carcinoma.

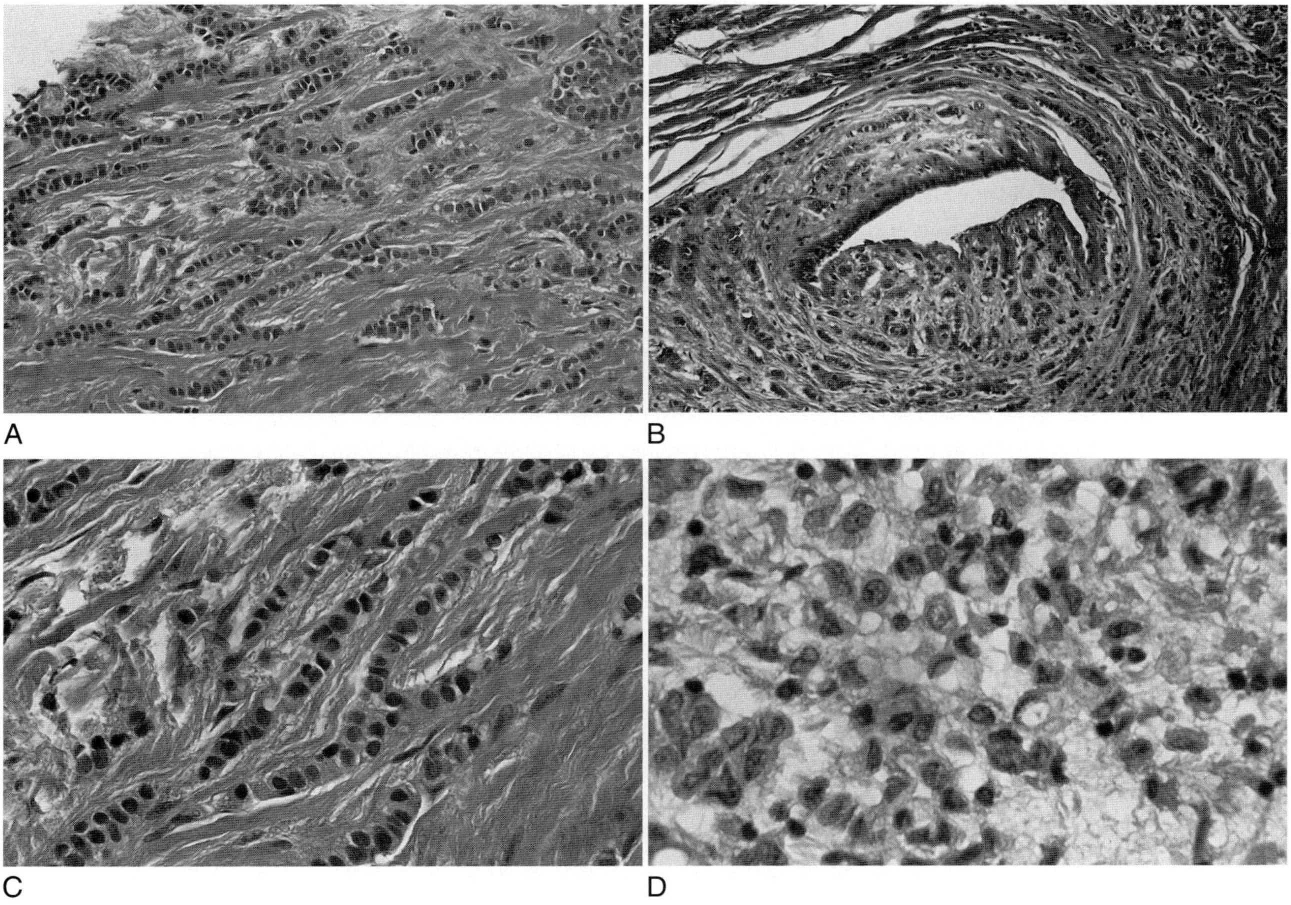

Figure 27–30. Infiltrating lobular carcinoma, classic type. **A,** Tumor cells are arranged in single files. **B,** A tagetoid pattern results from concentric arrangement of tumor cells around a benign duct. **C,** Tumor cells have small to medium-sized uniform nuclei. **D,** Signet-ring tumor cells.

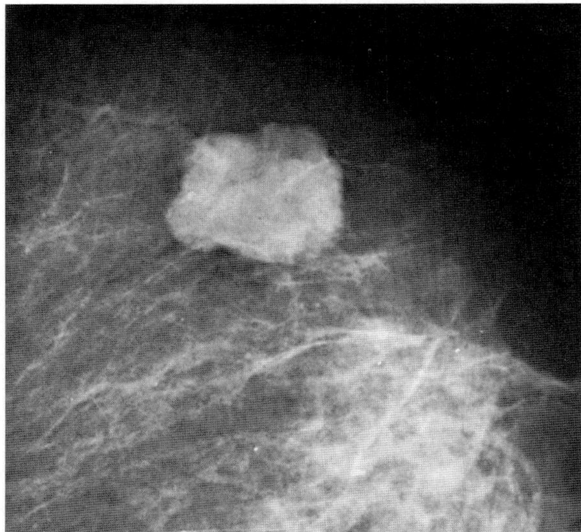

Figure 27–31. Medullary carcinoma, typical features. The patient complained of a palpable mass. Close-up view of tumor shows a lobulated shape and circumscribed margins.

borders; (2) prominent lymphoplasmacytic infiltration present diffusely within the tumor and involving at least 75% of the tumor periphery; and (3) tumor cells arranged in large solid nests and sheets with poorly defined cell borders, the so-called syncytial pattern (Fig. 27–33). Individual cells have large pleomorphic nuclei, prominent nucleoli, and high mitotic activity. They often express p53 but not the HER-2/neu oncogene.[58] The fibrous stroma should be scant. Tumors that have some but not all of these features are classified as atypical medullary carcinomas. A small portion of the tumor may undergo squamous metaplasia or may contain papillary, glandular elements. Typical medullary carcinomas meeting the strict criteria listed previously are associated with better outcome than the NOS type of invasive carcinoma. The prognosis is especially favorable for women whose tumors are smaller than 3 cm with "negative" nodes.[58] The prognosis with typical medullary carcinomas is only slightly better than or about the same as the prognosis with the NOS type.[59]

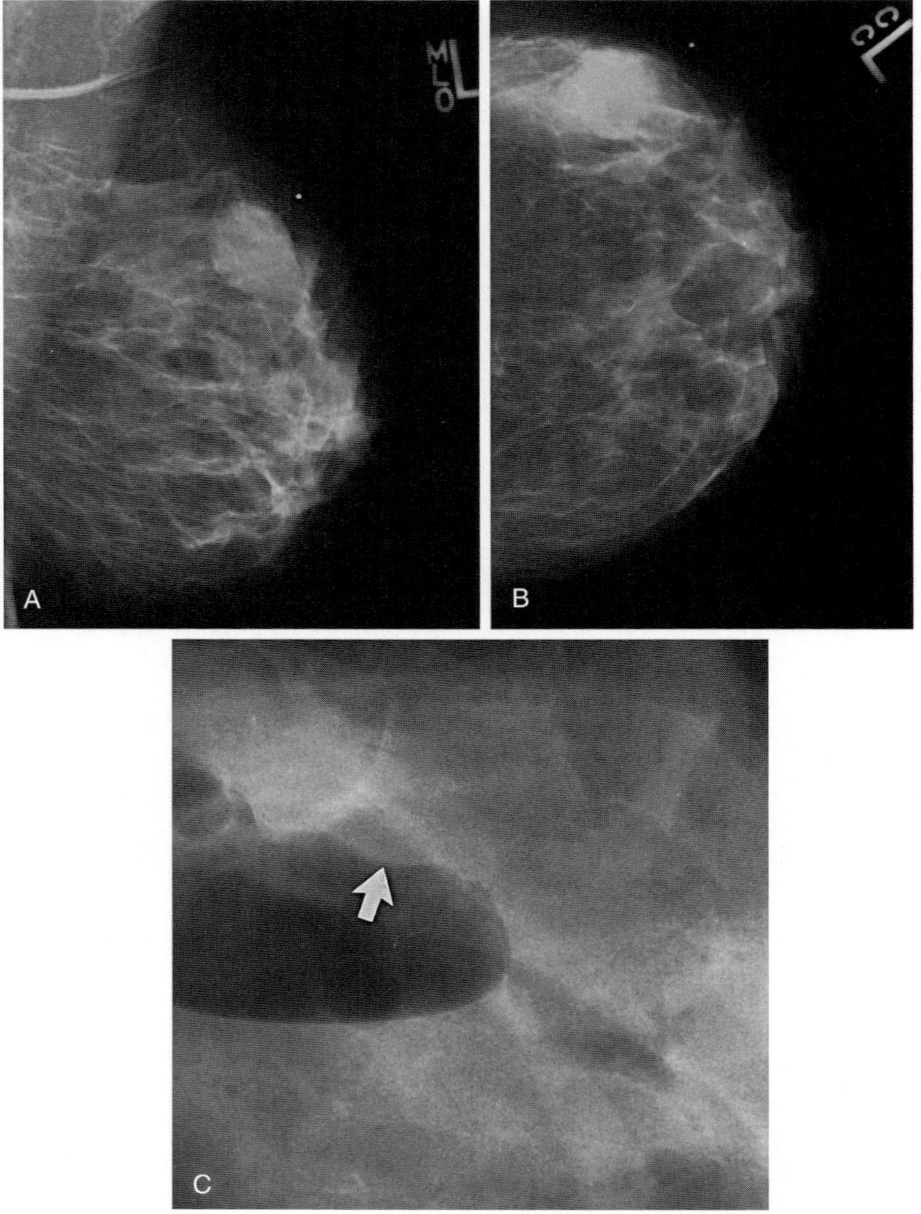

Figure 27–32. Medullary carcinoma. Left mediolateral oblique (**A**) and craniocaudal (**B**) views demonstrate a large, round circumscribed mass in the upper-outer quadrant. **C,** Pneumocystogram shows nodules (*arrow*) in the wall of the fluid-filled mass.

Colloid Carcinoma

Also called mucinous carcinoma and gelatinous carcinoma, colloid carcinoma makes up less than 5% of breast cancers. Colloid carcinoma tends to occur in older women and to grow slowly. It usually has a relatively good prognosis. This type is characterized by tumor cells floating within pools of mucin, so it is a soft mass at palpation. The expanding mass is enclosed by surrounding fibrous tissue, resulting in a circumscribed mass at clinical examination and mammography. However, it should be noted that elements of colloid carcinoma and ductal carcinoma of the NOS type may coexist in the same lesion. This mixed type of colloid carcinoma has a prognosis similar to that of the NOS type.[60]

Imaging Features

Colloid carcinoma characteristically has a spectrum of radiographic features. It may appear to have a round shape and circumscribed margins, suggesting a benign mass (Fig. 27–34). However, close inspection and the use of spot compression magnification films usually show that portions of the margins are indistinct (Fig. 27–35). Colloid carcinoma often has density that is equal to or lower than that of normal fibroglandular breast tissue, a finding that may contribute to a misdiagnosis of a benign mass. Ultrasonography is used to differentiate a circumscribed colloid carcinoma from a cyst (see Fig. 27–35B).

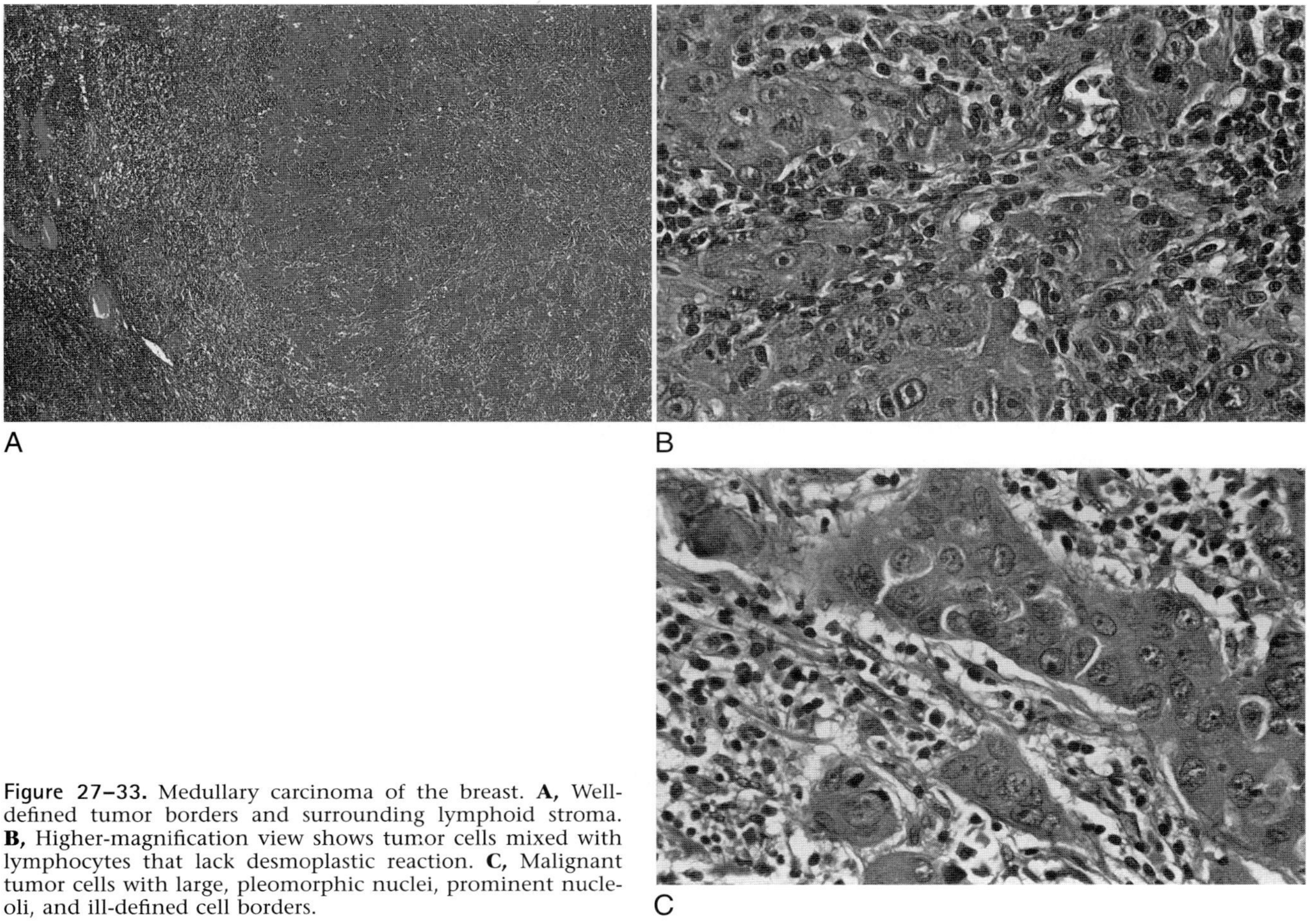

Figure 27–33. Medullary carcinoma of the breast. **A,** Well-defined tumor borders and surrounding lymphoid stroma. **B,** Higher-magnification view shows tumor cells mixed with lymphocytes that lack desmoplastic reaction. **C,** Malignant tumor cells with large, pleomorphic nuclei, prominent nucleoli, and ill-defined cell borders.

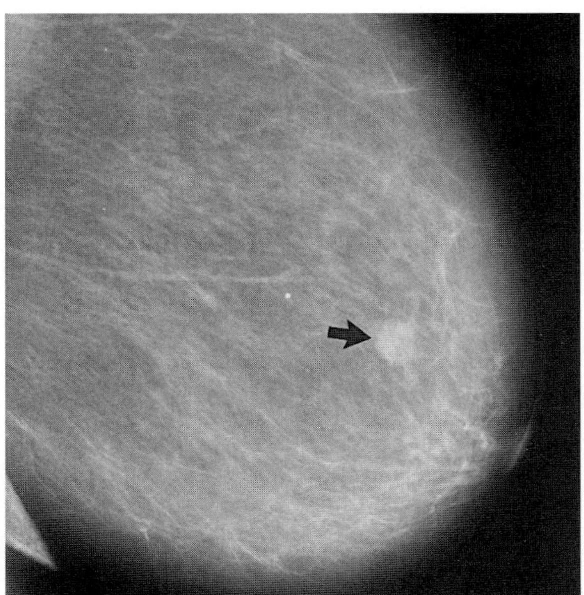

Figure 27–34. Colloid carcinoma. Mediolateral oblique view shows a round, circumscribed, low-density mass (*arrow*) in the subareolar area. Biopsy was performed because the mass was new, solitary, and solid on ultrasonography.

Pathology

Mucinous carcinoma is characterized by abundant extracellular mucin in which tumor cells form papillary clusters, glands, and, occasionally, sheets floating within the mucin (Fig. 27–36A). Individual cells have low-grade nuclear atypia (see Fig. 27–36B). Low-grade DCIS occurs in 75% of cases. For the designation of mucinous carcinoma, some pathologists require that either the entire tumor or at least 75% of it contain mucinous cells. Grossly, mucinous carcinomas often have circumscribed borders, soft consistency, and gelatinous, semitransparent cut surfaces. Because of these characteristics, mucinous carcinomas can be confused with benign tumors, such as fibroadenoma. Tumors having less than 75% mucinous component are classified as mixed carcinomas, which have a less favorable outcome than pure mucinous carcinoma.

An important differential diagnosis is mucocele-like lesions. Mammographically, these lesions have the appearance of well-circumscribed, lobulated nodules. Cysts containing abundant mucin rupture, and the extruded mucin results in fibrosis and histiocytic reaction. Coarse granular calcifications often occur in the cysts or cyst wall. The background pathologic changes are equally divided between benign and malignant diseases, such as ductal

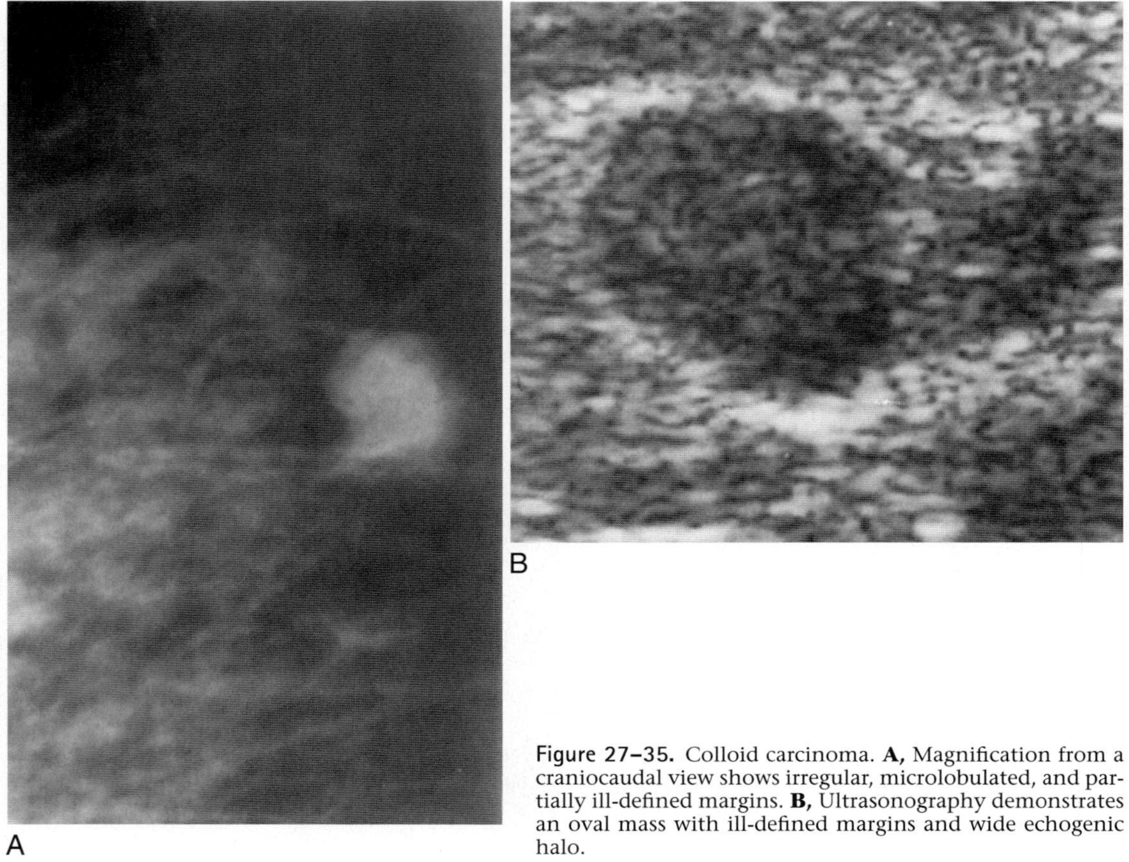

Figure 27–35. Colloid carcinoma. **A,** Magnification from a craniocaudal view shows irregular, microlobulated, and partially ill-defined margins. **B,** Ultrasonography demonstrates an oval mass with ill-defined margins and wide echogenic halo.

hyperplasia, atypical ductal hyperplasia, and in-situ and invasive ductal carcinomas.[61] In the benign mucocele-like lesions, the epithelial cells lining the cystic space do not become detached to form the cellular clusters seen in the mucinous carcinoma.

Tubular Carcinoma

Tubular carcinoma is named for its characteristic histologic tubule formation. It accounts for less than 5% of all invasive breast carcinomas.[62] The tumor is

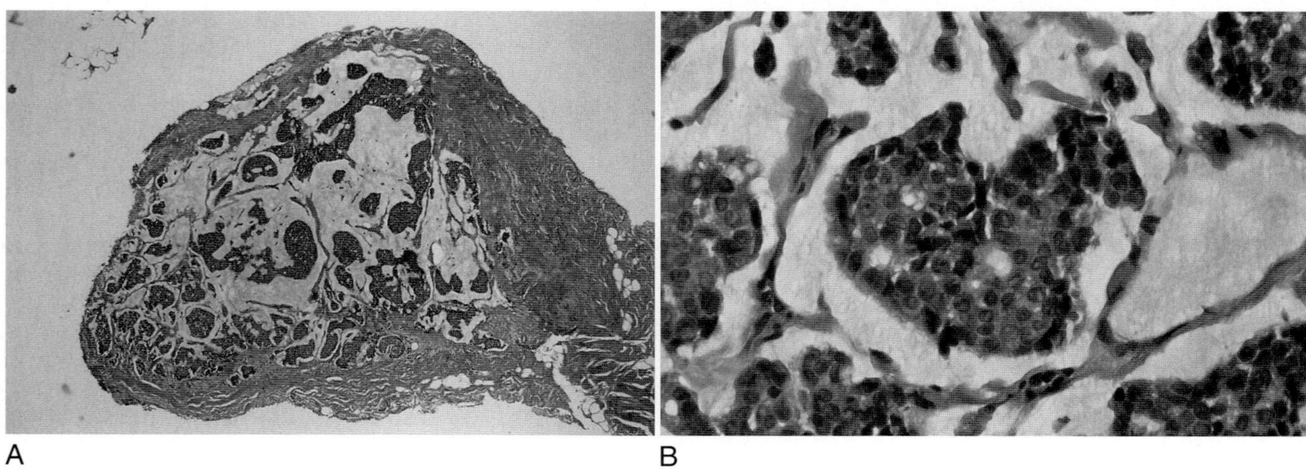

Figure 27–36. Mucinous carcinoma of the breast. **A,** Well-circumscribed smooth borders and abundant mucinous extracellular material. **B,** Nests of tumor cells with uniformly round to oval nuclei, inconspicuous nucleoli, and low mitotic activity.

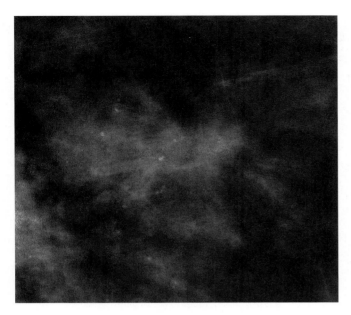

Figure 27–37. Tubular carcinoma. Close-up view shows an irregular mass with spiculated margins.

typically slow growing and small at the time of detection, and it has an excellent prognosis.[63,64] Because of the small size and slow growth, most tubular carcinomas are detected on mammography rather than on palpation. Although the rate of lymph node metastasis is lower than that for the NOS type of carcinoma, lymph node metastases can occasionally occur in tubular carcinoma.[65]

Imaging Features

Reflecting its slow growth, the tumor is usually small at the time it is identified. Because of its irregular shape and spiculated margins, tubular carcinoma is indistinguishable mammographically from invasive ductal carcinoma of the NOS type (Fig. 27–37). Tubular carcinomas do not manifest circumscribed margins.[66] Microcalcifications are reported to be uncommon, occurring in approximately 10% to 15% of cases.[67] Although tubular carcinoma does not have any distinctive radiographic features to differentiate it from the NOS type of carcinoma, tubular carcinoma should be suspected when a spiculated mass is noted retrospectively to be growing very slowly on serial examinations.

Pathology

Tubular carcinoma represents a highly differentiated form of infiltrating ductal carcinoma, usually less than 2 cm in dimension. The tumor cells form regular or sometimes angulated tubular glands surrounded by desmoplastic stroma and elastosis. Infiltration into the adjacent fat, when present, is a useful diagnostic feature (Fig. 27–38A). These glands are lined by a single layer of cells (see Fig. 27–38B) with minor nuclear atypia. Apocrine differentiation is commonly observed. In two thirds of the cases, noncomedo ductal carcinoma in situ is present. Some pathologists reserve the designation of "pure" tubular carcinoma for those in which 100% of the tumor is tubular,[50] whereas others require only 75% tubules.[52] If the tubular component is less than 75%, the tumor is classified as a mixed tubular carcinoma or ductal carcinoma with tubular features.[50] As might be expected, the pure type of tubular carcinoma has lower rates of lymph node metastasis and of recurrence after removal than the mixed type.[67,68]

Tubular carcinomas in core biopsy specimens can be difficult to distinguish from proliferating benign lesions such as sclerosing adenosis. However, tubular carcinomas can usually be distinguished by the following features: a single layer of cells lining the tubules, loss of lobular architecture, and local infiltration of surrounding tissues. A lack of myoepithelial cells can be confirmed by immunohistochemical staining for smooth muscle actin or S-100 protein.

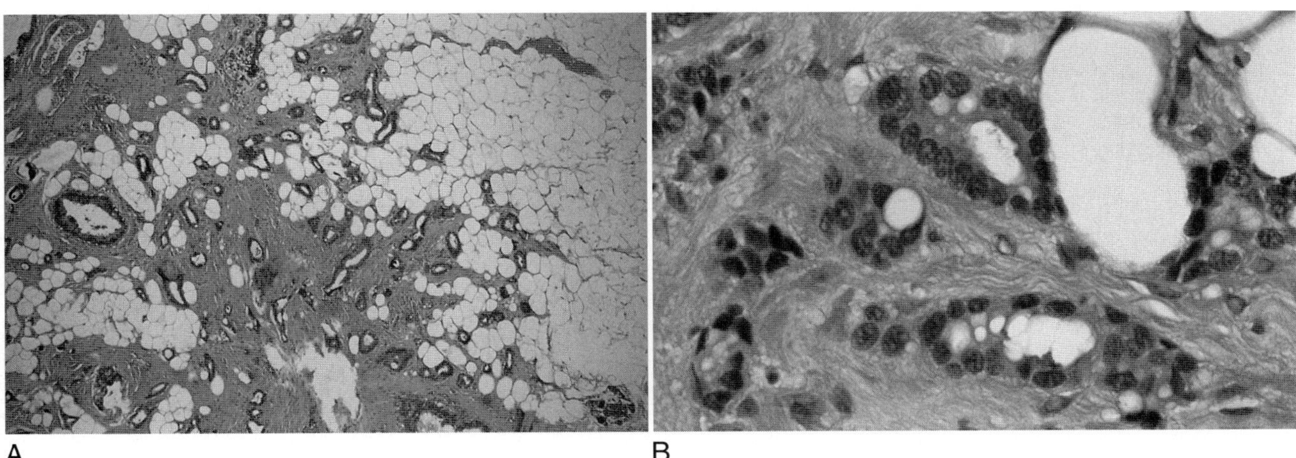

Figure 27–38. Tubular carcinoma of breast. **A,** Irregular neoplastic glands infiltrate into the adjacent adipose tissue. Notice the lack of lobular pattern. **B,** Neoplastic glands are lined by a layer of columnar to cuboidal cells with mild nuclear atypia, small nucleoli, and eosinophilic cytoplasm.

Sclerosing adenosis is characterized by glands with double cell layers consisting of epithelial and myoepithelial cells, and more important, sclerosing adenosis has a lobular pattern on low-power magnification. To avoid confusing these two lesions, the pathologist should follow the basic rule of requiring the presence of both local infiltration and nuclear abnormalities before designating a lesion as malignant.

Tubular carcinoma can also be confused with radial scar in which distorted ducts are surrounded by fibrosis and elastosis. Nevertheless, the ducts in radial scars have a lining of two cell layers, consisting of epithelial and myoepithelial cells, in contrast to the single–cell layer lining in tubular carcinoma.

Invasive Papillary Carcinoma

Invasive papillary carcinoma is a rare cancer with a relatively good prognosis. Lymph node metastases occur in slightly more than 30% of cases of invasive papillary carcinoma that undergo nodal dissection.[69] The tumor may have several mammographic manifestations, but a circumscribed mass is the most common (Fig. 27–39). Histologically, this tumor should be differentiated from noninvasive papillary carcinoma.

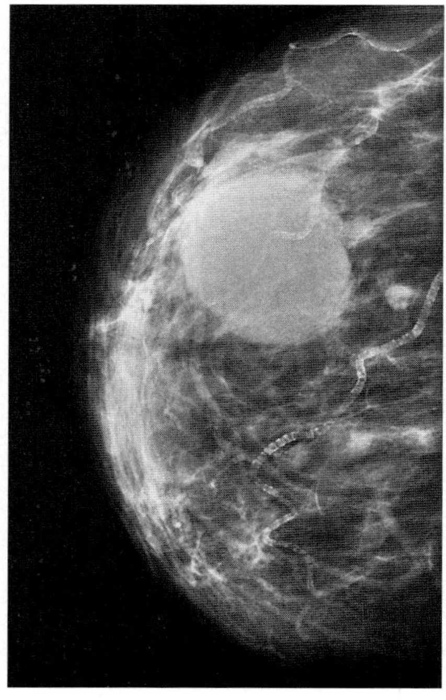

Figure 27–39. Invasive papillary carcinoma. The large tumor is predominantly circumscribed.

Pathology

Papillary carcinoma usually occurs in the central portion of the breast as a round, 2- to 3-cm nodule with areas of cystic change and hemorrhage. The diagnosis of papillary carcinoma is based on the presence of complex papillary projections and cribriform glands consisting almost entirely of epithelial cells (Fig. 27–40A). Individual cells have oval to elongated, hyperchromatic nuclei with mild irregularity in size and shape (see Fig. 27–40B). Nucleoli are generally small and inconspicuous. Mitotic activity is variable. Myoepithelial cells are few in number or are completely absent. In the solid variant, tumor cells proliferate in diffuse sheets with sclerotic vascular stalks in the background to indicate a papillary growth. The distinction between intraductal and invasive papillary carcinoma can be difficult because of the common occurrence of stromal fibrosis, hemorrhage, and chronic inflammation. The best evidence of invasion is the presence of irregular aggregates of papillae and glands involving the adjacent breast and fibroadipose tissue with an associated desmoplastic reaction. The prognosis of patients with papillary carcinoma is excellent, with a low frequency of lymph node metastasis and tumor recurrence.[70]

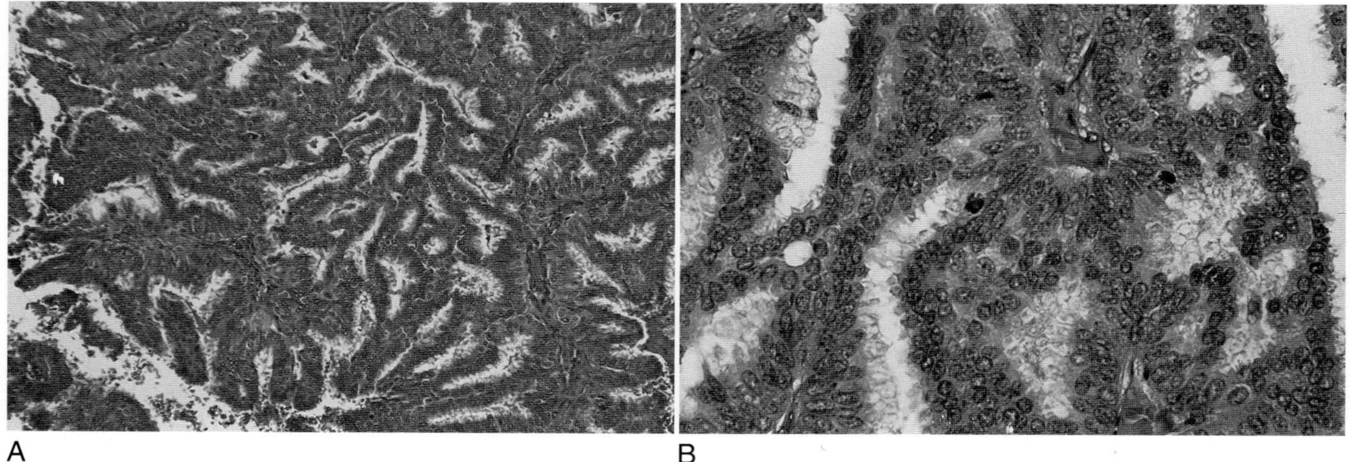

Figure 27–40. Papillary carcinoma. **A,** Complex papillary projections, some of which have fibrovascular cores. **B,** Tumor cells with uniform nuclei and multiple mitotic figures.

More recently, a micropapillary variant of papillary carcinoma was reported. The mean age of patients was 50 to 59 years.[71,72] The histologic features were characterized by invasive papillary aggregates surrounded by clear empty spaces without desmoplastic stroma. Many of the papillae did not have fibrovascular cores. The histologic grade determined by modified Bloom-Richardson method was 2 or 3.[71,72] Other findings were psammoma bodies in 64%, lymphatic invasion in 71%, and p53 expression in 75% of tumors.[71] In the series reported by Walsh and Bleiweiss,[72] 72.3% of patients had lymph node metastasis, including tumors smaller than 5 mm. An aggressive behavior was also indicated by the development of local recurrence in the skin and chest wall in 9 (82%) of 11 women.[71]

Rare Variants of Invasive Carcinoma

Rare variants of invasive carcinoma include metaplastic carcinoma, adenoid cystic carcinoma, and small cell carcinoma. In metaplastic carcinoma, poorly differentiated ductal carcinoma contains malignant squamous cells, bone, cartilage, or spindle cells that simulate sarcoma. Adenoid cystic carcinoma is indistinguishable from that seen in the salivary gland, rarely occurs in the breast, and has an excellent prognosis. In a series of 31 patients with adenoid cystic carcinoma, one woman experienced local recurrence 6 years after lumpectomy. All patients were alive and well, and none had experienced lymph node metastasis after lumpectomy or mastectomy.[73]

Small cell carcinoma similar to that of the lung rarely involves the breast. A series of nine women reported as having small cell carcinoma ranged from 43 to 70 years. The tumors varied from 1.3 to 5.0 (mean 2.6) cm in size; 67% of tumors expressed neuroendocrine markers, such as chromogranin, synaptophysin, or peptide hormones. Lymph node metastasis occurred in four of eight women undergoing lymph node dissection. All women lived for 3 to 35 months after diagnosis, including two (22%) patients with metastases. The prognosis, although poor, appears to be better than with similar tumors of the lung.[74]

Multifocal and Multicentric Carcinoma

We are using the term *multifocal* to refer to two or more foci of breast cancer in the same quadrant of the breast, and the term *multicentric* to refer to two or more foci of carcinoma in different quadrants. Lesions in the subareolar area can be evaluated as a separate unit or placed in whatever quadrant is closest. The importance of the clarification of these terms lies in their implications for treatment and prognosis.[75] One study of more than 650 mastectomy specimens found that 90% of secondary foci were in close proximity to the primary.[76] This finding suggests that most secondary foci represent spread from one primary rather than multicentric origin. Multifocal lesions are usually amenable to breast conservation treatment, whereas multicentric lesions are usually treated with mastectomy. Multicentricity increases the likelihood of recurrence after breast-conserving therapy. The incidence of multicentric *invasive* cancer (Fig. 27–41) in the same breast is low, and multicentric carcinoma involves a combination of an invasive breast cancer and a noninvasive carcinoma (Fig. 27–42).

The exact incidence of multifocal carcinoma is not known. It has been estimated that somewhere between 25% and 50% of cancers are multifocal.[77] Approximately 15% of breast cancers demonstrate multifocal lesions on mammography. Multicentricity, which is far less common, has been said to be associated with subareolar location of tumors,[78] the presence of an extensive intraductal component,[79] DCIS greater than 25 mm,[80] invasive lobular carcinoma,[47] and tubular carcinoma.[63]

Bilateral Carcinomas

Bilateral carcinoma is uncommon. Bilateral carcinoma is usually divided into two types, synchronous and metachronous. *Synchronous carcinoma* refers to detection of simultaneous bilateral carcinomas at the

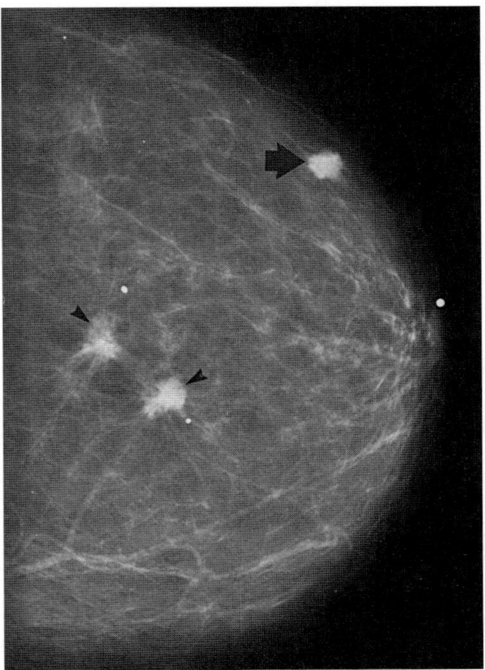

Figure 27–41. Multifocal and multicentric invasive breast carcinoma. Two irregular, spiculated carcinomas (*arrowheads*) are present in one quadrant, representing "multifocal" carcinoma. The presence of a third lesion (*arrow*) in another quadrant leads to the designation "multicentric."

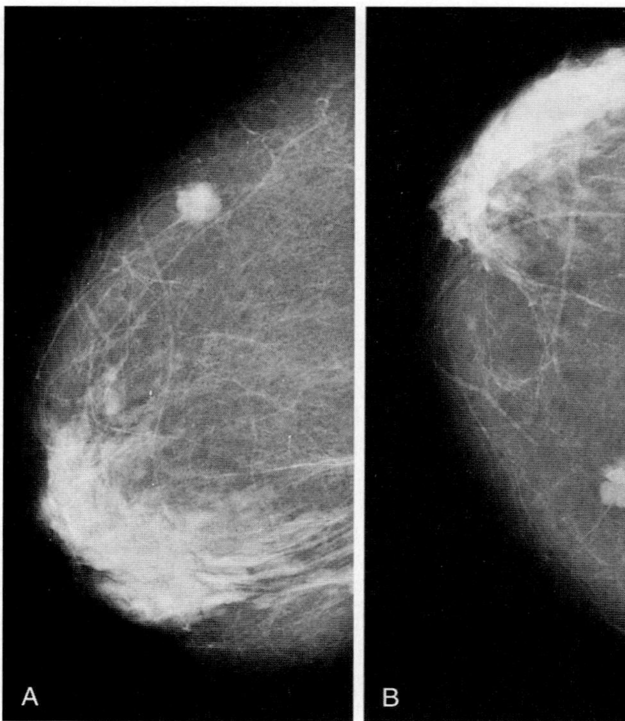

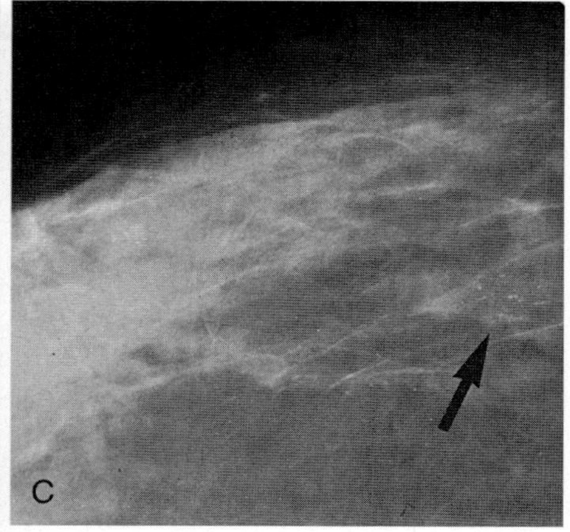

Figure 27–42. Multicentric carcinoma. Right mediolateral (**A**) and craniocaudal (**B**) mammograms show an irregular, spiculated, dense mass in the upper-inner quadrant. **C,** Magnification view in craniocaudal projection shows clustered calcifications (*arrow*) in the lower-outer quadrant. Biopsy of the calcifications revealed intraductal carcinoma. Mastectomy was performed.

same examination (Fig. 27–43). *Metachronous* carcinomas are nonsimultaneous carcinomas of the contralateral breast; they are found during follow-up, sometimes many years later. The exact incidence of bilateral breast carcinoma is difficult to determine because contralateral lesions can sometimes be metastases. It is known, however, that the likelihood of bilaterality depends on the histologic type of the cancer. Invasive lobular carcinoma has a higher likelihood of bilaterality than other cancers, with reported rates up to 30%.[47,75] Invasive ductal carcinoma has a lower reported incidence of bilaterality, the contralateral focus of cancer usually being intraductal carcinoma.[81] Overall, the risk of development of cancer in the other breast after mastectomy is reported to be 1% per year, about six times higher than in the general population.[82]

MALIGNANCIES OF THE BREAST NOT ARISING FROM DUCTAL TISSUES

Malignant lesions arising from the stromal tissues are rare. However, primary lymphomas and various types of sarcomas do occur.

Primary Non-Hodgkin's Lymphoma of the Breast

Primary lymphoma of the breast is rare and should be distinguished from metastatic lymphoma from an extramammary primary tumor. Primary lymphoma of the breast usually manifests as a palpable mass that may have associated skin changes, such as retraction, erythema, and peau d'orange. Axillary nodes are involved in 30% to 40% of cases.[6] Bilateral disease is present in approximately 13% of cases. If the tumor is small, it can be treated with lumpectomy and irradiation.

The majority of primary lymphomas manifest as solitary uncalcified masses on mammography.[83] Almost 30% are circumscribed, the remaining showing incompletely circumscribed margins (Fig. 27–44). Typically, they are not spiculated lesions. Primary lymphoma may manifest as multiple masses (<10% of cases), making it impossible to distinguish primary from metastatic lymphoma on mammography. Histologically, the majority are non-Hodgkin's lymphoma, predominantly B-cell type. T-cell lymphoma is rare.[84]

Sarcoma of the Breast

Various types of sarcomas have been reported to arise from the stromal tissues of the breast. These rare stromal lesions include angiosarcoma, phyllodes tumor (described later), liposarcoma, and osteosarcoma (Figs. 27–45 and 27–46).[1,85] Histologic diagnosis of angiosarcoma, especially the poorly differentiated epithelioid type, can be challenging and requires immunohistochemical confirmation by the presence of factor VIII and other endothelial cell markers (Fig. 27–47). The prognosis of stromal sarcoma is closely related to the extent of differentiation. Angiosarcoma and osteosarcoma of the breast are highly malignant.[58,85]

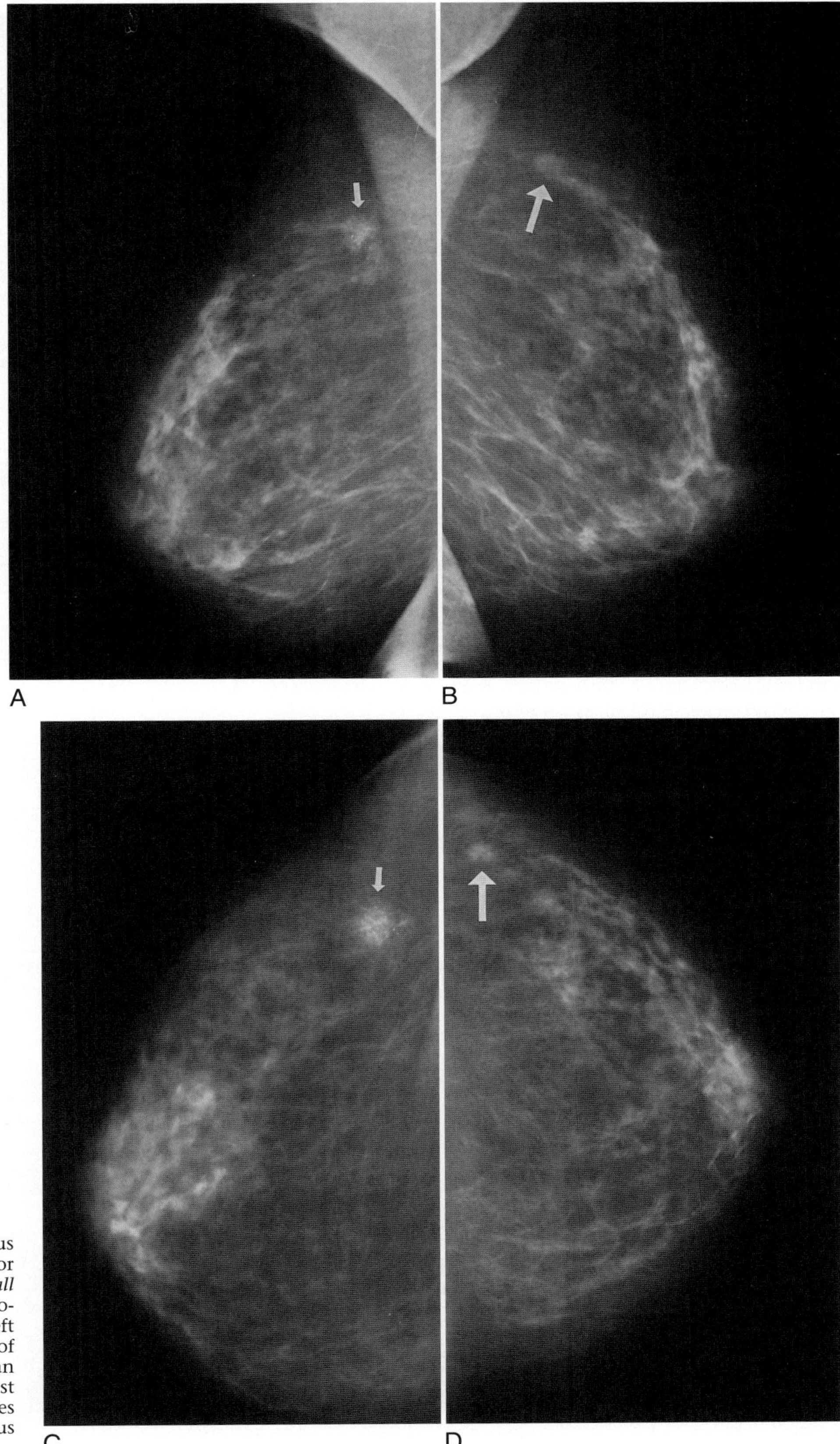

Figure 27–43. Bilateral synchronous carcinoma. The patient was referred for localization of a right breast mass (*small arrows*). Right (**A**) and left (**B**) mediolateral oblique views; right (**C**) and left (**D**) craniocaudal views. Review of outside mammograms showed an unexpected small suspicious left breast mass (*large arrows*). Excisional biopsies demonstrated bilateral synchronous carcinoma.

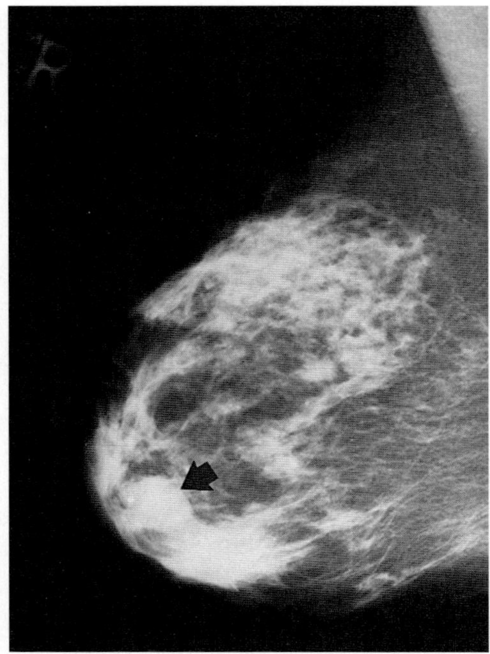

Figure 27–44. Primary non-Hodgkin's lymphoma of the breast. A 72-year-old woman felt a lump under the nipple. Right mediolateral oblique mammogram shows a partially circumscribed mass (*arrow*) at the site of the palpable abnormality. A radiopaque lead marker (BB) was placed on the skin over the palpable abnormality. Ultrasonography showed a solid mass.

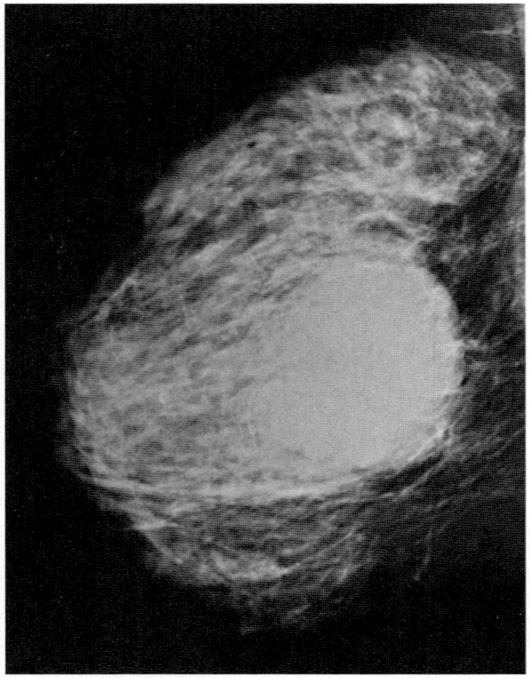

Figure 27–45. Primary osteosarcoma of the breast. Right mediolateral oblique view shows large, lobulated, dense mass.

Malignant Phyllodes Tumor

The most common malignancy of the breast not of ductal origin is phyllodes tumor. This lesion was once termed "cystosarcoma phyllodes." Approximately 10% of all phyllodes tumors are malignant and metastasize. These tumors usually manifest as rapidly growing palpable masses that may be attached to the skin or adjacent tissues.

Imaging Features

Malignant phyllodes tumors usually are round or lobular with circumscribed margins, without spiculation or calcifications. They grow rapidly and are large at the time of presentation. They cannot be distinguished mammographically from benign phyllodes tumors. On ultrasonography, malignant tumors tend to have low-level echoes and circumscribed margins and, occasionally, cystic regions. The

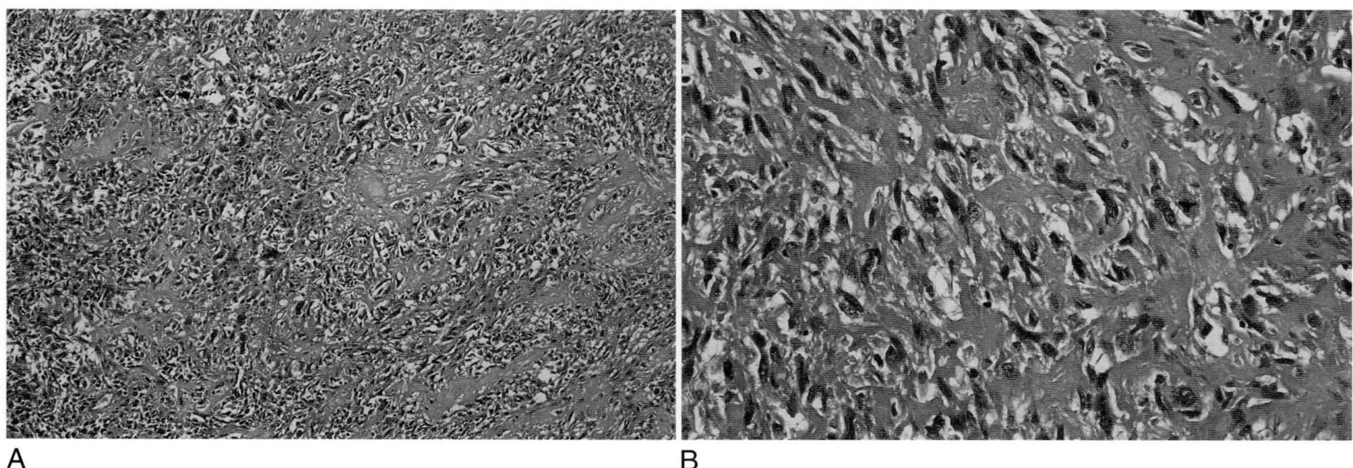

Figure 27–46. Osteosarcoma of breast. **A,** Malignant cells and osteoid stroma. **B,** Higher-magnification view reveals malignant spindle cells surrounded by eosinophilic osteoid material.

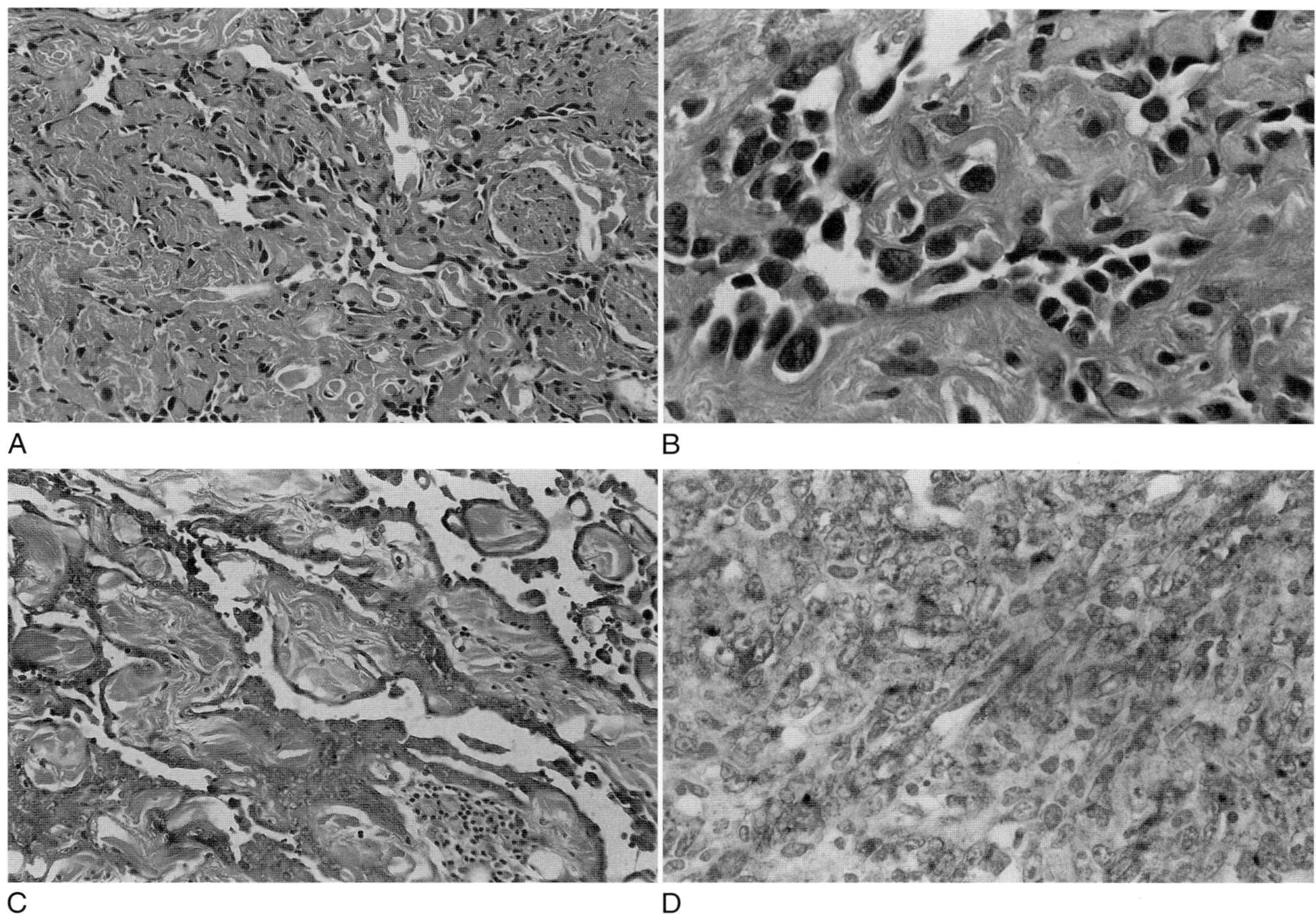

Figure 27–47. **A** and **B,** Well-differentiated angiosarcoma. **A,** Tumor cells form irregular vascular spaces. **B,** Large, irregular, hyperchromatic nuclei. **C** and **D,** Poorly differentiated angiosarcoma. **C,** Tumor cells form solid sheets and irregular spaces sometimes simulating carcinoma. **D,** Response to immunohistochemical stain for factor VIII is positive and dark, confirming the diagnosis of angiosarcoma.

determination whether a phyllodes tumor is benign or malignant is based on histologic, rather than imaging, features.

Pathology

Phyllodes tumor has a lobulated, leaflike appearance and varies in size from 1 cm to more than 15 cm. Microscopically, it consists of both epithelial and stromal elements. The branching, hyperplastic benign ducts are compressed by stromal tissue. On the basis of the appearance of the latter, phyllodes tumor is divided into benign and malignant groups.

The benign group is characterized by smooth, circumscribed borders, hypercellular stroma, minimal nuclear atypia, and low mitotic activity, usually less than one mitosis per 10 high-power field (HPF). Occasional stromal cells have hyperchromatic multiple nuclei.

In contrast, malignant phyllodes tumors have infiltrative borders, nuclear atypia, and higher mitotic activity (Fig. 27–48). In the low-grade malignant phyllodes tumor, the stromal elements resemble well-differentiated fibrosarcoma with mitotic activity in the range of 2 to 5 mitoses per 10 HPFs. High-grade malignant phyllodes tumor has a higher mitotic activity, exceeding 5 per 10 HPFs. Necrosis is common. In addition, the stromal components may contain liposarcoma, leiomyosarcoma, rhabdomyosarcoma, malignant fibrous histiocytoma, angiosarcoma, chondrosarcoma, and osteosarcoma.

With both benign and malignant phyllodes tumors, wide excision is needed to minimize the risk of local recurrence. Hematogenous spread is less than 5% for low-grade malignant phyllodes tumor but close to 25% for high-grade phyllodes tumor. Axillary lymph node metastasis is rare (<1%).[86-88]

Metastases from Extramammary Malignancies

Metastatic disease to the breast from extramammary primary lesions is unusual. The largest reported single source of such metastases is melanoma (Fig. 27–49), but a wide variety of other tumors may secondarily involve the breast.[88-92] The autopsy

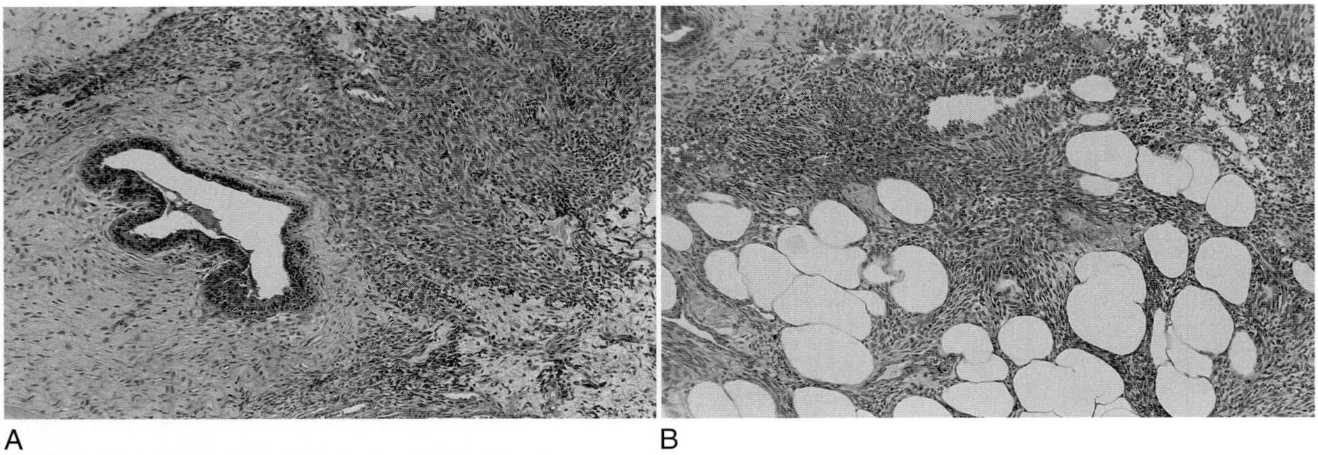

A B

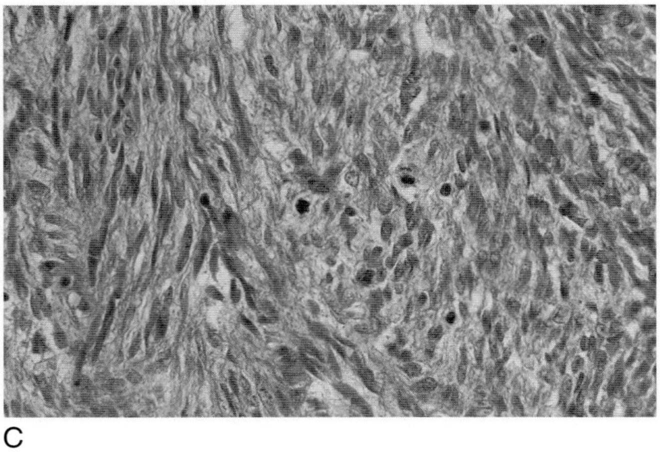

C

Figure 27–48. Malignant phyllodes tumor. **A,** Hyperplastic duct and highly cellular stroma. **B,** Infiltration into adjacent adipose tissue. **C,** Fibrosarcomatous cells with moderate nuclear atypia and multiple mitotic figures.

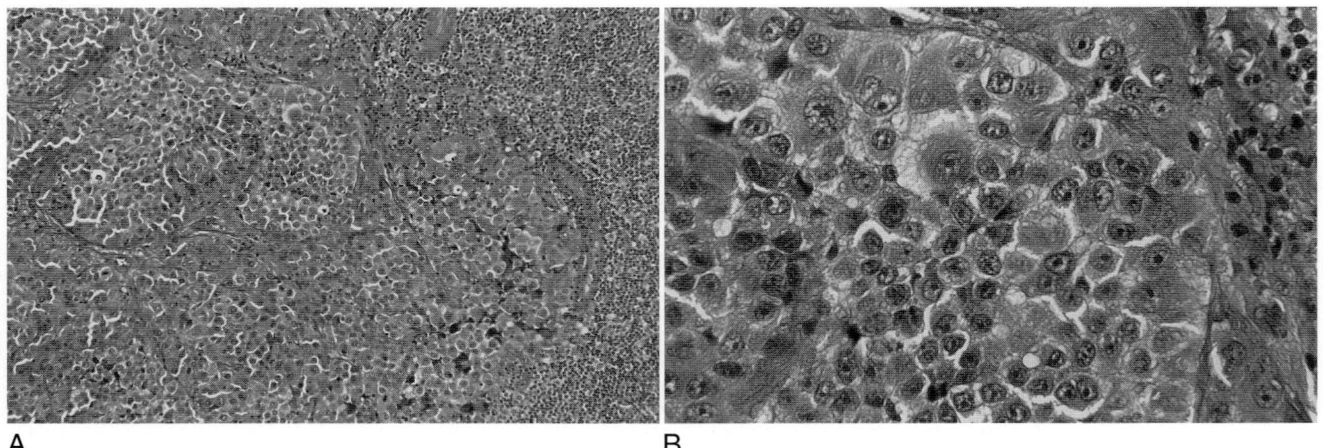

A B

Figure 27–49. Metastatic malignant melanoma. **A,** Diffuse sheets of tumor cells resemble poorly differentiated carcinoma. **B,** Loosely cohesive tumor cells have abundant eosinophilic cytoplasm, large nuclei, and prominent nucleoli.

incidence of metastasis to the breast from malignant neoplasms other than primary breast carcinoma varies from 1.7% to 6.6%.[93,94] In contrast, the clinically observed rate ranges from only 0.5% to 1.3%.[95] A metastatic nodule in the breast is rarely the initial sign of an extramammary malignancy.

Metastatic lesions tend to have the same size on palpation as they appear to have on mammography. In contrast, the usual infiltrating ductal carcinoma shows a discrepancy, feeling larger on clinical examination than on mammography. This discrepancy reflects the proliferation of fibrous connective tissue associated with invasive ductal carcinomas. In addition, metastatic lesions do not cause thickening or retraction of the skin or nipple. Because metastatic lesions are not intraductal, they are not associated with nipple discharge.

Imaging Features

Mammographically, metastases to the breast tend to be round, with circumscribed to ill-defined margins, lacking the spiculation characteristic of the usual infiltrating ductal carcinoma (Fig. 27–50). They usually range in size from 1 to 3 cm at the time of detection.[88] Although such metastases are usually solitary, multiple lesions may be seen (Fig. 27–51).

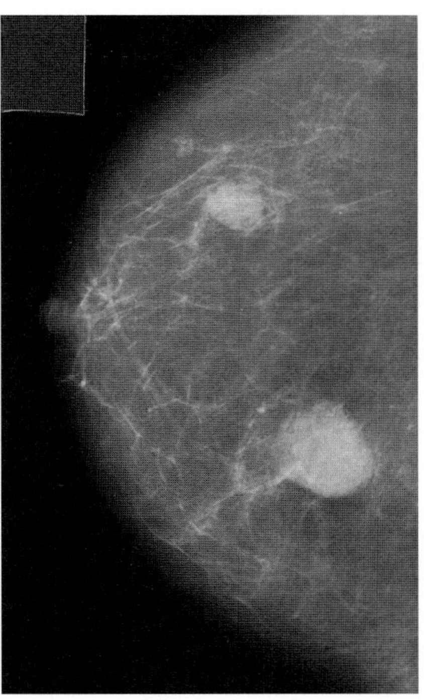

Figure 27–51. Multiple metastases to the breast in a woman with lung carcinoma and a palpable mass in the upper-inner quadrant of the right breast. Craniocaudal mammogram shows circumscribed masses. Biopsy of the palpable mass demonstrated metastasis.

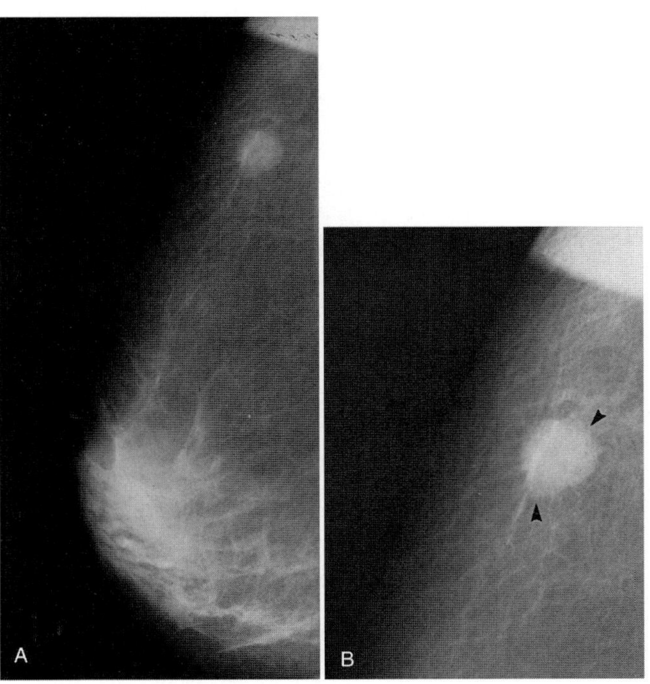

Figure 27–50. Palpable solitary metastasis to the breast in a woman with lung carcinoma. **A,** Right mediolateral view shows round mass in the upper hemisphere of the breast. **B,** Close-up reveals ill-defined margins (*arrowheads*).

References

1. Page DL, Anderson TJ, Connelly JL, Schnitt SF: Miscellaneous features of carcinoma. In Page DL, Anderson TJ (eds): Diagnostic Histopathology of the Breast. Edinburgh, Churchill Livingstone, 1987.
2. Cutler M: Diagnosis and differential diagnosis. In Cutler M: Tumors of the Breast. Philadelphia, JB Lippincott, 1962, pp 168-176.
3. Bearhs OH, Shapiro S, Smart C, et al: Report of the Working Group to Review the National Cancer Institute–American Cancer Society Breast Cancer Detection Demonstration Projects. J Natl Cancer Inst 1979;62:639-698.
4. Bassett LW, Liu TH, Giuliano AE, Gold RH: The prevalence of carcinoma in palpable vs impalpable, mammographically detected lesions. AJR Am J Roentgenol 1991;157:21-24.
5. Arcari FA, Wilson GS: Clinical diagnosis of breast masses. GP 1961;23:82-92.
6. Donegan WL, Spratt JS (eds): Cancer of the Breast, 4th ed. Philadelphia, WB Saunders, 1995.
7. Kaiser JS, Helvie MA, Blacklaw RL, Roubidoux MA: Palpable breast thickening: Role of mammography and US in cancer detection. Radiology. 2002;223:839-844.
8. Haagaensen CD: Diseases of the Breast, 3d ed. Philadelphia, WB Saunders, 1986.
9. Taylor GW, Meltzer A: Inflammatory carcinoma of the breast. Am J Cancer 1938;33:33-49.
10. Lee BJ, Tannenbaum NE: Inflammatory carcinoma of the breast. Surg Gynecol Obstet 1924;29:580-595.
11. Devitt JE: Management of nipple discharge by clinical findings. Am J Surg 1985;149:789-792.
12. Chaudary MA, Millis RR, Davies GC, et al: Nipple discharge: The diagnostic value of testing for occult blood. Ann Surg 1982;196:651-655.

13. Copeland MM, Higgins TG: Significance of discharge from the nipple in nonpuerperal mammary conditions. Ann Surg 1960; 151:638.
14. Halsted WS: A clinical and histologic study of certain adenocarcinomas of the breast. Ann Surg 1898;28:557-576.
15. Ashikari R, Rosen PP, Urban JA, et al: Breast cancer presenting as an axillary mass. Ann Surg 1976;183:415-417.
16. American College of Radiology: Breast imaging reporting and data system (BI-RADS). Reston, VA, American College of Radiology, 1995.
17. Sickles EA: Nonpalpable, circumscribed, noncalcified solid breast masses: Likelihood of malignancy based on lesion size and age of patient. Radiology 1994;192:439-442.
18. Jackson VP, Dines KA, Bassett LW, et al: Diagnostic importance of radiographic density of noncalcified breast masses: Analysis of 91 lesions. AJR Am J Roentgenol 1991;157:25-28.
19. Kalisher L, Chu AM, Peyster RG: Clinicopathological correlations of xeroradiography in determining involvement of metastatic axillary nodes in female breast cancer. Radiology 1976;121:333-335.
20. Andersson I, Marsal L, Nilsson B, et al: Abnormal axillary lymph nodes in rheumatoid arthritis. Acta Radiol [Diagn] 1980;21:645-649.
21. Sickles EA: Mammographic features of "early" breast cancer. AJR Am J Roentgenol 1984;143:461-464.
22. Bassett LW, Shayestehfar B, Hirbawi I: Obtaining previous mammograms for comparison: Usefulness and costs. AJR Am J Roentgenol 1994;163:1083-1086.
23. Bassett LW, Hendrick RE, Bassford TL, et al: Quality Determinants of Mammography. (Clinical Practice Guideline, N. 13. AHCPR Publication No. 95-0632.) Rockville, MD, Agency for Health Care Policy and Research, Public Health Service, U.S. Department of Health and Human Services, October 1994.
24. Mendelson E: Evaluation of the postoperative breast. Radiol Clin North Am 1992;30:107-138.
25. Hassell P, Klein-Parker H, Worth A, Poon P: Radial sclerosing lesions of the breast: Mammographic and pathologic correlation. Can Assoc Radiol J 1999;50:370-375.
26. Fisher ER, Gregorio RM, Fisher B, et al: The pathology of invasive breast cancer: A syllabus derived from findings of the National Surgical Adjuvant Breast Project (Protocol No. 4). Cancer 1975;36:1-85.
27. Fisher B, Bauer M, Wickerham L, et al: Relation of number of positive axillary nodes to the prognosis of patients with primary breast cancer: NSABP update. Cancer 1983;52:1551-1557.
28. Fisher B, Slack NH, Bross IDJ, et al: Cancer of the breast: Size of neoplasm and prognosis. Cancer 1969;24:1071-1080.
29. Elston CW, Ellis IO: Pathological prognostic factors in breast cancer. I: The value of histological grade in breast cancer: Experience from a large study with long term follow-up. Histopathology 1991;19:403-410.
30. Whiteside TL, Miescher S, Hurlimann J, et al: Clonal analysis and in situ characterization of lymphocytes infiltrating human breast carcinomas. Cancer Immunol Immunother 1986;23:169-173.
31. Rosen PP, Saigo PE, Braun DW Jr, et al: Predictors of recurrence in stage I (T1N0M0 breast carcinoma). Ann Surg 1981;193:15-25.
32. Rosen PP, Saigo PE, Braun DW, et al: Prognosis in stage II (T1N0M0) breast cancer. Ann Surg 1981;194:576-584.
33. Lauria R, Perrone F, Carlomagno C, et al: The prognostic significance of lymphatic and blood vessel invasion in operable breast cancer. Cancer 1995:76:1772-1778.
34. Schnitt SJ, Connolly JL, Harris JR, et al: Pathologic predictors of early local recurrences in stage I and II breast cancer treated by primary radiation therapy. Cancer 1984;53:1049-1057.
35. Wong JH, Kopald KH, Morton DL: The impact of microinvasion on axillary node metastases and survival in patients with intraductal breast carcinoma. Arch Surg 1990;125:1298-1302.
36. Silver SA, Tavassoli FA: Mammary ductal carcinoma in situ with microinvasion. Cancer 1998;82:2382-2390.
37. Hermanek P, Hutter RVP, Sobin LH, et al: TNM Atlas: Illustrated Guide to the TNM/p TNM Classification of Malignant Tumors, 4th ed. Berlin, Springer-Verlag, 1997, pp 201-212.
38. Prasad ML, Osborne MP, Giri DD, Hoda SA: Microinvasive carcinoma (T1mic) of the breast: Clinicopathologic profile of 21 cases. Am J Surg Pathol 2000;24:422-428.
39. Silverstein MJ, Lewinsky BS, Waisman JR, et al: Infiltrating lobular carcinoma: Is it different from infiltrating duct carcinoma? Cancer 1994;73:1673-1677.
40. Dixon JM, Anderson TJ, Page DL, et al: Infiltrating lobular carcinoma of the breast: An evaluation of the incidence and consequence of bilateral disease. Br J Surg 1983;70:513-516.
41. Tan SM, Behranwala KA, Trott PA, et al: A retrospective study comparing the individual modalities of triple assessment in the pre-operative diagnosis of invasive lobular breast carcinoma. Eur J Surg Oncol 2002;28:203-208.
42. Uchiyama N, Miyakawa K, Moriyama N, Kumazaki T: Radiographic features of invasive lobular carcinoma of the breast. Radiat Med 2001;19:19-25.
43. Mendelson E, Harris KM, Doshi N, Tobon H: Infiltrating lobular carcinoma: Mammographic patterns with pathologic correlation. AJR Am J Roentgenol 1989;153:265-271.
44. Sickles EA: The subtle and atypical mammographic features of invasive lobular carcinoma. Radiology 1991;178:25-26.
45. Krecke KN, Gisvold JJ: Invasive lobular carcinoma of the breast: Mammographic findings and extent of disease at diagnosis in 184 patients. AJR Am J Roentgenol 1993;161:957-960.
46. Chapellier C, Balu-Maestro C, Bleuse A, et al: Ultrasonography of invasive lobular carcinoma of the breast: Sonographic patterns and diagnostic value: Report of 102 cases. Clin Imaging 2000;24:333-336.
47. Lesser ML, Rosen PP, Kinne DW: Multicentricity and bilaterality in invasive breast carcinoma. Surgery 1982;92:234-240.
48. White JR, Gustafson GS, Wimbish K, et al: Conservative surgery and radiation therapy for infiltrating lobular carcinoma of the breast: The role of preoperative mammograms in guiding treatment. Cancer 1994;74:640-647.
49. DiCostanzo D, Rosen PP, Gareen I, et al: Prognosis in infiltrating lobular carcinoma: An analysis of "classical" and variant tumors. Am J Surg Pathol 1990;14:12-23.
50. Rosen PP, Oberman HA: Tumors of the Mammary Gland: Atlas of Tumor Pathology, 3rd Series, Fascicle 7. Washington, DC, Armed Forces Institute of Pathology, 1993.
51. Steinbrecher JS, Silverberg SG: Signet-ring cell carcinoma of the breast: The mucinous variant of infiltrating lobular carcinoma. Cancer 1976;37:828-840.
52. Tavassoli FA: Pathology of the Breast. New York, Elsevier, 1992.
53. Fisher ER, Kenny JP, Sass R, et al: Medullary cancer of the breast revisited. Breast Cancer Res Treat 1990;16:215-229.
54. Ridolfi RL, Rosen PP, Post A, et al: Medullary carcinoma of the breast. Cancer 1977;40:1365-1385.
55. Rosen PP, Lesser ML, Kinne DW, et al: Breast carcinoma in women 35 years of age or younger. Ann Surg 1984;199:133-142.
56. Meyer JE, Amin E, Lindfors KK, et al: Medullary carcinoma of the breast: Mammographic and sonographic appearance. Radiology 1989;170:79-82.
57. Moore OS Jr, Foote FW Jr: The relatively favorable prognosis of medullary carcinoma of the breast. Cancer 1949;2:635-642.
58. Rosen PP: Breast Pathology: Diagnosis by Needle Core Biopsy. Philadelphia, Lippincott Williams & Wilkins, 1999.
59. Wargotz ES, Silverberg SG: Medullary carcinoma of the breast: A clinical pathologic study with appraisal of current diagnostic criteria. Hum Pathol 1988;19:1340-1346.
60. Rasmussen BB: Human mucinous breast cancers and their lymph node metastasis: A histologic review of 247 cases. Pathol Res Pract 1985;180:377-382.
61. Hamele-Bena D, Cranor ML, Rosen PP: Mammary mucocele-like lesions: Benign and malignant. Am J Surg Pathol 1996; 20:1081-1085.
62. Boring CC, Squires TS, Tony T: Cancer statistics, 1991. CA Cancer J Clin 1991;41:19-36.
63. Lagios MD, Rose MR, Margolin FR: Tubular carcinoma of the breast associated with multicentricity and bilaterality, and family history of mammary carcinoma. Am J Clin Pathol 1980;73:25-30.
64. Tobon H, Salazar H: Tubular carcinoma of the breast: Clinical, histological and ultrastructural observations. Arch Pathol Lab Med 1977;101:310-316.

65. Elson BC, Helvie MA, Frank FS, et al: Tubular carcinoma of the breast: Mode of presentation, mammographic appearance, and frequency of nodal metastases. AJR Am J Roentgenol 1993;161:1173-1178.
66. Feig SA, Shaber GS, Patchefsky AS, et al: Tubular carcinoma of the breast. Radiology 1978;129:311-314.
67. McDivitt RW, Boyce W, Gersell D: Tubular carcinoma of the breast: Clinical and pathological observations concerning 135 cases. Am J Surg Pathol 1982;6:401-411.
68. Peters GN, Wolff M, Haagensen CD: Tubular carcinoma of the breast: Clinical pathologic correlations based on 100 cases. Ann Surg 1981;193:138-149.
69. Fisher ER, Palekar AS, Redmond C, et al: Pathologic findings from the National Surgical Adjuvant Breast Project (Protocol No. 4). VI: Invasive papillary cancer. Am J Clin Pathol 1980; 73:313-322.
70. Maluf HM, Koerner FC: Solid papillary carcinoma of the breast. Am J Surg Pathol 1995;19:1237-1244.
71. Middleton LP, Tressera F, Sobel ME, et al: Infiltrating micropapillary carcinoma of the breast. Mod Pathol 1999;12:499-504.
72. Walsh MM, Bleiweiss IJ: Invasive micropapillary carcinoma of the breast: Eighty cases of underrecognized entity. Hum Pathol 2001;32:583-589.
73. Kleer CG, Oberman HA: Adenoid cystic carcinoma of the breast. Am J Surg Pathol 1998;22:569-575.
74. Shin SJ, DeLellis RA, Ying L, Rosen PP: Small cell carcinoma of the breast. Am J Surg Pathol 2000;24:1231-1238.
75. Lagios MD, Westdahl PR, Rose MR: The concept and implications of multicentricity and bilaterality in invasive breast carcinoma. Pathol Ann 1981;16:83-102.
76. Gump FE, Habif DV, Logergo P, et al: The extent and distribution of cancer in breasts with palpable primary tumors. Ann Surg 1986;204:384-388.
77. McDivitt RW, Boyce W, Gersell D: Breast cancer multicentricity. In McDivitt RW, Oberman HA, Ozello L, Kaufman N (eds): The Breast. Baltimore, Williams and Wilkins, 1984, p 139.
78. Rosen PP, Fracchia AA, Urban JA, et al: "Residual" mammary carcinoma following simulated partial mastectomy. Cancer 1975;35:739-747.
79. Holland R, Connolly JL, Gelman R, et al: The presence of an extensive intraductal component (EIC) following a limited excision correlates with prominent residual disease in the remainder of the breast. J Clin Oncol 1990;8:113-118.
80. Lagios MD, Rose MR, Margolin FR: Multicentricity of breast carcinoma demonstrated by routine correlated serial subgross and radiographic examination. Cancer 1977;40:1726-1734.
81. Urban JA: Bilaterality of cancer of the breast. Cancer 1967; 20:1867-1870.
82. Chaudary MA, Millis RR, Hoskins EOL, et al: Bilateral primary cancer: A prospective study of disease incidence. Br J Surg 1984;71:711-714.
83. Liberman L, Giess CS, Dershaw DD, et al: Non-Hodgkin's lymphoma of the breast: Imaging characteristics and correlation with histopathologic findings. Radiology 1994;192:157-160.
84. Aguilera NSI, Tavassoli FA, Chu W-S, Abbondanzo SL: T-cell lymphoma presenting in the breast: A histologic, immunophenotypic and molecular genetic study of four cases. Mod Pathol 2000;13:599-605.
85. Silver SA, Tavassoli FA: Primary osteogenic sarcoma of the breast. Am J Surg Pathol 1998;22:925-933.
86. Hart WR, Bauer RC, Oberman HA: Cystosarcoma phyllodes: A clinicopathologic study of 26 hypercellular periductal stroma tumors of the breast. Am J Clin Pathol 1978;70:211-216.
87. Pietrusz M, Barnes L: Cystosarcoma phyllodes: A clinicopathologic analysis of 42 cases. Cancer 1978;41:1974-1983.
88. Bohman LG, Bassett LW, Gold RH, Voet R: Breast metastases from extramammary malignancies. Radiology 1982;144;309-312.
89. Charache H: Metastatic tumors in the breast with a report of 10 cases. Surgery 1953;33:385-390.
90. Ibach JR: Carcinoma of the ovary, metastatic to the breast: A case report and review of the literature. Arch Surg 1964;88: 410-414.
91. Moncada R, Cooper RA, Garces M, Badrinath K: Calcified metastases from malignant ovarian neoplasm: Review of the literature. Radiology 1974;113:31-35.
92. Toombs BD, Kalisher L: Metastatic disease to the breast: Clinical, pathologic, and radiographic features. AJR Am J Roentgenol 1977;129:673-676.
93. Abrams HL, Spiro R, Goldstein N: Metastases in carcinoma: Analysis of 1000 autopsied cases. Cancer 1950;3:74-85.
94. Sandison AT: Metastatic tumors in the breast. Br J Surg 1959;47:54-58.
95. Hadju SI, Urban JA: Cancers metastatic to the breast. Cancer 1972;29:1691-1696.

Chapter 28

The Clinically Abnormal Breast

Lusine Tumyan and Lawrence W. Bassett

Breast disease in women encompasses a spectrum of benign and malignant disorders. With intensive public education about breast cancer and the growing acceptance of routine breast self-examination (BSE), an increasing number of women can be expected to seek consultation for the evaluation of breast symptoms. Breast carcinoma is diagnosed in about 4% of patients with breast symptoms, indicating the importance of proper evaluation and management of patients' symptoms.[1] Appropriate imaging evaluation varies with the type of clinical problem as well as the patient's age and risk status.

PALPABLE MASS

In 2004, an estimated 192,200 new cases of female breast cancer will have been diagnosed, and a breast mass will have been the most common surgical indication.[2] A palpable breast mass may become evident during BSE or clinical breast examination (CBE) or retrospectively after screening mammography.

Clinical Examination

It is often difficult to determine by physical examination whether a true mass exists, because all breasts have variable combinations of glandular tissue, fibrosis, and fat. In addition, normal structures like a prominent rib or costochondral junction, the inframammary ridge, or a firm margin at the edge of biopsy site can at times be mistaken for masses.[3] True masses generally differ in character from the surrounding tissue and are asymmetrical in relation to the other breast. Dominant masses may be cystic or solid, and a true mass should persist throughout the menstrual cycle. Suspicious masses tend to be firm and to have attachments to the skin or deep fascia, at times creating dimpling of the overlying skin or nipple retraction. Benign lesions typically are discrete and mobile. However, the accuracy of physical examination alone in detecting carcinoma is limited, because clinical characteristics of benign and malignant masses are not absolute. In one study, four surgeons performed physical examination independently and agreed on the need for biopsy of only 73% of 15 masses subsequently proven malignant.[4] Overall, physical examination is correct in 60% to 85% of cases.[5,6]

Imaging evaluation is necessary in almost all cases, not only to characterize palpable lesions but also to screen the remainder of each breast for multicentric or multifocal lesions. It is estimated that multifocal carcinomas—carcinomas that become invasive at multiple locations within the same duct system—represent 25% to 50% of cancers. Multicentric carcinoma represents cancers of different duct system origin, and the incidence of simultaneous multicentric cancers is only 3%, with as many as 65% of these being found by mammography alone (Fig. 28–1).[7,8] Unfortunately not all palpable lesions are visualized with conventional imaging techniques. In the Breast Cancer Detection Demonstration Project (BCDDP), which began in the 1970s, 9% of cancers were found solely through CBE.[9] With current imaging techniques, this percentage should be considerably lower. Nevertheless, a normal imaging evaluation in cases of suspicious CBE should not defer tissue diagnosis.

Imaging Evaluation in Women 30 Years or Older

The American College of Radiology advocates the use of multiple modalities in the diagnosis of palpable masses as a measure to improve the true-positive rate.[2] In one study comparing physical examination, mammography, and ultrasonography for palpable masses, physical examination and ultrasonography formed the optimal preoperative test combination. In addition, mammography was necessary to detect subclinical multifocal and multicentric cancers.[10] Furthermore, when strict guidelines are used for benign and malignant features, a 99.8% negative predictive value of ultrasonography and mammography can be achieved in patients with palpable masses.[11] In another study, a 100% negative predictive value was attained when both ultrasonography and mammography results were normal in the presence of a palpable breast mass with a clinical follow-up period of 43 months.[12] Other imaging techniques are rapidly emerging and show promise in evaluation of palpable masses. Magnetic resonance imaging (MRI) shows great promise for diagnosis and staging of breast cancer. Although the sensitivity of MRI approaches 100%, its specificity is problematic, with many false-positive results.[13] However, many new MRI sequences aimed at increasing specificity while maintaining sensitivity are being evaluated.[14]

The purposes of an imaging evaluation of a palpable mass are (1) to define the nature of the mass, (2) to detect unexpected multicentric or multifocal cancers, and (3) to identify a nonpalpable extensive intraductal component (Fig. 28–2). A basic algorithm guideline for the evaluation of a palpable mass is

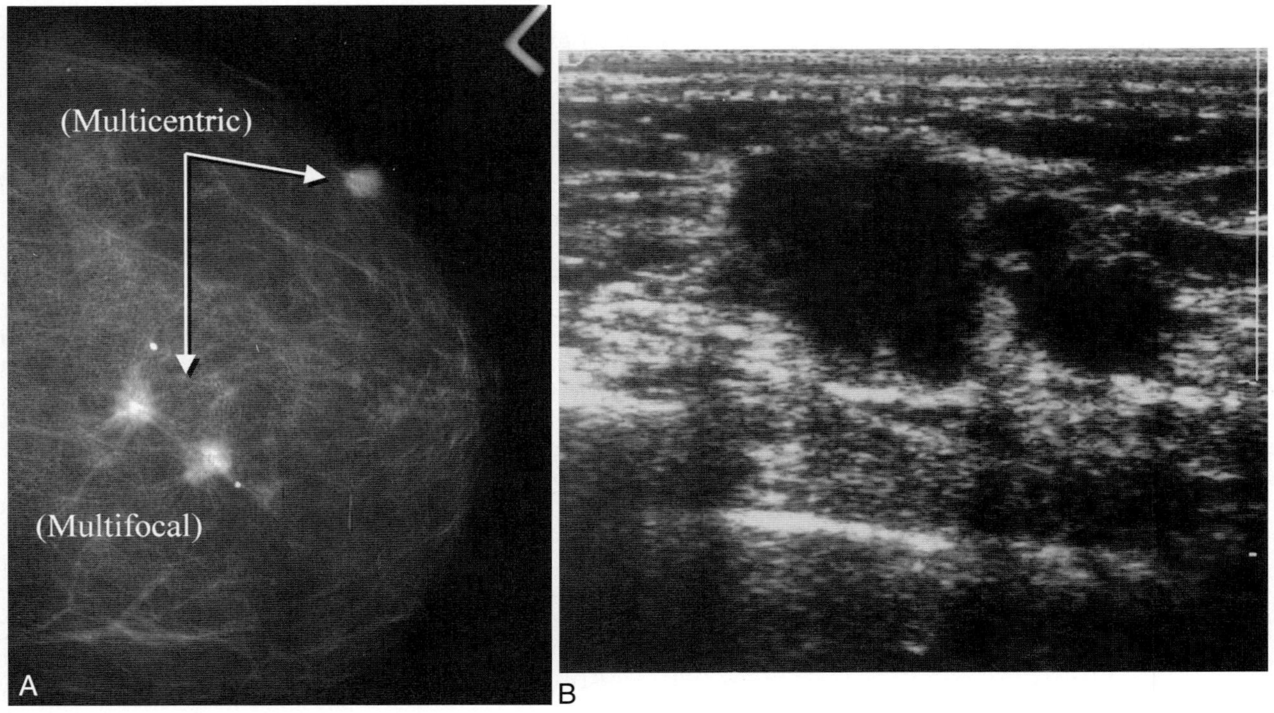

Figure 28–1. **A,** Multifocal and multicentric carcinoma. Multifocal carcinoma arises from the same duct system; the multicentric component is in a different duct system. (Courtesy of James Brenner.) **B,** Ultrasonogram of the multifocal carcinoma, with the foci of cancer in the same duct system.

shown in Figure 28–3. Before mammography is done, a correlative breast examination should be performed. The examination should be directed specifically to the area of concern.

Once the examination verifies the presence of a mass, a radiopaque marker (BB) is placed on the surface of the breast so as to lie directly over the mass on the mammogram. The position of the BB should be adjusted for each projection so that the BB and the mass are superimposed on the film in each of the mammographic projections (Fig. 28–4). Additionally, spot compression or tangential views may

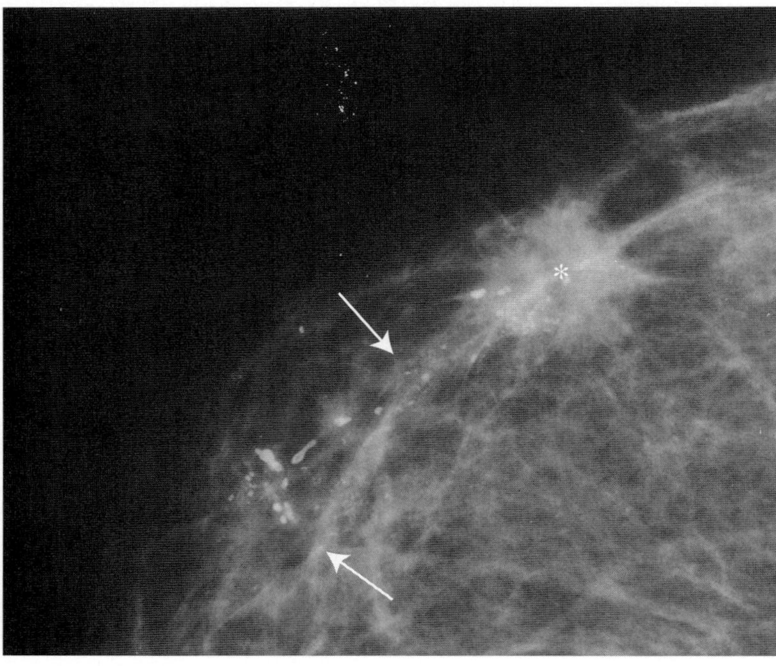

Figure 28–2. Palpable carcinoma with extensive intraductal carcinoma. The palpable mass *(asterisk)* is irregular and spiculated, leading to a final assessment highly suggestive of malignancy. The mammogram also showed extensive calcifications of ductal carcinoma in situ *(arrows)*, which was not palpable. Adequate treatment mandated removal of all the mammographically detected calcifications as well as the palpable carcinoma.

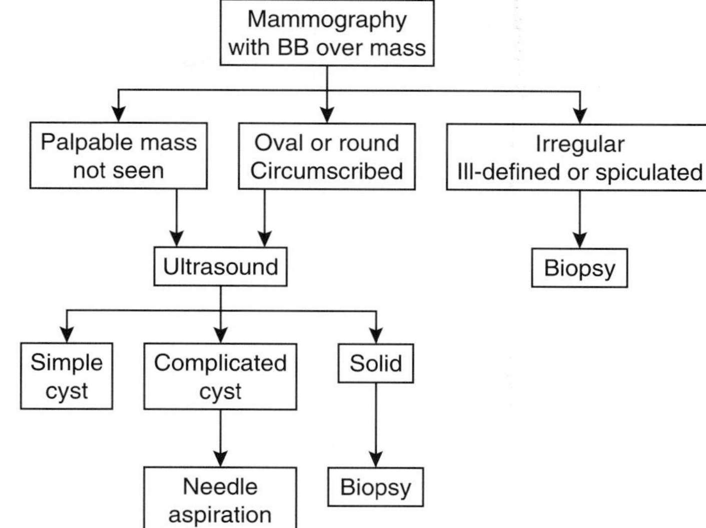

Figure 28–3. Algorithm for evaluation of a palpable mass in a woman 30 years of age or older.

be required when the mass is superimposed on dense glandular tissue. If the palpable mass is not seen on mammography or the mass is oval or round with circumscribed margins, the patient should be evaluated with ultrasonography. Once the mass is determined to be a simple cyst with ultrasonography, the patient can be managed with a routine screening protocol based on her age or risk profile (Fig. 28–5).[15] However, if the cyst is painful, is a concern to the patient, contains internal echoes (echogenic), or has features that suggest an internal solid component, cyst aspiration can be performed (Fig. 28–6). Cytologic evaluation of cyst fluid is not recommended unless it is bloody or dark red.[16]

If the palpable mass is solid on ultrasonography, a tissue diagnosis is usually recommended. There are several options for tissue diagnosis; each has its advantages and disadvantages, which should be carefully considered on a case-per-case basis. Fine-needle aspiration under the guidance of palpation is one

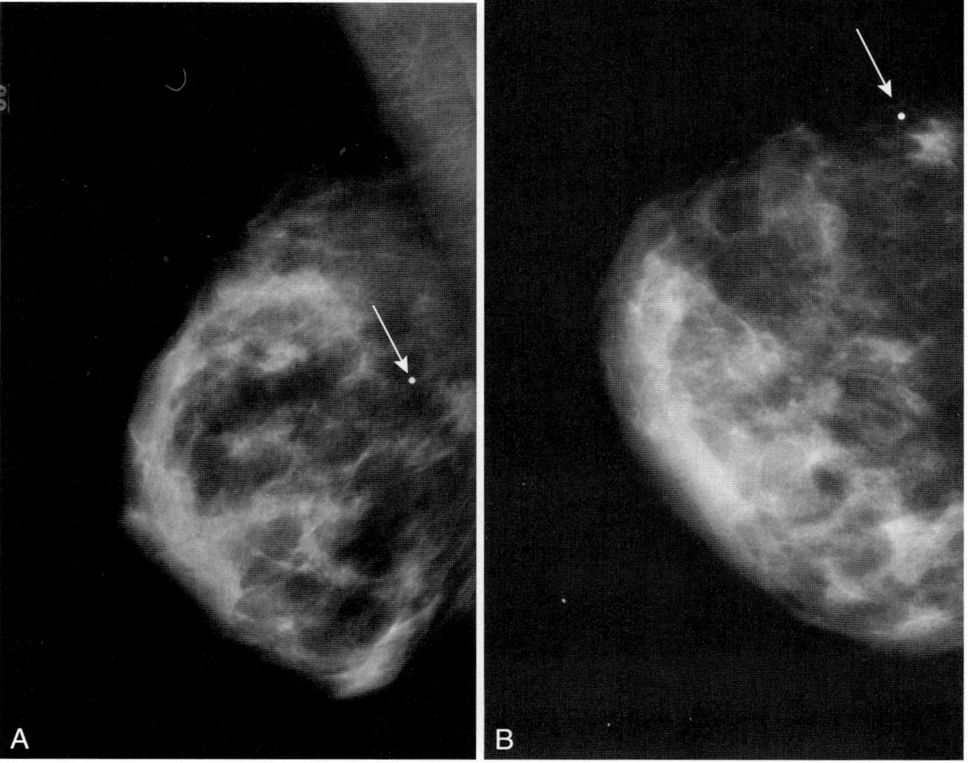

Figure 28–4. Radiopaque marker (BB) placed on the surface of the breast to identify the exact location of a palpable mass. **A,** Mediolateral oblique view. The BB is placed on the medial surface of the breast so it will be as close as possible to the palpable mass *(arrow)*. **B,** Craniocaudal view. The BB is placed on the superior surface of the breast directly over the palpable mass *(arrow)*.

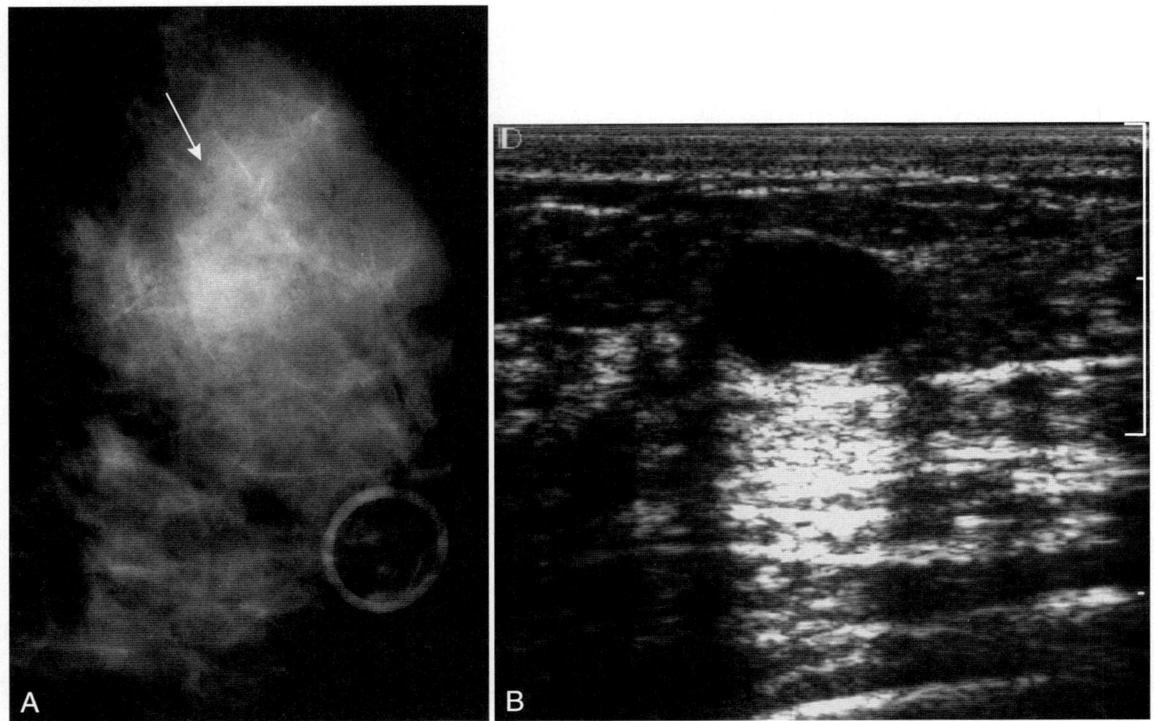

Figure 28–5. Simple cyst in woman with a palpable mass. **A,** Craniocaudal mammogram shows a palpable circumscribed mass *(arrow)*. Note the ring around a mole. **B,** Ultrasonogram directly over the mass shows an oval, circumscribed mass with sharply delineated anterior and posterior borders. The mass is anechoic, and there is enhancement of echoes posterior to it.

option. This procedure has a false-negative rate of 6% to 13%, a false-positive rate of 0 to 2%, and an insufficient sample rate of 6% to 15%.[17-20] Core needle biopsy can improve diagnostic yield and reduce or eliminate the false-positive rate, but it has a false-negative rate of 7% to 11% and an insufficient sample rate of 2% to 10%.[21-23] Stereotactic (x-ray) or ultrasonography-guided needle or core needle biopsy can also be performed if the mass is vaguely palpable, small, deep, mobile, or multiple or if attempts using palpation to biopsy the mass have been unsuccessful.[24] When choosing either procedure, the physician should keep in mind how the results will affect the overall management of the patient. For instance, if the patient or the physician has decided to have an imaging-benign mass excised regardless of needle biopsy results, then needle biopsy merely adds to the cost without significant contribution to the overall management. If the mass is suspected on imaging to be malignant, a core needle biopsy can provide important information, including confirmation of invasion and histochemical tests. For a mass that appears benign on mammography, ultrasonography, or both, the patient and physician may opt for needle biopsy to confirm benignity of the lesion and hence avoid the expense and risk of open biopsy. An example is a circumscribed, oval mass that proves to be a fibroadenoma at needle biopsy (Fig. 28–7).

For irregular masses with ill-defined or spiculated margins, the management depends on the protocol employed by the surgeon. In a one-step procedure, open biopsy and frozen section analysis are followed by an appropriate surgical treatment. In a two-step procedure, the biopsy is performed first followed by surgery at a later date. With the latter protocol, biopsy can provide information as to histologic type, invasion, tumor grade, and hormone receptor status and can better guide the management of the patient. In addition, biopsy confirms that the lesion is indeed malignant and must be removed, decreasing the rate of false-positive results. Preoperative needle localization can also be performed to localize a mass that is difficult to palpate but is clearly visualized on imaging.

Imaging Evaluation in Women 30 Years or Younger

A modified algorithm for management of a palpable mass in women younger than 30 years is suggested because of the low incidence of cancer (<1%) and lower sensitivity of mammography in such women (Fig. 28–8).[25] Considerable documentation shows that mammography is less effective in younger women because of the greater likelihood of dense breast tissue composition. Only about 20% to 35% of women younger than 35 years exhibit considerable fatty replacement.[25-28] Therefore, ultrasonography is

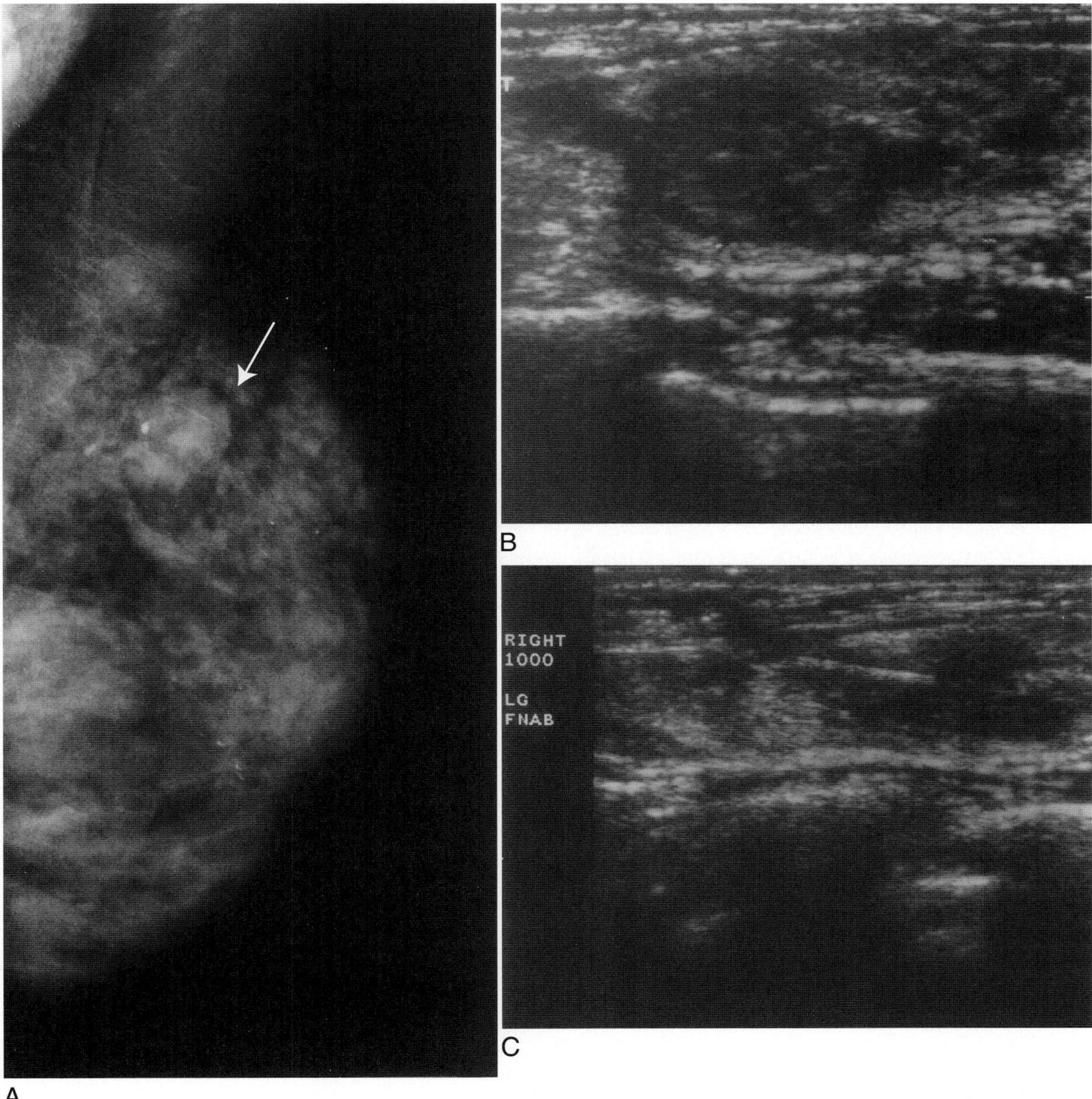

Figure 28–6. Complex cyst in a woman with a palpable mass. **A,** Mediolateral oblique view shows a palpable circumscribed mass *(arrow)*. **B,** Ultrasonogram directly over the mass shows an oval, circumscribed mass with internal echoes and posterior enhancement. **C,** A needle was placed into the lesion, which is partially evacuated in this image; when fluid was aspirated, the lesion completely disappeared.

the preferred initial imaging modality for evaluation.[25,29] If the mass turns out to be a simple cyst, routine clinical follow-up is recommended. For a benign-appearing solid mass, tissue diagnosis is recommended. If the mass has suspicious ultrasonographic features, mammography should be performed before a biopsy to identify possible multicentric or multifocal lesions or an intraductal component of the invasive tumor. As for any age group, a negative imaging finding in a patient with suspicious clinical findings should not delay tissue diagnosis.

NIPPLE DISCHARGE

Nipple discharge is a common symptom but an uncommon presentation of patients with carcinoma. In fact, nipple discharge occurs in 10% to 50% of women with benign breast diseases.[30,31] Only about 10% to 13% of all cases of pathologic discharge are secondary to carcinoma, and in only 1% to 5% of all breast cancers is nipple discharge the main clinical feature.[32-38] Nipple discharge is considered clinically significant or pathologic when it is spontaneous,

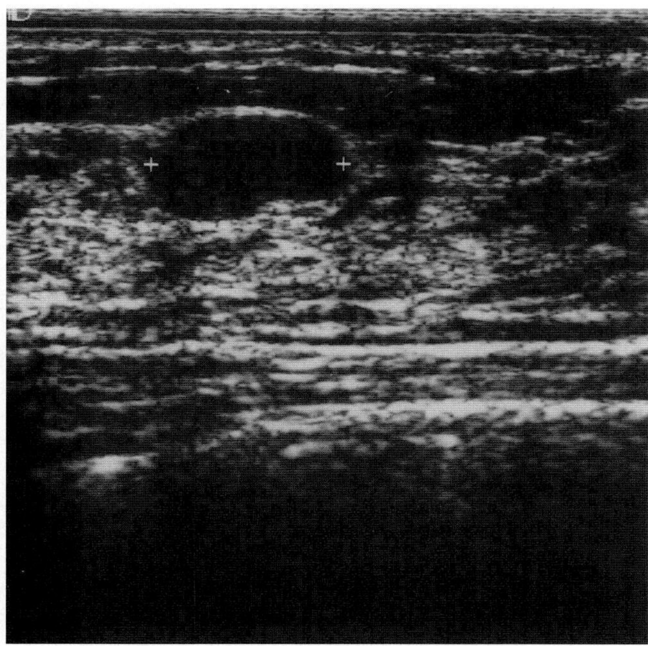

Figure 28–7. Fibroadenoma. Shown is a real time ultrasonogram of an oval circumscribed mass that is wider than tall and has fewer than three gentle lobulations.

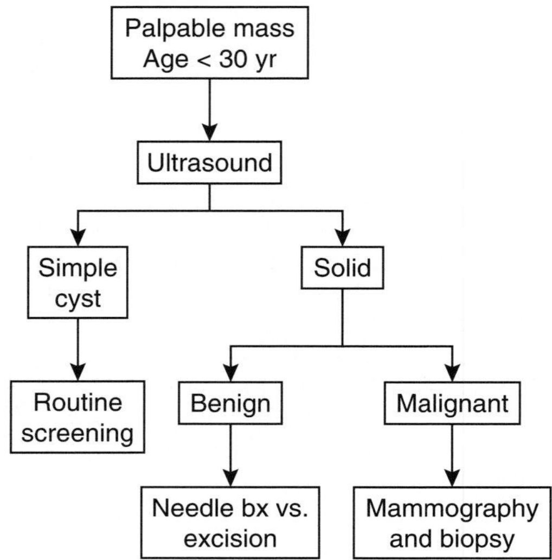

Figure 28–8. Algorithm for evaluation of a palpable mass in a woman 30 years or younger.

unilateral, localized to a single duct, persistent, and nonlactational.[33]

In general, the following four types of nipple discharge are suspicious: clear or watery, yellow or serous, pink, and bloody (Fig. 28–9). However, even these types of discharge are mostly due to benign breast disorders, the most common being intraductal papilloma and papillomatosis.[34-36] Factors that add to the suspicion of cancer are age greater than 55 years, bloody discharge, and the presence of a mass.[35,40] In one study, 32% of women older than 60 years who presented with nipple discharge were found to have underlying carcinoma, compared with 7% of women younger than 60 years with a similar diagnosis.[37] In another study, the mean age of women with breast carcinoma manifesting as nipple discharge was 56 years, with a range of 30 to 78 years.[38]

Clinical Evaluation

A detailed history should be obtained to determine whether the discharge is physiologic, pathologic, or consistent with galactorrhea. Spontaneous discharge

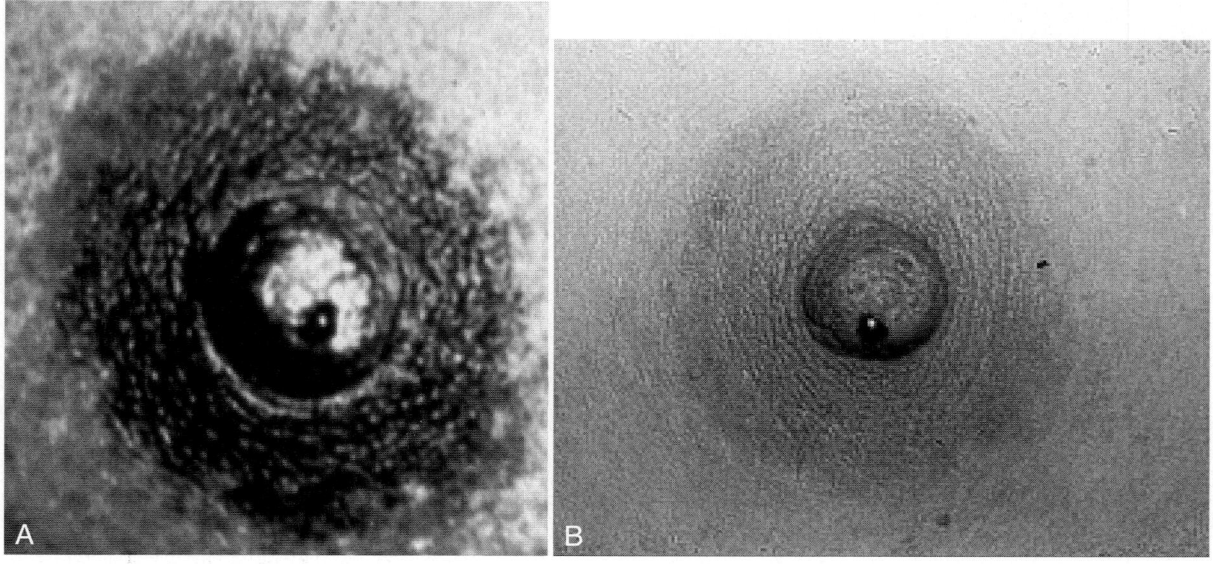

Figure 28–9. Indications for ductography include a persistent and spontaneous bloody (**A**) or serous (**B**) nipple discharge that originates from one or two ducts.

should be distinguished from discharge secondary to manipulation. It is also important to determine whether the discharge is bilateral or unilateral. Systemic and physiologic changes usually result in bilateral discharge and can be treated medically.[33] A thorough physical examination should be conducted, noting any pathologic physical findings, such as retraction of the nipple, dimpling of the skin, breast mass, or inflammatory changes. It is also helpful to ascertain the quadrant where the discharge originates and to determine whether the discharge comes from one or several ducts of the nipple. If discharge is produced on compression of the quadrant, the type of discharge should be assessed by observation of the color and consistency and by testing for occult blood.[32,41]

Imaging Evaluation

Mammography is recommended for any patient who presents with pathologic discharge. Mammography can reveal an occult mass, fibrocystic changes, fat necrosis, and microcalcifications. In particular, duct ectasia appears as dilated ducts, and carcinoma may show up as a mass, microcalcifications, or architectural distortion. However, a normal mammogram does not exclude breast cancer. In one study, only half of the patients who presented with nipple discharge and were diagnosed with breast cancer had an abnormal mammogram.[39] In another study, there was a 10.4% false-negative rate and a 1.4% false-positive rate in patients examined for pathologic nipple discharge.[32] The high false-negative rate could be due to the fact that mammography is poor at portraying lesions that are very small, contain no microcalcifications, and are completely intraductal.[36] Therefore, negative mammographic findings in clinically suspicious cases should not delay tissue diagnosis.

Ultrasonography is used as an adjunct to mammography. Breast ultrasonography is useful in determining not only the nature of the lesion (cystic versus solid) but also its relationship with the ductal system (single versus multiple ducts) and the transportation route of the pathologic discharge to the nipple.[42] Ultrasonography is poor at the detection of microcalcifications and is not very accurate in detection of peripheral small masses without ductal dilation and small lesions in excessively fatty breasts.[43]

Galactography or *ductography* is a mammographic study involving the injection of water-soluble contrast material into a duct (Fig. 28–10). The procedure is indicated for evaluation of spontaneous, unilateral, single-duct nipple discharge.[44] Circumscribed defects, wall irregularity, abrupt luminal changes, and cutoff of the contrast column are findings that can be associated with carcinoma. One or more circumscribed round, oval, lobulated defects and duct dilatation are due to secretions that are commonly observed with papillomas (Fig. 28–11).[45]

Galactography is more sensitive than mammography in the detection of intraductal lesions, but it cannot accurately distinguish between benign and malignant ductal tumors.[36,42,45] Furthermore, galactography cannot distinguish multiple lesions or

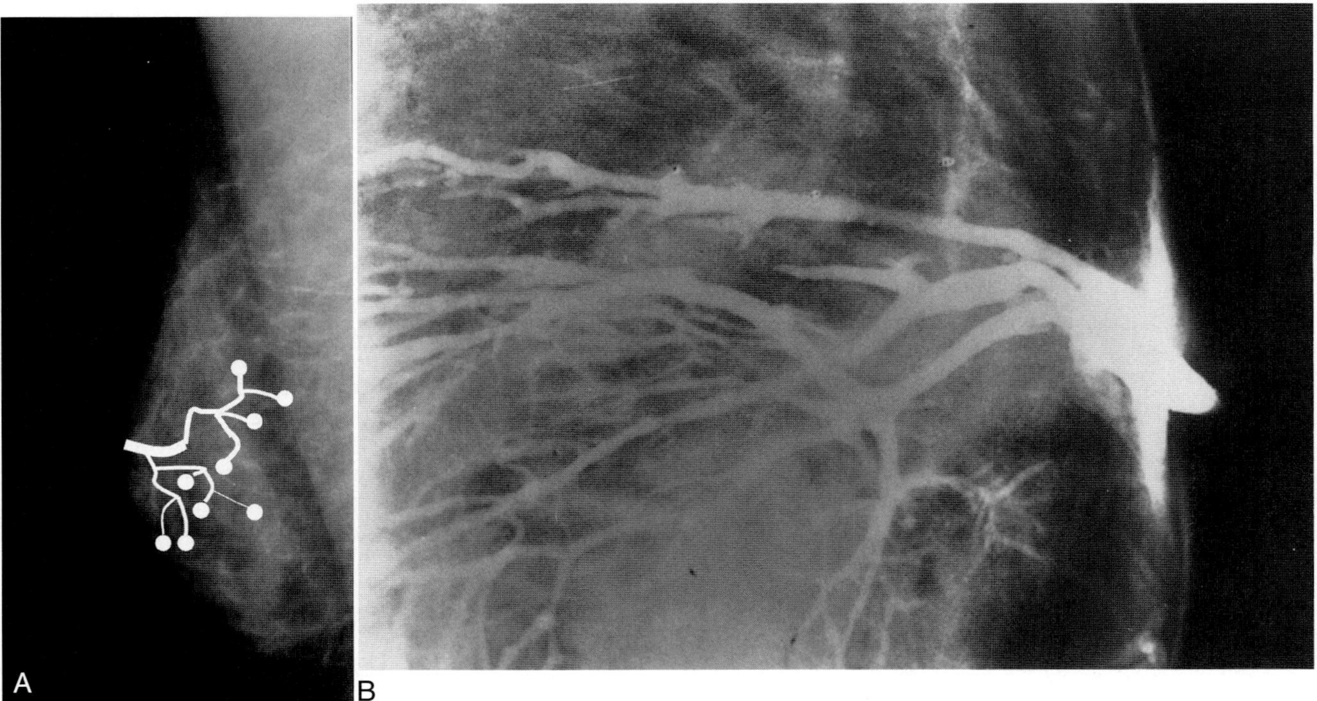

Figure 28–10. Normal ductography. **A,** Mediolateral view of normal arborization of the ductal systems. **B,** Magnified view of the ductogram demonstrating filling of the ductal system. *Continued*

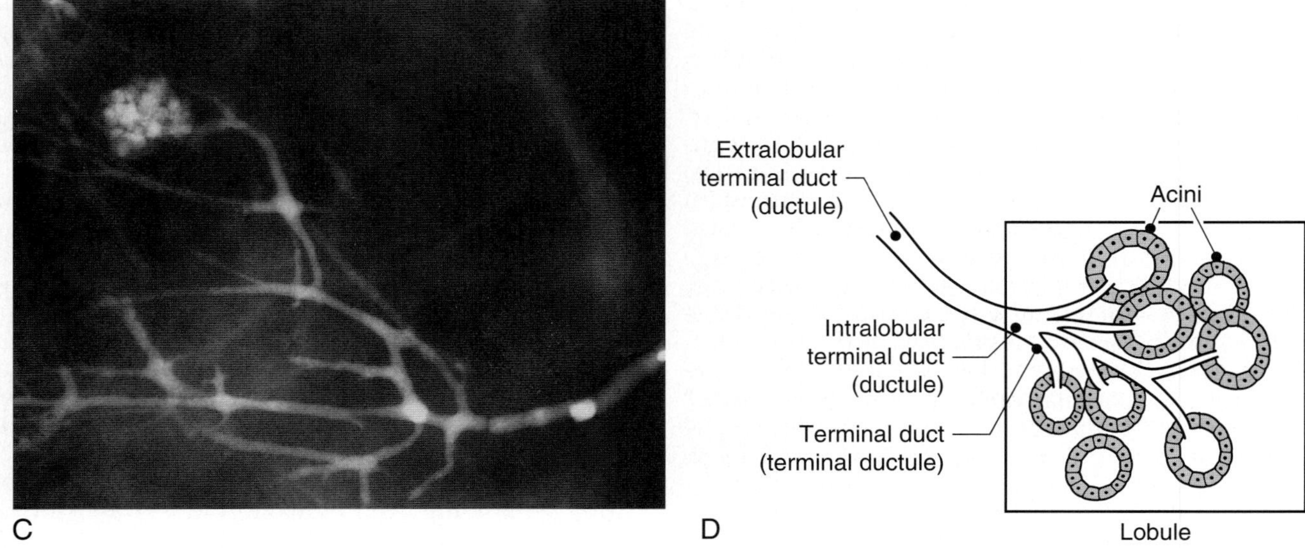

Figure 28–10, cont'd. C, Magnified view of the ductogram with filling of the lobule. **D,** Normal anatomy of the duct system.

lesions in multiple ducts. The most important role played by galactography is the identification and localization of the source of nipple discharge and, therefore, determination of the appropriate surgical therapy.[46,47] Accurate localization is particularly important in a woman with large breasts, in whom the lesion may not be resected during a routine duct excision, or the woman in whom the lesion is located in the peripheral ductal system.[35,46] Accurate localization may also decrease the amount of ductal system that is removed, allowing women of child-bearing age to retain the ability to lactate after terminal duct excision.[48]

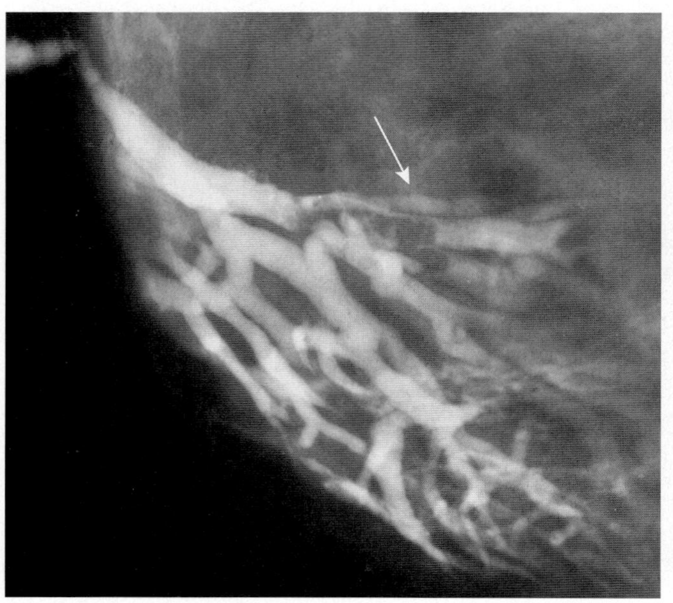

Figure 28–11. Filling defect. This magnification view demonstrates a filling defect *(arrow)* with irregularities.

Nipple Discharge Cytology

Exfoliative cytology of the breast is inherently difficult, because breast carcinoma cells are generally smaller and less pleomorphic than those arising in other organs. In addition, malignant cells are not always present in the discharge and are found more frequently if a tumor is located in a major duct. In one study, only 14 of 31 patients with breast cancer manifesting as nipple discharge had suspicious cytologic findings.[49] In general, cytologic results in nipple discharge analysis have a false-negative rate of 16% to 18%.[33,34] Furthermore, positive cytologic findings do not differentiate between ductal carcinoma in situ and invasive carcinoma.[49] Because of its low sensitivity, nipple discharge cytology should not be relied on for therapeutic decisions.

SKIN CHANGES

Skin changes represent a constellation of signs, including skin retraction, nipple retraction, and skin thickening. They are often vague physical findings with large interobserver variability, even among experienced specialists. In one study of 100 consecutive symptomatic women, the interobserver agreement among four experienced breast surgeons that a physical breast abnormality was present at CBE was only 25%.[50] Given the vagueness of the complaint, the management of the breast skin changes is not uniform.

Clinical Evaluation

Skin retraction consists of a spectrum of changes from local dimpling of the skin to shrinkage of the entire breast. Skin retraction can be a sign of underlying cancer that has attached to the suspensory ligaments, leading to shortening and thickening of the ligaments and overlying skin. This symptom may be hard to notice in the early stages of development. Therefore, a careful examination of the breast in several positions, including comparison of the two breasts for contour or skin asymmetries, should be part of every CBE. Symmetrical skin changes often represent the normal attachment of suspensory ligaments to the skin. This is especially common in the axillary region, where the skin is closely attached to the tail of the breast tissue.

Nipple retraction can be due to thickening and shortening of subareolar ducts. A thorough clinical history should be part of the evaluation of nipple retraction. If the nipple changes are progressive or of recent onset, the likelihood of underlying breast cancer is greater. In addition, it is important to differentiate nipple retraction from benign nipple inversion, which can be corrected by applying manual pressure that draws out the nipple and is not a recent finding. Nipple retraction can also be due to fat necrosis, plasma cell mastitis, and Mondor disease.

Skin thickening could have variety of causes, ranging from obstruction of the superior vena cava, pemphigus, nephrotic syndrome, congestive heart failure, lymphoma, post-irradiation changes, and inflammation to inflammatory carcinoma. Therefore, clinical examination with a thorough history is essential in the management of skin thickening.

Imaging Evaluation

Skin changes may represent a multitude of disorders, including carcinoma. Mammographic examination is essential because it can reveal an underlying mass and malignant microcalcifications. In addition, mammography can show inflammatory changes, such as skin and trabecular thickening, and increased breast density. In some cases, mammography may not offer additional information because of dense breast tissue. In these cases, ultrasonography becomes a useful tool in the detection of masses as well as the depiction of skin and pectoral invasion by carcinoma.[51] Ultrasonography is also more sensitive in the detection of metastatic axillary lymph nodes than is palpation or mammography. In one study, mammography showed only 24% of lymph node invasion, whereas ultrasonography showed 73%.[52] Thus, ultrasonographic evaluation is useful for mapping the extent of the disease so that appropriate treatment can be planned.

PAGET'S DISEASE OF THE NIPPLE

Clinical and Imaging Evaluation

Paget's disease of the nipple is an uncommon manifestation of breast cancer in which malignant cells from intraductal or invasive ductal carcinoma migrate to the nipple or areola. This results in characteristic presentation of a chronic, moist, scaly, or erythematous eruption with symptoms of itching, burning, oozing, or bleeding (Fig. 28–12). Mammographic findings in Paget's disease include nipple and areolar thickening, nipple calcifications, and a retroareolar breast mass. In some cases, however, mammographic findings are normal even though clinical findings suggest Paget's disease of the nipple. In one study, despite high-quality mammography, a tumor was detected in only 71% of the 17 cases of

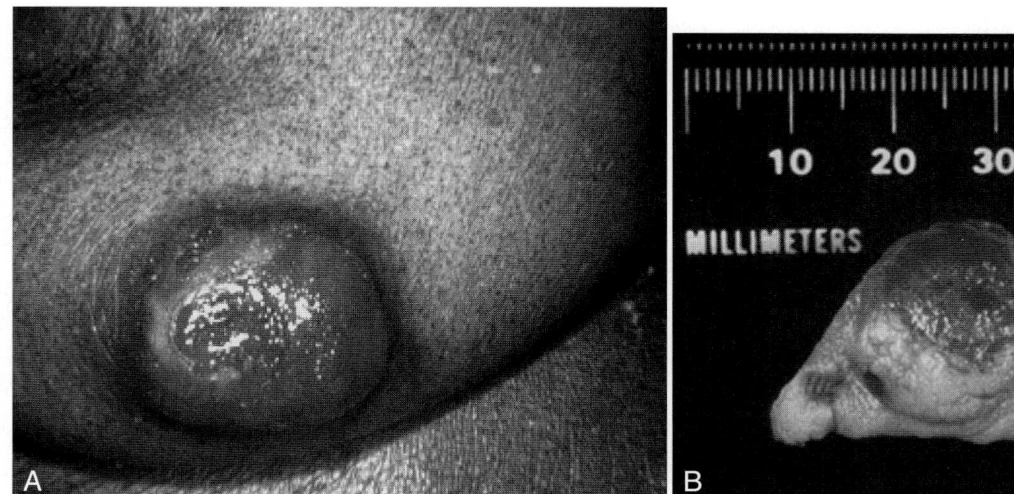

Figure 28–12. Paget's disease. **A,** Paget's disease is manifested by crusting, oozing, and erythema of the nipple, which are caused by tumor within the nipple. **B,** Pathologic specimen from a patient with Paget's disease demonstrating the characteristic crusting, oozing and bleeding of the nipple.

Paget's disease.[53] In another study, only 50% of 34 patients with Paget's disease of the nipple had abnormal mammographic findings.[54] Therefore, treatment should not be delayed in clinically suspicious cases with normal mammographic findings.

References

1. Barton NF, Elmore JG, Fletcher SW: Breast symptoms among women enrolled in a health maintenance organization: Frequency, evaluation, and outcome. Ann Intern Med 1999; 130:651-657.
2. Evans WP 3rd, Mendelson E, Bassett L, et al: Appropriate imaging work-up of palpable breast masses. American College of Radiology: ACR Appropriateness Criteria. Radiology 2000; 215 (Suppl):961-964.
3. Donegan LW: Evaluation of palpable breast mass. N Engl J Med 1992;327:937-942.
4. Boyd NF, Sutherland HJ, Fish EB, et al: Prospective evaluation of physical examination of the breast. Am J Surg 1981;142: 331-334.
5. Layfield LJ, Giasgow BJ, Cramer H: Fine-needle aspiration in the management of breast masses. Pathol Annu 1989;24:23-62.
6. Shabot MM, Goldberg IM, Schick P, et al: Aspiration cytology is superior in Tru-Cut needle biopsy in establishing the diagnosis of clinically suspicious breast masses. Ann Surg 1982;196:122-126.
7. Sterns EE, Fletcher WA: Bilateral cancer of the breast: A review of clinical, histologic, and immunohistologic characteristics. Surgery 1991;110:617-622.
8. Tinnemans JGM, Wobbes T, Hendricks JHCL, et al: The role of mammography in the detection of bilateral primary breast cancer. World J Surg 1988;12:382-388.
9. Baker LH: Breast Cancer Detection Demonstration Project: Five-year summary report. CA Cancer J Clin 1982;32:194-225.
10. van Dam PA, van Goethem ML, Kersschot E, et al: Palpable solid breast masses: Retrospective single and multimodality evaluation of 201 lesions. Radiology 1988;166:435-439.
11. Soo MS, Rosen EL, Baker JA, et al: Negative predictive value of sonography with mammography in patients with palpable breast lesions. AJR Am J Roentgenol 2001;177:1167-1170.
12. Dennis MA, Parker SH, Klaus AJ, et al: Breast biopsy avoidance: The value of normal mammograms and normal sonograms in the setting of palpable lump. Radiology 2001;219:186-191.
13. Orel SG, Schnall MD: MR imaging of the breast for detection, diagnosis and staging of breast cancer. Radiology 2001;220:13-30.
14. Kvistad KA, Rydland J, Vainio J, et al: Breast lesions: Evaluation of dynamic contrast enhanced T1-weighted MR imaging and with T2*-weighted first-pass perfusion MR imaging. Radiology 2000;216:545-553.
15. Denshaw DD: Mammographic screening of the high risk women. Am J Surg 2000;180:288-289.
16. Ciatto S, Cariaggi P, Bularesi P: The value of routine cytologic examination of breast cyst fluids. Acta Cytol 1987;31:301-304.
17. Howat AJ, Stringfellow HF, Briggs WA, Nicholson CM: Fine needle aspiration cytology of the breast: A review of 1,868 cases using the Cytospin method. Acta Cytol 1994;38:939-944.
18. Wills SL, Ramzy I: Analysis of false results in a series of 835 fine needle aspirates of breast lesions. Acta Cytol 1995;39:858-864.
19. O'Neill S, Castelli M, Gattuso P, et al: Fine-needle aspiration of 697 palpable breast lesions with histopathologic correlation. Surgery 1997;122:824-828.
20. Rubin M, Horiuchi K, Joy N, et al: Use of fine needle aspiration for solid breast lesions is accurate and cost-effective. Am J Surg 1997; 174:694-698.
21. Florentine BD, Cobb CJ, Frankel K, et al: Core needle biopsy: A useful adjunct to fine-needle aspiration in select patients with palpable breast lesions. Cancer 1997;81:33-39.
22. Cusick JD, Dotan J, Jaecks RD, Boyle WT: The role of Tru-Cut needle biopsy in the diagnosis of carcinoma of the breast. Surg Gynecol Obstet 1990;170:407-410.
23. Vega A, Garijo F, Ortega E: Core needle aspiration biopsy of palpable breast masses. Acta Oncol 1995;34:31-34.
24. Liberman L, Erberg LA, Heerdt A, et al: Palpable breast masses: Is there a role for percutaneous imaging-guided core biopsy? AJR Am J Roentgenol 2000;175:779-787.
25. Bassett LW: Imaging of breast masses. Radiol Clin North Am 2000;38:669-691.
26. Kerlikowske K, Grady D, Barclay J, et al: Effect of age, breast density, and family history on the sensitivity of first screening mammography. JAMA 1996;276:33-38.
27. Bassett LW, Ysrael M, Gold RH, Ysrael C: Usefulness of mammography and sonography in women less than 35 years of age. Radiology 1991;180:831-835.
28. Meyer JE, Kopans DB, Oot R: Breast cancer visualized by mammography in patients under 35. Radiology 1983;147:93-94.
29. Williams SM, Kaplan PA, Petersen JC, Lieberman RP: Mammography in women under age 30: Is there clinical benefit? Radiology 1986;161:49-51.
30. Gulay H, Bora S, Kilicturgay S, et al: Management of nipple discharge. J Am Coll Surg 1994;178:471-474.
31. Newman HF, Klein M, Northrup JD, et al: Nipple discharge: Frequency and pathogenesis in an ambulatory population. N Y State J Med 1983;83:928-933.
32. Leis HP Jr, Greene FL, Cammarata A, Hilfer SE: Nipple discharge: Surgical significance. South Med J 1988;81:20-26.
33. Fiorica IV: Nipple discharge. Obstet Gynecol Clin North Am 1994;21:453-460.
34. Leis HP Jr: Management of nipple discharge. World J Surg 1989;13:119-122.
35. Jardines L: Management of nipple discharge. Am Surg 1996; 62:119-122.
36. Sickles EA: Galactography and other imaging investigations of nipple discharge. Lancet 2000;356:1622-1623.
37. Seltzer MH, Perloff LJ, Kelley RI, Fitts WT Jr: The significance of age in patients with nipple discharge. Surg Gynecol Obstet 1970;131:519-22.
38. Fung A, Rayter Z, Fisher C, et al: Preoperative cytology and mammography in patients with single-duct nipple discharge treated by surgery. Br J Surg 1990;77:1211-1212.
39. Tabar L, Dean PB, Pentek Z: Galactography: The diagnostic procedure of choice for nipple discharge. Radiology 1983;149: 31-38.
40. Murad TM, Contesso G, Mouriesse H: Nipple discharge from the breast. Ann Surg 1982;195:259-264.
41. Sakorafas GH: Nipple discharge: Current diagnostic and therapeutic approaches. Cancer Treat Rev 2001;27:275-82.
42. Chung SY, Lee KW, Park KS, et al: Breast tumors associated with nipple discharge: Correlation of findings on galactography and sonography. Clin Imaging 1995;19:165-171.
43. Bassett LW, Kimme-Smith C: Breast sonography. AJR Am J Roentgenol 1991;156:449-455.
44. Cardenosa G, Doudna C, Eklund GW: Ductography of the breast: Technique and findings. AJR Am J Roentgenol 1994; 162:1081-1087.
45. Rongione AJ, Evans BD, Kling KM, McFadden DW: Ductography is a useful technique in evaluation of abnormal nipple discharge. Am Surg 1996;62:785-788.
46. Chow JS, Smith DN, Kaelin CM, Meyer JE: Case report: Galactography-guided wire localization of an intraductal papilloma. Clin Radiol 2001;56:72-73.
47. Slawson SH, Johnson BA: Ductography: How to and what if? Radiographics 2001;21:133-150.
48. Scott S, Morrow M: Breast cancer: Making the diagnosis. Surg Clin North Am 1999;79:991-1005.
49. Ciatto S, Bravetti P, Cariaggi P: Significance of nipple discharge clinical patterns in the selection for cytologic examination. Acta Cytol 1986;30:17-20.

50. Boyd NF, Sutherland HJ, Fish EB, et al: Prospective evaluation of physical examination of the breast. Am J Surg 1981;142: 331-334.
51. Kaiser JS, Helvie MA, Blacklaw LR, Roubidoux MA: Palpable breast thickening: Role of mammography and US in cancer detection. Radiology 2002;223:839-844.
52. Gunhan-Bilgen I, Ustun EE, Memis A: Inflammatory breast carcinoma: Mammographic, ultrasonographic, clinical, and pathologic findings in 142 cases. Radiology 2002;223:829-838.
53. Sawyer RH, Asbury DL: Mammographic appearances in Paget's disease of the breast. Clin Radiol 1994;49:185-188.
54. Ikeda DM, Helvie MA, Frank TS, et al: Paget disease of the nipple: Radiologic-pathologic correlation. Radiology 1993; 189:89-94.

Chapter 29 The Male Breast

Prem K. Chantra, Mark S. Shiroishi, George J. So, Jerome S. Wollman, and Lawrence W. Bassett

Mammography of the male breast accounts for less than 1% of mammographic examinations in most breast imaging centers.[1,2] Because of the very low incidence of breast cancers in men, the great majority of mammographic diagnoses should be benign, with most of these being gynecomastia. Therefore, it is important to recognize the features of benign conditions such as gynecomastia to reduce the number of unnecessary surgical biopsies performed in men. By the same token, suspicious lesions should be recognized and thoroughly evaluated.

Indications for mammography in men include evaluation of a palpable mass, recent onset of breast enlargement or tenderness, nipple-areolar skin changes or discharge, and a history of previous breast cancer. Screening mammography is not generally indicated for men. However, mammographically detected nonpalpable cancers have been reported in the contralateral breast of men with a history of breast cancer, suggesting that such men are in a high-risk category and justifying screening.[3,4] Nonetheless, the incidence of either synchronous or metachronous bilateral breast carcinoma in men is reported to be less than 2%.[5]

THE MAMMOGRAPHIC EXAMINATION

The standard mammographic views, craniocaudal (CC) and mediolateral oblique (MLO), of each breast are routinely performed in men. The majority of male breasts are small, making positioning difficult. In muscular patients, the prominent pectoral muscle can obscure the posterior breast tissue much as a breast implant does. In some cases, the "from below" (FB), caudocranial (CC), or reversed CC view shows more of the male breast than the standard CC (Fig. 29–1).[6] However, the FB view is not effective if the patient has a protruding abdomen because of obesity or ascites. Nipple markers are useful, especially when the nipples cannot be positioned in profile. Magnification views and spot compression views may be used, particularly when proliferative fibroglandular tissue associated with gynecomastia is present. Ultrasonography of the breast may be used when a mass is suspected but is difficult to visualize in a man with gynecomastia.[7,8]

NORMAL MALE BREAST

The breast tissues of both sexes are identical at birth and remain relatively quiescent until puberty, when further differentiation takes place under hormonal influences. Estrogens stimulate breast tissue, whereas androgens antagonize these effects. In the peripubertal period in boys, a 30-fold increase in the concentration of testosterone and a 3-fold rise in estrogen levels occur. The majority of boys undergo transient proliferation of the ducts and stroma during the period of rapid sexual maturation, followed by involution and, ultimately, atrophy of the ducts. Therefore, the normal adult male breast is characterized mammographically by radiolucent fat and a few strandlike subareolar densities representing residual ducts and fibrous tissue (Fig. 29–2). The pectoral muscle may be prominent (Fig. 29–3). Intramammary lymph nodes can also be found in normal male breasts (Fig. 29–4).

ABNORMAL MALE BREAST

Table 29–1 lists the most common malignant and benign conditions found with mammography in male patients.

Male Breast Carcinoma

Table 29–2 lists the malignant lesions of the male breast.

Breast cancer in men accounts for 0.2% to 0.9% of all reported breast cancers and less than 1.0% of all cancers in men in the United States.[1,2] Male breast cancer is rare before the age of 40 years, but thereafter the risk increases exponentially with time.[9] The mean age of men with breast cancer is 59 years, about 6 to 11 years older than the mean age in women. Bilateral breast cancer is seen in only 1.4% of cases.[10-12] Incidence rates around the world are less than 1 case per 100,000 man-years and have largely remained stable in the United States and Europe in the last few decades.[13-17] In the United States, approximately 1500 new cases are diagnosed annually, about 400 of which result in death.[18] The relationship of breast cancer to gynecomastia is controversial, but most evidence suggests that the two conditions are not related.[19-25] The reported coexistence of gynecomastia with breast cancer varies in different series from 2% to 35%, probably reflecting the differences in the patient populations studied. Fifty percent of male breast cancer patients have ipsilateral axillary adenopathy at the time of first presentation.

Although most cases of male breast cancer are sporadic, a number of risk factors have been identified (Table 29–3). Klinefelter syndrome is the strongest

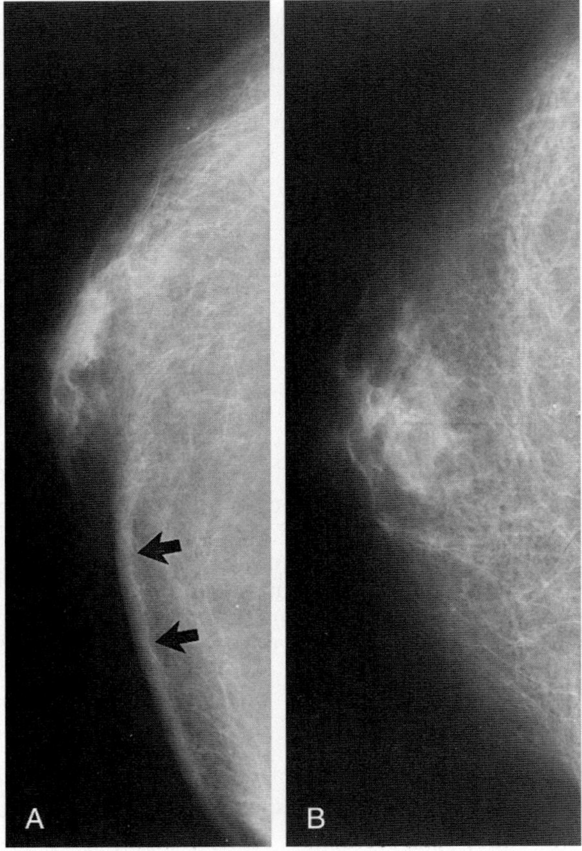

Figure 29–1. The "from below" (FB) view can eliminate unwanted chest wall skin folds and include more breast tissue. **A,** Right craniocaudal (CC) view of a man with gynecomastia shows skin fold *(arrows)* from upper chest wall. **B,** FB, or reversed CC, view includes more breast tissue without skin folds.

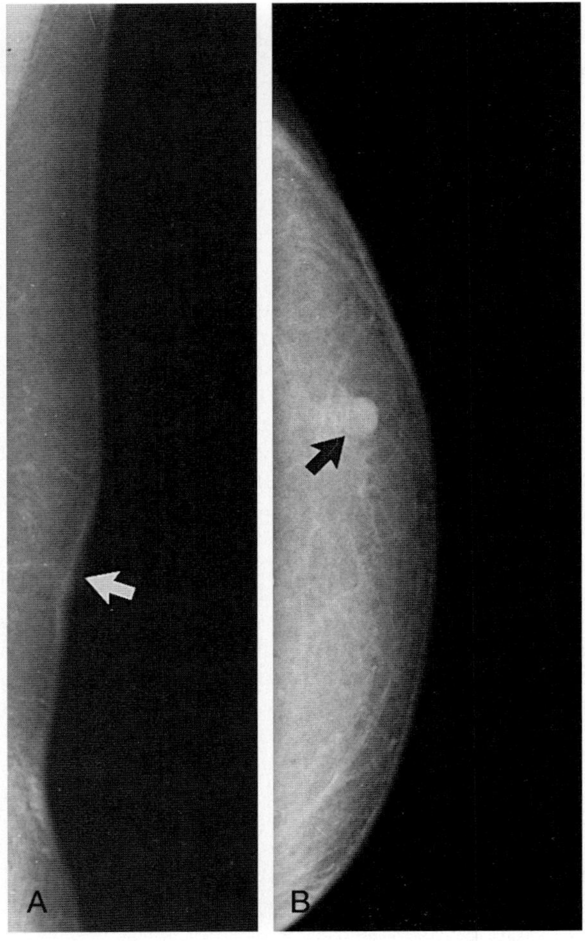

Figure 29–2. Normal left mammograms of a thin 67-year-old man with unilateral right breast gynecomastia. Mediolateral oblique (**A**) and craniocaudal (**B**) mammograms of the non-enlarged left breast show only radiolucent fat. No ductal or glandular opacities were present. Note that no Cooper ligaments are present. *Arrow* indicates nipple. (From Chantra PK, So GJ, Wollman JS, Bassett LW: Mammography of the male breast. AJR Am J Roentgenol 1995;164:853-858.)

Table 29–1. Mammographic Diagnoses in Men

Report*	No. of Examinations	Gynecomastia	Pseudogynecomastia	Carcinoma	Other Diagnoses
Chantra et al[73]	118	96 (81%)	12 (10%)	3 (3%)	5 lipomas, 1 cyst, 1 fat necrosis
Cooper et al[3]	263	213 (81%)	42 (16%)	6 (3%)	2 epidermal cysts, 2 metastases
Dershaw[75]	49	40 (80%)	5 (10%)	3 (6%)	
Quimet-Oliva et al[†]	171	139 (81%)	20 (12%)	20 (12%)	4 mastitis, 4 lipomas, 3 abscesses
Forman[107]	125	98 (78%)		8 (6%)	7 inflammatory lesions, 2 papillomas, 4 benign cases, 6 normal cases

* Superscript numbers indicate chapter references.
† Quimet-Oliva D, Hebert G, Ladouceur J: Radiographic characteristics of male breast cancer. Radiology 1978;129:37-40.

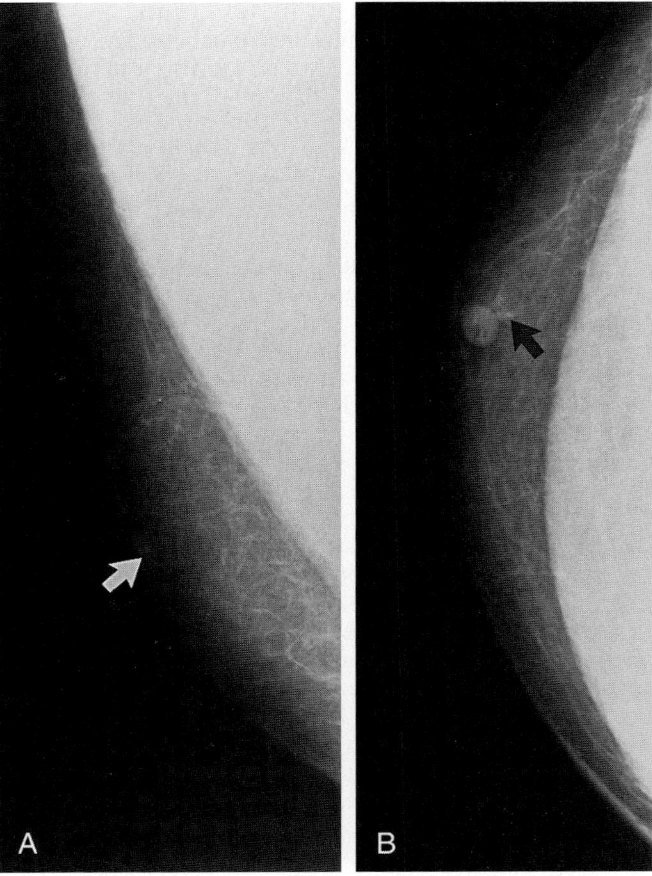

Figure 29–3. Normal right mammograms of a 40-year-old muscular man with contralateral breast tenderness. Mediolateral oblique (**A**) and craniocaudal (**B**) views show a prominent pectoralis muscle obscuring the posterior aspects of the breast, similar to the effect of a breast implant in a woman's breast. The small amount of ductal density *(arrow)* just beneath the nipple was normal. (From Chantra PK, So GJ, Wollman JS, Bassett LW: Mammography of the male breast. AJR Am J Roentgenol 1995; 164:853-858.)

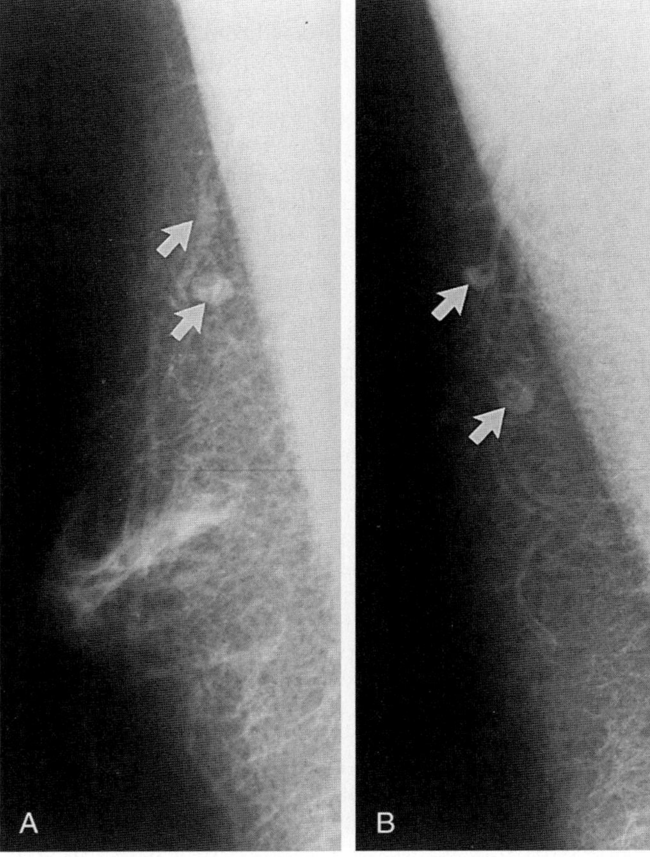

Figure 29–4. Right mediolateral oblique view (**A**) and close-up (**B**) show two benign intramammary lymph nodes (*arrows*) with typical lucent center.

Table 29–2. Malignant Lesions in the Male Breast

Carcinomas
Infiltrating ductal carcinoma (85%)
Ductal carcinoma in situ
Intraductal papillary carcinoma
Others
Metastasis
Prostate carcinoma
Melanoma
Renal cell carcinoma
Lung carcinoma
Lymphoma
Leukemia, chloroma
Phyllodes tumor

Table 29–3. Risk Factors for Male Breast Cancer*

Klinefelter syndrome (strongest risk factor)[16,26]
History of breast cancer in first-degree relative, especially male breast cancer[35]
Inguinal herniorrhaphy[13]
Mumps orchitis[116]
Undescended testes[116]
Testicular injury[116]
African men, black men in Western nations[117,118]
Ionizing radiation[10,42]
Electromagnetic fields[119,120]
Occupational heat exposure[121]
Head trauma (increased prolactin production)[122]
Local chest trauma[123]
Obesity[124]
Treatment with estrogenic hormones, such as for prostatic cancer[112]
Unclear risk: male-to-female transsexuals receiving long-term estrogen therapy

*Superscript numbers indicate chapter references.

risk factor (50-fold increase) for male breast cancer.[16,26] In addition to a higher risk of cancer, patients with this syndrome commonly have coexistent gynecomastia.[27-29]

In the patient undergoing estrogenic treatment for prostate cancer, determining whether a malignancy in the breast is a primary breast carcinoma or a metastasis from prostatic carcinoma can be difficult. For this reason, it is recommended that prostatic-specific antigen (PSA) immunohistochemical staining be performed on the histologic sections of male breast tumors.[30]

Male-to-female transsexuals who are receiving long-term estrogen therapy could be at increased risk for development of breast cancer, although several studies have not shown exogenous estrogen to be a causal factor.[10,31,32] Full acinar and lobular formation will occur in these patients, who are treated with progestative chemical castration combined with feminizing estrogen therapy.[33] Transsexuals should be followed closely for the possible development of breast cancer.[34] Baseline mammograms have been recommended, with additional studies performed when clinical indications are present. However, only four cases of breast cancer have been reported in transsexuals.[33] The precise role of estrogen as an etiologic factor in breast cancer in men is still unknown.

Several cases of early-onset female breast cancer seem to occur with most cases of familial disease, which include male breast cancer. This is seen most often with BRCA2 mutations and, to a lesser degree, with BRCA1 mutations.[35] Although women with the BRCA2 mutation have an 80% chance of experiencing breast cancer, men with this mutation have only a 5% chance.[36,37] The carrier risk of germline BRCA2 mutations is higher in Jewish and Icelandic populations.[38,39] Because daughters of men with breast cancer are at increased risk for development of breast cancer, BRCA gene mutation screening may be indicated.[40]

Biologic Characteristics

Male breast cancer seems to be biologically different from female breast cancer, and its cause is no better understood.[41] Estrogen and progesterone receptors are more common in male breast cancer, findings that may correlate with response to hormone therapy.[42-45] However, one study concluded that high estrogen receptor positivity correlated with a poor prognosis.[46] The use of HER-2/neu (c-erb-B2)/p53 status, ploidy status, and S-phase fraction as a predictor of outcome is unclear.[46-49] Investigators from Spain determined that apolipoprotein D expression was associated with a favorable outcome.[50]

Clinical Management

In general, the underlying cause of breast enlargement in men younger than 45 years of age is much more likely to be gynecomastia. Clinically, male breast cancer resembles female breast cancer, but distinguishing *early* breast cancer from gynecomastia may be difficult.[51] This difficulty may lead some surgeons to proceed directly to surgery if proper diagnostic evaluation is not performed.

Breast cancer typically manifests as a firm, painless mass in the subareolar region, eccentric to the nipple.[52] Nipple retraction or inversion, skin thickening, encrustation, and ulceration are the presenting symptoms in approximately one third of male patients with breast cancer. Nipple discharge in men can be due to benign conditions such as papilloma, duct ectasia, and gynecomastia. Amoroso and coworkers[53] reported that in about 2% of benign male breast diseases, nipple discharge was a symptom. About half of the benign lesions manifesting as nipple discharge are papillomas, and nearly all instances of bloody discharge are caused by papillomas. However, nipple discharge occurs in 14% of men with breast cancers, and this discharge is likely to be serosanguineous. In fact, bloody nipple discharge has a stronger association with underlying carcinoma in men than in women. Ipsilateral axillary adenopathy at presentation is common in male breast carcinoma, and its presence as the only sign has been reported.[48,54] In 5% of cases, male breast cancer manifests as Paget's disease, with erythema, inflammation, skin nodules, and satellite lesions.[44]

The diagnosis of male breast cancer can usually be confirmed with fine-needle aspiration and cytology (FNAC), the findings being similar to those seen in female breast cancer.[55] However, in cases of ductal carcinoma in situ (DCIS) in men, FNAC findings may be inconclusive, and core needle biopsy may be necessary to establish a diagnosis.[56] Because the male breast contains only ducts, most cancers tend to be infiltrating ductal carcinoma or DCIS.[57] Lobule formation rarely occurs in men. However, all other histologic types of breast cancer seen in females have been reported in males, including rare cases of invasive lobular carcinoma.[58,59] Ductography can be performed to diagnose cancer and to establish preoperative localization for surgical treatment of the discharging duct. A slight predilection of male breast cancer for the left breast has been reported.[44]

Owing to the rarity of this disease, most treatment regimens follow those already established for female breast cancer.[13] Most authorities believe that modified radical mastectomy is the best means to achieve locoregional control unless there is chest wall extension, in which case more radical resection, radiation therapy, or both can be used.[60-63] Thus far, no studies have demonstrated the efficacy of systemic adjuvant treatment in male breast cancer.[47] Generally, however, men with node-positive cancers or with node-negative cancers and a significant risk of recurrence undergo adjuvant treatment.

Metastatic spread of male breast cancer parallels that seen in women, the majority of lesions

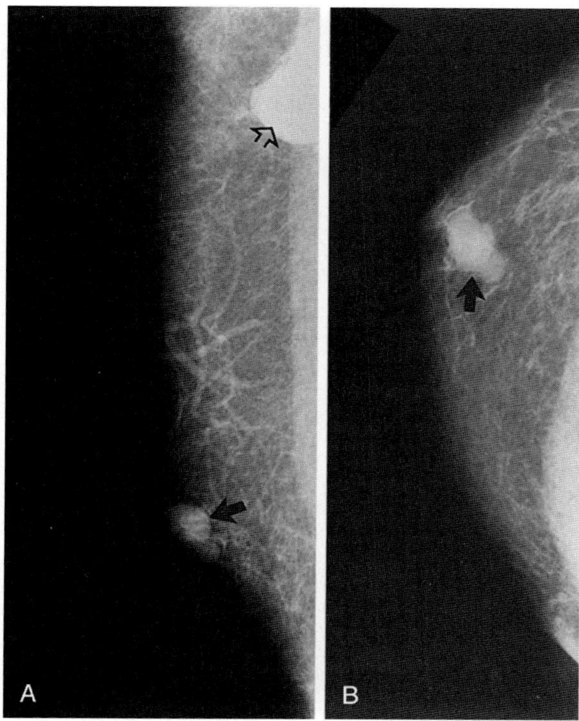

Figure 29–5. Metastatic melanoma. A 51-year-old man with a known history of melanoma presented with a complaint of a palpable mass in the right breast and right axilla. Right mediolateral oblique (**A**) and craniocaudal (**B**) views show a lobular mass *(arrows)* in the subareolar area. In addition, a large axillary lymph node *(open arrow)* was also present. Biopsy of the subareolar mass demonstrated metastatic melanoma.

occurring in the lung and bone.[61] Liver lesions tend to occur less commonly in men.

Metastases to the breast from extramammary malignancies can occur, and most arise from prostatic carcinoma. In addition, metastases arising from melanoma (Fig. 29–5), renal adenocarcinoma, leukemia, lymphoma, urothelial carcinoma, and lung carcinoma also occur.[35,64,65]

There are also two primary lesions in male breast cancer patients, with a disproportionately high percentage (41%) of colon and rectal carcinomas occurring simultaneously with breast carcinoma.[66,67] In contrast, the overall incidence of two primaries is only 3% in female breast cancer.

Stage for stage, the survival rate of male breast carcinoma is similar to that of women. The overall prognosis for men with breast cancer is worse than for women and has been attributed to a number of factors—delayed diagnosis,[60] anatomic factors,[48] inappropriate staging,[58] later stage of disease at presentation,[68,69] and older age at diagnosis.[68] The prognosis largely depends on lymph node status and tumor size, although histologic grade and duration of symptoms also appear to be significant. The presence of a family history of breast cancer does not seem to affect outcome.[70] The overall 5-year survival for male breast cancer is approximately 50%.[35,68] The 5-year survival rate is approximately 53% for men with carcinomas smaller than 2 cm, 44% for those with tumors 2 to 5 cm, and only 25% for those with tumors larger than 5 cm.[4,71] Furthermore, associated comorbid medical conditions also result in worse outcomes in men.

Imaging

Mammography

In younger men, mammography is reserved for those with compelling clinical indications, such as skin changes and nipple discharge.[3] Although mammography is not a replacement for clinical examination, Evans and colleagues[72] found that the modality was able to accurately distinguish between malignant and benign male breast disease. In the absence of overt clinical signs of cancer, a mammographic diagnosis of gynecomastia does not warrant a tissue diagnosis.[3,73]

Male breast cancer can present as a spiculated, ill-defined (Figs. 29–6 and 29–7), or circumscribed mass (Fig. 29–8).[74] Eccentric masses are highly suspicious for carcinoma. Gynecomastia may show some adherence of the skin but never causes ulceration or encrustation. Skin retraction and ulceration are helpful secondary signs and poor prognostic signs. In addition, skin thickening, nipple retraction, and axillary adenopathy may be present.[3,73-75] Calcifications are uncommon in male breast carcinoma (Figs. 29–9 and 29–10). If calcifications are seen, however, they can appear pleomorphic, large, round, and scattered.[76]

Ultrasonography

Very few reports detail the ultrasonographic features of male breast cancer,[7,77-79] which are similar to those found in female breast cancer.[7] Lesions appear as hypoechoic with irregular margins, and sound transmission may vary from dense distal acoustic shadowing to acoustic enhancement.[80] Complex cystic masses are also suggestive of malignancy, particularly papillary DCIS.[56] Secondary signs of malignancy may be important and can include architectural distortion of normal breast tissue and disruption of the subcutaneous fat layer.[81] Although nonspecific, the presence of axillary lymph nodes, especially those without normal fatty hilum, can also indicate malignancy.

Nuclear Medicine

The use of technetium Tc 99m (^{99m}Tc) tetrofosmin and ^{99m}Tc sestamibi scintimammography has been described in male breast cancer and classically demonstrates intense focal uptake of radiotracer.[82,83]

Pathology

The majority of primary male breast cancers are infiltrating ductal carcinomas of the "not otherwise

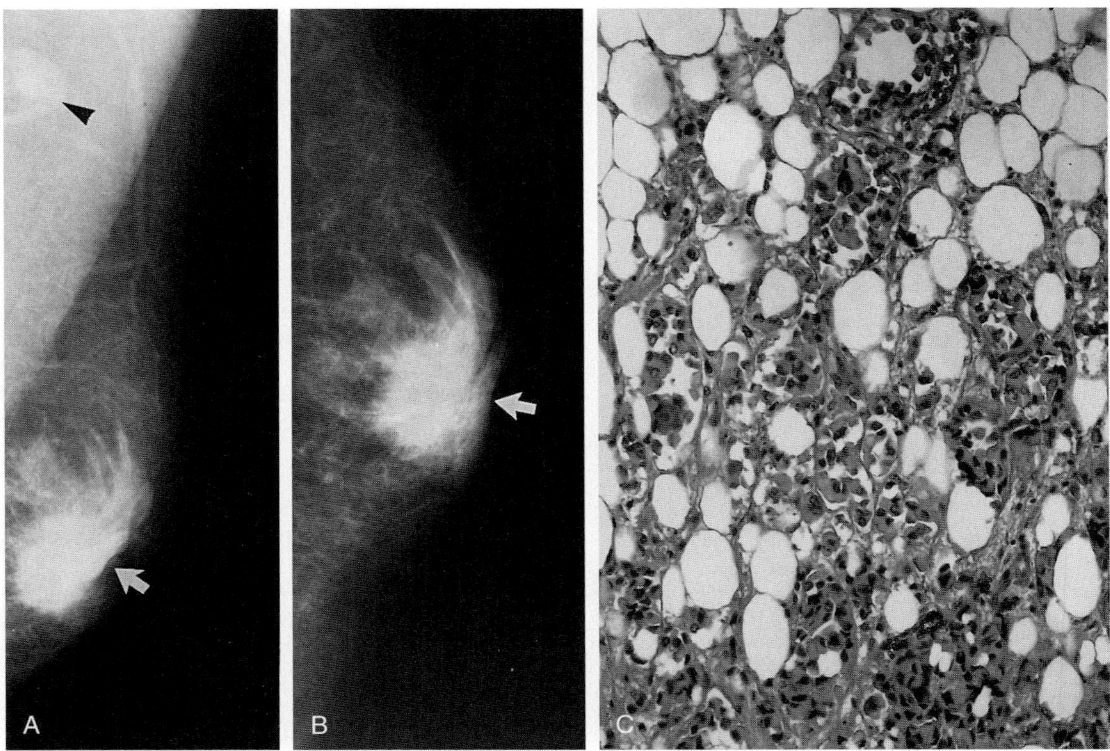

Figure 29–6. Male breast cancer. A 47-year-old man who had noticed a painless enlarging mass in his left breast for 3 years presented with a complaint of the onset of nipple crusting and discharge. Left mediolateral oblique (MLO) (**A**) and craniocaudal (**B**) views show a large spiculated mass directly under the nipple. The nipple is retracted *(arrow)*, and the overlying skin is thickened. An enlarged axillary lymph node *(arrowhead)* is seen on the MLO view. Surgery revealed infiltrating ductal carcinoma with 2 of 35 axillary nodes showing metastases. **C,** Photomicrograph shows pleomorphic tumor cells infiltrating between lipocytes (original magnification, ×100). The patient underwent a modified radical mastectomy and 9 months of chemotherapy and has been symptom free for 2 years. (From Chantra PK, So GJ, Wollman JS, Bassett LW: Mammography of the male breast. AJR Am J Roentgenol 1995;164:853-858.)

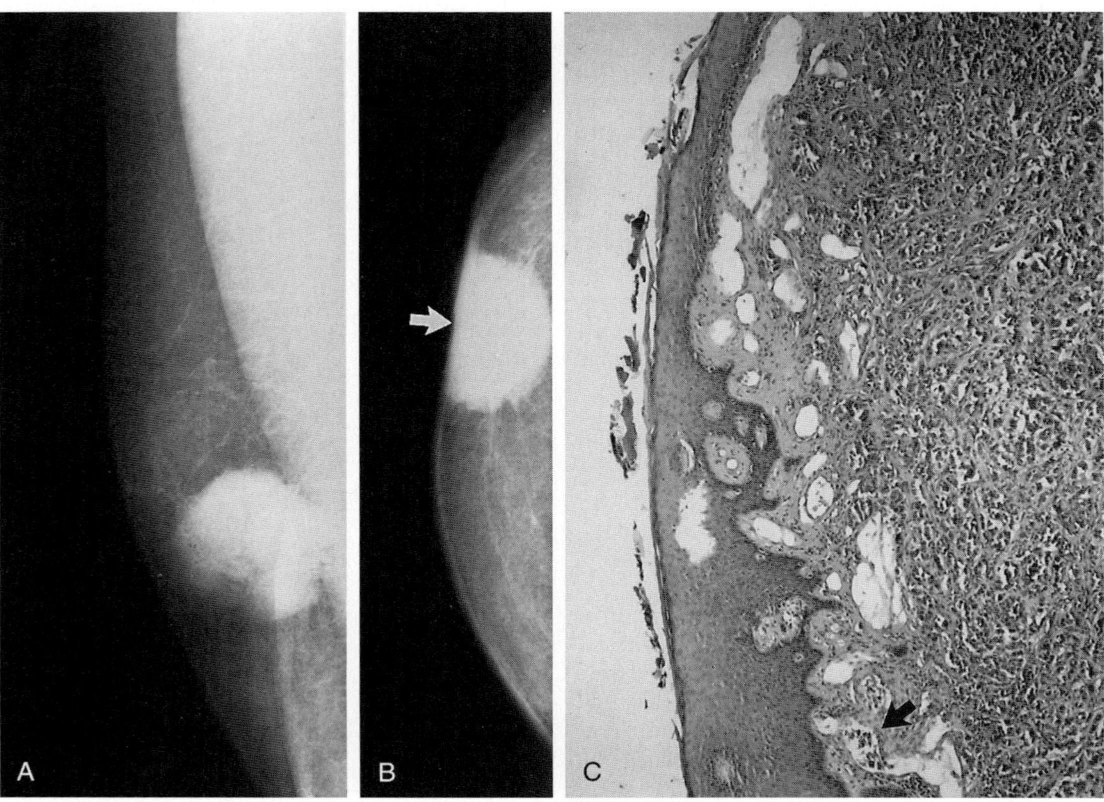

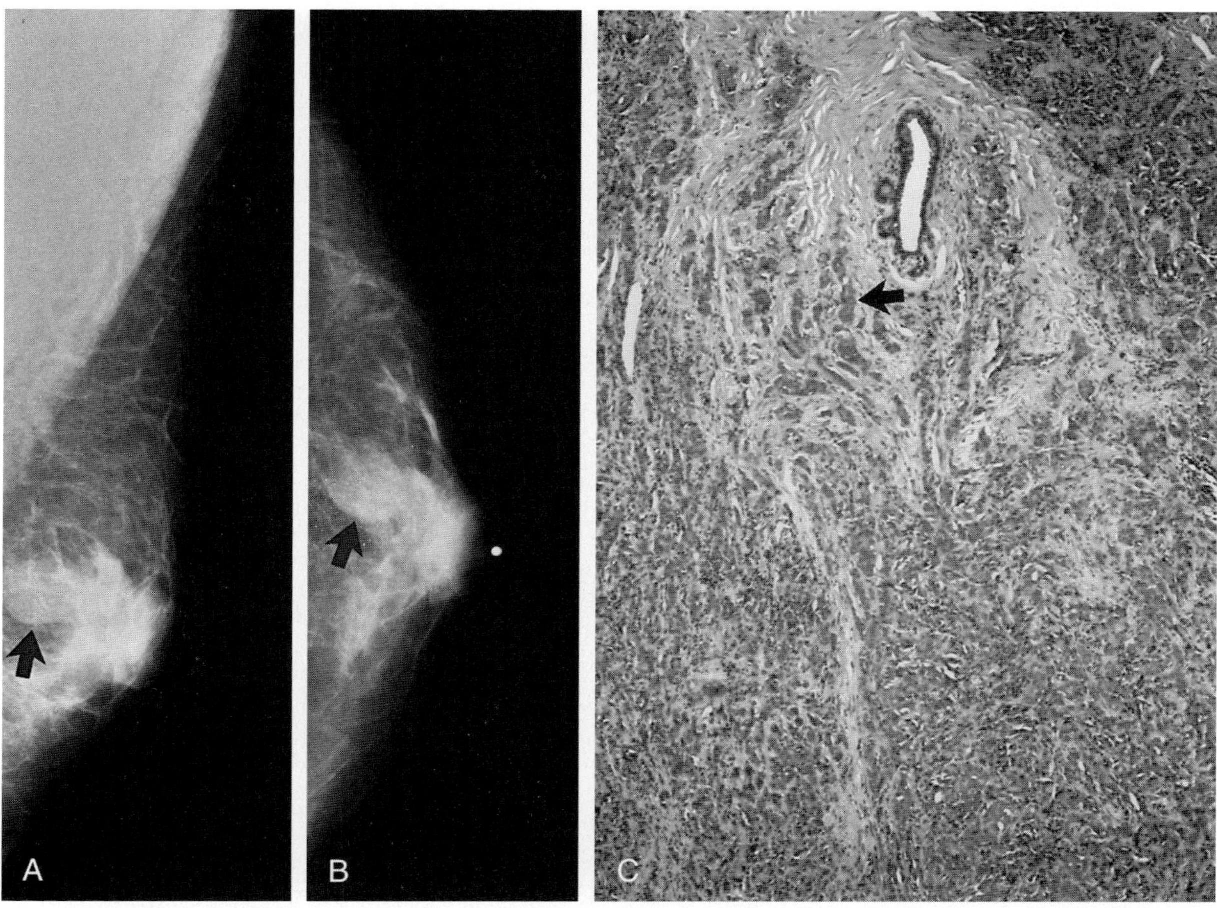

Figure 29–8. Male breast cancer. A 74-year-old man had had a painless, hard mass underneath his left nipple for 2 years. No nipple discharge or skin thickening was seen. Left mediolateral oblique (**A**) and craniocaudal (**B**) views show mild dendritic gynecomastia. In addition, a circumscribed, retroareolar mass is seen projecting posterior to the gynecomastia into the surrounding fatty tissue. **C,** Surgical specimen photomicrograph demonstrates solid and linear arrangement of neoplastic cells infiltrating the fibrotic stroma *(arrow)* (original magnification, ×10). The diagnosis was high-grade infiltrating ductal carcinoma.

Figure 29–7. Male breast cancer. A 56-year-old man had an enlarging nontender mass in his right breast for 2 years. **A** and **B,** Right mammograms show a radiodense, ill-defined subareolar mass extending to the edge of the pectoral muscle on the mediolateral oblique view (**A**). The craniocaudal view (**B**) shows flattening and retraction at the area around the nipple *(arrow)* and skin thickening. **C,** Photomicrograph shows high-grade ductal carcinoma involving the overlying skin. Note small anaplastic cells infiltrating the dermis and dilated lymphatics *(arrow)* (original magnification, ×40). Axillary node dissection revealed no metastases.

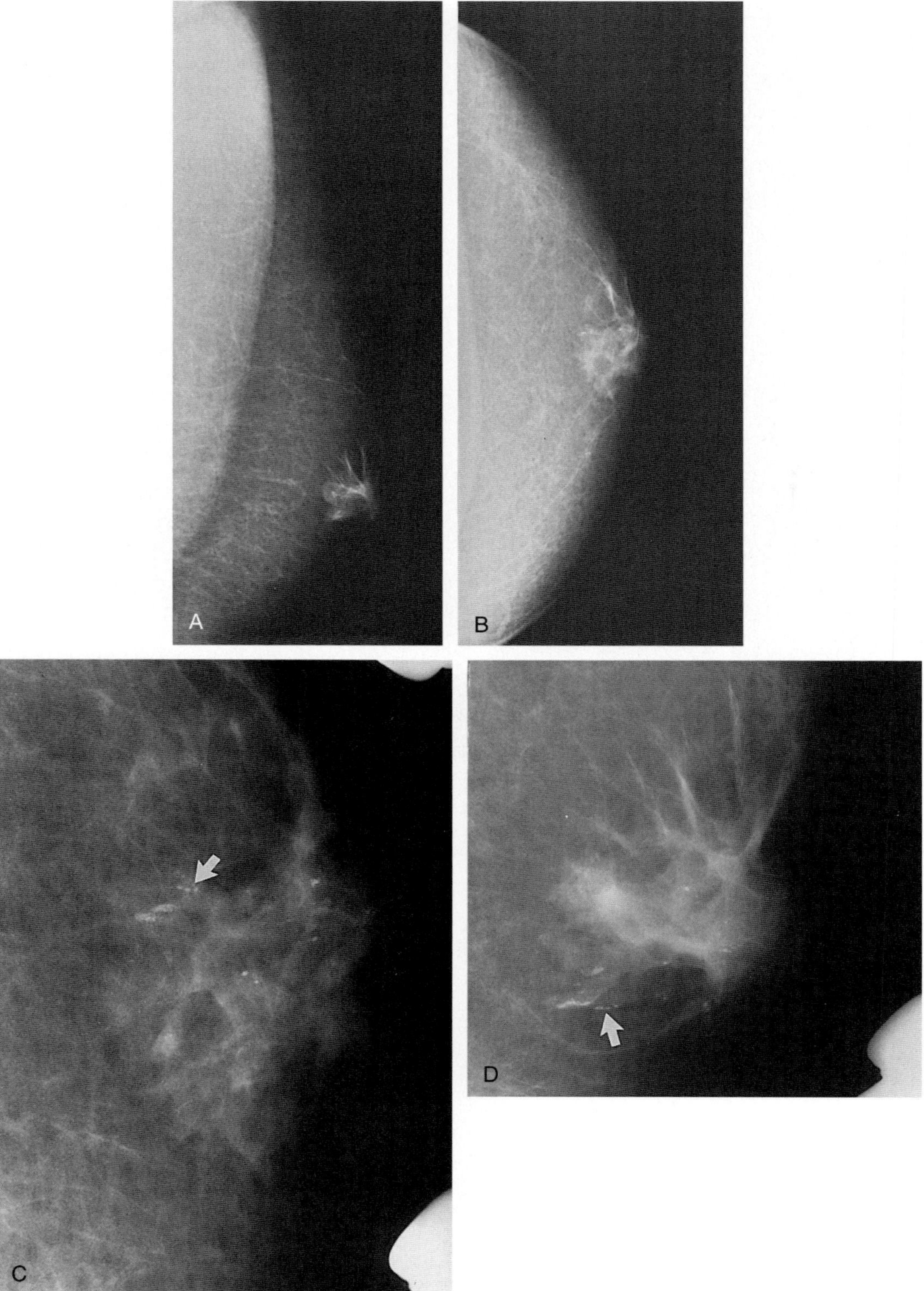

Figure 29–9. Calcifications in male breast carcinoma. A 50-year-old man complained of a mass under his left nipple. Mediolateral oblique (**A**) and craniocaudal (**B**) mammograms show increased density under the nipple. **C** and **D,** Magnification views of the density demonstrate heterogeneous microcalcifications *(arrow)*, some of which were in a linear and branching distribution. Biopsy revealed invasive carcinoma.

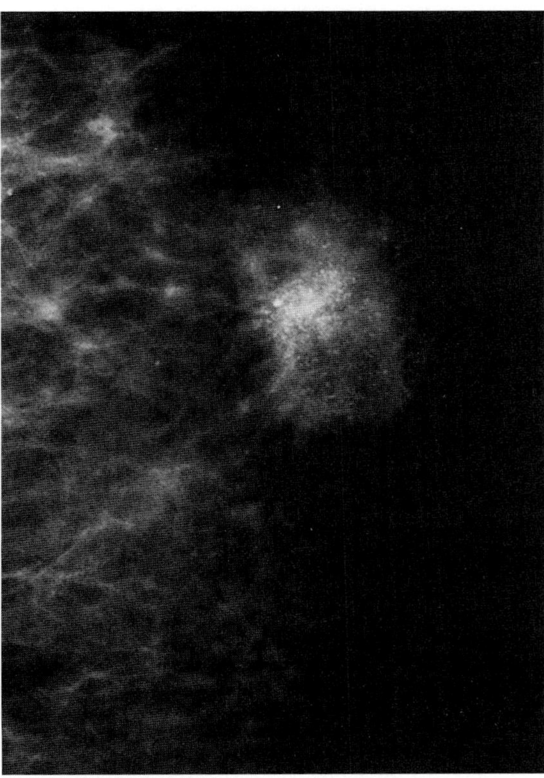

Figure 29–10. Male breast cancer with microcalcifications. The calcifications in this case were numerous, clustered, and varying in size and shape.

specified" (NOS) type.[53,77,84] Medullary and papillary carcinomas account for approximately 5% of cases. Most cases of DCIS (papillary subtype) in males have been associated with 35% to 50% of invasive carcinomas.[85,86] However, pure DCIS without an invasive component is very rare, representing about 7% of all breast cancers treated in men.[87] Intracystic papillary carcinoma accounts for about 5% to 7.5% of the cases, a larger proportion than that reported in women.[69,88] Therefore, malignancy should be considered in the diagnosis of breast cysts in men.[77,84] Small cell carcinomas and a rare case of lobular carcinoma in a patient with Klinefelter syndrome have also been reported.[89] Pure mucinous, medullary, papillary, and tubular histologic types have a somewhat more favorable prognosis than infiltrating ductal carcinoma.[13] Rare fibrosarcoma can manifest in the breast like the more common ductal adenocarcinoma (Fig. 29–11).

Gynecomastia

Gynecomastia is enlargement of the male breast due to benign ductal and stromal proliferation so that the breast takes on a female form (Greek *gyne*, pertaining to women; *mastos*, breast). Approximately 85% of male breast masses are due to gynecomastia, which is the most common disorder in the male breast that may be detected incidentally at the time of a routine physical examination as either a painful tender mass beneath the nipple or a progressive painless enlargement of the breast.[73] Most cases of gynecomastia can be managed conservatively; however, the disorder must be differentiated from malignant processes and can occasionally be the presenting clinical sign of a significant underlying disease.[90] Among men 17 years and older in the general population, the prevalence of gynecomastia has been reported to be between 32% and 65%.[91] In hospitalized patients, a prevalence of 72% has been reported in male veterans aged 50 to 69 years.[92] Gynecomastia is seen in more than 60% of men in the seventh decade of life.[93]

The development of gynecomastia is believed to be due to hormone imbalance, with a relative excess of female hormone.[91] Pathophysiologic mechanisms resulting in gynecomastia can be divided into the following four categories: (1) estrogen excess, (2) androgen deficiency, (3) androgen receptor defects, and (4) enhanced sensitivity of breast tissue to estrogenic hormones. Gynecomastia can be physiologic or due to underlying diseases, including medication effect (Table 29–4). Braunstein[91] reported that 25% of patients seeking consultation for gynecomastia are found to have idiopathic gynecomastia; another 25% have pubertal gynecomastia; 10% to 20% of cases are drug related; and 8% are associated with cirrhosis or malnutrition. A number of rare causes of gynecomastia have been reported in the literature. These include environmental occupational exposure to estrogen during the manufacture of oral contraceptives and exposure to estrogen secondary to contact with a sexual partner's vaginal estrogen cream.[94,95]

Physiologic Gynecomastia

Physiologic gynecomastia has three distinct peaks in age distribution—neonatal, pubertal, and senescent. Neonatal gynecomastia is thought to be secondary to transplacental passage of estrogens. Palpable breast tissue transiently develops in 60% to 90% of all newborns.[91] Considerable breast enlargement may occur, occasionally in association with a clear or cloudy colostrum-like nipple discharge termed "witch's milk." The nodule usually involutes spontaneously within days or weeks but may persist for months in breastfed infants. Other than reassurance of the parents, no treatment is required.

Pubertal gynecomastia occurs in adolescent boys during the transition from the prepubertal to the postpubertal stage, when a surge in pituitary gonadotropins results in a transient increase in the estrogen-to-testosterone ratio.[90] This proliferation of the ducts and stroma manifests during the period of rapid sexual maturation, within 1 to 2 years of enlargement of the testes (ages 12 to 15 years). The prevalence of pubertal gynecomastia ranges from 4%

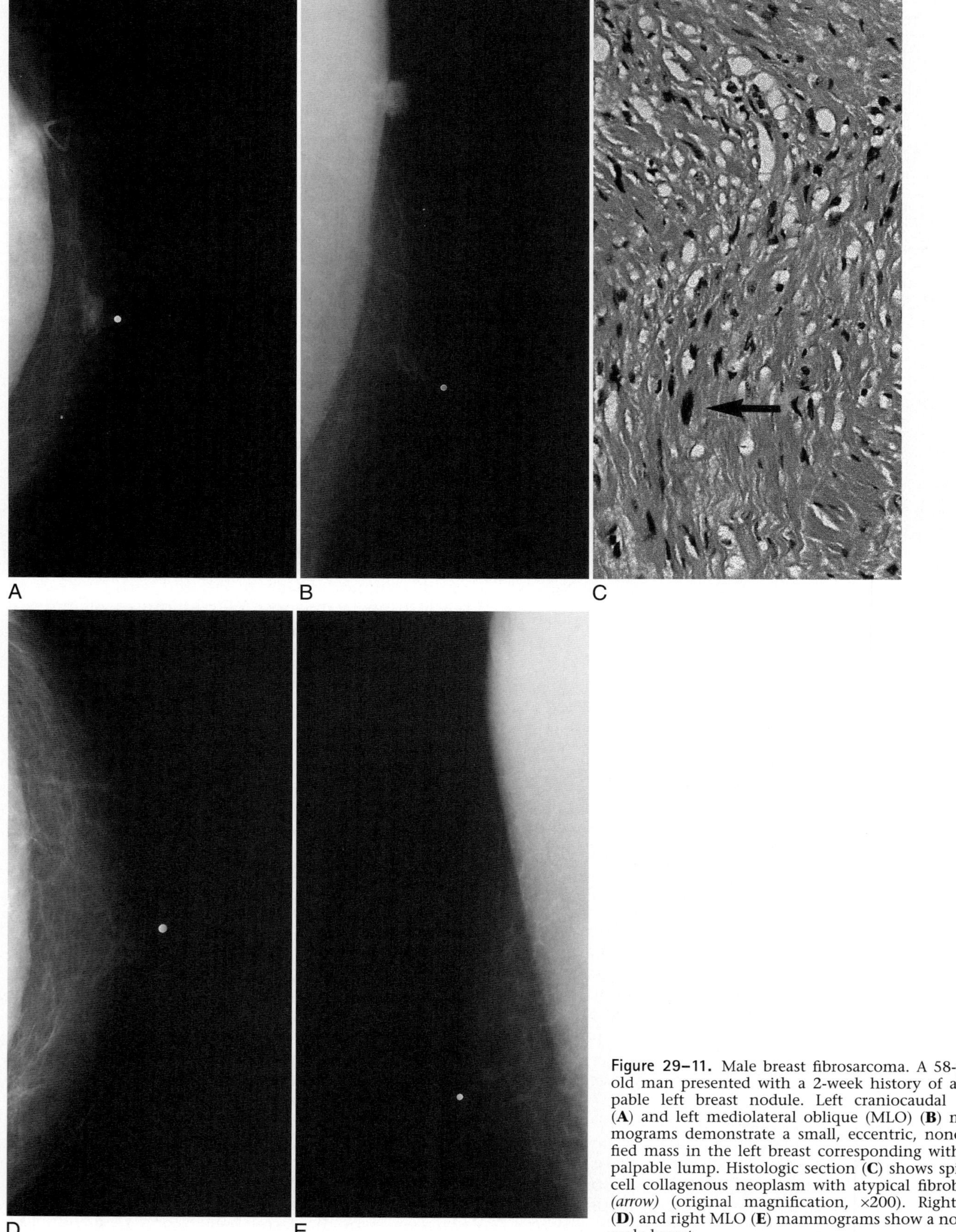

Figure 29–11. Male breast fibrosarcoma. A 58-year-old man presented with a 2-week history of a palpable left breast nodule. Left craniocaudal (CC) (**A**) and left mediolateral oblique (MLO) (**B**) mammograms demonstrate a small, eccentric, noncalcified mass in the left breast corresponding with the palpable lump. Histologic section (**C**) shows spindle cell collagenous neoplasm with atypical fibroblasts *(arrow)* (original magnification, ×200). Right CC (**D**) and right MLO (**E**) mammograms show a normal male breast.

Table 29–4. Conditions Associated with Gynecomastia

Predisposing conditions	
Estrogen excess	Gonadal origin
	True hermaphroditism
	Testicular estrogen-producing tumors
	Nontesticular tumors
	Adrenal cortical neoplasm
	Lung carcinoma
	Hepatocellular carcinoma
	Liver disease
	Nonalcoholic and alcoholic cirrhosis
Androgen deficiency	Aging
	Hypoandrogen states
	Primary testicular failure
	Klinefelter syndrome (XXY)
	Kallman syndrome
	Secondary testicular failure
	Trauma
	Orchitis
	Cryptorchidism
	Irradiation
	Hydrocele
	Varicocele
	Spermatocele
	Renal failure
Drug-related conditions	
Drugs with estrogenic or estrogen-related activity	Anabolic steroids
	Digitalis
	Estrogens
	Heroin
Drugs that inhibit the action and/or synthesis of testosterone	Antineoplastic agents (vincristine, nitrosoureas, methotrexate)
	Cimetidine
	D-Penicillamine
	Diazepam
	Flutamide
	Ketoconazole
	Phenytoin
	Spironolactone
Drugs with unknown mechanisms for induction of gynecomastia	Amiodarone
	Busulfan
	Furosemide
	Isoniazid
	Methyldopa
	Reserpine
	Theophylline
	Tricyclic antidepressants
	Verapamil

Adapted from Bland KI, Page DL: Gynecomastia. In Bland KI, Copeland EM III (eds): The Breast: Comprehensive Management of Benign and Malignant Diseases. Philadelphia, WB Saunders, 1991.

to 69%, depending on the diagnostic criteria used in the studies.[89] Pubertal gynecomastia is usually bilateral and asymptomatic, but it may have disturbing psychologic aspects involving body image and personality adaptation. This type of gynecomastia normally resolves spontaneously within a few months or up to 2 years after onset. A complete physical examination, including careful palpation of the testicles to exclude the nonphysiologic causes of gynecomastia, is recommended. If history and physical examination are normal, reassurance and periodic follow-up are adequate for clinical management. In some pubertal male subjects, gynecomastia may be pronounced and protracted because of an imbalanced ratio between estrogens and androgens or an inherent hypersensitivity of the breast tissues to estrogenic stimulation. Severe and progressive cases of pubertal gynecomastia may require medical or surgical treatment.

Senescent gynecomastia, which occurs in men older than 60 years, is common and thought to be secondary to a decrease in testicular function. The serum free testosterone level drops, but estradiol levels continue to be normal. Gynecomastia in older men may be accentuated owing to increased serum estradiol levels secondary to conversion of peripheral adipose tissue.[96] In obese elderly men, aromatization of androgens to estrogens in the adipose tissue increases. The extent of breast enlargement in these cases is directly correlated with body mass index (BMI) and with advancing age. In persons with a BMI greater than 25 kg/m^2, the prevalence of gynecomastia is 85%, compared with 40% in a group of nonobese men.[92] Senescent gynecomastia often regresses spontaneously within 6 to 12 months of onset, although physical examination commonly reveals persistent enlargement of the breast disc.[97] If gynecomastia has been present for more than 1 year, irreversible hyalinization and fibrosis of the stroma occur along with a reduction of epithelial proliferation.[98]

Clinical Management

When a patient is referred for evaluation of possible gynecomastia, a careful drug history should be taken. The breast and regional lymph nodes should be palpated, and physical signs of hyperthyroidism, liver failure, and testicular atrophy or tumor should be excluded.[90] Hormonal investigation (measurements of serum testosterone, estradiol, human chorionic gonadotropin [hCG], luteinizing hormone [LH], prolactin, liver function, thyroid-stimulating hormone, and thyroxine) should be reserved for patients with recent breast enlargement and no identifiable cause. Depressed LH or increased hCG and estradiol values are indications for testicular ultrasonography; if ultrasonographic findings are normal, chest radiography and abdominal computed tomography should be considered.

Gynecomastia can be unilateral or bilateral, and bilaterally symmetrical or asymmetrical. There is currently no standard method to define and grade the severity of this condition.[98] The Marshall Tanner breast stages used to record pubertal changes in girls have often been used.[99] Some investigators have suggested that gynecomastia is always a bilateral process and that unilateral presentations are actually the early stage in the development of a bilateral involvement. A 40% incidence of gynecomastia was found in a histologic study of male breasts in 447 consecutive autopsy cases, only 4 of which had obvious gross enlargement of the breasts.[100] All of the cases showed bilateral histologic changes consistent with gynecomastia, with the changes sometimes more marked in one breast than in the other.

Clinical breast examination for suspected gynecomastia should be performed with the patient supine. The physician places the thumb and the index finger at the opposite poles of the breast (e.g., 2 o'clock and 8 o'clock positions) and elevates the breast tissue up from the chest wall in a pinching fashion. In adolescent boys, different criteria have been used in various studies to diagnose gynecomastia. In adult men who are not obese, at least 2 cm of firm subareolar breast tissue should be present before the diagnosis of gynecomastia is made. In the early phase, the subareolar tissue is rubbery with a discrete subareolar disc, which is freely mobile and unattached to the skin. A hallmark of gynecomastia is its central, symmetrical location under the nipple. Therefore, the presence of an eccentric mass in relation to the nipple should be viewed with suspicion for malignancy. Patients with gynecomastia are generally asymptomatic, but breast tenderness, the symptom that usually leads them to seek medical attention, is reported in 20% of cases. Nipple discharge should be viewed with suspicion because a much higher percentage of cases of male breast cancer demonstrate this feature compared with cases of gynecomastia.[90] In the Western literature, gynecomastia is reported not to be causally related to the development of male breast cancer, although the two conditions can coexist because of a high prevalence of gynecomastia in older men and patients with Klinefelter syndrome.[20,21,23-25,96]

The physical appearance of the breasts of obese men may simulate gynecomastia through deposition of adipose tissue *(pseudogynecomastia)*. Physical examination of the fatty breast reveals the absence of a mound of firm or rubbery subareolar tissue, and the entire breast has the same consistency as the fatty tissue of the axillary fold.

Surgical treatment of gynecomastia involves a subtotal subcutaneous mastectomy performed through an areolar or periareolar incision.[101] Medical treatment consists of danazol or tamoxifen therapy.[102-105] Prophylactic low-dose radiotherapy can be considered for a patient who will be undergoing therapy with a drug strongly associated with gynecomastia.[106]

Imaging

Mammography

The mammographic hallmark of gynecomastia is the presence of a subareolar density concentrically distributed around the nipple, representing various degrees and stages of ductal and stromal proliferation.[75] Mammography of the normal breast shows a homogeneously radiolucent appearance with minimal strands of ductal or interlobar connective tissue.[73,81] Three mammographic patterns of gynecomastia have been described (Table 29–5).[75,107,108]

The first pattern is the *early nodular pattern* (florid phase on histopathology), which is seen in patients with gynecomastia of less than 1 year's duration (Fig. 29–12).[109] In this type, a relatively well-demarcated nodule under the nipple extends into the posterior fatty tissue of the breast in a fanlike configuration, evenly distributed above and below the midplane of the nipple (Fig. 29–13). In more severe cases, the nodule becomes triangular in appearance with the nipple at the vertex of the triangle or becomes a subareolar, disc-shaped mass (Fig. 29–14).

Table 29–5. Patterns of Gynecomastia

Early NODULAR or triangular pattern (florid phase on histopathology)
DENDRITIC pattern (fibrous or quiescent phase)
Diffuse GLANDULAR pattern

A later *dendritic pattern* (quiescent fibrous phase on histopathology) features a flame-shaped central subareolar opacity with prominent linear projections (dendrites) radiating into the deeper adipose tissue toward the upper-outer quadrant of the breast (Figs. 29–15 and 29–16). Williams[100] and Michels and colleagues[110] reported cases of chronic gynecomastia of many years' duration that featured combined pathologic and mammographic characteristics of both the triangular and dendritic types.

A *diffuse glandular* pattern features diffuse, dense nodular parenchyma in an enlarged breast that mimics the density seen in a dense female breast. This pattern of gynecomastia is commonly seen in patients who receive exogenous estrogen, such as men who undergo a sex change operation and those who are treated for advanced prostatic carcinoma (Figs. 29–17 and 29–18). In these situations, the relatively rapid breast enlargement usually has a conical or pyramidal contour, unlike the rather rounded or hemispherical shape found in women. Severe gynecomastia can also be distinguished from a dense female breast by the lack of Cooper ligaments. The high doses of estrogens given to patients with prostatic carcinoma often cause gynecomastia, which can be painful and psychologically distressing. A low dose of radiotherapy administered to the breasts prior to estrogen administration has been reported to reduce the incidence of gynecomastia from 85% to 11%.[111] Tamoxifen and LH-releasing hormone analogues have largely replaced estrogens in first-line hormonal therapy for prostatic cancer.[112]

Pseudogynecomastia, an enlargement of the breast due to obesity, is readily differentiated from true gynecomastia by means of the preponderance of radiolucent fat and the absence of dense retroareolar tissue in pseudogynecomastia (Fig. 29–19).

Ultrasonography

The ultrasonographic appearance of gynecomastia demonstrates breast tissue in the subareolar palpable area and often mimics the ultrasonographic findings

Text continued on p. 549

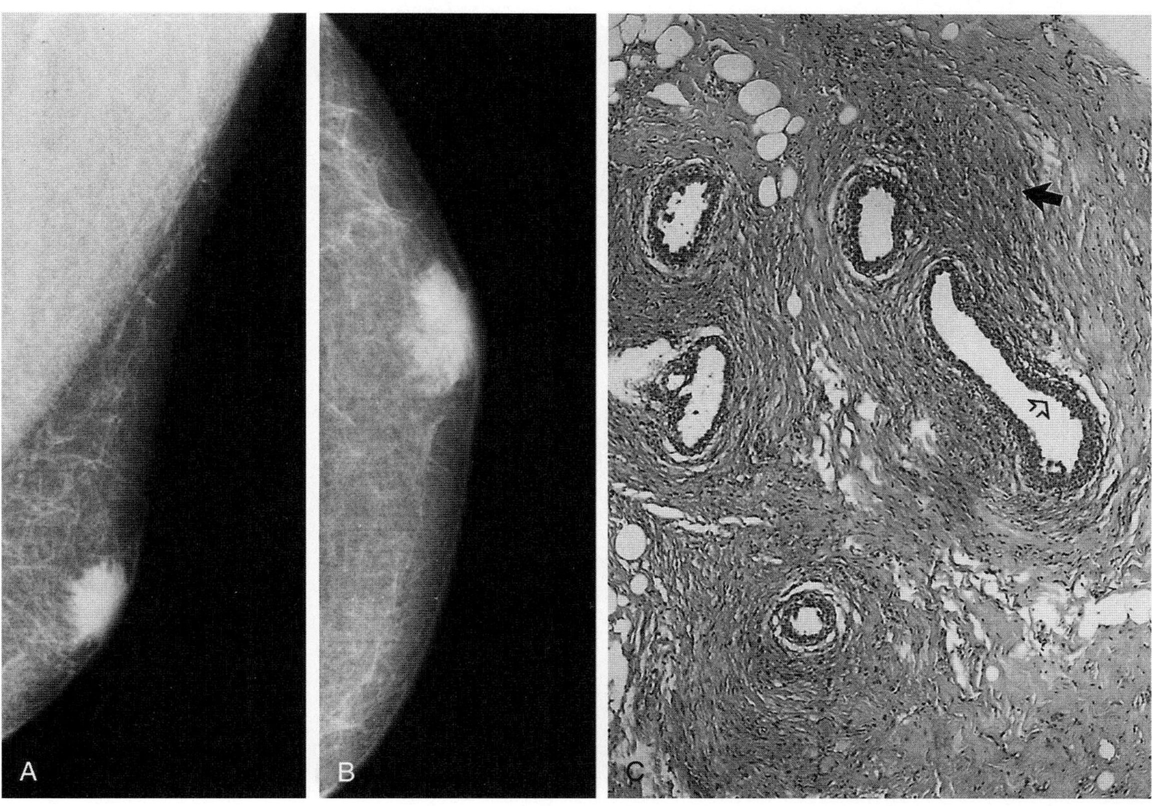

Figure 29–12. Early gynecomastia, nodular pattern (florid histopathologic phase). A 69-year-old man presented with a 2-week history of a tender retroareolar left breast mass. Left mediolateral oblique (**A**) and craniocaudal (**B**) mammograms show a discoid opacity beneath the nipple. No nipple retraction or skin thickening is seen. No calcification was noted. **C,** Photomicrograph of biopsy specimen demonstrates early-stage gynecomastia; note the dilated ducts with epithelial hyperplasia *(open arrow)* and periductal edema *(closed arrow)* with surrounding cellular, early fibrous tissue (original magnification, ×40). (From Chantra PK, So GJ, Wollman JS, Bassett LW: Mammography of the male breast. AJR Am J Roentgenol 1995;164:853-858.)

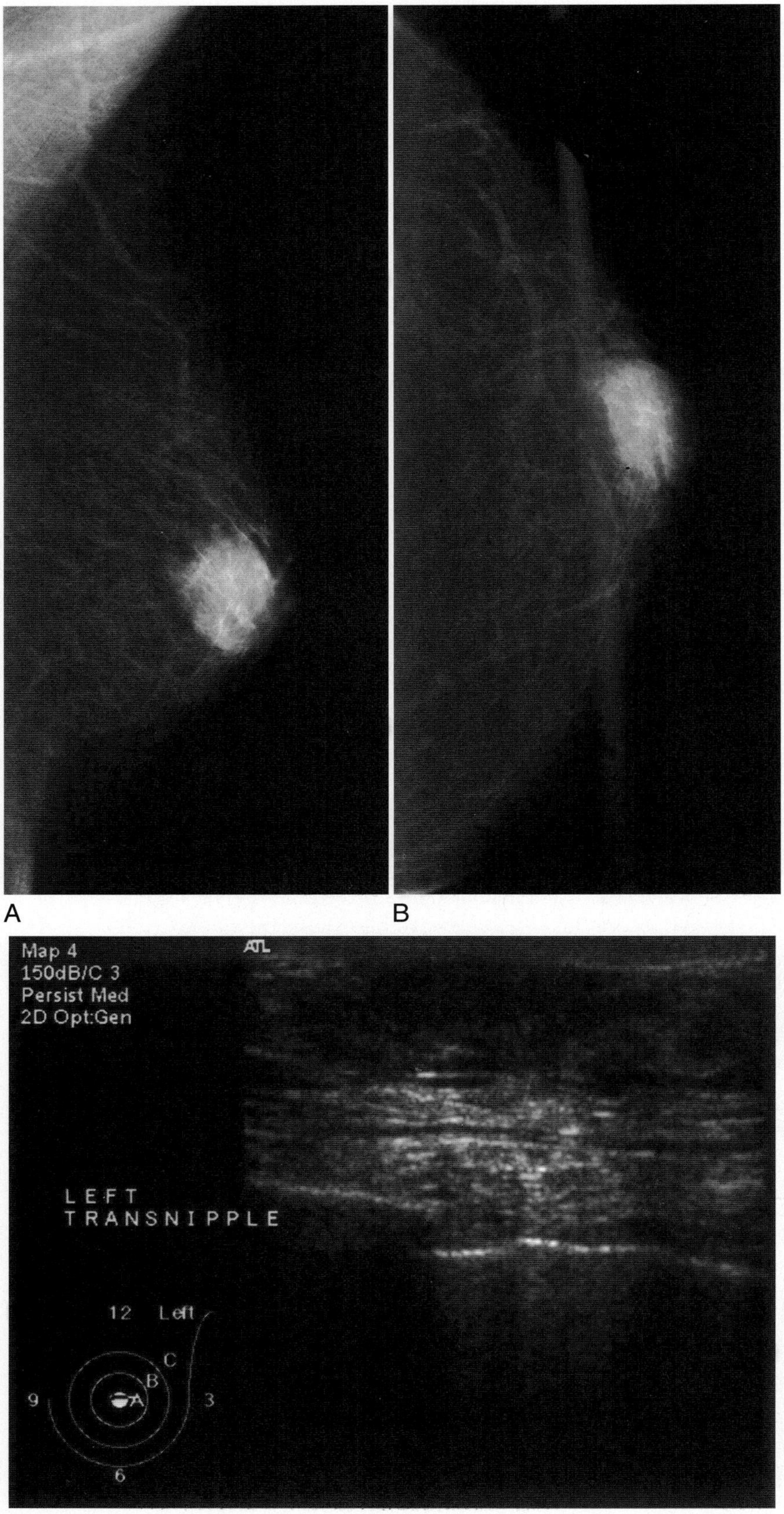

A B

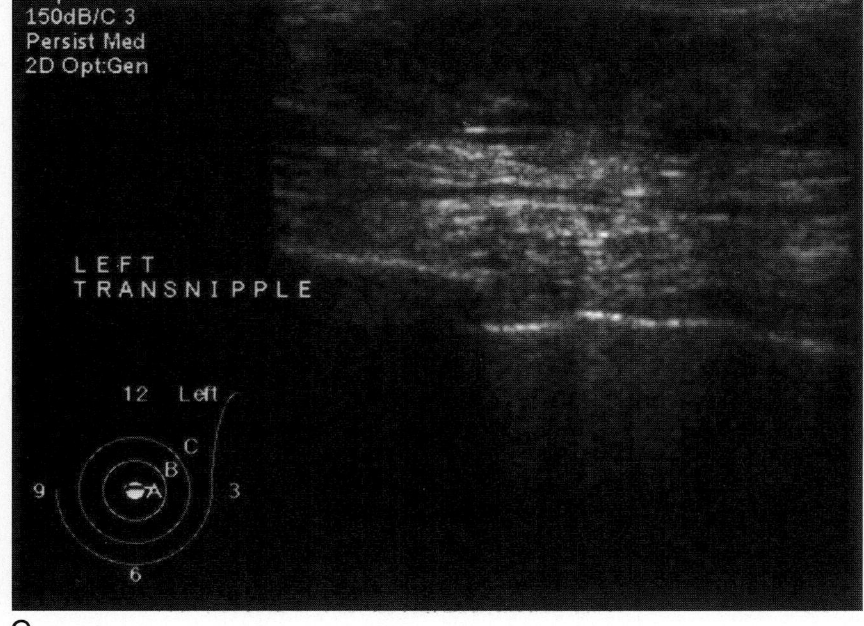

C

Figure 29–13. Nodular, triangular pattern of gynecomastia. A 70-year-old man who had been taking diuretics for hypertension presented with a history of bilateral breast tenderness for 1 month. Left mediolateral oblique (**A**) and craniocaudal (**B**) mammograms show a symmetrical triangular, fanlike opacity in the retroareolar area. Left breast ultrasonogram (**C**) demonstrates a fan-shaped subareolar hypoechogenicity with a fairly definable posterior border correlated with the mammographic finding of nodular gynecomastia.

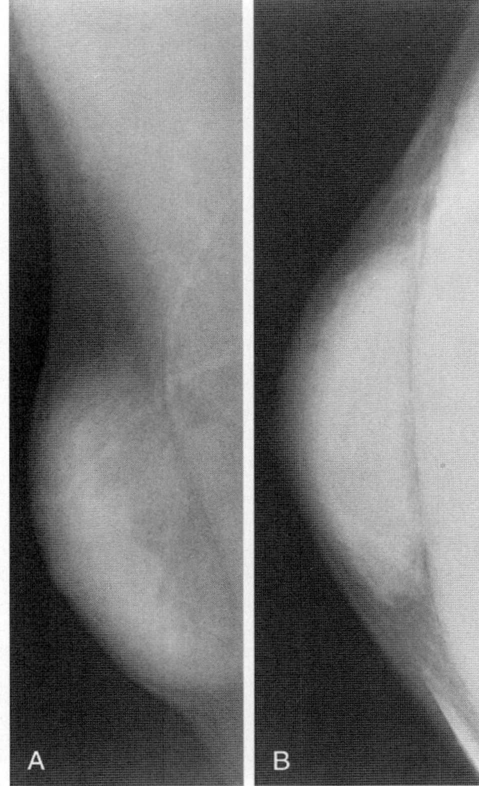

Figure 29–14. Severe disc-shaped gynecomastia. A 60-year-old man complained of having a painful right breast for approximately 1 year. Right mediolateral oblique (**A**) and craniocaudal (**B**) mammograms show a large disclike mass occupying almost the entire breast. Fine-needle aspiration revealed gynecomastia.

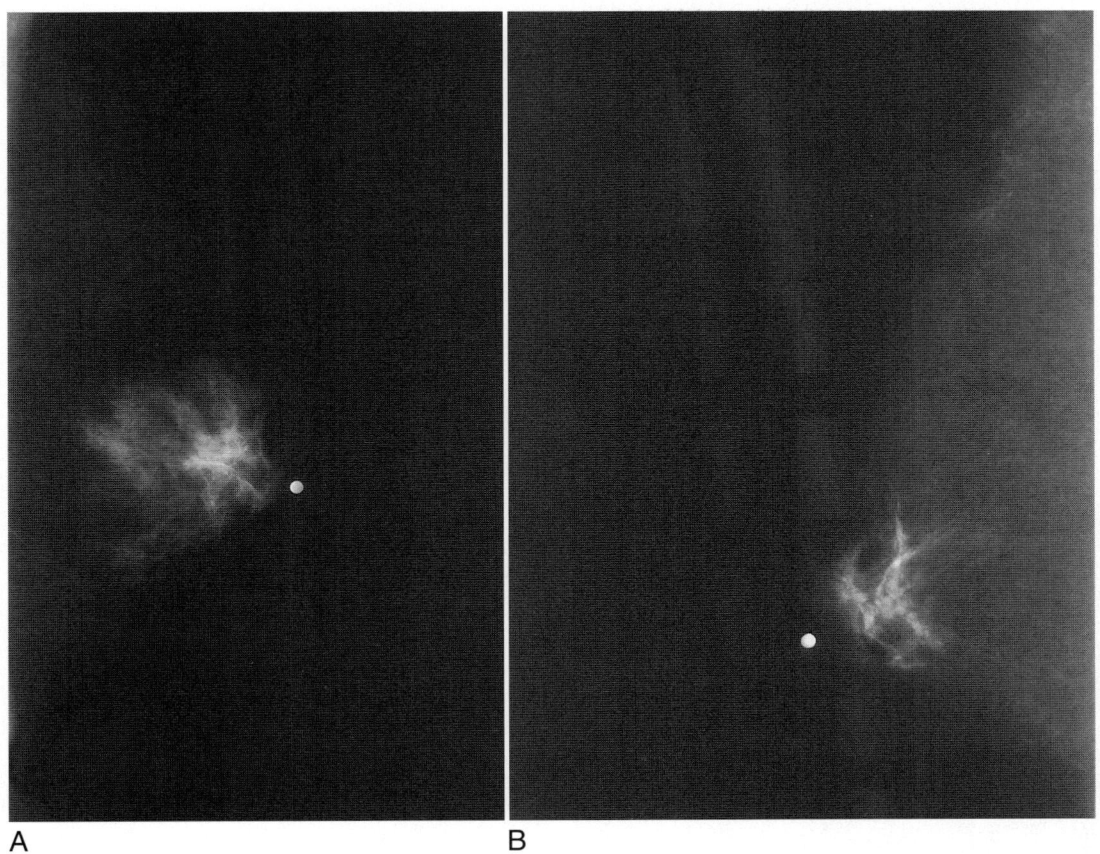

Figure 29–15. Late gynecomastia, dendritic pattern (fibrous or quiescent histopathologic phase). **A,** Left mediolateral oblique mammogram of a 71-year-old man with bilateral (right > left) breast tenderness for 9 months. **B,** Right mediolateral oblique mammogram of a 76-year-old man with chronic bilateral breast pain. Both images show an opacity radiating from behind the nipple into the fatty tissue in a "dendritic pattern." Note the symmetrical distribution of the ductal proliferation posterior to the nipple.

Continued

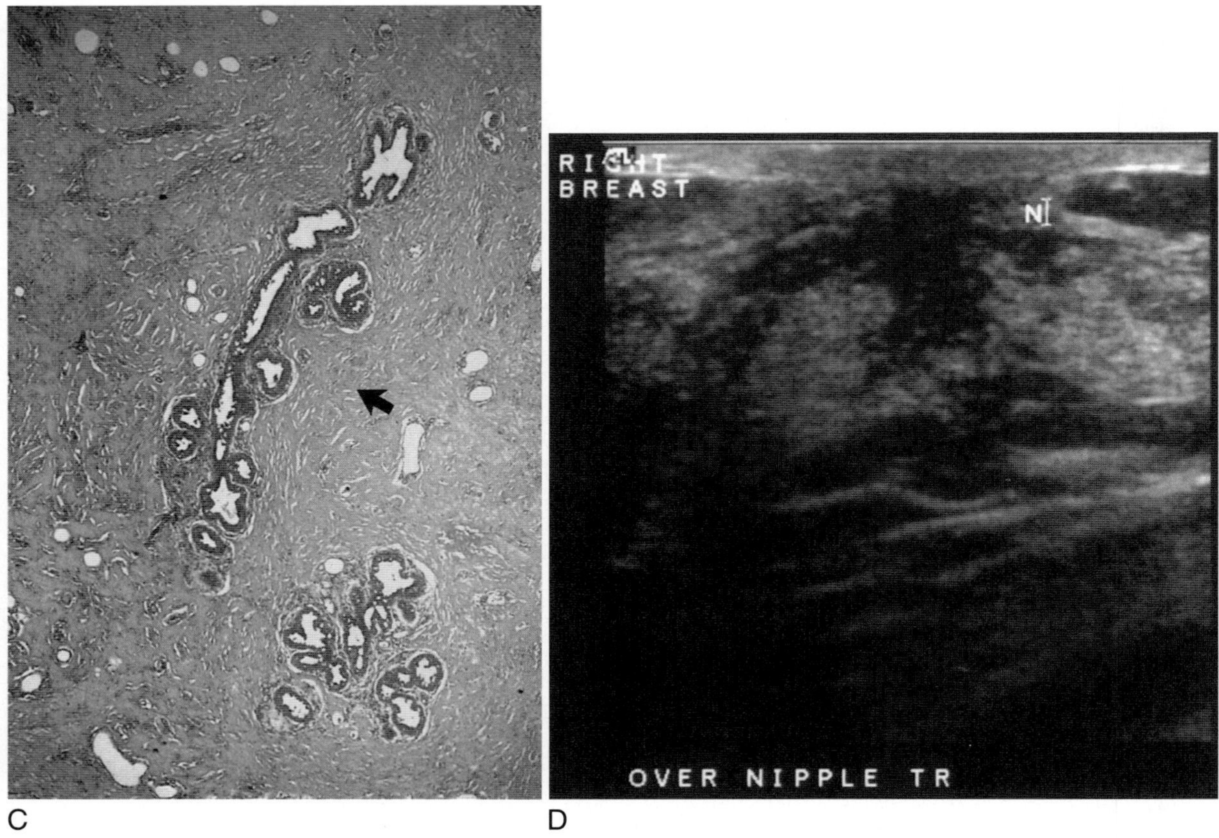

Figure 29–15, cont'd. C, Photomicrograph shows extensive dense hyaline fibrosis *(arrow)* surrounding ducts with hyperplastic ductal epithelium (original magnification, ×20). (From Chantra PK, So GJ, Wollman JS, Bassett LW: Mammography of the male breast. AJR Am J Roentgenol 1995; 164:853-858.) **D,** Sonogram shows subareolar hypoechogenicity with a stellate posterior border, extending into the surrounding echogenic fibrous tissue.

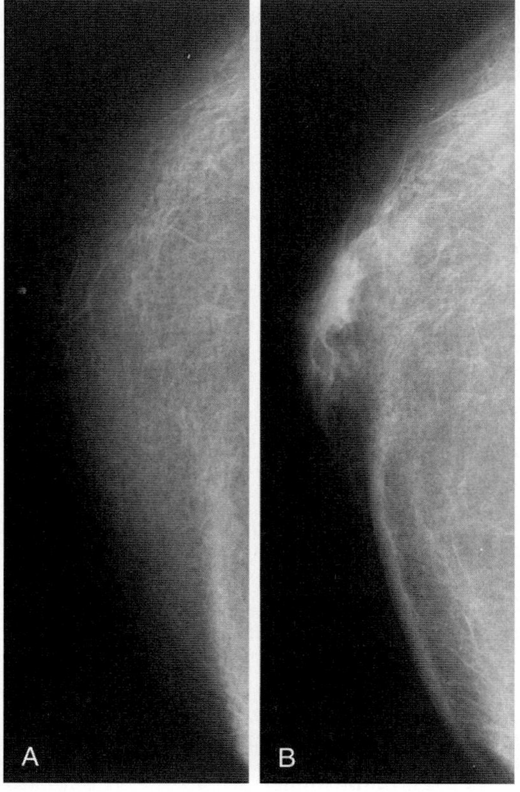

Figure 29–16. Evolving gynecomastia. A 68-year-old man undergoing cimetidine therapy for peptic ulcer disease complained of enlargement and intermittent pain in the left breast. **A,** Right craniocaudal (CC) mammogram at original presentation shows a normal appearance. **B,** Right CC mammogram taken 15 months later demonstrates development of dendritic gynecomastia in the interval.

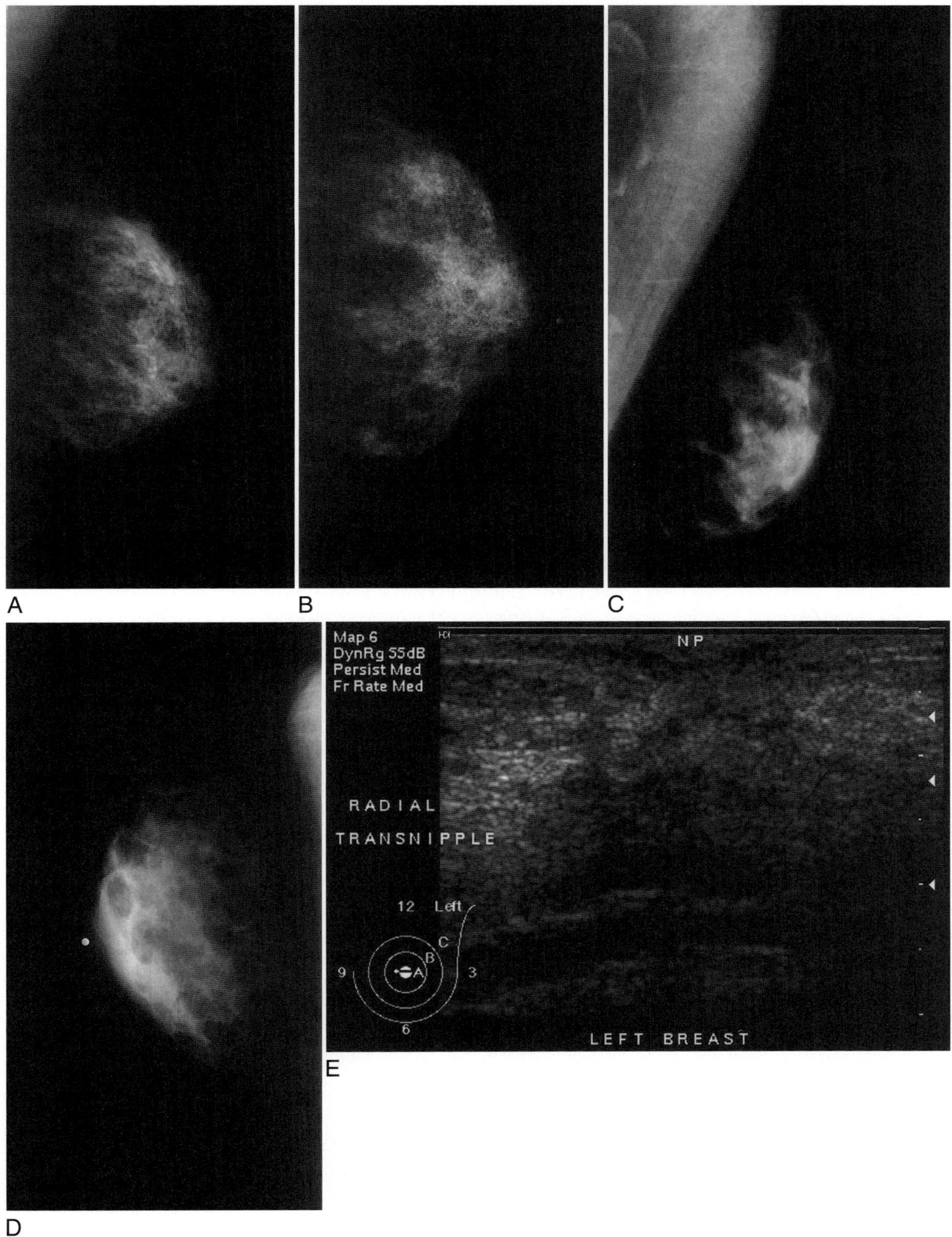

Figure 29–17. Severe gynecomastia, glandular pattern. Left mediolateral oblique (MLO) (**A**) and craniocaudal (CC) (**B**) mammograms of a 52-year-old man who has been taking spironolactone (Aldactone) for 5 years and presented with chronic breast enlargement. Left MLO (**C**) and CC (**D**) mammograms of a 53-year-old male-to-female transsexual who had been taking estrogen for 15 years. Clinical breast examination revealed large lumpy breasts with no dominant masses. Mammograms show diffuse breast enlargement with dense parenchyma mimicking the appearance of a female breast. In both patients, the other breast had a similar appearance. Note the lack of Cooper ligaments on the MLO. **E,** Ultrasonogram of the first patient demonstrates overall increased echogenicity in the breast, simulating fibroglandular tissue.

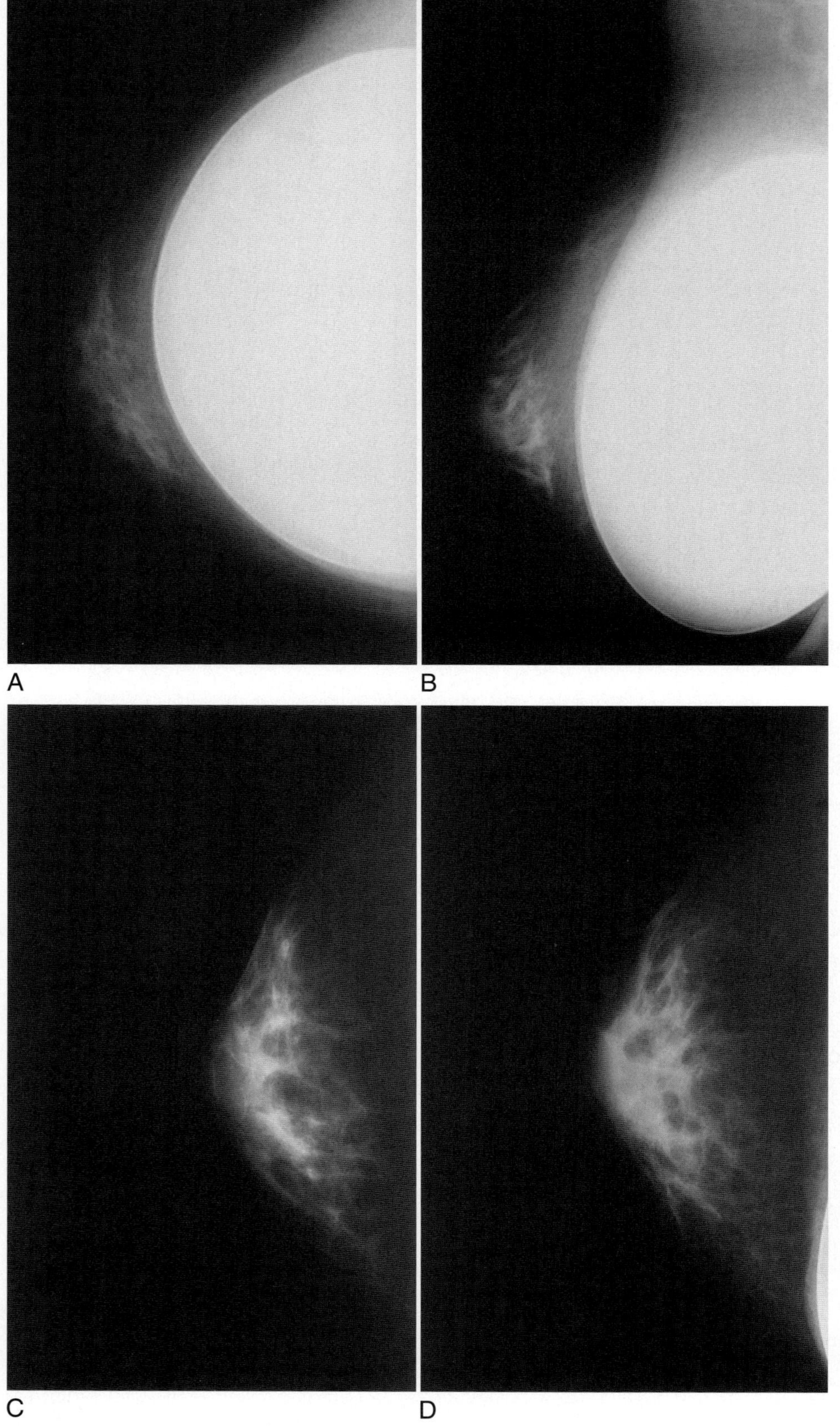

Figure 29–18. Gynecomastia, glandular pattern, with breast implants. A 48-year-old male-to-female transsexual with bilateral breast implants who had received estrogen treatment for 2 years. Right craniocaudal (**A**) and right mediolateral oblique (**B**) mammograms include the implants. Right CC (**C**) and right MLO (**D**) taken with implants displaced. Note markedly better depiction of glandular gynecomastia on the implant-displaced images.

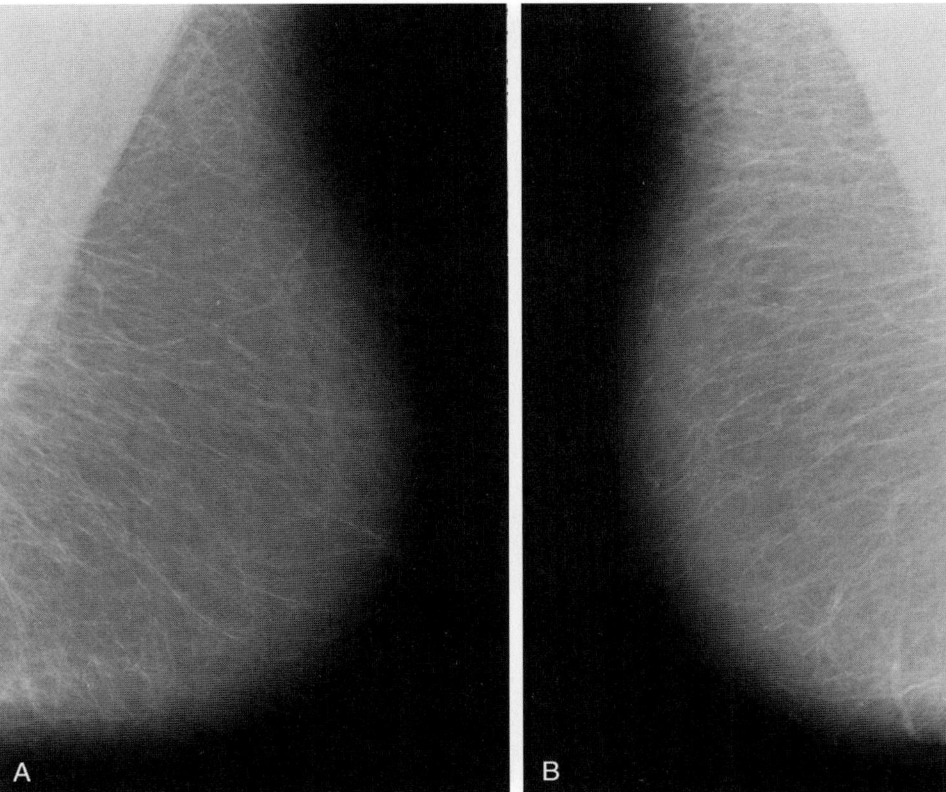

Figure 29–19. Pseudogynecomastia in an obese man. **A** and **B,** Bilateral mediolateral oblique mammograms show only fat, blood vessels, and supporting stroma. The absence of retroareolar ductal opacities ruled out true gynecomastia. (From Chantra PK, So GJ, Wollman JS, Bassett LW: Mammography of the male breast. AJR Am J Roentgenol 1995;164:853-858.)

in developing female breasts.[113] The ultrasonographic appearance of gynecomastia can be directly correlated with the findings on mammographic and histologic examinations. Initially, there is small subareolar hypoechogenicity with a definable, slightly lobulated posterior border representing ductal hyperplasia of the nodular phase (see Fig. 29–13C). In the dendritic phase, the posterior border of the subareolar hypoechoic change becomes stellate or finger-like projections (see Fig. 29–15D). Occasionally, it may be difficult to differentiate between early carcinoma and nodular gynecomastia because both conditions are hypoechoic. However, changes in gynecomastia are always subareolar in location and the hypoechogenicity is not associated with acoustic shadowing, a finding often seen in carcinoma. In the late stage, when more fibrosis develops, there is an increase in the echogenicity of the breast parenchyma, almost similar to the fibroglandular echogenicity in the female breast (Fig. 29–20).

Pathology

Histologically, the normal male breast has only major mammary ducts, which rarely branch. In early gynecomastia, or the florid histopathologic phase, proliferation of the ducts and formation of a loose, cellular, and richly vascular stroma with scattered mononuclear cells occur. The ductal system dilates and lengthens with an increase in the number of branches and typically shows epithelial hyperplasia. With time, the number of the ducts and the extent of epithelial hyperplasia become less prominent as fibrosis and hyalinization slowly replace the ductal system. The later fibrous quiescent phase takes place about a year after the onset of gynecomastia. Most cases of gynecomastia are idiopathic and resolve spontaneously. In other cases, gynecomastia is reversible if the causative factors are removed in the early stages of development. However, once gynecomastia has evolved to the stage of extensive fibrosis, the process may be irreversible.

Other Benign Conditions in the Male Breast

Table 29–6 lists a variety of benign conditions that can occur in the male breast. Among the more common are lipomas (Fig. 29–21), duct ectasia, simple cysts (Fig. 29–22), intraductal papillomas, fat necrosis (Fig. 29–23), abscess (Fig. 29–24), foreign bodies (Fig. 29–25), and epidermal inclusion cysts. Epidermal cysts are more commonly seen in the male breast than previously thought. They are clinically distinctive lesions because of their fixation to the overlying skin. Most often they arise from obstructed or occluded hair follicles.[114] Many also arise from previous skin trauma such as a surgical wound or insect bites. "Cyst" is a misnomer, because all such lesions are solid and composed of laminated keratin

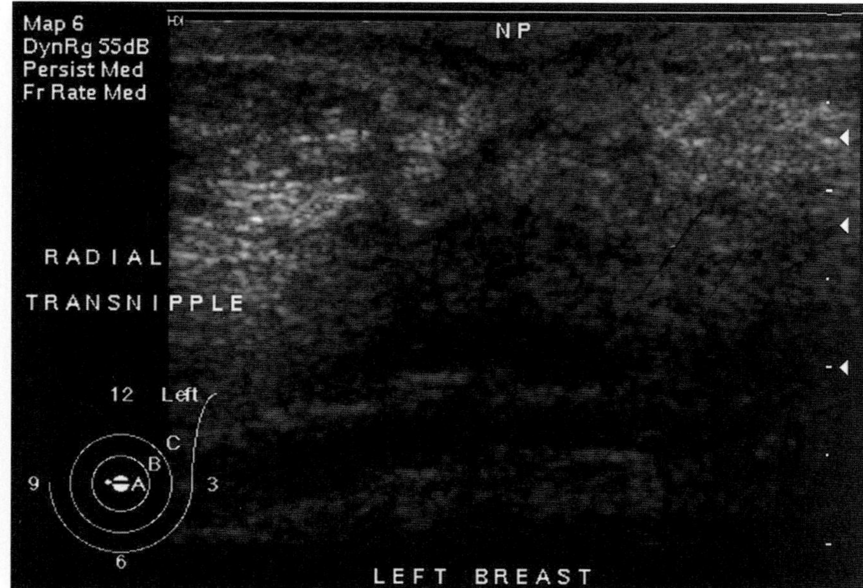

Figure 29–20. Ultrasonogram of late gynecomastia. Development of fibrosis in late gynecomastia leads to an increase in echogenicity of the breast parenchyma.

surrounded by stratified squamous epithelium (Fig. 29–26). Spontaneous rupture of such a cyst can occur, and the release of the keratin leads to inflammation and possibly abscess (Fig. 29–27).

It has been stated that all of the conditions that are found in the female breast can also be found in the male breast. Biphasic tumors (lesions composed of epithelial and mesenchymal elements), such as fibroadenoma and phyllodes tumor, are rare in men because of the absence of lobules in the male breast.[115] Lobular development, which requires both estrogen and progesterone stimulation in women, is not frequently observed in men, even in those with severe gynecomastia. Prolonged estrogen, spironolactone, and chlordiazepoxide therapies have been noted to cause the induction of lobule formation in

Table 29–6. Benign Male Breast Lesions Other than Gynecomastia

Lipoma
Papilloma
Epidermal inclusion cyst
Duct ectasia
Fibroadenoma
Sclerosing adenosis
Simple cyst
Inflammatory conditions
Abscess
Mastitis
Granulomatous disease
Tuberculosis
Syphilis
Hematoma
Contusion
Foreign bodies

Adapted from Stelling CB, Powell DE: Inflammatory, granulomatous, and male breast disorders. In Powell DE, Stelling CB (eds): The Diagnosis and Detection of Breast Disease. St. Louis, Mosby-Year Book, 1992.

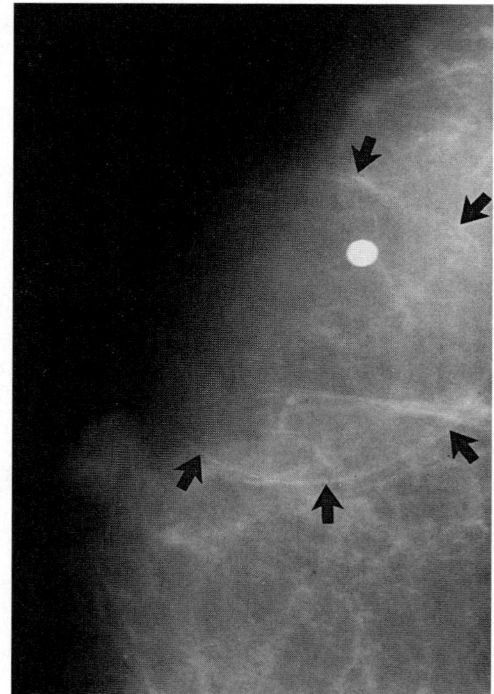

Figure 29–21. Lipoma. A 65-year-old man had noticed a soft, palpable lump in his left breast for 4 years. Mammogram shows a radiolucent mass with a thin wall *(arrows)* at the site of the palpable mass consistent with a lipoma. The lead marker (BB) indicates the site of the palpable finding. The patient had multiple other lipomas on his chest and abdomen. (From Chantra PK, So GJ, Wollman JS, Bassett LW: Mammography of the male breast. AJR Am J Roentgenol 1995;164:853-858.)

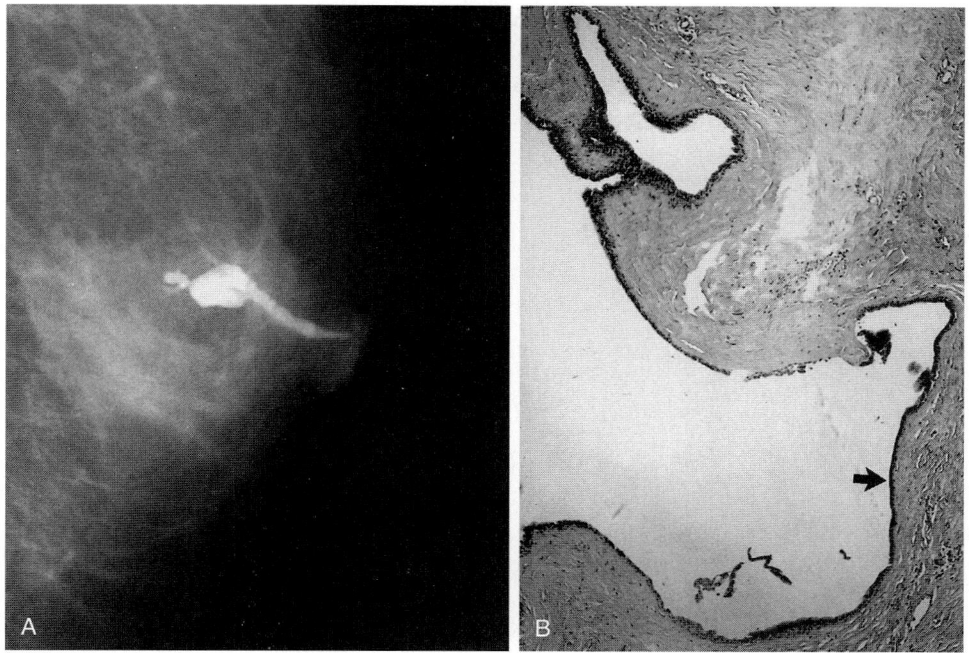

Figure 29–22. Benign cyst. A 72-year-old man with a 3-year history of intermittent bloody discharge from the left breast had mild tenderness directly over the nipple. **A,** Ductogram shows a slightly dilated but irregular duct with a large cystic blind end. Typical subareolar density of gynecomastia is present. The patient underwent surgical excision of the duct system after the ductogram. Pathologic analysis revealed a benign cyst. **B,** Photomicrograph correlates with the ductogram. Note the flattened epithelial lining *(arrow)* surrounded by a zone of fibrosis (original magnification, ×40). The patient has had no recurrence of symptoms. (From Chantra PK, So GJ, Wollman JS, Bassett LW: Mammography of the male breast. AJR Am J Roentgenol 1995;164:853-858.)

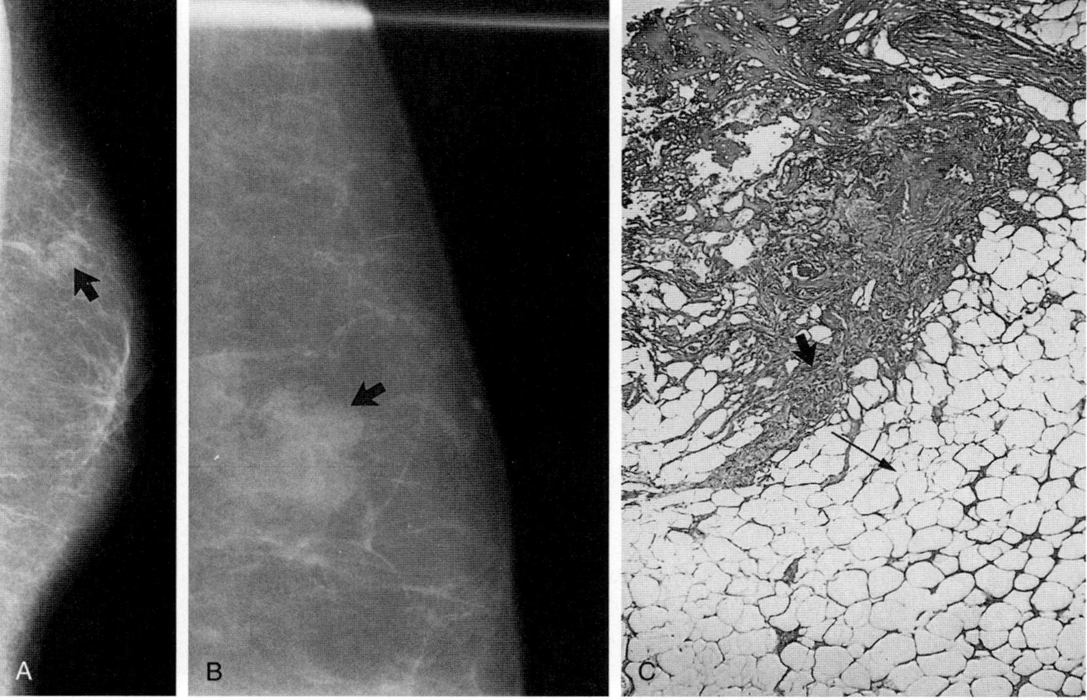

Figure 29–23. Fat necrosis and fibrosis. A 60-year-old man was noted to have a palpable, nontender, mobile mass in the left breast. The left nipple was flattened. Left mediolateral oblique (**A**) and magnification craniocaudal (**B**) mammograms show a lobulated mass *(arrow)* in the upper-outer quadrant. No associated calcification or skin thickening was present. **C,** Photomicrograph revealed mammary fat necrosis and adjacent fibrosis *(short arrow)*; note the anucleated lipocytes *(long arrow)* (original magnification, ×40). (From Chantra PK, So GJ, Wollman JS, Bassett LW: Mammography of the male breast. AJR Am J Roentgenol 1995;164:853-858.)

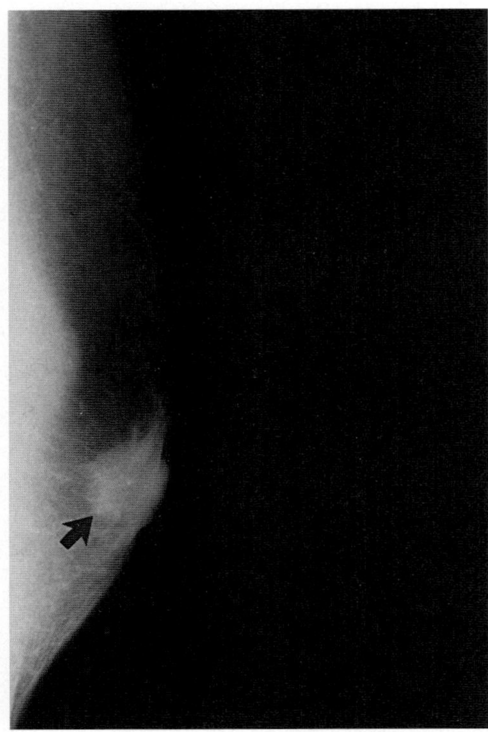

Figure 29–24. Organizing abscess. A 42-year-old man presented with a painful left breast mass. A left mediolateral oblique mammogram shows the mass. Fine-needle aspiration of the mass revealed an abscess.

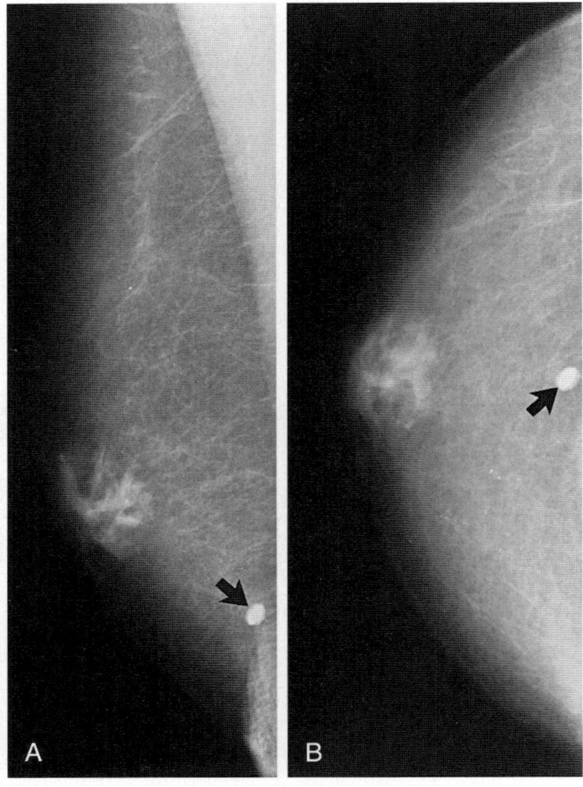

Figure 29–25. Foreign body. A 67-year-old male carpenter complained of enlarging breasts with mild right areolar tenderness. Clinical breast examination revealed an unexpected 4 × 5–mm, hard nodule deep within the breast, near the chest wall. Right mediolateral oblique (**A**) and craniocaudal (**B**) mammograms confirmed mild gynecomastia. A small metallic foreign body *(arrows)* was seen in the right pre-pectoral region corresponding to the palpable nodule, which was related to a work injury. (From Chantra PK, So GJ, Wollman JS, Bassett LW: Mammography of the male breast. AJR Am J Roentgenol 1995;164:853-858.)

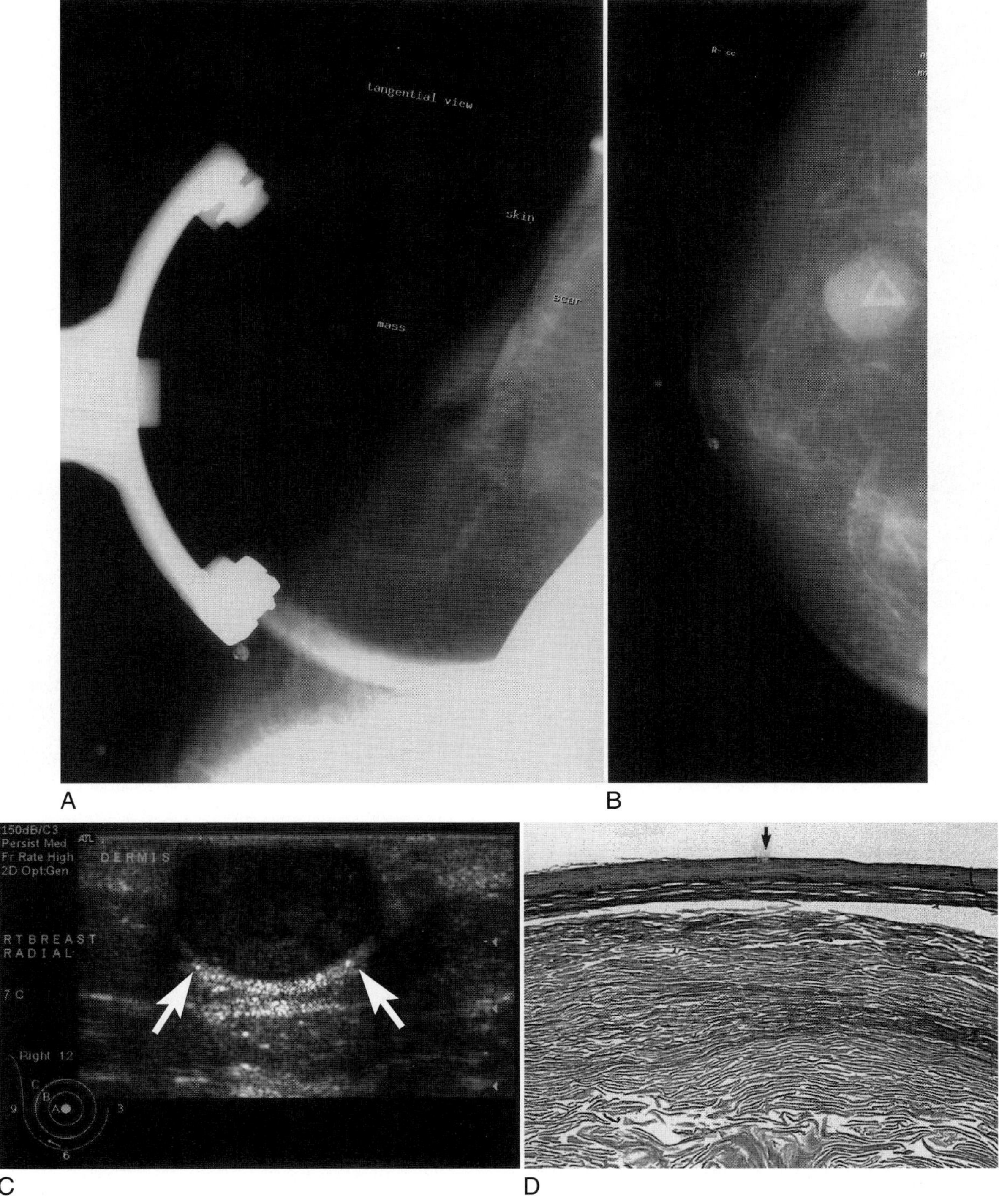

Figure 29–26. Epidermal inclusion cyst. A 67-year-old man who had undergone bilateral reduction mammoplasty 6 years earlier noticed the gradual development of a lump along the scar in the right breast. **A,** Craniocaudal mammogram shows a circumscribed, 2-cm, noncalcified mass. **B,** A tangential view reveals the mass abutting the surgical scar. **C,** Ultrasonogram of the mass demonstrates a circumscribed, homogeneously hypoechoic, solid lesion with its posterior margin enveloped by the deep layer of the skin, dubbed "claw sign," which is pathognomonic of epidermal cyst *(arrows)*. **D,** Histopathologic specimen shows stratified squamous epithelial lining *(arrow)* and keratotic content within its lumen (original magnification, ×100).

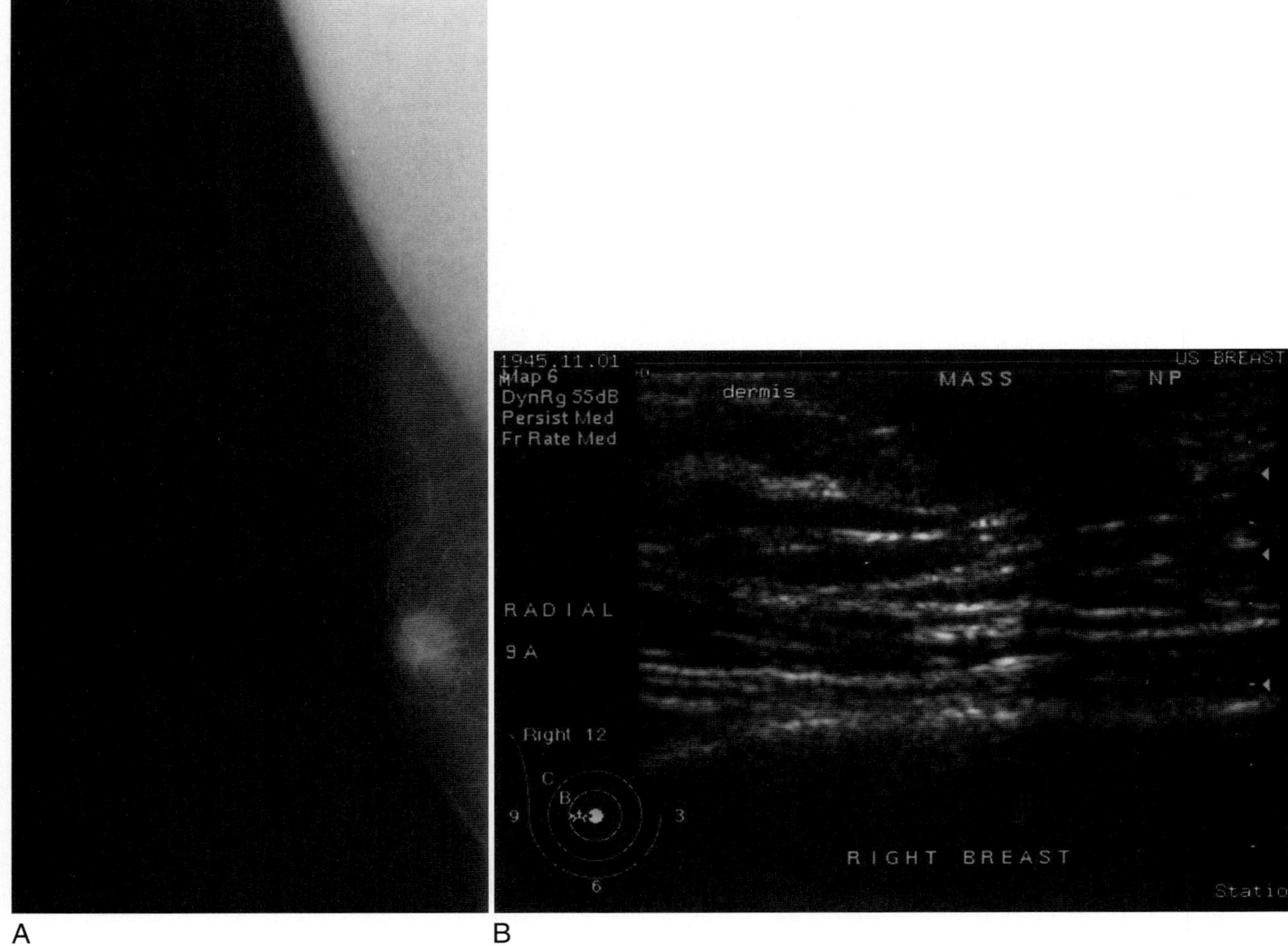

Figure 29–27. Epidermal inclusion cyst, ruptured. A 56-year-old man noticed an enlarging mass near the right nipple a week ago that was associated with mild skin redness. **A,** Right mediolateral oblique mammogram shows a 1.5-cm, noncalcified mass lateral to the nipple. The border of the mass is slightly ill-defined. **B,** Ultrasonogram demonstrates a heterogeneous hypoechoic mass adjacent to the nipple with a smooth but poorly defined border. Note the connection of the mass to the overlying skin, which is slightly thickened. The mass was excised after a course of oral antibiotics. Pathologic analysis revealed a ruptured and inflamed epidermal cyst.

men, some of whom go on to have multiple fibroadenomas.[115] Mammography in these patients often shows diffuse glandular patterns.

References

1. American Cancer Society: Cancer Facts and Figures—1991. New York, American Cancer Society, 1991.
2. Boring C, Squires T, Tony T: Cancer statistics 1991. CA Cancer J Clin 1991;41:19-36.
3. Cooper R, Gunter B, Ramamurthy L: Mammography in men. Radiology 1994;191:651-656.
4. Yap H, Tashima C, Blumenschein G, Eckles N: Male breast cancer: A natural history study. Cancer 1979;44:748-754.
5. Scheike O: Male breast cancer. 5: Clinical manifestations in 257 cases in Denmark. Br J Cancer 1973;28:552-561.
6. Hendrick R, Bassett L, Dodd G, et al: Patient positioning. Mammography Quality Control. Reston, VA, American College of Radiology, 1992, pp 57-98.
7. Jackson VP, Gilmor RL: Male breast carcinoma and gynecomastia: Comparison of mammography with sonography. Radiology 1983;149:533-536.
8. Wigley K, Thomas J, Bernardino M, Rosenbaum J: Sonography of gynecomastia. AJR Am J Roentgenol 1981;136:927-930.
9. Jaiyesimi IA, Buzdar AU, Sahin AA, Ross MA: Carcinoma of the male breast. Ann Intern Med 1992;117:771-777.
10. Crichlow RW: Carcinoma of the male breast. Surg Gynecol Obstet 1972;134:1011-1019.
11. Donegan WL, Perez-Mesa CM: Carcinoma of the male breast: A 30-year review of 28 cases. Arch Surg 1973;106:273-279.
12. Ribeiro G: Male breast carcinoma: A review of 301 cases from the Christie Hospital & Holt Radium Institute, Manchester. Br J Cancer 1985;51:115-119.
13. Donegan WL, Redlich PN: Breast cancer in men. Surg Clin North Am 1996; 76(2): 343-63.
14. Ewertz M, Holmberg L, Karjalainen S, et al: Incidence of male breast cancer in Scandinavia, 1943-1982. Int J Cancer 1989; 43:27-31.
15. La Vecchia C, Levi F, Lucchini F: Descriptive epidemiology of male breast cancer in Europe. Int J Cancer 1992;51:62-66.
16. Sasco AJ, Lowenfels AB, Pasker-de Jong P: Epidemiology of male breast cancer: A meta-analysis of published case-control studies and discussion of selected aetiological factors (review article). Int J Cancer 1993;53:538-549.

17. van Geel AN, van Slooten EA, Mavrunac M, Hart AA: A retrospective study of male breast cancer in Holland. Br J Surg 1985;72:724-727.
18. Giordano SH, Buzdar AU, Hortobagyi GN: Breast cancer in men. Ann Intern Med 2002;137(8):678-687.
19. Ajayi D, Osegbe D, Ademiluyi S: Carcinoma of the male breast in West Africans and a review of world literature. Cancer 1982;50:1664.
20. Azzopardi J: Problems in Breast Pathology. Philadelphia, WB Saunders, 1979.
21. Cole F, Quizilbash A: Carcinoma in situ of the male breast. J Clin Pathol 1979;32:1128.
22. Liechty R, Davis J, Gleysteen J: Cancer of the male breast: Forty cases. Cancer 1967;20:1617.
23. McDivitt R, Stewart F, Berg J: Atlas of Tumor Pathology, 2nd Series, Fascicle 2: Tumors of the Breast. Washington, DC, Armed Forces Institute of Pathology, 1968.
24. Treves N: Gynecomastia: The origins of mammary swelling in the male: An analysis of 406 patients with breast pathology. Cancer 1958;11:1083.
25. Wainwright J: Carcinoma of the male breast: Clinical and pathological study. Arch Surg 1927;14:836.
26. Hultborn R, Hanson C, Kopf I, et al: Prevalence of Klinefelter's syndrome in male breast cancer patients. Anticancer Res1997;17:4293-4298.
27. Coley G, Otis R, Clark WI: Multiple primary tumors including bilateral breast cancers in a man with Klinefelter's syndrome. Cancer 1971 27:1476.
28. Cuenca C, Becker K: Klinefelter's syndrome and cancer of the breast. Arch Intern Med 1968;121:159.
29. Moshakis V, Fordyce M, Griffiths J: Klinefelter's syndrome associated with breast carcinoma and Paget's disease of the nipple. Clin Oncol 1983;9:257.
30. Bland K, Buchanan J, Wisebar B, et al: The effects of exogenous estrogen replacement therapy of the breast: Breast cancer risk and mammographic parenchymal patterns. Cancer 1980;45:3027.
31. Crichlow RW, Galt SW: Male breast cancer. Surg Clin North Am 1990;70:1165-1177.
32. Rose DP: Endocrine epidemiology of male breast cancer (review). Anticancer Res 1988;8:845-850.
33. Kanhai RC, Hage JJ, van Diest PJ, et al: Short-term and long-term histologic effects of castration and estrogen treatment on breast tissue of 14 male-to-female transsexuals in comparison with two chemically castrated men. Am J Surg Pathol 2000;24:74-80.
34. Pritchard T, Pankowsky DA, Crowe JP, Abdul-Karim FW: Breast cancer in a male-to-female transsexual, a case report. JAMA 1988;259:2278-2280.
35. Carmalt HL, Mann LJ, Kennedy CW, et al: Carcinoma of the male breast: A review and recommendations for management. Aust N Z J Surg 1998;68:712-715.
36. Couch FJ, Farid LM, DeShano ML, et al: BRCA2 germline mutations in male breast cancer cases and breast cancer families. Nat Genet 1996;13:123-125.
37. Stratton MR, Ford D, Neuhasen S: Familial male breast cancer is not linked to the BRCA1 locus on chromosome 17q. Nat Genet 1994;7:103-107.
38. Casey G: The BRCA1 and BRCA2 breast cancer genes. Curr Opin Oncol 1997;9:88-93.
39. Struewing JP, Hartge P, Wacholder S, et al: The risk of cancer associated with specific mutations of BRCA1 and BRCA2 among Ashkenazi Jews. N Engl J Med 1997;336:1401-1408.
40. Storm HH, Olsen J: Risk of breast cancer in offspring of male breast-cancer patients. Lancet 1999;353(9148):209.
41. Meijer-van Gelder ME, Look MP, Bolt-de Vries J, et al: Clinical relevance of biologic factors in male breast cancer. Breast Cancer Res Treat 2001;68:249-260.
42. Borgen PI: Male breast cancer. Semin Surg Oncol 1991;7:314-319.
43. Cutuli B, Lacroze M, Dilhuydy JM, et al: Male breast cancer: Results of the treatments and prognostic factors in 397 cases. Eur J Cancer 1995;31A:1960-1964.
44. Ravandi-Kashani F, Hayes TG: Male breast cancer: A review of the literature. Eur J Cancer 1998;34:1341-1347.
45. Ribeiro GG: Tamoxifen in the treatment of male breast carcinoma. Clin Radiol 1983;34:625-628.
46. Bruce DM, Heys SD, Payne S, et al: Male breast cancer: Clinico-pathological features, immunocytochemical characteristics and prognosis. Eur J Surg Oncol 1996;22:42-46.
47. Clark JL, Nguyen PL, Jaszca WB, et al: Prognostic variables in male breast cancer. Am Surg 2000;66:502-511.
48. Joshi MG, Lee AK, Loda M, et al: Male breast carcinoma: An evaluation of prognostic factors contributing to a poorer outcome. Cancer 1996;77:490-498.
49. Willsher PC, Leach IH, Ellis IO, et al: Male breast cancer: Pathological and immunohistochemical features. Anticancer Res 1997;17:2335-2338.
50. Serra Diaz C, Vizoso F, Lamelas ML, et al: Expression and clinical significance of apolipoprotein D in male breast cancer and gynaecomastia. Br J Surg 1999;86:1190-1197.
51. Volpe CM, Raffetto JD, Collure DW, et al: Unilateral male breast masses: Cancer risk and their evaluation and management. Am Surg 1999;65:250-253.
52. Langlands A, Maclean N, Kerr G: Carcinoma of the male breast: Report of a series of 88 cases. Clin Radiol 1976;27:21-25.
53. Amoroso WL Jr, Robbins, GF, Treves N: Serous and serosanguinous discharge from the male nipple. Arch Surg 1956; 73:319-329.
54. Balich SM, Khandekhar JD, Sener SF: Cancer of the male breast presenting as an axillary mass. J Surg Oncol 1993;53: 68-70.
55. Bhagat P, Kline TS: The male breast and malignant neoplasms: Diagnosis by aspiration biopsy cytology. Cancer 1990;65:2338-2341.
56. Yang WT, Whitman GJ, Yuen EHY, et al: Sonographic features of primary breast cancer in men. AJR Am J Roentgenol 2001; 176:413-416.
57. Appelbaum AH, Evans GFF, Levy KR, et al: Mammographic appearances of male breast disease. Radiographics 1999;19: 559-568.
58. Salvadori B, Saccozzi R, Manzari A, et al: Prognosis of breast cancer in males: An analysis of 170 cases. Eur J Cancer 1994;30A:930-935.
59. Thomas D: Breast cancer in men. Epidemiol Rev 1993;15: 220-331.
60. Borgen PI, Wong GY, Vlamis V, et al: Current management of male breast cancer: A review of 104 cases. Ann Surg 1992;215:451-457.
61. Digenis AG, Ross CB, Morrison JG, et al: Carcinoma of the male breast: A review of 41 cases. South Med J 1990;83:1162-1167.
62. Lefor AT, Numann PJ: Carcinoma of the breast in men. N Y State J Med 1988;88:293-296.
63. Winchester DJ: Male breast cancer. Semin Surg Oncol 1996; 12:364-369.
64. Cappabianca S, Grassi R, D'Alessandro P, et al: Metastasis to the male breast from carcinoma of the urinary bladder. Br J Radiol 2000;73:1326-1328.
65. Toombs BD, Kalisher L: Metastatic disease to the breast: Clinical, pathologic, and radiographic features. AJR Am J Roentgenol 1977;129:673-676.
66. Huggins C, Taylor G: Carcinoma of male breast. Arch Surg 1955;70:303-308.
67. Keddie N, Morris P: Male breast tumours. Surg Gynaecol Obstet 1967;124:332-336.
68. Donegan WL, Redlich PN, Lang PJ, et al: Carcinoma of the breast in males: A multiinstitutional survey. Cancer 1998;83: 498-509.
69. Heller KS, Rosen PP, Schottenfeld D: Male breast cancer: A clinicopathologic study of 97 cases. Ann Surg 1978;188:60-65.
70. Hill A, Yagmur Y, Tran KN, et al: Localized male breast carcinoma and family history: An analysis of 142 patients. Cancer 1999;86:821-825.
71. Scheike O: Male breast cancer: Factors influencing prognosis. Br J Cancer 1974;30:261-271.
72. Evans GF, Anthony T, Appelbaum AH, et al: The diagnostic accuracy of mammography in the evaluation of male breast disease. Am J Surg Pathol 2001;181:96-100.

73. Chantra PK, So GJ, Wollman JS, et al: Mammography of the male breast. AJR Am J Roentgenol 1995;164:853-858.
74. Dershaw D, Borgen P, Deutch B, Liberman L: Mammographic findings in men with breast cancer. AJR Am J Roentgenol 1993;160:267-270.
75. Dershaw D: Male mammography. AJR Am J Roentgenol 1986;146:127-131.
76. Kapdi CC, Parekh NJ: The male breast. Radiol Clin North Am 1983;21:137-148.
77. Fallentin E, Rothman L: Intracystic carcinoma of the male breast. J Clin Ultrasound 1994;22:118-120.
78. Imoto S, Hasebe T: Intracystic papillary carcinoma of the breast in male: Case report and review of the Japanese literature. Jpn J Clin Oncol 1998;28:517-520.
79. Madden CM, Reynolds HE: Intracystic papillary carcinoma of the male breast. AJR Am J Roentgenol 1995;165:1011-1012.
80. McSweeney MB, Murphy CH: Whole-breast sonography. Radiol Clin North Am 1985;23:157-167.
81. Stewart RAL, Howlett LC, Hearn FJ: Pictorial review: The imaging features of male breast disease. Clin Radiol 1997;52:739-744.
82. Liu M, Husain SS, Hameer HR, et al: Detection of male breast cancer with Tc-99m methoxyisobutyl isonitrile. Clin Nucl Med 1999;24:882-883.
83. Marwah A, Kumar R, Sasan B, et al: Tc-99m tetrofosmin uptake in male breast cancer. Clin Nucl Med 2001;26:77-78.
84. Stebbings W, George B, Boyle S, et al: Malignant cysts of male breast. Postgrad Med J 1987;63:985-987.
85. Hittmair AP, Lininger RA, Tavassoli FA: Ductal carcinoma in situ (DCIS) in the male breast: A morphologic study of 84 cases of pure DCIS and 30 cases of DCIS associated with invasive carcinoma—a preliminary report. Cancer 1998;83:2139-2149.
86. Visfeldt J, Scheike O: Male breast cancer. I: Histologic typing and grading of 187 Danish cases. Cancer 1973;32:985-990.
87. Cutuli B, Dilhuydy JM, De Lafontan B, et al: Ductal carcinoma in situ of the male breast. Analysis of 31 cases. Eur J Cancer 1997;33:35-38.
88. Wolff M, Reinis MS: Breast cancer in the male: Clinicopathological study of 40 patients. In Fenoglio C, Wolff M (eds): Progress in Surgical Pathology. New York, Masson Publishing, 1981, p 3.
89. Sanchez A, Villanueva A, Redondo C: Lobular carcinoma of the breast in a patient with Klinefelter syndrome: A case with bilateral, synchronous, histologically different breast tumors. Cancer 1986;57:1181-1183.
90. Macmillan D, Dixon M: Gynaecomastia: When is action required? Practitioner 2000;244:785-787.
91. Braunstein G: Gynecomastia. N Engl J Med 1993;328:490-495.
92. Niewoehner C, Nuttall F: Gynecomastia in a hospitalized male population. Am J Med 1984;77:633-638..
93. Simon BE, Hoffman S, Kahn S: Classification and surgical correction of gynecomastia. Plast Reconstr Surg 1973;51:48-52.
94. Harrington JM, Stein GF, Rivera RO: The occupational hazards of formulating oral contraceptives: A survey of plant employees. Arch Environ Health 1978;33:12-15.
95. Vierhapper H, Nowotny P: Gynaecomastia and raised oestradiol concentrations. Lancet 1999;353(9153):640.
96. Vermeulen A: Testicular hormonal secretion and aging in males. In Grayhack J, Wilson J, Scherbenske M (eds): Benign Prostatic Hypertrophy. Washington, DC, National Institutes of Health, 1976, pp 76-111.
97. Webster DJ: The male breast. Br J Clin Pract Symp Suppl 1989;68:137-142.
98. McLeod DG, Iversen P: Gynecomastia in patients with prostate cancer: A review of treatment options. Urology 2000;56:713-720.
99. Marshall WA, Tanner JM: Variations in pattern of pubertal changes in girls. Arch Dis Child 1969;44:291-303.
100. Williams M: Gynecomastia, its incidence, recognition and host characterization in 447 autopsy cases. Am J Med 1963; 34:103-112.
101. Webster JP: Mastectomy for gynecomastia through a semicircular intra-areolar incision. Ann Surg 1946;124:557-575.
102. Alagaratnam TT: Idiopathic gynecomastia treated with tamoxifen: A preliminary report. Clin Ther 1987;9:483-487.
103. Jones DJ, Holt SD, Surtees P: A comparison of danazol and placebo in the treatment of adult idiopathic gynaecomastia: Results of a prospective study in 55 patients. Ann R Coll Surg Engl 1990;72:296-298.
104. McDermott MT, Hofeldt FD, Kidd GS: Tamoxifen therapy for painful idiopathic gynecomastia. South Med J 1990;83:1283-1285.
105. Parker LN, Gray DR, Lai MK, Levin ER: Treatment of gynecomastia with tamoxifen: A double-blind crossover study. Metabolism 1986;35(8):705-708.
106. Brown JS, Rubenfeld S: Irradiation in preventing gynecomastia induced by estrogens. Urology 1974;3:51-53.
107. Forman M: Roentgenology of the male breast. AJR Am J Roentgenol 1962;88:1126-1134.
108. Panzarola P, Bosso P, Ercolani S: Mammography and echography in male breast pathology. Radiol Med (Torino) 1992; 84:32-35.
109. Bannayan GA, Hajdu SI: Gynecomastia: Clinicopathologic study of 351 cases. Am J Clin Pathol 1972;57:431-437.
110. Michels L, Gold R, Arndt R: Radiography of gynecomastia and other disorders of the male breast. Radiology 1977;122: 117-122.
111. Waterfall N, Glaser M: A study of the effects of radiation on prevention of gynecomastia due to oestrogen therapy. Clin Oncol 1979;5:257-260.
112. Dearnaley D: Cancer of the prostate. BMJ 1994;308:780-784.
113. Weinstein SP, Conant EF, Orel SG, et al: Spectrum of US findings in pediatric and adolescent patients with palpable breast masses. Radiographics 2000;20:1613-1621.
114. Chantra PK, Tang JT, Stanley TM, et al: Circumscribed fibrocystic mastopathy with formation of an epidermal cyst. AJR Am J Roentgenol 1994;163:831-832.
115. Ansah-Boateng Y, Tavassoli F:. Fibroadenoma and cystosarcoma phyllodes of the male breast. Mod Pathol 1992;5:2114-2115.
116. Axelsson J, Andersson A: Cancer of the male breast. World J Surg 1983;7:281-287.
117. Bhagwandeen SB: Carcinoma of the male breast in Zambia. East Afr Med J 1972;49:89-93.
118. Simon MS, McKnight E, Schwartz A, et al: Racial differences in cancer of the male breast: 15 year experience in the Detroit metropolitan area. Breast Cancer Res Treat 1992;21:55-62.
119. Demers PA, Thomas DB, Rosenblatt KA, et al: Occupational exposure to electromagnetic fields and breast cancer in men. Am J Epidemiol 1991;134:340-347.
120. Matanoski GM, Breysse PN, Elliott EA: Electromagnetic field exposure and male breast cancer. Lancet 1991;337(8743): 737.
121. Rosenbaum P, Vena J, Zielezny M, Michalek A: Occupational exposures associated with male breast cancer. Am J Epidemiol 1994;139:30-36.
122. Olsson H, Ranstam J: Head trauma and exposure to prolactin-elevating drugs as risk factors for male breast cancer. J Natl Cancer Inst 1988;80:679-683.
123. Raviglione MC, Graham PE: Breast carcinoma in a man following local trauma. N Y State J Med 1987;87:186-187.
124. Hsing AW, McLaughlin JK, Cocco P, et al:. Risk factors for male breast cancer (United States). Cancer Causes Control 1998;9:269-275.

Section **VII**

Management of Breast Diseases and Post-Treatment Evaluation

Chapter 30 Treatment of Breast Disease

Susan M. Love, Helena R. Chang, and Robert S. Bennion

As the most visible physical evidence of a woman's sexuality and femininity, the human breast has acquired deep emotional significance. It is unfortunately also the most common site of newly discovered cancer in American women. It is estimated that in the year 2003, approximately 1,334,100 new cancer cases and 556,500 cancer deaths occurred in the United States. Breast cancer has been projected to have accounted for 212,600 new cases of cancer and 40,200 cancer deaths in 2003.[1] Therefore, women have become increasingly concerned that pain, tenderness, a new lump, nipple discharge, or a change in breast size may reflect the presence of breast cancer. Fortunately, the vast majority of breast disorders with these signs or symptoms are benign.

TREATMENT OF BENIGN BREAST DISEASE

Historically, the term *fibrocystic disease of the breast* has been used to describe almost any noninfectious benign process affecting the breast. This practice has resulted in considerable confusion for both physicians and patients and a significant concern for patients who believe that they have a "disease" in their breasts. With the exception of a histologic diagnosis of moderate to severe hyperplasia with atypia, no increased risk of subsequent cancer is associated with the microscopic description of changes formerly called "fibrocystic disease." Therefore, the term should be abandoned in favor of the more precise descriptors of benign breast complaints proposed in 1987.[2] These are as follows:

- Physiologic cyclic swelling and tenderness
- Nodularity
- Mastalgia
- Nipple discharge
- Infection
- Dominant mass

Physiologic Cyclic Swelling and Tenderness

The cyclic swelling and tenderness of a woman's breasts represent normal physiologic variations in size, shape, and tenderness that occur in relation to the menstrual cycle. Because these changes are hormonally governed, they occur during the reproductive years or later from the stimulation of exogenous estrogen. These variations are not always equally manifested in the two breasts, and the changes in one breast often predominate over those in the other. In the vast majority of women, these complaints are mild, and reassurance that they are normal is the appropriate management. The distinction between these physiologic variants and mastalgia or nodularity depends on their severity and persistence.

Nodularity

Nodularity throughout the breasts varies from finely granular to truly lumpy. Although the two breasts may be affected equally, the changes may predominate in one breast. Haagensen[3] believed that the decision clinicians were most frequently required to make regarding the breast was to distinguish increased physiologic nodularity from true disease. Because physiologic nodularity requires no treatment, the key decision to be made is whether the nodularity represents a dominant mass. If the clinician is unsure whether a dominant mass is present, the patient should be observed through one or two menstrual cycles and reexamined, preferably in midcycle when breast engorgement is minimal. Persistence of the nodule or any suspicion about its character mandates a further diagnostic evaluation.

Mastalgia

Breast pain is a common complaint in premenopausal women and may be either cyclic or noncyclic. Occurring in up to 40% of women, pain may be present in nodular regions of the breast, although most commonly it is independent of any anatomic changes. In fact, nodules documented by ultrasonography have been shown to have no relationship to breast pain.[4] The vast majority of women who present with breast pain, especially cyclic pain, can be treated with reassurance alone after a thorough examination, including appropriate imaging studies. Occasionally, a woman describes pain in one specific location that is unrelated to the menstrual cycle. If the mammographic findings are normal, the physician may be tempted to perform a biopsy of that area. However, this urge should be resisted because significant disease is encountered very rarely in such cases despite the persistence of pain.

For only a small number of patients with mastalgia (about 5%) is some form of specific therapy required. Various regimens have been suggested. Withholding or significantly limiting caffeine ingestion traditionally has been stated to be of benefit in treating breast pain and nodularity. In randomized trials, however, consumption of caffeine or the other methylxanthines has not been shown to have any relationship to either pain or nodularity.[5] Likewise, the use of vitamin E has not been shown to have any effect on breast pain.[6]

Estrogen blockade has been used to treat patients with severe mastalgia in whom all other treatment modalities have failed. Danazol, a 17-ethinyltestosterone that suppresses both follicle-stimulating hormone (FSH) and luteinizing hormone (LH), has been used most commonly. A dose of 100 mg to 400 mg per day often results in a significant decrease in pain within a month or two. Unfortunately, nearly half of the patients demonstrate recurrence of symptoms within a year after therapy is stopped. Danazol is quite expensive and has significant side effects, such as weight gain, acne, menstrual disturbances (from spotting to amenorrhea), and hirsutism (which may persist after cessation of therapy). Other agents that have been used to treat mastalgia are bromocriptine (a dopaminergic agonist that inhibits the release of prolactin), progesterone,[7,8] and tamoxifen.[9]

Other causes of mastalgia that must be excluded include costochondritis and some forms of cervical radiculopathy,[10] disorders that are generally treated with nonsteroidal anti-inflammatory agents. Thrombophlebitis of the superficial veins of the breast (Mondor syndrome) is yet another rare source of localized pain commonly occurring after trauma to the breast (surgical or nonsurgical). It commonly manifests as pain along the periphery of the breast radiating to the epigastrium. Dimpling or retraction of the skin along the course of the vein may be seen. The process is self-limited, and therapy consisting of nonsteroidal anti-inflammatory agents and, perhaps, ice packs is all that is required.

Nipple Discharge

It is normal for breast tissue to secrete some fluid, and in fact, in nearly 85% of all women, regardless of age or menstrual status, nipple discharge can be induced by manual compression of the nipple.[2] Thus, nipple discharge is the second most common complaint of women seeking consultation for breast problems. In one large series, nipple discharge was the presenting symptom in 9.1% of patients who underwent operations for benign breast lesions and in 3.1% of patients who underwent operations for malignant disease.[11] Varying in color from nearly clear to very dark green or brown and in consistency from watery to thick, the discharge is usually of benign origin or is the result of systemic neuroendocrine causes or drugs. Although bilateral discharge is almost always benign, bilateral milky discharge in a nonlactating woman (galactorrhea) demands a specific evaluation. Hyperprolactinemia resulting from a pituitary adenoma is most easily diagnosed from the presence of elevated serum prolactin values. If elevated prolactin values are found, imaging evaluation of the pituitary gland is required. If no specific cause of copious galactorrhea can be found, bromocriptine, 0.5 mg to 2.5 mg per day, may be useful to control it.

Spontaneous unilateral nipple discharge that is either clear and sticky or persistently bloody (or guaiac positive) may be pathologically significant. The causes of the discharge and the frequency of its occurrence in a series of more than 500 women have been reported as follows: intraductal papillomas, 45.9%; fibrocystic changes (mammary dysplasia), 36.0%; carcinoma (either in situ or invasive), 13.3%; and severe ductal ectasia, 4.8%.[11] Intraductal papillomas are the most common cause of bloody discharge and are rarely palpable, averaging only 2 to 3 mm in diameter. The peak age of incidence of discharging papillomas is the 40s, and more than 92% of such lesions are located within 1 cm of the areolar complex.[12] Although gentle stroking toward the areola in a clockwise fashion until the discharge has been induced usually allows the quadrant of the breast containing the papilloma to be identified, the use of ductography is more sensitive and more precise. Once localized, the duct containing the papilloma can be easily excised through a circumareolar incision with the use of local anesthesia. If neither ductal ectasia nor papillomas are seen on ductography, it is necessary to excise the central ducts with a surrounding wedge of breast tissue from the quadrant to which the origin of the discharge has been localized. This can usually be performed via a circumareolar incision using local anesthetic agent with good cosmetic results. Any further treatment is dictated by the pathologic findings and may range from no further treatment to definitive surgery if cancer is found.

Infection

Acute bacterial infections of the parenchyma of the breast are uncommon in nonlactating women. They generally occur in the actively lactating breast in the first month or two after delivery. The portal of entry of the bacteria is a cracked or abraded nipple. The best treatment is prevention—the breastfeeding woman should carefully clean and dry her nipples after each nursing. If a localized area of inflammation develops, she should stop nursing and should take oral antibiotics that are effective against skin flora, especially *Staphylococcus aureus*. Progression of acute bacterial mastitis to a breast abscess is not common, but if it occurs, surgical drainage is required. The best approach is through a curvilinear incision over the most dependent portion of the abscess. After drainage of the pus, a drain is placed or the wound is packed, depending on the size of the abscess cavity. Small abscesses can sometimes be localized, aspirated, and drained under ultrasonographic guidance. Oral antibiotics are given only during the perioperative period, and the wound is allowed to heal by secondary intent.

An infection in the breast that is particularly difficult to deal with is a chronic subareolar abscess. It often appears as a focus of erythema and tenderness along the areolar border and is more common in women with inverted nipples. It is caused by blockage of an outflow track of a sebaceous gland in the nipple or areola.[13] Although blockage of the lactiferous ducts themselves was once thought to contribute to the problem, later evidence indicates that infection of a sebaceous gland is the main cause.[14] Even after appropriate surgical drainage, a subareolar abscess can evolve into a chronic fistula.

As with treatment of infected sebaceous glands elsewhere, it is imperative that the entire gland be removed to guarantee eradication of the infection. A circumareolar incision is inadequate and is often followed by recurrence. A radial incision encompassing the entire infected gland is preferred, including excision of a wedge of nipple if necessary. If a secondarily involved lactiferous duct or an infected gland opens at the nipple, placement of a lacrimal duct probe before excision may be helpful in delineating the extent of any fistulous tract between the gland and the duct. With the use of either monitored anesthetic care or light general anesthesia, excision of the infected duct and tract is carried out down into the subareolar tissues. Careful reapproximation of the wound edges using nonabsorbable suture is essential for a reasonable cosmetic result (especially if the nipple is partially excised). If the volume of the tissue is so great that excision would significantly deform the breast or nipple, widely opening the infected duct or tract may help resolve the inflammation so that a smaller excision may suffice if required in the future.

The primary complication after treatment of chronic subareolar abscess is recurrence, which has been reported to occur in as many as 25% to 40% of patients.[15] If the initial recurrence is localized, treatment of the process, as outlined previously, may be repeated. However, after multiple recurrences, it may be best to recommend that the patient consider having the nipple and areolar complex excised and rebuilt by a plastic surgeon.

Dominant Mass

A *dominant mass* is best defined as a palpable breast lesion that is distinct from surrounding breast nodularity, persistent through at least two or three menstrual cycles, and relatively unchanging. Although most often benign, such a mass must be evaluated to exclude malignancy. Once a dominant mass has been identified by physical examination, an attempt at aspiration in the office with a syringe connected to a 22-gauge needle or an ultrasonographic examination should be performed to determine whether the mass is cystic or solid. If it is cystic, the contents should be aspirated so that the cyst collapses. If the mass is solid, microscopic evaluation of the mass is required.

The most common types of benign dominant masses are gross cysts, fibroadenoma, and galactoceles. *Gross cysts* are fluid-filled, epithelium-lined structures that are distinguished from microcysts (a normal condition) by being more than 3 mm in diameter. It is estimated that 10% to 12% of women have gross cysts, and more than 95% of cysts are encountered in women between the ages 30 and 55 years.[16] Cysts range from asymptomatic to very painful and have no "typical" clinical presentation. In fact, cysts are not infrequently found incidentally on otherwise normal mammograms or ultrasonograms obtained for another reason. Nonpalpable gross cysts found on mammography or ultrasonography need no further evaluation or aspiration unless there is some question about the diagnosis. Palpable cysts are usually well circumscribed and tend to move under the examiner's fingers in relation to the surrounding tissue. When they are aspirated, the fluid typically varies in consistency from thin to thick and in color from straw-colored to a dark gray-green (almost blackish brown) and contains formless debris and occasional degenerating epithelial cells. Nothing is gained by sending the fluid for cytologic analysis. A cytologist unfamiliar with cyst fluid may mistake degenerating epithelial cells with hyperchromatic nuclei for carcinoma cells.

The indications for further investigation of a cyst include a complex cyst, a mass that does not completely resolve on aspiration, aspirated fluid that resembles old blood (being dark red and thicker than fresh blood), and a complex cyst on ultrasound. An excision is the usual means of investigation.

Fibroadenomas are the most common benign solid masses in the breast. Occurring almost exclusively in women between the ages of 15 and 45 years, these masses are hormonally sensitive and occasionally may become quite large, although it is uncommon for them to exceed 3 cm in diameter. They are painless and usually well circumscribed, are somewhat mobile, and feel round, discoid, or lobulated. A fibroadenoma cannot be distinguished from a gross cyst on physical examination, and because both lesions occur in premenopausal women, determination whether a mass is solid or cystic by aspiration or ultrasonography is an important initial diagnostic step. Once the mass has been shown to be solid, further evaluation depends on the patient's age. Breast cancer is extremely unlikely in a woman younger than 25 years, so if the ultrasonographic features of the mass are characteristic of a fibroadenoma, reassurance of the patient is probably all that is required. Biopsy is often necessary to confirm the diagnosis in patients older than 25 years. For women with fibroadenomas that are larger or growing and women who are anxious, excisional biopsy may be the procedure of choice.

A *galactocele* is nothing more than a milk-filled cyst occurring in a breast that is actively lactating or in which lactation was established and abruptly terminated. A galactocele has all the physical characteristics of a gross cyst, except that only rarely is it tender. It is thought to be caused by inspissated milk blocking one of the ducts and thereby obstructing flow. Once a galactocele has been proven by ultrasonography to contain fluid, complete aspiration is curative.

DIAGNOSTIC SURGERY

As noted previously, the primary reason for surgical intervention in benign breast disease is to document that the process is truly benign and not malignant. Nipple discharge and a dominant mass are the most common conditions that justify surgery. Several other diagnostic procedures may be used in appropriate circumstances.

Cyst Aspiration

Any physician who treats a significant amount of breast disease should have facility with aspiration of a dominant mass. Although direct puncture of the mass is possible without anesthesia, prior injection of intradermal lidocaine is an option, especially for anxious patients. With the fingers of one hand holding the mass firmly in place, the physician punctures the mass with a 22-gauge needle attached to a 12-mL syringe and applies gentle suction. The use of a large syringe (15 mL or bigger) or too vigorous suction may result in aspiration of little or no fluid. If the mass is resolved completely and the aspirated fluid was not bloody, the fluid should *not* be sent for cytologic analysis. If no fluid can be aspirated, ultrasonography should be considered, if it has not already been performed, to document whether the mass is solid or cystic.

Fine-Needle Aspiration and Cytology

During the last decade, interest in fine-needle aspiration and cytology (FNAC) has grown. Because it does not deform the breast in any way, FNAC does not limit further surgical options. It has also been projected to be cost effective, even if in some cases the procedure is followed by open biopsy for confirmation of results.[17] In a review of nearly 11,000 cases, Grant and colleagues[18] concluded that FNAC could provide an added measure of confidence in the diagnosis of benign breast lesions, act as an additional safeguard against the misdiagnosis of malignant lesions, and reduce the cost of managing breast cancer. Although an extensive review of the literature found that the overall accuracy of FNAC was generally greater than 95%, the extent of both false-positive results (up to 18%) and false-negative results (up to 35%) was disconcerting.[19] In addition, the same review noted that from 1% to 68% of specimens were unsatisfactory for evaluation. These findings point out the primary disadvantages of FNAC: A definite learning curve occurs before the technique is mastered, and the slides must be evaluated by an experienced cytopathologist who is familiar with breast cytology.[19] In addition, the rule of "concordance" must be followed to avoid false-negative results—that is, the histologic diagnosis must correspond with the imaging and clinical findings.

The technique used for FNAC of a palpable mass is important. As in simple cyst aspiration, the physician fixes the mass with the fingers of one hand and infiltrates the skin overlying the mass with local anesthesia. He or she then uses a 12-mL syringe to which a 22-gauge needle has been attached to puncture the mass while applying suction to the syringe. The physician passes the needle in several directions to sample as much of the mass as possible. He or she then releases suction and withdraws the needle. The syringe is then either passed to a cytologist or cytopathologist or expelled directly onto glass slides. The smears are fixed according to the standard routine for a Papanicolaou smear. Because it is now possible to analyze FNAC specimens for estrogen receptor activity by immunocytochemical methods[20] as well as by flow cytometry, a decision whether to use these modalities must be made at the time of the FNAC, because if they are to be used, special fixatives are required.

With the exception of insufficient sampling of a lesion, the only potential complications related to FNAC are hematoma formation and pneumothorax. Inadequate sampling may be minimized with the use of ultrasonographic or mammographic guidance.[21] The most significant limitation of FNAC is an inability to distinguish invasive from noninvasive carcinomas. Epithelial proliferations, ductal papilloma, fibroadenoma, fat necrosis, mastitis, gynecomastia, and radiation changes have all led to false-positive diagnoses.[19]

Core Needle Biopsy

In the past, core needle biopsy (CNB) was considered inferior to FNAC because FNAC required no special equipment or needles, was quicker and less invasive, and could sample a larger area.[22] However, because of problems related to specimen insufficiency, lack of widespread expertise in breast cytopathology in the United States, and the inability of FNAC to determine whether a lesion is invasive, CNB is once again becoming the popular alternative to open biopsy.[23,24] As with FNAC, the rule of concordance must be followed.

For palpable lesions, CNB is performed with the use of a handheld true-cut–style needle. After the skin has been infiltrated with local anesthesia, the physician holds the mass fixed to the chest wall with the fingers of one hand and makes a small nick in the skin to allow passage of the needle. For nonpalpable lesions, a CNB can be done with ultrasound or stereotactic guidance. To decrease sampling error, at least three good cores should be obtained through the same skin opening. Although the insertion and movement of the needle are often uncomfortable for the patient, the procedure is usually tolerable, and sedation or postprocedure analgesia is rarely required. The most commonly encountered complication of CNB is hematoma formation or bruising, especially in patients who are taking nonsteroidal anti-inflammatory medicine.

Incisional Biopsy

Although used extensively in the past, incisional biopsy of a breast mass is now an uncommon procedure. At present, its primary indication is to obtain tissue than cannot be obtained with certainty by CNB in a patient who has a large (>5 cm) and poorly defined breast lesion and for whom preoperative chemotherapy or radiation therapy is being considered. With the use of local anesthesia or managed anesthetic care, a wedge of tissue is excised from the mass, often with the overlying skin, and a clip is placed to mark the site of tissue removal. Because necrosis may interfere with biochemical and histologic analysis, care must be taken not to sample tissue that is extensively necrotic. A small pressure dressing is helpful in decreasing the potential of hematoma formation. Because incisional biopsy is usually the precursor for definitive local treatment, specific orientation and marking of the specimen for the pathologist are not required.

When an incisional or excisional biopsy is planned, thought must be given at the time of surgery as to placement of the wound. It not only must be cosmetically acceptable but also must not interfere with the performance of a definitive procedure should one be required. Therefore, incisions following the lines of tension of the breast should be used at all times, because an incision along these lines usually results in a thin, cosmetically acceptable scar. In the United States, the majority of breast biopsy findings are benign.[25] It should be emphasized that a biopsy incision must always be within the boundaries of potential total or segmental mastectomy incisions that may be required in the future.

Excisional Biopsy

An excisional biopsy of a mass is indicated when its diagnosis, either by FNA or by CNB, is inconclusive or whenever a dominant mass must be completely removed. Because, as noted previously, the vast majority of all breast biopsy findings are benign, it is important to remove only the mass with little, if any, surrounding normal tissue. If the pathology report indicates the presence of only benign tissue, nothing more is required. If malignancy is present, definitive local treatment, either segmental mastectomy or total mastectomy, is indicated. It is important to remember that an area that is incompletely excised can always be reexcised but that tissue that is removed cannot be replaced.

The location and size of the incision are of great importance. As indicated previously, incisions must be placed parallel to the lines of natural skin tension. If the lesion is within 1 or 2 cm of the areola, it can be removed through a circumareolar incision. This approach should not be used with a lesion more than 2 cm from the areola, which would require a larger incision and subcutaneous tunneling, with increased risk of hematoma and infection. Placement of a small incision directly over such a lesion, with the lines of skin tension used as a guide, is the procedure of choice. The incision is usually cosmetically acceptable, requires less dissection, and marks the location of the lesion if reexcision is necessary.

Like incisional biopsies, excisional biopsies are usually performed with the use of either local anesthesia or monitored anesthetic care; only very rarely is general anesthesia required. It is helpful to mark the skin not only at the site of incision but also over the mass with a sterile marker before proceeding further. The skin and subcutaneous tissue are then infiltrated with local anesthetic, and the incision is made. Every effort should be made to remove the mass intact. All excised breast specimens should be sent to the pathologist in the fresh state for gross examination. The specimen should be oriented in at least two directions (i.e., lateral and superior) with sutures so that its margins can be accurately assessed. Improper handling of the tissue, such as removing the specimen in pieces, can lead to significant problems in pathologic interpretation.

Once the biopsy specimen has been removed, meticulous hemostasis should be obtained. If desired, the breast tissue may or may not be reapproximated, and the wound is closed. (Subcuticular sutures and sterile strips are usually appropriate.) Drains are seldom indicated. Complications generally encountered include wound infection and hematoma or seroma formation. Because the risk of wound infection is small for excisional biopsy, prophylactic antibiotics are not indicated. A double-blind, randomized, placebo-controlled trial of prophylactic antibiotics in breast surgery demonstrated no difference between placebo and antibiotics on wound infection rates for either excisional biopsy or simple mastectomy.[26] The risk of hematoma or seroma is also small, especially with use of a pressure dressing, and should either lesion occur, no specific therapy is required.

Needle (Wire)–Localized Biopsy

As mammography screening for breast lesions gains popularity, clinicians are increasingly faced with the problem of a patient who has a nonpalpable breast abnormality that requires biopsy. These abnormalities range from suspicious microcalcifications to nonpalpable masses. According to a review of 5500 biopsies culled from 17 reported series of 100 or more cases each, indications for biopsy include suspicious microcalcifications in 45%, masses in 43%, masses containing microcalcifications in 6%, and asymmetrical tissue density in 5% of cases.[27] In one report, the predicted cancer yield for these abnormalities was nearly 13% for microcalcifications, 74% for masses thought to be malignant on mammographic morphology, and just over 5% for masses thought to be benign.[28] If ultrasonography-guided core biopsy or stereotactic CNB of nonpalpable abnormalities is not performed for technical reasons or because of lack of equipment, or if a question exists about the adequacy of the specimen, a needle (or wire)–localized biopsy must be performed.

Although several needle and wire combinations are available for wire-localized breast biopsy, the most commonly used ones are the Homer, Kopans, and Sadowsky varieties. The Homer wire is a curved J-wire that has the advantage of being able to be repositioned if the initial placement is not optimal. Its disadvantage is that the wire is too thin to be palpated through the breast tissue. Therefore, the needle is usually left in place over the wire as a guide. Because the Kopans and Sadowsky wires have a distinct hook at the end that fixes them in position, they cannot easily be repositioned. The Sadowsky wire comes with stiffeners of varying length, aiding the surgeon in finding the lesion. The injection of methylene blue dye through the needle before placement of a wire is a helpful means of marking the area of concern. It is critical that the radiologist place the wire within 0.5 cm of the lesion. Inadequate radiologic localization may lead to the removal of an excessively large amount of tissue—not an optimal result of a diagnostic procedure on a nonpalpable lesion that may turn out to be benign.

Once the wire localization has been performed, the surgery is performed with the use of monitored anesthetic care. The surgeon must think about the operative approach for the biopsy. To avoid excision of a large volume of normal tissue, tissue should not be excised along the entire length of the wire, although this step may be required if the needle is not left in place over a Homer wire or if a stiffener apparatus has not been used to reinforce a Sadowsky wire. Very rarely has there been evidence that a wire track may be seeded with cancer cells and must therefore be excised. Otherwise, it is better to palpate the wire or needle tip and place the incision directly over it. Thus, if the lesion is malignant, the area is well marked for future reexcision or radiation, and if it is benign, the smallest amount of tissue will have been excised. With the use of local anesthesia or monitored anesthetic care, the incision is made, and dissection is carried to the shaft of the wire, with care being taken not to disturb it. Once it has been dissected free, the shaft of the wire is carefully passed through the skin and into the wound. The tissue surrounding the wire is then dissected free from the normal adjacent breast tissue, with no blue-stained tissue being left behind, and the lesion is removed. To ensure that the abnormality is included in the specimen, the specimen with the wire in place is sent to radiology for specimen radiography. Because specimen radiography cannot determine whether the entire lesion, including calcifications, has been removed, a benign diagnosis for calcifications can be followed by mammography within 6 to 8 weeks to document any residual microcalcifications or other abnormalities. This mammogram also serves as a new baseline mammogram if postoperative changes occur.

Although complications may follow a breast biopsy, failure to excise the lesion is the most disconcerting problem for the patient and her physicians. The surgeon relies on a high level of radiologic precision in a wire-localized breast biopsy. Compensating for poor localization by the excision of additional tissue defeats the purpose of wire-localized biopsy. If the lesion is missed, the best tactic is to repeat the procedure in 2 to 3 months. This provides time for the tissue to heal sufficiently to allow relocalization. Patients undergoing wire localization must be informed that although every effort is made to sample the abnormality, missing the lesion is a potential risk.

A serious problem that may be associated with wire-localized biopsy is the excision of so much tissue that reexcision becomes impossible. Because most biopsy findings are benign, removal of only the tissue around the tip of the wire is generally sufficient for diagnosis. Undue worry should not be expended on the chance of obtaining clear margins for the lesion. If the lesion is malignant and breast conservation is elected, reexcision is required to obtain clear margins. Another serious problem arising from inadequate preoperative planning occurs when the biopsy incision is placed far from a lesion that is malignant, and reexcision is required. The clinician must then attempt to mentally reconstruct the precise location of the primary lesion, a daunting task at best. On occasion, scar tissue can be found to help solve this dilemma, but it cannot be relied on. To avoid these problems, the incision should be made as close to the wire tip and lesion as possible, and the smallest amount of tissue required to make the diagnosis should be removed.

Ductography/Ductectomy

In the past, identifying the quadrant of the breast that contained the duct responsible for a bloody discharge from the nipple was accomplished by radially "milking" each quadrant and then, through a circumareolar incision, excising all of the subareolar ductal tissue in that quadrant. On pathologic examination, the specimen may or may not have demonstrated an abnormality, even though the discharge had ceased because the external communication of the ducts had been severed. Ductography is currently the initial procedure of choice in the evaluation of a nipple discharge. It is helpful in localizing both the abnormal duct and the lesion within it, allowing precise placement of the skin incision. Lesions that are found by ductography to be distant from the areola or that are found within a duct that extends into a second quadrant are sampled for biopsy after radiologic wire localization.

With the patient under monitored anesthetic care, ductal excision is usually performed through a circumareolar incision, because the vast majority of lesions are found within 1 cm of the areolar border. Installation of methylene blue dye into the abnormal duct at the beginning of the procedure or passage of a probe into the involved duct is helpful in demonstrating both the affected duct and the extent of resection required. The primary pitfall of ductal excision is failure to excise the lesion, which probably occurs more commonly than is generally appreciated. A pathologic diagnosis of ductal ectasia may, in fact, represent a case in which the dilated duct has been excised but not the obstructing lesion. In addition, if the lesion is located at some distance from the areola, the duct may be resected with resolution of the nipple discharge but the lesion remains. Preoperative ductography permits the avoidance of both situations by precisely localizing the lesions. Another potential sequela is nipple and areolar deformity or necrosis secondary to excessive undermining of the areola during the procedure. This complication can also be minimized by the accurate preoperative assessment of the location of the lesion with ductography and by limiting the amount of tissue excised to the area that is actually involved.

Special Circumstances

Biopsy during Lactation

It is not uncommon for the surgeon to be called on to perform an excisional breast biopsy in a lactating woman. In general, lactation should not be viewed as a contraindication to surgery, nor should it require that the woman stop breastfeeding completely before the biopsy. The patient should be instructed to either breastfeed or pump the breast just before the procedure to empty it of as much milk as possible. As with most excisional biopsies, the procedure is performed with the use of local anesthesia using lidocaine, preferably without epinephrine. To decrease the potential for a milk leak, the skin incision is placed directly over the lesion and the amount of dissection is limited to what is absolutely necessary.

After surgery, the patient should be instructed to pump the breast for 24 hours rather than use it for nursing, to prevent the baby from ingesting any residual lidocaine. She should also be told that there may be a bloody tinge to the milk from that breast for 24 to 48 hours after the biopsy. The primary complication of surgery is leakage of milk from the transected ducts, resulting in a galactocele or cutaneous milk fistula. A galactocele can be left to resorb or, if symptomatic, can be aspirated. A cutaneous milk fistula generally continues to leak milk until lactation ceases.

Silicone or Saline Breast Implants

Performance of a biopsy in a patient with a breast implant requires planning to avoid damage to the prosthesis. It is important to ascertain the size of the prosthesis before the operation, and a replacement (and a plastic surgeon, if appropriate) should be available if needed. This is one circumstance in which it is advisable to use electrocautery to perform most of the dissection, because cautery is less likely than scissors or a knife to damage the implant.

Prepubescent Female

Because the possibility of breast cancer in a prepubescent female is essentially zero, the indications for biopsy of a breast mass in this age group are very few, and watchful waiting is the best tactic. If a biopsy is deemed absolutely necessary, it is vital not to remove the breast bud completely. If the bud is completely removed, the breast will not develop on that side.

TREATMENT OF MALIGNANT BREAST DISEASE

Carcinoma of the breast is the most common cancer in women and the leading cause of death from cancer in those 15 through 54 years old.[29,30] The disease accounts for nearly one third of all cancers in women and is responsible for one in six of the cancer-related deaths in all women. It has been determined from cancer registry data in the United States that the age-adjusted incidence of new breast cancer has been steadily rising since 1940. The probability that a woman in the United States will have breast cancer during her lifetime is now 1 in 8, considerably greater than the 1980s probability of 1 in 13. An annual report to the nation on the status of cancer demonstrated that breast cancer and melanoma continued to rise when the other top eight cancers were leveling or declining in incidence rates. Part of this increase in breast cancer frequency may be due to early detection. The percentage of patients with stage IV disease has remained constant during the same period.

The natural history of breast cancer is characterized by a long duration of tumor latency and marked differences both within and among different groups of patients. Breast cancer is among the more slow-growing of human cancers; the time before diagnosis as well as that after diagnosis, even after the appearance of metastases, is often measured in years and even decades. However, a wide variation in presentation is seen. Some patients present with very aggressive cancers and do exceedingly poorly, whereas others are noted to have such indolent cancers that it is difficult to demonstrate that therapy has any effect at all on their long-term survival.

The staging of breast cancer is an attempt to predict potential survival rates from objective data. It consists of grouping patients according to the extent of their disease and is useful for determining the treatment of individual patients, for estimating prognosis, and for comparing the results of different programs of management. Staging is performed at two separate times. Initially, staging is performed clinically, on the basis of results of physical laboratory and imaging evaluations. Later, the patient's disease is restaged after surgical treatment, on the basis of the histologic evaluation of the resected specimen. Pathologic staging is the most accurate predictor of the prognosis for the individual patient. The most widely used staging system is the one adopted by the Union Internationale Contre Cancer (UICC) and the American Joint Committee on Cancer (AJCC) Staging and End Results Reporting. It is based on the tumor-nodes-metastasis (TNM) system, as detailed in the AJCC's 2002 *Manual for Staging of Cancer.*[31]

New American Joint Committee on Cancer Staging System for Breast Cancer

The original staging system served its purpose during the past decade, but advancements in breast cancer detection, innovative treatment, and prognostic evaluation called for an update of breast cancer staging systems to reflect current knowledge. The AJCC[31,32] revised the staging system and published the official adaptation in January 2003. The focus of the revision is reclassification of nodal staging. The changes include refinement of size-based minimal nodal metastasis and the inclusion of nodal metastasis detected by sentinel lymph node, immunohistochemical (IHC) staining, reverse transcriptase–polymerase chain reaction (RT-PCR), and the number and site of metastatic nodes. The revised TNM staging for breast cancer is summarized in Table 30–1.

Table 30–1. TNM Staging System for Breast Cancer

Primary tumor (T)	
TX	Primary tumor cannot be assessed
T0	No evidence of primary tumor
Tis	Carcinoma in situ
Tis (DCIS)	Ductal carcinoma in situ
Tis (LCIS)	Lobular carcinoma in situ
Tis (Paget)	Paget disease of the nipple with no tumor*
T1	Tumor ≤ 2 cm in greatest dimension
T1mic	Microinvasion ≤ 0.1 cm in greatest dimension
T1a	Tumor > 0.1 cm but not > 0.5 cm in greatest dimension
T1b	Tumor > 0.5 cm but not > 1 cm in greatest dimension
T1c	Tumor > 1 cm but not > 2 cm in greatest dimension
T2	Tumor > 2 cm but not > 5 cm in greatest dimension
T3	Tumor > 5 cm in greatest dimension
T4	Tumor of any size with direct extension to (a) chest wall or (b) skin, only as described below
T4a	Extension to chest wall, not including pectoralis muscle
T4b	Edema (including peau d'orange) or ulceration of the skin of the breast, or satellite skin nodules confined to the same breast
T4c	Both T4a and T4b
T4d	Inflammatory carcinoma
Regional lymph nodes (N)	
NX	Regional lymph nodes cannot be assessed (e.g., previously removed)
N0	No regional lymph node metastasis
N1	Metastasis in movable ipsilateral axillary lymph node(s)
N2	Metastases in ipsilateral axillary lymph nodes fixed or matted, or in clinically apparent† ipsilateral internal mammary nodes in the absence of clinically evident axillary lymph node metastasis
N2a	Metastasis in ipsilateral axillary lymph nodes fixed to one another (matted) or to other structures
N2b	Metastasis only in clinically apparent† ipsilateral internal mammary nodes and in the absence of clinically evident axillary lymph node metastasis
N3	Metastasis in ipsilateral infraclavicular lymph node(s), or in clinically apparent† ipsilateral internal mammary lymph node(s) and in the presence of clinically evident axillary lymph node metastasis; or metastasis in ipsilateral supraclavicular lymph node(s) with or without axillary or internal mammary lymph node involvement
N3a	Metastasis in ipsilateral infraclavicular lymph node(s) and axillary lymph node(s)
N3b	Metastasis in ipsilateral internal mammary lymph node(s) and axillary lymph node(s)
N3c	Metastasis in ipsilateral supraclavicular lymph node(s)

Table 30–1. TNM Staging System for Breast Cancer—cont'd

Regional lymph nodes (pN)‡	
PNX	Regional lymph nodes cannot be assessed (e.g., previously removed or not removed for pathologic study)
PN0	No regional lymph node metastasis on histologic examination, no additional examination for isolated tumor cells§
pN0(i–)	No regional lymph node metastasis on histologic examination, negative IHC result
pN0(i+)	No regional lymph node metastasis on histologic examination, positive IHC result, no IHC cluster > 0.2 mm
pN0(mol–)	No regional lymph node metastasis on histologic examination, negative molecular results (RT-PCR)
pN0(mol+)	No regional lymph node metastasis on histologic examination, positive molecular results (RT-PCR)
pN1mi	Micrometastasis (> 0.2 mm, none > 2.0 mm)
pN1	Metastasis in one to three axillary lymph nodes and/or in internal mammary nodes with microscopic disease detected by sentinel lymph node dissection but not clinically apparent¶
pN1a	Metastasis in 1 to 3 axillary lymph nodes
pN1b	Metastasis in internal mammary nodes with microscopic disease detected by sentinel lymph node dissection but not clinically apparent¶
pN1c	Metastasis in 1 to 3 axillary lymph nodes and in internal mammary lymph nodes with microscopic disease detected by sentinel lymph node dissection but not clinically apparent¶‖
pN2	Metastasis in 4 to 9 axillary lymph nodes, or in clinically apparent† internal mammary lymph nodes in the absence of axillary lymph node metastasis
pN2a	Metastasis in 4 to 9 axillary lymph nodes (at least one tumor deposit > 2.0 mm)
pN2b	Metastasis in clinically apparent† internal mammary lymph nodes in the absence of axillary lymph node metastasis
pN3	Metastasis in 10 or more axillary lymph nodes, or in infraclavicular lymph nodes, or in clinically apparent† ipsilateral internal mammary lymph nodes in the presence of one or more "positive" axillary lymph nodes; or in more than 3 axillary lymph nodes with clinically "negative" microscopic metastasis in internal mammary lymph nodes; or in ipsilateral supraclavicular lymph nodes
pN3a	Metastasis in 10 or more axillary lymph nodes (at least one tumor deposit > 2.0 mm), or metastasis to the infraclavicular lymph nodes
pN3b	Metastasis in clinically apparent† ipsilateral internal mammary lymph nodes in the presence of one or more "positive" axillary lymph nodes; or in more than 3 axillary lymph nodes and in internal mammary lymph nodes with microscopic disease detected by sentinel lymph node dissection but not clinically apparent¶
pN3c	Metastasis in ipsilateral supraclavicular lymph nodes
Distant metastasis (M)	
MX	Distant metastasis cannot be assessed
M0	No distant metastasis
M1	Distant metastasis

DCIS, ductal carcinoma in situ; IHC, immunohistochemical staining; LCIS, lobular carcinoma in situ; RT-PCR, reverse transcriptase–polymerase chain reaction.
*Paget disease associated with a tumor is classified according to the size of the tumor.
†"Clinically apparent" is defined as detected by imaging studies (excluding lymphoscintigraphy) or by clinical examination.
‡Classification is based on axillary lymph node dissection with or without sentinel lymph node dissection. Classification based solely on sentinel lymph node dissection without subsequent axillary lymph node dissection is designated "(sn)" for "sentinel node"—e.g., pN0(i+)(sn).
§"Isolated tumor cells" are defined as single tumor cells or small cell clusters no greater than 0.2 mm that are usually detected only by immunohistochemical or molecular methods but that may be verified on hematoxylin and eosin stains. Isolated tumor cells do not usually show evidence of metastatic activity (e.g., proliferation or stromal reaction).
¶"Not clinically apparent" is defined as not detected by imaging studies (excluding lymphoscintigraphy) or by clinical examination.
‖If associated with more than 3 "positive" axillary lymph nodes, the internal mammary nodes are classified as pN3b to reflect greater tumor burden.
Adapted from American Joint Committee: Cancer Staging Manual, 6th ed. New York, Springer-Verlag 2002, with permission of the American Joint Committee on Cancer, Chicago, IL.

After a long and heavy debate during the revision process, it was decided that the revised TNM staging would not incorporate histologic grade. The most commonly used histologic grading system is the modified Bloom and Richardson system prepared by Elston and Ellis.[33] It quantitatively measures nuclear grade, tubular formation, and number of mitotic cells in a defined microscopic field. This system was found to be reproducible[34-36] and predictive for long-term survival. However, histologic grading information alone does not affect treatment. Similarly, other biomarker-based prognostic analyses are not part of the AJCC staging system. Because the emerging data suggest their potential use, both grading information and biomarkers should be continually included in pathology reports for all breast cancer cases.

Treatment of In-Situ Carcinoma

As a result of the greater use of screening mammography and the heightened awareness of breast cancer, breast malignancies are being encountered at earlier stages now more than ever before. Carcinoma in situ of the breast arises from duct epithelium, is confined within the lumen of the ducts or lobules, and is classified as either ductal or lobular depending on the cytologic features and pattern of growth. Both ductal carcinoma in situ (DCIS), also known as intraductal carcinoma, and lobular carcinoma in situ (LCIS), also known as lobular neoplasia, are characterized by a proliferation of malignant epithelial cells confined to the mammary ducts or lobules, without microscopic evidence of invasion through the basement membrane into the surrounding stroma. The histologic distinction between DCIS and LCIS is usually not difficult, but overlap exists.

Lobular Carcinoma In Situ

Arising within the blunt ending ducts of the lobule, LCIS is almost impossible to diagnose through clinical examination. In most instances, the diagnosis is made incidentally in a biopsy specimen obtained from a patient with an unrelated palpable mass or mammographic abnormality. LCIS rarely forms masses and rarely calcifies. It is frequently multifocal and can be widely scattered in both breasts.

LCIS is considered a marker of greater risk for the development of invasive breast cancer, and occasionally a premalignant lesion that may become the nidus of an invasive cancer. The cumulative risk for the development of an invasive cancer in the ipsilateral breast at 25 years is 22% (slightly less than 1% per year), and the risk for the contralateral breast is 15%.[37] It is interesting to note that more than half of the invasive cancers that develop after a diagnosis of LCIS are in fact ductal rather than lobular. Because LCIS represents a diffuse bilateral process and very rarely becomes cancerous itself, ipsilateral total mastectomy or reexcision of the original biopsy site to obtain clear margins is not indicated. Nor do radiation therapy and axillary nodal dissection have any role in the management of LCIS. Five years of tamoxifen therapy has been shown to reduce the risk of developing breast cancer by 56%. Careful surveillance through physical examination and yearly mammography is the most reasonable course of management of patients with LCIS. It is important to point out to the patient that this close follow-up is not to detect recurrent LCIS but rather to detect an invasive carcinoma at the earliest possible stage. Prophylactic bilateral mastectomy is appropriate for only a select group of patients with LCIS whose emotional well-being is at stake.

Ductal Carcinoma In Situ

Infrequently diagnosed in the past, DCIS is now being detected more commonly because of the widespread use of screening mammography. Today, DCIS is the most rapidly growing type of breast cancer. On the basis of its morphology, DCIS is broadly classified into comedo and noncomedo (cribriform, micropapillary, and solid) subtypes. In contradistinction to LCIS, DCIS is viewed as a true preinvasive or premalignant lesion. Studies have shown that invasive cancer develops in approximately 30% of patients with untreated DCIS, always in the area of the original DCIS lesion.[38,39] Comedo DCIS appears to be the most aggressive form but is also the one type that tends to form microcalcifications that delineate its extent on mammograms. Noncomedo DCIS is generally less aggressive, less well characterized by microcalcifications, and frequently more extensive.

The treatment of DCIS is controversial. Total mastectomy was the standard treatment in the past because of its efficacy in local control. Treatment of DCIS with total mastectomy results in cure rates exceeding 98%.[40,41] However, treatment of this noninvasive cancer by such aggressive local therapy appeared to be excessive, prompting consideration of less aggressive therapeutic approaches. Lagios and associates[42] found that wide excision alone of DCIS lesions less than 2.5 cm in diameter on mammograms with clear margins at surgery was associated with a 10% recurrence rate; 50% of the recurrences were invasive carcinoma. Schwartz and coworkers,[43] also using wide excision alone, demonstrated a 15% local recurrence rate; 27% of the recurrences were invasive. The local recurrence rate increases with the duration of the follow-up.[40] Recurrences typically appear at or near the site of the initial lesion and, as just mentioned, contain invasive cancer in up to 50% of cases. The addition of whole-breast irradiation to wide local excision reduces the rate of recurrence by more than one half[40,44] and is particularly effective in preventing invasive recurrences (Fig. 30–1).[45] Comedo-type DCIS appears to recur more frequently than the noncomedo type.[43] Achievement of clear margins is the best predictor of successful local control.[44]

DCIS is treated by both local excision with clear margins and whole-breast irradiation or mastectomy. Recent studies have demonstrated an additional benefit for 5 years of tamoxifen therapy. In selected cases, women in whom small noncomedo DCIS lesions were removed by surgery achieving clear margins can be followed without breast irradiation. All patients with DCIS associated with microcalcifications who have chosen breast conservation treatment must undergo a postlumpectomy

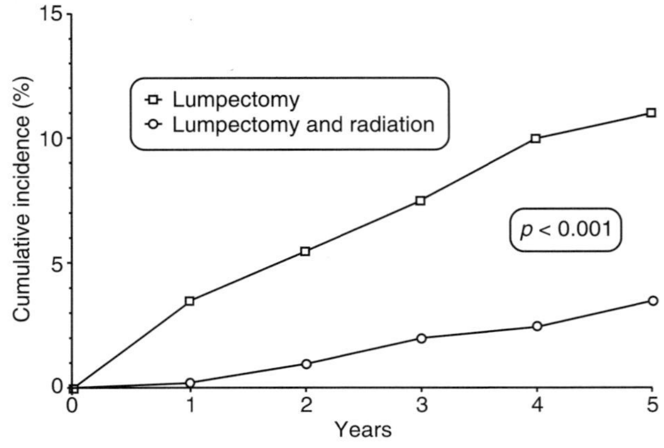

Figure 30–1. Cumulative incidence of ipsilateral recurrence of invasive breast cancer in patients with ductal carcinoma in situ treated by either lumpectomy alone or lumpectomy plus whole-breast radiation therapy. (Adapted from Fisher B, Costantino J, Redmond C, et al: Lumpectomy compared with lumpectomy and radiation therapy for the treatment of intraductal breast cancer. N Engl J Med 1993;328:1581-1586. Copyright 1993, Massachusetts Medical Society. All rights reserved.)

mammography to ensure complete removal of microcalcifications. DCIS lesions larger than 5 cm and recurrence of breast cancer after breast conservation surgery plus whole breast irradiation are probably best treated with total mastectomy. Because of the very low incidence of axillary node involvement associated with DCIS, an axillary node dissection is not indicated. Sentinel lymph node biopsy has been shown to identify axillary nodal metastasis in as many as 10% of patients with high-grade comedo DCIS. Therefore, sentinel lymph node biopsy may be helpful in this subset of patients.

Should a recurrence of either DCIS or invasive ductal carcinoma be detected in patients who have previously been treated by breast conservation, salvage is highly effective.[46-49] Salvage for patients treated initially with excision and radiation therapy usually consists of total mastectomy, whereas salvage for patients treated initially with excision alone may consist of either reexcision with radiation therapy or total mastectomy, depending on the size and extent of the lesion.

Local and Regional Treatment of Infiltrating Carcinoma

Although historically the treatment of invasive breast cancer has been primarily directed locally to the breast through surgical extirpation, current management is best considered in terms of local and regional therapies that are directed at the breast and the adjacent axillary lymph nodes. Eradication of the primary tumor is the goal of local treatment in patients without metastases. Unfortunately, occult micrometastases, which are unaffected by local management, have been found in a substantial number of women with apparently localized breast cancer. As a result, systemic therapy to eradicate these micrometastases has emerged as a vital arm of breast cancer treatment. Because breast cancer commonly metastasizes to the lymph nodes in the axilla, local treatment of the nodes, consisting of either surgical removal, radiation therapy, or a combination of the two, had been performed in the hope of improving survival. Data on the survival benefit resulting from treatment of axillae are conflicting, however.[50] Nevertheless, the presence and extent of axillary node metastases have been found to be the best predictors of overall survival in patients with breast cancer.[51,52] Thus, removal of the axillary lymph nodes is considered for both treatment and staging.

The two major options currently available for the local treatment of invasive breast cancer are (1) total mastectomy (with or without reconstruction) with axillary lymph node dissection and (2) breast-conserving surgery coupled with axillary lymph node dissection and postoperative whole-breast irradiation. Postoperative breast irradiation is essential because of the nearly 40% local recurrence rate associated with lumpectomy alone (Fig. 30–2). The results of five randomized, prospective trials comparing mastectomy with breast-conserving surgery (lumpectomy and irradiation) for the treatment of stage I and stage II breast cancer have demonstrated equivalence. As shown in Table 30–2, overall survival and relapse-free survival rates were not statistically different for the two modalities (Fig. 30–3). The local recurrence rate after breast conservation therapy ranged from 4% to 19%, whereas that after mastectomy ranged from 2% to 9%. No difference in the rate of development of distant metastases or in the development of contralateral breast cancer was seen. On the basis of these data, the 1990 National Cancer Institute Consensus Development Conference on the Treatment of Early-Stage Breast Cancer concluded that "breast conservation treatment is an appropriate method of primary therapy for the majority of women with stages I and II breast cancer and is preferable because it provides survival equivalent to

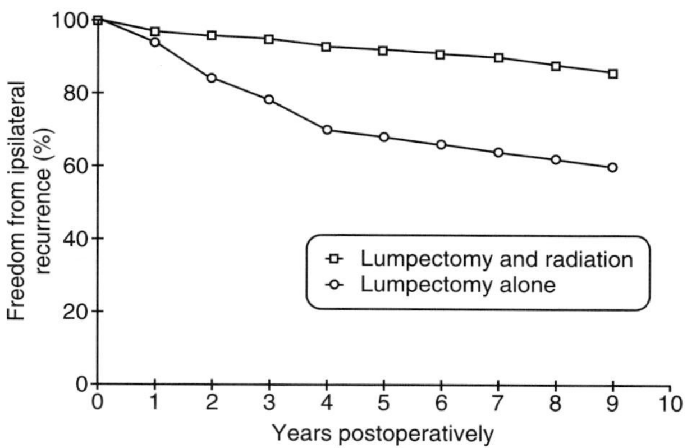

Figure 30–2. Rate of freedom from ipsilateral recurrence of invasive breast cancer after either lumpectomy alone or lumpectomy plus whole-breast radiation therapy. (Adapted from Fisher B, Costantino J, Redmond C, et al: Lumpectomy compared with lumpectomy and radiation therapy for the treatment of intraductal breast cancer. N Engl J Med 1993;328:1581-1586. Copyright 1993, Massachusetts Medical Society. All rights reserved.)

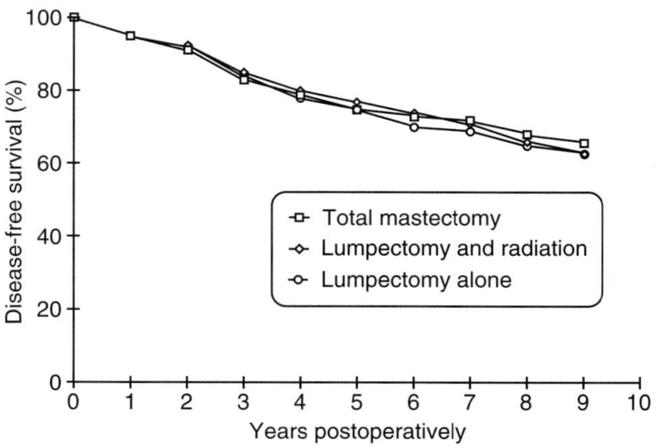

Figure 30–3. Rate of disease-free survival in patients with invasive breast cancer treated by total mastectomy, lumpectomy plus whole-breast radiation therapy, or lumpectomy alone. (Adapted from Fisher B: A biologic perspective of breast cancer: Contributions of the National Surgical Adjuvant Breast and Bowel Project clinical trials. CA Cancer J Clin 1991;41:97-111.)

Table 30–2. Comparison of Survival and Local Recurrence Rates for Breast-Conserving Treatment versus Mastectomy in Prospective, Randomized Trials

		Overall Survival (%)		Disease-Free Survival (%)		Local Recurrence Rate (%)	
Study	Years of Follow-Up	BC	M	BC	M	BC	M
Fisher et al*	8	76	71	59	58	10	8
Veronesi et al†	10	79	78	77	76	4	2
Sarrazin et al‡	10	78	79	65	56	7	9
Blichert-Toft et al§	6	79	82	70	66	4	3
Lichter et al¶	10	89	85	66	76	19	6

*Fisher B, Redmond C, Fisher ER, et al: Ten year results of a randomized clinical trial comparing radical mastectomy and total mastectomy with or without radiation. N Engl J Med 1985;312:674-681.
†Veronesi U, Banfi A, Del Vecchio M, et al: Comparison of Halsted mastectomy with quadrantectomy, axillary dissection, and radiotherapy in early breast cancer: Long-term results. Eur J Cancer Clin Oncol 1986;22:1085-1089.
‡Sarrazin D, Le MG, Arriagada R, et al: Ten-year results of a randomized trial comparing a conservative treatment to mastectomy in early breast cancer. Radiother Oncol 1989;14:177-184.
§Blichert-Toft M, Rose C, Andersen A, et al: Danish randomized trial comparing breast conservation therapy with mastectomy: Six years of life-table analysis. J Natl Cancer Inst 1992;11:19-25.
¶Lichter AS, Lippman ME, Danforth DN, et al: Mastectomy versus breast-conserving therapy in the treatment of stage I and II carcinoma of the breast: A randomized trial at the National Cancer Institute. J Clin Oncol 1992;10:976-983.
BC, breast conservation; M, mastectomy.

total mastectomy and axillary dissection while preserving the breast."[53]

Breast Conservation Surgery

Many terms have been used to describe the surgery involved in breast conservation—*lumpectomy, wide excision, segmental resection, quadrantectomy,* and *partial mastectomy*. Only *quadrantectomy* specifically defines the amount of tissue that is removed. It is important to remember that breast conservation has two goals: (1) removal of the cancer with a margin of normal tissue and (2) a good cosmetic result. The placement and performance of the skin incision are critical to the quality of cosmesis. Incisions in the resting skin tension lines generally achieve the best cosmetic result; however, it is also necessary to consider the size of the breast, the location of the cancer, and whether a previous biopsy scar must be encompassed by the incision.

Once the borders of the specimen have been palpated through the fat, resection is carried directly through the breast tissue to the level of the chest wall. To prevent inadvertent removal of more or less tissue than is required, care should be taken not to deviate from a line perpendicular to the chest wall. The specimen is removed, along with the pectoralis fascia at the deep margin of resection, just as in a total mastectomy. Once the tissue has been removed, it must be carefully oriented for the pathologist. Frozen-section analysis is not advised because one section through a 2-cm-thick specimen of tissue allows evaluation of only 1% of the margin. (Nearly 3000 sections would be needed to ensure that all of the margins are completely evaluated.) Once hemostasis is achieved, reapproximation of the remaining breast tissue becomes a challenge.

Although removal of only a small amount of tissue, especially from the lateral half of the breast, may produce little if any deformity, excision of tissue from the medial half of the breast or removal of a large amount of tissue can leave a noticeable dent. Some surgeons advocate concomitant mobilization and rotation of adjacent breast tissue to improve the cosmetic outcome of conservation surgery, but most surgeons believe that it is best to wait until after the procedure to judge the adequacy of the cosmetic result. If the cosmetic result is deemed unsatisfactory postoperatively, or if it is anticipated that a large defect will be created during breast conservation surgery in a small-breasted woman, the rotation of a small latissimus dorsi muscle flap can be advantageous. The skin is closed with a subcuticular suture material, and a dressing is left in place for 48 hours.

The primary and most frustrating problem in breast conservation surgery is the failure to obtain "clean" margins. As pointed out previously, it is impossible for the pathologist to absolutely guarantee pathologically clean (or clear) margins without the examination of thousands of slides. Therefore, at what point should the margins be considered "dirty"? The removal of larger amounts of tissue (quadrantectomy vs lumpectomy) has been shown to result in less common local recurrence.[54] Most surgeons accept a margin as being clean if normal breast tissue remains between the cancer and the inked margin. At this time, however, no consensus exists regarding the optimal extent of the surgical resection required before the patient undergoes radiation therapy. It is well recognized that the patient whose cancer has an extensive intraductal component (EIC) (defined as greater than 25% of the tumor) may have a higher rate of recurrence if the margins are not completely clean.[55]

Another common problem of breast conservation surgery is the formation of a seroma or hematoma. As with such lesions after breast biopsy, they are usually self-limited and, with reassurance of the patient, can be allowed to resolve on their own. However, a seroma that is large enough to cause significant discomfort should probably be aspirated. A single aspiration is usually sufficient to take care of the problem. An expanding hematoma demands reexploration of the wound.

Axillary Dissection

Axillary dissection (also called axillary lymph node dissection [ALND]) is defined as the surgical removal of lymph node–bearing tissue from an anatomically defined area of the axilla. It is different from *axillary sampling,* which consists of the non-anatomic removal of a variable and undefined amount of tissue. The performance of an axillary dissection is preferable to axillary sampling because the former allows evaluation of a larger and more consistent number of lymph nodes. One study showed that local recurrence rates were significantly higher in patients undergoing axillary sampling than in those undergoing axillary dissection.[56] Dissection is considered adequate when it contains at least 10 lymph nodes[57]—usually when the dissection encompasses all of the level I and some of the level II lymph nodes (see later).

The axillary dissection should be carried out in an orderly, anatomic manner that is the same whether it is performed as part of a modified radical mastectomy or as part of a breast-conserving surgical procedure. The only difference between the two procedures is whether the axillary dissection is done in continuity with the excision of the breast. When performed in conjunction with breast conservation surgery (unless the breast lesion is immediately adjacent to the axilla), the axillary dissection is usually performed through a separate incision. When it is performed in conjunction with a total mastectomy, it is done through the same incision. A transverse incision placed just lateral to the anterior axillary fold of the pectoralis muscle and extending to the posterior axillary fold of the latissimus dorsi muscle provides the best cosmetic result. Extension of the incision to the border of the pectoralis major muscle results in a scar that will be visible when the patient lowers her arms and that may be unsightly when she wears a sleeveless dress. The incision should be placed at the lower edge of the axillary hair line.

After the skin incision, the initial step of an axillary dissection is to create small skin flaps, either sharply or with an electrocautery unit. The lateral border of the pectoralis major muscle is next identified, and care is used to identify and preserve the medial pectoral nerve as it passes around the pectoralis minor muscle and into the undersurface of the pectoralis major muscle. The lymph node–bearing tissue between the pectoralis major and the pectoralis minor muscles is swept laterally to be removed as part of the surgical specimen. Identification of the lateral border of the pectoralis minor muscle and its elevation exposes the clavipectoral fascia, which is then entered and dissected laterally. The lymph nodes located infralateral to the lateral edge of the pectoralis minor muscle are designated as level I nodes. Those lying behind the pectoralis minor muscle are identified as level II nodes, and those lying between the superomedial edge of the pectoralis minor muscle and the subclavius muscle (or Halsted ligament) are the level III nodes.

The axillary vein is then identified, and the lymph node–bearing tissue is swept inferiorly and laterally along the chest wall. This step allows early identification of both the intercostobrachial nerve, which is seen emerging from the serratus anterior and passing into the axillary fat pad, and the long thoracic nerve, which courses along the chest wall just above the subscapular muscle. The intercostobrachial nerve is carefully dissected by opening of the axillary fat pad and dissection of the nerve free of the surrounding lymph node–bearing tissue. The nerve is occasionally noted to form two, or sometimes three, branches as it passes through the axilla, and attempts should be made to preserve as many branches as possible. The long thoracic nerve must be preserved. As tissue is swept inferiorly from the axillary vein, a superficial unnamed branch that passes into the axillary fat pad is identified and can be safely divided. Directly posterior to this branch, the subscapular artery and vein are identified. Just medial to these vessels, the thoracodorsal nerve runs along the anterior surface of the subscapular muscle; this nerve must also be preserved.

Once all three nerves have been identified and dissected free from the axillary contents, the axillary fat pad is dissected in a lateral and inferior direction to the anterior border of the latissimus dorsi muscle. There it is divided and removed. Specific orientation of the specimen for the pathologist, identifying the highest axillary nodes taken, is controversial and actually does not influence the prognosis or recommendations for further therapy. After meticulous hemostasis is achieved, it is helpful to inject a long-acting local anesthetic (0.25% to 0.50% bupivacaine hydrochloride) into the wound to diminish pain in the immediate postoperative period. Drainage of the axillary wound is controversial, and even placement of a closed suction drain does not completely eliminate the chance of seroma formation. The subcutaneous tissue is closed with an absorbable suture material, and the skin is closed with subcuticular absorbable sutures.

A complication of axillary dissection in addition to seroma or hematoma formation is nerve injury. Division of the intercostobrachial nerve may cause permanent numbness in the lateral axilla and medial portion of the upper arm, a distressing symptom to a woman when she shaves her underarms. Injury can also occur to the two motor nerves that run through the axilla. Injury to the long thoracic nerve, which may result in a winged scapula or palsy of the serratus anterior muscle, occurs in approximately 10% of cases. Injury to the thoracodorsal nerve, which innervates the latissimus dorsi muscle, can lead to temporary weakness; it usually resolves within 6 weeks to 6 months. The most serious and distressing complication of axillary dissection is arm edema, which may occur in as many as 10% to 20% of cases. A direct correlation appears to exist between the extent of axillary dissection and the development of edema. The addition of axillary irradiation further raises the risk.[58]

Sentinel Lymph Node Mapping

Sentinel lymph nodes (SLNs) are the first lymph nodes to receive drainage from the primary cancer. SLN mapping is a procedure to identify and to selectively remove these lymph nodes for pathologic assessment of nodal status. It differs from ALND in that SLN mapping removes significantly fewer lymph nodes (average 2 or 3 lymph nodes for SLN, compared with 20 lymph nodes for ALND) without compromising the accuracy of nodal staging. The less invasive nature and highly accurate staging proficiency makes SLN mapping a preferred procedure over the conventional ALND and axillary sampling procedures.

The concept of the SLN was first introduced by Cabanas in 1977 for the treatment of penile cancer.[59] The SLN procedure was popularized by Morton and associates[60] to assess lymph node metastases in patients with early stage melanoma. Giuliano and colleagues[61] and Krag coworkers[62,63] developed surgical techniques for using SLN mapping to stage lymph nodes in breast cancer. Many early studies reported in the 1990s, including the UCLA experience,[65] compared the accuracy of nodal staging with SLN and ALND by performing ALND in all patients after the initial SLN procedure.[61,63,64] These studies reported that the SLN procedure was successful in more than 90% of cases with a low false-negative rate.

Of many techniques used to identify sentinel lymph nodes, the use of a combination of technetium Tc 99m (^{99m}Tc)–labeled sulfur colloid (^{99m}Tc-SC) and lymphazurin dye is favored by many surgeons.[66] When the nonfiltered ^{99m}Tc-SC is used, the injection is performed at least 2 hours and up to 24 hours before the SLN procedure. When the filtered tracer is used, it is given immediately before the surgery. Preoperative lymphoscintigraphy can visually identify any unexpected draining basins, information that can be important in planning for radiation treatment (Fig. 30–4). The lymphazurin, 3 to 5 mL, is injected 5 to 10 minutes before the skin incision is made. The breast is massaged to promote lymphatic drainage. A small skin incision is made in the axilla along the premarked "hot spot "detected by a handheld gamma probe. The incision is frequently along the lowest axillary line. The SLN is first identified by following the blue lymphatic tract that leads to the SLN, blue or not. The removed SLN is individually checked for radioactivity. Once the visible SLNs are removed, the handheld gamma probe is used to ensure that there are no additional SLNs in the operative field or in the nonexposed area. Although routine intraoperative examination of the SLNs by the pathologist is not recommended, studies show that frozen-section[67] and touch-preparation cytology examinations[68] are useful in identifying nodal metastasis. Selective intraoperative pathology evaluation may be helpful in patients with either a high risk for nodal metastasis or suspicious SLNs found during surgery. Drainage is not used for the SLN procedure.

Choi and associates[66] reported on a group of 81 consecutive women with an average follow-up of 12 months after SLN procedures. At one week after surgery, 86% had full range of motion of the involved shoulder. The complication rate was low; 7.4% of the patients had axillary wound seroma, and 1.2% had wound infection. Measurable lymphedema was absent in all patients throughout the follow-up period.

In general, patients who have primary breast cancers that are not multicentric and have clinically normal axillary findings are candidates for SLN procedures. However, patients with locally advanced breast cancer (T3 and T4) should be considered for conventional axillary dissection because of the high incidence of multiple nodal metastases in this group of patients. Patients with large or comedo DCIS may also benefit from the SLN procedure, as a significant number of patients are found to have nodal metastasis by SLN. Patients with early breast cancer with hormonal receptor–negative tumors and evidence of lymphovascular invasion (LVI) have a markedly higher risk for nodal metastasis.[66] These patients should be made aware of their risk during the discussion of surgical options for lymph node staging, and selective intraoperative nodal evaluation may be worthwhile in these patients.

Axillary lymph node dissection is not necessary in patients with negative SLNs. Axillary dissection may have no added value in patients with small primary cancers (≤2 cm) and micrometastasis in SLN detected by IHC staining only.[69,70] Additional axillary dissection is recommended otherwise in all patients in whom SLNs test positive on hematoxylin and eosin staining.

Although the prospective nonrandomized studies provided information that guided the selection of patients for SLN procedures and the selection of the course of subsequent treatment, data from randomized studies are not available. The National Surgical Adjuvant Breast and Bowel Project (NSABP) trial B32 is being conducted to compare SLN and ALND in patients with operable breast cancer and clinically negative axillae. The American College of Surgeons Oncology Group (ACOSOG) Z 0010 trial is studying women with positive SLNs with or without subsequent ALND. These two prospective randomized studies will give us definitive evidence as to the efficacy of SLN in nodal staging, including the short-term and long-term morbidity, the incidence of recurrence after negative SLN results, the surgical recommendation after positive SLN results, and

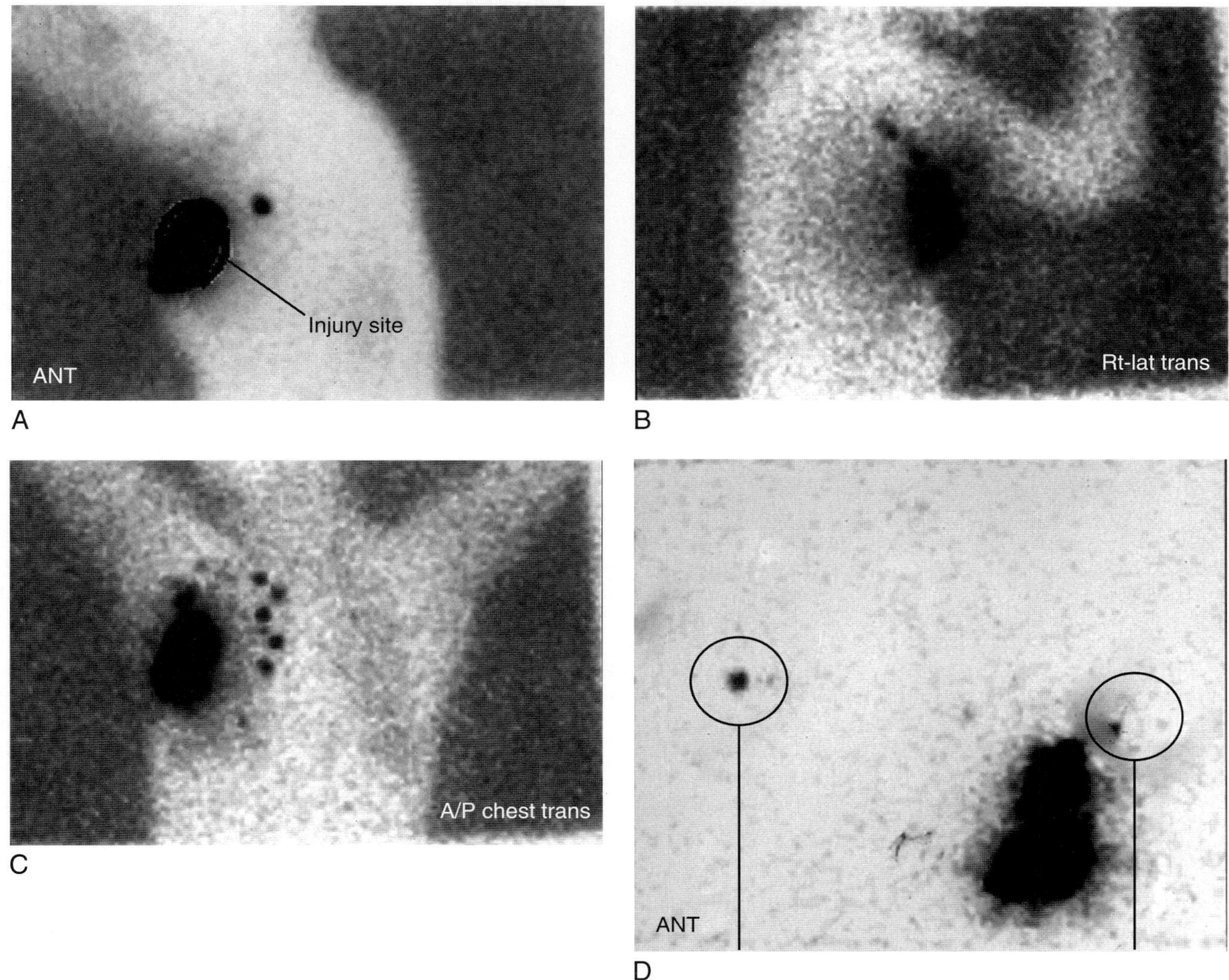

Figure 30–4. Sentinel lymph nodes (SLNs) detected by technetium Tc 99m–labeled sulfur colloid. **A,** Single SLN in axilla. **B,** Multiple SLNs in axilla. **C,** SLNs in both axilla and internal mammary area. **D,** Bilateral axillary drainage reflected by SLN in each axilla.

the clinical implications of IHC-detected SLN micrometastasis.

Total Mastectomy and Axillary Dissection

For almost 100 years, complete or en bloc removal of the breast and axilla was the standard treatment for breast cancer. From the time of its original description in 1894,[71] this so-called radical mastectomy remained the treatment of choice until approximately 20 years ago. Since the 1970s, a succession of operations that preserved more and more of the chest wall and axillary structures has now reached the point at which not even the term *modified radical mastectomy* adequately describes the operation. For that reason, the term *total mastectomy* is probably the best description of an operation that removes all breast tissue. For invasive adenocarcinoma of the breast, therefore, a total mastectomy with ALND describes most precisely the procedure that is actually performed.

As indicated previously, total mastectomy is most commonly used for large diffuse breast cancer and is also the treatment of choice when radiation therapy is undesirable or contraindicated. In addition, a small number of women desire removal of the breast regardless of the stage of their cancer. Total mastectomy has also been used for breast cancer prevention in women with high risk for development of breast cancer. If, for whatever reason, a total mastectomy is chosen as the treatment, the patient should be offered immediate breast reconstruction at the time of the original surgery, either with an autogenous tissue flap or by placement of a tissue expander. The patient's age should not deter a surgeon from offering reconstruction. However, immediate reconstruction may be contraindicated because of other medical problems.

The skin incision for a total mastectomy should be elliptical and placed in such a manner as to minimize scar visibility. Obviously, if immediate reconstruction is to be performed, placement of the incision should be discussed with the collaborating plastic surgeon to maximize cosmesis, and a circumareolar incision is frequently preferred. If an incisional scar from a previous cancer biopsy is present, it and the nipple should be excised. With dissection carried into the subcutaneous tissue, the skin flaps are developed. The plane of dissection is between the breast and the superficial fascia of the subcutaneous tissue, which contains the subdermal plexus of arteries and veins. In premenopausal women, the skin flaps are usually thin, whereas in postmenopausal women, they are thick. The dissection is carried superiorly to the clavicle, medially to the sternum, inferiorly to below the inframammary crease near the costal margin, and laterally to the anterior border of the latissimus dorsi muscle. The breast is then dissected from the underlying pectoralis musculature in a medial-to-lateral fashion, with the pectoralis fascia excised as part of the surgical specimen.

Once the lateral border of the pectoralis major muscle is identified, the node-bearing tissue between it and the pectoralis minor muscle is swept laterally to be included with the surgical specimen. Care should be taken not to injure the medial pectoral nerve, because injury to this nerve can result in atrophy of the lower portion of the pectoralis musculature, with resultant chest wall deformity. If no axillary dissection is to be performed, dissection is continued laterally from this point across the serratus anterior muscle to the anterior border of the latissimus dorsi muscle. The resected specimen is oriented for the pathologist and sent in a fresh state for pathologic examination. The wound is irrigated and meticulously inspected for hemostasis. Closed-suction drains are placed across the chest wall and into the axilla. The skin is then closed without tension, by means of interrupted absorbable sutures placed subcutaneously and a running absorbable subcuticular suture.

If an axillary dissection is performed in conjunction with total mastectomy, the contents of the axilla are left in continuity with the resected breast. The complications of the procedure, outlined in the previous section on breast conservation surgery, consist of seroma or hematoma formation and injury to the nerves in the axilla. An additional complication, partial necrosis of the skin flaps, may occur very close to the edge of the suture line but seldom requires débridement. Rarely, a large area of necrosis may require surgical débridement.

Breast Reconstruction

Unless the patient has a specific medical contraindication, breast reconstruction should be offered to any woman undergoing total mastectomy. No evidence has been found that reconstruction compromises adjuvant chemotherapy, increases the incidence of local recurrences, or delays the detection of locally recurrent cancer in the chest wall. Reconstruction has the advantage of helping restore the patient's perception of body image. It is important to point out to the patient that although reconstruction will not allow her to regain a normal breast, it will minimize the deformity created by the treatment. The actual timing of the performance of the reconstruction varies from immediately after the mastectomy to years later. Although in the past most reconstructions were delayed from 3 to 9 months after mastectomy to allow completion of adjuvant treatment, immediate reconstruction is now common. Currently, two major types of reconstruction are available. One involves the use of a tissue expander and prosthesis, and the other uses a myocutaneous flap, either free or with a pedicle. Each method has advantages and disadvantages, and one is not necessarily superior to the other.

The simplest form of breast reconstruction involves the placement of a tissue expander beneath the musculofascial layers. It can be performed at the time of mastectomy or postoperatively. After the wound has healed, the tissue expander is gradually filled with saline. Once the local tissues are stretched to the desired size, the tissue expander is removed under local or general anesthesia, and a permanent prosthesis is placed in the subpectoral muscle pocket. The tissue expander has the advantage of relatively rapid and easy placement and, therefore, can be used in a patient who otherwise might not tolerate the long operative time required for myocutaneous flap reconstruction. The disadvantages are those seen with any type of prosthesis: infection, capsular contraction, and overlying skin necrosis. However, because of the subpectoral placement of the prosthesis, skin necrosis is unlikely.

The myocutaneous flap for breast reconstruction is becoming increasingly popular because of the "natural feel" of the reconstructed breast as well as the low incidence of infection and the absence of capsular problems. The three types of flaps generally used for reconstruction are the transverse rectus abdominis myocutaneous (TRAM) flap from the lower abdomen, the lower latissimus dorsi myocutaneous flap from the back, and the gluteus maximus myocutaneous flap from the buttock. A myocutaneous flap consists of a section of muscle that is transposed with its overlying skin and subcutaneous tissue either as a rotational flap or as a completely detached free flap. Free flaps can also be performed without muscle removal in selected patients; such flaps are based on deep inferior epigastric perforator vessels. Flap reconstruction has the advantage of containing enough bulk to replace the breast mound and affords a better long-term cosmetic result than an implant. Because of the possibility of greater blood loss and prolongation of operating time, the decision to perform an immediate reconstruction should be discussed with all members of the surgical team. Of the three types of flaps, the TRAM flap operation does not require moving or manipulation of the patient during the operation, as do the latissimus dorsi and gluteus maximus flap procedures.

The technique for reconstruction of the nipple-areolar complex is identical for the two methods of reconstruction. It is important that the nipple-areolar complex be symmetrically positioned and similar in size and appearance to that of the normal breast. Regardless of the timing of breast reconstruction, reconstruction of the nipple-areolar complex is ordinarily delayed for 3 to 6 months to allow settling of the prosthesis and to ensure complete vascularity of the myocutaneous flap. The cosmetic results of nipple-areolar reconstruction are generally only fair to good, with the best cosmetic results obtained from the use of skin from the inner thigh.

Radiation Therapy after Lumpectomy

Although extensive local and regional surgery of the breast and axillary lymph nodes was for many years the "gold standard" for treatment of breast cancer, no difference in survival benefit has been found between total mastectomy and breast-conserving surgery coupled with whole-breast irradiation. Conservative surgery and radiation therapy imply the gross surgical removal of the invasive cancer with a margin of normal breast tissue and subsequent destruction of any residual microscopic disease in the breast with radiation therapy. In three large randomized, prospective trials, radiation therapy with opposed tangential fields in doses of at least 5000 cGy over 5 to 6 weeks, after completion of breast conservation surgery, yielded rates of disease-free survival and overall survival at 20 years' follow-up equivalent to those for mastectomy.[72,73] The 20-year follow-up study conducted by Veronesi and colleagues[73] indicated that patients who underwent breast-conserving therapy had higher local recurrence rates (8.8%) than those who had mastectomy (2.3%). In addition, the time to recurrence differed in the two groups. The majority of recurrences after mastectomy appeared in the first 3 years,[46-48] whereas those after conservative surgery and radiation therapy appeared later.[74] In the patients undergoing conservative surgery with irradiation, a recurrence rate of 2% to 3% per year was noted for the first 5 to 7 years, with a slowing in the rate thereafter.

In patients who underwent conservation surgery and radiation therapy, 75% of cancer recurrences seen in the first 5 years were at or near the original cancer site and probably represented a recurrence of the original cancer, whereas 13% appeared elsewhere in the breast and were most likely new cancers.[75] The remaining recurrences were in the skin of the breast. Salvage of these patients with recurrence after breast conservation therapy is more successful than salvage of patients with recurrence after mastectomy. Long-term disease-free survival has been reported to exceed 50% in women with recurrences after conservation surgery and radiation therapy,[74,76] compared with less than 30% in women who had chest wall recurrences after mastectomy.[8] Localized radiation therapy is now being studied as an alternative to whole breast treatment.

After radiation therapy, most patients have minimal to mild fibrosis throughout the breast, although it may be greater if a booster dose of radiation was given to the excision site, especially if radioactive implants were used. In addition to fibrosis after therapy, the breast can undergo retraction, edema, and telangiectasis.[77] Retraction of the breast may progress for 2 to 3 years after therapy but generally remains stable thereafter. Breast edema appears to be related to the extent of the axillary dissection as well as the radiation therapy. Moderate or severe edema nearly always resolves by a year after treatment, whereas mild edema that may include the skin can persist indefinitely or resolve slowly over years. Telangiectasis does not generally appear until about a year or more after treatment, reaching its maximum incidence and extent at about 4 years.

Postmastectomy Radiation Therapy

Postmastectomy radiation therapy (PMRT) is rarely used in patients with either in-situ or invasive breast cancer. There are several indications that might justify the use of PMRT[78] to reduce local-regional recurrence and improve survival. Patients with four or more positive axillary lymph nodes who received PMRT showed significantly better local-regional control and disease-free survival in the Southeastern Cooperative Study Group Trial.[49] Retrospective data also suggest that patients with operable T3 node-positive cancer have a local recurrence rate of 25% after modified radical mastectomy and systemic chemotherapy.[79,80] Two Danish studies showed that the local-regional control, disease-free survival, and overall survival were improved by PMRT in patients with large tumors (T3).[81,82] PMRT to the chest wall is considered beneficial for patients with the following:

- Four or more positive lymph nodes
- T3 or T4 breast cancers
- Positive surgical margins

In patients with T3 or T4 cancer or positive axillary lymph nodes, irradiation is extended to include the upper axillary (undissected) and supraclavicular areas. The internal mammary nodes are included if the internal mammary lymph nodes are involved or they are the SLN draining area with positive axillary nodes.

Systemic Treatment of Infiltrating Carcinoma

One of the major contributions of research into breast cancer treatment in the past 25 years has been the realization that more extensive surgery or radiation therapy or both have generally not improved patient survival. This realization not only ushered in the era of breast-conserving surgery but also formed the basis of the concept of breast cancer as a systemic disease frequently requiring systemic therapy. With the exception of patients with stage 0 and many with stage I cancers, systemic therapy forms an integral part of the treatment plan for patients with breast cancer. Usually employed after local treatment of the primary cancer ("adjuvant therapy"), systemic therapy is given with curative intent in many patients.[83] It is also used in patients with advanced or grossly metastatic disease in the hope of prolonging and improving the quality of their lives. Endocrine manipulation and cytotoxic chemotherapy represent the two accepted classes of systemic therapy used in these patients, and they can be used separately or together.

Endocrine Manipulation

The use of endocrine manipulation in the treatment of carcinoma of the breast was originally described about 100 years ago, when Beatson reported a response to bilateral oophorectomy in a patient with breast cancer.[84] Endocrine therapy consists of ovarian ablation—through surgery, drugs, or with pelvic irradiation—in premenopausal patients and of the medical blockade of cell surface receptors in both premenopausal and postmenopausal patients. Although early studies of ovarian ablation demonstrated only delayed recurrence and no improvement in overall survival, later studies have shown a prolongation of both relapse-free survival and overall survival, especially in women with positive axillary lymph nodes.[85] Although not as frequently employed in the United States as in Europe, surgical ovarian ablation may be relatively easily performed endoscopically. Medical ovarian ablation through the use of an LHRH (luteinizing hormone–releasing hormone) or GnRH (gonadotropin-releasing hormone) agonist, such as leuprolide acetate (Lupron) or goserelin acetate (Zoladex), is becoming an increasingly popular method of achieving the same results.

Tamoxifen is a nonsteroidal antiestrogen that competes with estrogen for binding sites in target tissues such as the breast. Because, in general, approximately 50% of premenopausal women and nearly 90% of postmenopausal women with breast cancer have been shown to have positive estrogen receptor (ER) activity in their cancers, tamoxifen has been firmly established as an effective adjuvant therapy. Tamoxifen alone has been shown to improve disease-free survival in patients with ER-positive, node-negative cancers regardless of menopausal status.[45] In addition, reduction in both ipsilateral and contralateral breast cancers with tamoxifen was also noted in these patients.[86] Tamoxifen has also been shown to be effective adjuvant therapy in postmenopausal patients with ER-positive, node-positive breast cancers.[50] The use of tamoxifen as adjunct therapy in postmenopausal patients with ER-negative cancers is not recommended because the response rate is only 5%. A duration of treatment of up to 5 years has been shown to significantly improve relapse-free survival.[87] Given the recognized risk of endometrial abnormalities, including cancer with tamoxifen therapy[88] and no added benefit, treatment for more than 5 years is not justified. Therefore adjuvant tamoxifen therapy for 5 years should be recommended to women whose breast cancers contain hormone receptor protein, regardless of age, menopausal status, involvement of axillary lymph nodes, and tumor size.[89,90]

The International Consensus Panel on the Treatment of Primary Breast Cancer added an ovarian suppression agent, goserelin, to tamoxifen in its recommendations for hormonal treatment in premenopausal patients with breast cancer. Furthermore, the panel also encouraged the testing of aromatase inhibitors, such as anastrozole, letrozole, and exemestane, in postmenopausal women with ER-positive tumors.[90]

Tamoxifen has also been successfully used in prevention for women who are at increased risk for development of breast cancer.[91,92] The success opens other target-directed preventive strategies and will give women with high risk choices beyond prophylactic mastectomy.

Cytotoxic Chemotherapy

With publication of the results of two seminal studies on the effectiveness of adjuvant cytotoxic chemotherapy in patients with breast cancer,[93,94] systemic chemotherapy has become an essential part of treatment. A study with a 20-year follow-up has shown a significant improvement in the survival of patients with node-positive disease who were treated with chemotherapy (Fig. 30–5).[95] The first adjuvant chemotherapy trials demonstrated an improvement in relapse-free survival only in premenopausal patients, particularly those with positive nodes. Although many regimens have been evaluated, the regimens that are currently accepted are (1) a combination of cyclophosphamide, methotrexate, and 5-fluorouracil (CMF) and (2) a doxorubicin-based combination (either doxorubicin [Adriamycin] and cyclophosphamide [AC] or doxorubicin, cyclophosphamide, and 5-fluorouracil [CAF]). Although CAF can be administered over a shorter period, the two combinations appear to be equally effective.[96] However, it is important to remember that although CMF can be administered simultaneously with postoperative

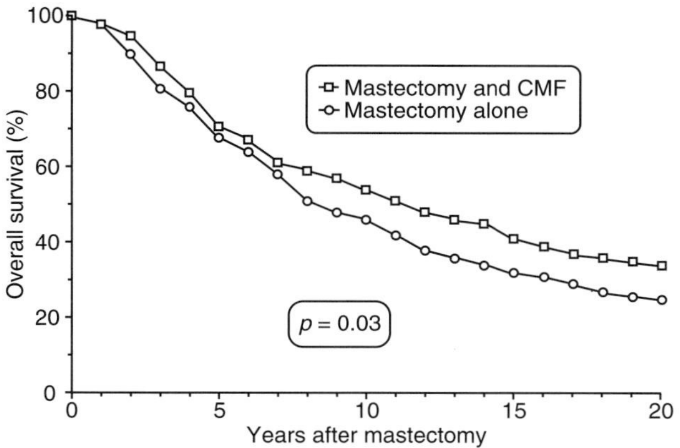

Figure 30–5. Overall survival of patients with node-positive breast cancer treated with either mastectomy alone or mastectomy plus a combination of cyclophosphamide, methotrexate, and 5-fluorouracil (CMF). (Adopted from Bonadonna G, Balagussa P, Moliterni A, et al: Adjuvant cyclophosphamide, methotrexate, and fluorouracil in node-positive breast cancer: The results of 20 years of follow-up. N Engl J Med 1995;332:901-906.)

whole-breast irradiation as part of breast-conserving surgical therapy, doxorubicin-based regimens cannot. In patients receiving doxorubicin-based chemotherapy, breast irradiation should be delayed until after completion of the chemotherapy.

The use of cytotoxic chemotherapy in postmenopausal patients with positive nodes and all patients with "negative" nodes is controversial. Although studies have shown that chemotherapy is beneficial in postmenopausal women with node-positive breast cancer,[50] chemotherapy is usually not offered to patients older than 70 years because of its toxicity and because tamoxifen therapy alone in these patients is highly effective. Questions regarding the usefulness of chemotherapy in patients with negative nodes, regardless of menopausal status, have led to its being recommended only for patients with a large primary tumor and unfavorable histopathologic features and biologic markers, such as ER status. Patients with negative nodes whose primary cancers are less than or equal to 1 cm, because of their excellent prognosis and negligible risk of metastasis, should not receive chemotherapy unless they are part of a clinical protocol.[53] Patients with negative nodes whose primary cancers are between 1 and 2 cm and who have "favorable" biologic markers also have an excellent prognosis and should probably not be started on systemic chemotherapy. Patients with "unfavorable" markers, such as ER negativity, elevated S-phase values, aneuploidy, or HER-2/neu oncoprotein overexpression, have a lifetime risk for metastasis of about 15% and should therefore probably be offered systemic therapy. Patients with node-negative cancers whose primary tumors are larger than 2 cm appear to have a more than 30% risk of metastasis and should therefore be offered systemic therapy. Examples of systemic therapy regimens according to cancer stage are given in Figure 30–6.

Most of the short-term toxic side effects of the two nonprotocol chemotherapeutic regimens for breast cancer (CMF and CAF or AC) are essentially identical in type and frequency. The common toxic effects are fatigue (95%), nausea (90%), leukopenia-thrombocytopenia (65%), nervousness-irritability (60%), and amenorrhea (55%).[93,97] Less common side effects are cystitis, vomiting, conjunctivitis, musculoskeletal pain, and deep vein thrombosis. The major difference in side effects between the two regimens is the occurrence of alopecia, which is seen in essentially all patients undergoing doxorubicin-containing regimens and in about 40% of patients receiving CMF (although rarely is the hair loss total). The primary long-term toxicity, cardiac dysfunction, is associated with doxorubicin-based regimens and is not seen with CMF. It includes progressive heart failure (which can be lethal), conduction abnormalities, and a subclinical decrease in the left ventricular ejection fraction. These complications may be compounded in patients receiving radiation therapy to the left side of the chest. Studies indicate that doxorubicin used at the cumulative doses in standard adjuvant programs does not cause excessive cardiac toxicity in patients without significant preexisting heart disease.

Anthracycline-based poly-chemotherapy is more effective in terms of disease-free survival and overall survival than CMF.[98] Four to six courses of treatment are considered to provide optimal benefit. Dose-intensive treatment regimens with stem cell support are not more effective than the poly-chemotherapy treatment and should not be used outside the setting of a randomized clinical trial.[99] Taxanes (docetaxel and paclitaxel) have also been shown to be effective in treating metastatic breast cancer. Their use is being expanded as part of the adjuvant poly-chemotherapy.

In addition to the need to develop new chemotherapeutic agents, target-directed nonchemotherapeutic treatment has attracted much interest. Trastuzumab (Herceptin) for HER-2/neu–overexpressing breast cancer represents a new class of treatment for breast cancer. Its use as adjuvant therapy in combination with chemotherapy is being investigated in patients with HER-2/neu–overexpressing breast cancer.

It is important for both the patient and the clinician to realize that despite these side effects, women who receive systemic chemotherapy enjoy improvement not only in their long-term survival but also in the overall quality of their lives compared stage for stage with women who do not receive systemic chemotherapy.[100]

Treatment of Locally Advanced Breast Cancer

Locally advanced carcinomas of the breast are primarily stage III cancers, which have no demonstrable distant metastases but carry a high risk of early relapse and mortality. This group consists of primary tumors

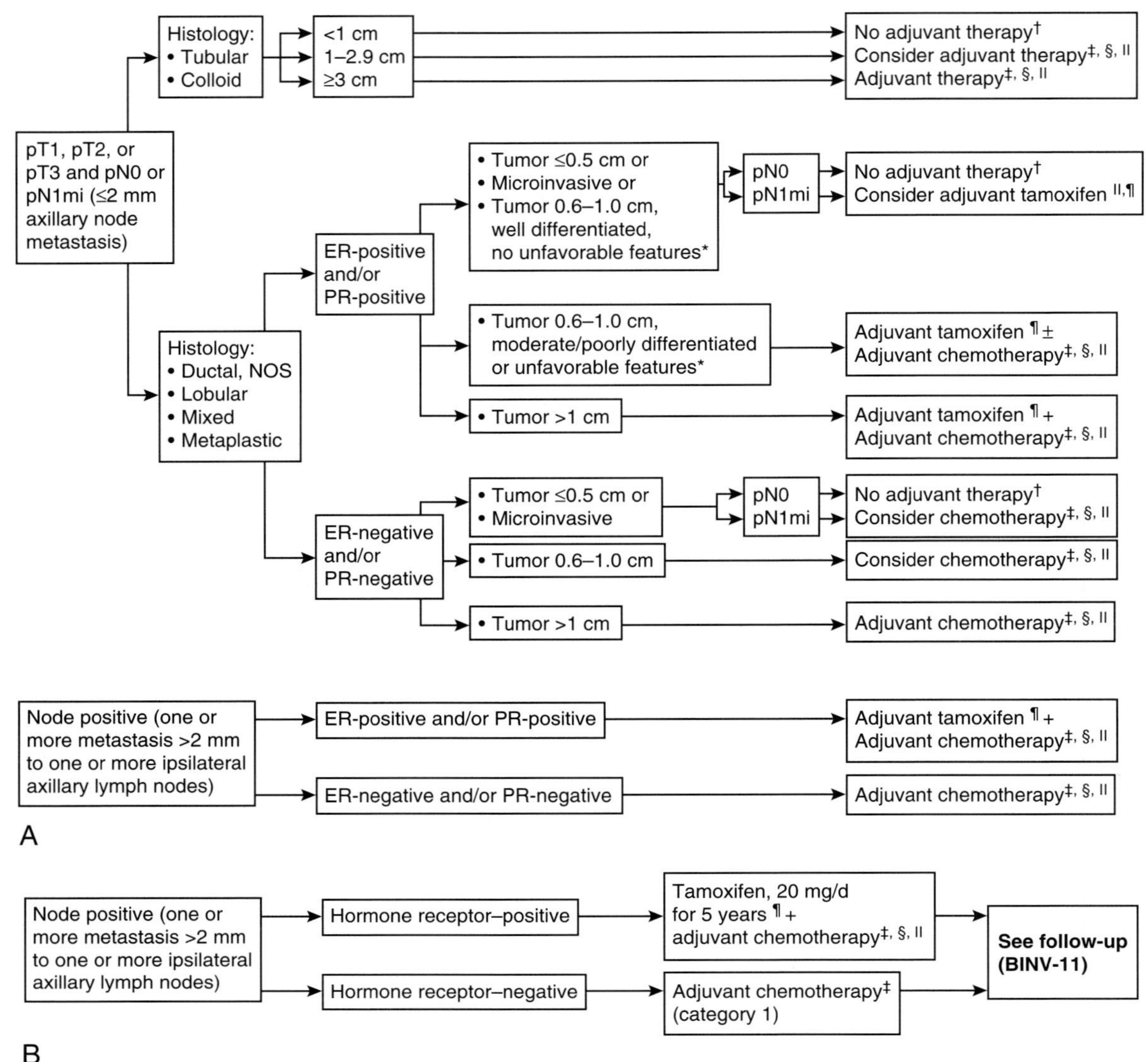

Figure 30–6. National Comprehensive Cancer Network (NCCN) practice guidelines for invasive breast cancer. Note: All recommendations are category 2A unless otherwise indicated. Clinical Trials: NCCN believes that the best management of any cancer patient is in a clinical trial. Participation in clinical trials is especially encouraged.

These guidelines are a work in progress that will be refined as often as new significant data become available.

The NCCN Guidelines are a statement of consensus of its authors regarding their views of currently accepted approaches to treatment. Any clinician seeking to apply or consult any NCCN guideline is expected to use independent medical judgment in the context of individual clinical circumstances to determine any patient's care or treatment. The National Comprehensive Cancer Network makes no warranties of any kind whatsoever regarding their content, use or application and disclaim any responsibility for their application or use in any way.

*Unfavorable features: angiolymphatic invasion, high nuclear grade, high histologic grade, HER-2 overexpression, hormone receptor–negative (category 2B).

†If ER-positive, consider tamoxifen for risk reduction and to diminish the small risk of disease recurrence.

‡There are insufficient data to make chemotherapy recommendations for those older than 70 years of age. Treatment should be individualized with consideration of comorbid conditions.

§Chemotherapy and tamoxifen used as adjuvant therapy should be given sequentially with tamoxifen following chemotherapy. The benefits of chemotherapy and of tamoxifen are additive. However, the absolute benefit from chemotherapy may be small. The decision to add chemotherapy to tamoxifen should be individualized, especially in those with a favorable prognosis and in women 60 years of age or older where the incremental benefit of chemotherapy may be smaller. Available data suggest that sequential or concurrent tamoxifen with RT is acceptable.

||Evidence supports that the magnitude of benefit from surgical or radiation overian ablation in premenopausal women with hormone-receptor–positive breast cancer is similar to that achieved with CMF alone. Early evidence suggests similar benefits from ovarian suppression (i.e., LHRH agonist or antagonist) as from ovarian ablation. The combination of ovarian ablation/suppression plus tamoxifen may be superior to suppression alone. The benefit of ovarian ablation/suppression in premenopausal women who have received adjuvant chemotherapy is uncertain.

¶Anastrozole, 1 mg/d for 5 years, may be considered an option to tamoxifen in women postmenpausal at the time of diagnosis. Women who have received approximately 5 years of tamoxifen and who are postmenopausal should consider sequential treatment with letrozole.

Reproduced with permission from The NCCN Invasive Breast Cancer Guideline, *The Complete Library of NCCN Clinical Practice Guidelines in Oncology* [CD-ROM]. Jenkintown, Pennsylvania; © National Comprehensive Cancer Network, June 2004. To view the most recent and complete version of the guideline, go online to www.nccn.org.

greater than 5 cm in size; tumors fixed to the skin, chest wall, or both; and tumors associated with skin edema (peau d'orange), skin ulceration, satellite nodules or infiltration, fixed and matted axillary lymph nodes, supraclavicular lymphadenopathy, or arm swelling. Included in this group is inflammatory carcinoma, which accounts for as much as 6% of all breast cancers and which is generally considered to be more aggressive and to have a poorer prognosis than other forms of locally advanced breast cancer.[101] Despite the lack of demonstrable distant metastases, the poor prognosis for patients with these tumors suggests that distant micrometastases are present at the time of the initial diagnosis and, therefore, that local and regional therapy alone will be unsuccessful. The lack of success of traditional therapeutic approaches for these patients, employing initial local control and later systemic therapy, has led to the development of multimodality therapy. An optimal multimodality treatment program is still being sought. Patients whose tumors are larger than 5 cm or that have invaded the skin or chest wall show good response to preoperative neoadjuvant chemotherapy.

Popularized initially as therapy for inflammatory breast cancer, induction chemotherapy is based on the premise that aggressive systemic therapy before local surgical treatment produces a survival advantage by eradicating micrometastases.[83,102-104] Four cycles of CAF or AC are given prior to surgical resection. The resection can be either total mastectomy or segmental resection, depending on the size of residual cancer and whether it is inflammatory breast cancer. Lymph node dissection is indicated in all patients with locally advanced breast cancer. Additional chemotherapy is given after resection. Postoperative irradiation is recommended to patients with T3 and T4 breast cancers, frequently after chemotherapy. Patients with ER-positive cancers can also be treated with tamoxifen in addition to the chemotherapy.

Aggressive multimodality therapy for locally advanced breast cancer has produced impressive response rates in terms of reduction in tumor volume. In fact, studies that evaluated pathologic response rates found that complete histologic responses, with no evidence of residual tumor in the mastectomy specimen, occurred in 3% to 18% of specimens.[103] Overall survival rates range from 38% to 65% at 5 years after initial presentation, with a median of 56%. The extent of response of the primary tumor is an important indicator of survival, with one study reporting an 85% 5-year survival rate if the tumor had responded substantially to induction chemotherapy.[104]

Treatment of Less Common Neoplasms and Special Cases

Contralateral Breast Cancer

The occurrence of cancer in the contralateral breast, either in patients with a history of prior breast cancer or in patients in whom the contralateral cancer is detected during initial screening, is not common. The incidence of contralateral breast cancer is between 3% and 6%, and for a metachronous cancer, the annual risk is approximately 0.5% to 0.7% per year from the time of diagnosis of the first carcinoma.[105,106] The risk factors most often associated with contralateral breast cancer are young age (especially in association with metachronous cancer), presence of invasive or in-situ lobular carcinoma, tubular carcinoma, and multicentricity.[107-109]

Metachronous contralateral breast cancer has traditionally been thought to manifest at a more favorable stage than the first carcinoma. One study indicates, however, that the method of discovery, not the specific nodal status of the first cancer, is the best predictor of the stage of the second lesion.[106] Because most patients with breast cancer are subjected to constant and rigorous ongoing screening, especially with mammography, the vast majority of metachronous contralateral lesions are discovered at an early stage and are easily treated by conventional breast-conserving techniques. Synchronous contralateral lesions are usually detected during the initial evaluation of the patient with breast cancer, illustrating the importance of obtaining a contralateral mammogram once the diagnosis of breast cancer is made, if mammography has not already been performed. Because mammograms are usually obtained routinely, synchronous cancers also are generally discovered at an early stage and, therefore, are easily treated by conventional breast-conserving techniques. Because of the low overall risk of bilateral breast cancer, whether metachronous or synchronous, and an overall prognosis that is similar to that for patients with unilateral carcinoma, routine prophylactic mastectomy is not justified.[107] Careful surveillance with yearly mammography and clinical examination is a more logical approach.

Paget's Disease of the Breast

Best described as an unusual presentation of an underlying ductal carcinoma, Paget's disease of the breast is characterized by ulceration, eczema, or bleeding of the nipple-areolar complex.[110] The underlying intraductal or invasive ductal carcinoma is diagnosed by a biopsy of the nipple-areolar complex, the epidermis of which will be found to contain large, clear intraepithelial Paget's cells. Although most patients with Paget's disease have a palpable mass beneath the nipple, more than one third have no mass. Architectural distortion or microcalcifications may be seen on mammograms, but their absence does not rule out the diagnosis. Therefore, clinical suspicion must be high, and any questionable area must undergo biopsy.

The traditional treatment of Paget's disease of the breast has been total mastectomy without axillary lymph node dissection, because the vast majority of these lesions represent an intraductal carcinoma. Today, however, breast conservation with wide, local excision of the nipple-areolar complex is an acceptable surgical alternative. Although the use of postoperative radiation therapy is controversial owing to the lack of experience with this rare tumor, such therapy may be indicated if breast conservation is undertaken, especially for a lesion larger than 5 cm.

Phyllodes Tumor

The most common breast neoplasm of nonepithelial origin, phyllodes tumor is unique in that it occurs exclusively in the female breast and appears in no other site in the body. Although such tumors have been historically called *cystosarcoma phyllodes*, the vast majority are benign. Thus, the World Health Organization classification of breast tumors uses the term *phyllodes tumor*, which carries no implication of biologic potential. If possible, a pathologic diagnosis of phyllodes tumor should be qualified by an indication of its malignancy or benignity, because this qualification may affect the treatment recommendation. Histologically, phyllodes tumors most closely resemble fibroadenomas, although the epithelium-lined clefts are scattered within a more cellular connective tissue stroma. Metaplastic changes can occur in the stroma, and focal areas of fat, bone, and cartilage have been described. Lesions with malignant potential tend to have greater stromal cellularity, with the cells being anaplastic and exhibiting large numbers of mitotic figures.

On physical examination, phyllodes tumors tend to be sharply demarcated and freely mobile, with a smooth contour similar to that of fibroadenomas. Although they may be of any size, phyllodes tumors are frequently large, one study demonstrating a median size of about 5 cm.[111] Although they may occur in patients of any age, the median age of presentation tends to be between 40 and 50 years, at least a decade older than the usual age of presentation for fibroadenomas. Mammographically, the phyllodes tumor usually appears as a round, oval, or lobulated mass with a circumscribed margin, often indistinguishable from a fibroadenoma. The diagnosis, generally suggested by the large size, rapid growth, and occurrence in an older patient, can be confirmed by CNB or excisional biopsy.

The biologic behavior of phyllodes tumors is difficult to predict with accuracy. Even histologically "low-grade" tumors have been known to metastasize. Factors that suggest malignant potential at biopsy include fixation to adjacent breast tissue, large size, and the presence of tumor cells in marginal breast tissue surrounding the mass. Wide local excision with a margin of normal breast tissue is appropriate therapy for those tumors that appear "benign" histologically (i.e., that do not exhibit stromal overgrowth and with few, if any, mitotic figures per high-power field), but patients must undergo careful follow-up because of a high incidence of local recurrence and a slight but real risk of distant metastases. Local recurrences appear only at the site of the original excision and are preferably treated with reexcision or total mastectomy, depending on the size and histologic characteristics of the recurrent tumor. When the histologic appearance of the primary tumor suggests malignancy or when the tumor is very large, total mastectomy, with or without immediate reconstruction, is warranted. Because the malignant element is a sarcoma, there is no indication for axillary lymph node dissection or the use of adjuvant chemotherapy. Metastases from phyllodes tumors most commonly arise in the lungs, mediastinum, and bones. The optimal treatment of metastatic disease has not been determined.

Breast Cancer during Pregnancy

Despite being the most commonly diagnosed cancer occurring during pregnancy,[112] breast cancer during pregnancy or lactation is relatively rare. Because the peak incidence of breast cancer is seen in women well into their 50s, a clinician should not expect to see the frequent coexistence of pregnancy and breast cancer. In one review of nearly 46,000 cases of breast cancer, less than 3% were found in pregnant or lactating women.[113] Other studies have placed the rate even lower, between 1% and 2%, and have calculated the incidence at about 3 per 10,000 pregnancies.[114] However, with the average age of pregnant patients with breast cancer being about 35 years, and with the current trend toward postponing child-bearing to well within the 30s, the incidence of breast cancer in women who are pregnant or lactating can be expected to rise.

Breast cancer diagnosed during pregnancy or lactation is generally considered to carry a worse prognosis than breast cancer diagnosed in nonpregnant patients, probably reflecting the delayed diagnosis of the former.[115-117] The duration of symptoms before diagnosis is significantly longer than in nonpregnant patients, approaching 15 months in some series, and can be attributed to both physician and patient neglect. During pregnancy, the breasts become engorged and tense, making the palpation of a discrete mass difficult. In addition, because the breasts frequently become even more nodular than usual, new masses may be ignored by both the patient and her physician, who believe them to be normal changes due to pregnancy. Even if a discrete mass is detected, most masses that arise during pregnancy spontaneously resolve, so evaluation is frequently delayed until after delivery. As a consequence, these patients tend to have a more advanced stage of breast cancer when diagnosed than nonpregnant women. Node-positive breast cancer is reported to be present at the time of initial diagnosis in 70% to 90% of pregnant or lactating women,[118,119] as opposed to about 40% of nonpregnant, nonlactating women.[120]

Although the performance of mammography during pregnancy is often avoided because of fears about the radiation risk to the fetus, one series of 368 pregnant women who underwent mammography showed no fetal damage.[121] Ultrasonography of a new dominant mass in a pregnant patient is probably the best method to begin the evaluation. If the mass is cystic, either aspiration or follow-up is considered appropriate. If the mass is solid, serious consideration should be given to obtaining a biopsy. In these patients, FNAC or CNB is the best initial method. If the result is nondiagnostic, proceeding to an open excisional biopsy with local anesthesia presents no undue risk to the mother or fetus.

Once the diagnosis of breast cancer has been made, one should proceed promptly to local therapy. The risk of spontaneous abortion from surgical resection, including total mastectomy, is low, even during the first trimester.[122] Although breast conservation should be offered to the patient if her cancer is clinical stage I or II, some mitigating factors should be considered. Patients in their first trimester who wish to keep their pregnancy should be advised to have a total mastectomy and axillary dissection because the postoperative radiation therapy required for breast conservation would have to be postponed at least 6 months to avoid irradiating the fetus. If the patient insists that breast conservation be performed, alternatives should be discussed, including delaying irradiation until after the delivery, although the delay increases the risk of recurrence. The patient must understand that a significant risk to the fetus from internal scattered radiation exists, even at low doses. Pregnant patients in the second or third trimester who desire breast conservation should have prompt surgical therapy, with postoperative radiation therapy delayed until after delivery.

In patients who are pregnant and who are diagnosed with stage II breast cancer, the fetus may be at risk from chemotherapy. As with stage I tumors, the time of greatest risk is the first trimester. Although the reported incidence of teratogenicity of chemotherapeutic agents is less than 15%,[123] it is generally agreed that the use of chemotherapy during the first trimester should be avoided. No reports of teratogenicity during the second or third trimesters have been made and chemotherapy can probably be given, but no long-term follow-up studies of the fetal consequences of chemotherapy are available. Because the majority of these women have node-positive disease, the chemotherapy may be started during the second and third trimesters of their pregnancies.

Because patients with stage III cancer are treated with induction chemotherapy, such women whose cancer is diagnosed in the first trimester should be advised to consider termination of the pregnancy. There is no evidence that termination of pregnancy improves the outlook for such patients, but it does permit the use of standard, aggressive therapy for advanced disease.

Breast Cancer in Men

Carcinoma of the breast in men is uncommon, accounting for only 0.6% of breast cancers in the United States and 0.2% of all malignant tumors in men.[124] The mean age at presentation is well into the 60s.[125,126] Less than 5% of male breast cancer occurs before age 40.[127] Unlike cancer of the female breast, no significant increase in the incidence of male breast cancer has occurred over the past 40 to 50 years.[29] Possible risk factors include a positive family history, advanced age, Klinefelter syndrome, gynecomastia, obesity, testicular injury, racial predisposition, and prior irradiation of the chest. However, there is no strong evidence of any specific factor that significantly increases risk.[128]

The primary presenting complaint of men with breast cancer is a painless, eccentric, ill-defined subareolar mass. Nipple abnormalities such as inversion, discharge, fixation, edema, and ulceration are noted in 25% to 35% of patients.[128] In contradistinction, gynecomastia is characterized by a tender, discoid, symmetrical, subareolar mass. Although both gynecomastia and male breast cancer may demonstrate some adherence to the overlying skin, fixation to the pectoral fascia and nipple abnormalities generally indicate cancer. Mammography may be less useful for men than for women, but it should still be performed to evaluate the contralateral breast. Diagnosis by FNAC represents a simple method of identifying breast cancer in men, but as in women, a negative result cannot exclude cancer.

Historically, male breast cancer had been thought to be more aggressive than female breast cancer, and therefore radical surgical therapy, including removal of the pectoralis muscles, had been recommended to treat it. Later studies, however, have indicated no difference in prognosis between men and women with comparable stages of disease.[126,129] For stage 0 disease, total mastectomy is the preferred therapy because breast conservation is usually impossible owing to the small size of the male breast. Stage I or II breast cancer in men should be treated to obtain local control with total mastectomy and axillary lymph node dissection. Evidence shows that stage III breast cancer in men, as in women, is best treated by induction chemotherapy followed by total mastectomy and chest wall irradiation.[129]

Systemic therapy for male breast cancer is similar to that for female breast cancer. Although the number of patients reported is low, patients with stage II, node-positive disease appear to benefit from systemic adjunctive chemotherapy with either CMF or CAF.[130,131] Treatment of either stage I or node-negative stage II disease is more controversial. Because breast cancer in men is ER positive in nearly 85% of cases, it has been suggested that tamoxifen may play a pivotal role as adjuvant therapy in such patients, especially because response rates in excess of 70% have been reported.[132] In addition, studies have shown that the response rate of metastatic disease to tamoxifen is equivalent to the response to orchiectomy. Tamoxifen, therefore, is replacing orchiectomy as the initial treatment of choice in men with metastatic disease.[126,129,133] Second-line therapy for men with metastatic disease consists of progestational agents such as megestrol or antiandrogen/luteinizing-releasing hormone analogues such as goserelin.

References

1. Jemal A, Murray T, Samuel A, Ghafoor A, Ward E, Thun MJ: Cancer statistics, 2003. CA Cancer J Clin 2003;53:5-26.
2. Love SM, Connolly JL, Schnitt SJ, Shirley RL: Benign breast disorders. In Harris JR, Hellman S, Henderson IC, Kinne DW (eds): Breast Diseases. Philadelphia, JB Lippincott, 1987, pp 22-30.
3. Haagensen CD: The normal physiology of the breasts. In Haagensen CD (ed): Diseases of the Breast, 3rd ed. Philadelphia, WB Saunders, 1986, pp 47-55.
4. Ayres JW, Gidwani GP: The "luteal breast": Hormonal and sonographic investigations of benign breast disease in patients with cyclic mastalgia. Fertil Steril 1983;40:779-785.
5. Allen SS, Froberg DG: The effect of decreased caffeine consumption on benign proliferative breast disease: A randomized clinical trial. Surgery 1987;101:720-730.
6. Ernester V, Goodson W, Hunt T, et al: Vitamin E and benign breast disease: A double-blind, randomized clinical trial. Surgery 1985;97:490-495.
7. Tye J, Mansel R, Hughs L: Clinical experience of drug treatments for mastalgia. Lancet 1985:2:373-375.
8. Aberizk WJ, Silver B, Henderson IC, et al: The use of radiotherapy for treatment of isolated locoregional recurrence of breast carcinoma after mastectomy. Cancer 1986;58:1214-1218.
9. Fentiman I, Caleffi M, Brane K, et al: Double-blind controlled trial of tamoxifen therapy for mastalgia. Lancet 1986;1:287-290.
10. Leban MM, Meerscharet JR, Taylor RS: Breast pain: A symptom of cervical radiculopathy. Arch Phys Med Rehabil 1979;60:315-320.
11. Leis HP, Greene FL, Cammarata A, Hilfer SE: Nipple discharge: Surgical significance. South Med J 1988;81:20-26.
12. Haagensen CD: Solitary intraductal papilloma. In Haagensen CD (ed): Diseases of the Breast, 3rd ed. Philadelphia, WB Saunders, 1986, pp 136-175.
13. Haagensen CD: Infections in the breast. In Haagensen CD (ed): Diseases of the Breast, 3rd ed. Philadelphia, WB Saunders, 1986, pp 384-393.
14. Maier WP, Berger A, Derrick BM: Periareolar abscess in the nonlactating breast. Am J Surg 1982;144:395-362.
15. Watt-Bollesen S, Ryegaard R, Blichert-Toft M: Primary periareolar abscess in the nonlactating breast: Risk of recurrence. Am J Surg 1987;153:571-575.
16. Haagensen CD: Gross cystic disease. In Haagensen CD (ed): Diseases of the Breast, 3rd ed. Philadelphia, WB Saunders, 1986, pp 250-266.
17. Lannin DR, Silverman JA, Pories WJ, Walker C: Cost-effectiveness of fine needle biopsy of the breast. Ann Surg 1986;203:474-480.
18. Grant CS, Goelliner JR, Welsh JS, Martin JK: Fine-needle aspiration of the breast. Mayo Clin Proc 1986;61:377-381.
19. Layfield LJ, Glasgow BJ, Cramer H: Fine-needle aspiration in the management of breast masses. Pathol Annu 1989;24:23-62.
20. Flowers JL, Cox EB, Geisinger KR, et al: Use of monoclonal antiestrogen receptor antibody to evaluate estrogen receptor content in fine needle aspiration biopsies. Ann Surg 1986; 203:250-254.
21. Giuliano AE, Jones RC, Brennan UI, et al: Sentinel lymphadenectomy in breast cancer. J Clin Oncol 1997;15:2345-2350.
22. Shabot MM, Goldberg IM, Schick P, et al: Aspiration cytology is superior to Tru-Cut needle biopsy in establishing the diagnosis of clinically suspicious breast masses. Ann Surg 1982;196:122-126.
23. Dronkers DJ: Stereotaxic core biopsy of breast lesions. Radiology 1992;183:631-634.
24. Parker SH, Lovin JD, Jobe WE, et al: Stereotactic breast biopsy with a biopsy gun. Radiology 1990;176:741-747.
25. Walt AJ: Screening and breast cancer: A surgical perspective. Bull Am Coll Surg 1990;75:96-100.
26. Platt R, Zaleznik DF, Hopkins CC, et al: Perioperative antibiotic prophylaxis for herniorrhaphy and breast surgery. N Engl J Med 1990;322:153-160.
27. Morrow M: Management of nonpalpable breast lesions. PPO Updates 1990;4:1-11.
28. Moskowitz M: The predictive value of certain mammographic signs in screening for breast cancer. Cancer 1993; 51:1007-1011.
29. Devesa SS, Silverman DT, Young JL, et al: Cancer incidence and mortality trends among whites in the United States, 1947-1984. J Natl Cancer Inst 1987;79:701-720.
30. Graves EJ: Detailed diagnoses and procedures. National Hospital Discharge Survey, 1992. Series 13: Data from the National Health Survey. Vital Health Stat 1994;13:1-281.
31. Singletary SE, Allred C, Ashley P, et al: Revision of the American Joint Committee on Cancer Staging System for Breast Cancer. J Clin Oncol 2002;20:3628-3636.
32. American Joint Committee on Cancer Prognostic Factors Consensus Conference. Cancer 1999;86:2436-2446.
33. Elston CW, Ellis IO: Pathological prognostic factors in breast cancer. I: The value of histologic grade in breast cancer: Experience from a large study with long-term follow-up. Histopathology 1991;19:403-410.
34. Dalton LW, Page DL, Dupont WD: Histologic grading of breast carcinoma: A reproducibility study. Cancer 1994;73: 2765-2770.
35. Friedson HF, Wolber RA, Bersan KW, et al: Interobserver reproducibility of the Nottingham modification of the Bloom & Richardson histologic grading scheme for infiltrating ductal carcinoma. Am J Clin Pathol 1995;103:195-198.
36. Robbins P, Pinder S, DeKlerk N, et al: Histologic grading of breast carcinomas: A study of interobserver agreement. Hum Pathol 1995;26:873-879.
37. Haagensen CD, Lane N, Lattes R, Bodian C: Lobular neoplasia (so-called lobular carcinoma in situ) of the breast. Cancer 1978;42:737-769.
38. Page DL, Dupont WD, Rogers LW, Landenberger M: Intraductal carcinoma of the breast: Follow-up after biopsy only. Cancer 1982;49:751-758.
39. Rosen PP, Braun DW, Kinne DE: The clinical significance of pre-invasive breast cancer. Cancer 1980;46(Suppl):919-925.
40. Chang HR, Soo C, Barsky SH: In situ breast cancer. In Haskell CM, Berek JS (eds): Cancer Treatment, 5th ed. Philadelphia, WB Saunders, 2001, pp 532-542.
41. Kinne DW, Petrick JA, Osbourne MP, et al: Breast carcinoma in situ. Arch Surg 1989;124:33-36.
42. Lagios MD, Margolin FR, Westdahl PR, Rose MR: Mammographically detected duct carcinoma in-situ. Cancer 1989;63: 618-624.
43. Schwartz GF, Finkel GC, Garcia JC, Patchefsky AS: Subclinical ductal carcinoma in situ of the breast: Treatment by local excision and surveillance alone. Cancer 1992;70:2468-2474.
44. Weng E, Julliard D, Parker R, et al: Outcomes and factors impacting local recurrence of ductal carcinoma in situ (DCIS). Cancer 2000;88:1643-1649.
45. Fisher B, Costantino J, Redmond C, et al: Lumpectomy compared with lumpectomy and radiation therapy for the treatment of intraductal breast cancer. N Engl J Med 1993;328: 1581-1586.
46. Di Pietro S, Bertario L, Piva L: Prognosis and treatment of locoregional breast cancer recurrences: Critical considerations on 120 cases. Tumori 1980;66:331-338.
47. Donegan WL, Perez-Mesa CM, Watson FR: A biostatistical study of locally recurrent breast carcinoma. Surg Gynecol Obstet 1966;122:529-540.
48. Karabali-Dalamaga S, Souhami RL, O'Higgins NJ, et al: Natural history and prognosis of recurrent breast cancer. Br Med J 1978;2:730-733.
49. Recht A, Schnitt SJ, Connolly JL, et al: Prognosis following local or regional recurrence after conservative surgery and radiotherapy for early stage breast carcinoma. Int J Radiat Oncol Biol Phys 1989;16:3-9.

50. Fisher B, Redmond C, Legault-Poisson S, et al: Postoperative chemotherapy and tamoxifen compared with tamoxifen alone in the treatment of positive-node breast cancer patients aged 50 years and older with tumors responsive to tamoxifen: Results from the National Surgical Adjuvant Breast and Bowel Project B-16. J Clin Oncol 1990;8:1005-1018.
51. Carter CL, Allen C, Henson DE: Relation of tumor size, lymph node status, and survival in 24,740 breast cancer cases. Cancer 1989;63:181-187.
52. Fisher B, Bauer M, Wickerham DL, et al: Relation of number of positive axillary nodes to the prognosis of patients with primary breast cancer. Cancer 1983;52:1551-1557.
53. NIH Consensus Conference: Treatment of early-stage breast cancer. JAMA 1991;265:391-395.
54. Veronesi U, Volterrani F, Luini A, et al: Quadrantectomy versus lumpectomy for small size breast cancer. Eur J Cancer 1990;26:671-673.
55. Vicini FA, Eberlein TJ, Connolly JL, et al: The optimal extent of resection for patients with stage I or II breast cancer treated with conservative surgery and radiotherapy. Ann Surg 1991; 214:200-204.
56. Benson EA, Thorogood J: The effect of surgical technique on local recurrence rates following mastectomy. Eur J Surg Oncol 1986;12:267-271.
57. Cady B, Sears HF: Usefulness and technique of axillary dissection in primary breast cancer. J Clin Oncol 1986;4:623-624.
58. Larson D, Weinstein M, Goldberg I, et al: Edema of the arm as a function of the extent of axillary surgery in patients with stage I-II carcinoma of the breast treated with primary radiotherapy. Int J Rad Oncol Biol Phys 1986;12:1575-1582.
59. Cabanas RM: An approach for the treatment of penile carcinoma. Cancer 1977;39:456-466
60. Morton DL, Wen DR, Wong JH, et al: Technical details of intraoperative lymphatic mapping for early stage melanoma. Arch Surg 1992;127:392-399.
61. Giuliano AE, Kirgan DM, Guenther M, et al: lymphatic mapping and sentinel lymphadenectomy for breast cancer. Ann Surg 1994;220:391-401.
62. Krag DN, Ashikaga T, Harlow SP et al: Development of sentinel node targeting technique in breast cancer patients. Breast J 1998;4:67-74.
63. Krag DN, Weaver D, Ashikaga T, et al: The sentinel lymph node in breast cancer: A multicenter validation study. N Engl J Med 1998;339:941-946.
64. Borgstein PJ, Pijpers R, Comans EF, et al: Sentinel lymph node biopsy in breast cancer: Guidelines and pitfalls of lymphoscintigraphy & gamma probe detection. J Am Coll Surg 1998;186:275-283.
65. Offodie R, Hoh C, Barsky S, et al: Minimally invasive breast carcinoma staging using lymphatic mapping with radiolabeled dextran. Cancer 1998;82:1704-1708.
66. Choi S-H, Barsky S, Chang, HR: Clinicopathological analysis of sentinel lymph node mapping in early breast cancer. Breast J 2003;9:153-162.
67. Tanis PJ, Boom RPA, Koops HS, et al: Frozen section investigation of sentinel node in malignant melanoma and breast cancer. Ann Surg Oncol 2000;8:222-226.
68. Henry-Tillman RS, Korourian S, Rubio IT, et al: Intraoperative touch preparation for sentinel lymph node biopsy: A 4-year experience. Ann Surg Oncol 2002;9:333-339.
69. Chu KU, Turner RR, Hansen NM, et al: Do all patients with sentinel node metastasis from breast carcinoma need complete axillary node dissection? Ann Surg 1999;229:536-541.
70. Reynolds C, Mick R, Donohue JH, et al: Sentinel lymph node biopsy with metastasis: Can axillary dissection be avoided in some patients with breast cancer? J Clin Oncol 1999;17: 1720-1726.
71. Halsted WS: The results of operations for the cure of cancer of the breast performed at the Johns Hopkins Hospital from June, 1889 to January, 1894. Johns Hopkins Hosp Bull 1894;4:297.
72. Fisher B, Anderson S, Bryant J, et al: Twenty-year follow-up of a randomized trial comparing total mastectomy, lumpectomy and lumpectomy plus irradiation for the treatment of invasive breast cancer. N Engl J Med 2002;347:1233-1241.
73. Veronesi U, Cascinelli N, Mariani L, et al: Twenty-year follow-up of a randomized study comparing breast-conserving surgery with radical mastectomy for early breast cancer. N Engl J Med 2002;347:1227-1232.
74. Recht A, Silen W, Schnitt SJ, et al: Time-course of local recurrence following conservative surgery and radiotherapy for breast cancer. Int J Radiat Oncol Biol Phys 1988;15:255-261.
75. Kurtz JM, Amalric R, Brandone H, et al: Local recurrence after breast-conserving surgery and radiotherapy: Frequency, time course, and prognosis. Cancer 1989;63:1912-1917.
76. Leung S, Otmezguine Y, Calitchi E, et al: Locoregional recurrences following radical external beam irradiation and interstitial implantation for operable breast cancer: A twenty-three year experience. Radiother Oncol 1986;5:1-10.
77. Rose MA, Olivotto I, Cady B, et al: Conservative surgery and radiation therapy for early breast cancer: Long-term cosmetic results. Arch Surg 1989;124:153-157.
78. Recht A, Edge SB, Solin LJ, et al: Postmastectomy radiotherapy: Clinical practice guidelines of the American Society of Clinical Oncology. J Clin Oncol 2001;19:1539-1569.
79. Recht A, Gray R, Davidson NE, et al: Local-regional failure ten years after mastectomy and adjuvant chemotherapy in women with or without tamoxifen without irradiation: Experience of The Eastern Cooperative Oncology Group. J Clin Oncol 1999;17:1689-1700.
80. Stefanik D, Goldgerg R, Byrne P, et al: Local-regional failure in patients treated with adjuvant chemotherapy for breast cancer. J Clin Oncol 1985;3:660-665.
81. Overgaard M, Jensen MJ, Overgaard J, et al: Postoperative radiotherapy in high risk post menopausal breast cancer patients given adjuvant tamoxifen: Danish Breast Cancer Cooperative Group DBCG 82c randomized trial. Lancet 1999;353:1641-1648.
82. Overgaard M, Hansen PS, Overgaard J, et al: Postoperative radiotherapy in high-risk premenopausal women with breast cancer who receive adjuvant chemotherapy. N Engl J Med 1997;337:949-955.
83. Loprinzi C, Carbone PP, Tormey DC, et al: Aggressive combined modality therapy for advanced local-regional breast carcinoma. J Clin Oncol 1984;2:157-163.
84. Beatson GT: On the treatment of inoperable cases of carcinoma of the mamma: Suggestions for a new method of treatment, with illustrative cases. Lancet 1896;2:104-107.
85. Gelber RD, Goldhirsch A, Coates AS: Adjuvant therapy for breast cancer: Understanding the overview. J Clin Oncol 1993;11:580-585.
86. Early Breast Cancer Trialists Collaborative Group: Tamoxifen for early breast cancer: an overview of the randomized trials. Lancet 1998;352:98-101.
87. Fisher B, Costantino J, Redmond C, et al: A randomized clinical trial evaluating tamoxifen in the treatment of patients with node-negative breast cancer who have estrogen-receptor-positive tumors. N Engl J Med 1989;320: 479-484.
88. Keder RP, Bourne TH, Powles TJ, et al: Effects of tamoxifen on uterus and ovaries of postmenopausal women in a randomised breast cancer prevention trial. Lancet 1994;343: 1318-1321.
89. NIH Consensus Development Conference: Adjuvant Therapy for Breast Cancer. Bethesda, Maryland, USA. November 3, 2000. J Natl Cancer Inst Monogr 2001;30:1-152.
90. Goldhirsch A, Glick JH, Gelber RD, et al: Meeting highlights: International Consensus Panel on the Treatment of Primary Breast Cancer. J Clin Oncol 2001;19:3817-3827.
91. Fisher B, Costantino JP, Wickerham DL, et al: Tamoxifen for prevention of breast cancer: Report of National Surgical Adjuvant Breast & Bowel Project P-1 study. J Natl Cancer Inst 1998;90:1371-1388.
92. Cuzick J, Forbes J, Edwards R, et al: First results from the International Breast Cancer Intervention Study (IBIS-I): A randomized prevention trial. Lancet 2002;360:817-824.
93. Bonadonna G, Brusamolino E, Valagussa P, et al: Combination chemotherapy as an adjuvant treatment in operable breast cancer. N Engl J Med 1976;294:405-410.
94. Fisher B, Carbone P, Economou SG, et al: L-Phenylalanine mustard (L-PAM) in the management of primary breast

cancer: A report of early findings. N Engl J Med 1975;292: 117-122.
95. Bonadonna G, Valagussa P, Moliterni A, et al: Adjuvant cyclophosphamide, methotrexate, and fluorouracil in node-positive breast cancer: The results of 20 years of follow-up. N Engl J Med 1995;332:901-906.
96. Fisher B, Brown AM, Dimitrov NV, et al: Two months of doxorubicin-cyclophosphamide with and without interval reinduction therapy compared with six months of cyclophosphamide, methotrexate, and fluorouracil in positive-node breast cancer patients with tamoxifen-nonresponsive tumors: Results from NSABP B-15. J Clin Oncol 1990;8:1483-1496.
97. Meyerowitz B, Sparks FC, Spears IK: Adjuvant chemotherapy for breast cancer: Psychosocial implications. Cancer 1979;43: 1613-1618.
98. Polychemotherapy for early breast cancer: An overview of the randomized trials. Early Breast Cancer Trialists Collaborative Group. Lancet 1998;352:930-942.
99. Weiss RB, Rifkin RM, Stewart FM, et al: High-close chemotherapy for high risk primary breast cancer, an on-site review of the Bigwoda Study. Lancet 2000;355:999-1003.
100. Gelber RD, Goldhirsch A: A new endpoint for the assessment of adjuvant therapy in postmenopausal women with operable breast cancer. J Clin Oncol 1986;4:1772-1779.
101. Lucas F, Perez-Mesa C: Inflammatory carcinoma of the breast. Cancer 1978;41:1595-1605.
102. De Lana M, Zucali R, Viganotti G, et al: Combined chemotherapy-radiotherapy approach in locally advanced (T3b-T4) breast cancer. Cancer Chemother Pharmacol 1978; 1:53-59.
103. Heys SD, Eremin JM, Sarkar TK, et al: Role of multimodality therapy in the management of locally advanced carcinoma of the breast. J Am Coll Surg 1994;179:493-504.
104. Schwartz GF, Cantor RI, Biermann WA: Neoadjuvant chemotherapy before definitive treatment for stage III carcinoma of the breast. Arch Surg 1987;122:1430-1434.
105. Schell SR, Montague ED, Spanos WJ, et al: Bilateral breast cancer in patients with initial stage I and II disease. Cancer 1982;50:1191-1194.
106. Singletary SE, Taylor SH, Guinee VF, et al: Occurrence and prognosis of contralateral carcinoma of the breast. J Am Coll Surg 1994;178:390-396.
107. Fisher ER, Fisher B, Sass R, Wickerham L: Pathologic findings from the National Surgical Adjuvant Breast Project (Protocol No. 4). XI: Bilateral breast cancer. Cancer 1984;54:3002-3011.
108. Lagios MD, Rose MR, Margolin FR: Tubular carcinoma of the breast: Association with multicentricity, bilaterality, and family history of mammary carcinoma. Am J Clin Pathol 1980;73:25-30.
109. Leis HP: Managing the remaining breast. Cancer 1980;46: 1026-1030.
110. Paone J, Baker R: Pathogenesis and treatment of Paget's disease of the breast. Cancer 1981;48:825-829.
111. Page DL, Anderson TJ, Johnson RJ: Sarcomas of the breast. In Page DL, Anderson TJ (eds): Diagnostic Histopathology of the Breast. Edinburgh, Churchill Livingstone, 1987.
112. Donegan WL: Cancer and pregnancy. CA Cancer J Clin 1983;33:194-201.
113. White TT, White WC: Breast cancer and pregnancy: A report of 49 cases followed 5 years. Ann Surg 1956;144:384-390.
114. Wallack MK, Wolf JA, Bedwinek J, et al: Gestational carcinoma of the female breast. Curr Probl Cancer 1983;7:1-75.
115. Anderson JM: Mammary cancers and pregnancy. Br Med J 1979;1:1124-1144.
116. King RM, Welch JS, Marten JK, et al: Carcinoma of the breast associated with pregnancy. Surg Gynecol Obstet 1985;160: 228-232.
117. Nugent P, O'Connell TX: Breast cancer in pregnancy. Arch Surg 1985;120:1221-1224.
118. Holleb AI, Farrow JH: The relation of carcinoma of the breast in pregnancy in 283 patients. Surg Gynecol Obstet 1962;115: 65-70.
119. Ribeiro GG, Palmer MK: Breast carcinoma associated with pregnancy: A clinician's dilemma. Br Med J 1977;2:1524-1526.
120. Harris JA, Morrow M, Bonadonna G: Cancer of the breast. In DeVita VT, Hellman S, Rosenberg SA (eds): Cancer. Principles and Practice of Oncology, 4th ed. Philadelphia, JB Lippincott, 1993, pp 1264-1332.
121. Lippman ME, Lichter AS, Danforth DN: Breast cancer occurring during pregnancy. In Diagnosis and Management of Breast Cancer. Philadelphia, WB Saunders, 1988, pp 414-420.
122. Byrd BF, Bayer DS, Robertson JC, et al: Treatment of breast tumors associated with pregnancy and lactation. Ann Surg 1962;155:940-945.
123. Schapira DV, Chudley AE: Successful pregnancy following continuous treatment with combination chemotherapy before conception and throughout pregnancy. Cancer 1984; 54:800-804.
124. Wingo PA, Tong T, Bolden S: Cancer statistics, 2002. CA Cancer J Clin 2002;45:8-30.
125. Erlichman C, Murphy KC, Elhaim T: Male breast cancer: A 13-year review of 89 patients. J Clin Oncol 1984;2:903-907.
126. Sandler B, Carman C, Perry RR: Cancer of the male breast. Am Surg 1994;60:816-820.
127. Holleb AI, Freeman HP, Farrow JH: Cancer of the male breast. N Y State J Med 1968;68:656-660.
128. Crichlow RW, Galt SW: Male breast cancer. Surg Clin North Am 1990;70:1165-1177.
129. Borgen PI, Wong GY, Vlamis V, et al: Current management of male breast cancer: A review of 104 cases. Ann Surg 1992;215:451-459.
130. Bagley CS, Wesley MN, Young RC, et al: Adjuvant chemotherapy in males with cancer of the breast. Am J Clin Oncol 1987;10:55-60.
131. Patel HZ, Buzdur AU, Hortobagyi GN: Role of adjuvant chemotherapy in male breast cancer. Cancer 1989;64:1583-1585.
132. Kinne D, Hakes T: Male breast cancer. In Harris J, Hellman S, Henderson C, Kinne D (eds): Breast Diseases. Philadelphia, JB Lippincott, 1991, pp 782-790.
133. Manni A: Tamoxifen therapy of metastatic breast cancer. J Lab Clin Med 1987;109:290-299.

Chapter 31

The Conservatively Treated Breast

D. David Dershaw

The traditional roles of breast imaging, particularly mammography, have been the detection of breast cancer and the assessment of clinically evident breast disease. In the past, when the treatment of breast cancer was predominantly removal of the breast, breast imaging did not contribute to the care of the patient after her initial operation, and the breast imager did not participate in the cancer treatment plan. The use of breast-conserving techniques to treat primary breast cancer has dramatically altered the role of the radiologist in this process.

Unlike mastectomy, in which the sole goal of treatment is to cure the patient of her disease, breast-conserving therapy has two goals: cure and an acceptable cosmetic result. Before a patient can be offered breast-conserving therapy, it must be possible to resect the cancer without causing unacceptable breast deformity. Because the radiologist is often able to determine the extent of tumor before surgery more accurately than the surgeon, the radiologist is integral to the decision-making process about treatment options. Cancer can recur in the treated breast and early detection of recurrence can improve the likelihood of survival, so the radiologist also has a responsibility to monitor the breast after therapy to detect recurrences as early as possible. Additionally, the breast imager must be able to discuss the appropriate issues because he or she is often confronted with questions from patients and surgeons about the possibility of breast conservation. This chapter reviews the principles involved in breast-conserving treatment and describes the role of breast imaging in the care of patients who undergo these procedures. It should be remembered that although the efficacy of breast conservation has been proven and is widely accepted, areas of controversy remain, and some details of treatment continue to evolve.

CLINICAL TRIALS OF BREAST-CONSERVING THERAPY

Breast-conserving therapy has been tested in large numbers of controlled, prospective clinical trials, and its results have been reported in multiple retrospective single-institution studies. Of these investigations, seven randomized clinical trials are the most important.[1-10] In these trials, women with stage I or stage II breast cancers (invasive tumors no larger than 5 cm in greatest diameter) were treated. These women had no evidence of distant metastases and did not have fixed axillary lymph nodes. Presence of nonfixed but clinically involved axillary nodes at the time of enrollment into a study was not considered a reason for exclusion. In these randomized trials, women were treated either with mastectomy or with resection of the breast cancer and total breast irradiation of 45 to 50 Gy. In all trials but the National Surgical Adjuvant Breast and Bowel Project (NSABP) trial,[5] an additional boost dose was given at the site of the original cancer, raising the total dose in that area to more than 60 Gy. The boost dose was not given in the NSABP trial because surgical excision of the cancer had to include margins with no histologic evidence of tumor. In the NSABP trial and the Guy's Hospital (London) trial,[7] radiation to the axillary lymph nodes, which was routinely performed in the other five trials, was not given. Of the other five studies, four were conducted in Europe and include the National Tumor Institute in Milan,[11] the Danish Breast Cancer Group,[3,4] the Institut Gustave Roussy,[8] and the European Organization for Research and Treatment of Cancer (EORTC).[2,8] Along with NSABP, the National Cancer Institute (NCI) conducted the other randomized, prospective American study.[1,6]

From these trials, follow-up data are available for a minimum of 8 years. Survival rates for women treated with breast conservation versus mastectomy are comparable for overall disease-free survival. The occurrence of distant metastases and of contralateral breast cancer is also the same for the two groups. Women treated with breast conservation, however, have a risk for local treatment failure (recurrence of tumor in the treated breast), which cannot occur in the woman treated with mastectomy. Reports of the incidence of local failure have ranged from 3% at 8 years in the Danish study to a locoregional failure rate of 19% at 8 years in the National Cancer Institute study.[3] The EORTC reported a 13% local recurrence rate at 8 years.[9] For women in high-risk groups, local recurrence rates of 20% to 40% have been reported.[12] The high-risk factors for local recurrence are discussed in this chapter.

The randomized controlled trials included a total of approximately 4400 women. The results of treatment of another 5600 women reported in retrospective data from single institutions show an overall survival at 10 years of 63% to 86%, with a disease-free survival of 63% to 74%.[11] Among those institutions reporting 15-year data, overall survival has been 45% to 79%. The 10-year rate of local recurrence in the treated breast has ranged from 8% to 20%, and the 15-year rate from 17% to 18%. These studies reinforce the data of the randomized controlled trials on the efficacy of breast-conserving therapy for the treatment of primary breast cancer, yielding results comparable to those achieved with mastectomy.

SELECTION OF WOMEN FOR BREAST-CONSERVING THERAPY

Because of the ability to detect nonpalpable breast cancer with mammography and the use of imaging-guided breast biopsy to make a definitive histologic assessment, the radiologist may be the first physician to confront the patient regarding her diagnosis of breast cancer. In this setting, it is not uncommon for the patient to initiate a discussion about the possibility of breast-conserving therapy. The determination of the appropriateness of this type of treatment depends on an assessment of the extent of tumor within the breast to ascertain whether the cancer can be resected without causing unacceptable breast deformity. The determination of the extent of local disease is made by the surgeon, pathologist, and radiologist, each using different modalities to identify the extent of tumor within the breast. Therefore, any of these physicians can recommend mastectomy as the appropriate therapy if the physical findings, histologic assessment of tumor margins, or size of tumor as determined on imaging studies indicated that it is too large to be resected without significant deformity of the breast.

When discussing the possibility of breast conservation with a patient or her physician, the radiologist needs to be familiar with the contraindications, both absolute and relative, to this treatment. Absolute contraindications, which can be determined by discussion with the patient, include first or second trimester of pregnancy and a history of prior therapeutic irradiation to the breast. Women in early pregnancy must have the pregnancy terminated if they wish to undergo breast-conserving therapy. Women in late pregnancy may elect to delay therapy until after delivery. For women who have had prior therapeutic irradiation to the breast, additional radiation is not possible because the total dose would be excessive. Therefore, women who have undergone previous breast-conserving therapy with radiation and those who have been treated for Hodgkin disease with a mantle-type field of radiation are not eligible for breast-conserving therapy. In instances in which conservative treatment did not include radiation, such as for small foci of ductal carcinoma in situ (DCIS), a second attempt at conservation is possible.

Women should be queried about a history of collagen vascular disease, a relative contraindication to breast-conserving therapy. If the disease is quiescent, the radiotherapist may determine that treatment may proceed. Active collagen vascular disease, however, often leads to significant complications after radiation therapy and may make the patient ineligible for such treatment.[11]

The completion of radiation therapy usually takes 4 to 6 weeks. Women who have difficulty traveling to a radiation treatment center because of distance or because of infirmity that makes traveling a problem, as well as women who may not be sufficiently responsible to complete their course of therapy, may not be appropriate candidates for breast conservation.

Tumor size is an important determinant of whether a woman can undergo breast-conserving therapy, but absolute measurements of tumor size are not used. The determining factor is the ratio of the size of the tumor to the size of the breast. In a large breast, a large tumor can be resected with good cosmetic results. In a small breast, a large tumor may be impossible to excise without causing such severe deformity as to make breast-conserving therapy inappropriate. Although the large size of a tumor is not an absolute contraindication, because randomized prospective studies included only tumors up to 5 cm in diameter, data are not available on the appropriateness of therapy for larger cancers.

As has been noted previously, the presence of clinically involved axillary lymph nodes has not precluded the inclusion of women in randomized series comparing breast-conserving therapy with mastectomy unless the nodes were matted on physical examination. Nonmatted axillary nodal metastases should therefore not be considered a contraindication to breast-conserving therapy. When a tumor is subareolar in location, the patient should be advised that surgery will involve sacrifice of the nipple-areolar complex. However, survival rates appear to be identical to those for similar-sized tumors in other areas of the breast.[13] Modern radiotherapy techniques have allowed women with large, pendulous breasts to be successfully treated without the fibrosis that often resulted when older techniques were used. To provide homogeneity of the dose delivered to the breast, these women should be treated with equipment having the capability of delivering greater than 6 MeV of photon beam irradiation.[11]

The patient presenting with multiple cancers requires special consideration. Single, bilateral cancers, whether synchronous or metachronous, can be treated conservatively if they meet the criteria outlined previously. However, the ability to successfully treat multiple, synchronous, unilateral breast cancers with breast-conserving therapy is problematic. If the lesions occupy more than one quadrant, successful resection results in considerable deformity of the breast, and mastectomy is probably preferable. If two cancers are located in the same quadrant, especially if they are in close proximity to each other, resection may be possible with adequate cosmetic results. However, because these women are at much greater than normal risk for future breast cancer in the treated breast, mastectomy may be required at a later date.[14] Thus, these women might be better served if their original cancers are treated with mastectomy. A dense parenchymal pattern or the presence of extensive, indeterminate microcalcifications may make it difficult for the radiologist to detect tumor recurrence with mammography. Women with these radiologic findings should be advised that a local recurrence may not be detectable until the lesion has become palpable.

PRETREATMENT ASSESSMENT WITH BREAST IMAGING TECHNIQUES

The size and extent of the cancer may not always be obvious from physical examination or even on histologic assessment of the lumpectomy specimen and should be estimated by mammography. Because skip areas of tumor can result in falsely negative histologic assessment of tumor margins, multiple foci of tumor may be evident only in mammograms. A coexistent fibrotic reaction may lead to an overestimation of the extent of the tumor on physical examination, and nonpalpable tumor may result in its being underestimated. High-quality mammography is essential to evaluate the extent of disease. Spot compression views and microfocus magnification may be useful in this setting. The other breast should be studied to exclude bilateral cancer.

The radiologist should be aware of the limitations of mammography in mapping the extent of tumor. DCIS, especially noncomedo DCIS, may form a large volume of tumor that is noncalcified and that therefore is not evident on a mammogram.[15] This appears to be increasingly true with increasing size of the lesion.[16] The radiologist, surgeon, and patient must be aware that the mammogram may significantly underestimate the extent of this nonpalpable lesion. Areas of DCIS larger than 2.5 cm, and especially tumors extending over more than 4 cm, are highly likely to involve the breast more extensively than is evident in the mammogram.[17] It may not be possible to sterilize with radiation an extensive burden of DCIS that remains after surgery, increasing the risk of recurrence. Therefore, it may be appropriate to consider mastectomy for women with extensive DCIS.

In a growing number of reports, it has become obvious that in some cases ultrasonography and magnetic resonance imaging (MRI) have been shown to be capable of demonstrating the local extent of breast cancer more accurately than mammography.[18-20] In two studies, ultrasonography detected foci of carcinoma that were not seen on mammography in 14% of cases.[21,22] In another report, MRI findings correctly changed patient treatment in 14% of study patients, but another 4% underwent unnecessary biopsy (Fig. 31–1).[23] MRI has also been found to be valuable in determining tumor extension into the pectoralis major, a finding that does not contraindicate breast conservation but alters the extent of surgery that might be performed (Fig. 31–2).[24] Investigators have also suggested that technetium Tc 99m (^{99m}Tc) sestamibi radionuclide scanning may also be useful, but this imaging technique has not been widely incorporated into the breast imaging armamentarium.[25] No consensus has developed over whether nonmammographic imaging techniques should be routinely incorporated into the preoperative assessment of women who are considering breast conservation.[26]

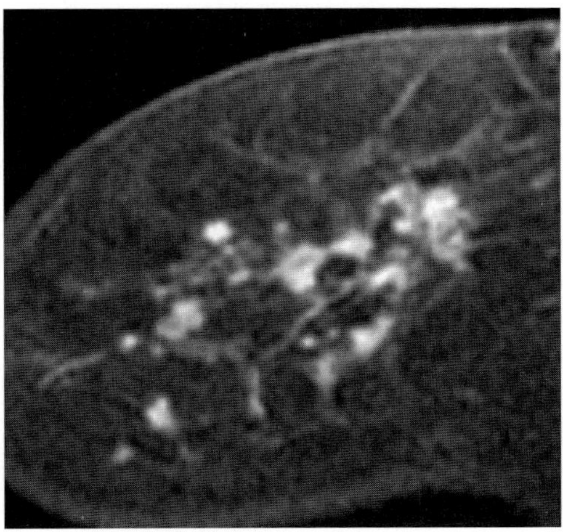

Figure 31–1. Post-contrast magnetic resonance image shows multiple enhancing lesions throughout the breast due to multicentric carcinoma. Breast conservation is not possible in this patient.

For the patient in whom imaging studies suggest the possibility of multiple sites of carcinoma in the breast, percutaneous imaging-guided breast biopsy can be valuable in evaluating the extent of tumor. If multiple cancers are found, breast conservation may be inappropriate. This preoperative evaluation assists the surgeon and patient in choosing the correct therapeutic procedure. Diagnosis of multiple, suspicious areas can be made with core needle biopsy. The biopsy can be performed with stereotactic or ultrasonographic guidance, avoiding open surgical biopsy. Technology has also been developed to permit

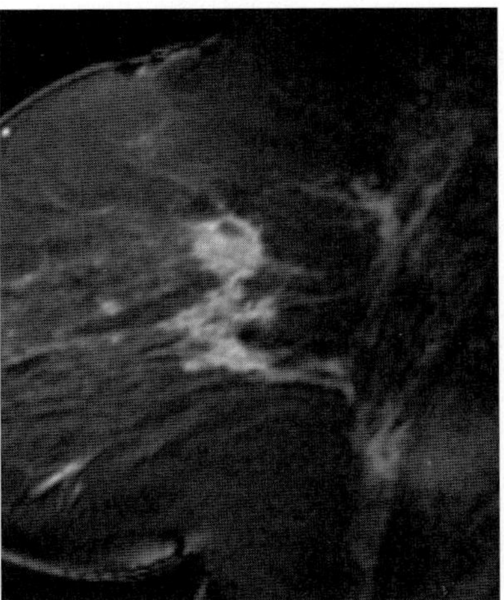

Figure 31–2. Post-contrast magnetic resonance image shows a central, enhancing carcinoma with areas of enhancement in the pectoralis. This finding indicates tumor involvement of the chest wall musculature and modifies the surgical approach to the carcinoma.

MRI biopsy guidance, enabling lesions apparent only with MRI to undergo core needle biopsy without open surgery.[27]

INTRAOPERATIVE EVALUATION OF ADEQUACY OF TUMOR RESECTION

The goal of surgical resection is to remove at least all gross tumor—palpable disease as well as tumor identified only on mammography (or other imaging techniques). For women with nonpalpable lesions, adequate surgical resection is assisted by preoperative needle localization performed by the radiologist. A variety of techniques are available for this procedure.[28] The method chosen at any institution should be that with which the surgeon and radiologist are the most comfortable. The localizing wire or dye should be positioned within 1 cm of the lesion, even closer if possible. For large tumors, localization of the margins of the lesion with more than one wire or dye injection may be valuable.

During surgery, specimen radiography is performed to determine whether the lesion has been sampled and whether the tumor extends to the margin of the specimen. It is sometimes possible to determine from the specimen radiograph that not all of the cancer has been removed and that further excision is necessary. However, use of the specimen radiograph to assess the completeness of the excision is not reliable.[29] The specimen radiograph is also important in directing the pathologist to the site of the lesion within the specimen.

Specimen radiography can be performed with either conventional mammography equipment or a tabletop x-ray unit that can be kept in the pathology department or near the surgical suite. When uncalcified masses have been excised, compression of the specimen during the x-ray exposure can be useful to improve the depiction of the lesion.[30] In addition to determining that the lesion has been removed, the specimen radiograph should be assessed to identify whether the lesion extends to the margin of resection (Fig. 31–3). If it does, residual tumor may have been left within the breast. To obtain this information, two orthogonal views are useful.[31] Some surgeons mark the specimen with surgical clips to identify the superior and deep margins, thereby directing the area of further resection, if this is needed. The specimen radiograph should be compared with the lesion in the preoperative mammogram while the patient is still on the operating table. It is important that the specimen not be dissected before specimen radiography, so that an accurate comparison with the preoperative mammogram can be made. The specimen radiograph is most valuable for confirmation of excision when the lesion contains calcifications or is a discrete mass. It is least helpful in cases of architectural distortion or for a lesion characterized only as a focal asymmetry.[32]

Determination of the adequacy of excision depends not only on the specimen radiograph but also on the histologic evaluation of the specimen and, in some instances, on the postoperative mammogram. When findings are positive, the specimen radiograph is reliable in showing tumor extension to the margin of resection; however, when this extension is not seen on specimen radiography, the finding is not reliable in excluding tumor extension to the resected margin.[33] Evaluation also includes histologic assessment of margins, aided by the pathologist's inking of

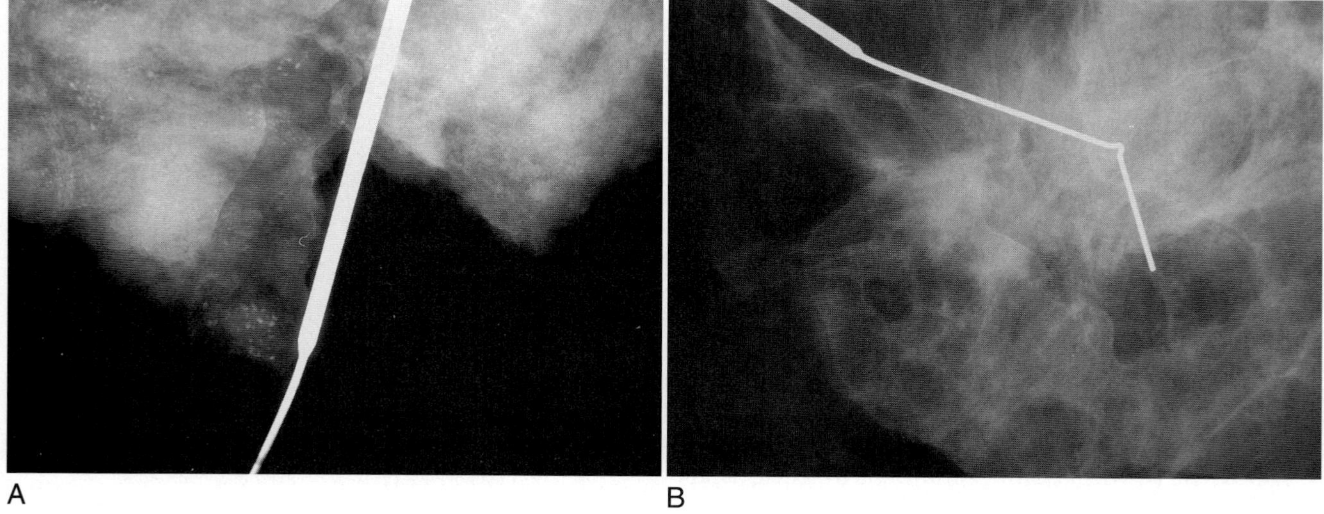

Figure 31–3. **A,** Specimen radiography shows calcium at the margin of the excised specimen. Calcium was due to ductal carcinoma in situ. Its presence at the margin of the specimen resulted in excision of more tissue to attempt to clear the breast of cancer. **B,** A spiculated carcinoma is seen in this specimen. Spicules and mass extend to the resected margin because of transection of tumor. Additional tissue was excised to clear the breast of cancer.

the outer margins of the resected tissue before histologic sectioning.[34] The outer margin of the specimen can therefore be appreciated during microscopic evaluation, and its relationship to the margin of the tumor can be ascertained.

POSTOPERATIVE DETERMINATION OF THE COMPLETENESS OF TUMOR RESECTION

Because the mammographic changes of surgical distortion and hematoma formation that occur at the surgical site obscure findings related to unresected uncalcified carcinoma, postoperative preradiation mammography need not be performed. However, the calcifications of carcinoma are not obscured by these immediately postoperative findings, and postoperative mammography is worthwhile to seek evidence of incomplete resection of a calcified tumor in the form of residual calcifications (Fig. 31–4). Because microscopic residual tumor will presumably be sterilized by postoperative radiotherapy,[35] evidence of minimal residual tumor may not require further surgery. However, large volumes of residual tumor will not be adequately treated by postoperative irradiation and will have to be excised.[36] In addition to determining whether a reexcision may be necessary, the postoperative preradiation mammogram is useful in establishing a new baseline image of the calcifications remaining in the breast. If the residual calcifications at the lumpectomy site are not reexcised, it is important to be able to determine on later mammograms whether the pattern of calcifications is stable or they have increased in number or extent.

Magnification views are useful to determine more accurately the number and extent of residual calcifications. Occasionally, when routine views of the lumpectomy site do not show residual calcium, this finding might be evident on magnification imaging.[37] Therefore, the routine use of magnification in at least one view may be desirable in postoperative imaging. Punctate microcalcifications can be seen postoperatively at the lumpectomy site. Therefore, comparison with the preoperative mammogram should be made to be certain that calcium at this site is residual tumoral calcium and not postoperative benign calcification.

The precise number of residual microcalcifications that require a reexcision has not been determined. One or two calcifications suggests the presence of minimal residual tumor. Although this residual tumor may be sterilized with radiation, some surgeons routinely reexcise any residual microcalcifications.[38] A large number of residual calcifications indicates a large volume of tumor that must be surgically excised. The histologic assessment of the margins of the resected specimen should also be considered in the determination of the need for reexcision.

Postoperative mammography to exclude residual calcifications that may necessitate reexcision may be performed at any time before the start of radiotherapy. After a reexcision, another postoperative mammogram should be obtained to determine the adequacy of reexcision and to establish a new baseline. Because the breast may be tender after reexcision, compression to immobilize the breast during the two standard x-ray exposures should be no greater than the patient can tolerate.

Residual microcalcifications at the lumpectomy site do not invariably imply the presence of residual tumor. In one study of 29 women who underwent reexcision of a focus of mammographically evident residual microcalcifications, only 69% were found to have residual carcinoma.[39] The women who were

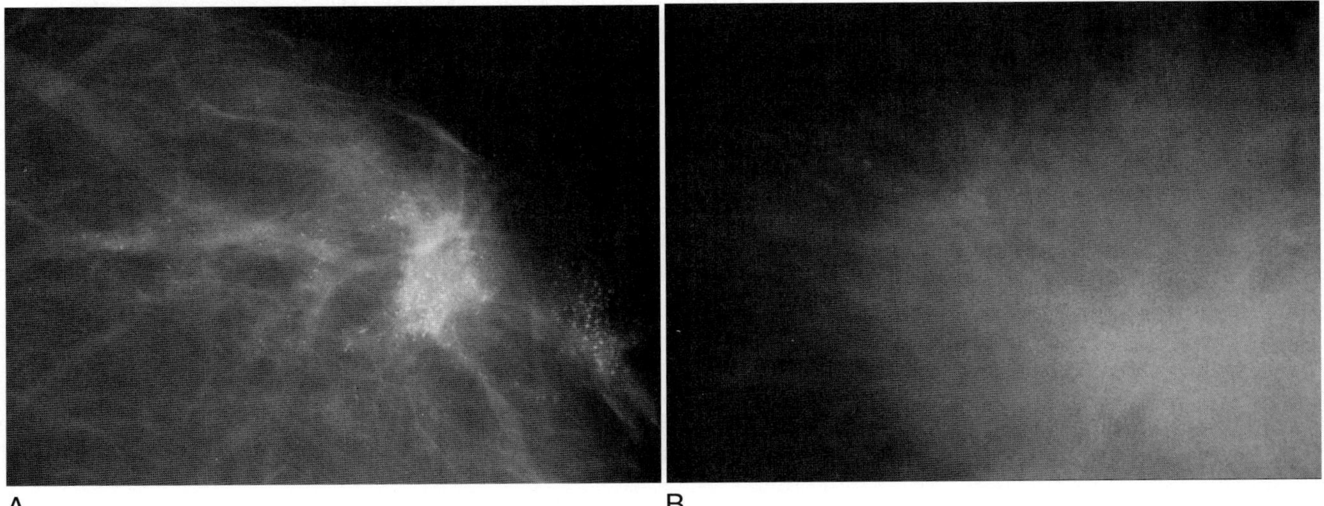

Figure 31–4. **A,** Preoperative mammogram shows calcifications due to ductal carcinoma in situ (DCIS). **B,** A postoperative mammogram shows a spiculated scar. Residual tumoral calcifications are present because of incomplete excision of DCIS. Additional tissue was removed to clear the breast of tumor calcium.

found not to have residual cancer were usually those in whom small numbers of residual calcifications had been seen. Although the calcifications were pleomorphic, they were found to be associated with sclerosing adenosis, fat necrosis, and foreign body reaction. In the same study, 64% of 14 women in whom tumor-associated calcifications had been completely excised had no residual tumor at reexcision. Because a carcinoma may not have calcifications throughout its entire extent, it is not surprising that the removal of all calcifications does not always result in complete excision of the tumor.[40,41] Thus, the removal of all tumor-associated calcifications does not ensure the total removal of the tumor.

In women with positive margins histologically, MRI has been found to be able to demonstrate the extent of residual carcinoma in the breast that might otherwise be unsuspected.[42,43] A pattern of smooth enhancement around the lumpectomy site due to granulation tissue is normal, but clumped or irregular enhancement can be found in women with residual carcinoma (Fig. 31–5). Accurate mapping of the extent of residual tumor can spare the patient multiple trips to surgery, for procedures that only "chip away" at the cancer, by demonstrating the extent of tumor requiring resection or treatment with mastectomy.

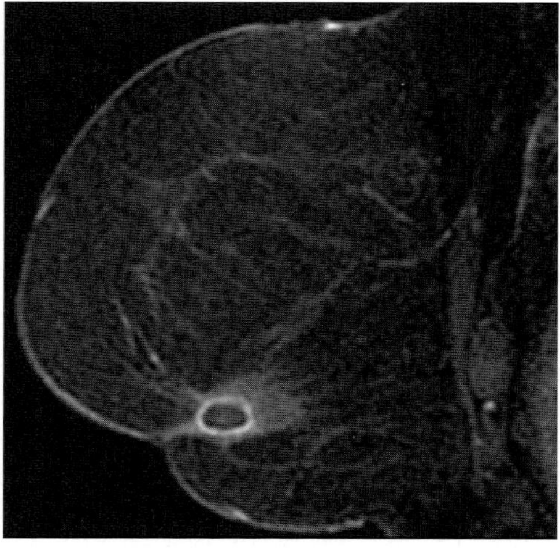
A

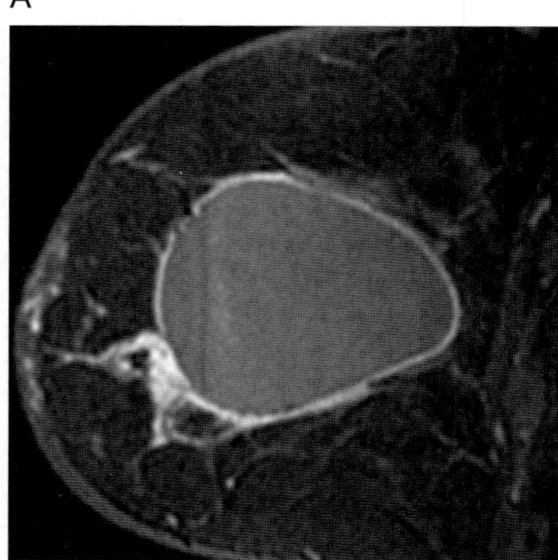
B

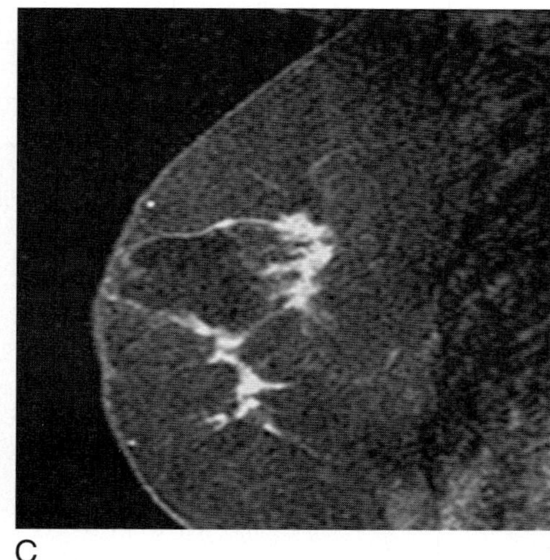
C

Figure 31–5. A, Shortly after lumpectomy, a contrast-enhanced magnetic resonance (MR) image shows a ring of enhancement in the wall of the seroma that has formed at the operative site. **B,** Clumped enhancement at the anterior seroma margin was due to residual tumor. The lumpectomy specimen showed tumor extension to the anterior margin of the removed tissue. **C,** The posterior and inferior margins of the seroma are contaminated by residual tumor. MR imaging is helpful in this case in mapping the extent of carcinoma left in the breast.

ROUTINE MAMMOGRAPHY AFTER RADIATION THERAPY

After the completion of radiation therapy, routine mammography is performed to detect recurrent tumor as early as possible, to characterize any palpable abnormality that develops in either breast, and to screen for cancer in the untreated breast. Mammography of the untreated breast should be performed annually. The treated breast requires a baseline mammogram after the completion of radiotherapy and routine follow-up thereafter. It has been the policy at my institution to perform the initial post-treatment mammogram of the irradiated breast 3 to 6 months after completion of therapy. If the breast becomes red, firm, and tender, the mammogram is delayed for 6 months, at which time the breast is usually less tender, allowing for more effective compression. For those women in whom only minimal radiation reaction is seen on physical examination, the mammogram is performed 3 months after the completion of radiation therapy.

Routine mediolateral oblique and craniocaudal views are obtained. It is important that the tumorectomy site be imaged as completely as possible, because that is the area at greatest risk for recurrent cancer. Because a recurrence may be manifest merely as a subtle change in the scar, additional images of the lumpectomy site, including spot cone views, are often obtained to document the post-treatment size and configuration of the scar. Whatever additional views are needed at the time of this initial post-treatment mammogram to fully image the surgical bed are routinely included in follow-up mammograms to screen for tumor recurrence. If the original tumor contained microcalcifications, and magnification views were not obtained before radiation therapy, it is the policy at my institution to obtain these views as part of the post–radiation therapy baseline study to allow any calcifications near the scar to be fully documented. If later in the course of follow-up a patient is seen at my institution for the first time and magnification views have not yet been obtained or are unavailable, and either the original tumor contained calcifications or its mammographic appearance is unknown, a magnification view of the lumpectomy site is obtained as part of the initial assessment of the patient.

The timing of further mammograms is a source of debate. Some authorities have suggested follow-up mammograms at 6-month intervals for the first 2 to 5 years.[44,45] However, no existing data suggest that routine follow-up at intervals shorter than 1 year result in a diagnosis of recurrence at an earlier stage. It has been the policy at my institution to perform mammography within 6 months of completion of radiation therapy, at 1 year after treatment, and annually thereafter (Table 31–1). For women who do not undergo radiation therapy, the initial mammogram is performed within a few months of surgery to establish a new baseline, and thereafter mammography follows the same schedule as for patients who have undergone radiation therapy.

The changes seen in the mammogram after breast-conserving therapy include focal alterations at the lumpectomy site resulting from surgery and more diffuse changes caused by radiation therapy. All, some, or none of the following changes may be present in any individual case.

Seromas and Hematomas

In the initial postoperative period, a new round or oval mass at the lumpectomy site usually represents a seroma or hematoma (Fig. 31–6).[46] The seroma occasionally contains a fat-fluid or air-fluid level that is visible on a 90-degree lateral view. These masses are clinically unimportant, tend to resolve slowly (sometimes over a period of a year), and may be replaced by a scar in the form of a spiculated mass that should not be mistaken for recurrent cancer.[37]

Scars

Scars and areas of parenchymal distortion are often evident at the lumpectomy site. It is imperative that the radiologist know the location of this site to be certain that the spiculated mass is consistent with a scar. Surgical clips that are placed at the lumpectomy site to accurately target the boost dose of radiation are helpful in defining the lumpectomy bed for the radiologist (Fig. 31–7). The surgical site can also localized by reference to the preoperative mammogram (if it showed the cancer) or the postoperative mammogram. Although some radiologists have suggested the placement of radiopaque skin markers at the cutaneous scar to localize the area of resection, the skin incision is often far removed from the site of resection.

Table 31–1. Memorial Sloan-Kettering Schedule for Mammography in Patients Treated with Breast-Conserving Therapy

Timing	Study	Technique	Comments
Preoperative	Bilateral mammogram	Routine views; use magnification and coned views as needed to assess full extent of tumor	Determine presence and extent of multiplicity of tumor to assess possibility of breast conservation; evaluate other breast
Intraoperative	Specimen radiography	May require at least two orthogonal views and magnification view; compression useful for masses	Determine whether lesion of interest has been sampled; if malignant, determine whether tumor extends to margins of resection, requiring further surgery
Before radiation therapy	Unilateral mammogram for women whose tumors contained calcifications	If no calcifications present at lumpectomy site, perform magnification view; if calcium present, perform magnification view to determine extent	Assess completeness of tumor excision by mammographic criteria; if reexcision performed, repeat this study
Post-therapy baseline	Unilateral mammogram	Do at 3–6 month after radiation therapy; if calcium was present in original cancer and magnification view was not previously performed, do it now	Reestablish baseline mammographic pattern
Routine follow-up	Annual bilateral mammogram	Additional views as clinically indicated	To detect early recurrence
Area of clinical concern	Diagnostic mammogram	Two-view mammogram with additional views as need	Evaluate new area of concern

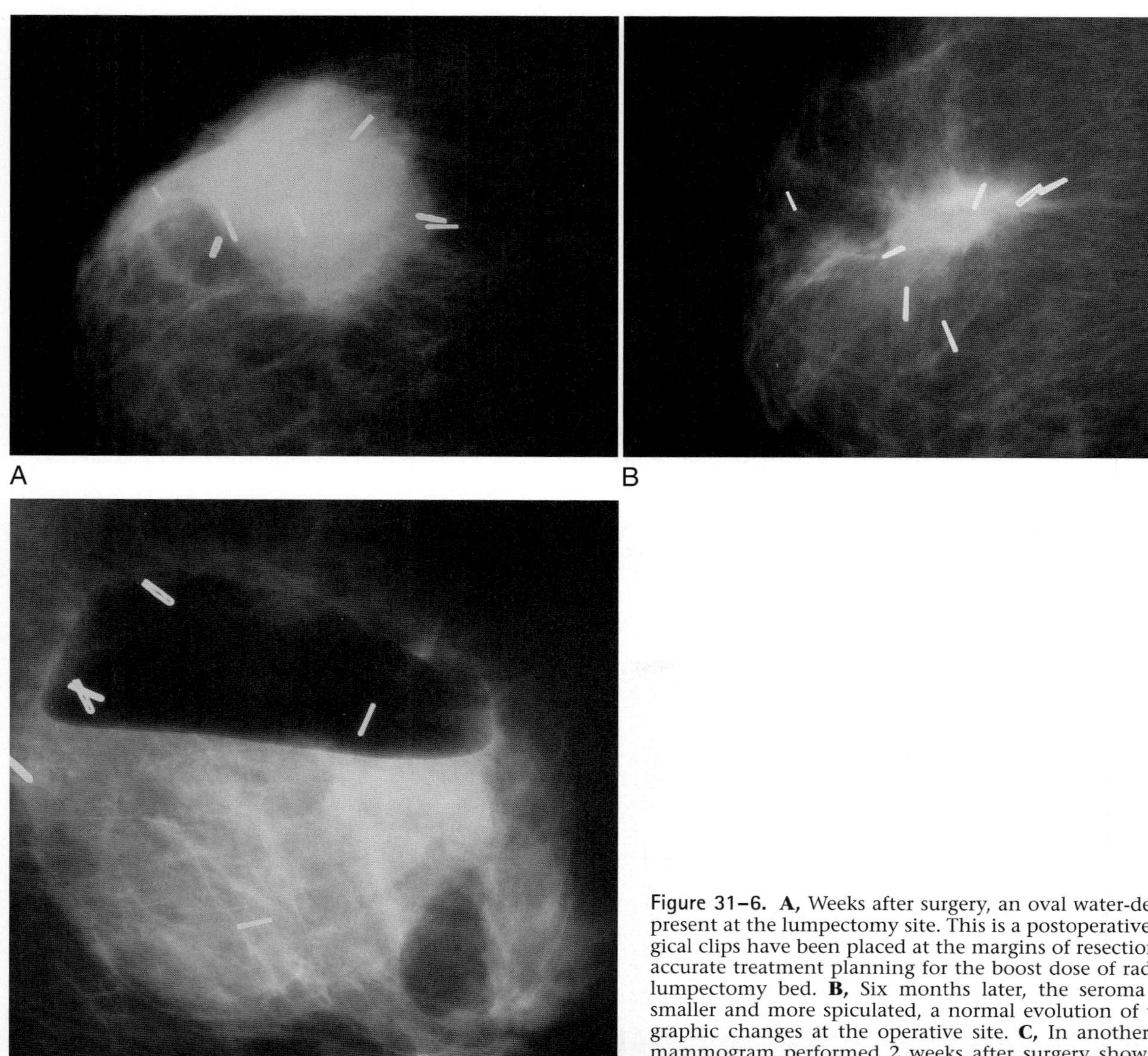

Figure 31–6. **A,** Weeks after surgery, an oval water-density mass is present at the lumpectomy site. This is a postoperative seroma. Surgical clips have been placed at the margins of resection to facilitate accurate treatment planning for the boost dose of radiation to the lumpectomy bed. **B,** Six months later, the seroma has become smaller and more spiculated, a normal evolution of the mammographic changes at the operative site. **C,** In another patient, the mammogram performed 2 weeks after surgery shows an air-fluid level at the lumpectomy site on the mediolateral oblique view. This finding, due to acute changes, is a normal pattern shortly after lumpectomy.

The scar may be associated with a contour deformity and focal skin thickening, which can also be useful in localizing the surgical site. In the early postoperative period, edema may obscure the scar, which then becomes increasingly apparent as the edema subsides. Careful attention to the earlier mammogram may show that an increasingly apparent spiculated mass is the scar that was "silhouetted" by the edema on earlier studies and does not represent a new lesion. The scar may also be characterized by a pattern that is more prominent on one orthogonal view than on the other. Although cancer occasionally may look similar, this pattern supports the diagnosis of a scar. Scars may contain a central focus of fat owing to the herniation of fat into the lumpectomy site and the occurrence of fibrosis around it. Finally, in some conservatively treated breasts, no scar may be evident in mammograms. In one series, a scar was evident on the mammograms in only one fourth of the women who underwent breast-conserving therapy.[47]

Diffuse Mammographic Changes

Superimposed on the focal changes at the surgical site are diffuse alterations in the mammogram that are due to radiation. Histologically, the early changes resulting from radiation therapy result from edema, and the more chronic alterations are caused by fibrosis.[48] Mammographically, these changes are manifested as skin thickening, trabecular thickening, increase in the density of the parenchyma, and diffuse increase in the density of the breast (Fig. 31–8).[49]

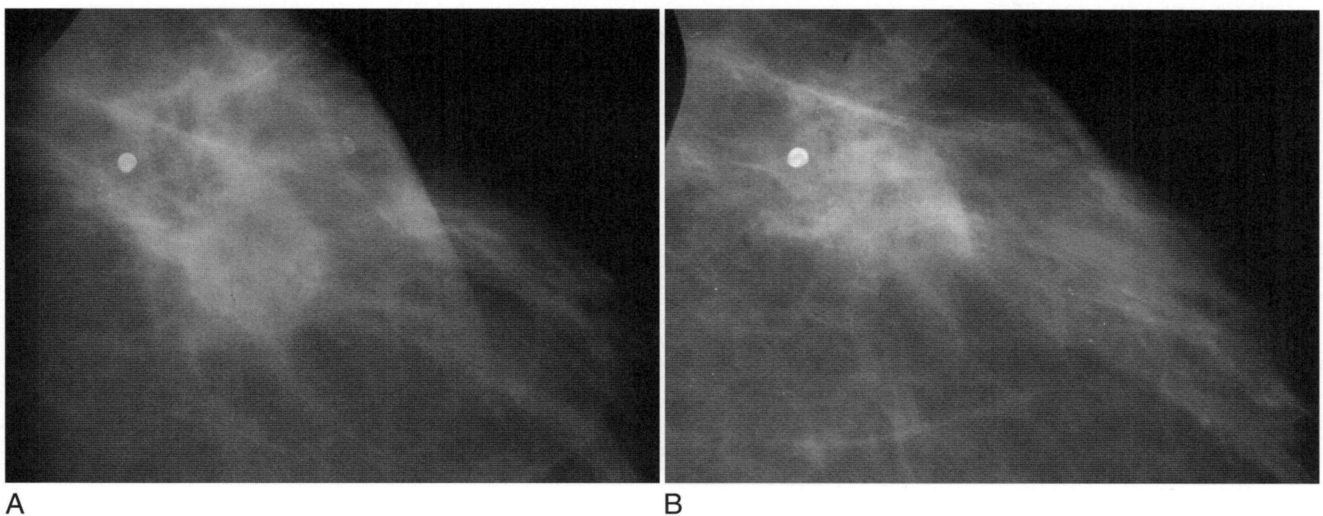

Figure 31–7. **A,** Within the first few months after lumpectomy, the scar is as large as it should ever be. An oval mass at the lumpectomy site on this mammogram is a small seroma. Note the tethered contour of the skin due to surgical deformity. **B,** One year later, the scar is smaller, and spiculation is slightly more prominent. This is a normal pattern of scar formation.

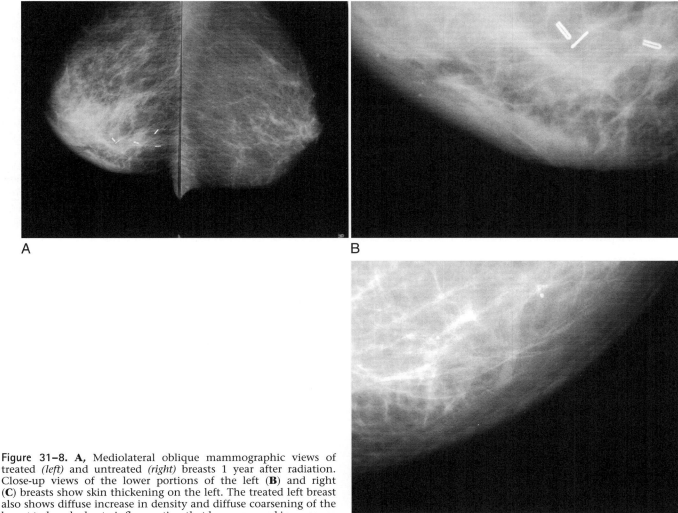

Figure 31–8. **A,** Mediolateral oblique mammographic views of treated *(left)* and untreated *(right)* breasts 1 year after radiation. Close-up views of the lower portions of the left (**B**) and right (**C**) breasts show skin thickening on the left. The treated left breast also shows diffuse increase in density and diffuse coarsening of the breast trabecula due to inflammation that have occurred in response to radiation.

These changes are identical to those that result from inflammatory breast cancer, mastitis, lymphoma, and obstructed lymphatic or venous drainage. A patient may have none, some, or all of these findings, and their occurrence is not related to radiation dose.[50] On serial examinations, these findings may remain unaltered, may decrease, or may completely resolve. After the initial baseline mammogram, any progression of findings is worrisome and should lead to an investigation of the cause.

Skin Changes

Thickening of the skin may be diffuse or localized to the surgical site or dependent portion of the breast.[47] Skin changes are more common in women who have also undergone axillary node dissection. Diffuse skin thickening may be apparent only on comparison of the mammogram of the treated breast with that of the breast before treatment or with the mammogram of the other breast. Skin thickening is the most common change on the mammogram after breast-conserving therapy, being reported in up to 90% of cases.[47,51] The radiologist should remember that this finding is more conspicuous on mammograms performed with full breast digital imaging than with screen-film technique. Thickened skin returns to normal by 2 to 3 years after therapy in 46% to 60% of cases.[47,52,53]

Parenchymal Changes

Postirradiation changes of the parenchyma include coarsening of the fibrous supportive tissues of the breast (thickening of the trabeculae), an increase in the density and bulk of the ductal and glandular elements, and a diffuse increase in the density of the entire breast. In addition to the edema and fibrosis caused by radiation, increased flow through the lymphatic channels and small blood vessels causes them to become distended, contributing to this pattern.[54] In the dense breast, trabecular thickening may be most apparent in the subdermal fat, especially when the mammogram is examined with bright light. Although these changes may be nonexistent or subtle in some women,[49] they may be accentuated in women undergoing chemotherapy.[47]

Calcifications

Calcifications develop in one third to one half of women who have undergone breast radiation therapy, sometimes after a delay of up to 5 years.[47,52-55] Calcified suture material and coarse calcifications of fat necrosis are commonly apparent in the irradiated breast, particularly at the site of tumorectomy and the boost dose of radiotherapy (Fig. 31–9). The calcifications of fat necrosis tend to be round, may have radiolucent centers, and usually do not develop sooner than 2 years after treatment. They reflect the trauma of radiotherapy and surgery. Radiopaque surgical clips may also be present at the surgical site. Microcalcifications, if not fully excised at surgery, may increase, decrease, or remain stable in number. The calcifications that decrease in number are presumably associated with cancer that has responded to radiotherapy. An increase in number of microcalcifications raises the concern about an associated viable growing tumor, and biopsy is indicated. The radiologist should be aware that nonmalignant processes can also cause microcalcifications to develop; these are discussed later. Microcalcifications that remain stable may reflect viable tumor whose growth has been retarded by radiotherapy. Such stable calcifications followed for several years with mammograms to confirm that they remain unchanged do not signal the presence of viable tumor.

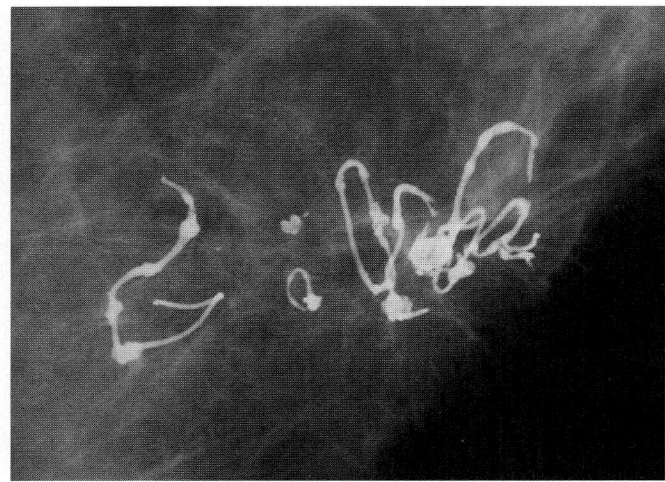

Figure 31–9. Linear calcifications are due to calcified suture material at the lumpectomy site. Clumped, eggshell calcifications and punctate calcifications are foci of fat necrosis.

TUMOR RECURRENCE IN THE IRRADIATED BREAST

Mammographic follow-up after breast-conserving therapy is undertaken to detect recurrent tumor in the treated breast (local treatment failure) as early as possible. Local treatment failure is reported to occur at a rate of 5% at 5 years and of 10% to 15% at 10 years after completion of therapy.[56] Because the stage of tumor recurrence is related to the likelihood of survival, the early diagnosis of recurrence is of extreme importance.[57,58] The woman whose recurrent cancer is diagnosed while it is still intraductal or whose invasive cancer is less than 2 cm in diameter has the best prognosis. Survival rates decrease with increasing tumor size.[59]

Although local treatment failure can occur in any woman who has undergone breast-conserving therapy, certain women are at a higher risk. Some risk factors remain controversial but include younger age at the time of treatment, an extensive intraductal component of the tumor, and vascular invasion by the tumor.[12] Also implicated in increasing the likelihood of recurrence are multiple cancers at the time of the original treatment, tumor involvement at the margin of resection, lymphatic invasion by tumor, high histologic grade, larger tumor size, nonductal histologic type, and monocellular reaction to the tumor.[60] Chemotherapy has been reported to lower the incidence of recurrence.[60]

The ability of mammography to identify recurrent cancer after breast-conserving therapy is compromised compared with its ability to detect cancer in the untreated breast. This is due to the surgical distortion and increased breast density that result from treatment. Mammography reportedly has been unable to detect 19% to 50% of local recurrences.[57,61-63] However, 29% to 42% of local recurrences have been reported to be detected only by mammography. Compared with local recurrences detected on physical examination, those found by mammography are more often DCIS, whereas those found on physical examination are more often invasive.[61,64] Recurrences consisting of invasive lobular histology can be extremely difficult to detect mammographically.

To optimize the efficacy of mammography of the treated breast, it is extremely important that careful communication between the clinician and the radiologist occurs and that subtle mammographic signs of tumor recurrences be vigorously sought. The signs are those of breast cancer superimposed on the findings characteristic of an irradiated breast. They include the development of new, pleomorphic microcalcifications or a new mass (Fig. 31–10). Enlargement of the scar may signal the recurrence of tumor (Fig. 31–11). Enlargement of axillary nodes can result from metastatic tumor, causing an axillary recurrence (Fig. 31–12). As noted previously, an increase in breast density or in skin thickening should be viewed with suspicion, and the cause should be investigated. The other breast must also be monitored, as it is always at risk for cancer.

In the event of failure of local treatment, the site in the breast at which the new tumor occurs is related to the time from completion of treatment. A carcinoma that arises within 4 to 6 years after therapy is usually the result of failure to eradicate the original tumor. The tumor recurrence usually occurs at or near the site of the original cancer.[44,61,65] Recurrences rarely occur earlier than 18 months after adequate therapy. It is important during this follow-up period that the lumpectomy site be fully imaged. Treatment for the patient's original cancer usually sterilizes undetected sites of tumor within the breast. It usually takes at least 4 to 6 years for new cancers to grow in the breast and become detectable. Therefore, starting at 4 to 6 years after therapy, the breast is at risk for the development of a new cancer, usually arising in a different quadrant from that in which the original cancer developed.

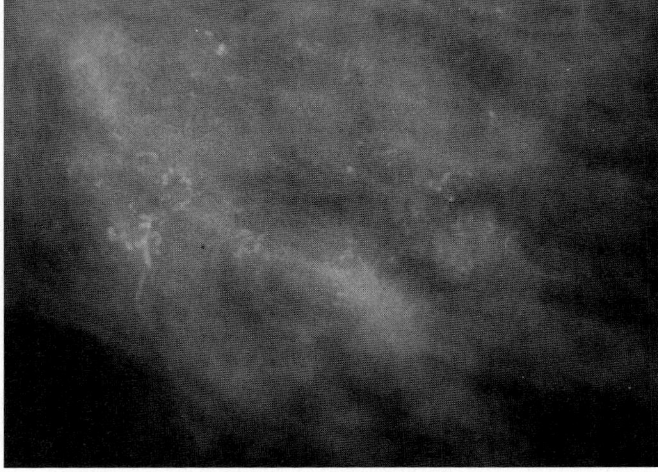

Figure 31–10. Pleomorphic, BI-RADS category 5 microcalcifications developed at the lumpectomy site of this women owing to local recurrence of ductal carcinoma in situ.

BENIGN SEQUELAE MIMICKING RECURRENCE

Although the development of a palpable mass or mammographic abnormality after breast-conserving therapy raises the specter of recurrent carcinoma, complications of treatment can mimic recurrent cancer and yet be clinically innocent. Fat necrosis and fibrosis can be caused by surgery or radiation, and radiation can produce a new mass and pleo-

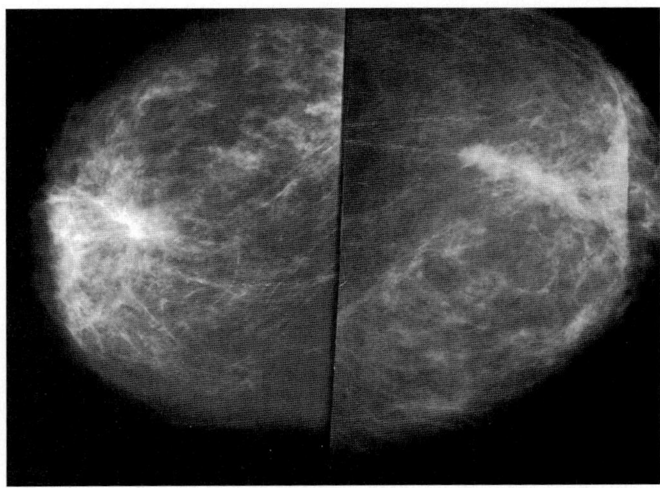

Figure 31–11. *Left,* the mammogram performed 2 years after treatment shows baseline changes. *Right,* A year later, the central scar has become elongated and lobulated. This change was due to recurrence of invasive ductal carcinoma.

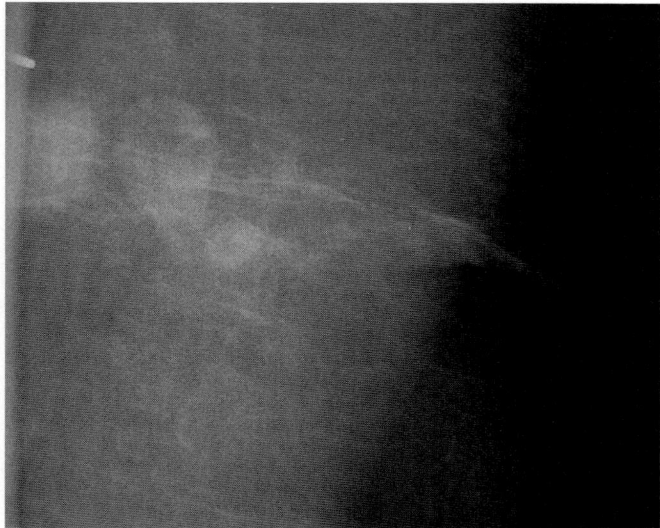

A

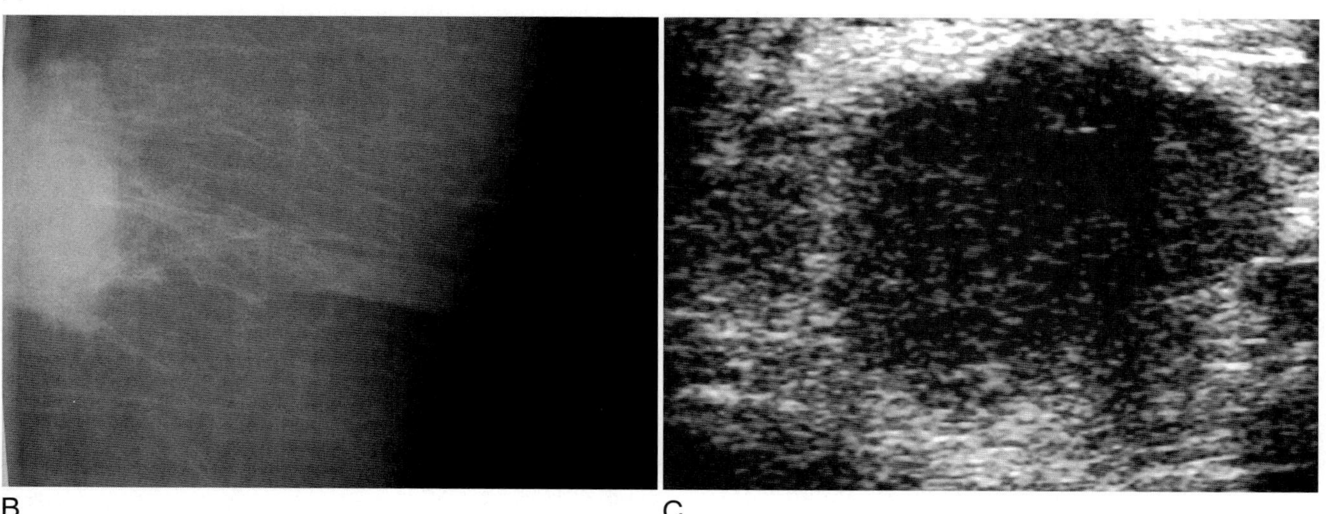

B C

Figure 31–12. **A,** A mammogram performed 1 year after treatment shows normal axillary nodes. **B,** A year later, nodal enlargement and irregularity, due to an axillary recurrence, are present. **C,** Ultrasonogram of the adenopathy shows an irregular node. Ultrasonography was used to perform fine-needle aspiration, which led to diagnosis of carcinoma in the axilla.

morphic microcalcifications, findings identical to those of recurrent tumor. In one reported series of patients treated with breast-conserving therapy, 19 of 29 women who underwent breast biopsy for suspected recurrence had benign disease.[66]

It is important to attempt to differentiate fat necrosis and fibrosis from recurrent tumor. Surgical biopsy can compromise the cosmetic result of breast-conserving surgery, and scarring may be worsened because of damage to microvasculature that occurs during radiation therapy.[37] The mammographic changes that suggest fat necrosis include its location at the tumorectomy site within 3 years after the completion of therapy.[66,67] Fat necrosis may produce a palpable mass in the absence of mammographic findings (Fig. 31–13).[66] The calcifications of fat necrosis usually represent a sequela of irradiation, tend to occur at the site of the boost dose, and are usually punctate microcalcifications (Fig. 31–14). They do not have the pleomorphism characteristic of carcinoma, nor do they have a branching pattern.[66] Benign calcifications can also arise in an incidental benign disorder such as sclerosing adenosis. Coexistent benign and malignant findings can occur, so the radiologist needs to carefully assess all findings (Fig. 31–15).

When it is not possible to determine whether the findings are due to carcinoma, fibrosis, or other benign processes, biopsy should be performed. Percutaneous needle biopsy may be useful in differentiating tumor from scar. Data from one series of women treated with breast-conserving therapy showed that differentiation was possible with the use of stereotactically guided fine-needle aspiration.[68] Six patients had malignant aspirates, and one had an atypical aspirate. Examination of the surgical specimens showed all seven to be malignant.

MRI of the lumpectomy site has also been shown to be reliable in differentiating scar from tumor recurrence. Because breast cancers are vascular and scars are hypovascular or avascular, the enhancement of the cancers after the intravenous administration

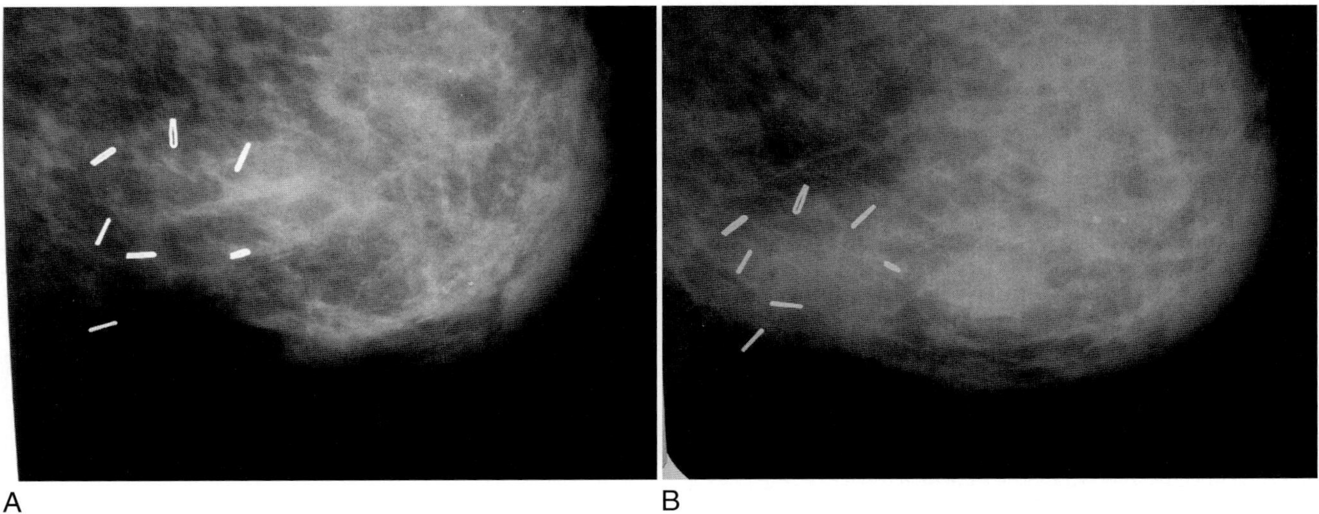

Figure 31–13. **A,** One year after treatment, baseline changes are evident on a mammogram. **B,** A year later, increased density is surrounded by the surgical clips at the lumpectomy site. A palpable mass had also developed here. Biopsy revealed fat necrosis.

Figure 31–14. Calcifications evident on the mammogram developed as a new finding at the lumpectomy site. Biopsy was done, and histological examination showed only dystrophic calcifications.

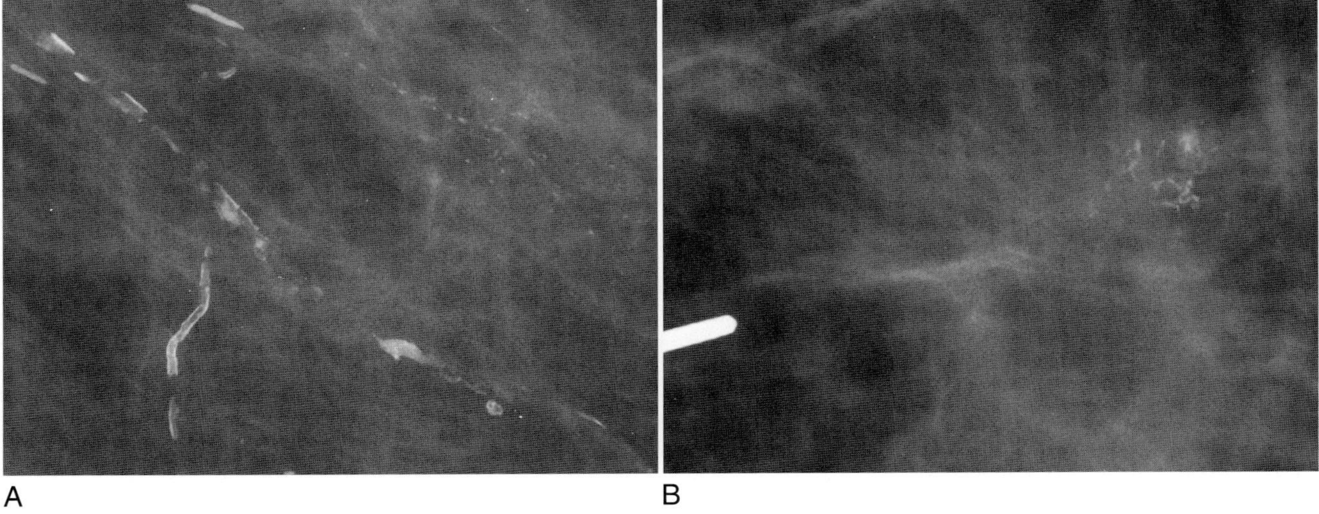

Figure 31–15. **A,** Multiple patterns of calcifications are present at the lumpectomy site in this patient. There are vascular calcifications as well as an eggshell calcification due to fat necrosis. Additionally, pleomorphic microcalcifications have formed because of recurrent ductal carcinoma. **B,** Against a background pattern of architectural distortion from previous lumpectomy, a coarse dystrophic calcification is seen along with multiple, pleomorphic calcifications due to recurrent carcinoma.

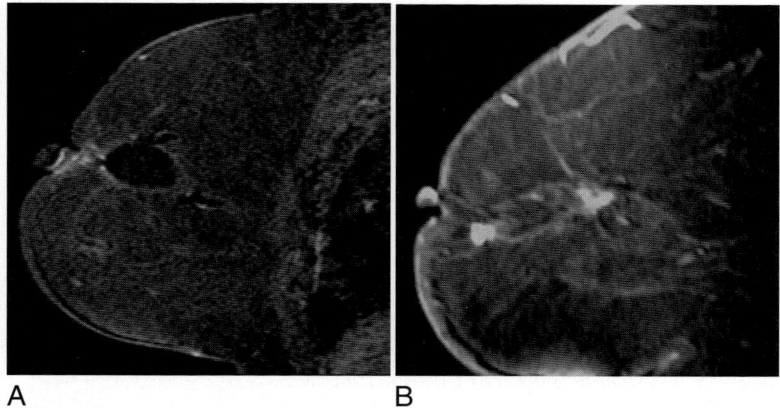

Figure 31–16. **A,** Two years after surgery, there is no enhancement on contrast-enhanced magnetic resonance imaging (MRI) of a seroma. Note the artifact from clips next to the seroma and normal enhancement of the nipple. **B,** Three years after treatment, enlargement of the surgical scar was further evaluated with contrast MRI. Clumped enhancement is due to recurrent invasive carcinoma.

of gadolinium has enabled them to be distinguished from nonenhancing scars (Fig. 31–16).[69,70] However, during the first 18 months after therapy, both scars and cancers tend to enhance with administration of a contrast agent, and MRI patterns are not reliable during this period. Fortunately, recurrences are rare this early. Also, enhancing scars have been reported more than 18 months after treatment, although they also seem to be unusual.

References

1. Bader J, Lippman ME, Swain SM, et al: Preliminary report of the NCI early breast cancer (BC) study: A prospective randomized comparison of lumpectomy (L) and radiation (XRT) to mastectomy (M) for Stage I and II BC [abstract]. Int J Radiat Oncol Biol Phys 1987;13(Suppl 1):160.
2. Bartelink H, van Dongen JA, Aaronson N, et al: Randomized clinical trial to assess the value of breast-conserving therapy (BCT) in stage II breast cancer; EORTC Trial 10801 [abstract]. In Proceedings of the 7th Annual Meeting of the European Society for Therapeutic Radiology and Oncology (ESTRO). Den Haag, 1988, p 211.
3. Blichert-Toft M: A Danish randomized trial comparing breast conservation with mastectomy in mammary carcinoma. Br J Cancer 1990;62(Suppl 12):15.
4. Blichert-Toft M, Brincker H, Andersen JA, et al: A Danish randomized trial comparing breast-preserving therapy with mastectomy in mammary carcinoma: Preliminary results. Acta Oncol 1988;27:671-677.
6. Glatstein E, Straus K, Lichter A, et al: Results of the NCI early breast cancer trial [abstract]. In Proceedings of the NIH Consensus Development Conference, June 18-21. Bethesda, MD: National Institutes of Health, National Cancer Institute, 1990, pp 32, 33.
7. Habibollahi F, Fentiman IS, Chaudary MA, et al: Conservation treatment of operable breast cancer [abstract]. Proceedings of the American Society of Clinical Oncology 1987;6:A231.
8. Sarrazin D, Le MG, Arriagada R, et al: Ten-year results of a randomized trial comparing a conservative treatment to mastectomy in early breast cancer. Radiother Oncol 1989;14:177-184.
9. van Dongen JA, Bartelink H, Aaronson H, et al: Randomized clinical trial to assess the value of breast-conserving therapy in stage I and stage II breast cancer; EORTC Trial 10801 [abstract]. In Proceedings of the NIH-Consensus Development Conference, June 18-21. Bethesda, MD, National Institutes of Health, National Cancer Institute, 1990, pp 25-27.
10. Veronesi U, Banfi A, Del Vecchio M, et al: Comparison of Halsted mastectomy with quadrantectomy, axillary dissection, and radiotherapy in early breast cancer: Long-term results. Eur J Cancer Clin Oncol 1986;22:1085-1089.
11. Winchester DP, Cox JD: Standards for breast-conservation treatment. CA Cancer J Clin 1992;42:134-162.
12. Borger J, Kemperman H, Hart A, et al: Risk factors in breast-conservation therapy. J Clin Oncol 1994;12:653-660.
13. Clarke DH, Le M, Sarrazin D, et al: Analysis of local regional relapses in patients with early breast cancers treated by excision and radiotherapy: Experience of the Institut Gustave Roussy. Int J Radiat Oncol Biol Phys 1985;11:137-145.
14. Kurtz JM, Jacquemier J, Amalric R, et al: Breast-conserving therapy for macroscopically multiple cancers. Ann Surg 1991; 212:38-44.
15. Holland R, Hendricks J, Verbeek AL, et al: Extent, distribution and mammographical/histological correlations of breast ductal carcinoma in situ. Lancet 1990;335:519-522.
16. Dershaw DD, Abramson A, Kinne DW: Ductal carcinoma in situ: Mammographic findings and clinical implications. Radiology 1989;170:411-415.
17. Lagios MD, Westdahl PR, Margolin FR, et al: Duct carcinoma in situ: Relationship of occult invasion, multicentricity, lymph node metastases and short term treatment failures. Cancer 1982;50:1309-1314.
18. Davis PL, Staiger MJ, Harris KB, et al: Accuracy of breast cancer measurements with MR imaging, US, and mammography [abstract]. Radiology 1994;193:267.
19. Gordon PB: Malignant breast masses detected only with US [abstract]. Radiology 1994;193(P):177.
20. Orel SG, Schnall MD, Hochman MG, et al: Impact of MR imaging and MR-guided biopsy on detection and staging of breast cancer [abstract]. Radiology 1994;193(P):318.
21. Berg WA, Gilbreath PL: Multicentric and multifocal cancer: Whole-breast US in preoperative evaluation. Radiology 2000; 214;59-66.
22. Moon WK, Noh DY, Im JG: Multifocal, multicentric, and contralateral breast cancers: Bilateral whole breast US in the preoperative evaluation of patients. Radiology 2002;224:569-576.
23. Fischer U, Kopka L, Grabbe E: Breast carcinoma: Effect of preoperative contrast-enhanced MR imaging on the therapeutic approach. Radiology 1999;213:881-888.
24. Morris EA, Schwartz LH, Drotman MB, et al: Evaluation of pectoralis major muscle in patients with posterior breast tumors on breast MR images: Early experience. Radiology 2000;214: 67-72.
25. Fisher B, Redmond C, Poisson R, et al: Eight-year results of a randomized clinical trial comparing total mastectomy and lumpectomy with or without irradiation in the treatment of breast cancer. N Engl J Med 1989;320:822-828.
25. Khalkhali I, Cutrone JA, Mena IG, et al: Scintimammography versus mammography: Complimentary role of Tc-99m sestamibi breast imaging in the prone position for the diagnosis of breast carcinoma [abstract]. Radiology 1994;193(P):158.
26. Morrow M. Strom EA, Bassett LW, et al: Standard for breast conservation therapy in the management of invasive breast carcinoma. CA Cancer J Clin 2002;52:277-300.
27. Fischer U, Vosshenrich R, Doler W, et al: MR imaging-guided breast intervention: Experience with two systems. Radiology 1995;195:529-532.

28. Kinne DW, Dershaw DD, Rosen PP: Needle localization. In Harris JR, Hellman S, Henderson IC, Kinne DW (eds): Breast Diseases, 2nd ed. Philadelphia, JB Lippincott, 1991, pp 113-117.
29. Lee CH, Carter D: Detecting residual tumor after excisional biopsy of impalpable breast carcinoma: Efficacy of comparing preoperative mammograms with radiographs of the biopsy specimen. AJR Am J Roentgenol 1995;164:81-86.
30. Chilcote WA, Davis GA, Sucky P, et al: Breast specimen radiography: Evaluation of a compression device. Radiology 1988; 168:425-427.
31. Rebner M, Pennes DR, Baker DE, et al: Two-view specimen radiography in surgical biopsy of nonpalpable breast masses. AJR Am J Roentgenol 1987;149:283-285.
32. Stomper PC, David SP, Sonnenfeld MR, et al: Efficacy of specimen radiography of clinically occult noncalcified breast lesions. AJR Am J Roentgenol 1988;151:43-47.
33. Graham RA, Homer MJ, Sigler CJ, et al: The efficacy of specimen radiography in evaluating the surgical margins of impalpable breast carcinoma. AJR Am J Roentgenol 1994;162: 33-36.
34. Rosen PP: The pathology of invasive breast cancer. In Harris JR, Hellman S, Henderson K, Kinne DW (eds): Breast Diseases, 2nd ed. Philadelphia, JB Lippincott, 1991, p 281.
35. Hellman S, Harris JR: Breast cancer: Considerations in local and regional treatment. Radiology 1986;164:593-598.
36. Harris JR, Lippman ME, Veronesi U, et al: Medical progress: Breast cancer (2). N Engl J Med 1992; 327:390-398.
37. Dershaw DD: Mammography in patients with breast cancer treated by breast conservation (lumpectomy with or without radiation). AJR Am J Roentgenol 1995;164:309-316.
38. Morrow M, Strom EA, Bassett LW, et al: Standard for the management of ductal carcinoma in situ of the breast. CA Cancer J Clin 2002;52:256-267.
39. Gluck BS, Dershaw DD, Liberman L, et al: Microcalcifications on postoperative mammograms as an indicator of adequacy of tumor excision. Radiology 1993;188:469-472.
40. Gefter WB, Friedman AK, Goodman RL: The role of mammography in evaluating patients with early carcinoma of the breast for tylectomy and radiation therapy. Radiology 1982; 142:77-80.
41. Homer MJ, Schmidt-Ulrich R, Safaii H: Residual breast carcinoma after biopsy: Role of mammography in evaluation. Radiology 1989;170:75-77.
42. Orel SG, Reynolds C, Schnall MD, et al: Breast carcinoma: MR imaging before reexcision. Radiology 1997;205:429-436.
43. Sonderson CE, Harms SE, Farrell RS Jr, et al: Detection with MR imaging of residual tumor in the breast soon after surgery. AJR Am J Roentgenol 1997;168:485-488.
44. Hassell PR, Olivotto IA, Mueller HA, et al: Early breast cancer: Detection of recurrence after conservative surgery and radiation therapy. Radiology 1990;176:731-735.
45. Rebner M, Pennes DR, Adler DD, et al: Breast microcalcifications after lumpectomy and radiation therapy. Radiology 1989;170:691-693.
46. Harris KM, Costa-Greco MA, Baratz AB, et al: The mammographic features of the postlumpectomy, postirradiation breast. Radiographics 1989;9:253-268.
47. Dershaw DD, Shank B, Reisinger S: Mammographic findings after breast cancer treatment with local excision and definitive irradiation. Radiology 1987;164:455-461.
48. Schmitt SJ, Connolly JL, Harris JR, et al: Radiation induced changes in the breast. Hum Pathol 1984;15:545-550.
49. Amalric R, Santamaria R, Robert F, et al: Radiation therapy with or without primary limited surgery for operable breast cancer: A 20-year experience at the Marseilles Cancer Institute. Cancer 1982;49:30-34.
50. Bloomer WD, Berenberg AL, Weissman BN: Mammography of the definitely irradiated breast. Radiology 1976;118:425-428.
51. Hohenberg G, Wolf G: Mammographisch fassbare veranberungen bei der teiloperierten und machbesstrahletn Brust. Strahlentherapie 1983;159:622-625.
52. Libshitz HI, Montague ED, Paulus DD: Calcifications and the therapeutically irradiated breast. AJR Am J Roentgenol 1977; 128:1021-1025.
53. Roebuch EJ: The subcutaneous reaction: A useful mammographic sign. Clin Radiol 1984;35:311-315.
54. Berenberg AL, Levene MB, Tonnesen GL: Mammographic evaluation of the postirradiated breast. In Harris JR, Hellman S, Silen W (eds): Conservative Management of Breast Cancer: New Surgical and Radiotherapeutic Techniques. Philadelphia, JB Lippincott, 1983, pp 265-272.
55. Buckley JH, Roebuch EJ: Mammographic changes following radiotherapy. Br J Radiol 1986;59:337-344.
56. Osborne MP, Borgen PL: Role of mastectomy in breast cancer. Surg Clin North Am 1990;70:1023-1046.
57. Fowble B, Solin LJ, Schultz DJ, et al: Breast recurrence following conservative surgery and radiation: Patterns of failure, prognosis and pathologic findings from mastectomy specimens with implications for treatment. Int J Radiat Oncol Biol Phys 1990;19:833-842.
58. Hietner P, Miettinen M, Makinen J: Survival after first recurrence in breast cancer. Eur J Cancer Clin Oncol 1986;22:913-919.
59. Kurtz JM, Spitalier JM, Almaric R, et al: Results of wide excision for local recurrence after breast-conserving therapy. Cancer 1989;61:1969-1972.
60. Harris JR, Recht A: Conservative surgery and radiotherapy. In Harris JR, Hellman S, Henderson IC, Kinne DW (eds): Breast Diseases, 2nd ed. Philadelphia, JB Lippincott, 1991, pp 388-419.
61. Dershaw DD, McCormick B, Osborne MP: Detection of local recurrence after conservative therapy for breast carcinoma. Cancer 1992;70:493-496.
62. Locker AP, Hanley P, Wilson AR, et al: Mammography in the pre-operative assessment and post-operative surveillance of patients treated by excision and radiotherapy for primary breast cancer. Clin Radiol 1990;41:388-391.
63. Stomper PC, Recht A, Berenberg AL, et al: Mammographic detection of recurrent cancer in the irradiated breast. AJR Am J Roentgenol 1987;148:39-43.
64. Orel SG, Fowble BL, Solin LJ, et al: Breast cancer recurrence after lumpectomy and radiation therapy for early-stage disease: Prognostic significance of detection method. Radiology 1993;188:189-194.
65. Kurtz JM, Amalric R, Brandone H, et al: Local recurrence after breast-conserving surgery and radiotherapy: Frequency, time course and prognosis. Cancer 1989;63:1912-1917.
66. Dershaw DD, McCormick B, Cox L, et al: Differentiation of benign and malignant local tumor recurrence after lumpectomy. AJR Am J Roentgenol 1990;155:35-38.
67. Rostom AY, El-Sayed ME: Fat necrosis of the breast: An unusual complication of lumpectomy and radiotherapy in breast cancer. Clin Radiol 1987;38:31.
68. Mitnick JS, Vazquez MF, Roses DF, et al: Recurrent breast cancer: Stereotaxic localization for fine-needle aspiration biopsy. Radiology 1992;182:103-106.
69. Dao TH, Rahmouni A, Campana F, et al: Tumor recurrence versus fibrosis in the irradiated breast: Differentiation with dynamic gadolinium-enhanced MR imaging. Radiology 1993; 187:751-755.
70. Gilles R, Guinebretiere JM, Shapeero LG, et al: Assessment of breast cancer recurrence with contrast-enhanced subtraction MR imaging: Preliminary results in 26 patients. Radiology 1993;188:473-487.

Chapter 32

The Augmented Breast

Nanette D. DeBruhl, Dawn Michael, David P. Gorczyca, and Lawrence W. Bassett

METHODS OF BREAST AUGMENTATION AND RECONSTRUCTION

During the last century, many different methods were used for augmentation and reconstruction of the breast. Unfortunately, the majority of the methods attempted were disappointing and were sometimes associated with adverse complications.[1-3] Methods for augmentation and reconstruction of the breast can be divided into the following three different groups: (1) autogenous tissue transplantation, (2) injectable materials, and (3) implanted prostheses. This chapter deals with the latter two types of augmentation.

Injectable Materials

In the early 1900s, a variety of different materials were injected into the breast for augmentation purposes. Paraffin was one of the earliest such materials to meet with success. Several other materials were also injected but had unacceptable cosmetic outcomes and complications. The complications of injected materials have ranged from granulomatous and inflammatory reactions to necrosis, pulmonary embolism, and even death. The injection of liquid silicone into the breast was first attempted in the 1950s, and this method also eventually was associated with complications similar to those identified for paraffin injections.[2,3] Silicone injections into the breast over time resulted in palpable masses that mimicked carcinoma. The problem of differentiating these silicone granulomas from cancerous tumor was further complicated by the limited visualization of the parenchyma on mammograms of patients with silicone injections (Fig. 32–1). Contrast-enhanced magnetic resonance imaging (MRI) may be the method for screening women for breast cancer in whom the other imaging modalities are not effective. For further discussion, please refer to Chapter 14.

Implantable Prosthesis

The 1950s also saw the first use of synthetic implantable sponge prostheses. The first implantable prosthesis was composed of polyvinyl alcohol (Ivalon). The results of this new method of breast augmentation were initially promising. However, the development of abundant reactive scar tissue caused these implants to have a hard consistency and to actually shrink over time. Undaunted, investigators tried other synthetic materials, such as etheron, polyether polyurethane, polypropylene, and even polytef (Teflon). All of these implants eventually had complications, including undesirable cosmetic effects.

In 1963, Cronin and Gerow[4] described the first use of a silicone gel prosthesis. This method revolutionized plastic surgery of the breast. The majority of silicone implants are composed of an outer membrane made of silicone that surrounds and contains the silicone gel. The composition of the silicone membrane is an elastic polymer of silicone. It is the "liquid" silicone gel within the membrane that gives the implant its desirable feel and movability. Today the majority of the estimated 2 million American women with breast implants have some type of silicone gel prosthesis.

These implants have been used for both augmentation and reconstruction purposes. A large number of different types of silicone gel implants have been manufactured. There are two major types of silicone gel implants: single-lumen and double-lumen. The single-lumen implant (Fig. 32–2) has a smooth or textured outer silicone membrane coating that contains the silicone gel. The double-lumen type usually consists of a saline outer chamber surrounding the inner silicone gel implant.

For augmentation mammoplasty, implants are placed either anterior (subglandular) or posterior (subpectoral) to the pectoralis major muscle. Insertion of a subglandular implant requires less complicated and less expensive surgery. The surgical insertion of subpectoral implants is technically more difficult, but subpectoral implants interfere less with visualization of the breast tissue at mammography, have a lower incidence of capsular contractures, and are associated with less obvious surgical scars.

Silicone Breast Implants

As indicated previously, silicone breast prostheses have been manufactured for more than 40 years. Despite their vast improvement over previous methods of breast augmentation, however, complications with silicone implants have been frequent. These complications include rupture and leakage, fibrous or calcific contracture of the tissue capsule that forms around the implant, localized pain, paresthesias, and possibly even generalized autoimmune disorders.[5-7] As a result of reported complications, in

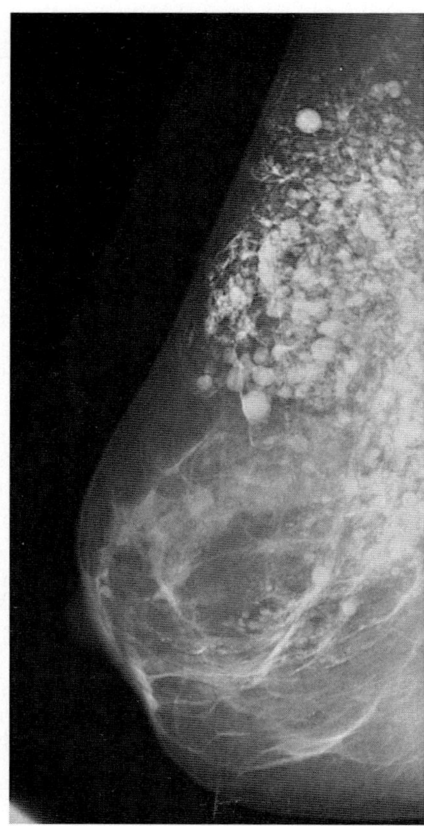

Figure 32–1. Silicone injections. Mediolateral mammogram demonstrating silicone granulomas, most of which have migrated to the uppermost aspect of the breast.

1992 the U.S. Food and Drug Administration (FDA) held hearings about the possible complications of the use of silicone gel implants. After hearing the evidence, the FDA restricted the use of silicone gel implants.[8] Silicone gel–filled implants were allowed on the market only under controlled clinical adjunct studies for reconstruction after mastectomy, correction of congenital deformities, or replacement of silicone gel–filled implants that were ruptured for medical or surgical reasons. These adjunct studies were developed to enable continued availability of silicone gel breast implants for what was considered a public need. The use of implants for cosmetic enhancement or augmentation was postponed until the results of the adjunct studies were reported.

The manufacturers of saline-filled breast implants were notified by the FDA in January 1993 that the agency would require data on their products' safety and effectiveness. While the manufacturers were conducting the required studies, saline-filled breast implants remained on the market.

In 1998, research conducted by individual manufacturers allowed a limited number of patients to participate in breast augmentation with silicone implants through investigational device exemption (IDE) studies. These studies required informed consent from women who would receive the implants through a protocol or plan that had been approved by a research site's review board, which was to be composed of scientists, health professionals, and community members. The FDA approved the IDE studies before their implementation to help ensure that the resulting data will be meaningful and that patients will not be exposed to unreasonable risks. By the year 2000, saline implants were given premarket approval by the FDA. This allowed the approved manufacturers to market implants without informed consent of consumers. Silicone implants are still being evaluated through IDE studies.[9]

Encapsulation of Silicone Gel Implants

A fibrous capsule invariably forms around a breast implant after it is placed in the breast. The capsule may be soft and impalpable or hard and resistant. If the capsule becomes hardened, the breast is likely to have an undesirable contour and feel.[1] Closed capsulotomy, a procedure by which the surgeon uses vigorous manual compression to disrupt a hard fibrous capsule, was once used to restore the more natural feeling of the augmented breast.[10] Closed capsulotomy is no longer performed because of its association with significant herniations and ruptures of silicone breast implants.[11]

Rupture

Implant rupture can be divided into two major categories: intracapsular and extracapsular.[12] *Intracapsular rupture,* the most common type, is a rupture of the implant membrane (elastomer envelope) that allows the release of silicone gel, which is then contained by an intact fibrous capsule. *Extracapsular rupture* is defined as rupture of both the implant membrane and the fibrous capsule, which leads to extravasation of the silicone into the surrounding breast tissues.

Gel Bleed

Gel bleed is an interesting phenomenon. It represents microscopic silicone leakage through an intact implant membrane.[13] This leakage across the silicone membrane undoubtedly accounts for the sticky feel on the surface of older intact implants. It is believed that most if not all implants eventually have some gel bleed but that the bleed is usually not extensive enough to be detectable. Therefore, a patient can be exposed to silicone leakage into the breast and throughout the body even when her silicone implants are intact. Whether gel bleed is ever great enough to be detectable by imaging methods is controversial. Some investigators have reported visualization of silicone outside the membrane on MRI and computed tomography (CT) without evidence of a rupture of the silicone membrane and have

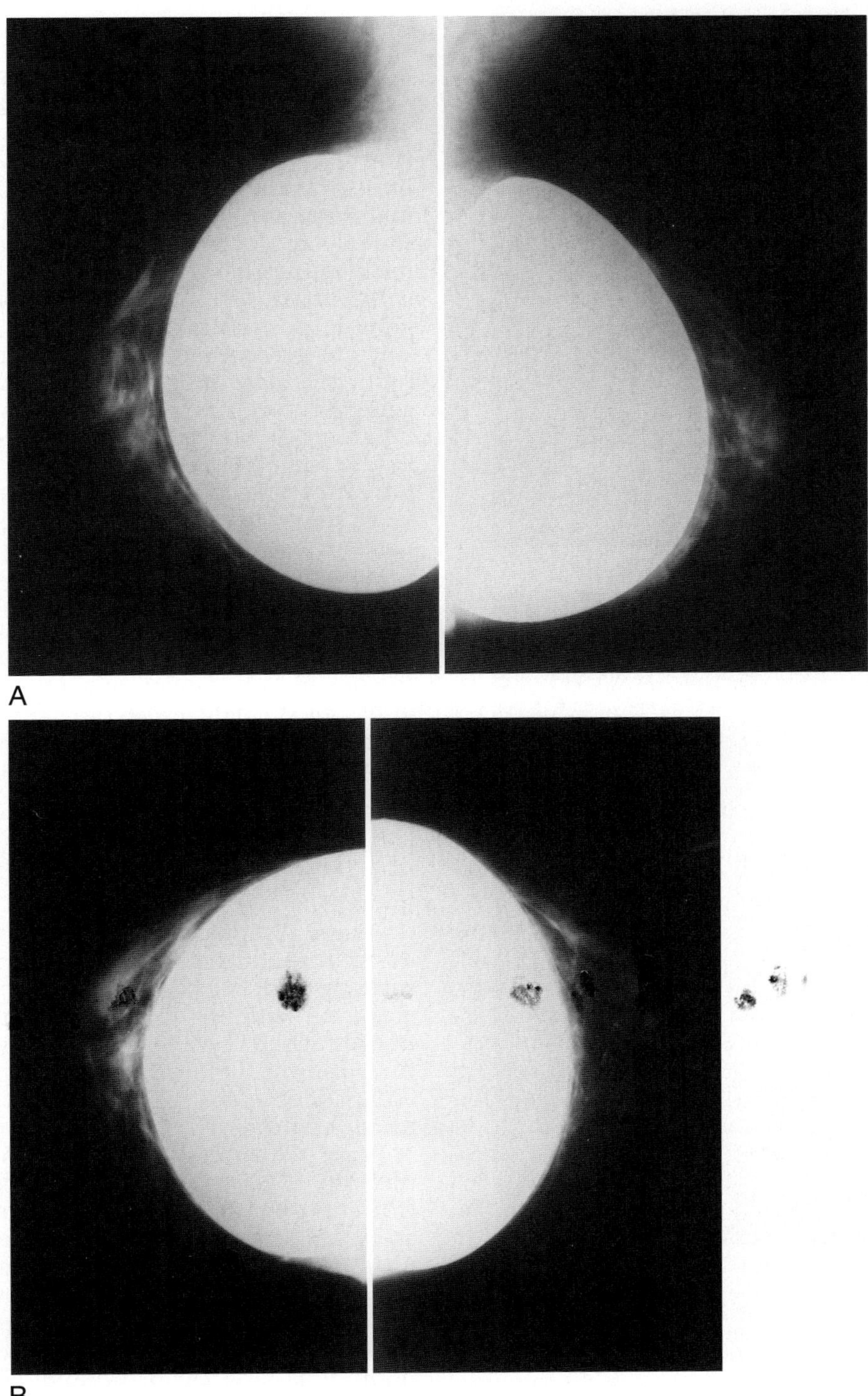

Figure 32–2. Subglandular silicone implants. Implant-included mammograms, mediolateral oblique (MLO) (**A**) and craniocaudal (CC) (**B**) mammographic views performed with moderate compression, required manual technique because the implants were over the photocell.

Continued

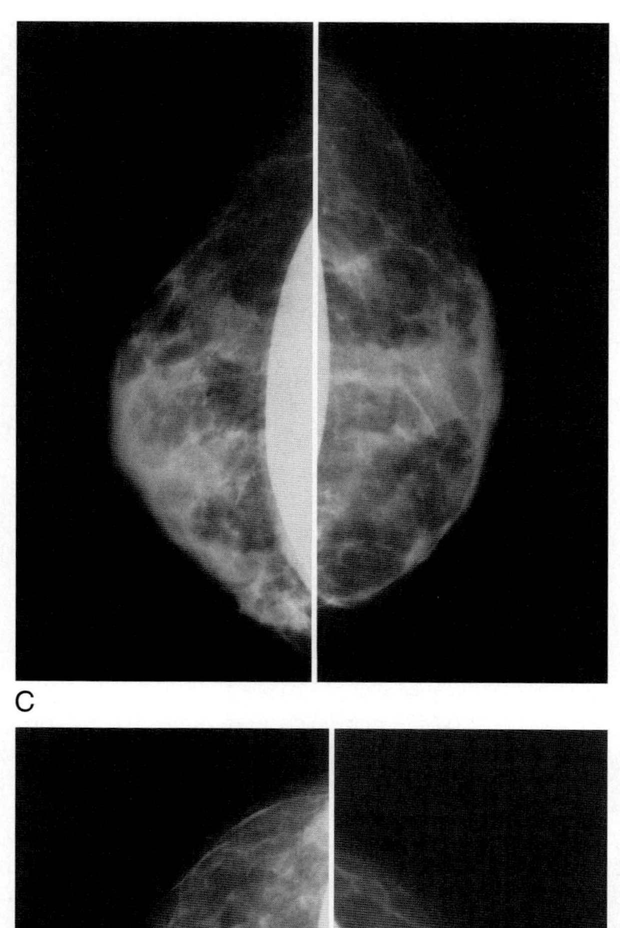
C

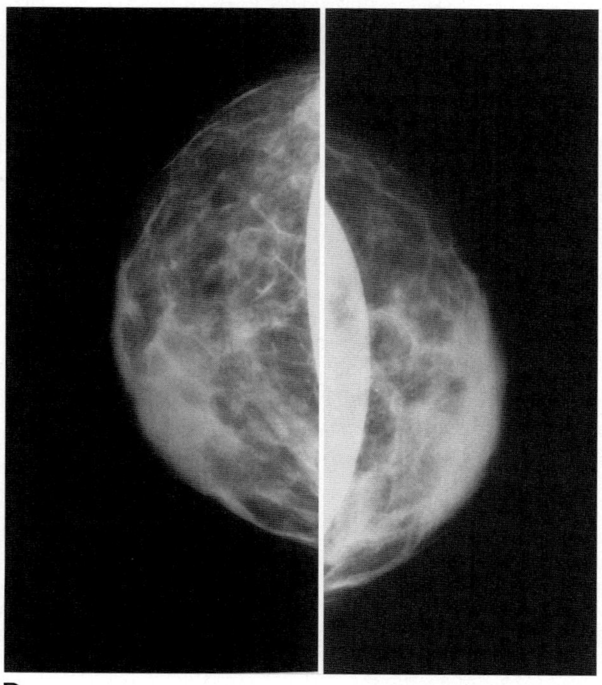
D

Figure 32–2, cont'd. Ninety-degree lateral (LM) (**C**) and CC implant-included (**D**) mammographic views allow for compression of tissue anterior to implants and can be done with automatic exposure control as long as the breast tissue covers the photocell completely.

attributed this finding to excessive gel bleed.[14] Other investigators believe that occult tears in the silicone membrane are present whenever this phenomenon occurs and that these tears can be found if the surgeon looks carefully enough.[15] The imaging features are described in the following section.

IMAGING AFTER BREAST IMPLANTS

Mammography

The woman with silicone breast implants is not at increased risk for development of breast cancer, so regular mammography screening is recommended at intervals appropriate for the woman's age.[16,17] However, the presence of silicone implants usually limits the amount of tissue that can be visualized on mammograms. Clinical reports have suggested a possible delay in breast cancer diagnosis, but epidemiologic studies have not supported these claims.[17-20] It is important to emphasize that the proper mammographic positioning of the breasts of women with silicone gel implants requires that radiologic technologists have special training and experience. In general, more tissue can be visualized in the mammograms of women with subpectoral implants than in the mammograms of women with subglandular implants. Special views called implant-displaced (ID) views have been developed to better visualize the breast tissue anterior to a silicone breast implant.[21]

Mammography of women with subglandular implants requires the use of the ID views, or "push-back" views, whenever possible (see Fig. 32–2).[22,23] Implant-included views are performed first through the use of only moderate compression. ID views are done next. The posterior displacement of the implant during the ID maneuvers allows for greater compression of the tissue anterior to the implants and also provides an opportunity to visualize more breast tissue.[21] ID views cannot be performed if an implant is hard and fixed, a change due to changes in the fibrous capsule that prevent mobility of the implant.

Imaging implants with digital mammography has markedly reduced the number of additional exposures needed, because the modality enables the operator to "window" and level the post-acquisition images at the console and at the work station.[24] The surrounding tissue and implants can be evaluated independently with the window and leveling technique, improving overall visualization (Fig. 32–3).

There are no well-documented cases of implant rupture due to mammography compression. However, we are aware of several unsubstantiated cases of rupture attributed to mammography. Although new, non-implanted silicone gel implants can withstand considerable mammographic compression, it is suspected that over time, implanted silicone gel implants may be subject to fatigue and trauma, making them more vulnerable to mammographic compression. Therefore, radiologists should at least be aware of the *potential* for implant rupture during mammography and should have a protocol within their facilities to deal with any complications that may arise. Clinical signs of implant rupture include palpable silicone nodules, decreased breast size, asymmetry, tenderness, and a change in texture of the implant. Breakage of the fibrous capsule

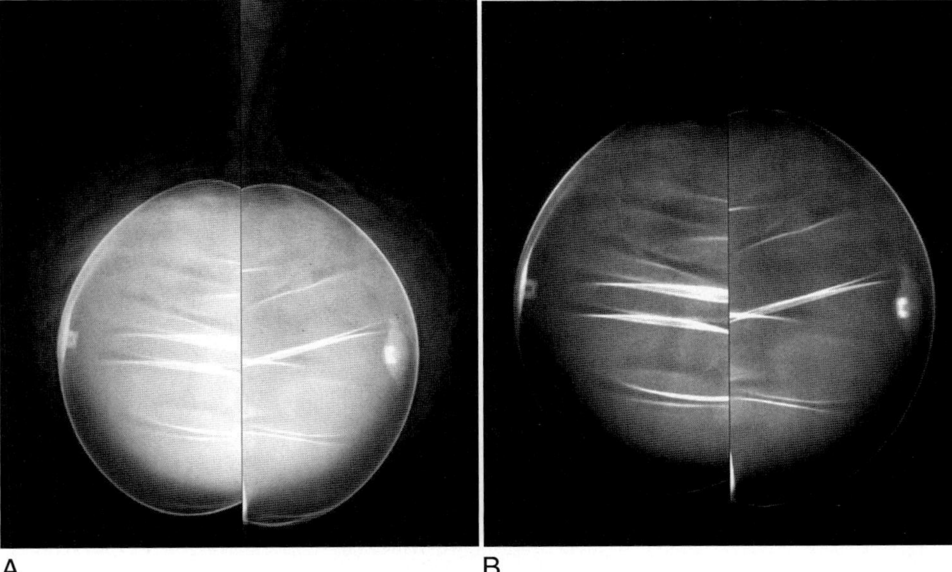

Figure 32–3. Subpectoral implants. **A,** Digital mammographic image of saline implants (mediolateral oblique view) in the implant-included view optimized for imaging soft tissues. **B,** Digital mammogram with windowing and leveling, which optimized the image of the implant.

around the implant may occur with compression and may be accompanied by an audible "pop." Thus, mammographic compression can potentially convert an intracapsular rupture—one contained by the fibrous capsule—to an extracapsular rupture if the fibrous capsule is broken.

The American College of Radiology does not recommend that written informed consent be obtained for mammography of women with breast implants but does encourage the giving of educational information to such women.[25]

Mammographic Findings

Mammographic findings that may be encountered in women with implants are (1) a measurable periprosthetic dense band or rim of tissue that corresponds to the fibrous capsule around the implant, (2) periprosthetic calcification, (3) peri-implant fluid collections, (4) asymmetry of implant size or shape, (5) focal herniation of the implant, and (6) implant rupture with deflation of the envelope and extravasation of silicone beyond the membrane.[26-29] Free silicone in the breast may manifest as a dense mass, linear streaks, or lymph node opacification (Figs. 32–4 to 32–8).

Mammography for the Evaluation of Implant Rupture

Rupture of a saline implant is clinically obvious, because the implant deflates immediately. The saline is quickly absorbed by the body, so that by the time a woman undergoes imaging, only a collapsed outer membrane is visible on mammography. Ultrasonography and MRI are not required for the diagnosis of a saline implant rupture.

Because clinical examination may fail to disclose an implant rupture and its extent, radiologists are often requested to evaluate the integrity of breast prostheses. In our experience, mammography has not been useful in the detection of intracapsular implant rupture, the more common type of rupture. Although mammography can identify free silicone after an extracapsular silicone implant rupture, the silicone may be obscured by the overlying implant. After the removal of ruptured silicone implants, residual silicone granulomas may be visualized in the breast tissue (see Fig. 32–8). These granulomas may be confused with breast lesions.

Because of the limitations of clinical breast examination and mammography in the evaluation of breast implants, MRI and ultrasonography have been investigated as adjunctive methods for the evaluation of implants, especially for the identification of rupture.

Magnetic Resonance Imaging

MRI has proved to be the most accurate method for the detection of breast implant ruptures.[30,31] Familiarity with the MRI characteristics of silicone is helpful to an understanding of the different MRI sequences that can be used to differentiate silicone from surrounding breast parenchyma. The chemical composition of most medical-grade silicones is dimethyl polysiloxane with varying degrees of polymerization.[32] The MRI signal is derived from the protons of the methyl groups. The implant membrane is also composed of silicone but differs from the gel in chemical structure because of the many additional cross-linkages between the methyl groups, resulting in an elastic solid. Although the implant membrane is composed of silicone, only minimal MRI signal is produced from the silicone membrane

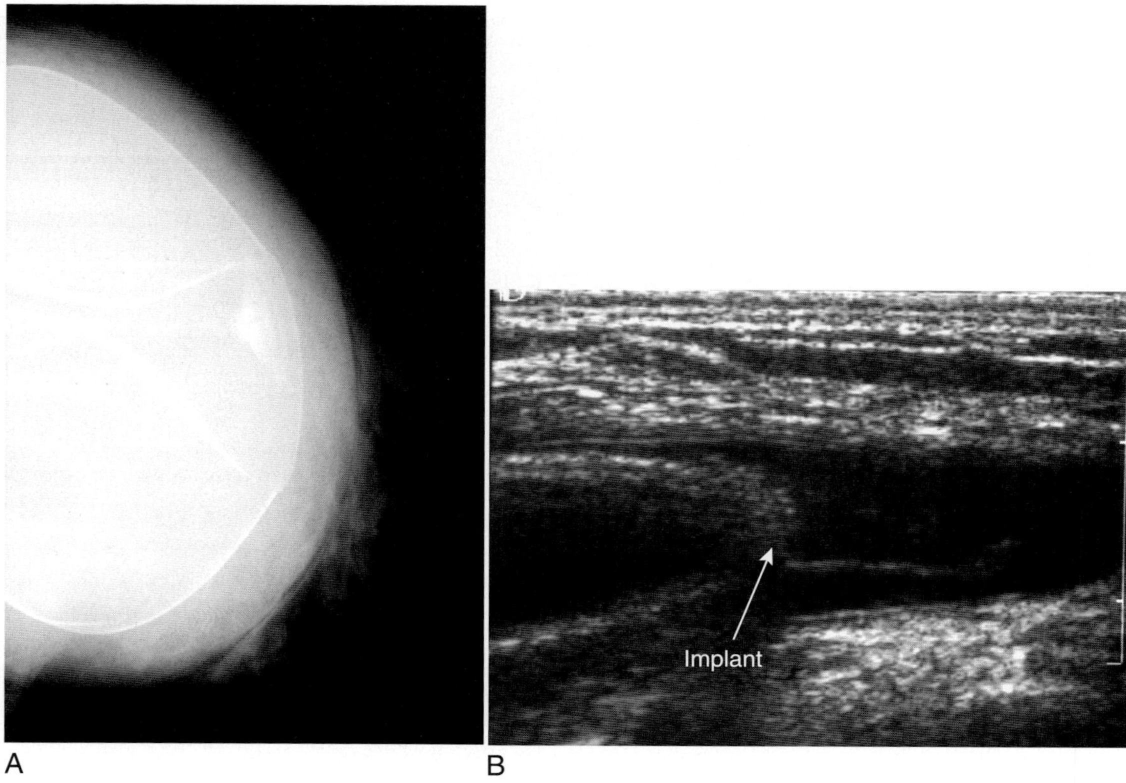

Figure 32–4. Reactive fluid. **A,** Mediolateral oblique mammogram of a single-lumen implant with peri-implant fluid collection of serous fluid due to inflammation. Fluid surrounding the implant expands the fibrous capsule. **B,** Ultrasonogram confirms that the fluid collection is external to the implant and adjacent to the implant edge.

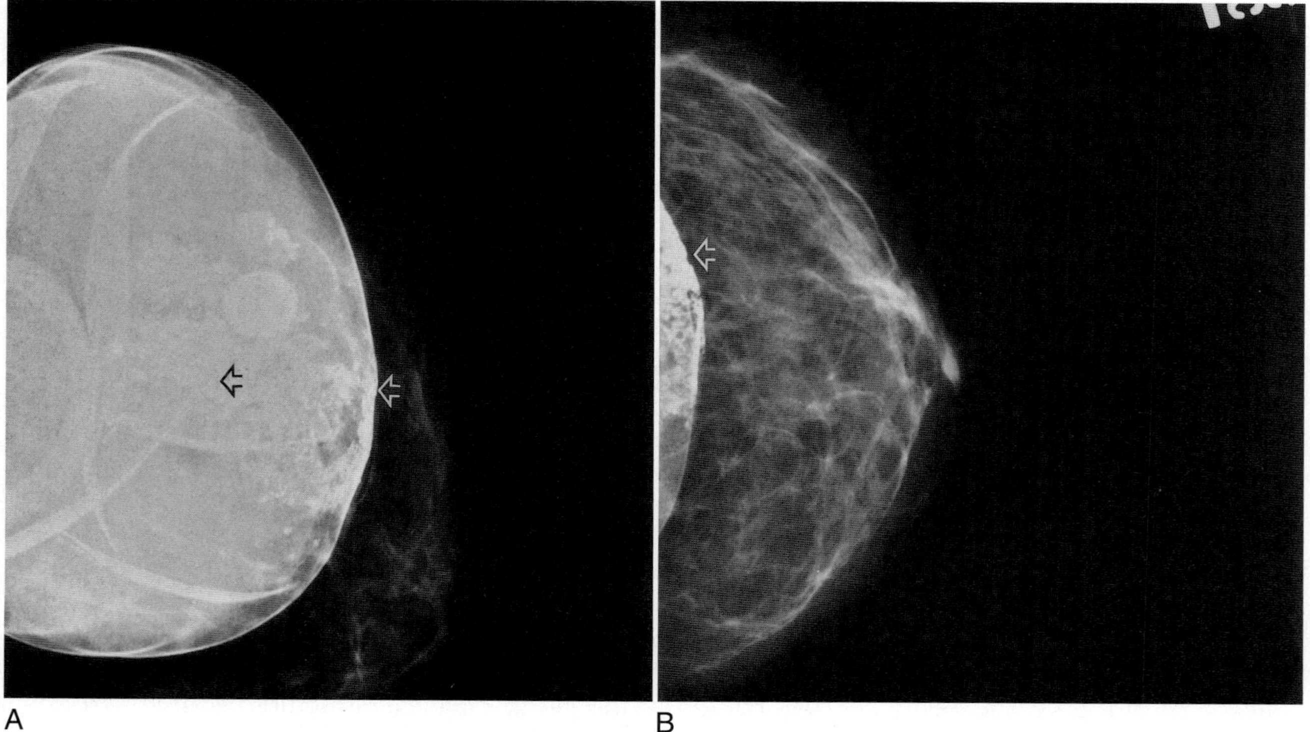

Figure 32–5. Peri-implant calcifications. **A,** Mediolateral oblique mammogram of a saline implant shows dense calcifications circumferentially involving the anterior aspect of the implant (*arrows*). **B,** Implant-displaced craniocaudal mammogram improves visualization of the dense calcium deposition (*arrow*).

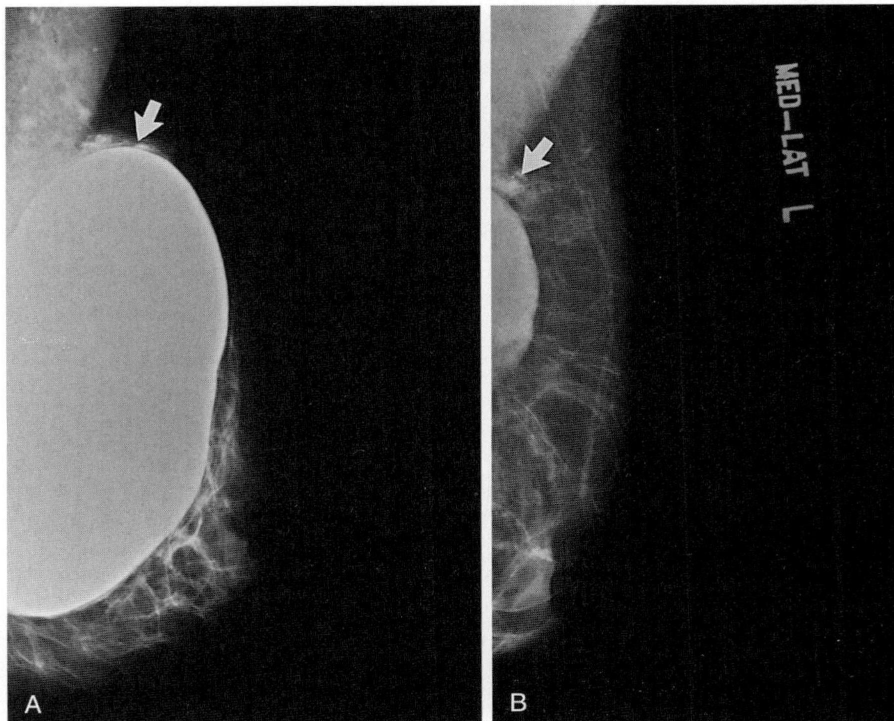

Figure 32–6. Ruptured subglandular implant. **A,** Free extracapsular silicone (*arrow*) anterior and superior to the implant. **B,** Implant-displaced mediolateral view confirms presence of free silicone in the breast parenchyma (*arrow*).

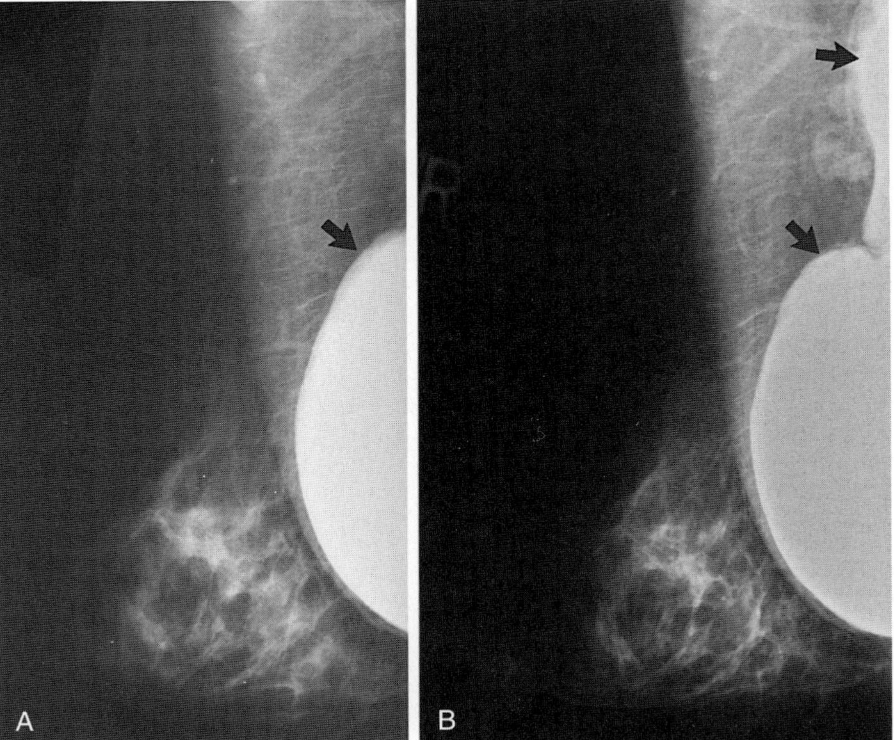

Figure 32–7. Ruptured subpectoral implant. **A,** Original implant-included mediolateral oblique (MLO) mammogram suggests free silicone gel (*arrow*) at the superior aspect of the implant. **B,** A second MLO mammogram that includes more pectoral muscle shows free silicone (*arrows*) migrating into the axilla.

A

B

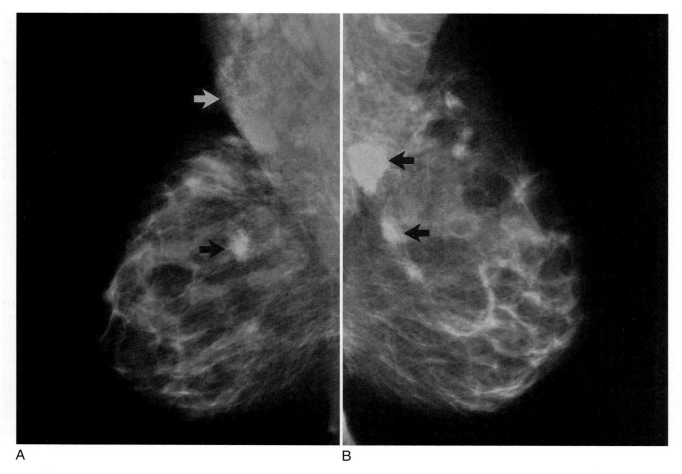

Figure 32–8. Residual silicone after removal of ruptured implants. Right (**A**) and left (**B**) mediolateral oblique mammograms obtained several years after explantation show multiple dense, irregular masses (*black arrows*), which are silicone granulomas. Silicone can be seen to have extended into the axilla on the right (*white arrow*).

because of the many additional cross-linkages between the methyl groups.

Technical Factors

A variety of pulse sequences are available for imaging silicone implants. In general, the selection of MRI pulse sequences used to image breast implants is determined by the relative Larmor precessional frequencies, as well as the T1 and T2 properties of the tissues (fat, muscle, and silicone). The relative resonance frequency of silicone is approximately 100 Hz lower than that of fat and 320 Hz lower than that of water at 1.5 Tesla (T) (Fig. 32–9). Because the resonance frequency of silicone is close to that of fat, the MRI signal from silicone behaves similarly to that from fat when chemical suppression techniques (chemical fat or water suppression) are used. As a result, the silicone signal is high when chemical water suppression is used and low when chemical fat suppression is used (Table 32–1).

One can use MRI sequences that selectively emphasize the signal from silicone by taking advantage of the different relative relaxation times of fat, silicone, and water. The relaxation time of fat is shorter than that of silicone. Therefore, one can use this difference to suppress the fat signal while maintaining a strong signal from silicone. It has been found that the use of an inversion recovery sequence with a short inversion time (short-tau inversion recovery [STIR]) suppresses the signal from fat while maintaining high signal from silicone.[14,33,34] The use of a chemical

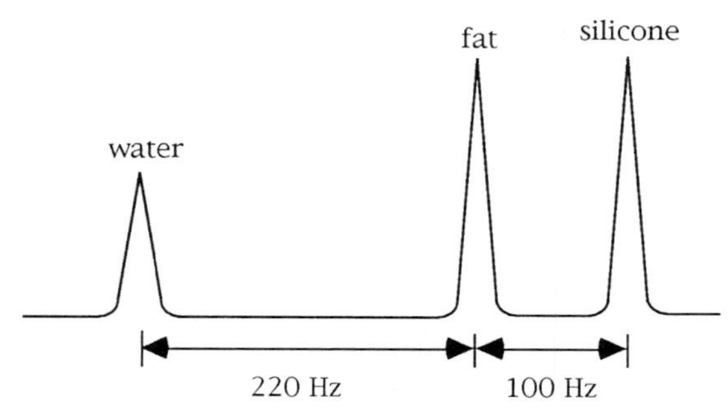

Figure 32–9. Relative resonance frequencies of water, fat, and silicone at 1.5 T. The resonance frequency of silicone is approximately 320 Hz lower than that of water and 100 Hz lower than that of fat.

Table 32–1. Signal Intensities of Silicone, Fat, and Water with Different Magnetic Resonance Imaging (MRI) Pulse Sequences for Evaluation of Silicone Implants

	Signal Intensity		
MRI Sequence	Silicone	Fat	Water
Fast spin echo (FSE) T2-weighted (TR/TE > 5000/200)	High	Medium	Very high
FSE with water suppression	High	Medium	Low
Inversion recovery FSE (IRFSE) (TR/TE >5000/90, TI = 150)	High	Low	Very high
IRFSE with water suppression	High	Low	Low
Three-point Dixon (3PD)—silicone only	High	None	None

water-suppression pulse in conjunction with a STIR sequence results in a silicone-selective sequence.

Chemical shift imaging (CSI) provides another method to selectively image silicone.[35-37] This method uses the differences among the Larmor frequencies of silicone, fat, and water to separate the MRI signal of silicone from the signal of fat and water. An example of a CSI sequence is the modified three-point Dixon technique.[36,37] This sequence produces a silicone-only image and a simultaneous fat/water image with a single MR sequence.

Imaging Protocols

In our practice, the patient undergoing MRI lies prone with the breasts in a dedicated dual-breast coil.[38] The 1.5-T superconducting magnet is used to acquire an axial scout image—fast spoiled gradient-recalled acquisition (SPGR)—followed by an axial T2-weighted fast spin echo (FSE) or STIR sequence without water suppression and a sagittal STIR T2-weighted with water-suppression sequences. A 256 × 192 matrix, 2 NEX with slice thickness between 3 and 5 mm, with a 1-mm skip, is used to cover the entire implant. Frequency direction is anterior to posterior (AP) on axial images and right to left (RL) for sagittal images to reduce the artifact created by heart motion in the phase-encoding direction. The STIR sequence, designed to suppress signal from fat, increases the conspicuity of the silicone implant and the extravasation of silicone gel within the tissues. When heavily T2-weighted FSE images are used, the TE is set at approximately 200 to decrease the signal from the breast adipose tissue while keeping the signal from the silicone fairly high. This examination requires 20 to 30 minutes to complete, depending on the number of sequences performed. Contrast agent is usually not given if the study is performed for the evaluation of the implants only. This protocol has been optimized for the evaluation of silicone and not breast parenchyma. Other imaging techniques have been reported in the literature.[34,39,40]

Table 32–1 presents a summary of the relative signal intensities of silicone, fat, and water with different pulse sequences.

Appearance of Normal Implants

On MRI, a normal single-lumen silicone implant contains homogeneous high-signal-intensity silicone (Fig. 32–10). A double-lumen silicone implant typically has an inner lumen of high-signal-intensity silicone surrounded by a smaller outer lumen that contains saline with different signal intensities, depending on the pulse sequence (see Table 32–1) (Fig. 32–11). A variety of other types of implantable prostheses are occasionally encountered that alter the MRI appearance; they include expander implants, reverse double-lumen implants (saline in the inner lumen, silicone in the outer lumen), multicompartmental implants, foam implants, and single-lumen silicone implants into which saline was injected directly at the time of surgery.

Two or more implants placed in one breast, one on top of the other, are commonly known as "stacked implants." Some implants have a coating of polyurethane covering the surface of the silicone envelope. Such an implant is typically surrounded by a moderate to large amount of reactive fluid. Saline implants have become more popular since the FDA limited the use of silicone gel implants in 1992.

One of the most commonly encountered mammographic findings in normal implants is the presence of prominent radial folds, normal infoldings of the Silastic elastomer membrane (Fig. 32–12A). These folds may be prominent enough to suggest an appearance of implant rupture. However, even very prominent radial folds can be recognized as such because they extend to the periphery of the implant and are relatively few in number (Fig. 32–12B).

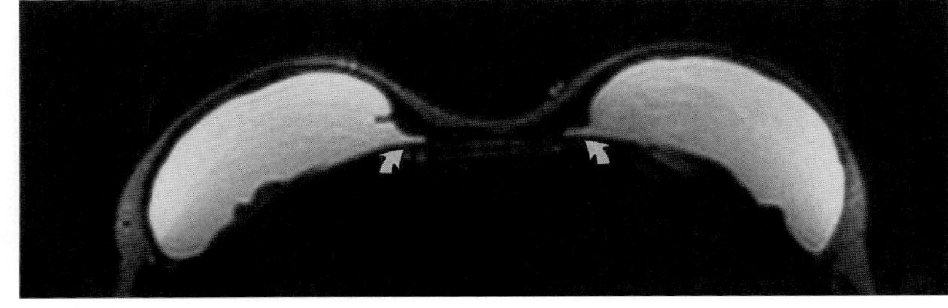

Figure 32–10. Axial T2-weighted magnetic resonance images showing intact subpectoral single-lumen silicone implants. Finger-like projections are shown medially. This finding, which has been reported as the "rat-tail sign" (*curved arrows*), is not associated with implant rupture.

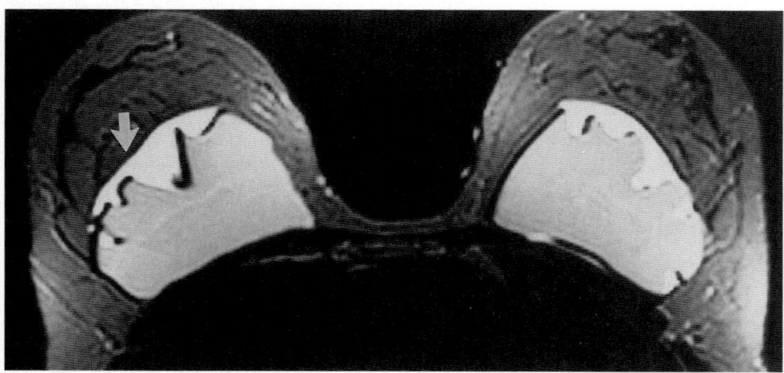

Figure 32–11. Axial T2-weighted magnetic resonance image (without water suppression) of breasts with bilateral intact double-lumen implants. The saline outer chambers (*arrow*) have higher signal intensity than the inner chambers containing silicone gel.

Signs of Intracapsular Rupture

Linguine Sign

The most reliable sign of intracapsular rupture on MRI is the presence of multiple, curvilinear low-signal-intensity lines within the high-signal-intensity silicone gel, the so-called linguine sign (Fig. 32–13).[31] These curvilinear lines represent the collapsed implant membrane floating within the silicone gel.[41] In the very early stages, the curvilinear lines may be found close to the periphery of the implant rather than floating in the center of it (see Fig. 32–16).

Teardrop Sign

The teardrop sign is sometimes the only indication of implant rupture. This sign represents silicone that has leaked out of the ruptured silicone implant and entered one of the radial folds on the exterior of the implant (Fig. 32–14). It can be an early sign of

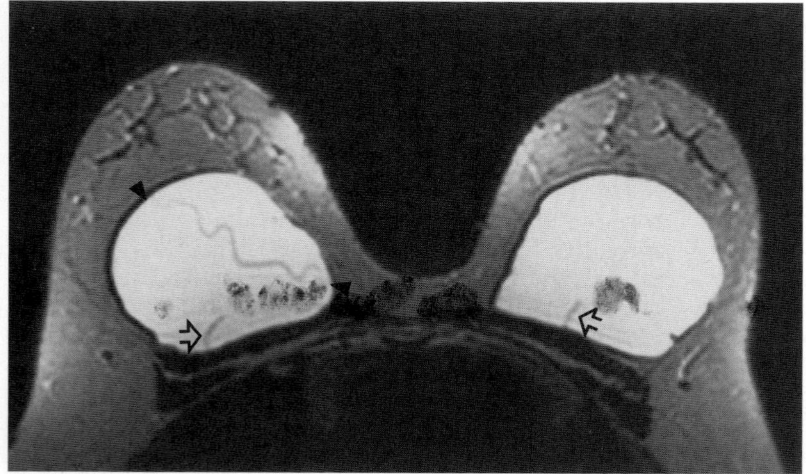

A

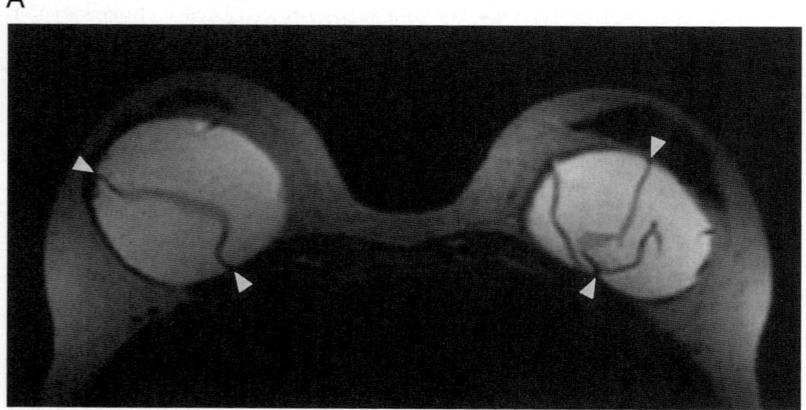

B

Figure 32–12. Radial folds. **A,** Axial T2-weighted fast spin echo (FSE) image with water suppression shows a normal implant with bilateral low-signal-intensity radial folds (*arrows*) that extend to the periphery of the implant. **B,** Axial T2-weighted FSE image with water suppression shows prominent radial folds in a single-lumen implant. Radial folds can be distinguished from a collapsed implant shell because the folds extend to the periphery of the implant and are usually few in number (*arrowheads*).

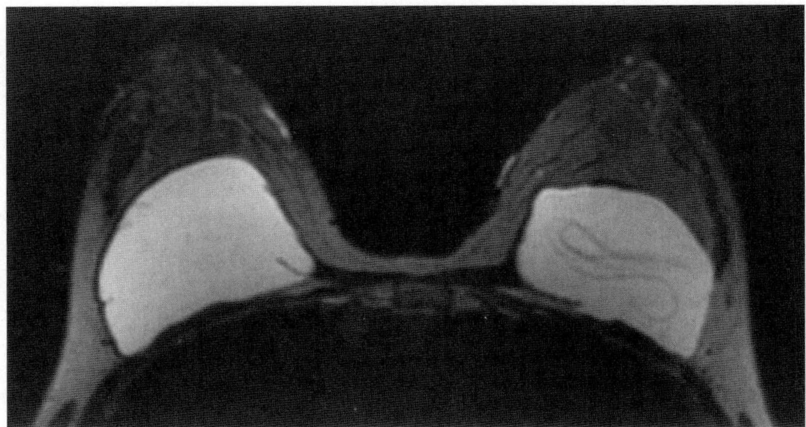

Figure 32–13. Intracapsular rupture. Axial T2-weighted magnetic resonance image shows multiple curvilinear low-signal-intensity lines within the left implant (linguine sign), which represent the collapsed implant shell. The right implant is intact with a normal radial fold.

implant rupture. Whether this finding may result from extensive gel bleed or whether a small tear is invariably present is controversial.

Unreliable Signs of Intracapsular Rupture

Water Droplets

Rarely, intracapsular rupture may be associated with the appearance of multiple hyperintense foci within the implant lumen on T2-weighted images or multiple hypointense foci on water-suppression images. We have seen numerous cases in which these small water droplets have been present in patients with intact implants. Therefore, when only a few (usually fewer than six) of these water droplets are seen within a silicone implant, we do not make the diagnosis of ruptured implant unless other supporting evidence of rupture is present.

Contour Deformities

Bulges and other contour deformities are not reliable signs of implant rupture and may be seen with intact implants (see Fig. 32–10). Finger-like medial projections along the chest wall—the "rat-tail sign," indicated by the arrows on Figure 32–10—can be mistaken for signs of implant rupture.[39]

Fluid on the Periphery of the Implant

Fluid may be seen around the periphery of intact implants and therefore is not considered a sign of rupture. This fluid may represent saline in the outer component of a double-lumen implant or, possibly, reactive fluid in surrounding tissue (Fig. 32–15).

Signs of Extracapsular Rupture

The presence of free silicone in the breast parenchyma is the definitive sign of an extracapsular rupture. On MRI, free silicone appears as focal areas of high signal intensity outside the confines of the implant (Figs. 32–16 and 32–17).[14,34] Because of its multiplanar capabilities and its ability to identify even small foci of silicone, MRI can provide precise localization of free silicone deposits in the breast and surrounding structures. However, previous silicone injections or silicone remaining from a previous rupture of a silicone implant that has been removed can give rise to the same finding, so careful history-taking is essential before the diagnosis of extracapsular implant rupture is made.

Signs of intracapsular rupture are expected to be present in extracapsular rupture. For example, the linguine sign, the most reliable sign of intracapsular

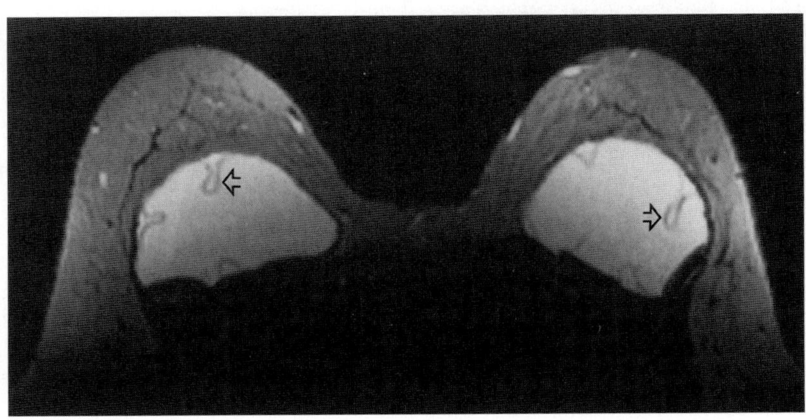

Figure 32–14. Teardrop sign. Axial T2-weighted image shows bilateral subpectoral implants with radial folds (*open arrows*) containing silicone gel. At surgery, silicone gel was seen outside the implant shells. Careful inspection revealed a small tear in each implant shell.

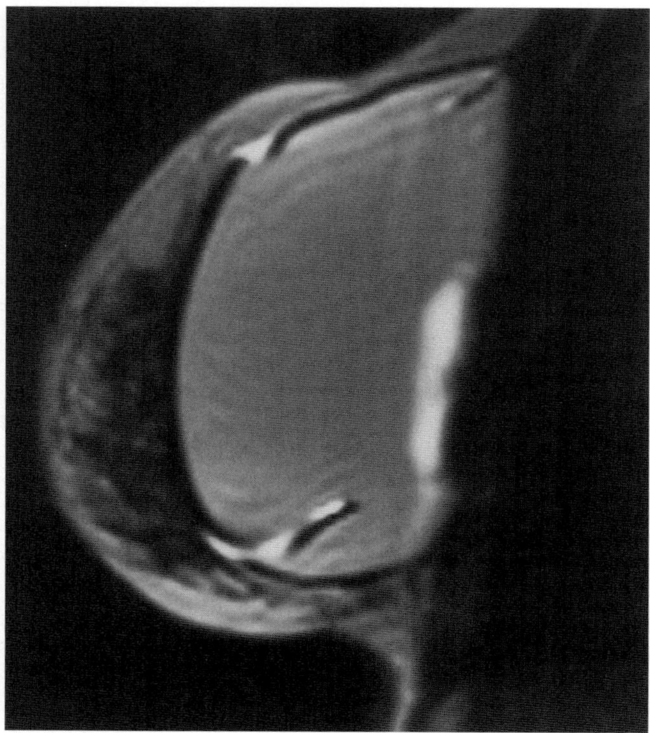

Figure 32–15. Fluid on the periphery of the implant. Sagittal magnetic resonance image of a breast implant with high signal intensity around the circumference of the implant representing reactive fluid.

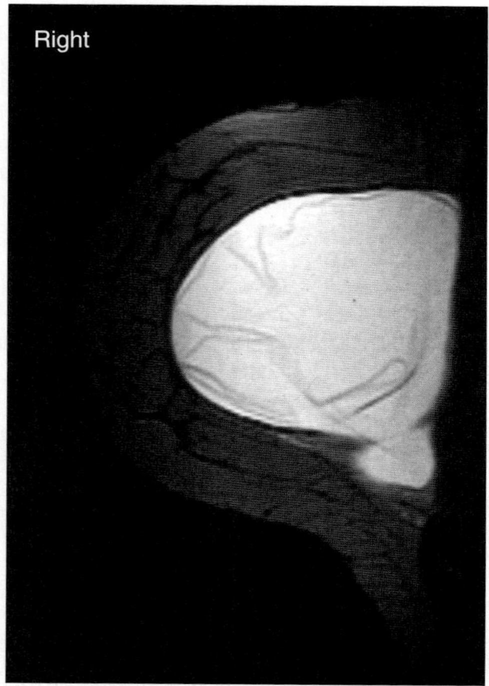

Figure 32–16. Extracapsular rupture. Sagittal STIR (short-tau inversion recovery) magnetic resonance image shows extravasated silicone migrating along the inferior aspect of the implant. The edges of the collapsed implant shell can be seen in the center and peripheral regions of the implant.

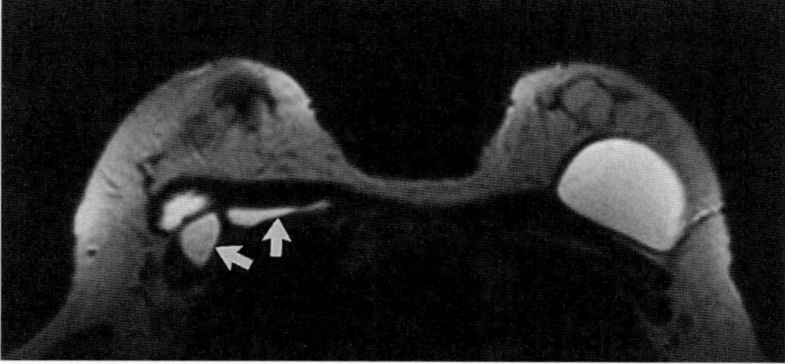

Figure 32–17. Extracapsular rupture. Axial T2-weighted magnetic resonance image at the superior aspect of the breasts demonstrates silicone granuloma formation (*arrows*) above the right implant. The left implant is intact.

rupture, is almost always seen in extracapsular rupture (see Fig. 32–16).

Gel Bleed

Gel bleed is microscopic leakage of silicone through an intact implant membrane.[13] Most if not all implants eventually have gel bleed; however, the majority of gel bleeds are so small that they cannot be detected on MRI. Only when gel bleed is extensive can silicone gel be detected outside the silicone membrane, manifesting as a teardrop sign when the silicone enters a radial fold. Even this finding is controversial, and some investigators believe that a small hole in the implant can be found if the evaluator is persistent in looking for one.[15] In fact, a focal or early intracapsular rupture can have a similar appearance to that of an extensive gel bleed, and it may be difficult if not impossible to differentiate these two entities on MR images (see Fig. 32–14).[36]

Ultrasonography

Investigations into the usefulness of ultrasonography in detecting implant ruptures have reported conflicting results.[42-44] The variation in these results may reflect the technical factors employed. In our experience, the accuracy of ultrasonography is operator dependent, and the best results are achieved with on-site, real-time evaluation by an experienced radiologist.[45] A 7.5- to 12-MHz transducer is recommended to evaluate the integrity of a silicone implant. High resolution is needed to identify subtle implant abnormalities; however, a 5-MHz transducer may be required to show the posterior aspects of the implant or adequately depict a subpectoral implant. The ultrasonography examination should be done systematically to ensure that all aspects of the implant are seen, including the surrounding breast and axilla. Clockwise scanning of the breast is used in our practice to ensure that the examination is complete. Selected hard-copy images are obtained for documentation.

Table 32–2. Ultrasonographic Signs of 57 Surgically Removed Silicone Breast Implants

	Ultrasonographic Sign (No.)					
Surgical Finding (No.)	Anechoic Interior	Anterior Reverberations	Stepladder Sign	Heterogeneous Aggregates	Discontinuity of Envelope*	Echogenic Noise†
Ruptured (20)	0	15	14	5	2	2
Intracapsular (16)	0	12	10	4	0	0
Extracapsular (4)	0	3	4	1	2	2
Intact (37)	8	25	3	1	4	0

*Numbers given are the number of implants that displayed the sign of discontinuity of the echogenic representation of the boundary between the implant shell and the tissue anterior to it.
†Homogeneous echogenic appearance due to silicone gel leakage, which prevents visualization of tissues posterior to it (Rosculet et al[44]).
From DeBruhl ND, Gorczyca DP, Ahn CY, et al: Silicone breast implants: US evaluation. Radiology 1993;189:95-98.

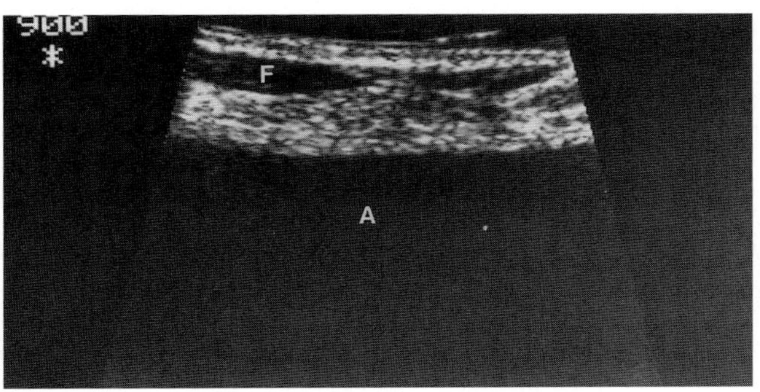

Figure 32–18. Ultrasonography of intact subglandular implant: A, anechoic implant interior; F, subcutaneous fat.

Normal Ultrasonographic Findings

Table 32–2 reports the common ultrasonographic findings in 57 surgically proven normal or ruptured breast implants.[45] The most reliable sign of an intact implant is an anechoic interior (Fig. 32–18). However, reverberation artifacts can be encountered in the anterior aspects of intact implants, and these echoes should not be considered abnormal (Fig. 32–19). As a general rule, the reverberation artifacts should be no thicker than the breast tissue anterior to the implant. The implant membrane, sometimes visualized as a thin echogenic line at the parenchymal tissue-implant interface, should be intact throughout.

On ultrasonography, radial folds are depicted as echogenic lines extending from the periphery of the implant to the interior (Fig. 32–20). Radial folds are normal infoldings of the implant membrane into the silicone gel, but they may be more prominent in association with capsular contracture.

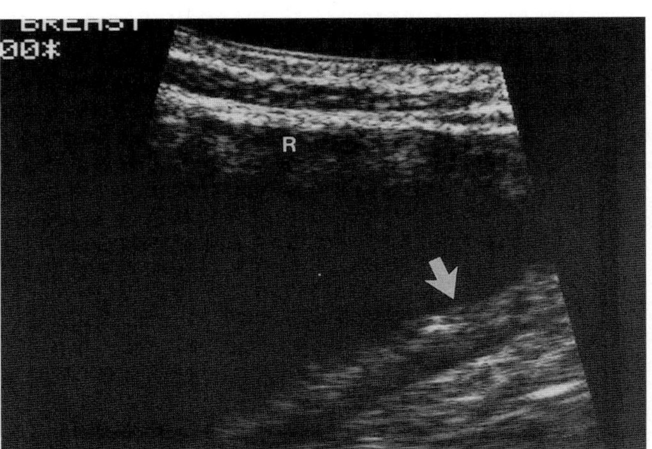

Figure 32–19. Reverberation artifact (R), which is commonly seen at the anterior border of implants on ultrasonography, should not be mistaken for evidence of rupture. The implant is otherwise anechoic. *Arrow* indicates the posterior border of the implant.

Ultrasonographic Signs of Implant Rupture

The reported ultrasonographic signs of implant rupture include hyperechoic or hypoechoic masses, dispersion of the ultrasonographic beam ("snowstorm" or "echogenic noise"), discontinuity of the implant membrane, multiple parallel echogenic lines within the implant interior (stepladder sign), and aggregates of medium- to low-level echoes in the interior of the implant.[44-46]

Intracapsular Ruptures

In our experience, the stepladder sign is the most reliable ultrasonographic evidence of an intracapsular

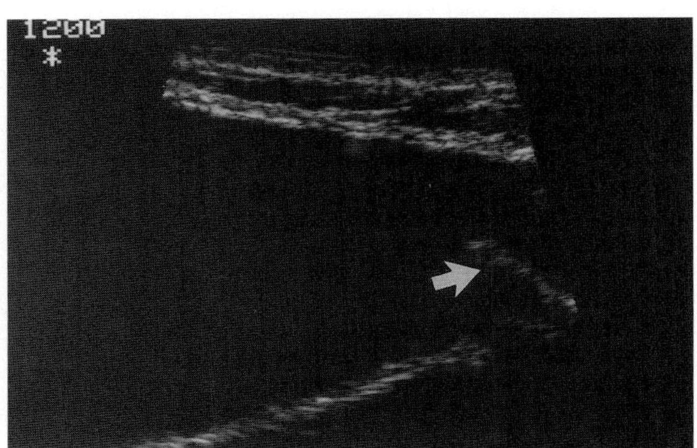

Figure 32–20. Ultrasonography of an intact silicone implant with radial fold (*arrow*), manifested as a single echogenic line that extends to the periphery of the implant.

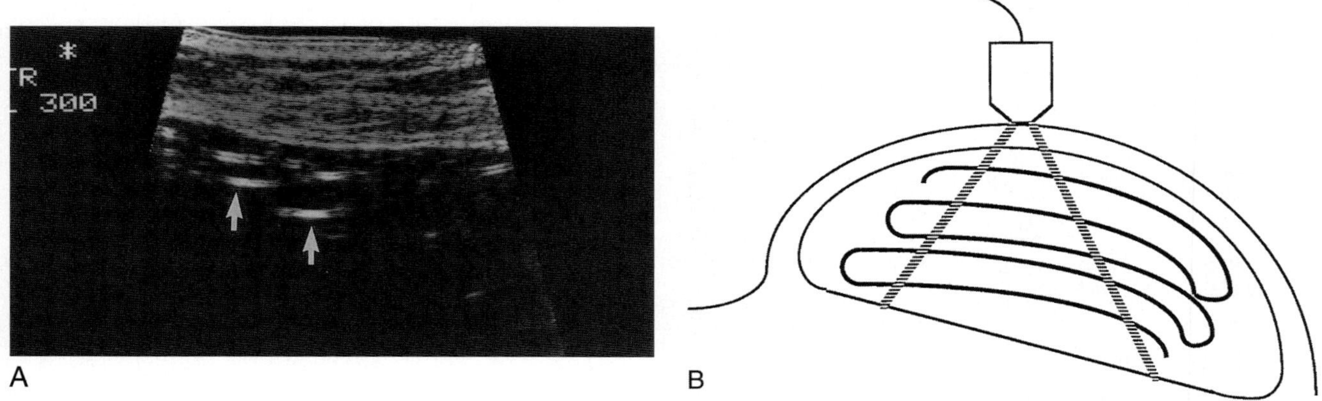

Figure 32–21. Ultrasonography of intracapsular rupture of a breast implant. **A,** The collapsed implant shell is signified by the stepladder sign, multiple horizontal echogenic lines (*arrows*) that are roughly parallel to one another. **B,** The diagram shows how the stepladder sign of ultrasonography is related to the linguine sign seen on magnetic resonance imaging.

rupture (see Table 32–1).[45] As previously mentioned, the stepladder sign consists of a series of horizontal echogenic straight or curvilinear lines, somewhat parallel, traversing the interior of the implant (Fig. 32–21). This sign represents the collapsed implant membrane floating within the silicone gel and is analogous to the linguine sign seen on MRI (see later). The continuity of these echogenic lines is usually not obvious on ultrasonography, as it is on MRI, because of the narrow field of view of the ultrasonographic image. However, the continuity of the lines representing the floating membrane can usually be visualized with scanning along the lateral and medial aspects of the implant.

In our experience, the presence of aggregates of low- to medium-level echoes within the implant has not been a reliable sign of intracapsular rupture. The etiology of these aggregates of echoes is uncertain, but they have been hypothesized to be related to chemical and physical changes of the silicone gel secondary to its exposure to tissue fluids.

Extracapsular Rupture

The most reliable ultrasonographic sign of an extracapsular rupture is the presence of hyperechoic or hypoechoic nodules, often surrounded by a hyperechoic border within the parenchyma (Figs. 32–22 and 32–23). The nodules represent silicone granulomas outside the confines of the fibrous capsule. The hyperechoic border around the nodules is believed to reflect the surrounding fibrous tissue reaction.[46] The granulomas have been associated with distal loss of ultrasonographic information, a phenomenon termed "echodense noise"[44] (see Fig. 32–22). This

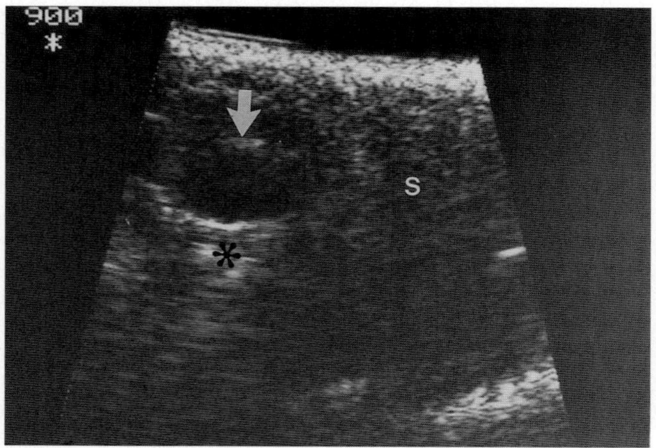

Figure 32–22. Ultrasonography of breast after silicone injections. Dispersion of the ultrasound beam is referred to as a "snowstorm" appearance (S). A hypoechoic silicone granuloma (*arrow*) is identified in the parenchyma. A hyperechoic interface (*asterisk*) is seen directly posterior to the granuloma.

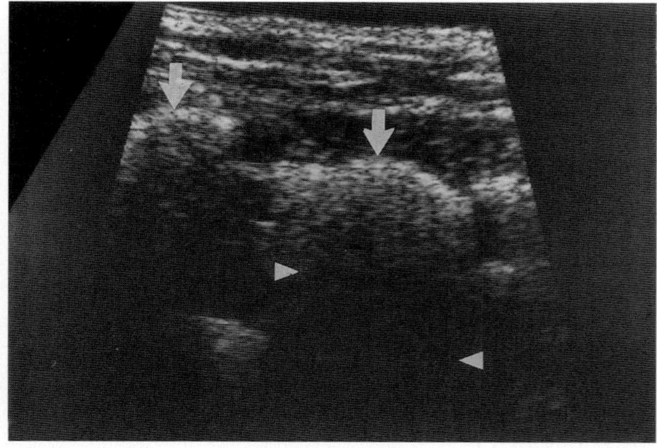

Figure 32–23. Ultrasonography of silicone granulomas formed in the breast after extracapsular rupture. There are hyperechoic nodules of granuloma formation around extravasated silicone (*arrows*). Note the loss of ultrasonographic information posterior to the implants due to beam absorption by the silicone granuloma (*arrowheads*).

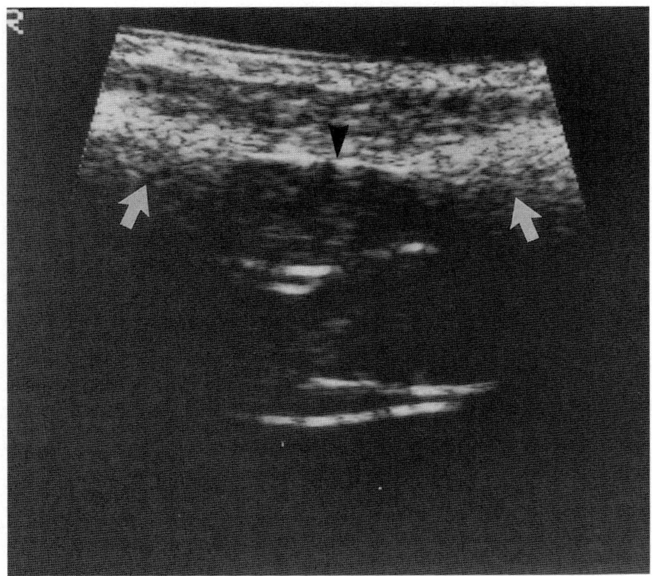

Figure 32–24. Ultrasonographic findings for an implant with extracapsular rupture: Discontinuity of the echogenic breast-implant fibrous capsule interface along the anterior border of the implant (*arrows*) due to extracapsular implant rupture. Note the stepladder sign (multiple parallel echogenic lines) in the posterior aspect of the implant.

noise is often present without any recognizable nodules.[43] The granulomas are differentiated from breast tumors through the correlation of clinical, mammographic, and ultrasonographic findings. Occasionally, extracapsular rupture is associated with discontinuity of the breast-implant fibrous capsule interface along the anterior border of the implant (Fig. 32–24). This discontinuity may represent the extrusion of silicone through the ruptured fibrous capsule and into the anterior breast tissue.

Ultrasonographic signs of intracapsular rupture, specifically the stepladder sign, can be expected to accompany extracapsular ruptures (see Fig. 32–24). When ultrasonographic signs of intracapsular rupture are present, a thorough search for extracapsular rupture should be performed, including careful scanning of the axilla to look for silicone granulomas.

Limitations of the Ultrasonographic Evaluation of Implants

We have identified some significant limitations to the ultrasonographic evaluation of silicone implants. Because of the marked attenuation of the ultrasound beam by silicone, ultrasonography is of limited use in the evaluation of the posterior wall of the implant as well as the tissue posterior to it. Another limitation is the prominent reverberation artifacts that are encountered and that can be confused with implant abnormalities. If a woman had silicone injections before undergoing placement of silicone implants, ruling out extracapsular rupture with ultrasonography may be impossible. In addition, if the silicone injections are extensive, it can be extremely difficult to evaluate the interior of a subsequently placed silicone implant because of attenuation of the ultrasound beam by residual injected silicone and granuloma formation. In the same way, residual silicone granulomas from a previous extracapsular rupture of explanted silicone implants can compromise the evaluation of new implants.

Comparison of Different Imaging Modalities

Mammography, ultrasonography, MRI, and CT have all been used to evaluate the integrity of silicone breast implants.[14,30,39,47,48] To better understand the relative roles and efficacy of these different imaging methods for the evaluation of silicone implants, we have compared them in an animal model.[49] The images of the animals were evaluated by a number of breast imagers through review of the hard copy images. Our study showed that MRI and CT were more accurate than ultrasonography and mammography for detection of intracapsular silicone implant rupture.

Overall, MRI appears to be the most accurate method for evaluating the integrity of breast implants, with a reported sensitivity of 94% and specificity of 97% when two orthogonal sequences are used to evaluate the implant.[36]

CT is also accurate in detecting intracapsular rupture and is capable of depicting the linguine sign originally described on MR images.[48,49] The ability of CT to detect extracapsular rupture needs further investigation. CT is not the modality of choice for imaging a young woman with implants because of the radiation exposure entailed. However, it is worthwhile for radiologists to become familiar with the CT findings of implant rupture, because silicone implants may be encountered during CT examinations of the chest and upper abdomen.

As indicated earlier, mammography has only a limited ability to detect silicone rupture and leakage and is not appropriate for the evaluation of intracapsular rupture.[27] Ultrasonography is capable of detecting both intracapsular and extracapsular ruptures, with a reported sensitivity of 70% and specificity of 92%.[45] We have found, however, that the success of ultrasonography in this endeavor depends largely on the individual operator. A steep learning curve is needed for the development of proficiency in the ultrasonographic evaluation of silicone implants. Thus, the sensitivity of ultrasonography in the detection of implant rupture approaches that of MRI only when the ultrasonography examination is performed by an experienced operator who evaluates and records the findings at the time of actual scanning.

References

1. Bridges AJ, Vasey FB: Silicone breast implants: History, safety, and potential complications. Arch Intern Med 1993;153:2638-2644.
2. Letterman G, Schurter M: History of aesthetic breast surgery. In Lewis JR (ed): The Art of Aesthetic Plastic Surgery, Vol 1. Boston: Little, Brown, 1989, pp 21-27.
3. Steinbach BG, Hardt NS, Abbitt PL, et al: Breast implants, common complications, and concurrent breast disease. Radiographics 1993;13:95-118.
4. Cronin TD, Gerow F: Augmentation mammoplasty: A new "natural feel" prosthesis. In Transactions of the Third International Congress of Plastic Surgeons. Amsterdam: Excerpta Medica, 1964.
5. Marik PE, Kark AL, Zambakides A: Scleroderma after silicone augmentation mammoplasty: A report of two cases. S Afr Med J 1990;77:212, 213.
6. Spiera H: Scleroderma after silicone augmentation mammoplasty. JAMA 1988;260:236-238.
7. Weiner SR: Silicone augmentation mammoplasty and rheumatic disease. In Stratmeyer ME (ed): Silicone in Medical Devices: Proceedings of a Conference Held in Baltimore, MD, February 1-2, 1991. (Publication FDA 92-4249.) Bethesda, MD: Department of Health and Human Services, 1991, pp 81-102.
8. Kessler DA: The basis of the FDA's decision on breast implants. N Engl J Med 1992;326:1713-1715.
9. Center for Devices and Radiological Health, US Food and Drug Administration: Breast Implants. 2000. Available at: www.fda.gov/cdrh/breastimplant/
10. Baker JL, Bartels RJ, Douglas WM: Closed compression technique for rupturing a contracted capsule around a breast implant. Plast Reconstr Surg 1976;58:137-141.
11. Gruber RP, Jones HW: Review of closed capsulotomy complications. Ann Plast Surg 1981;6:271-275.
12. Ahn CY, Shaw WW, Narayanan K, et al: Definitive diagnosis of breast implant rupture using magnetic resonance imaging. Plast Reconstr Surg 1993;94:681-691.
13. Brody GS: Fact and fiction about breast implant "bleed." Plast Reconstr Surg 1977;60:615-616.
14. Mund DF, Farria DM, Gorczyca DP, et al: MRI of the breast in patients with silicone-gel implants: Spectrum of findings. AJR Am J Roentgenol 1993;161:773-778.
15. Middleton MS: Does silicone gel really bleed? Radiology 1995; 197(P):370-371.
16. Berkel H, Birdsell DC, Jenkins H: Breast augmentation: A risk factor for breast cancer? N Engl J Med 1992;326:1649-1653.
17. Pukkala E, Boice JD Jr, Hovi SL, et al: Incidence of breast and other cancers among Finnish women with cosmetic breast implants, 1970-1999. J Long Term Eff Med Implants 2002; 12:271-279.
18. Holmich LR, Mellemkjaer L, Gunnarsdottir KA, et al: Stage of breast cancer at diagnosis among women with cosmetic breast implants. Br J Cancer 2003;88:432-835.
19. Fajardo LL, Harvey JA, McAleese KA, et al: Breast cancer diagnosis in women with subglandular silicone gel-filled augmentation implants. Radiology 1995;194:859-862.
20. Skinner KA, Silberman H, Dougherty W, et al: Breast cancer after augmentation mammoplasty. Ann Surg Onc 2001;8:138-144.
21. Eklund GW, Busby RC, Miller SH, et al: Improved imaging of the augmented breast. AJR Am J Roentgenol 1988;151:469-473.
22. American College of Radiology Committee on Quality Assurance in Mammography: Patient positioning. In Mammography Quality Control. Reston, VA: American College of Radiology, 1992, pp 57-99.
23. Bassett LW, Hendrick RE, Bassford TL, et al: Quality Determinants of Mammography. (Clinical Practice Guideline, N. 13. AHCPR Publication No. 95-0632.) Rockville, MD: Agency for Health Care Policy and Research, Public Health Service, US Department of Health and Human Services, 1994.
24. Diekmann S, Diekmann F, Hauschild M, Hamm B: Digital full field mammography after breast augmentation. Radiology 2002;42:275-9
25. Bassett LW, Brenner RJ: Considerations when imaging women with breast implants. AJR Am J Roentgenol 1992;159:979-981.
26. Dershaw DD, Chaglassian TA: Mammography after prosthesis placement for augmentation or reconstructive mammoplasty. Radiology 1989;170:69-74.
27. Destouet JM, Monsees BS, Oser RF, et al: Screening mammography in 350 women with breast implants: Prevalence and findings of implant complications. AJR Am J Roentgenol 1992; 159:973-978.
28. Leibman AJ, Kruse B: Breast cancer: Mammographic and sonographic findings after augmentation mammoplasty. Radiology 1990;174:195-198.
29. Young VL, Bartell T, Destouet JM, et al: Calcification of breast implant capsule. South Med J 1989;82:1171-1173.
30. Berg WA, Caskey CI, Hamper UM: Diagnosing breast implant rupture with MRI, US, and mammography. Radiographics 1993;13:1323-1336.
31. Gorczyca DP, Sinha S, Ahn C, et al: Silicone breast implants in vivo: MRI. Radiology 1992;185:407-410.
32. Habal MB: The biologic basis for the clinical application of the silicones. Arch Surg 1984;119:843-848.
33. Mukundan S, Dixon WT, Kruse BD, et al: MRI of silicone gel-filled breast implants in vivo with a method that visualizes silicone selectively. J Magn Reson Imaging 1993;3:713-717.
34. Berg WA, Nguyen TK, Middleton MS, et al: MRI of extracapsular silicone from breast implants: Diagnostic pitfalls. AJR Am J Roentgenol 2002;178:465-472.
35. Garrido L, Kwong KK, Pfleiderer B, et al: Echo-planar chemical shift imaging of silicone gel prostheses. Magn Reson Imaging 1993;11:625-634.
36. Gorczyca DP, Schneider E, DeBruhl ND, et al: Silicone breast implant rupture: Comparison between three-point Dixon and fast spin-echo MRI. AJR Am J Roentgenol 1994;162:305-310.
37. Schneider E, Chan TW: Selective MRI of silicone with the 3-point Dixon technique. Radiology 1993;187:89-93.
38. Sinha S, Gorczyca DP, DeBruhl ND, et al: MRI of silicone breast implants: Comparison of different coil arrays. Radiology 1993;187:284-286.
39. Ikeda DM, Borofsky HB, Herfkens RJ, et al: Silicone breast implant rupture: Pitfalls of magnetic resonance imaging and relative efficacies of magnetic resonance, mammography, and ultrasound. Plast Reconstr Surg 1999;104:2054-2062.
40. Harms, SE, Jensen RA, Meiches MD, et al: Silicone -suppressed 3D MRI of the breast using rotating delivery of off-resonance excitation. J Comput Assist Tomogr. 1995;19:394-349.
41. Gorczyca DP, DeBruhl ND, Mund DF, Bassett LW: Linguine sign at MRI: Does it represent the collapsed silicone implant shell? Radiology 1994;191:576-577.
42. Ganott MA, Harris KM, Ilkhanipour ZS, Costa-Creco MA: Augmentation mammoplasty: Normal and abnormal findings with mammography and US. Radiographics 1992;12:281-295.
43. Harris KM, Ganott MA, Shestak KC, et al: Silicone implant rupture: Detection with US. Radiology 1993;187:761-768.
44. Rosculet KA, Ikeda DM, Forrest ME, et al: Ruptured gel-filled silicone breast implants: Sonographic findings in 19 cases. AJR Am J Roentgenol 1992;159:711-716.
45. DeBruhl ND, Gorczyca DP, Ahn CY, et al: Silicone breast implants: US evaluation. Radiology 1993;189:95-98.
46. Levine RA, Collins TL: Definitive diagnosis of breast implant rupture by ultrasonography. Plast Reconstr Surg 1991;87:1126-1128.
47. Everson LI, Parantainen H, Detlie T, et al: Diagnosis of breast implant rupture: Imaging findings and relative efficacies of imaging techniques. AJR Am J Roentgenol 1994;163:57-60.
48. Scott IR, Muller NL, Fitzpatrick DG, et al: Ruptured breast implant: Computed tomographic and mammographic findings. J Can Assoc Radiol 1988;39:152-154.
49. Gorczyca DP, DeBruhl ND, Ahn CY, et al: Silicone breast implant ruptures in an animal model: Comparison of mammography, MRI, US, and CT. Radiology 1994;190:227-232.

Chapter

33 Reduction Mammoplasty

Valerie P. Jackson

Reduction mammoplasty is a plastic surgical procedure performed for the treatment of macromastia or to achieve symmetry in women with congenital hypoplasia or aplasia in one breast or after mastectomy of one breast with reconstruction, large segmental resection for breast cancer, or severe trauma to the contralateral breast. Macromastia may lead to a number of problems, including poor posture, kyphosis, back pain, deep grooves and skin ulceration in the shoulders from the pressure of brassiere straps, brachial plexus pressure symptoms, and chronic intertrigo under the breasts. Of women with breast carcinoma treated with mastectomy and reconstruction, 6% to 36% undergo reduction mammoplasty to achieve symmetrical breast size.[1]

A number of surgical techniques for reduction mammoplasty have been described.[2,3] All involve removal of breast tissue and repositioning of the nipple-areolar complex (Figs. 33–1 and 33–2). Nipple repositioning may be achieved by two types of procedures: use of a pedicle flap with dermal nipple transposition, in which the nipple remains connected to the subareolar ducts, or use of a pedicle flap with full-thickness nipple-areolar grafts, in which the ducts are severed (see Figs. 33–1 and 33–2).[4] The most commonly used surgical techniques lead to a characteristic scar in the circumareolar region, which extends down the inferior aspect of the breast and along the inframammary fold (Fig. 33–3).

INDICATIONS FOR IMAGING

Many plastic surgeons recommend preoperative mammography for all women undergoing reduction mammoplasty, particularly those older than 35 years.[3,5-12] The major value of the preoperative mammogram is to detect any lesion that requires further investigation or removal at the time of the reduction procedure. Ozmen and colleagues[13] recommend specimen radiography of the removed breast tissue to evaluate for abnormalities such as breast carcinoma, but this step is probably unnecessary if preoperative mammography has been performed. Because major imaging changes occur after the surgical procedure, the preoperative mammogram is of little value after the reduction procedure. Many plastic surgeons advocate establishing a new baseline with mammography 3 to 12 months after the reduction procedure,[5-9,12] and my colleagues and I have found this principle to be extremely useful in our own practice. It is often helpful to wait at least 6 months after surgery to minimize patient discomfort during the mammogram and to allow the postoperative changes within the breasts to diminish.[8]

Early complications of reduction mammoplasty include seromas, hematomas, areolar necrosis, infection, and delayed skin healing. Most of these complications are handled clinically and do not require imaging.[14] Imaging is indicated if a woman has a new clinical abnormality later after reduction mammoplasty. Many benign breast masses occur as a result of the surgery, including hematomas, fat necrosis, and fibrous scars.[9] Mammography can definitively diagnose many of these lesions, which should not be assumed to be benign on the basis of clinical breast examination.

There is evidence that women have a somewhat lower risk of breast cancer after reduction mammoplasty.[15] Their prognosis and mortality rates are the same as for women with breast cancer in the general population.[16] Nonetheless, it is important to remember that all women older than 40 years should undergo annual screening mammography. A woman who has reduction mammoplasty to achieve symmetry after treatment for contralateral breast carcinoma is at increased risk for development of additional breast cancer and requires annual imaging of the reduced breast regardless of age.

MAMMOGRAPHIC FINDINGS AFTER REDUCTION MAMMOPLASTY

A number of characteristic mammographic changes have been reported after reduction mammoplasty (Table 33–1). Regardless of the exact type of reduction procedure performed, the changes reflect the removal and repositioning of breast tissue and the nipple-areolar complex. The commonly encountered mammographic findings are as follows:

- *Alteration of breast contour:* The breasts tend to be higher and flatter in contour than normal breasts (Fig. 33–4).[6]
- *Elevation of the nipple:* There is less skin above the nipple and more below the nipple than in normal breasts for a person of the same age (see Fig. 33–4).[4,6,7]
- *Displacement of breast parenchyma:* All of the surgical procedures involve movement of breast tissue, usually with displacement of tissue from the upper portions to the lower aspects, leading to movement of fibroglandular tissue, which is normally most prominent in the upper-outer quadrant, to the inferior aspect of the breast.[4,6,7,17] This is best seen on the mediolateral oblique (MLO) and lateral

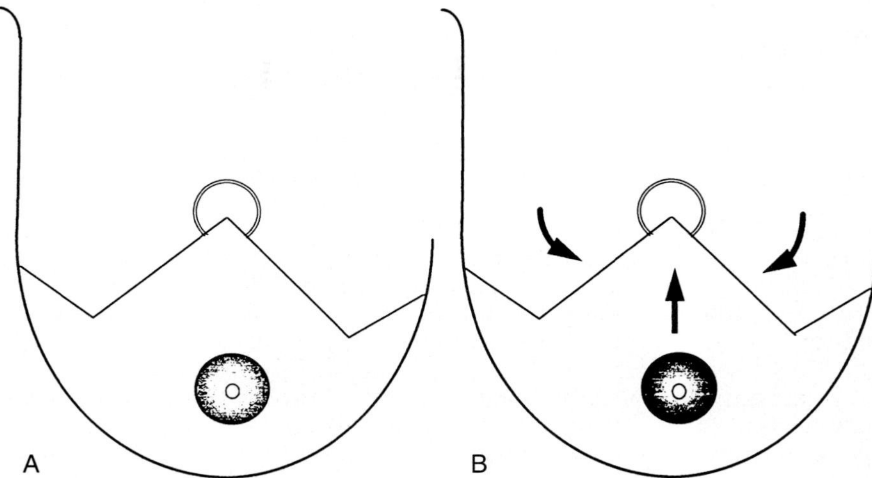

Figure 33–1. Typical pattern of excision for reduction mammoplasty with nipple transplantation. **A,** The inferior, medial, and lateral breast tissues are resected with removal of the nipple. **B,** The upper aspects of the breast are brought inferiorly *(curved arrows)* and the nipple-areolar complex is transplanted superiorly as a full-thickness graft *(straight arrow)*.

(mediolateral [ML] or lateromedial [LM]) views (Fig. 33–5). The pattern of fibroglandular density is often asymmetrical (see Fig. 33–5).[6]

- *Architectural distortion:* Postoperative scarring and displacement of fibroglandular tissue usually lead to distortion of the normal breast architecture.[4,17] This is more prominent in breasts with fibroglandular tissue than in breasts that are almost completely fatty. One of the most common findings is a "swirled" pattern of architectural distortion or lines seen inferiorly on the MLO or lateral (ML or LM) views (Figs. 33–5 through 33–7).[17]
- *Fat necrosis:* Fat necrosis is a common sequela of extensive surgery such as reduction mammoplasty. The most common findings are oil cysts, often with spherical lucent-centered, eggshell, or dystrophic calcifications (see Fig. 33–5).[6,7,17-20]
- *Suture calcifications:* Suture material used in the surgical procedure may calcify, leading to small ringlike calcifications in the regions of surgical anastomoses.[17] Knots are occasionally seen.
- *Skin thickening:* Thickening of the skin is most commonly seen in the areolar region and the inferior aspect of the breast, in the areas of surgical anastomosis (see Fig. 33–7).[4,6,7]
- *Retroareolar fibrotic band:* A radiopaque band less than 0.5 cm thick that runs parallel to the skin line,

Table 33–1. Mammographic Changes after Reduction Mammoplasty

Alteration of breast contour
Elevation of the nipple
Displacement of breast parenchyma
Architectural distortion
Fat necrosis
Suture calcifications
Skin thickening
Retroareolar fibrotic band
Disruption of subareolar ducts

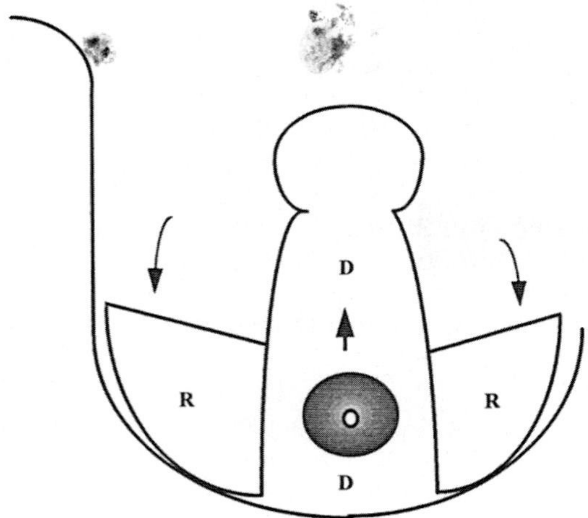

Figure 33–2. Typical pattern of excision for reduction mammoplasty with nipple transposition. The skin and parenchymal tissue within the triangular areas (R) are resected. The nipple-areolar complex remains intact, but the surrounding region (D) is deepithelialized. When the nipple is transposed superiorly into the "keyhole," it remains attached to the underlying ducts and vascular pedicle. The upper aspects of the breast are brought inferiorly as shown by the *curved arrows*.

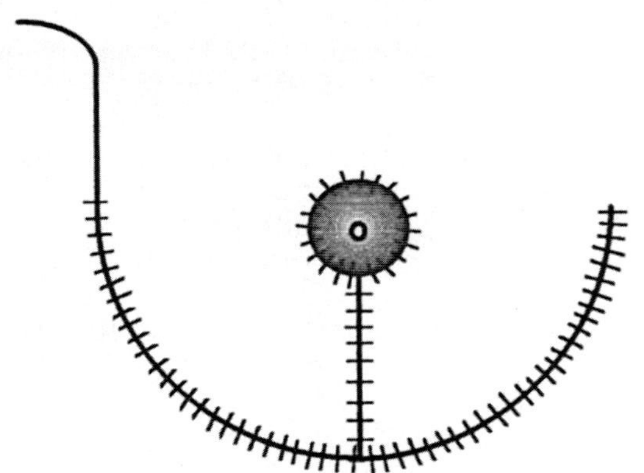

Figure 33–3. Typical postoperative appearance after reduction mammoplasty. Surgical scars are found in the circumareolar region, inframammary fold, and at the 6 o'clock position *(cross-hatched lines)*.

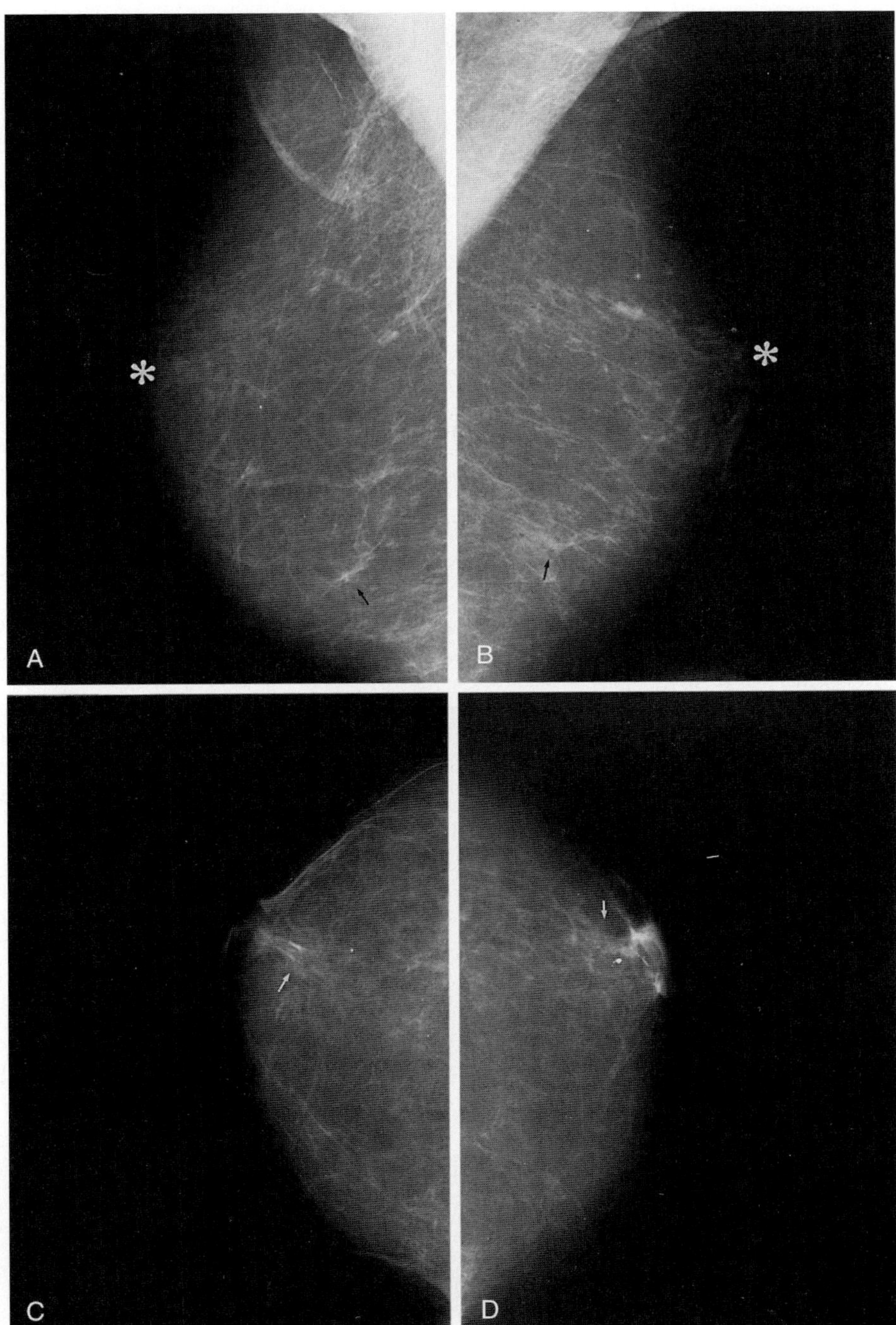

Figure 33–4. Right and left mediolateral oblique (MLO) (**A** and **B**) and craniocaudal (**C** and **D**) mammograms taken 2 years after reduction mammoplasty in a 50-year-old woman. This patient was difficult to position for the MLO views, leading to suboptimal visualization of the pectoralis muscles. The breasts are higher and flatter in contour than normal breasts, and the nipples *(asterisks)* are elevated. Minimal scar tissue is present inferiorly *(arrows)*.

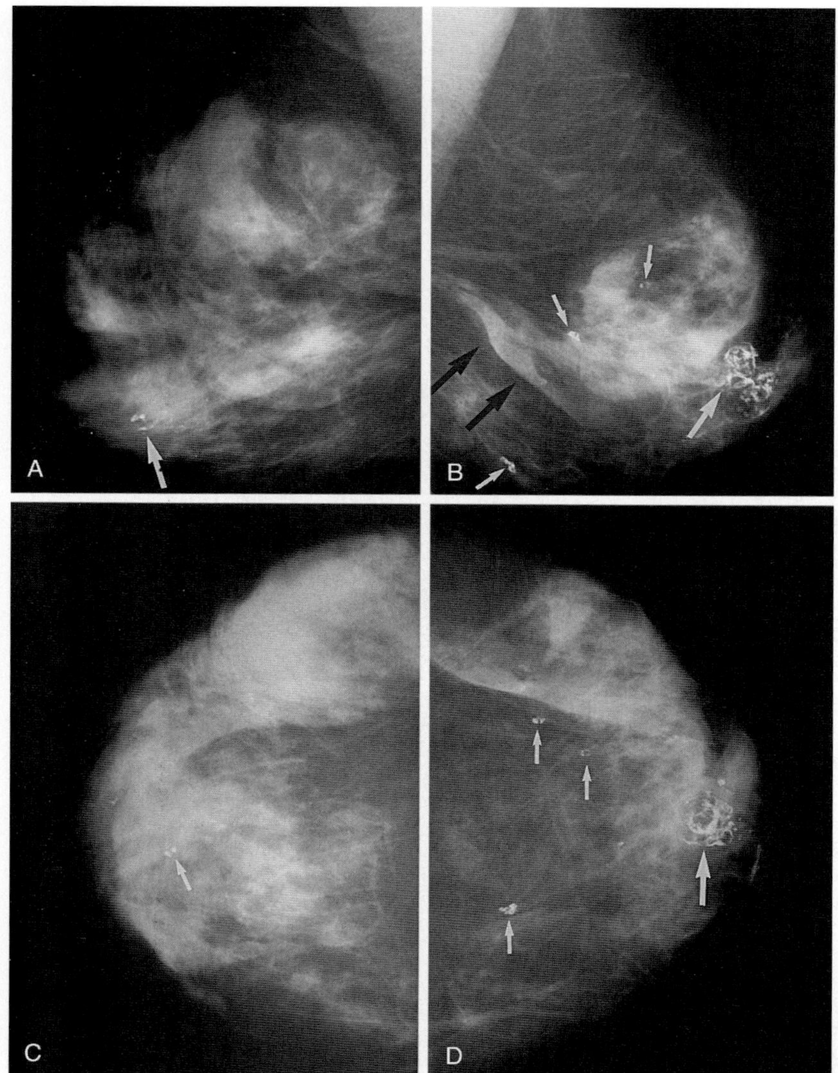

Figure 33–5. Right and left mediolateral (MLO) (**A** and **B**) and craniocaudal (**C** and **D**) mammograms taken 4 years after reduction mammoplasty in a 45-year-old woman. Displacement and distortion of fibroglandular tissue are present bilaterally. This is most prominent on the left MLO view (**B**). The swirled pattern of architectural distortion is present in the inferior aspect of the left breast (**B,** *black arrows*). Typical findings of fat necrosis with calcifications are present bilaterally *(white arrows).*

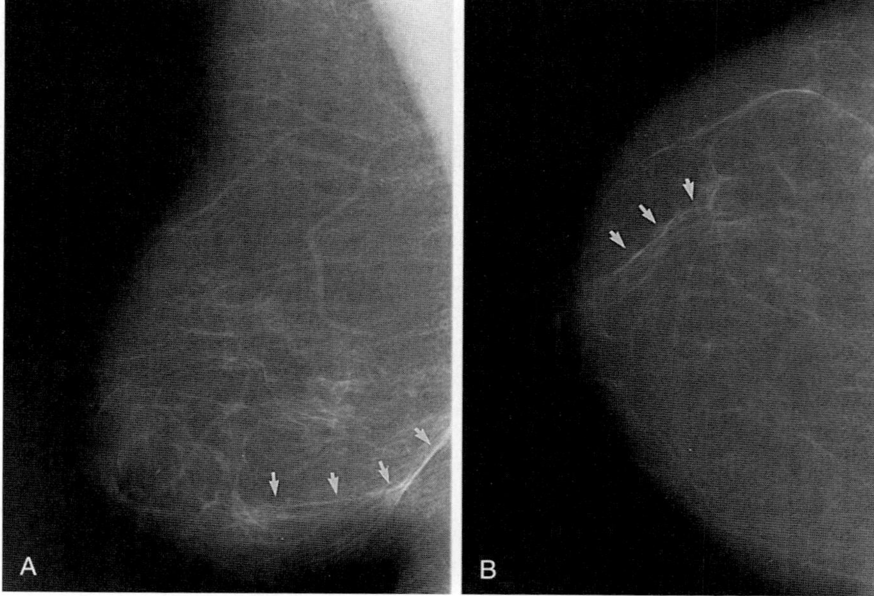

Figure 33–6. Swirled lines of architectural distortion at the inferior aspect of the breast 5 years after reduction mammoplasty *(arrows).* **A,** Right mediolateral oblique mammogram; **B,** right craniocaudal mammogram.

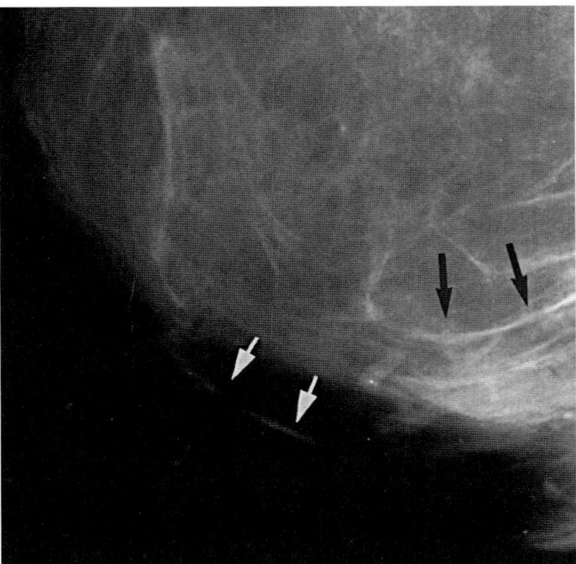

Figure 33–7. Skin thickening at inferior aspect of breast on right mediolateral mammogram *(white arrows)*. Note the swirled pattern of architectural distortion posteriorly *(black arrows)*.

the retroareolar fibrotic band is best seen on the craniocaudal (CC) view.[4,6,7] It occurs in women undergoing nipple-areolar transposition procedures (Fig. 33–8).[4]

- *Disruption of subareolar ducts*[4,6]*:* The subareolar ducts are preserved when a nipple-areolar transposition procedure is done (Fig. 33–9). However, when a transplantation type of reduction mammoplasty is performed, the ducts are severed and appear disrupted on mammography.[4] This finding is not apparent in women with breasts that are almost completely fatty.[4]

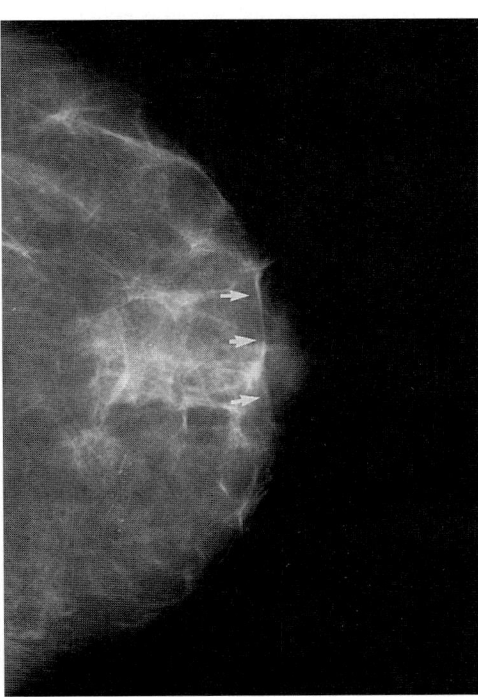

Figure 33–8. Left craniocaudal mammogram demonstrating retroareolar fibrotic band *(arrows)* in a woman who had undergone reduction mammoplasty with a nipple transposition procedure 2 years previously.

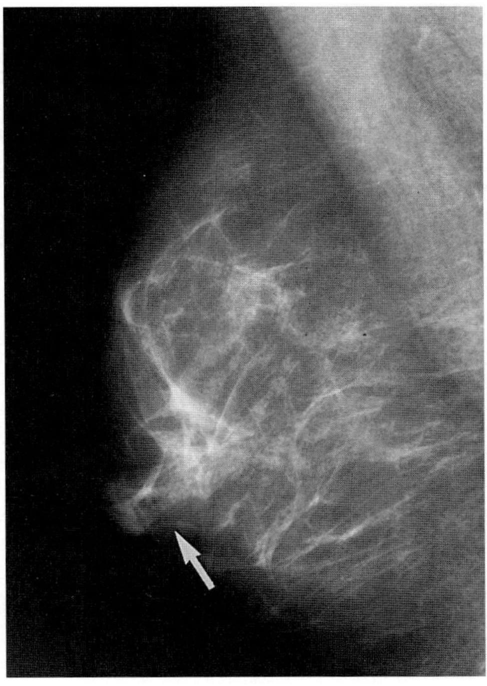

Figure 33–9. Preservation of subareolar ducts *(arrow)* in a woman with a nipple-areolar transposition type of reduction mammoplasty.

Unusual mammographic findings include spiculated scars[17] and epidermal inclusion cysts related to the surgical procedure.[21]

Brown and colleagues[6] monitored women with serial mammography after reduction procedures and found that the architectural changes, such as periareolar and inferior breast alterations, were most prominent on the first postoperative mammogram and usually diminished over time. In none of their patients did these changes increase on subsequent mammograms. Asymmetrical densities were found in 50% of women in the first year after surgery but in only 25% of women after 2 years. In patients in whom they persisted, the asymmetrical densities usually reduced in size and prominence and did not enlarge. Calcifications tended to develop later and therefore could represent more of a diagnostic problem. Only 3% of women had calcifications within the first year, 20% by the second year, and more than 40% after 2 years. Although the number and extent of calcifications increased over time, the calcifications were usually coarse and therefore obviously benign. However, early fat necrosis calcifications may be fine and pleomorphic and therefore may mimic malignant microcalcifications.

Breast cancer in women with prior reduction mammoplasty has the same imaging features as that in normal women. However, the changes from reduction mammoplasty may cause confusion, particularly if previous mammograms are not available for comparison. If one is aware of the typical changes of reduction mammoplasty and careful to compare current with previous mammograms, it is possible to detect early breast carcinoma in these women.[22] In cases with indeterminate findings, imaging-guided fine-needle aspiration biopsy[23,24] or core or vacuum-assisted needle biopsy can be used to differentiate postoperative changes from malignancy.

References

1. Greco RJ, Dascombe WH, Williams SL, et al: Two-staged breast reconstruction in patients with symptomatic macromastia requiring mastectomy. Ann Plast Surg 1994;32:572-579.
2. Hidalgo DA, Franklyn EL, Palumbo S, et al: Current trends in breast reduction. Plast Reconstr Surg 1999;104:806-815.
3. Strombeck JO: Reduction mammaplasty. In Strombeck JO, Rosato FE (eds): Surgery of the Breast: Diagnosis and Treatment of Breast Diseases. New York, Georg Thieme, 1986, pp 277-311.
4. Miller CL, Feig SA, Fox JW: Mammographic changes after reduction mammoplasty. AJR Am J Roentgenol 1987;149:35-38.
5. Beer GM, Kompatscher P, Hergan K: Diagnosis of breast tumors after breast reduction. Aesthetic Plast Surg 1996;20:391-397.
6. Brown FE, Sargent SK, Cohen SR, Morain WD: Mammographic changes following reduction mammaplasty. Plast Reconstr Surg 1987;80:691-698.
7. Danikas D, Theodorou SJ, Kokkalis G, et al: Mammographic findings following reduction mammoplasty. Aesthestic Plast Surg 2001;25:283-285.
8. Howrigan PJ: Reduction and augmentation mammoplasty. Obstet Gynecol Clin North Am 1994;21:539-549.
9. Isaacs G, Rozner L, Tudball C: Breast lumps after reduction mammaplasty. Ann Plast Surg 1985;15:394-399.
10. Keleher AJ, Langstein HN, Ames FC, et al: Breast cancer in mammoplasty specimens: Case reports and guidelines. Breast J 2003;9:120-125.
11. Perras C, Papillon J: The value of mammography in cosmetic surgery of the breasts. Plast Reconstr Surg 1973;52:132-137.
12. Spear SL, Antoine GA: Surgery for mammary hypertrophy. In Nonne RB (ed): Plastic and Reconstructive Surgery of the Breast. Philadelphia, BC Decker, 1991, pp 189-194.
13. Ozmen S, Yavuzer R, Latifoglu O, et al: Specimen radiography: An assessment method for reduction mammaplasty materials. Aesthetic Plast Surg 2001;25:432-435.
14. Lejour M: Vertical mammaplasty: Early complications after 250 personal consecutive cases. Plast Reconstr Surg 1999;104:764-770.
15. Brown MH, Weinberg M, Chong N, et al: A cohort study of breast cancer risk in breast reduction patients. Plast Reconstr Surg 1999;103:1674-1681.
16. Tang CL, Brown MH, Levine R, et al: A follow-up study of 105 women with breast cancer following reduction mammaplasty. Plast Reconstr Surg 1999;103:1687-1690.
17. Swann CA, Kopans DB, White G, et al: Observations on the postreduction mammoplasty mammogram. Breast Dis 1989;1:261-267.
18. Baber CE, Libshitz HI: Bilateral fat necrosis of the breast following reduction mammoplasties. AJR Am J Roentgenol 1977;128:508-509.
19. Bassett LW, Gold RH, Cove HC: Mammographic spectrum of traumatic fat necrosis: The fallibility of "pathognomonic" signs of carcinoma. AJR Am J Roentgenol 1978;130:119-122.
20. Mendelson EB: Imaging the post-surgical breast. Semin Ultrasound CT MR 1989;10:154-170.
21. Fajardo LL, Besson SC: Epidermal inclusion cyst after reduction mammoplasty. Radiology 1993;186:103-106.
22. Leibman AJ, Kruse BD: Imaging of breast cancer after reduction mammoplasty. Breast Dis 1991;4:261-270.
23. Mitnick J, Roses DF, Harris MN: Differentiation of postsurgical changes from carcinoma of the breast. Surg Gynecol Obstet 1988;166:549-550.
24. Mitnick JS, Vazquez MF, Plesser KP, et al: Distinction between postsurgical changes and carcinoma by means of stereotaxic fine-needle aspiration biopsy after reduction mammaplasty. Radiology 1993;188:457-462.

Index

Note: Page numbers in italics indicate figures; those with a *t* indicate tables.